Handbuch der experimentellen Pharmakologie

Handbook of Experimental Pharmacology

Heffter-Heubner New Series

Herausgegeben von / Edited by

O. Eichler
Heidelberg

A. Farah
Syracuse, N.Y.

Vol. XIX

Springer-Verlag · Berlin · Heidelberg · New York 1966

5-Hydroxytryptamine and Related Indolealkylamines

Contributors

H. Blaschko · W. P. Burkard · A. Carlsson · L. H. Cohen · V. Erspamer
K. F. Gey · L. Gyermek · P. B. Hagen · A. Hanson · W. G. Levine
P. Mantegazzini · A. Pletscher · R. S. Stacey · M. Vialli

Sub-Editor

Vittorio Erspamer

With 109 Figures and 2 Plates

Springer-Verlag New York Inc. 1966

ISBN 978-3-642-85469-9 ISBN 978-3-642-85467-5 (eBook)
DOI 10.1007/978-3-642-85467-5

Softcover reprint of the hardcover 1st edition 1966

Library of Congress Catalog Card Number AGR 25–699

Titel-Nr. 5724

Preface

The study of biogenic amines, which from the beginning of modern pharmacology has always attracted the enthusiastic attention of research workers and has led to some of the most brilliant and illuminating experimental results in biology, has been unexpectedly extended in the last fifteen years. With the discovery of 5-hydroxytryptamine (enteramine, serotonin), in fact, the vast field of indolealkylamines has been opened up for research.

In a decade of intensive and dedicated work, an immense amount of experimental data has been collected, the significance of which, having rapidly overrun the limits of pharmacology, physiology, and biochemistry, has spread into all fields of biology and medicine, as previously occurred with choline esters, catecholamines and imidazolealkylamines. Thus, the study of indolealkylamines, especially that of their metabolism, has led not only to explanation of the mechanism of action, formerly largely obscure, of some important drugs, to clarification of the pathogenesis of some morbid syndromes and to a parallel flourishing of research on other biogenic amines, but also to surprising achievements in the field of therapeutics. The discovery of monoamineoxidase and dopadecarboxylase inhibitors, and of drugs which block the storage of biogenic amines in the body depots are among the most striking results of research on the indolealkylamines.

The present volume of the "Ergänzungswerk" attempts to offer the reader the best of about 4000 papers which have appeared in the field of the indolealkylamines up till the end of 1963. Many of the data reported in the volume can already be considered to be firmly established; others still require confirmation. Some of the problems herein posed can be considered solved, while others need elucidation by future research. First and foremost among these is the problem of the biological significance of 5-hydroxytryptamine and related indolealkylamines in their various localizations. It will be an adequate reward for our efforts and those of our collaborators if this volume proves to be of even little help towards research progress in this field of endeavour, to which each of us has dedicated some of his best years.

I should like to express my gratitude to Prof. Oskar Eichler for the testimony of esteem he as shown me in selecting me as Sub-Editor of this volume and my warmest thanks to all the collaborators who have taken a share in the labour of this enterprise by adding to it the contributions of their exceptional competence. Thanks are particularly due to Dr. A. Hanson and Dr. L. Gyermek who agreed to write their chapters under difficult conditions owing to the late withdrawal of other collaborators. I also beg to be permitted (since I shall probably never have another similar opportunity) to thank Professors M. Vialli and P. di Mattei, who gave me so much encouragement in the study of "enteramine" at a time when it could certainly not have been said that this study would lead to success or immediate satisfaction. And finally I should like to thank my dear ones (my wife, who has also been very helpful to me in the compilation of the bibliography and the subject index, and my children, Francesco and Maria Luisa) for having made it possible, by creating a quiet atmosphere in which to work, to carry on even under conditions that were not always easy.

V. Erspamer

List of the most usual abbreviations

ACH Acetylcholine
ACTH Adrenocorticotropic hormone
AMP Adenosine monophosphate
ATP Adenosine triphosphate
BAB 1-Benzyl-2-methyl-5-methoxy-N,N-dimethyltryptamine (benzyl analogue of bufotenine)
BAS 1-Benzyl-2-methyl-5-methoxytryptamine (benzyl analogue of serotonin)
BOL 2-Bromo-D-lysergic acid diethylamide
CNS Central nervous system
CPZ Chlorpromazine
DAO Diamine oxidase
DCA Decarboxylase of aromatic L-amino acids
DOCA Desoxycorticosterone acetate
DHE Dihydroergotamine
DMPP 1,1-Dimethyl-4-phenylpiperazinium bromide
DOPA 3,4-Dihydroxyphenylalanine
DPN Oxidized diphosphopyridine nucleotide
EC Enterochromaffin cell(s)
EDTA Ethylenedinitrile tetraacetic acid tetrasodium salt
EEG Electroencephalogram
GABA γ-Aminobutyric acid
GFR Glomerular filtration rate
5-HIAA 5-Hydroxyindoleacetic acid
5-HT 5-Hydroxytryptamine
5-HTP 5-Hydroxytryptophan
4-HIAA 4-Hydroxyindoleacetic acid
4-HT 4-Hydroxytryptamine
4-HTP 4-Hydroxytryptophan
6-HIAA 6-Hydroxyindoleacetic acid
6-HT 6-Hydroxytryptamine
6-HTP 6-Hydroxytryptophan
7-HIAA 7-Hydroxyindoleacetic acid
7-HT 7-Hydroxytryptamine
7-HTP 7-Hydroxytryptophan
IAA Indoleacetic acid
LSD D-Lysergic acid diethylamide
LSM D-Lysergic acid morpholide
MAO Monoamine oxydase
MBL 1-Methyl-2-bromo-D-lysergic acid diethylamide
MSH Melanocyte-stimulating hormone
NE Norepinephrine, noradrenaline
PIH β-Phenylisopropylhydrazine
PAS Paraaminosalicylic acid
RPF Renal plasma flow
STH Somatotropic hormone
T Tryptamine
TMA Tetramethylammonium bromide
TP Tryptophan
TPNH Reduced triphosphopyridine nucleotide
UML 1-Methyl-D-lysergic acid butanolamide, methysergide

List of Contributors

HERMANN BLASCHKO, Dr., Dept. of Pharmacology, University of Oxford, Oxford, Great Britain.

WILLY PAUL BURKARD, Dr. phil., F. Hoffmann-La-Roche & Co. Ltd., Basel, Switzerland.

ARVID CARLSSON, Professor of Pharmacology, Department of Pharmacology, University of Göteborg, Göteborg, Sweden.

LEONARD H. COHEN, PH. D., Associate Member, Institute for Cancer Research, Fox Chase, Philadelphia, Pa., USA.

VITTORIO ERSPAMER, Professor of Pharmacology, Department of Pharmacology, University of Parma, Parma, Italy.

KARL FRIEDRICH GEY, Dr. med., F. Hoffmann-La-Roche & Co. Ltd., Basel, Switzerland.

LASZLO GYERMEK, M. D., Associate Director, Biological Research, Syntex Laboratories, Palo Alto, California, USA.

PAUL B. HAGEN, Dr., Professor of Biochemistry, Queen's University Kingston, Ontario, Canada.

ARNE HANSON, Dr., Department of Clinical Chemistry, General Hospital, Malmö, Sweden.

WALTER, G. LEVINE, Department of Pharmacology, Albert Einstein College of Medicine, New York 61, N.Y., USA.

PAOLO MANTEGAZZINI †, Dr., Laboratori Ricerche Farmitalia S. p. A.Milano, Italy.

ALFRED PLETSCHER, Professor Dr. med. et phil., F. Hoffmann-La-Roche & Co. Ltd., Basel, Switzerland.

REGINALD STEPHEN STACEY, Professor of Pharmacology and Therapeutics, St. Thomas's Hospital Medical School, London S.E. 1, Great Britain.

MAFFO VIALLI, Professor, Direttore dell'Istituto di Anatomia Comparata dell' Università di Pavia e Centro di Studio per l'Istochimica del C.N.R., Pavia, Italy.

Contents

Chapter 1

Histology of the enterochromaffin cell system

By

MAFFO VIALLI

With 10 figures and 2 plates

I. Introduction

The histological problems of interest to the pharmacologist, when he studies substances occuring naturally in organisms, are extremely varied. Besides questions of a more general nature, which arise in the study of any substance of pharmacological import, there are some peculiar to this particular type of investigation (VIALLI 1962, 1964). In the first place it bears essentially on the localization of the substance and on the determination of its nature; as such it is common to the general field of histological investigation, or more specifically to its histochemical branch.

In the writer's opinion, questions of this type may be classified into seven topics:

I. the histochemical characterization of the substance directly concerned, and secondarily of other substances which may be more or less correlated to it;

II. the morphological characteristics of the elements in which histochemical methods have shown the substance to be present;

III. the physical characteristics of the elements in which the histochemical reactions prove the presence of the substance;

IV. the distribution of the substance in the organism studied at a level which would be impossible in normal biochemical procedures;

V. the presence and consequently the distribution of the substance in a series of organisms; this comparative method often provides a broader outlook on the problem than that attainable even by an extremely refined study limited to only a few species, as in paragraph II;

VI. the embryological origin of the elements containing the substance and the ways it may manifest itself in them;

VII. the modifications observable at the histological level when quantitative variations in the substance are induced by particular functional conditions, either normal or experimental; this last type of data coincides, to a certain extent, with that obtainable by the traditional methods of bio-pharmacological investigation.

However, it is not often that the pharmacologist or the biochemist can offer the histologist completely new a field of investigation, at least as far as normally-occurring substances are concerned; there is usually already a certain body of knowledge more or less connected with the problem concerned.

At times, as for instance in the case of 5-HT (5-hydroxytryptamine), it appears, from the way research on a subject develops, that the histological and, even more, the histochemical parts of the investigation have not only preceded the discovery of the substance but have actually conditioned it.

A historical study of the development of the histological and histochemical questions concerning 5-HT is not given in this paper for two reasons. First, it would burden the discussion and hinder the schematic presentation of the proposed subject matter, and also, since the question has been examined quite recently from this point of view (VIALLI 1962), it would only mean unnecessary repetition.

II. The elements of the enterochromaffin cell system

In the study of 5-HT, the relationship between biochemistry, pharmacology, histology in general, histochemistry in particular and, most important of all, the fact that most research is the work of the same scientists, explains the existence of a homogeneous body of knowledge directly connected with the question and also the fact that, to a great extent, it has been gathered following the pattern previously discussed.

In 1954 ERSPAMER published a monographical survey of what was then known about 5-HT under the title "The enterochromaffin cell system and enteramine (5-hydroxytryptamine)" (1954), thus stressing the importance that histological questions may have in the solution of a great variety of biological problems. The first part of this paper is totally based upon histological and comparative data which, too often, biochemists, physiologists and pharmacologists do not take into consideration, thus greatly reducing the scope of the conclusions which may be reached.

In the first few pages, which are dedicated to histology, ERSPAMER briefly outlines the principal characteristics of the elements of the enterochromaffin cell system. In his opinion the system includes all those cells in which, after formalin fixation, it is possible to demonstrate the presence of chromaffin and argentaffin granules which are capable of coupling with diazonium salts and fluoresce in WOOD's light[1]. In all these cells the specific substance present is enteramine, often together with its parent substances or its derivatives.

As early as 1954 the writer commented upon some considerations concerning the nature of the enterochromaffin cell system; more recently, in 1960 and 1962, he had occasion to deal with this subject more fully. We will come back to it later. At present it will suffice to recall the elements of the system, following ERSPAMER:

a) enterochromaffin cells, both intra- and extra-intestinal. In his monograph of 1961, ERSPAMER (1961) subdivides this category, distinguishing between the various localizations and placing the enterochromaffin cells of *Amphioxus* and *Ascidia* in different sections;

b) the chromaffin cells of the posterior salivary glands of *Octopoda*;

c) the giant chromaffin cells of the hypobranchial gland of *Muricidae*;

d) the secreting cells of amphibian granulous cutaneous glands, when these cells are producers of a chromaffin secretion.

In his work of 1962 the writer considered the system to be still open to future additions, both of histochemically correspondent cellular elements in which the presence of enteramine could be shown and also of biochemically demonstrable localizations of 5-HT for which a histological substrate could subsequently be found.

---

[1] Actually, since the development of fluorescence techniques for the study of adrenaline and noradrenaline carried out by FALCK (1962), it would be more correct to say "give characteristic fluorescence".

Thus the following may be included in the system:

e) the chromaffin cells of *Calliactis parasitica*;

f) the poison-gland cells of some scorpions.

ERSPAMER (1961), re-examining and modifying his 1954 classification, has added:

g) the mast cells of the rat and the mouse,

in which it is occasionally possible to demonstrate the presence of 5-HT histochemically. This classification undoubtedly offers many advantages, being, as already mentioned, open to the new elements which future research may discover.

The basic criterion for the inclusion of an element in the system is the possibility of demonstrating the presence of 5-HT histochemically. As ERSPAMER (1961) points out, a substantial increase in the sensitivity of the reactions may permit the inclusion of elements in which the concentration of the substance is below the threshold of sensitivity of the methods available at present. However, ERSPAMER's classification obviously omits any concept of morphological unity and each element or group of elements generally appears to be independent of the others.

Leaving aside the enterochromaffin cell system for the time being, let us consider what situations may be encountered in the study of 5-HT.

We may find:

a) localizations, such as those previously mentioned, in which the presence of 5-HT may be demonstrated both histologically and biologically;

b) localizations more or less similar to those of enteramine, in which a physiological demonstration of 5-HT is lacking or else the reactions are attributable to other substances;

c) localizations in which the presence of 5-HT has been proven biologically but for which histological data are lacking or incomplete.

What we have said stresses the importance of the relationship between histochemical, biological, physico-chemical and pharmacological tests for 5-HT in the search for new elements and even more so for a better understanding of the many other unsolved problems.

The principal purpose of this review is the study of the elements listed under a); the elements under b) and c) will also be mentioned because of their obvious relationship.

Because of the lack of morphological unity in the enterochromaffin system, the descriptive part, that is the answers to questions II—III—IV—V—VI—VII, previously listed will require a comprehensive study of the system section by section. The qualitative histochemical questions on the other hand, which are the basis for the unification into a single system of this heterogeneous set of elements, may be treated as a whole and, in a sense, may be considered to be the necessary premise for our discussion.

The histochemical data of interest to us are closely related to the class of reactions for the assay of phenolic and indolic compounds; in fact it is impossible with certainty to separate these two fields of investigation (VIALLI, 1960, 1963a).

The part of the enterochromaffin cell system of greatest interest to the pharmacologists is obviously that of the enterochromaffin cells. Therefore this subject will be explored in greater detail in the present paper. However, for a complete understanding of the biological importance of 5-HT, it is also necessary to have some knowledge of the other elements of the system. With good reason, both ERSPAMER (1954, 1961) and the present writer (1954, 1960, 1962) have repeatedly stressed the necessity of a complete rational knowledge and evaluation of all the elements involved; probably many incomplete, or even mistaken, interpretations could have been avoided if other Authors had taken into account all the elements available.

The enterochromaffin cell itself is not, in our opinion, a single completely independent entity but, to judge its importance properly, should also be viewed as part of an organic and systematic whole. The histological viewpoint, in particular, requires the inclusion of other elements also and the discussion of their relationship with the typical cell.

III. Histochemical characteristics of 5-HT of diagnostic importance

ERSPAMER's (1954) summary outline of the histochemical characteristics of the enterochromaffin cell system clearly indicates that a histochemical diagnosis based on one reaction alone is impossible: for the identification of 5-HT one must employ a series of reactions. On the other hand, the writer (1960, 1962) has already pointed out that often a histochemical diagnosis to be truly unequivocal, at least at the present state of our knowledge, must also be integrated with criteria from other types of research.

In their treatises on histochemistry particular attention is awarded to 5-HT by PEARSE (1960), LISON (1960) and LILLIE (1954).

PEARSE entitles the paragraph on this substance "Enterochromaffin (KULTSCHITSKY) Cell Granules" and discusses it in a more comprehensive chapter on pigments. LILLIE discusses 5-HT in a paragraph "Enterochromaffin or Argentaffin cells" from the chapter "Amino-acid End Groups, etc". LISON, however, entitles his paragraph "Serotonine (5-hydroxytryptamine, enteramine)" and places it in a section on catecholalkylamines and indolalkylamines; it should be noted that, following the new arrangement of the subject matter, LISON in the latest edition of his book considers in a general chapter "Noyaux et fonctions aromatiques et hétérocycliques" the various histochemical possibilities of diagnosis offered by phenolic, pyrrolic, and indolic substances. A paper by the present writer (1963a) is also devoted to a critical review of the histochemistry of phenolic and indolic compounds, but with particular attention to enterochromaffin cells.

In a recent classification of histochemical techniques the writer (1962a) has distinguished between "non-destructive" methods and "destructive" methods. In the system under consideration most of the techniques are non-destructive. It should be pointed out though that the study of incongruous fixations, which has been given such great importance in the research of ERSPAMER and the writer (VIALLI and ERSPAMER, 1937, 1937a, 1937b, 1937c, 1937d, 1937e, 1937f, 1937g, 1938) on the extraction and identification of enteramine, may be considered an "in situ" destructive method; but the homogenization and differential centrifugation methods for the separation of specific granules are included among the "extra situm" methods.

Without strictly following the classification just mentioned we may consider chemical and physical methods of determination; they will now be discussed in this sense. First of all though we must make a general remark: 5-HT, because of its formula, should obviously show the phenol, pyrrol and indol reactions; however, as we shall see in the case of formalin fixation, 5-HT is denaturated and consequently some reactions which should be positive are negative, while the response to others goes beyond those which are considered its normal limits. Obviously the positive or negative response is also affected, as already mentioned, by the sensitivity of the reaction; this factor, therefore, may explain some of the apparently paradoxical results.

A. Fixability characteristics

The fixability characteristics of the granules may be used as preliminary criteria for discriminating between elements belonging to the complex group of phenolic and indolic substances. For instance, (VIALLI 1935) it was possible to exclude in various sections of the system the possibility that the granules were made up of adrenalin, on the basis of their fixability with formalin; on the other hand, a distinction is also possible on the basis of a greater fixability spectrum, as for example in the case of phenolic granules of the vitellogen cells of *Platyhelmintha* (VIALLI, 1933) or the vitelline granules of *Polyclada* (VIALLI, 1934).

It is generally stated that the materials containing enteramine present in various localizations may be fixed only with formalin. Actually, this statement is not strictly true, in fact some substances, which work simultaneously both as fixatives and as reagents, may permit the fixation of 5-HT (CHRISTIE, 1955a, VIALLI, 1960). Furthermore, the granules may be preserved by freezing-drying; in this case, of course, they are unaltered even after inclusion in paraffin, and fixation must be carried out on the sections. This technique is particularly important since it permits a study of the true physical and chemical characteristics of un-denaturated 5-HT (GHIRINGHELLI, 1960). Thus previous observations of CORDIER (1926) and of HAMPERL (1925a, 1927), confirmed also by ERSPAMER and the writer (VIALLI and ERSPAMER, 1936), show that by fixation of enterochromaffin cells with potassium bichromate alone, instead of with formolbichromic mixtures, the chromaffin reaction is no longer localized in the granules but is diffuse.

CHRISTIE (1955a) points out that, among some of the first observations of enterochromaffin cells, those of NUSSBAUM (1870) and GRÜTZNER and MENZEL (1879) concern material fixed with osmic acid; he describes his own positive results, obtained also by electron microscopy, on guinea-pig intestine fixed with a 1% solution of osmium tetroxide maintained at pH 7,3—7,5 with a sodium — acetate sodium veronal buffer. Many other recent ultrastructural data confirm this result.

GHIRINGHELLI (1960) has observed that material treated with the freezing-drying method permits subsequently the fixation of the granules with osmic acid vapours.

In any case, formalin is undoubtedly the best fixative for 5-HT; one may employ greatly varied concentrations and times of reaction: generally, 10% for 24 hours or more; however, granules are at least partially fixed and histochemically denaturated even after very brief periods of fixation (2—3 hours) (LANERI, unpublished observations, GHIRINGHELLI, 1960).

After freezing-drying an excellent fixation may be obtained by the action of formalin vapours on tissues still impregnated with paraffin or from which it has been removed (GHIRINGHELLI, 1960).

Quite recently, FALCK and TORP (1961) and FALCK (1962) have introduced a modification of the method of fixation during freezing-drying which, at least for adrenaline and nor-adrenaline, has provided some extremely interesting results. FALCK carries out the formalin treatment for 1 hour on previously lyophilized pieces of an organ by means of formaldehyde gas developed from paraformaldehyde at 80° C. The tissue is then paraffin-embedded in a vacuum.

In certain cases it is best to employ a neutral formalin or one buffered near neutrality. A basic solution of formalin preserves the granules until its alkalinity destroys the tissue; acid solutions have a harmful effect on the fixation of the granules. It is impossible to preserve them even when as little as a 2—3% solution of HCl has been added to the fixative (VIALLI and ERSPAMER, 1936). Usually, a good fixation may be obtained, as long as the formalin concentration is sufficient, with a variety of solutions which may or may not include reactive substances (such as, for example, bichromate). In the case of mixtures with ethyl alcohol, methyl alcohol or acetone, such as SCHAFFER's formalin-alcohol solution (2:1 ethyl alcohol:formalin), fixation is only possible when the solvents have been diluted with water (VIALLI and ERSPAMER, 1936).

In 1940 VIALLI and ERSPAMER (1940, 1942) were able to show that the reaction characteristics of crude extracts containing 5-HT appeared to be different from some of the histochemical characteristics of enterochromaffin cells. After it was recognized that enteramine corresponds to 5-HT, it was possible to verify this incomplete congruity of response on the pure substance also; in fact, most of the disagreement over the true value of histochemical reactions on fixed material was due to the denaturation which is known to occur during fixation.

An interpretation of the chemical mechanism of formalin fixation was formulated by BARTER and PEARSE (1953, 1955), and later by PEARSE (1956, 1960): 5-HT, by closure of the lateral chain upon the CH situated in α of the pyrrolic nucleus, would form a β-carbolinic compound. This question, moreover has been amply discussed by LEMBECK and KLEMEMTSCHITZ (1955) who also made some tests on paper. According to VIALLI and TRAVERSO (1960) the β-carbolinic compound postulated is not an end-product but by further oxidation may form other substances; this would explain the more or less intense yellow colour one observes in individual localizations within the fixed material and which is particularly bright in the posterior salivary glands of *Octopus* (VIALLI and ERSPAMER, 1938a) and in the hypobranchial gland of *Murex* (VIALLI, 1934a).

BARTER and PEARSE's interpretation with a few modifications has been confirmed experimentally in test-tube and paper tests. We may say that it explains the fixability of the granules but does not prove that 5-HT will always be fixed by formalin; in fact: a) the process of formation of the β-carbolinic derivative is rather slow; b) after homogenation and differential centrifugation of the granules fixed proportions of 5-HT and ATP are found, as will be discussed later, and the factors which determine this coexistence are unknown; c) there are localizations of 5-HT, such as for instance those in the central nervous system, of which a histotopochemical demonstration is lacking, a fact that cannot be explained solely by an insufficient sensitivity of reaction. Finally, it seems worth while pointing out that the observation that ethyl alcohol and acetone do not permit fixation of the granules induced VIALLI and ERSPAMER (1936, 1937) to follow what we may call the principle of incongruous fixation; this procedure made it possible to obtain extracts of enteramine for the first time.

B. Colour reactions

In the study of colour reactions which may be employed in research on 5-HT one obviously must take into account all that is known about the fixation procedures. There are reasons for believing that reactions will be different in non-fixed material (freezing-drying) and in material fixed with formalin, and also that mixtures of formalin with other substances may carry on the denaturation of 5-HT to a higher degree and possibly in a different manner.

As a purely empirical datum which follows from what we have said and may be useful in our discussion, we will list some of the types of reaction response that may be observed:

a) reactions which are consistent both in fixed material and with pure 5-HT;

b) reactions which although positive show different behaviour in the two cases;

c) reactions with pure 5-HT which do not take place in fixed material;

d) reactions which take place in fixed material but not with pure 5-HT.

It seems appropriate to begin our review of the various reactions by listing those which ERSPAMER (1954) considers characteristic of the elements which belong to the enterochromaffin system and which are also the most commonly used: chromaffin, argentaffin reactions and the diazo-reaction.

1. Chromaffin reaction

This was the histochemical reaction most commonly used in the past for the study of enterochromaffin cells. The limits of reaction, at first considered to be restricted to adrenaline, were well defined by VERNE (1923) and later by GERARD, CORDIER and LISON (1930), CORDIER and LISON (1930); and LISON (1931). On various occasions VIALLI proposed an extension to indolic substances (1934a, 1940); an exhaustive discussion on this subject may be found in VIALLI (1963a).

According to LISON (1931) the polyphenols, the aminophenols and the polyamines ortho- and para- are chromaffin. On the other hand, as VIALLI (1963a) pointed out elsewhere the contemporaneous presence of an OH in position 5 and of the NH of the pyrrol ring explains the positive reaction of both the non-denaturated substance and the β-carbolinic derivative.

LISON (1960) in the latest edition of his book admits the possibility that the formation of quinone-imine may permit the reaction to take place with 5-HT.

The reaction is carried out jointly with fixation by employing formalin-bichromic solutions (e.g. REGAUD's solution), either directly by treatment with bichromate alone in fixation or by carrying out the reaction on tissues fixed in formalin and included in paraffin. The best results are obtained when the reaction and the fixation are carried out concurrently; post-treatment of fixed material with bichromate seldom provides appreciable results.

It is worth while pointing out that LISON (1932, 1933a) considers the possibility of obtaining a false reaction (pseudochromaffinity) in the case of the lateral portions of the hypobranchial gland of *Murex*.

2. Argentaffin reactions and argentophily

This subject is somewhat more complex since, particularly in the case of research on enterochromaffin cells, a clear distinction has not always been made between typical cells which show the reaction and pre-enterochromaffin argentophil cells in which it is lacking. The distinction between argentaffinity and argentophily is fundamental, although the terms do not show the meaning of this difference. Argentaffinity occurs with substances which are capable, by themselves, of reducing silver salt solutions in a way similar to that which occurs when a photographic film is developed. In the case of argentophily, on the other hand, the substance concerned retains silver compounds from the solution and reduction to metallic silver is obtained later, by means of an appropriate developer (CORDIER 1927, HAMPERL 1932). From this definition it should follow that argentaffin substances are also argentophil; actually though, according to HAMPERL (1952) and HELLWEG (1952) a certain percentage of the argentaffin cells is not argentophil.

The present writer (1954) has already made critical comments on these findings from the theoretical point of view. Quite recently SINGH (1963, 1963a, 1964) mapped out and counted the enterochromaffin cells on sections treated with the silver urotropine technique. Successively the same sections have been tested by the Bodian reaction and every argentaffin cell has been demonstrated to be argentophil, in contrast with the above mentioned affirmation of HAMPERL (1952) and HELLWEG (1952).

While the theoretical distinction between argentaffinity and argentophily is clear-cut, this does not hold in practice. In fact, if procedures which would normally be indicative of argentaffinity are carried out for too long, or on pieces of tissue instead of sections, false argentaffin reactions may be obtained which are actually due to argentophily alone. Also some techniques which have been proposed as specific for argentaffinity may actually work partly as argentophil reactions. Thus, for instance, in GOMORI's silver-methenamine reaction for argentaffinity the formation of formaldehyde from methenamine, which has a well-known activity as a developer, may occur (VIALLI 1963a, LEWIS 1962).

While it is fairly easy to determine the limits of positivity of the argentaffin reaction which has a well-known chemical mechanism, it is not so easy to define the exact histochemical value of argentophily. The fact is that the argentaffin reaction is positive whenever the chromaffin reaction is positive. But the argentaffin reaction is also positive with numerous substances that are not chromaffin. LISON (1960) in a table lists the principal compounds of histochemical interest which are capable of reducing silver solutions; they are: ortho- and para-polyphenols, aldehydes, uric acid, urates, ascorbic acid, hexoses and 5-HT.

In all these cases one may speak of primary argentaffinity; there are numerous other cases, of which here we will only mention the mucopolysaccharides and the polysaccharides, in which, by chemical means, it is possible to produce reducing groups and which therefore have what we may call a secondary argentaffinity.

Even if we limit our discussion to substances reducing in themselves, we find that this capacity, and hence their argentaffinity, varies greatly. In the first place, the differences in reactivity allow the reduction of silver reagents of different constitution: for instance, only ascorbic acid can reduce an acid solution of silver nitrate (GIROUD and LEBLOND 1936, 1937). Furthermore, according to various authors, the different reducing capacity should also imply different reaction times. On the basis of just this property GOMORI (1948, 1950, 1952), assuming that the argentaffin reaction occurs rather slowly in the granules of the enterochromaffin cells, postulated, in opposition to the then current diagnosis of an ortho- or para-, di- or poly-phenol, that the substance was a meta-diphenol. Actually, after ERSPAMER's discovery that enteramine corresponds to 5-HT, GOMORI (1954) himself recognized that 5-HT may have a relatively low reducing power, implying a fairly long reaction time. One should also bear in mind that the argentaffinity of the granules, as it is normally assayed, does not depend directly on 5-HT but on its β-carbolynic derivative; in a sense, therefore, we may speak of a secondary argentaffinity. Reaction tests on paper imbued with 5-HT show much lower reactivity after treatment with formalin vapours (BENDITT and WONG, 1957, GHIRINGHELLI, 1960). On the other hand, in enterochromaffin cells too, the reaction takes place fairly quickly. In fact LANERI's unpublished observations show that, at room temperature, a certain number of cells react after only three hours of treatment.

In spite of its low specificity, one may say that the argentaffin reaction is the one most commonly used. This is particularly true in the study of enterochromaffin cells — of which all the histochemical characteristics are now well known — when it is necessary to individuate cells present in very small numbers or to perform cell counts. It is convenient because the reaction is easy to perform and because the black granules stand out clearly against a practically colourless background.

There would be no need even to mention argentophily here if it were not for the close relationship existing, as we shall see, between the typical enterochromaffin cell and the argentophil pre-enterochromaffin cell. Certainly, in many cases argentophily may be a characteristic completely independent of argentaffinity and as such it should be normally interpreted. However, one cannot exclude the possibility that, at times, argentaffin substances, when present in concentrations below the limit of sensitivity, may still respond to argentophil reactions.

The fact is that one may still obtain an argentophil reaction after fixation with alcohol, which is certainly incompatible as far as 5-HT is concerned. Argentophil techniques may be employed on fragments of an organ, as for instance in CAYAL's photographic method or on free sections as in the original Gross-Schultze technique.

Whenever very precise observations or counts are required, or in any case for comparisons, it is very useful to carry out the reaction on sections attached to a slide; for this reason, various modifications of the original free-section methods have been studied. Today, a large number of these types of technique are available, not only because they are useful in research on argentophil cells, but also because they are employed in the study of the nervous system and the reticular fibres. The great number of modifications carried out on the classical techniques indicate a certain difficulty in obtaining good and repeatable results, not only when work is done on different species, but also on material quite homogeneous from this point of view. Most of the observations have been made with BODIAN's method (MARCOLI 1949) or with modifications of it.

FEYRTER (1953) and many others employ instead a modification of the Gross-Schultze technique. In spite of all these precautions, the demonstration of argentophily often does not work, or worse still, provides results which are only apparently positive; one notices this when counts performed on correspondding sections appear to be very similar in preparations treated with argentaffin and argentophil methods indicating that the reaction is positive only for the former. Obviously the argentaffin cells in this case, will give positive results even in the first stage of the treatment independently of subsequent chemical development.

3. Diazo reactions

We may say that the use of these reactions in histochemistry began with the work of GERARD, CORDIER and LISON (1930) on the adrenal medulla and of CORDIER and LISON (1930) on the enterochromaffin cells. A more detailed study of the reaction may be found in LISON (1931). The reaction is usually performed in a basic medium, but to exploit its discriminative possibilities fully one should not neglect the reaction in an acid medium or in a basic medium when the reaction product is later strongly acidified (VIALLI and ERSPAMER 1939). The diagnostic meanings of these three reaction modalities are very different; all three give a positive diazoreaction with 5-HT; indeed, VIALLI and ERSPAMER obtained positive responses of the three reactions from crude extracts of rabbit stomach (VIALLI and ERSPAMER 1942) and of the posterior salivary gland of *Octopus*, (VIALLI and ERSPAMER 1940) suggesting to them that enteramine was of a pyrrolic or indolic nature. On the other hand the applications of histochemical techniques gave them at first negative results with an acid diazoreaction: this seemed to suggest that formalin fixation had modified the reactivity; their acid solutions were rather concentrated (2.25 equivalents to 2) and thus it was impossible to obtain any histochemically demonstrable reaction; they later found though, that by reducing the acidity somewhat (pH 5.2—5.4), it was possible to get the positive reaction as expected. The only data in the literature on a basic-medium diazoreaction followed by strong acidification concern the posterior salivary gland of *Octopus* (VIALLI and ERSPAMER 1938a).

The diazonium compounds for the reaction may be prepared from appropriate amines; the choice of the amine to diazotate depends on a number of factors, according to what one wishes to obtain. The most important distinction is between diazotates and tetrazotates because of the presence of one or two azo groups respectively. The latter case is of particular importance since of the two azogroups one may combine with the substance to be identified and the other with a reactive compound; thus a tetra-diazo-compound is obtained which has a much more intense colour than the corresponding diazo-compound. In the diazo-safranin reaction of LILLIE, BURTNER and GRECO HENSON (1953) we have a particular kind of diazoreaction which may be prepared expressly. Finally, it is worth while pointing out that fluorescent diazonium salts may be prepared from appropriate amines (VIALLI, unpublished observations). Stabilized diazotate salts were introduced into histochemistry by CLARA (1934) who used *Nitrazol-CF* and *Nitrosaminrot*. As with all stains carrying factory names there is a very intricate synonymy. Recently, in the Journal of Histochemistry and Cytochemistry (LILLIE 1959) and in an appendix of GURR's (1960) book we find a fairly complete list of these stains with their formulae and a rich synonymy. Although, using these commercial stains, one does not always obtain results equal to those with expressly-made diazo-compounds, in the wide gamut of reagents available there are compounds to satisfy most needs.

4. Pearse's thyo-indoxyl reaction

To the three above-mentioned reactions which ERSPAMER (1954) in his 1954 monograph considers to be capable of identifying bodies containing 5-HT, the author himself, in his 1961 monograph, adds the thyo-indoxyl reaction proposed by PEARSE in 1956 and used with good results by VIALLI and QUARONI (1956). The mechanism of the reaction, which occurs also on the β-carbolinic compound formed during formalin fixation, takes place in two stages: in the first, by weak iodine or sodium-iodate oxidation the corresponding quinonimine should form; in the second stage a substituted thyo-indoxyl is used which determines the formation of a thyo-indigo stain. On the basis of this reaction, in the writer's opinion (1963), PEARSE's reaction may be put among the indophenol reactions of GIBB's classification (1927, 1927a). The reaction is highly specific, but PEARSE himself believes that it should not be used as a routine technique.

5. Other reactions

In addition to these four reactions, which ERSPAMER (1954, 1961) considers to be the most indicative, PEARSE (1960) ascribes a good deal of importance to the indophenol reaction and to GIBB's reaction with 2:6 dichloroquinonechlorimine. There are numerous others, of different significance, which show a positive response; on the other hand, their mechanism is not always known: some are analogous to the chromaffin reaction, others to the argentaffin and some do not bear any resemblance to other reactions.

We must now go on to make some brief analytical remarks about some of the more important reactions. The iodaffin reaction proposed by LISON (1931) should correspond completely, in its range of positivity, to the chromaffin reaction when REGAUD's type formulae are used; an advantage is that the reaction products of the iodate which eventually form are completely colourless. It has been employed with particular formulae by HILLARP and HÖKFELT (1955) for the demonstration of noradrenaline and by CATTANEO (1958, 1960, 1960a) for the differential demonstration of adrenaline and noradrenaline. On the other hand, although it has not, as yet, found a histochemical application, an iodate reaction according to FEARON and BOGGUST (1950) is known in biochemistry, which forms coloured products with tryptophan also, in the absence therefore of a phenolic OH.

SCHMORL's reaction recommended by GOMORI (1948, 1952), LILLIE (1954) and LILLIE and BURTNER (1953) for enterochromaffin cells corresponds rather well to the argentaffin reaction, thus indicating the presence of reducing agents. It depends on the reduction of ferric to ferrous iron, which is revealed as Turnbull-blue. It is a reaction of high sensitivity but low specificity; in fact, under various names, numerous reactions based on this reduction have been proposed for substances which have nothing in common with indols or phenols.

Another reduction reaction is PEARSE's (1954, 1960) formazan reaction. It is also worth while recalling the osmic acid reaction, since the first observations of enterochromaffin cells were made with it and because it is still employed in electron microscopy. The COUJARD-CHAMPY (1943) reaction is a modification of greater sensitivity but less specificity.

For more complete information on these various reactions and their classification see VIALLI and ERSPAMER (1936), VIALLI (1963).

6. Reactions which do not give the expected positive response

There are a certain number of reactions which, although excellent for 5-HT in vitro, provide no appreciable histochemical results. The general explanation for this phenomenon is based on the fact that what actually reacts is the β-carbolynic derivative. Some of these reactions are quite important, being commonly used in the quantitative assay of 5-HT; among them we may recall EHRLICH's para-dimethyl-amino-benzaldehyde reaction (LILLIE 1956), the xanthydrol reaction (LILLIE 1957), GERNGROSS's, VOSS's and HERFELD's (1933) α-nitroso-β-naphthol reaction, Folin-Ciocalteu's reaction (VIALLI and ERSPAMER 1940, 1942), the di-methyl-para-phenylene-diamine reaction (LILLIE 1956) and MOREL-SISLEY's (LILLIE 1957a) reaction. It may be that the negative response obtained with some of these procedures is simply due to insufficient sensitivity; in fact, it is well known that in certain reactions, the sensitivity for the β-carbolynic derivative is greatly inferior to that for 5-HT.

7. Various procedures

Of some importance in the study of 5-HT are some procedures based on chemical or enzymatical denaturation; in part they belong to the so-called block reactions. Some are worth while recalling: for instance, the deamination treatment of ZORZOLI and LILLIE (1956) and the blocking of the OH by diazo-methane described by VIALLI and TRAVERSO (1960a). The pepsin demolition described by GLENNER and LILLIE (1959) is also of interest.

C. Fluorescence as a diagnostic criterion

The appearance of a secondary fluorescence due to the β-carbolynic compound formed during formalin fixation is well known and quite distinctive. After FALCK's (1962) treatment, a similar type of fluorescence also develops for adrenalin and nor-adrenalin, with slightly different characteristics in the two substances, which are apparent even by direct observation under the fluorescence-microscope. However, according to FALCK (1962) one must be extremely cautious in employing fluorescence as a criterion for distinguishing between these various amines. The remarkable differences in fluorescence-colours one observes at times in different localizations of 5-HT may possibly be explained by the presence of interfering substances as in the cutaneous glands of Amphibians; however, in the writer's opinion, this limits even more the usefulness of fluorescence in chemical diagnosis.

D. Limits of histochemical diagnosability of 5-HT

As we have seen, none of the four reactions listed by ERSPAMER (1954) are sufficient for a strictly specific diagnosis of 5-HT, nor is there any other particular reaction capable of this. An over-all examination of all four reactions, or even, on a wider basis, of all procedures employing blocks does not provide sufficient results for an unequivocal diagnosis. In this context, we may recall the fifth procedure considered by ERSPAMER (1961) for the identification of elements belonging to the enterochromaffin system: the fluorescence in WOOD's light of material fixed in formalin. Clearly this is a diagnostic characteristic of great importance and its limits will be described later on among the physical characteristics of the granules.

However, not even this provides what may be considered a complete diagnosis and it is necessary to integrate the histochemical data (VIALLI 1963, LEWIS 1962) with other elements taken mostly from biochemistry and pharmacology. In the analysis of the data this integration is necessary on two distinct levels: in fact, the histochemical requirements will be different according to whether preceding biochemical or pharmacological data have indicated the presence of 5-HT in a given localization, or whether the histochemical data must be collected as a guide for future biochemical or pharmacological work. The positive or negative results one may thus obtain may be useful in evaluating and correlating histochemical data which in themselves would be insufficient.

E. Histochemical data obtained by destructive extra-situm methods

All the reactions considered up to now, following VIALLI's recent classification (1962a), belong to the group of non-destructive or destructive "in-situ" methods. However, data of great interest have been collected also by "extra-situm" destructive methods; they deserve our attention, since they offer many interesting possibilities of future development not only to the histologist, but also to the biochemist and pharmacologist. Essentially, they are methods of separation by means of homogenization and differential centrifugation, including density gradient centrifugation; both techniques are well known also to the non-histologist. Up to now, they have been applied to the study of the intestinal mucosa by BAKER (1958, 1958a, 1959) and PRUSOFF (1960), but the method should also be applicable, for instance, to the posterior salivary glands of *Octopus*. On the other hand, still in the field of "extra situm" histochemical assay, one may consider as a direct mechanical method the squeezing of the poison glands, feasible in certain species of Amphibians.

Let us also recall the separation of isolated "Mast cells" in the peritoneal fluid of the rat, by means of the techniques of GLICK, BONTING and DEN BOER (1956); in fact, according to ERSPAMER (1961) the "Mastzellen" of the rat should be included in the enterochromaffin cell system. Obviously the material collected by these "extra-situm" methods lends itself to many usages which in a strict sense may be partly outside the field of histochemistry; they may provide completely new results, such as, for instance, the discovery of the presence of ATP. in enterochromaffin cells, which we will discuss later.

IV. The enterochromaffin cell system

A. Enterochromaffin cells

As the writer has already had occasion to say, the enterochromaffin cell is not a unit in itself but must be included in a wider picture comprising other cell types which according to ERSPAMER (1937), may be classified together in the system of the enterochromaffin cells, in a broad sense.

It includes:

a) clear, non-argentophil pre-enterochromaffin cells;

b) argentophil pre-enterochromaffin cells;

c) enterochromaffin cells in a strict sense;

d) empty enterochromaffin cells.

Not all these types are equally well known and, actually, the existence of types a) and d) is admitted for the sake of completeness although they have not yet been identified unequivocally.

A knowledge of these different cell types is of fundamental importance for the reconstruction of the developmental cycle of the enterochromaffin cells, and for considerations on comparative anatomical and embryological data and on extra-intestinal localizations. Even if we neglect the necessity, for the topic we are discussing, of taking this aspect into account, we find that it is still of the utmost importance because all these elements more or less correspond to that morphological picture which, as a whole, FEYRTER (1953) calls the peripheric endocrine glands, and which many authors, including PAGÈS (PAGÈS 1955, PAGÈS and PAGÈS 1957), call the "system of clear cells".

We may say that a typical enterochromaffin cell may be identified by the presence of granules of particular shape and disposition, the fact that fixation is possible only with formalin solutions and finally by all those histochemical and histophysical characteristics which, according to ERSPAMER (1954), indicate that the cell belongs to the enterochromaffin system; moreover the granules are obviously also argentophil.

The argentophil pre-enterochromaffin cell has the same morphological characteristics as the typical enterochromaffin cell, only its granules are provided with a much wider fixation spectrum and, though argentophil, they lack the histochemical and histophysical characteristics of the typical cell. If one does not resort to particular devices, which on the other hand do not necessarily guarantee precision, preparations fixed with 10% formalin and treated with argentophil techniques provide an over-all picture which does not discriminate between argentophil cells and typical enterochromaffin cells; to distinguish between the two types counts are made on contiguous sections treated with the two methods. In this connection the technique of SINGH (1963, 1964) above mentioned may be used. If typical enterochromaffin cells are totally lacking, as may often be the case, or as may occur with alcoholic fixation, a clear cut datum on argentophil cells alone is obtained.

One must thus suppose that the actual enterochromaffin cell is the only element of the enterochromaffin cell system, in its broader sense, which contains 5-HT in a form and quantity that can be revealed by histochemical methods; therefore we must now concentrate essentially on this type and leave till later any attempt to discuss and put into perspective the other problems.

As for the intestine, we must recall that the enterochromaffin cell, in its broader sense, does not represent the only epithelial element present and is accompanied by: the columnar cell, the goblet cell and PANETH's cell. It does not seem worth while at this point to list the various differences between these and the enterochromaffin cell since this information may easily be obtained from any good text-book on microscopical anatomy. For further details consult PATZELT (1936) for the intestine and PLENK (1932) for the stomach. Obviously, in the case of other intestinal tracts or organs, it is for other cell types that one must find criteria of discrimination.

1. The typical enterochromaffin cell

Synonymy. — The term enterochromaffin cell has been employed by us from the very beginning of our research because it refers to one of the first characteristics demonstrated and because CIACCIO (1907), the first Italian author to mention this cell type, also used it.

Leaving out the numerous designations based on the names of various authors, which should be discarded anyhow. let us recall the following names: argentaffin cells (CORDIER) silver-reducing cells (MASSON), enterochrome cells (MASSON), chromargentaffin cells (CORDIER), chromoenteroargentaffin cells (BÚLLÓN-RAMÍREZ et al.), yellow cells (SCHMIDT, HAMPERL), basal granulated cells (KAUFMANN-WOLF, CLARA and his school).

Morphological data. — As early as 1870, HEIDENHAIN (1870) described these cells in the fundus glands of the rabbit and dog stomach on the basis of their positive chromaffinity; he discussed the possibility of having to distinguish between them and the chief and parietal cells. Generally, the first clear-cut description of them as a distinct cell type is attributed to NICOLAS (1891) who discusses them in detail for the intestinal epithelium of the lizard.

A chapter on the enterochromaffin cells in the above-mentioned treatise by PATZELT (1936) and three monographs by CLARA (1933), BARRY (1943), BROUSSY and BARRY (1944), although somewhat dated, summarize the available data fairly well.

The shape of the cells is somewhat variable probably because they adapt themselves, in response to mutual pressure, to the space available between adjacent cells. Anyhow, in general, they are larger at the base, where the nucleus is situated, than at the apex. Often the base protrudes somewhat with respect to the neighbouring cells ("bourgeonment" according to MASSON, "Einsprossung" or "Endophytia" according to FEYRTER) modifying at times the arrangement of the basement membrane.

This phenomenon is more conspicuous in pathological conditions; however, SIMARD (1933, 1934) has described in normal conditions too a few cases in which the cells detach themselves completely from the intestinal epithelium of *Phoca vitulina* and calf embryo.

Towards the apical extremity, however, the cell always becomes more or less narrow and in many cases does reach the outer limit of the other cells; when it does reach it, a brush border may be present as mentioned by CLARA (1933) and VIALLI (1929).

The dimension and the shape of the nucleus do not always distinguish it from the adjacent cells. Its position, although generally basal, is also variable. One or two nucleoli may be present (though not always). In normal or pathological conditions rare binucleate and even tri- and quadrinucleate cells have been described (HAMPERL 1927, VETTER 1939, ERSPAMER 1936, FRIEDMAN 1934) however no mitotic or amitotic figures have ever been observed following colchicine treatment (VIALLI and GHIRINGHELLI 1960).

The undifferentiated cytoplasm is clear and homogeneous, only slightly stainable and, within it, other cytoplasmic organelles are more or less evident. The centrosome often appears as a diplosome and is located apically with respect to the nucleus and the GOLGI internal reticular apparatus. This is not always easy to demonstrate, because, at least with some colourations, it may be confused with the specific granulations present. The GOLGI internal reticular apparatus is of limited size and presents itself quite clearly as a negative image if the staining of the granules is sufficiently intense. Its typical appearance in the intestinal cells is that of a "lacunoma"; its position is always super-nuclear. GILLMAN (1942) regards this disposition of the Golgi apparatus as proof of the endodermic origin of the enterochromaffin cells. It is very difficult to get a good representation of the chondrioma; however, besides granular images which, with most colourations, are indistinguishable from the specific granulations, one may sometimes also observe more or less flexuous filaments which must certainly represent the chondriosomes. In any case the presence of elements of the chondrioma is unequivocally attested by electron microscopy.

Apart from extreme cases of endophytia the enterochromaffin cells show connections with the nervous fibres of the periglandular plexus. This has been exactly demonstrated by SIMARD (1934). A figure of his concerning the foetal intestine of a calf is reproduced (Plate 1, Fig. f).

a) Specific granules

Morphological and staining characteristics. — The specific granules are the most important characteristic of the enterochromaffin cells. Even from the morphological point of view they are perfectly distinguishable from the granules present in other cell types, such as PANETH's cells and the muciparous cells of the gastric epithelium. The granules are very minute and stand out more or less clearly, according to the stain employed, against an undifferentiated cytoplasm.

Their arrangement is typical too: normally they cluster more densely in the infra-nuclear portion of the cell, surround the nucleus, and in the super-nuclear region mark the boundary of the internal reticular apparatus; further towards the apex they may or may not be present. In the latter situation their density is always lower and, in any case, when the distal extremity of the cell reaches the intestinal lumen, one always observes, even if the presence of a brush border cannot be demonstrated, an undifferentiated region of protoplasm in which the granules are missing. Usually, there is a certain variation in the arrangement of the granules, even within cells of the same preparation. However, there are some aspects peculiar to a given species, such as in the guinea-pig, where the cells are very often extremely rich in granules even in the super-nuclear region.

For material fixed in formalin or, in many cases, even with other fixatives, the granules are distinctly acidophil: in this respect the results obtained with eosin or erythrosin are particularly indicative. When a preparation stained with iron haematoxylin is differentiated, the granules mantain a strong colouration even after the nuclear chromatin begins to bleach. In material fixed with formalin-bichromic solutions, in preparations by KULL's modification of ALTMANN's method the granules are stained by aurantia.

Distribution and quantity of the granules. — For functional and comparative anatomical studies of the enterochromaffin cells, the most important data concern the quantity of the granules present and their distribution within the cells. It is well known that the quantity of the granules is extremely variable and may be expressed in terms of granule concentration and estimated cell-area occupied.

For a detailed analysis, on a factual basis, of these characteristics one should refer to the situations as they occur in a given species. YAMASAKI (1940), on the basis of observations on the rat fixed with REGAUD's solution and stained by KULL's method, distinguishes three types of cells which, in his opinion, represent different functional stages. Again with regard to the intestine of the rat, MARKS, SORGEN and HAYES (1958) and GHIRINGHELLI and MIRA (1959, 1959a) have proposed a classification based on the number and distribution of the granules. The most frequently quoted classification is that of GHIRINGHELLI and MIRA who distinguish eight types, taking into account separately the granulosity of the infra- and super-nuclear regions. Usually the granules are studied on material prepared with MASSON's method. By counting the different cell types separately one obtains a weighted granular index which appears to correspond better to the biochemical data than the over-all cell count. Obviously, the numbers obtained represent only a morphological evaluation, since the content in 5-HT probably varies from granule to granule. Naturally, to apply these criteria to cells of other species, one must adapt the classification to their particular type of granule distribution. On the basis of considerations by GERZELI and GHIRINGHELLI (1961), GHIRINGHELLI (1961) has elaborated, for material treated with the Masson-Hamperl technique, a method of objective evaluation by photometry, with the use of the integrating microdensitometer according to DEELEY.

α) Histochemical characteristics. In addition to the reactions which ERSPAMER (1961) considers to be characteristic of the enterochromaffin cell-system: argentaffinity (Plate II, Fig. b), chromaffinity, diazo- (Plate I, Fig. a) and Pearse- (Plate I, Fig. d) reactions, the granules also respond positively to a group of reactions which: a) depend in part on the presence of 5-HT; Schmorl reaction (Plate I, Fig. c); b) are based on what may be called the non-enteraminic component; moreover c) give a negative result although they should be positive in the presence of 5-HT. Questions concerning reactions of type a) and c) have already been discussed in general terms in the chapter devoted to the various reactions. The series of data one may obtain, completed by the reaction block tests (LILLIE 1958, ZORZOLI and LILLIE, 1956, VIALLI and TRAVERSO 1960a), may be compatible with the assumption of the presence of 5-HT, but cannot provide the critical proof of it. The reactions of type b) deserve particular mention; the question, up to now, has been insufficiently studied.

As far as the presence of a lipidic component is concerned, the question has been amply discussed, taking into account all the preceding data also, by GHIRINGHELLI and BOTTINO (1960). The apparently most convincing assay is by CHRISTIE (1954) who observed a positive response to BAKER's test and, on the basis of this alone, concludes that a phospholipine is present in the granules.

GHIRINGHELLI and BOTTINO (1960), however, on the basis of a series of controls, and also of a lipid specific test, believe it to be a false reaction due to the fact that 5-HT, following treatment with bichromate, becomes stainable with haematein. The problem is treated also by PEARSE (1960).

As for the presence of a polysaccharide or muco-polysaccharide component, the most complete data are again those of BOTTINO and GHIRINGHELLI (1958, 1958a) and of GHIRINGHELLI and BOTTINO (1959), who have shown a positive Hotchkiss reaction, also supported by a spectrophotometric analysis capable of discriminating between the effects on the coloration due to oxidation of 5-HT by periodic acid and to SCHIFF's reagent.

JACOBSON (1939), considering the results of other reactions, believes a carbohydrate to be present. He interprets the positive result obtained by nitric acid oxidation, followed by alkalinization, as due to the murexide reaction, characteristic for substances containing a pyrimidinic ring. However, this result may also be interpreted as the expression of a xanthoproteic reaction.

We may also mention a few indirect data on the enzymes by GERZELI, GHIRINGHELLI and MIRA (1962) who, studying the extremities of the fundus glands of a rabbit, which are particularly rich in enterochromaffin cells, were not able to observe a difference in enzyme content between the enterochromaffin cells certainly present and the delomorphous that are much poorer in the enzymes assayed. The Authors have studied: isocitrate DH, succinate DH, lactate DH, glucose-6-phosphate DH, α-glycero-phosphate DH, diaphorase, DPN, diaphorase-TPN and cytochrome-oxydase.

PEARSE and PEPLER (1957) were unsuccessful in demonstrating peptidase in normal cells but found it in the cells of a carcinoid. Quite recently LOJDA and FRIČ (1964) and LOJDA, VEČEREK and PELICHOVÁ, who also recall some preceding data by KOJECKY and KODOUSEK (1961) and by KOJECKÝ, BENÝŠEK, KODOUSEK and MALINSKÝ (1963) have described, in human bioptic material, histotopochemical images of alkaline phosphatase, adenosintriphosphatase, acid phosphatase, unspecified esterase, DPN and TPN diaphorase and lactate DH, malate DH, isocitrate DH, glucose-6-phosphate DH, succinate DH, β-hydroxybutyrate DH and α-glycerophosphate DH.

The results obtained, partly from modifications of the common techniques, deserve to be extended and verified. It is an interesting fact that the ferments are often localized in the apical part of the cell.

The determination of the apparent isoelectric point performed by CASTOLDI (1960) following PISCHINGER's method probably depends on the over-all physicochemical conditions in the granules.

It is also necessary to recall here the assertion, upon which JACOBSON (1939, 1954), JACOBSON and GOOD (1949), JACOBSON and SIMPSON (1946, 1946a) have been insisting for some time now, that the granules contain a pterinic substance. On this subject, JACOBSON wrote in 1954: "The failure to establish positive evidence that the yellow pigment of the argentaffin cells is a known derivative of serotonin does not exclude the possibility of serotonin being present in these cells and that both the yellow pigment and serotonin might occur independently in the cytoplasm." However, JACOBSON considers as a serious objection to this hypothesis a series of grossly erroneous data on the quantitative distribution of the enterochromaffin cells. Most Authors do not believe a pterin to be present.

β) Histophysical characteristics. The most well known histophysical characteristic of the enterochromaffin cells is the typical fluorescence exhibited after excitation with WOOD's light. It is clear now that this is a secondary fluorescence due to the β-carbolynic compound formed by formalin fixation (REGGIANI 1946, BARTER and PEARSE 1953, PEARSE 1956, VIALLI 1960, GHIRINGHELLI 1960). CASELLA and REGGIANI (1946, 1949) with a photographic spectro-photometric technique have obtained the emission curve of the fluorescent light and have determined the peak to be at $\lambda = 535$ mμ (Fig. 1a and b). The numerous data of JACOBSON (1939, 1954) of JACOBSON and SIMPSON (1946, 1946a) and of JACOBSON and GOOD (1949) are not very trustworthy since they were not obtained by single cell determinations. JACOBSON considers these data to be one of the proofs of the presence of a pterin. According to CHRISTIE (1955), the granules of material treated by freeze-drying and excited with light of wavelength $\lambda = 275$ mμ emit a clearly visible primary green yellow fluorescence of lower intensity. Again according to CHRISTIE the strong absorption at 275 mμ that may be observed in non-fixed (frozen-dried) material cannot be further revealed photographically after fixation with formalin. Instead, the granules show no appreciable absorption at $\lambda = 257$ mμ either in formalin-fixed or in frozen-dried material. Preliminary measurements by VIALLI and GERZELI (1955) on the dry-mass of the granules indicate a value of 36,75%. In electron-microscopy, the granules show a very strong contrast probably due to osmic fixation (CHRISTIE 1955a).

γ) Ultrastructural data. After CHRISTIE's (1955a) first investigation in 1955, there has been a proliferation of work with the electron microscope on enterochromaffin cells: TAYLOR and HAYES (1961), KUROSUMI, SHIBASAKI, UCHIDA and TANAKA (1958), BULLÓN-RAMÍREZ, LANGER and SCHULTZ (1960), WETZSTEIN and DOERFLER (1962), WESTZTEIN, DOERFLER and SCHWINK (1962), HELANDER (1961, 1962), ITO and WINCHESTER (1963). The species studied were the guinea pig the mouse and the bat; research concerned the gastric and intestinal enterochromaffin cells and, in certain cases, one cannot exclude the possibility that together with the enterochromaffin cells some argentophil cells were included; HELANDER (1961) explicitly considers the latter type too. The enterochromaffin cell as a whole has not revealed any peculiarity worth mentioning (Plate II, Fig. a). Some elements — pigment bodies, according to HELANDER (1962) — have been described which appear to be surrounded by a variable number of double membranes. LUSE and LACY (1960) and ITO and WINCHESTER (1963) have also succeeded in observing cells whose apex reaches the intestinal lumen and have come across terminal bars and microvilli, thus, in a sense, confirming some of the data obtained by optical microscopy. The principal datum though, concerns the specific granules. The estimate of their average dimensions varies from Author to Author μ 0,3 according to CHRISTIE (1955a), WETZSTEIN et al. (1961, 1962) μ 0,18 according to HELANDER (1962). The data available are insufficient to determine whether these differences are species-specific or depend on topographical location; a question which would be of great interest. HELANDER's (1962) description mentions a central core of higher density surrounded by a thin region of low density limited by a surface membrane. A different description of the granules is provided by BULLÓN-RAMÍREZ, LANGER and SCHULTZ (1960), in preparations treated with MASSON's argentaffin technique. The granules are not homogeneously impregnated, but present in their interior an extremely fine deposit of silver grains and often a central region in which the grains are lacking. WETZSTEIN and DOERFLER (1962) have not confirmed the findings of BULLÓN-RAMÍREZ et al. They observed, on the contrary, that the granules were surrounded by a limiting membrane about 50 Å tick. These data, however incomplete, represent an important contribution, since they show that the granules are endowed with a multiplicity of structure and consequently also of chemical composition.

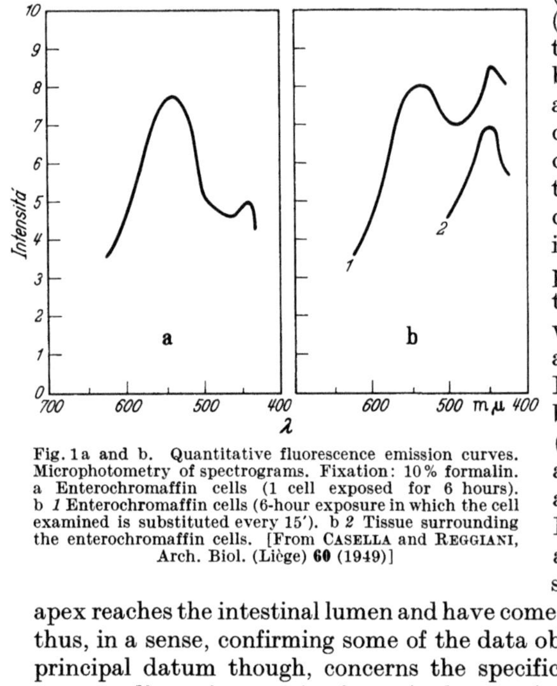

Fig. 1a and b. Quantitative fluorescence emission curves. Microphotometry of spectrograms. Fixation: 10% formalin. a Enterochromaffin cells (1 cell exposed for 6 hours). b *1* Enterochromaffin cells (6-hour exposure in which the cell examined is substituted every 15'). b *2* Tissue surrounding the enterochromaffin cells. [From CASELLA and REGGIANI, Arch. Biol. (Liège) **60** (1949)]

δ) Data obtained by homogenization and differential centrifugation. The histochemical data discussed so far are based on direct histomorphological and histochemical methods; we will now consider some data which are obtained by what, in the present writer's recent classification (1962a), are called destructive *extra-situm* histochemical methods; some biochemists believe them, incorrectly in the writer's opinion, to by outside the scope of histology. Following some preliminary work by BLASCHKO (1956), BAKER (1958, 1958a, 1959), by homogenization and density gradient centrifugation, separated from the mitochondrial fraction a portion showing a high concentration of 5-HT. The electron-microscopy data which distinguish between the specific granules and the mitochondria, are thus confirmed. This is in contrast with the findings of BOGDANSKI, WEISSBACH and UDENFRIEND (1957) who believe that 5-HT cannot be localized in any particular fraction. Later data obtained by PRUSOFF (1960), employing the same technique, provide a further important contribution; 5-HT is always accompanied by ATP and the quantitative ratio between the two substances is fairly constant; the mean content in 5-HT of the dense granule fraction is 4.1 ± 0.9 m.mole, that in ATP is 1.6 ± 0.4 m.mole, the molar ratio being 2.6.

These data are very important, in the first place, because they extend to 5-HT what is known about the relationship between ATP, adrenaline and noradrenaline the relative proportions being not very different. One may thus infer that, in this aspect also, the three amines behave in a similar way. In the second place, from a different point of view they attest once more the multiplicity of the constitution of the specific granules.

b) Topographical distribution

α) Intestinal distribution. As regards their topographical distribution, the enterochromaffin cells are normally found in the intestine (Fig. 2a and b); but numerous other localizations have been described outside the intestine, which may be more or less directly related to the latter. Most of the data on the cells present in the digestive tube concern the intestine proper; however, there are some gastric localizations which, for instance in the rabbit, are particularly important (ERSPAMER 1935). In the lower vertebrates the cells may also be extremely numerous

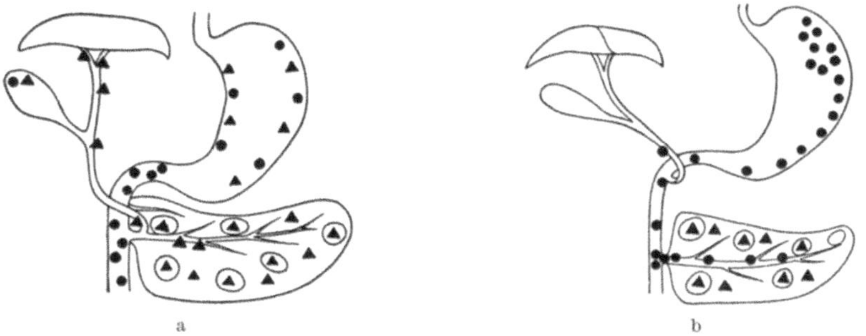

Fig. 2a and b. Schematic diagram of the distribution of typical enterochromaffin cells (●) and argyrophil cells (▲) in the stomach, pancreas and biliary ducts of a Man and b Rabbit. [From ERSPAMER, Z. Anat. Entwickl.-Gesch. **109** (1939)]

in the oesophagus, while in birds and mammals they are rare or even undetectable there. Their distribution in the various tracts of the intestine proper usually shows some fairly similar general characteristics; in some cases, however, we may observe species-specific peculiarities.

The salient characteristics is the way they almost always cluster in the very first portion of the duodenal tract extruding more or less to the adjacent gastric portion. Mostly, the data in the literature are based on subjective evaluations of the cells' density; but there are also various types of quantitative data. These numerical data may be obtained by studying either longitudinal or cross-sections. The two methods have slightly different meanings.

The first, employed mostly by Clara's school, has furnished numerous data in normal and in various experimental conditions. Of particular interest are the

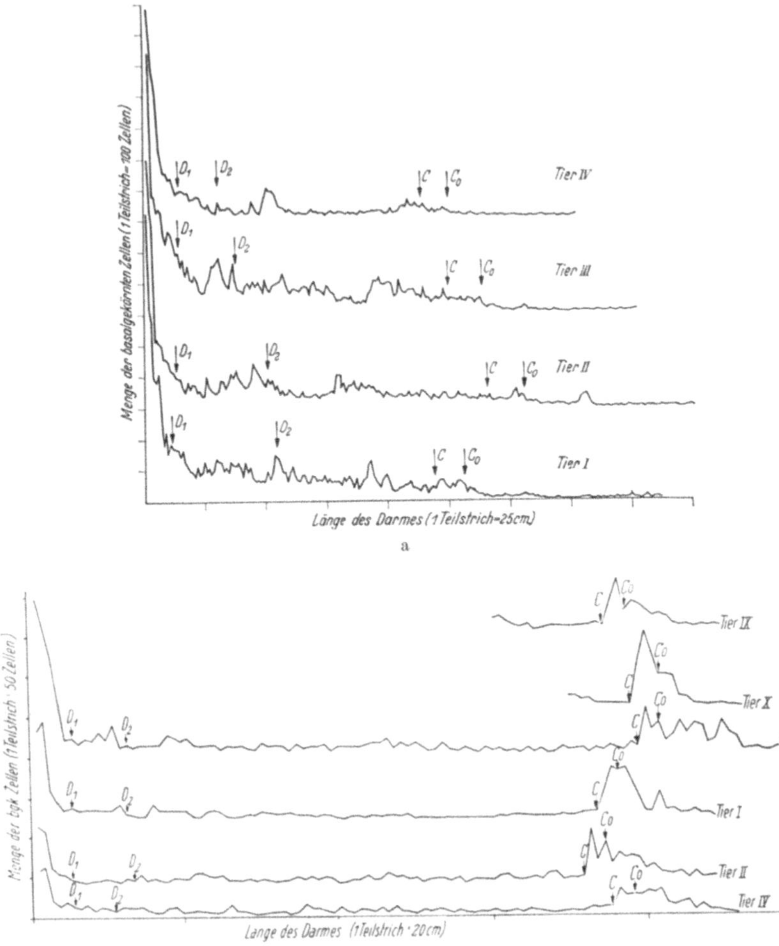

a

b

Fig. 3a and b. Graphical representation of the quantity and distribution of the enterochromaffin cells in individual intestinal tracts. D_1 Microscopic limit of the duodenum. D_2 Histological limit of the duodenum. *C* Beginning of the coecum. *Co* Beginning of the colon. a In the guinea-pig [from Hoeschen, Z. Zellforsch. **27** (1938); b in the rat [from Münch, Z. mikr.-anat. Forsch. **45** (1939)]

data of Hoeschen (1938) on the guinea-pig and of Münch (1939) on the rat for which the entire intestine was studied inch by inch. The concluding diagrams (Fig. 3a and b) drawn by the two Authors clearly show a likeness between the two species in the way the cells cluster in the very first portion of the duodenum and rapidly become more and more scarce in the rest of the tract. In the case of the rat, though, a secondary less-developed concentration of the cells is observed in the coecum and in the beginning of the colon. From Hoeschen's data, Barry (1943) tentatively estimated the number of cells in the guinea pig to be 15.10^6.

Data obtained from cross-sections provide information, which in some aspects is more detailed, when, as in our laboratory, the entire intestinal ring is considered. In fact, it is much easier to distinguish the cells according to their location in the positive or negative part of the relief and also to show possible differences of behaviour in the ventral and dorsal portions. From these data it is possible to obtain more or less refined and complete evaluations according to the requirements of the investigation. In cross-sections also the estimate of the weighted granularity index, according to GHIRINGHELLI and MIRA (1959a), is greatly facilitated (Fig. 4). A final advantage is the possibility of obtaining a continuous set of distribution data from the bottom of the glandular invaginations to the apex of the villi. In the stomach, when it is impossible to obtain complete cross-sections, the quantitative numerical evaluation is more difficult. Obviously all

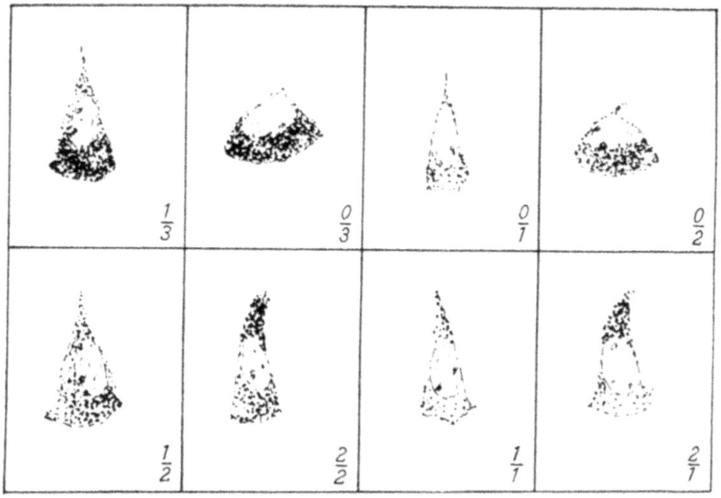

Fig. 4. Diagrammatic representation of the eight types of enterochromaffin cells in the rat, classified according to the estimate of the weighted granularity index. [From GHIRINGHELLI and MIRA, Arch. Biol. (Liège) **70** (1959)]

these quantitative data represent only numerical estimates; for more precise values, of volume for instance, it is necessary to estimate an average volume, which acquires its full significance only when calculated as a relative quantity, i.e. as its ratio to the volume of the remaining part of the intestine.

Similarly, it is possible to compare various estimates obtained by biochemical assay, when they are related to the weight of the intestine or of a portion of it. By integrating these data with the above-mentioned weighted index of granularity, an even more refined determination is possible (GHIRINGHELLI and BERTACCINI 1961). For the datum to be completely meaningful, it would, however, be necessary to measure the degree to which the granules participate in the make-up of the cell and the concentration of 5-HT in the granules (VIALLI 1963a).

β) **Extra-intestinal localization.** First of all, we will consider the localizations which are, more or less directly, connected to the intestine. Enterochromaffin cells may be present: a) in the biliary ducts (ERSPAMER 1936), b) in the pancreas (ducts, acini and islets) (ERSPAMER 1937, ARCHETTI 1936, 1938, UGGERI 1938) c) in the vitelline caecum of birds (CITTERIO 1932), d) in the bursa of Fabricius of birds (CITTERIO 1931, 1936), (PERRONE and ACOSTA FERREIRA 1950), e) in the rectal gland of *Latimeria* (VIALLI 1962, 1963) (Fig. 5). Among these localizations connected to the intestine, one may also classify the cells described by FIORENTINI and MIRA (1963) in the buccal epithelium and *aditus ad laryngem* of certain species of *Amphibia*. In certain cases, as for instance the pancreas, the cells are regularly encountered, in other cases their occurence is sporadic, limited to very small numbers, and possibly in one species alone. Also indirectly connected to the intestinal epithelium, are cells found in the thymus of birds (Fig. 6) and reptiles (CIACCIO 1906, REGGIANI 1946, PERRONE and ACOSTA FERREIRA 1948, QUARONI 1956, VIALLI and QUARONI 1956a); the presence of the cells in two lympho-epithelial glands, such as the bursa of Fabricius and the thymus, is rather suggestive. A fairly common localization, also in Man, is in the prostate and urethra (PRETL 1944, GHIRINGHELLI 1956, ARRIGONI, CALAFATI and LONGO 1956). Finally, we will recall that these cells have been reported by VIALLI and CERIOTTI (1939) in the epithelium of the oviduct of *Lacerta muralis* and of the urinary bladder of *Rana esculenta* and *Triton cristatus* (1939a). Certainly, these cases of extra-intestinal localization will increase in number, as soon as an accurate and systematic survey is carried out; the fact remains, though, that they have never been found in certain epithelia — even of endodermic derivation — such as the tracheobronchial epithelium; carcinoids though are known to occur in the tracheobronchial epithelium. One should keep in mind that when enterochromaffin cells are encountered in certain localizations of a given species, while in another species they are absent, often, argentophil pre-enterochromaffin cells may be present in their place.

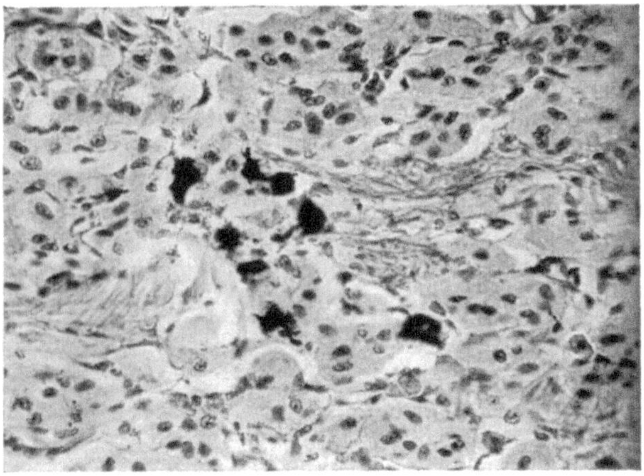

Fig. 5. Rectal gland of *Latimeria chalumnae*. Fixation: Bouin. MASSON-HAMPERL's reaction; haematoxylin

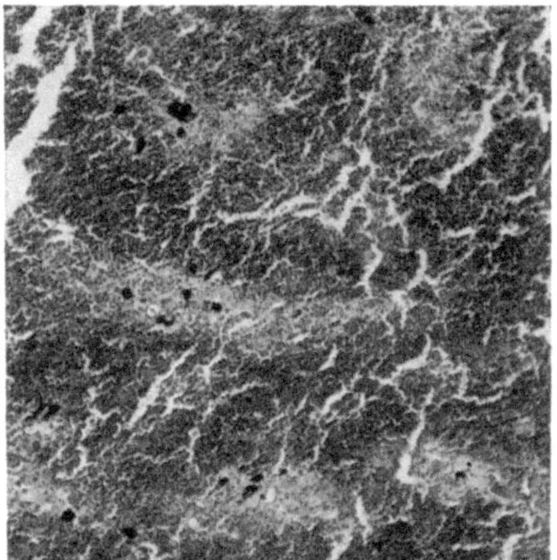

Fig. 6. Chicken thymus gland. Fixation: 10% formalin. Bodian technique. 132 ×

c) Taxonomical distribution

Information on the taxonomical distribution of enterochromaffin cells is of particular interest. As far as we know today, the enterochromaffin cell is characteristic of the Chordates. Although most of the information available concerns the vertebrates, we now have some data on its presence also in the tunicates and *Cephalochordata*. That typical enterochromaffin cells are present in the *Ascidia*, was observed in *Ciona intestinalis* by LISON (1933a), who also briefly described their characteristics. Quite recently, GERZELI (1962b) has re-examined the question and has come across these cells in various species of *Ascidiaceae* and *Thaliaceae*, only in the oesophagus, however. A study of the enterochromaffin cells in *Amphioxus* is also due to GERZELI (1961); in this organism they present all the morphological and histochemical characteristics of the cells found in vertebrates. In the posterior part of the mid gut and in the hind gut they are found only in the ciliated tracts.

The taxonomical distribution shows that the enterochromaffin cells are present in all classes, excepting *Cyclostomata*. In fishes, they have been observed in *Selachii*, in *Holocephali*, in *Chondrostei*, in *Holostei* and in *Crossopterygii*. For a certain period of time, all studies on *Teleostei* were negative, but now some unpublished results produced by ERSPAMER (1961) indicate the presence of enterochromaffin cells in the teleostean fish *Amiurus catus*. Naturally, this brings up the problem of how far the question can be generalized and shows the need for a more detailed investigation, not only in *Teleostei* but also in *Cyclostomata*. In amphibians, reptiles, birds and mammals the cells are universally present. One may say that the few negative data in the literature, especially those concerning the lower vertebrates, have always been contradicted by later observations. We must conclude, therefore, that except for *Cyclostomata* and *Teleostei*, which require further study, the enterochromaffin cells occur constantly throughout the vertebrates. BARRY (1943) lists in a table the percentages of species, within various groups, in which enterochromaffin cells have been observed; there are remarkable differences compared with those in which they are not observed and the percentages are lower in poikilothermous than in homothermous vertebrates. The table, at present, must be discarded in its entirety, with a few possible doubts in the case of *Teleostei* and *Cyclostomata*. There are differences, in frequency and extension, in the distribution of the cells along the digestive tube; these, in part, reflect species-specific and, in part, group-specific characteristics. It has also been assumed that the chemical nature of the granules may vary from one taxonomical group to another. Thus CLARA (1933, 1936), working on amphibians and reptiles (1932), came to the conclusion that it was possible to demonstrate a different reactivity of the granules; these observations are in disagreement with the findings of VIALLI and ERSPAMER (1933) who show that the reactions in *Holocephali*, *Selachii*, *Ganoidei*, Amphibians, Reptiles, Birds and Mammals are perfectly concordant, and, therefore — the Authors conclude — the constitution of the specific substance must also be homogeneous. Besides by later histological investigations, this point of view is also confirmed by the results of biochemical research on intestinal extracts carried out by ERSPAMER (1954); in every case the presence of 5-HT was shown. More recently, on the basis of differences in the resistance to deamination, ZORZOLI and LILLIE (1956) have proposed the existence of species-specific differences among Mammals in the constitution of the granules. Even without considering ZORZOLI's and LILLIE's data inaccurate, in the writer's opinion they may be subjected to a different interpretation.

2. Brief notes on the argentophil pre-enterochromaffin cells

As already has been mentioned, this cell type is histomorphologically indistinguishable from the typical cell. Its distinctive characteristic is argentophily. By employing fixatives other than formalin, one limits the observable histological picture to the argentophil cells alone; formalin fixation, on the other hand, may be employed to study them in the intestinal tract of those species which lack enterochromaffin cells. With the exception of the negative response to the typical reactions for enterochromaffin cells, histochemical data are completely lacking and their study represents one of the most serious problems still awaiting solution in the field of enterochromaffin cell research. In the pancreas it is particularly difficult to discriminate argentophil cells; undoubtably, since typical enterochromaffin cells are present in the pancreatic islets of a few species, one must assume that, at least part of what is classified as argentophil actually consists of typical pre-enterochromaffin cells; on the other hand, again in the islets, the A-cells too, believed to be secretors of glucagon, are typically argentophili therefore, if nothing else, we have the problem of distinguishing between these two cell types (CAVALLERO, MALANDRA and MOSCA 1957, MOSCA 1958). Of greater importance, though, is the problem of the relationship between the two cell types; ERSPAMER (1939), in answer to FERNER'S (1938, 1939) objections. proposes the following scheme: the pluripotent argentophil cell (pre-enterochromaffin or insulopotent, according to its topographical situation) would develop either into an insulogenic B-type cell or into an enteraminogenic enterochromaffin cell as was to be supposed at that time. Now that so much is known on the relationship between A and B type islet cells, the proposed developmental pattern must be confirmed by further experimental investigations; however, since it is based on a rather substantial body of available evidence, one may consider it to be rather well grounded in fact, although, in some parts, it may possibly have to be modified. In any case, one must always take into account the fact that, in some cases, typical enterochromaffin cells are surely present in the islets.

A general characteristic of the distribution of the pre-enterochromaffin cells, within a given species, is that its topographical distribution is somewhat wider than that of typical enterochromaffins. This fact is particularly evident for extra-intestinal localizations; for instance, in the pancreas of Amphibians GARDOSI (1938) found only argentophil pre-enterochromaffin cells, while in other groups, in various sections of the exocrine and endocrine pancreas, the argentophil pre-enterochromaffin cells are also accompanied by typical enterochromaffins. Until ERSPAMER (1961) discovered typical enterochromaffin cells in a short tract of the stomach of *Amiurus*, *Teleostei* represented a group in which, throughout the intestine, only argentophil cells could be demonstrated (UGGERI 1938). As far as we know today the same situation occurs in *Cyclostomata* (UGGERI 1938).

A wide gamut of fixatives may be employed for the granules of the pre-enterochromaffin argentophil cells, which are even satisfactorily fixed in alcohol. The characteristic argentophily does not provide any clue as to the nature of the substance present in the granules; the fixability in alcohol suggests, in a general way, a protein make-up.

When we consider our incomplete knowledge about the results of other reactions, it is extremely difficult to reach more precise conclusions. Better known are some histochemical characteristics of the A-type islet cells.

FEYRTER (1934, 1938, 1953), PAGÈS (1955) and PAGÈS and PAGÈS (1957) have made some important contributions on the subject of argentophil cells; however, in general the question as a whole has never been exhaustively examined. There have been some attempts to obtain and interpret precise comparisons between the A-type cells and the argentophil cells in the intestine. For instance, SUTHERLAND and DE DUVE (1948) believe that the intestinal argentophil cell is also capable of producing glucagon; but DAVIS (1954), HARTROFT, WRENSHALL and WILSON (1954) believe otherwise. The former Author bases his conclusions on detailed staining and experimental (treatment with synthalin-A) comparisons between A-type islet cells and what he calls the X cells, in the fundus glands of a rabbit stomach. However what DAVIS calls the X cells corresponds in the writer's opinion to typical enterochromaffin cells therefore the comparison is not fitting.

LACY (1957) has carried out an accurate ultrastructural study to compare pancreatic A-cells with enterochromaffin cells and has found that they have several characteristics in common.

The question of the relationships between A-cells and the argentophil cells of the islets is seen to have different aspects following the recent research by HELLER-

STRÖM and HELLMAN (1960), PETERSSON, HELLERSTRÖM and HELLMAN (1962), HELLMAN, ROTHMAN and HELLERSTRÖM (1962), SOLCIA (1962), CAVALLERO and SOLCIA (in press). The work of these Authors shows how it is possible to distinguish, in the complex of A-cells, two types of elements, some argentophil and others not argentophil, or only so under certain particular conditions. In the latter there seem to be phenomena of "luminescence" in the dark field, and histochemical characteristics which might point them out to be responsible for the secretion of glucagon.

At this point, we should also consider the non-argentophil pre-enterochromaffin clear cells and the empty cells, but as already explained, the information available is too scarce.

3. Embryology of the enterochromaffin cell

The data on embryonic development may be grouped under three different chapters: a) time of appearance and characteristics of the first identifiable cells, b) experimental embryology, c) discussion on the origin of the enterochromaffin cells.

a) Time of appearance of the enterochromaffin cells

This question has been treated by many Authors for both chicken and mammal embryos, however, not all the data, especially the less recent, are immune to serious criticism. The principal reasons are: a) the fixatives employed; b) the use of techniques which are either insufficiently specific (stains) or are not sensitive enough to assure identification of the cells when they are present in small numbers; c) the use of a technique which is not sufficiently reliable in discriminating between argentaffinity and argentophily; d) the use of either an argentaffin or argentophil reaction alone, which makes it impossible to determine separately the time of appearance of the typical enterochromaffin cells and of the argentophil pre-enterochromaffin cells. The latter distinction is obviously of great theoretical interest. The data thus collected are often contradictory, even within the same species. Generally, the work of the various Authors concerns one species alone and therefore, is useless for comparative purposes; moreover, from the results obtained, inferences are made which turn out to be untenable in the face of a rigorous comparative analysis. This, for instance, is the case of PARAT's (1924) views on the concomitance between the appearance of the enterochromaffin cells and the beginning of pancreatic secretion.

It is worth while discussing in greater detail GHIDINI's (1940) and MONESI's (1959, 1960) data on the chicken embryo and those of CORDIER (1926), PATZELT (1931), CLARA (1934), COLE and MCKALEN (1962) and SINGH (1963) on human embryos.

GHIDINI (1940) studied formalin-fixed embryonic intestine, treated with the Masson-Hamperl reaction (argentaffin cells) and with the Roger-Simard method (argentophil cells) every 12 hours, beginning at the 144th, he was able to show, after 241 hours of development, the appearance in the small intestine of argentaffin and argentophil cells, which formerly were lacking. Subsequently, the number of cells increased continuously and the intestinal tracts, in which the cells could be found, expanded. It is not possible to show, on the basis of GHIDINI's observations, that there is any asynchrony in the development of the enterochromaffin and of the argentophil pre-enterochromaffin cells. According to MONESI (1959, 1960), who employed the Masson-Hamperl and the Bodian techniques, it is possible to demonstrate argentophil pre-enterochromaffin cells after 14 days of incubation (336 hrs.), that is 36 to 48 hours before the appearance of the enterochromaffin cells; during the first few days after the appearance of the two cell types, the argentophil cells are 3 to 4 times the number of the argentaffins; later, the ratio stabilizes at 1:2 and remains at this value in the chick and the adult. The discrepancy between GHIDINI's and MONESI's results is difficult to explain, at least as regards the time of appearance. The fact that GHIDINI was unable to show any asynchrony in the appearance of the two cell types may be due to some malfunction of the argentophil technique employed; in fact, he mentions an equal number of argentaffin and argentophil cells. Besides, the present writer has come across conditions of this sort, due to defective silver impregnation, which, in any case is rather erratic. In such situations one finds that leaving out the last part of the argentophil technique (i.e. the development), the same number of cells can show a positive reaction.

Obviously, this leads one to think that the appearance of the argentophil pre-enterochromaffin cells occurs earlier than the 241st hour. On the other hand, GHIDINI's observations are in greater accord than MONESI's with the data of SIMARD and VAN CAMPENHOUT (1932) who by "en masse" silver impregnation found that argentaffin cells appear on the 264th hour. Again, DAWSON (1948), in the surface epithelium of the glandular portion of the stomach of a chicken embryo, observed an even earlier appearance (8th day of incubation) of argentophil cells. Therefore, if we integrate hypothetically GHIDINI's data with DAWSON's, we find that the time of appearance of the two cell types is asynchronous and that it occurs at an earlier date than that proposed by MONESI (1959, 1960). All these discrepancies stress the importance, of further research.

As for human embryos, the data of CORDIER (1926), PATZELT (1931), and CLARA (1934) are in good agreement, placing the time of appearance of the enterochromaffin cells at the twelfth week. CLARA (1934) points out that the appearance of the goblet cells (9th week) precedes that of the enterochromaffin cells while the appearance of PANETH's cells follows it (17th week).

Recent research by SINGH (1963) has led to a detailed report on the quantitive distribution of argentaffin and argentophil cells in numerous human embryos and foetuses.

Finally, it seems worth while to stress the fact that all the Authors agree that enterochromaffin cells show all the characteristic reactions when they appear.

b) Experimental embryological data

Experimental embryological research on the chicken has been performed by SIMARD and VAN CAMPENHOUT (1932) and by GHIDINI (1940) employing chorio-allantoic grafts and by MONESI (1960a, 1960b) with organotypic cultures (BORGHESE 1961). In all three series of experiments the development of the enterochromaffin cells was observed in fragments of intestinal tissue under various experimental conditions. From MONESI's observations it appears that also "in vitro" there is an asynchrony between the appearance of the enterochromaffin and the argentophil pre-enterochromaffin cells; nor is their number significantly different from that observed "in vivo". Grafting very precocious embryos, SIMARD and VAN CAMPENHOUT (1932) are led to believe that their experiments show that the enterochromaffin cells are not of nervous origin; GHIDINI (1940) adds to this the demonstration that differentiation takes place without the conveyance of any material through the intestine; it follows that the specific substance or the precursors must either be formed directly in the cells or arrive there through the blood stream. Finally, this last possibility is excluded by MONESI's (1960a, 1960b) experiments, which prove that the substance originates within the cells themselves: therefore they are true organs of elaboration and not merely of deposit or excretion of 5-HT (Borghese 1961).

Lastly, alongside these findings in the field of experimental embryology, mention should be made of the recent research by Andrew (1963), who, using chorioallantoic grafts of chicken embryo preceding the stage with 22 somytes and operated on for ablation of the neural crests and the neural plate, noticed enterochromaffin cells developing normally in the graft. This has led to the conclusion that enterochromaffin cells are not derived from the neural crests.

As a whole, these studies on the experimental embryology of the cells have provided clearly interpretable results of great importance; of course, there still are many points which require clarification, especially that of the numerical ratio between argentaffin and argentophil cells observed by Monesi in organotypic cultures.

c) Origin of the enterochromaffin cells

For a complete understanding of the data available on the origin of the enterochromaffin cells, it seems necessary, first of all, to present some data on their renewal in the adult. Mitotic or amitotic figures have never been observed in enterochromaffin cells, not even in colchicin-treated animals (Vialli and Ghirinchelli 1960, Castoldi 1963). Hamperl (1925, 1927) and many Authors describe binucleate enterochromaffin cells, which may be assumed to have originated by karyodieresis without an accompanying plasmodieresis; on the other hand, there is no evidence that, when the division of the nucleus occured, the cells were already differentiated. Since, undoubtedly, cell renewal does occur, we must assume that differentiation takes place from proliferating stem-cells which up to now, have been indistinguishable from the principal cells (Vialli and Ghiringhelli, 1960).

Although it is quite clear that the renewal of the cells must proceed in this manner, we cannot say at the moment that all the stages between the undifferentiated cell and the typical enterochromaffin cell are well known. However, differentiation should proceed, more or less following the pattern proposed by Erspamer. If we were to admit that in the adult the enterochromaffin cells originate from elements other than the principal cells, we should also have to assume the persistance, throughout the life of the organism, of cells not of common endodermic origin. On the other hand, we might point out that the other two cell types, the muciparous and Paneth's cells, behave quite similarly; therefore, for the time being there is no reason to imagine a different situation in the case of the enterochromaffin cells. Again, clearly the prospectic capacity of the embryonic intestinal epithelial cell cannot be less than in the adult; consequently in the embryo differentiation must also follow the same pattern. Most Authors are of this opinion: for instance Cordier (1926), Patzelt (1931) and Clara (1934). Barry (1943), in particular, insists on the terminology employed in discussing this controversial issue. To some extent Masson's (1914) description — never confirmed — of an amitosis followed by differentiation is conducible to the scheme of events just described. As examples of points of view which disagree with the above, we could mention that of Danisch (1924) who believes that the enterochromaffin cells derive from cells present in the nerves and sympathetic ganglia, subsequently migrating to the epithelium and that of Kull (1913, 1925) who assumes a migration from the connective tissue to the epithelium. It would seem that the idea of an allochthonous origin of the enterochromaffin cells is still favoured by some, so much so that recently Pearse and Pepler (1957) state that most Authors believe in the theory of their origin from the neural crests.

In the writer's opinion, these views are based principally on data from pathological anatomy, which it is not appropriate to discuss here. Of particular interest are data on carcinoids and their genesis, and on the state of cells in more or less inflamed appendixes,

ANDREW's (1963) experimental embryological research, mentioned above, clearly indicates the enterochromaffin cells as not originating from the neural crests.

Possibly a closer integration between data on normal and pathological conditions may provide a clearer and more complete picture. The idea of an autochthonous origin of the enterochromaffin cells implies, in most cases at least, an exclusively endodermic nature. Some of the extraintestinal localizations described, such as in the prostate and in the urethra (GHIRINGHELLI 1956) in the urinary bladder of Amphibians (VIALLI and CERIOTTI 1939a) and the oviduct of the lizard (VIALLI and CERIOTTI 1939), seem to extend the range of possible derivations to mesodermic epithelia. The recent data of FIORENTINI and MIRA (1963) on the presence of enterochromaffin cells in the buccal epithelium and in the *aditus ad laryngem* of Amphibians even raise the question of a possible origin from ectodermic epithelia.

The sum total of these partially contrasting data indicates that the question of embryological origin requires further study, possibly with emphasis on the experimental approach.

4. Various functional conditions of the enterochromaffin cell

Histological research, first revealed a certain number of functional conditions in the cell. Long before this was confirmed by biochemistry and pharmacology, the fact that in many cases the apical extremity of the cells does not reach the lumen of the intestine suggested the endocrine nature of their secretion. Also indicative was the fact that they are found in certain situations pancreatic islets (ERSPAMER 1937, ARCHETTI 1938), and thymus (CIACCIO 1906) where, while showing perfectly normal behaviour, they cannot possibly have an esocrine function. In the second place, also incompatible with an esocrine function during digestion, is the distribution of the cells along the gastroenteric tube; here, within a gross homogeneity, one may discern variations which — in the stomach for instance may be quite spectacular. The existence of functional stages as postulated by ERSPAMER (1937) with his four cell types, is a histomorphological and histochemical datum supported by a mass of anatomical and comparative-anatomical and embryological evidence; the direct proof, however, of this highly important concept is still of histological — normal and pathological — derivation. Even remaining within the context of typical enterochromaffin cells, the previously mentioned data of YAMASAKI (1940) represent facts which would have escaped any other method of investigation. Again, of great importance to the interpretation of functional stages and to that of the response to various agents is the classification of the cells on the basis of degree of granularity expressed, for instance, as a weighted index following the procedure of MARKS, SORGEN and HAYES (1958), or better of GHIRINGHELLI and MIRA (1959).

If to this we add cell-counts and the estimation of 5-HT content per granule, it is easily understood that the methods now available may provide results that may be considered clearer and more coherent than those attainable by biochemical analysis. It seems worth while mentioning, however that before the discovery that the granules contain 5-HT, numerous investigations — often with contrasting results — were carried out on the effect of diets and of various substances: pilocarpine and atropine, respectively the best known secretory stimulants and depressants acetylcholine, histamine, adrenaline, various hormones and vitamins. Many of these investigations were performed with uniform assay techniques and experimental conditions by CLARA's school, mainly in the period from 1930 to 1940.

It would certainly be worth continuing this co-ordinated line of investigation, especially now that biochemical methods are available which can confirm or disprove the histological data. Today, a new stimulus in this direction comes from the knowledge of various drugs capable of modifying the 5-HT content of the organism, especially in the intestine. Reserpine is certainly the most closely studied among these substances: the literature on this subject is quite abundant and the results are not only generally unequivocal but also concern species other than Mammals: Birds (VIALLI and QUARONI 1956a), Reptiles (CASATI 1958), Amphibians (VIALLI and QUARONI 1957). The most complete work concerns the mammals (ZBINDEN, PLETSCHER and STUDER 1957, 1957a, PLETSCHER 1957, MARKS, SORGEN and HAYES 1958, GHIRINGHELLI and MIRA, 1959a, LILLIE, WEISSBACH and GLENNER 1959).

DOERFLER, SCHWINK and WETZSTEIN (1963) and WETZSTEIN, DOERFLER and SCHWINK (1964) have studied the enterochromaffin cells of guinea-pig treated with reserpine by the use of electron microscopy. These cells, when observed by light microscope following specific reactions, appear to be devoid of granules; on the contrary, under the electron microscope, the specific granules are present and are normally osmiophilic. The authors postulate that osmic acid reacts in this case with the proteins of the granules instead of reacting with 5-HT.

Moreover differences are also observed when the cells of the negative and positive portion of the intestinal relief are considered separately. The data indicate, at times, a differential response of the intestine from segment to segment, both in terms of cell number and weighted index of granularity. Observations of PLETSCHER (1957) also concern the decrease in reactivity of the granules under the action of reserpine.

Recently, PRUSOFF (1960, 1961), applying the method of homogenization and centrifugation in density gradient mentioned earlier, found that, after treatment with reserpine, the fraction which normally contains 5-HT and ATP shows a lower content of 5-HT and lacks ATP; the quantity of the latter however does not diminish in the mitochondrial fraction.

Less studied is the typical enterochromaffin-cells: argentophil pre-enterochromaffin-cells ratio, considered by VIALLI and QUARONI (1956) in the chicken and in the Amphibians (1957): the results obtained by the Authors fit nicely into a scheme which assumes a genetic relationship between the two cell types. All these data offer possibilities of discrimination far beyond those attainable by biochemical assay, they also permit the investigation of some aspects of the physiology of the cell. Various other studies on the enterochromaffin cells have been partly carried out, following the same criteria of planning the techniques of investigation on the basis of previous biochemical assays. It has been found that benzoquinolizine (VIALLI and GHIRINGHELLI 1958, 1958a) and colchicin (VIALLI and GHIRINGHELLI 1960, GHIRINGHELLI and BERTACCINI 1961) determine a decrease in the number of cells and the weighted index of granularity. Hypophysectomy also brings about a decrease in both values (GHIRINGHELLI 1961) while if somatotropic hormone is administered in normal animals the opposite effect is observed (MIRA 1960). Finally, GHIRINGHELLI, MIRA and BERTACCINI (1961) have examined contemporaneously with appropriate controls the histological and the biochemical data on hypophysectomized rats and on rats which had been hypophysectomized and treated with STH. By referring to entire cross-sections they were able to confirm the preceding data of GHIRINGHELLI (1961) and MIRA (1960); however, when, to allow for size variations in the intestine, the cell counts and weighted indexes of granularity were calculated per unit tissue area, they found no significant difference between the controls and the two series of treated animals, as is the case when the results of biochemical assays are referred to unity of weight. The new method of examination, which certainly conforms to rational physiological criteria, shows what great caution must be used in evaluating the data in the literature, especially when they are not directly comparable. Considering also some more recent data on the relationship between 5-HT and the adrenal glands, GHIRINGHELLI, MIRA and BERTACCINI (1961) have pursued earlier investigations by ERÖS (1930) and ERSPAMER (1937a). They studied surrenectomized rats, fed on a standard diet and on a beverage made up of a 9% sodium chloride acqueous solution and treated by daily subcutaneous injections of 100 μg pro die D.O.C.A.

They found, in the duodenum, an increase in cell number and in the weighted index of granularity; in other parts of the intestine there were no significant variations. Biochemically, an increase in 5-HT in the small intestine can also be demonstrated. In rats, seven months after colectomy, GHIRINGHELLI, MIRA and BERTACCINI (1961b) demonstrated a compensating increase in cell number and weighted index of granularity in the duodenum; this was not observed in the ileum. On the basis of biochemical data showing the presence of 5-HT, noradrenaline, DOPA and tryptamine in bananas and that in monkeys, fed partially on bananas, the urinary excretion of 5-hydroxyindolacetic acid increases, GHIRINGHELLI and MIRA (1960) tried feeding rats exclusively on a banana diet; they observed an increase in the cell number and in the weighted index of granularity. We have considered here a few examples of particular interest, from a methodological point of view also, of histophysiological research on the variations observable in enterochromaffin cells subjected to diverse experimental conditions.

We must stress the fact that, in this case, the data are not always either unequivocal or clear. In an over-all view, we must keep in mind the completely different meaning to be assigned to histological research — which provides well defined topographical data on what are unfortunately, however, only very limited samples — when it is used to explain biochemically observed phenomena; in fact, in the latter case one is always concerned with the mean values of rather large samples, which in no way indicate the conditions existing in the individual cells; a knowledge of these conditions is necessary to understand the true mechanism underlying the observed variations. Obviously, the maximum information may be obtained by the integration of the two types of data in a properly planned experiment, such as some of those mentioned above. Certainly, any inference, even if its experimental basis is solely biochemical, must be fitted into the picture provided by histofunctional research.

B. Chromaffin cells of the posterior salivary glands of Octopoda

The presence of cells containing chromaffin granules in the posterior salivaries of the cephalopods *Octopoda* is not of general occurence in all species of this group; testing for 5-HT in extracts confirms this completely. The comparative anatomical picture of the species in which the cells are present is rather restricted at the moment and should be completed by the study of other species and genera; the cells have been found and described in *Octopus vulgaris* (VERNE 1923, VIALLI and ERSPAMER 1939a, VIALLI 1946a, VIALLI and QUARONI 1956), *Octopus appellyon* Barry (BENDITT and WONG 1957), *Eledone moschata* (LISON 1931, VIALLI 1946) and *Eledone cirrosa* (ROMANINI 1952). Repeated investigations on *Octopus macropus* (VIALLI 1946 and unpublished data), in which biochemical tests for 5-HT are negative, gave not only negative results with chromaffin reactions but also with reactions such as the diazo- which at least should demonstrate tyramine which HENZE (1913) has shown to be present. Also lacking is research which would permit us to extend our knowledge to groups, other than the *Octopoda*, which are also provided with posterior salivary glands. The most detailed histomorphological data on structure and cell types are those of AZZI (1917) in *Octopus macropus* which however lacks any cells containing chromaffin granules. The adenomeres of the posterior salivary glands of *Octopoda* contain many cell types; cells with chromaffin granules are present in numbers which vary from region to region of the gland and from species to species (Plate Ie, Plate IIe). Morphologically, the chromaffin cell is immediately distinguishable by the presence of fairly large granules situated in the cytoplasm above and below the nucleus. They are clearly visible in formalin-fixed material and show a distinct typical yellow to brown colouration, much stronger than that of the enterochrom affin cells. Because of this clearly distinguishable characteristic, it is unnecessary to go into further possibilities of differential diagnosis of this cell type. VERNE (1923) — although his interpretation was not entirely correct — described the chromaffinity of the granules as a histochemical characteristic. Later on, in *Eledone moschata* LISON (1931) found the three typical reactions for di- or poly-phenols. More detailed histochemical specifications were given by VIALLI and ERSPAMER (1938), VIALLI (1946) and ROMANINI (1952). VIALLI and QUARONI (1956) demonstrated that the granules also show a good PEARSE's reaction. The typical colouration we have just mentioned is accompanied by a weak, scarcely typical fluorescence with characteristics probably due in part to autoabsorption. Both are secondary characteristics which depend on formalin fixation and are missing in freeze-dried preparations (FIORENTINI 1960). According to PICCINELLI (1958) (who employs biochemical methods) the posterior salivaries are not depleted of their secretion by the action of reserpine.

5-HT is not the only indolic or phenolic substance present in extracts of the posterior salivaries of *Octopoda*; we need only mention tyramine and octopamine (ERSPAMER 1940, 1948). Recently, ERSPAMER and ANASTASI (1962) have also isolated an endecapeptide: eledoisin.

GHIRETTI (1959) has described a protein-like active substance, cephalotoxin which is not only present in the posterior salivaries of *Octopus vulgaris* and *macropus* but also in *Sepia officinalis*. Thus, the poison of the *Octopoda* is a rather complex secretion. In conclusion, the information on the histochemistry and, as a whole, on the histomorphology of the chromaffin cells of *Octopoda* is rather scarce, while on histophysiology it is practically nil; this is especially apparent when compared with the great mass of data on enterochromaffin cells.

C. Chromaffin cells in the hypobranchial gland of Muricidae

Since ancient times the *Muricidae* have been famous as producers of a purple dye: purpura. That this animal pigment corresponds to 6,6-dibromo-indigo was discovered by FRIEDLÄNDER (1922) in *Murex brandaris*. DUBOIS (1909) was able to trace the formation of the pigment to the action of an enzyme, purpurase on a pre-chromogen. A histological study of purpura secretion is due to GRYNFELTT (1909, 1913, 1913a). The hypobranchial gland may be divided into three portions: a medial one which secretes the dye, and two lateral ones, respectively branchial and rectal, which do not have this function (Fig. 7). The medial portion is made up of a mono-layered epithelium of tall cells of various kinds. Among

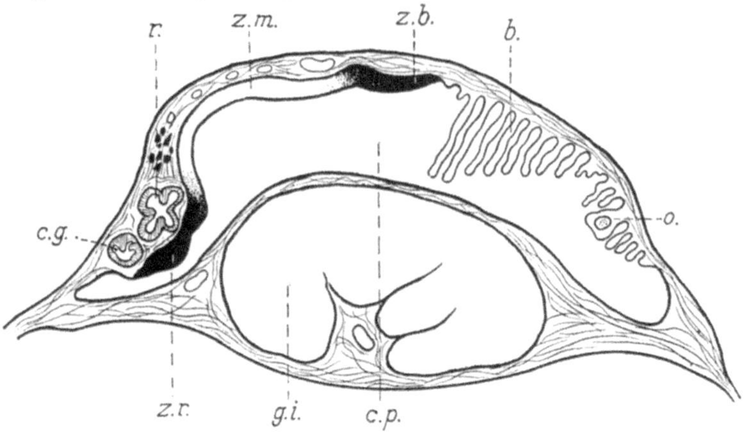

Fig. 7. Diagrammatic section through the pallcal cavity of *Murex*. *b* gill; *c.g.* genital duct; *c.p.* pallcal cavity; *g.i.* gland of anterior intestine; *o* osphradium; *r* rectum; hypobranchial gland: *z.b.* branchial zone; *z.m.* medial zone; *z.r.* rectal zone. [From LISON, J. Physiol. Path. gén. **31** (1933), according to GRYNFELTT]

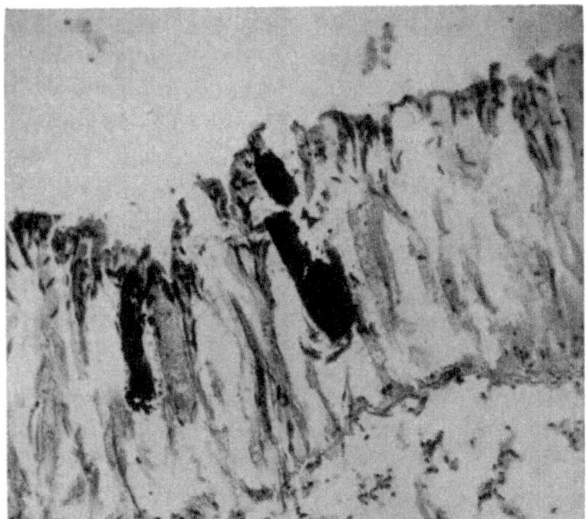

Fig. 8. Median portion of the hypobranchial gland of *Murex trunculus*. Fixation: 10% formalin MASSON-HAMPERL's reaction; haematoxylin. 66×

these, of interest to us are the cells which ERSPAMER (1954) calls the giant chromaffin cells. Cells showing a positive chromaffin reaction had been described in *Purpura lapillus* by ROAF (1911) who believed them to be secretors of adrenaline-like substances which he and ROAF and NIERENSTEIN (1907) had shown to be present in extracts. On the other hand, neither GRYNFELTT (1909) nor LISON (1933) were able to find this type of cell in *Murex trunculus*. LISON's (1933) observations led him instead to the conclusion that an indolic substance was present in the lateral portions. Some old work by VIALLI (1934), also on *Murex trunculus*, later extended to *M. brandaris*, confirmed ROAF's (1911) findings and showed that the granules of secretion are not only chromaffin but are also argentaffin and diazo-reaction positive (Fig. 8). To explain these properties, it was suggested at that time that the substance might be 6,6-dibromo-leuco-indigo or indoxyl; this was the first time that, in opposition to LISON's (1931) view, the three positive reactions were attributed also to an indolic substance. ERSPAMER's (1948) demonstration that the medial, pigment-secreting portion contains enteramine explains nicely the reactions observed, even if it cannot be directly related to purpurogenesis. We still have the problem of the genetic relationship between purpura and 5-HT. In the middle portion of the hypobranchial gland there are other substances besides 5-HT, the most important of which is a choline derivative, murexin (ERSPAMER 1948b). The chemical complexity of the secretion is in accord with the morphological complexity of this portion, formed by different cell types. The most important remaining problem, though, is that of the nature of the extremely abundant secretion of the lateral portions of the gland.

D. Cutaneous poison glands in Amphibians

The skin of the adult amphibian is rich in pluricellular glands of two distinct types: the granulous or poison glands and the mucous glands, the former secreting, in anurans, substances of indolic or phenolic nature. The distribution of the granulous glands varies in a typical way from species to species; they are generally found along the back, scattered irregularly or gathered in more conspicuous glandular packets, often characteristics for a given species, such as for instance the so called parotoids of the toad or the two lateral-dorsal crests typical of many species of frogs.

The glands are of the typical alveolar type and often exceed one millimetre in diameter. Their lumen is very wide and contains the secretion in the form of spheroidal granules up to a few microns in diameter, which occupy the glandular cavity almost completely without any form of differentiation. The opening to the exterior is more or less well defined. The granules can be conveniently fixed in formalin whereas, at least in *Rana esculenta* (VIALLI 1946), they do not withstand other fixatives. In the Urodeles, in which however there is no 5-HT secretion, the fixation spectrum is much wider. Furthermore, in the cavity of the gland one observes at times a typical structure, the so-called poison sacks, by means of which, during at least a part of the maturation period, the granules of poison remain included in the cell secreting them. In the anuran Amphibia on the other hand, it is only rarely possible to demonstrate granules, in the course of maturation, still to be expelled from the cytoplasm of the gland cells (VIALLI 1955). In this case, the granules show the same reactivity as the ones already secreted, but are usually of much smaller size (VIALLI 1946c, 1955).

At times, it is possible, within a given species, to demonstrate slightly different types of glands; the best known case is that of *Bombinator pachypus* (VIALLI 1934b and FARAGGIANA 1937, 1939) (Plate Id) and *B. igneus* (BERTOSSI 1938) in which one finds two types of glands easily distinguishable in size, intensity of reaction characteristics and fluorescence. Similar situations are also found in *Rana latastei* (CONRIERI 1960) with respect to granule size. while in various species of the genus *Bufo* (VIALLI 1940a) there are glands with different staining characteristics, and in *Rana esculenta* (VIALLI 1946b) (Plate If) and in *Discoglossus pictus* (ZANOTTI 1962) the glands differ in fluorescence (Fig. 9) and primary colour. Only to a small degree are these facts interpretable as different stages of the same maturation cycle. The known histochemical and histophysical data concern primarily the material secreted. The histochemical characteristics denoting the presence of phenolic or indolic substances are generally the same in all the anuran species studied with the exception of *Pelobates fuscus* (VIALLI 1934), a species in which not even biochemical analysis shows the presence of 5-HT. The chromaffin reaction was found for the first time in Amphibians in *Bufo agua* (ABEL and MACHT 1912) and in *Rana temporaria* (VOSS, 1929). The group of reactions for di- and poly-phenols was demonstrated by LISON (1932a) only in the species of the genus

Bufo while he erroneously excluded their presence in other Amphibians. VIALLI (1933a, 1934b) showed the generality of the reaction throughout the Anurans and the lack of it in the Urodeles. The poison granules also give the tyoindoxyl Pearse reaction (VIALLI and QUARONI 1956). In WOOD's light the poison granules show fluorescent colours which differ slightly from species to species, and also from one type of gland to the other (VIALLI 1937, 1946c). Up to now, it has been impossible to surely relate these differences to any constitutional characteristic of the granules themselves.

Biochemical analysis of poison squeezed manually from toad parotoids has demonstrated the presence of various indolic substances related to 5-HT: bufotenine, bufotenidine, bufothionine — of which the structural formulae are now well known (WIELAND, KONZ and MITTASCH 1934, WIELAND and WIELAND 1937, ERSPAMER 1963). Substances showing a cardiokinetic action also were found (GESSNER 1938). The demonstration by chromatography of 5-HT and other indolic and phenolic substances is due to ERSPAMER and VIALLI (1951, 1952). In some exotic species of the genus *Bufo* adrenaline has been found and quite recently, noradrenaline also.

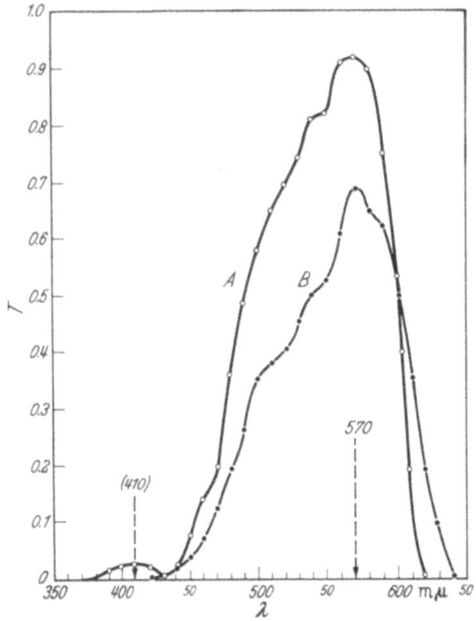

Fig. 9. Fluorescence emission curves of single poison granules of *Discoglosuss pictus*. Fixation: 10% formalin. Direct photometrical readings employing a photomultiplier (Universal Zanotti Histophotometer). *A*: granule showing yellow-orange fluorescence. *B*: granule showing whitish fluorescence. [From ZANOTTI, Ann. Histochim., Suppl. 2 (1962)]

Again in manually-squeezed poison, VIALLI and BOLOGNANI (1963) have demonstrated the presence of ATP in *Bufo vulgaris* and *Bufo viridis* thus widening the field of knowledge about relationships between ATP and 5-HT.

In numerous other anuran species, ERSPAMER and VIALLI (1952) have demonstrated 5-HT and several of its derivatives and have found that its distribution characteristics vary from species to species. Among the Urodeles, in *Salamandra maculosa* small quantities of 5-HT have also been demonstrated, besides tryptamine, the former being also present in *Triton cristatus*. Some of the substances which, in certain species, accompany 5-HT have not yet been defined chemically. Finally, from *Leptodactylus ocellatus* and *Leptodactylus pentadactylus* a pure substance called leptodactyline has been isolated which ERSPAMER (1959) has shown to be m-hydroxyphenylethyltrimethylammonium. Up to now though, there has been no histochemical research on the poison of *Leptodactylus*.

The degree of specificity attainable with our present histochemical reactions for phenolic and indolic substances does not enable us to demonstrate histochemical differences among species which can be referred certainly to a particular chemical constitution. Moreover, we cannot even determine, in those species in which adrenaline and noradrenaline are also present besides tryptophan derivatives, whether the former two substances enter into the reactions and, if so, to what degree. Now, one would imagine that the best analytical criteria are based on a fine analysis of the characteristics of fluorescence and of colouration obtained by the diazo-reaction. Unfortunately, up to now these techniques have provided no tangible results. Moreover, the general complexity of the composition of the poison makes it extremely difficult to find histological models capable of representing well-defined conditions adequately. Besides, the possibility of employing block reactions to demonstrate specific functions shows no promise for future development because the differences among the various substances mostly concern functions which cannot be used for diagnosis. Certainly, the elaboration of some of these substances may require different enzymic endowments; therefore a possible path to be followed in the solution of these problems might be that of studying the individual enzymes. For some of these, though, it will be necessary to seek out appropriate techniques of investigation following the well-known general criteria of enzyme histochemistry.

The poison of Urodeles is always distinguishable from that of Anura because the former lack the group of characteristic reactions and show a wider spectrum of fixability (VIALLI 1934b). While, in general, morphological data on the development of these glands are plentiful, the histochemical information is almost completely lacking.

The renewal of the poison after the glands have been squeezed manually has also been well studied (FARAGGIANA 1937a, 1938). There is no biochemical proof that the glands discharge their secretion under the action of reserpine (LIEBECQ-HUTTER and BACQ 1958, PICCINELLI 1958, LIEBECQ-HUTTER, RENSON and FISCHER 1959).

However, this matter has not been investigated histochemically and it may well be that, at the level of the individual secreting cells, a discharge of endocellular poison occurs in such small quantities, with respect to the poison already secreted, that it escapes detection by biochemical procedures. Summing up, we may say that 5-HT and other tryptophan derivatives in the poison of Amphibia represent a rather conspicuous deposit; however, they do not seem to to be strictly correlated either quantitatively or qualitatively to the degree of development of the enterochromaffin cells.

E. Chromaffin cells in Calliactis parasitica

The biochemical demonstration by MATHIAS, ROSS and SCHACHTER (1957) of the presence of enteramine in *Calliactis parasitica* was soon confirmed histochemically by VIALLI and CASATI (1958). In this species they found, scattered in the internal epithelial lining, among other types of cells, a certain number in which they believe 5-HT is localized. These cells are rather long (about 40 μ) and thin (about 5 μ), are present in fairly large numbers in the epithelium with a frequency which varies a good deal from region to region; their topographical distribution has not yet been studied exhaustively. After fixation in 10% formalin, the cells show rather large granules (about 1.4 μ), densely packed in the supernuclear region of the cell up to its distal limit; according to the Authors, one has at times the impression that they are extruded from the cell. Histochemically, the granules are chromaffin and iodaffin (even after formalin fixation), argentaffin and positive to an alkaline diazo-reaction. They also show various other typical reactions for 5-HT and, in particular, are positive to the 2,6-dichloro-quinone-chlorimide-Gibbs reaction and to the thyoindoxyl-Pearse's reaction.

As for physical characteristics, the granules always show, after formalin fixation, a very light yellow colouration and in WOOD's light a secondary, not very bright, yellow-brown fluorescence. There seems to have been no histochemical work on *Metridium senile*, a species in which PHILIPPS (1956), WELSH (1955) and WELSH and MOORHEAD (1960) have demonstrated the presence of 5-HT and bufotenine, particularly abundant in the acontia and tentacles. WELSH (1955) and WELSH and MOOREHEAD (1960) have found 5-HT in *Hydra oligactis*.

These histochemical findings in *Calliactis parasitica* appear to be particularly important because of the number of cells observed; a correspondingly high concentration of 5-HT is revealed by biochemical research. It is also interesting to note that, at least in some species, not only 5-HT but also other tryptophan derivatives may be found.

F. Poison gland cells of some scorpions

The most trustworthy data on the histochemistry of the chromaffin cells present in the poison glands of scorpions are those of ADAM and WEISS (1959)

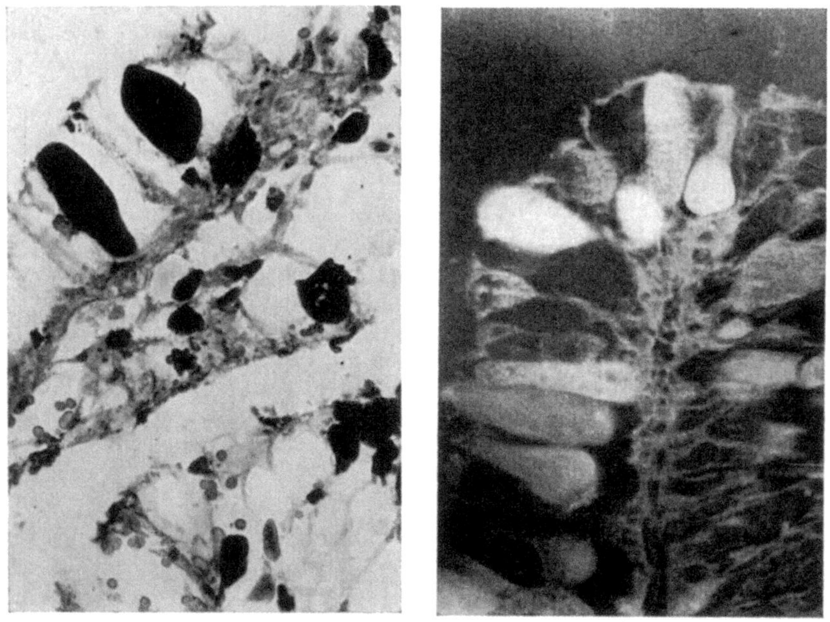

a b

Fig. 10a and b. Venom gland of *Leiurus quinquestriatus*. Fixation: formalin a Argentaffin reaction with ammoniacal silver nitrate; b Fluorescence in U.V. light (photograph by ADAM and WEISS)

on a scorpion from the Sudan, *Leiurus quinquestriatus*. In this species, the same Authors (1958) had previously demonstrated biochemically the presence of 5-HT and had accompanied the datum with a few histochemical observations, not completely probative as far as the group of characteristic reactions was concerned. In the poison gland cells one finds coarse granules showing the argentaffin reaction (Fig. 10a) and a positive diazo-reaction.

Fluorescence in ultraviolet light (*sic*) is yellow-green in a part of the granules, the typical ones (Fig. 10b). This is also observed however in some finely granulated cells. The reaction of indoles to paradimethyl-amino-benzaldehyde is positive but, according to the Authors, is not specific for the typical cells alone, occurring also in the finely-granulated cells and in some which show a positive Sakaguki-reaction. Similarly to some recent data of DE PAOLI (1962, 1963), on *Patella*, they find in

Leiurus, within the same organ but in different cell types, the characteristic reactions for 5-HT and, what may be called the general reactions for indoles. ADAM's and WEISS's (1959) interpretation that also indole reactions may indicate the presence of 5-HT or its precursors is hard to accept and should probably be rejected. The histochemical results of the dimethyl-amino-parabenzaldehyde reaction and of other similar ones, which are always negative in enterochromaffin cells and in other localizations particularly rich in 5-HT support this opinion; moreover, it is in accord with the reaction mechanism postulated to explain the positive results with non-denaturated 5-HT and the negative results with the β-carbolynic derivative formed during formalin fixation. ADAM and WEISS (1959) describe analogous but fainter reactions in *Parabuthus hunteri*, while in *Buthotus minox* (Likoch), a species in which the quantity of 5-HT biochemically demonstrable is about 100 times less than in *Leiurus quinquestriatus*, the reactions are extremely faint. ADAM and WEISS (1959, 1959a) believe that, besides undeniable specific differences, there must also be seasonal ones; to the latter they ascribe the results obtained in *Leiurus quinquestriatus* which are not always concordant.

G. Mast cells in the rat and mouse

The biochemical demonstration that the rat and mouse mast cells contain 5-HT — beside substances such as histamine and heparin present also in the mast cells of other species (BENDITT 1958) — has obviously raised the question of its histochemical demonstrability; this is complicated by the fact that histamine gives, in part, reactions similar to those of 5-HT. The problem of the histochemical demonstration of histamine has also been approached and recently solved by SCHAUER and WERLE (1959) and by LAGUNOFF, PHILLIPS and BENDITT (1961). In normal conditions, the presence of 5-HT in the mast cells cannot be histochemically demonstrated; in material included by freeze-drying and fixed in formalin vapours, the results obtained with some reactions: diazo, argentaffin, Schmorl reaction and a fluorescence reaction not completely comparable to that of enterochromaffin cells, according to LAGUNOFF, PHILIPPS and BENDITT (1961) may be due in part to the histamine present at a concentration ten times that of 5-HT.

FALCK (1962) presents some beautiful and unequivocal illustrations of fluorescence in rat mast cells after treatment according to his technique.

Under experimental conditions, however, there are also some data which should be considered indicative of the presence of 5-HT in the mast cells. In the skin of mice in a pre-cancerous state from treatment with 9,10-dimethyl-1,2-benzanthracene, RILEY (1958) and COUPLAND and RILEY (1960), after formolcalcium fixation, observed not only the characteristic fluorescence but also the group of reactions typical for 5-HT. On the other hand, EDER and SCHAUER (1959) after lengthy treatment with strong doses of 5-HT observed positive reactions for 5-HT in the mast cells. Finally, in a mastocytoma of a dog — on which, however, no biochemical assay of 5-HT had been performed — RICE and MITCHENER (1961) conclude that 5-HT is present on the basis of some reactions and of the characteristic fluorescence (Plate I, Fig. g). ERSPAMER (1961) however does not consider these last histochemical data to be completely persuasive.

Recently ENERBACK (1963) described mast cells, occurring in human carcinoid tumours, that exhibit histochemical reactions suggesting the presence of 5-HT. ENERBÄCK put the problem as to whether the mast cells in this case elaborate their own 5-HT or store 5-HT that has been elaborated by the tumour cells.

V. Localizations of phenolic and indolic substances which cannot be referred to 5-HT

As we stated at the beginning of our discussion, even the group of reactions characteristic for the enterochromaffin cell system cannot prove that the substance demonstrated is actually 5-HT or even related to it; moreover, if instead of considering the sum-total of the diagnostic characteristics, only a few are taken into consideration, those that are histochemical in a strict sense — diazo-reaction, chromaffinity, argentaffinity — many localizations of indolic or phenolic substances cannot be attributed to 5-HT.

A better specification is obtained by the response to formalin fixation (VIALLI 1935, 1940) and by secondary fluorescence (GHIRINGHELLI 1960, FIORENTINI 1960) due to formalin treatment. Without attempting to recall all the known localizations, we will concern ourselves only with those having some characteristics in common with 5-HT; we may mention the adrenal medulla, the paraganglia, the chromaffin cells of the nervous ganglia of the Anellids (POLL and SOMMER 1903, GASKELL 1914, VIALLI 1934c), the vitellogenes of the *Platyhelmintha* (VIALLI 1933, M. G. ROMANINI 1947), the vitelline granules of the *Polyclads* (VIALLI 1934, VALCURONE 1953, GERZELI 1960), the testaceous cells of the eggs of *Ascidians* (BIGNARDI 1935, PAULETTA 1942, GERZELI 1962), the chromaffin cells in the intestine and kidney of *Patella* (LISON 1932, BALLI 1936, DE PAOLI 1963), the connective cells of *Zonites algirus* (FROUTIN 1937), the dopamine cells of some Ruminants (FALCK, HILLARP and TORP 1959, 1959a).

Again with respect to this type of situation, we might also recall some other localizations in which even fewer characteristics are positive; it will suffice to mention as an example the well known argentaffinity of the melanoblasts. By considering characteristics which answer even less to the over-all diagnostic picture for 5-HT, we may associate, from this broader point of view, localizations positive to the Morel-Sisley reaction, to para-dimethyl-amino-benzaldehyde and to other similar reactions. It is absolutely improbable that there is any connection between these localizations and those of the enterochromaffin cell system, although in some cases they may co-exist. This, in fact, is the case of the association of the reactions between testaceous and enterochromaffin cells in Ascidians. Obviously therefore, every newly-discovered localization of a phenolic or indolic substance must, first of all, be thoroughly investigated to see whether it is assignable to the enterochromaffin cell system. Phenolic and indolic substances, within the broader picture drawn above, are connected to a large variety of morphological and functional situations. An analytical examination of these substances does not appear to provide, at the moment, any new element which would permit us to frame a better over-all picture of the various sections of the enterochromaffin cell system according to ERSPAMER (1954, 1961), which would not be based solely on the presence of 5-HT as a common denominator.

VI. Localizations of 5-HT which cannot be histochemically demonstrated

Many are the localizations of 5-HT which have been demonstrated biochemically but for which no positive response has been observed to the specific histochemical reactions, for the time being at least. In very general terms, applicable not only to 5-HT but also to any other substance, a negative response to the reactions may be assigned to two different types of causes: a) insufficient sensitivity of the reactions, b) impossibility of fixing the reactive material.

Concerning the former, one should keep in mind the demonstration by BENDITT and WONG (1957) that the sensitivity of histochemical reactions for 5-HT in formalin fixed material with respect to concentration, is much lower than in the test-tube. Furthermore, the use of a biochemically measured concentration is not a valid criterion; in fact, the material may be either uniformly distributed or else be concentrated within limited areas, as for instance in the case of the enterochromaffin cells, compared to the totality of intestinal tissues. The path to be followed is clearly indicated by the concepts expressed by ERSPAMER (1961) and VIALLI (1962) on the possibility of extending the enterochromaffin cell system to other elements by employing new, more sensitive reactions or by refining the sensitivity of the ones now available. The demonstration of the impossibility of fixing the reactive material offers more difficulties; of course the problem may be avoided by using the freeze-drying method and reactions or fixation in the vapour phase. On the other hand, we may consider other possibilities of more or less indirect "extra situm" histochemical demonstrations. Thus, for instance, we may say that the presence of 5-HT in the platelets has been demonstrated histochemically: in fact, the substance may be obtained by differential centrifugation from blood fractions which are made up almost exclusively of platelets.

Referring to some unpublished data, FALCK (1962) mentions the possibility of obtaining by his fluorescence method positive results with platelets when they contain more than 100 μg/ml of the substance.

The collection, from a nervous tissues homogenate, of a mitochondrial fraction rich in 5-HT may be also considered a histochemical demonstration (WALASZEK and ABOOD 1957). The same meaning may be attached to WELSH's (1954) data on the nervous ganglia of *Venus mercenaria*; not only was he able to separate by differential centrifugation a granular portion containing 5-HT, but also to demonstrate that, by chemical and physical actions, presumably capable of damaging the granule envelope, it is possible to obtain better responses to biological tests.

FALCK (1962) mentions some interesting data by DAHL, FALCK, LINDQUIST and v. MECKLENBURG (1962) on the demonstration by his fluorescence method of the presence of 5-HT or dopamine in some molluscan nervous ganglia. Finally, the demonstration mentioned by FALCK (1962) of the presence of 5-HT-containing cells in the thyroid of a rat would further widen the scope of the enterochromaffin cell system, providing a histochemical confirmation of PAASONEN's (1958) data. Another example we might mention concerns the electron microscope picture of the epiphysis after treatment with reserpine; it is an organ in which the presence of 5-HT and melatonin is known; in fact, according to PELLEGRINO DE IRALDI and DE ROBERTIS (1961) after treatment with reserpine, within 24 hours, the pluri-vescicular secretory activity of the pinealocytes disappears and reappears on the eighth day; this is in accord with the observed biochemical behaviour. On the other hand unfortunately, especially in some cases, the biochemical demonstration of 5-HT is not accompanied even by an attempt at histochemical research. This is the case, for example, with a datum by TWAROG (1954) on the presence of 5-HT in the retractor muscle of the byssus of *Mytilus edulis*.

Finally, it might be useful at this point to recall some notes, though incomplete, of histochemical demonstrations regarding localizations in which the presence of 5-HT is known, or at least supposed.

There are numerous data on the presence of 5-HT in the vegetable kingdom, together with other indolic substances (see, for example, ERSPAMER's tables 21—23 in chapter 4, and a preceding report by KIRBERGER and BRAUN (1961) on nuts). The only histochemical datum known to the present writer is the one by COLLIER

(1958) who recalls the unpublished research of JACOBSON on cells which are argentaffin but not diazopositive in nettle leaves.

FÄNGE (1960) speaks of cells which show enterochromaffin reactions (*sic*) in the salivary glands of the gastropod *Neptunea antiqua*. However, there are no hints of the presence of 5-HT in the biochemical part of the work.

COLLIER (1958) predicted that the poison of another kind of gastropod (*Conus*) might contain 5-HT. According to KOHN (1956) although there is no pharmacological or biochemical proof of the presence of 5-HT in the poison glands of species of the genus *Conus*, the histochemical proof is positive. KOHN, SAUNDERS and WIENER (1960) describe chromaffin granules in the poison glands of *Conus striatus*, while MARTOJA (1960) claims that 5-HT is probably present in *Conus mediterraneus*, mainly on the basis of noteworthy results obtained from the post-coupled *p*-dimethylaminobenzylidene reaction, which had previously given negative findings in the localizations of 5-HT.

MARCHE MARCHAD, GIONO, MAZER and LEMAIRE (1961), on the basis of pharmacological findings, point out the possible presence of 5-HT in the poison gland of *Cymbium patulum*, which belongs to the same group of gastropods as *Conus* and they, too, recall the histochemical observations of MARTOJA (1960.s It is likely that interesting suggestions may be obtained from the whole of this field of poisonous molluscan gastropods.

Still closer integration of the histochemical data — especially concerning "extra-situm" methods with the biochemical data — seems fairly easy to plan and would certainly be fruitful.

VII. Final considerations

The body of histological information on the enterochromaffin cell system we have gathered in this chapter, accompanying it when possible with indications on the corresponding biochemical data, lends itself to some considerations, partly of a general and partly of a special nature.

It is immediately evident from morphological considerations that the system defined biochemically by the common denominator, 5-HT, is made up of elements which differ greatly among themselves. It would be vain therefore to try to gather all the data into a unitary system; in this, morphological research confirms and supports the results of all other fields of investigation. On the other hand, it should also be obvious that any biological explanation of the over-all meaning of 5-HT cannot be upheld unless it accounts for all the elements of the system. With regard to this we should recall COLLIER'S (1958) incisive considerations. He distinguishes four conditions concerning distribution: a) taxonomical units (species, classes and phyla), b) the organs, c) particular cell types, d) endocellular localization. For the reasons we have given, when one studies the morphological data on the individual sections of the system, at least a series of partial considerations must be taken into account and one must judge the degree to which they are compatible or incompatible with more general criteria. Morphological and histological data enable us to consider the presence of 5-HT under many different aspects. As for the meaning of the organs elaborating the substances, they may be typically endocrine, as in the case of endocrine enterochromaffin cells, or esocrine and endocrine, as probably is the case with the posterior salivary glands of *Octopoda*, or even more typically esocrine such as the cutaneous poison glands of anuran Amphibia and the poison glands of Scorpions. Again, one should remember that in some cases the material elaborated may have the meaning of an excretion, in a narrow sense, while in other cases that of a deposit of storage material. The study of these conditions is a field in which morphological and histological research predominates. The differences in general or special characteristics, at times even profound, which may be found when the taxonomical distribution of certain conditions is studied, clearly indicate, at least in some sections, the need for a comparative study, not only histomorphological, but in its broadest sense. In fact, one is obliged to assume that the greater complexity of a secretion, such as the poison of Amphibia, requires more varied metabolic pathways than those of the enterochromaffin cells which secrete 5-HT alone. From the historical and other points of view one may say that the less refined type of morphological investigation, that concerning the organs as a whole, has represented the point of departure for every other type of research. Biochemical research at times has been the primary incentive for further investigation, at other times it has been stimulated by a histological study, intending the latter to be essentially histochemical and histofunctional. In any case, by repeated reciprocal integration both methodologies have acquired greater effectiveness. The writer mentioned at the beginning of this chapter that the subject has recently been treated from this point of view in a paper (VIALLI 1962) which may be referred to for more details. More specifically, there is a need for pharmacological, physiological, and physiopathological research as far as possible associated closely with other methods of investigation with a finely detailed study of morphological conditions; the purpose of this is to develop, as far as possible, the histochemical and histophysiological branches of histology. Even when this is impossible in a given investigation the results must always be interpreted by referring to the data furnished by the histologist; one cannot admit data which are in sharp disagreement with histological findings, unless of course the latter can be proved to be wrong.

VIII. Technical appendix

The technical data on the principal methods which may be useful in the histochemical study of the elements of the enterochromaffin cell system have been gathered here.

A. Fixations

1. Formalin fixation

This is the most useful technique in histochemistry because, besides, well preserving the morphological characteristics it is also compatible with most reactions. Generally, the slight acidity of formalin is not harmful, so it is unnecessary to neutralize it in any way. Various concentrations of formaldehyde may be employed; commonly the following solution is used:

1 part: commercial formalin (35—40% solution of formaldehyde).

9 parts: water.

The time of fixation is also not critical; a certain number of cells are fixed after only a few hours and fixation may be protracted for a whole month without any damage. Generally, we take 4 or 5 days but even 24 hours may suffice. After fixation and before dehydration, the tissue is washed at length in running water. If this has not been done beforehand — at least with rather delicate reactions — one should always wash the slides thoroughly after rehydratation.

2. Freezing drying

This is not a routine method and should only be employed in special cases when one wishes to study non-denaturated 5-HT. Embedding is carried out by the usual procedures, employing any vacuum-inclusion apparatus. Before attempting any further treatment one must remember that the tissue, and consequently also the 5-HT, is not fixed. Fixation and also some reactions may be carried out directly on tissue before embedding, or on sections with paraffin or from which paraffin has been removed with nonane. Among vapour-phase fixatives and fixative-reagents we may mention formaldehyde vapours, from formalin or paraformaldehyde, and iodine or osmic acid vapours. However, no positive results have been obtained up to now with cryostat sections.

3. Fixation for electron-microscopy

Most Authors (Christie 1955a, Kurosumi, Shibasaki, Uchida and Tanaka 1958, Helander, 1961, 1962) use the usual osmic-acid fixative buffered at pH 7.4 according to Palade. Only Bullón, Ramírez-Langer and Schultz (1960), without furnishing any details, mention some results obtained by applying directly the Masson-reaction with gold toning, on blocks of material fixed in 10% formalin before embedding. Fixation with osmic acid or osmium containing reagents has also been used for histological studies by electron-microscopy, being simultaneously also a specific reaction for granules. Palade's fixative is a solution — isotonic to the tissue to be fixed — of 1% osmic acid, buffered with Veronal buffer at pH 7.4. The pH is measured directly in the osmium solution with a pH meter. Some Authors, Wetzstein et al. (1962) for instance, when studying enterochromaffin cells, add 1% Zinc-iodide. Embedding is done in metacrylate or Vestopal.

B. Principal reactions

1. Chromaffin reactions

This reaction may be carried out during fixation or on sections fixed in 10% formalin and normally embedded.

There are many variants of the formol-bichromate fixatives, the most commonly employed being Regaud's solution.

a) Fixation for chromaffin reaction

Solutions:

A. Potassium bichromate 3%.

B. Formalin.

Method:

1. Fix tissue for 2—4 days in a mixture of solution A: 8 parts, solution B: 2 parts. The liquid darkens and forms a precipitate.
2. Place tissue for 4—8 days in solution A.
3. Wash at length in running water.
4. Pass through the alcohol scale and embed as usual in paraffin.
5. If necessary counterstain with a faint nuclear stain.

Results:

Localization of 5-HT and of any di- or poly-phenolic substances are coloured from yellow to a more or less well-defined brown. According to Falck and Hillarp (1959) the products of the chromaffin reaction are partially soluble during the paraffin-embedding. Material thus treated may be subjected to numerous other colourations but does not show, or rarely shows, the other characteristic reactions.

b) Reaction on sections

Solutions:

Potassium bichromate 5%.

Method:

1. Remove paraffin from the sections of tissue fixed in 10% formalin, then rehydrate and treat with the bichromate solution for a few days at room temperature.

2. Employ faint nuclear counterstain.

Results:

The reaction is always fainter than that carried out during fixation and at times may even be imperceptible.

2. Iodaffin reactions

It may be used in place of the chromaffin reaction and is generally carried out during fixation; one may vary the formula somewhat according to GERARD, CORDIER and LISON (1930).

Solutions:

CORDIER and LISON advise the following solution:

100 cm³ 10% Formalin, 3 g Potassium iodate.

We generally use a formula which exactly follows that of REGAUD's solution.

Method:

Carry out fixation for a few days in the chosen fixative and then wash the tissue in running water. Embed in paraffin wax.

Results:

The reaction specificity corresponds to that of the chromaffin reaction.

With regard to localizations of 5-HT the results correspond to those of the chromaffin reactions or are possibly slightly fainter. Substitution of iodate with bi-iodate or iodic acid provides less satisfactory results (VIALLI and ERSPAMER 1936).

3. Silver reactions

a) Argentaffin reaction according to MASSON-HAMPERL

Solutions:

A. Ammonia is cautiously added to a 5% solution of silver-nitrate: at first a good deal of brownish precipitate is formed but is dissolved by the addition of more ammonia. The solution must be brought to a slight opalescence. If the optimal point is surpassed one may correct by addition of silver-nitrate. The solution must be fresh.

B. 5% sodium-thiosulphate.

Method:

1. Formalin is preferable as a fixative. However other formalin-containing solutions will do as long as no reaction incompatible with the β-carbolynic condensation occurs: after sectioning remove paraffin and carefully rehydrate tissue in distilled water.
2. Place preparation in solution A for 12—24 hrs. in the dark.
3. Wash carefully in distilled water.
4. Treat with solution B for 3—5 minutes.
5. Wash in distilled water.
6. Counterstain very faintly with haematoxylin. If for special purposes another counterstain is required the appropriate times must be determined case by case.

Results:

The granules of the enterochromaffin cells show a brown to black colouration, according to the intensity of the reaction, and stand out clearly against an undifferentiated cytoplasm which is practically colourless in the best preparations.

b) *Argentaffin reaction according to* MASSON

This differs from the preceding only in that, after treatment with the silver solution, gold-toning is carried out.

Solutions:

A. and B. as in the preceding reaction.

C. 1,2 g gold chloride, 3 g ammonium thiocyanate, 3 g sodium thiosulphate, 98 ml H_2O (formula according to LILLIE 1954).

Method:

Up to stage 3. as in the Masson-Hamperl reaction.

4. 5 minutes in solution C.
5. Wash in distilled water.
6. Fix for one minute in solution B.
7. Wash in water.
8. If necessary, counterstain.

c) *Methenamine silver argentaffin reaction according to* GOMORI-BURTNER

Solutions:

A. WEIGERT's solution 1 part iodine, 2 parts potassium iodide, 100 parts H_2O.

B. 5% sodium thiosulphate.

C. Stock solution of methenamine silver.

Dissolve 3 g of methenamine (hexa-methylene-tetramine) in 100 cm³ of H_2O, add 5 cm³ of a 5% solution of silver nitrate in H_2O (the solution lasts for months if stored in a cool dark place).

D. HOLME's borate buffer at pH 7.8 16 parts M/5 H_3BO_3, 14 parts M/2 $Na_2B_4O_7 \cdot 10\,H_2O$.

E. The silver solution employed is made up of: 30 parts solution C, 8 parts solution D.

F. 0.1% gold chloride.

Method:

1. Treat rehydrated sections for ten minutes in solution A.
2. Treat for two minutes in solution B.
3. Wash in running water for 10 minutes.
4. Wash in two changes of distilled water.
5. Place sections in solution E for 3 to $3^1/_2$ hrs. at 60° C.
6. Wash in distilled water.
7. Tone in solution F for 10 minutes.
8. Wash in distilled water.
9. Fix in solution B.
10. Wash in running water for 5 minutes (counterstain if necessary).

d) *Bodian's argyrophil technique*

Solutions:

A. 5 g electrolytic copper (in sheet, treat or powder), 1 g Protargol, 100 cm³ H_2O.

The solution should be prepared carefully by slowly sprinkling Protargol on water containing the copper.

B. 1 g hydroquinone, 5 g sodium sulphite, 100 cm³ H_2O.

C. 1% gold chloride.

D. 2% oxalic acid.

E. 5% sodium thiosulphate.

Method:

1. Wash rehydrated sections thoroughly in distilled water.
2. Immerse sections in solution A for 25 hrs. in a thermostat regulated at 37° C.
3. Wash rapidly in distilled water.
4. Develop in solution B for 5—10 minutes.
5. Wash in three changes of distilled water.
6. Tone in solution C for 3—4 minutes.
7. Wash rapidly in distilled water.
8. Treat with solution D for 3—4 minutes.
9. Wash rapidly in distilled water.
10. Fix in solution E for 5—10 minutes.

Results:

The reaction is somewhat capricious and sometimes none of the numerous modifications provide any better results. Often the result is incomplete, only the typical enterochromaffins being impregnated, as can be seen from cell-counts and from the fact that similar results are obtained even if development in solution B is omitted.

e) Gross-Schultze's modification of the Bielschowski's argyrophil technique

This is the most commonly used technique before applying BODIAN's method. The principal disadvantage is that it is carried out on free floating sections cut with the freezing microtome and therefore does not permit any precise comparisons with argentaffin techniques: on the other hand however one has the advantage of following the impregnation under the microscope. Formalin fixed material is employed.

Solutions:

A. 20% silver nitrate.

B. 1 part formalin, 2 parts tap water.

C. Ammoniacal silver: add ammonia ($D = 0.91$) in drops to a 20% solution of silver nitrate, stirring all the time; a precipitate forms which redissolves immediately. The solution must be prepared fresh for every section.

D. Ammonia ($D = 0.91$).

E. 1% gold chloride.

F. 5% sodium thiosulphate.

Method:

1. Fix material in formalin, cut with the freezing microtome and then wash sections in distilled water.

2. Immerse for an hour or more in solution A.

3. Immerse in solution B: sections are placed one at a time in a watch glass containing formalin and must be kept in motion all the time. As soon as any murkiness is observed, transfer the sections to another watch glass until the murkiness disappears. Time required: about 10 minutes.

4. Add one drop of solution B per cm^3 of solution C prepared in the mean time: transfer sections to it and check impregnation under the microscope. If the results turn out to be unsatisfactory, also the nuclei and connective tissue being impregnated, repeat the operation on another section increasing the quantity of solution C to 2—3 drops per cm^3.

5. Transfer immediately for one minute to a mixture of 8 parts distilled water to 2 parts of solution D.

6. Rinse briefly in distilled H_2O.

7. Tone in 3—5 drops of solution E in 10 cm^3 of distilled water.

8. Fix in solution F for 1—2 minutes.

9. Wash thoroughly (1—2 hrs.) in running water.

f) Feyrter's adaptation of Gross-Schultze's argyrophil technique to paraffin embedded sections

Solutions:

A. 20% silver nitrate.

B. Ammoniacal silver solution. Add drop by drop concentrated ammonia to solution A until all the precipitate has dissolved, then add 0.6 cm^3 of concentrated ammonia for every 10 cm^3 of solution; Filter.

C. 100 cm^3 20% formalin, 1 cm^3 85% formic acid.

D. 1 part concentrated ammonia, 4 parts distilled H_2O.

E. 0.1 cm^3 acetic acid, 10 cm^3 distilled H_2O.

F. 10 drops 2% gold chloride, 10 cm^3 distilled H_2O.

G. 2.5% sodium thiosulphate.

Method:

Fix in 10% formalin for 24 hrs.; embed in paraffin wax. Attach sections, 10—15 μ thick, to slide with albuminated glycerine.

1. Rinse twice for five minutes the rehydrated sections in distilled water.
2. Immerse for half-an-hour in solution A in the dark.
3. Without passing through distilled water, blot the slide with a wad of filter paper.
4. Place for 10 minutes in solution B.
5. Remove and set aside the sections. To every 10 cm^3. of solution add 0.05 cm^3 of solution C.
6. Place the sections in the solution thus prepared and check them under the microscope until impregnation is apparent (about 10—20 minutes).
7. Blot with filter paper.
8. Place in solution D for 1—2 minutes.
9. Blot with filter paper.
10. Place in solution E for 1 minute.
11. Blot with filter paper.
12. Tone for about 15 minutes in solution F until the sections acquire a uniform grey colouration.
13. Blot with filter paper.
14. Place sections in solution G for 1 minute.
15. Wash twice for 15 minutes in tap water. Optional counterstain. Mount in Canada Balsam.

4. Schmorl's reaction

Solutions:

A. 1% ferric chloride or 1% ferric sulphate.

B. 1% potassium iron ferricyanide (must be fresh solution).

C. 3 parts solution A, 1 part solution B (solution must be used immediately).

Method:

1. Hydrate the sections.
2. Immerse sections for 5 minutes in solution C.
3. Wash in running water. Optional counterstain.

5. Diazoreactions

a) Diazoreactions with the diazotate of sulphanilic acid

α) In alkaline solution. Sulphanilic acid is one of the amines which provides the best results with the greatest ease. By calculating the stoichiometric values, numerous other amines may also be employed; among these the amines which form tetrazo-compounds by additional coupling.

Solutions:

A. 1 part 1 M solution of sulphanilic acid (19.12%), 1 part 2.25 M solution of hydrochloric acid (HCl d 1.19 sol. 50.57%).

B. 1 M solution of sodium nitrite (6.9%).

C. 1% sodium hydroxide.

D. Cool solutions A and B below 5° C. Add slowly and stirring solution B to solution A. Let the reaction go on for about 10 minutes. The solution is strongly acid and should be alkalinized with solution C before use.

Method:

1. Hydrate sections with great care.
2. Immerse sections in ice-cold water.
3. Treat sections for 1—2 minutes with solution D.
4. Place in water.

Or:

1.—2. As above.

3. Place sections in ice-cold water alkalinized with solution D diluted 1 to 4.

4. Remove slides from solution and without letting them drip, lay them flat and add a few drops of solution C (1—2 minutes).

5. Wash slide directly in water or if necessary immerse briefly first in alkalinized water without letting them drip. Optional counterstain.

Results:

The method always works well and provides a good contrast between the background and the reactive material.

β) In acid solution. Solution D prepared as above is too acid to permit a diazoreaction in acid conditions; acidity may be reduced by careful addition of alkali. In the latter case, substitute stage 3 with a passage in slightly acidified water or in a buffer at pH 5.2—5.4.

γ) In alkaline solution with subsequent strong acidification. Solutions: A., B., C., D. as in basic diazoreaction.

E. 50 parts HCl (D 1.19), 50 parts H_2O.

Method:

1., 2., 3., 4. as in preceding reaction.

5. Transfer slides directly to solution E for 2—5 minutes.

6. Wash in water. Optional counterstain.

b) Diazoreaction with stabilized diazotates

Numerous diazotates are now available. Their synonymy is extremely complicated because not all manufacturers assign the same name to the same compounds. In Gurr's book (1960) and in an article by Lillie (1959) in the J. of Histochem. and Citochem. there is a whole list of synonyms.

When in place of one azo-group there are two, the diazotates are called tetrazotates. We generally use tetrazotized di-ortho-anisidine, 3:3'-di-methoxy-diphenyl-4:4'-tetrazonium-chloride, known also as Fast Blue B salt and diazotized o-aminotoluene-2':3-dimethyl-benzene-4-diazonium-hydrogen-sulphate, also known as Fast Garnet GBC salt. Stabilized diazotates dissolve directly in the appropriate buffers used for basic or acid diazoreactions.

α) In alkaline solution:

Diazotate stabilized at 0.2—0.5% in a Veronal buffer at pH 9.4 (Lillie, 1954) (97.4 parts M Veronal sodium, 2.5 parts M/1 HCl).

Method:

As for diazoreaction with sulfanilic acid.

β) In acid solution:

Diazotate stabilized at 0.20—0.5% in acetate buffer at pH 5.2 (16 parts M/5 acetic acid 4 parts M/5 sodium acetate).

Method:

As for diazoreaction with sulfanilic acid.

c) Coupled tetrazonium reaction according to Pearse

Solutions:

A. Suspension of 2% benzidine in 2 NHCl.

B. Sodium nitrite 5%.

C. Ammonium sulphamate 5%.

D. Sodium carbonate, saturated aqueous solution.

E. To about 3 ml of solution A add 8 drops of cold solution B. Agitate rapidly for 10 min. Add 1 ml of solution C and 10 ml solution D. Add water to 50 ml. The solution should not be used more than an hour after preparation.

F. Saturated solution (1 g in 50 ml) of H acid (1-amino-8-naphthol-3:6-disulphonic acid) in veronal acetate buffer at pH 9.2.

Method:

1. Hydrate sections with care.
2. Immerse in solution E at 4° for 15 min.
3. Wash in water and in three changes of veronal acetate buffer at pH 9.2 for 2 min in each change.
4. Immerse in solution F for 15 min.
5. Wash in water for 3 min.

d) Diazosafranin method according to Lillie, Burtner and Henson

Solutions:

A. 360 mg Safranin 0 in 6 cm³ H_2O, 3 cm³ N HCl.

B. 1 N $NaNO_2$ 69 mg in 1 cm³.

C. Cool to less than 4° C solutions A and B, mix and let stand for 10—15 minutes.

D. Disodium phosphate.

E. N/10 HCl.

Method:

1. Hydrate sections and place them in H_2O.
2. Immerse in a chilled mixture of 1 part C to 40 parts D for 5 minutes.
3. Wash sections in three changes of solution E.

6. Gibbs's dichloroquinonechlorimide reaction

Solutions:

A. 20 mg 2-6-dichloroquinone-chlorimide, 20 ml Veronal buffer at pH 9.2 (the Veronal buffer at pH 9.2 is prepared by heating to 70° C: 95.2 parts M/10 Veronal sodium, 4.8 parts M/10 HCl. Cool and filter).

Method:

1. Hydrate the sections.
2. Treat sections for 10—15 minutes in solution A.
3. Wash at length in water and counterstain if necessary.

7. Pearse's thioindoxyl reaction

Solutions:

A. 2.5% sodium iodide.

B. 5% iodine in 90° alcohol.

C. 5% sodium thiosulphate.

D. 0.2 M buffer of triaminomethane at pH 8.5 (25 cm^3 0.2 M tris-hydroxy-methyl-amino-methane, 15 cm^3 0.1 M HCl bring to 100 cm^3 with H_2O).

E. Dissolve 10—15 g of 4-methyl-6-chlorothioindoxyl in 2.5 cm^3 of acetone and add 35 cm^3 of solution D. Solution must be fresh and filtered before use.

Method:

1. Rehydrate sections.
2. Oxidize sections for 10 minutes in solution A or for 10 minutes in solution B.
3. If solution B has been employed, transfer sections to water and treat for two minutes in solution C.
4. Rinse briefly in water.
5. Incubate in solution E either for 30 minutes at 56° C or for 2—4 hrs. at 37° C.
6. Wash in water and counterstain if necessary.

C. Estimation of the weighted index of granularity in the rat according to Ghiringhelli and Mira

As already mentioned the enterochromaffin cells have been classified into eight categories on the basis of the degree of supernuclear and infra-nuclear granularity. The granularity is expressed by number from 0 to 3: in the infra-nuclear region where the granules are usually prevalent we have the values 1—2—3 while in the supra-nuclear region the values are 0—1—2. These eight classes are then reduced arbitrarily to four by considering the sum-total of the two numbers representing respectively the super-nuclear and the infra-nuclear granularity: thus 1 (0.1)—2 (1.1, 0.2)—3 (0.3, 1.2, 2.1)—4 (1.3, 2.2) (Fig. 4).

Given a well-defined tract of the intestine, one considers a certain number of complete cross-sections, of known and constant thickness; after treatment with Masson-Hamperl reaction, all the cells present are counted (C. N. = number of cells) assigning to each, one of the four values which are equal to the sums of the possible combinations of paired values (0 to 3) denoting the eight cell categories. Each one of these sums represents the weighted index of granularity (W.I.G.) for a given cell. The sum of these values per cell gives the comprehensive weighted index of granularity in the localization under consideration. For a more detailed analysis in which the percentages of each of the 8 cell categories are considered separately see Ghiringhelli and Mira (1959a); other methods of classification are also employed. First, the estimation of the index is made separately for the cells of the glandular bottoms and for those situated on the villi, then a total estimate is made for all the cells. From these values, by the ratio W.I.G./C.N. one computes the *mean index of granularity*. A difference between the glandular bottoms and the villi is immediately apparent. By comparing different tracts of the intestine or the results of different treatments on the same tract it is possible to follow the increase or decrease of each of the three values C.N., W.I.G. and W.I.G./C.N. The data thus obtained may then be compared with those collected by biochemical procedures in analogous conditions. If a more precise comparison is desired, one must also take into account the variation in the mean section-area. Obviously, the comparison becomes more meaningful because quantitative biochemical assays are always referred to the weight of the tissue analyzed (Ghiringhelli, Mira and Bertaccini 1961). A table by Ghiringhelli, Mira and Bertaccini seems to me worth while reproducing below; it may in fact be useful as an outline of the procedure employed in our laboratory which, to facilitate comparisons, should be followed when possible in future estimations.

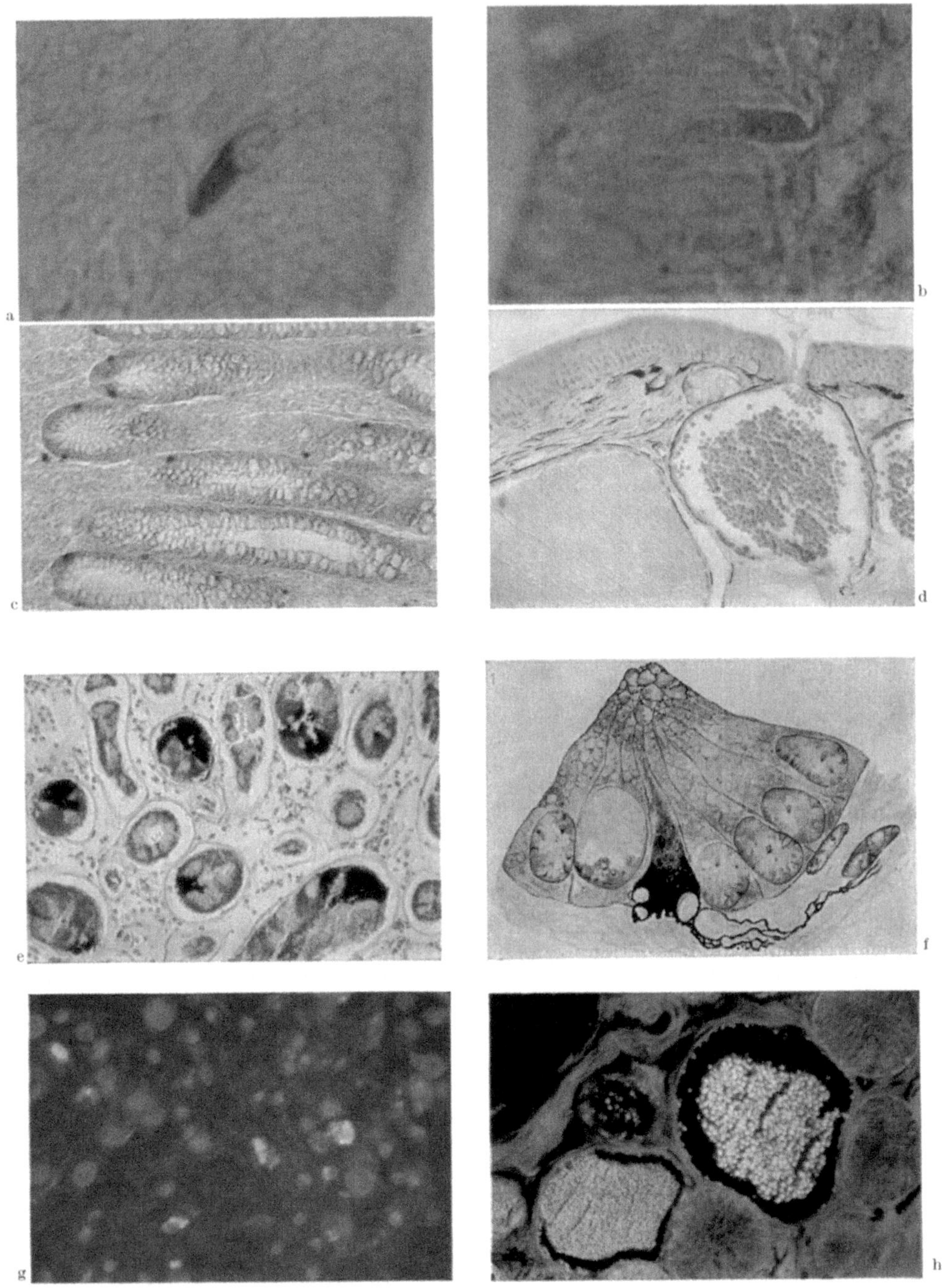

Plate I

Fig. a. Chicken duodenum. Fixation: 10% formalin. Alkaline diazoreaction. Fast blue B salt 250. 1300×

Fig. b. Chicken duodenum. Fixation: 10% formalin. PEARSE's thioindoxyl reaction. 1300×

Fig. c. Human rectum. Fixation: 10% formalin. SCHMORL's reaction. 132×

Fig. d. Skin of *Bombinator pachypus*. Fixation: 10% formalin. Alkaline diazo-reaction (para-nitro-aniline), haematoxylin. Portions of a gland with larger and of one with small granules. 100×

Fig. e. Posterior salivary gland of *Eledone moschata*. Fixation: 10% formalin. MASSON-HAMPERL's reaction; haematoxylin

Fig. f. Intestine of an ox foetus. Innervation of an enterochromaffin cell. ROGER's method (from SIMARD 1934, Arch. Anat. Microscop. **30**)

Fig. g. Dog mastocytoma: fluorescent mast cells. Photograph by RICE and MITCHENER

Fig. h. Skin of *Rana esculenta*. Fixation: 10% formalin. Fluorescence reaction: one gland showing yellow fluorescence and another showing whitish fluorescence. 80×

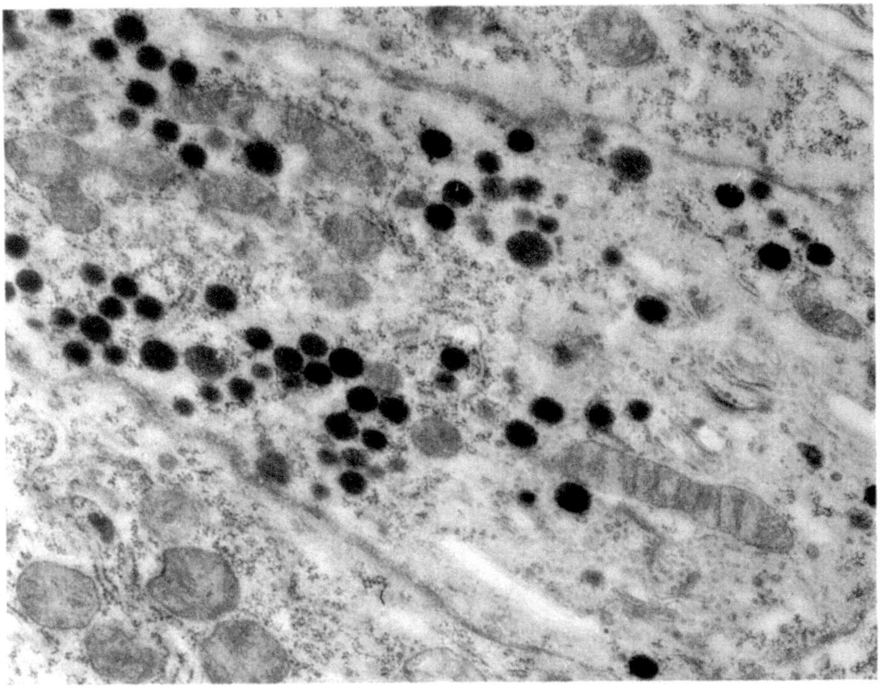

a

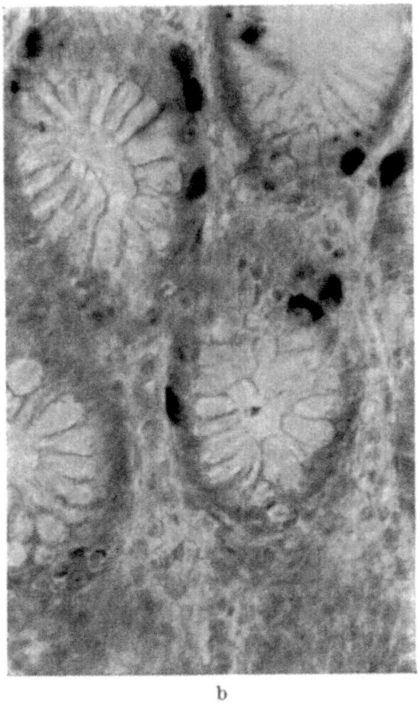

b

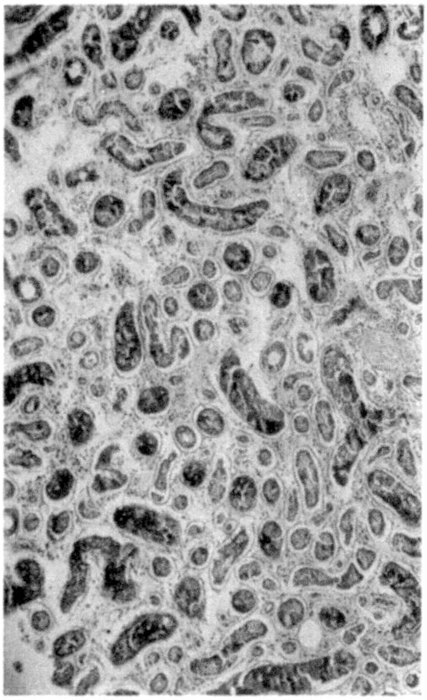

c

Plate II

Fig. a. Electron microphotograph of a portion of a rat enterochromaffin cell. Fixation by OsO_4 according to Millonig meth. B. Staining according to KARNOWSKY. 20200 ×. (Negative by RAVIOLA)

Fig. b. Enterochromaffin cells of the human rectum. Fixation: 10% formalin. MASSON-HAMPERL's reaction; haematoxylin. 395 ×

Fig. c. Posterior salivary gland of *Eledone moschata*. Fixation: 10% formalin. MASSON-HAMPERL's reaction; haematoxylin. 65 ×

Table 1. *Masson-Hamperl reaction on a normal rat*

	Duodenum			Ileum		
	Gland bottom	Villi	Bottom + villi	Gland bottom	Villi	Bottom + villi
a) Cell no	2087	1211	3298	503	280	783
Distribution of percentages of cell no	63%	37%	100%	64%	36%	100%
b) Granularity index	3732	2450	6182	831	546	1377
Percentage distribution of granularity index.	60%	40%	100%	60%	40%	100%
c) Ratio: W.I.G./C.N.	1,78	2,02	1,87	1,65	1,95	1,75

d) Mean weight of small intestine . . . . g 6,94 ± 0,55
e) Mean content of 5-HT in the small intestine . . . . µg/g 1,07 ± 0,07
[From Arch. Biol. (Liège) **72** (1961)].

Obviously, all data must be tested statistically for significance.

References

Abel, A., and D. J. Macht: Two cristalline pharmacological agents obtained from the tropical toad Bufo agua. J. Pharmacol. exp. Ther. **3**, 319—377 (1912).

Adam, K. R., and C. Weiss: The occurrence of 5-hydroxytryptamine in Scorpion venom. J. exp. Biol. **35**, 39—42 (1958).

— — Distribution of 5-hydroxytryptamine in Scorpion venoms. Nature (Lond.) **183**, 1398—1399 (1959).

— — Scorpion venom. Z. Tropenmed. u. Parasit. **10**, 334—339 (1959a).

Andrew, A.: A study of the developmental relationship between enterochromaffin cells and the neural crest. J. Embryol. exp. Morph. **11**, 307—324 (1963).

Archetti, I.: Sulla presenza di cellule enterocromaffini nel pancreas degli Uccelli. Nota preventiva. Boll. Zool. **7**, 181—187 (1936).

— Cellule enterocromaffini e cellule argentofile nel pancreas degli Uccelli. Arch. Biol. **49**, 569—604 (1938).

Arrigoni, G., F. Calafati e T. Longo: Cellule e materiale argentaffine nella prostata umana normale e patologica (Studio preliminare). Atti Soc. lombarda Sci. med.-biol. **11**, 55—58 (1956).

Azzi, A.: Sulla fine struttura della ghiandola salivare posteriore di Octopus macropus. Arch. It. Anat. Embriol. **16**, 246—258 (1917).

Bacq, Z. M., et F. Ghiretti: La sécrétion externe et interne des glandes salivaires postérieures des céphalopodes octopodes. Arch. int. Physiol. **59**, 288—314 (1951).

Baker, R. V.: Observations on the localization of 5-hydroxytryptamine. J. Physiol. (Lond.) **142**, 563—570 (1958).

— The intracellular localization of 5-hydroxytryptamine (5-HT) in relation to mitochondrial enzymes. J. Physiol. (Lond.) **143**, 80P (1958a).

— Mitochondria and storage granules for 5-hydroxytryptamine. J. Physiol. (Lond.) **145**, 473—481 (1959).

Balli, A.: Le cellule a granuli cromaffini dell'intestino di Patella vulgata. Boll. Zool. **7**, 25—32 (1936).

Barry, J.: La cellule argentaffine. Thèse de Medecine Lyon 1943, pp. 9—165. Lyon: Imprimerie du Salut Public 1943.

Barter, R., and E. A. G. Pearse: Detection of 5-hydroxytryptamine in mammalian enterochromaffin cells. Nature (Lond.) **172**, 810 (1953).

— — Mammalian enterochromaffin cells as the source of serotonin (5-hydroxytryptamine). J. Path. Bact. **69**, 25—31 (1955).

Benditt, E. P.: 5-hydroxytryptamine and 5-hydroxytryptophan decarboxylase in rat mast cells. In: G. P. Lewis, Hydroxytryptamine, pp. 26—31. London: Pergamon Press 1958.

— and R. L. Wong: On the concentration of 5-hydroxytryptamine in mammalian enterochromaffin cells and its release by reserpine. J. exp. Med. **105**, 509—524 (1957).

— — M. Arase and E. Roeper: 5-hydroxytryptamine in mast cells. Proc. Soc. exp. Biol. (N.Y.) **90**, 303—304 (1955).

Bertler, A., B. Falck, N. Å. Hillarp, E. Rosengren and A. Torp: Dopamine and chromaffin cells. Acta physiol. scand. **47**, 251—258 (1959).

Bertossi, F.: Sulle ghiandole granulose cutanee di Bombinator igneus Laur. Monit. zool. ital. **48**, 341—344 (1938).

BIGNARDI, C.: Contributo alla conoscenza istochimica delle cellule testacee di Ciona intestinalis. Pubbl. Staz. zool. Napoli **15**, 194—197 (1935).
— Cellule enterocromaffini e cellule argentofile nel pancreas dei Rettili. Arch. Biol. Liège **50**, 535—558 (1939).
BLASCHKO, H.: Biochemical principles in relation to hypotensive-drug action. In: Hypotensive Drugs, ed. M. HARINGTON, London and New York: Pergamon Press 1956.
BOGDANSKI, D. F., H. WEISSBACH and S. UDENFRIEND: The distribution of serotonin 5-hydroxytryptophan decarboxylase and monoamine oxidase in brain. J. Neurochem. **1**, 272—278 (1957).
BORGHESE, E.: Die Organkultur als Methode der kausalen Embryologie und ihre Anwendung in der Strahlenbiologie. Embryologia (Nagoya) **6**, Mangold Festschrift, 159—168 (1961).
BOTTINO, D., e F. GHIRINGHELLI: Osservazioni istochimiche sulla componente non enterami nica delle cellule enterocromaffini. Riv. Istochim. norm. pat. **4**, 325 (1958).
— — Ricerche istochimiche sul sistema cellulare enterocromaffine. Nota I. Sulla presenza di una componente mucopolisaccaridica nelle cellule enterocromaffini tipiche di alcuni Vertebrati. Riv. Istochim. norm. pat. **4**, 73—79 (1958a).
— — Ricerche istochimiche sul sistema cellulare enterocromaffine. Nota III. Rivelazione delle cellule enterocromaffini tipiche con sali di rame. Acta Histochem. (Jena) **8**, 199—206 (1959).
BOUCHILLOUX, S., et J. ROCHE: Contribution à l'étude biochimique de la pourpre des Murex. Bull. Soc. Chim. biol. (Paris) **37**, 37—53 (1955).
BRACCO, M., e P. C. CURTI: La 5-ossitriptamina enteramina-serotonina. Recenti Progr. Med. **25**, 425—459 (1958).
BROUSSY, J., et J. BARRY: La cellule entéro-chromo-argentaffine. Biol. méd. (Paris) **34**, 1—19 (1944).
BULLÓN-RAMÍREZ, A., E. LANGER y H. SCHULTZ: La visualizacion de los granulos de las celulas cromoenteroargentafines mediante el microscopio electronico. Rev. clin. esp. **79**, 321—328 (1960).
BURSTONE, M. S.: An evaluation of histochemical methods for protein groups. J. Histochem. Cytochem. **3**, 32—49 (1955).
CARLSSON, A., B. FALCK, N.-Å. HILLARP, G. THIEME and A. TORP: A new histochemical method for visualization of tissue catechol amines. Med. exp. (Basel) **4**, 123—125 (1961).
— N.-Å. HILLARP and B. WALDECK: A Mg^{++}-ATP dependent storage mechanism in the amine granules of the adrenal medulla. Med. exp. (Basel) **6**, 47—53 (1962).
CASATI, C.: Azione della reserpina sul sistema delle cellule enterocromaffini in Lacerta viridis. Riv. Istochim. norm. pat. **4**, 47—58 (1958).
CASELLA, C., e M. REGGIANI: Spettro di fluorescenza delle cellule enterocromaffini di cavia. Boll. Soc. ital. Biol. sper. **22**, 480—481 (1946).
— — Istospettrografia di fluorescenza. Arch. Biol. (Liège) **60**, 207—234 (1949).
CASTOLDI, G. L.: Determinazione del punto isoelettrico apparente delle cellule enterocromaffini mediante colorazione a vari pH. 1st Internat. Congr. of Histochem. and Cytochem. Abstracts, pp. 140—141, Paris 1960.
— Chromosome preparations from the intestinal mucosa. Experientia (Basel) **19**, 549—551 (1963).
CATTANEO, L.: Ricerche istochimiche sulla midollare del surrene. 1. Reazioni allo jodato di potassio per la dimostrazione selettiva delle cellule ad adrenalina e delle cellula a nor-adrenalina. Riv. Istochim. norm. pat. **4**, 85—116 (1958).
— Ricerche istochimiche sulla midollare del surrene. 2. Reattività in vitro allo jodato di potassio di precursori della nor-adrenalina e della adrenalina. Riv. Istochim. norm. pat. **6**, 209—228 (1960).
— Sulla realizzazione di metodi allo jodato di potassio per la colorazione delle cellule ad adrenalina e delle cellule a nor-adrenalina della midollare del surrene. Atti Accad. naz. Lincei. Rend., Classe sci. fis., mat. e nat. **28**, 509—512 (1960a).
CAVALLERO, C., B. MALANDRA e L. MOSCA: Isole pancreatiche e glucagone. Relazione VII. Congr. Soc. Ital Endocrinol., Belforte, Livorno, pp. 3—283, 1957.
—, and E. SOLCIA: Cytological and cytochemical studies on the pancreatic islets. In: S. BROLIN, ed., Wenner-Gren Symposium no. 3, p. 83—97. London: Pergamon Press 1964.
CHRISTIE, A. C.: A histochemical property of the argentaffin (KULSCHITZKY) cells. Nature (Lond.) **173**, 589 (1954).
— A study of the argentaffin (KULTSCHITZKY) cells im frozen-dried tissue by phase-contrast microscopy and ultra-violet light. Quart. J. micr. Sci. **96**, 289—293 (1955).
— A study of the Kultschitzky (argentaffin) cell with the electron-microscope, after fixation by osmium tetroxide. Quart. J. micr. Sci. **96**, 295—299 (1955a).

CIACCIO, C.: Ricerche istologiche e citologiche sul timo degli Uccelli. Anat. Anz. **29**, 597—600 (1906).
— Sopra speciali cellule granulose della mucosa intestinale. Arch. ital. Anat. Embriol. **6**, 482—498 (1907).
— Contributo all'istochimica delle cellule enterocromaffini. II. Cellule cromaffini del timo di Gallus domesticus. Boll. Soc. ital. Biol. sper. **17**, 619—620 (1942).
CITTERIO, V.: Presenza di enterocromaffini nella borsa di Fabricio. Boll. Zool. **2**, 39—46 (1931).
— Il cieco vitellino degli Uccelli. Atti Soc. ital. Sci. nat. **71**, 145—168 (1932).
— Nuove ricerche sulle cellule enterocromaffini nella borsa del Fabricio. Boll. Zool. **7**, 189—194 (1936).
CLARA, M.: Untersuchungen über die chemische Natur der Körnchen in den basalgekörnten Zellen des Darmepithels bei den Sauropsiden. Z. Anat. Entwickl.-Gesch. **98**, 516—526 (1932).
— Über die basalgekörnten Zellen des Darmepithels bei den Amphibien nach Untersuchungen an Salamandra maculosa Laur. Z. Anat. Entwickl.-Gesch. **100**, 76—89 (1933).
— Die basalgekörnten Zellen im Darmepithel der Wirbeltiere. Ergebn. Anat. Entwickl.-Gesch. **30**, 240—340 (1933a).
— Über die Diazokuppelungsreaktion zum Nachweis der ortho- und para-Phenole in der histologischen Technik. Z. wiss. Mikr. **51**, 316—337 (1934).
— Über die Entwicklung der basalgekörnten Zellen beim Menschen. Z. Anat. Entwickl.-Gesch. **103**, 131—139 (1934a).
— Untersuchungen über die „spezifische" Substanz in den basalgekörnten Zellen der Amphibien. Z. Zellforsch. **24**, 241—247 (1936).
— Über die Morphologie und Histochemie der basalgekörnten Zellen. Acta neuroveg. (Wien) **16**, 294—312 (1957).
COLE, J. W., and A. MCKALEN: Argentaffin cells in the intestinal epithelium of human embryos. Nature (Lond.) **193**, 198 (1962).
COLLIER, H. O. J.: The occurrence of 5-hydroxytryptamine (HT) in nature. In: G. P. LEWIS, 5-Hydroxytryptamine, p. 5—19. London: Pergamon Press 1958.
CONRIERI, C.: Caractéristiques histomorphologiques et histochimiques des glandes granuleuses de Rana latastei. 1st Internat. Congr. of Histochem. and Cytochem. Abstracts, p. 143, Paris 1960.
CORDIER, R.: Recherches morphologiques et expérimentales sur la cellule chromoargentaffine de l'épithélium intestinal des Vertébrés. Arch. Biol. (Liège) **36**, 427—463 (1926).
— L'argentaffinité en histologie. Bull. Histol. appl. **4**, 161—169 (1927).
—, et L. LISON: Etude histochimique de la substance chromoargentaffine de la cellule de KULTSCHITZKY. Bull. Histol. appl. **7**, 140—148 (1930).
CORONA, L. E.: Sostanze fenoliche dei vitellogeni di *Distoma hepaticum*. Ann. Histochim. **9**, 227—232 (1964).
COUJARD, R., et CHR. COUJARD CHAMPY: Essais sur une réaction des terminaisons et des cellules nerveuses surtout du système sympatique. Arch. Zool. exp. gén. **82**, 47—74 (1943).
COUPLAND, R. E., and J. F. RILEY: Mast cells and 5-hydroxytryptamine in precancerous mouse skin. Nature (Lond.) **187**, 1128—1129 (1960).
DAHL, E., B. FALCK, M. LINDQVIST and C. v. MECKLENBURG: Monoamines in mollusc neurons. Kungl. fysiogr. Sällsk. Lund Förh. **32**, 89—92 (1962).
DANISCH, F.: Zur Histogenese der sogenannten Appendixkarzinoide. Beitr. path. Anat. **72**, 687—709 (1924).
DAVIS, J. C.: The relation between the pancreatic alpha cells and certain cells in the gastric mucosa. J. Path. Bact. **67**, 237—240 (1954).
DAWSON, A. B.: Argentophile and argentaffin cells in the gastric mucosa of the rat. Anat. Rec. **100**, 319—329 (1948).
—, and S. L. MOYER: Histogenesis of the argentophile cells of the proventriculus and gizzard of the chicken. Anat. Rec. **100**, 493—515 (1948).
DE PAOLI, A. M.: Contributo alla conoscenza istochimica delle cellule a granuli fenolici dell'epitelio intestinale di Patella. Riv. Istochim. norm. pat. **9**, 192—193 (1963).
— Contributo alla conoscenza istochimica dei tipi cellulari presenti nell'epitelio intestinale di Patella coerulea L. Monit. Zool. ital. **70/71**, 320—325 (1962—1963).
DOERFLER, W., A. SCHWINK u. R. WETZSTEIN: Der Einfluß von Reserpin auf die Zellen der Lieberkühnschen Krypten. Anat. Anz. **112** Erg.-H., 222—223 (1963).
DUBOIS, R.: Recherches sur la pourpre et sur quelques autres pigments animaux. Arch. Zool. exp. gén. **42**, 471—590 (1909).
EDER, M., H. MARKUS u. K. LOEWE: Zur Funktion des enterochromaffinen Zellsystems des Darms im Experiment. Beitr. pathol. Anat. **121**, 50—63 (1959).

EDER, M., u. A. SCHAUER: Morphologische und experimentelle Untersuchungen zur Fibrosierung beim Carcinoid. Beitr. path. Anat. 121, 375—405 (1959).
— H. WILLE u. O. MIDORIKAWA: Der Einfluß der Fixation bei histochemischen Untersuchungen an enterochromaffinen Zellen und Panethschen Körnerzellen. Histochemie 3, 54—64 (1962).
ENERBACK, L.: Serotonin in human mast cells. Nature (Lond.) 197, 610—611 (1963).
ERÖS, G.: Über die Bedeutung der argentaffinen Zellen. Frankfurt. Z. Path. 40, 155—160 (1930).
— Eine neue Darstellungsmethode der sogenannten „gelben argentaffinen Zellen des Magen-Darmtraktes". Zbl. allg. Path. path. Anat. 54, 385—391 (1932).
ERSPAMER, V.: Le cellule enterocromaffini nel coniglio. Boll. Soc. med.-chir. Pavia 9, 877—887 (1935).
— Die enterochromaffinen Zellen der Gallenwege in normalen und pathologischen Zuständen. Virchows Arch. path. Anat. 296, 70—92 (1936).
— Cellule enterocromaffini e cellule argentofile nel pancreas dell'uomo e dei mammiferi. Z. Anat. Entwickl.-Gesch. 107, 574—619 (1937).
— Ricerche sperimentali sul significato biologico delle cellule enterocromaffini. Arch. Fisiol. 37, 156—169 (1937a).
— Il sistema enterocromaffine ed i suoi rapporti con il sistema insulare. Z. Anat. Entwickl.-Gesch. 109, 586—608 (1939).
— Caratterizzazione biologica di una nuova amina di- o polifenolica negli estratti acetonici di ghiandola salivare posteriore di "Octopus vulgaris". Arch. Sci. biol. (Bologna) 26, 295—340 (1940).
— Presenza di enteramina o di una sostanza enteraminosimile negli estratti gastrointestinali e splenici dei pesci e negli estratti gastroenterici delle Ascidie. Experientia (Basel) 2, 369—371 (1946).
— Active substances in the posterior salivary glands of Octopoda. II. Tyramine and octopamine (Oxyoctopamine). Acta pharmacol. (Kbh.) 4, 224—247 (1948).
— Ricerche chimiche e farmacologiche sugli estratti di ghiandola ipobranchiale di Murex trunculus, Murex brandaris e Tritonalia erinacea. IV. Presenza negli estratti di enteramina o di una sostanza enteraminosimile. Arch. int. Pharmacodyn. 76, 308—326 (1948a).
— Osservazioni preliminari, chimiche e farmacologiche, sulla murexina. Experientia (Basel) 4, 226—228 (1948b).
— Ricerche preliminari sulla moschatina. Experientia (Basel) 5, 79—81 (1949).
— Wirksame Stoffe der hinteren Speicheldrüsen der Octopoden und der Hypobranchialdrüse der Purpurschnecken. Arzneimittel-Forsch. 2, 253 (1952).
— Über den 5-Hydroxytryptamin-(Enteramin-)Gehalt des Magen-Darmtraktes bei den Wirbeltieren. Naturwissenschaften 40, 318—319 (1953).
— Il sistema cellulare enterocromaffine e l'enteramina (5-idrossitriptamina). Rend. Sci Farmitalia 1, 1—193 (1954).
— Pharmacology of indolealkylamines. Pharmacol. Rev. 6, 425—487 (1954a).
— Observations on the fate of indolalkylamines in the organism. J. Physiol. (Lond.) 127, 118—133 (1955).
— Osservazioni critiche sulle ipotesi concernenti il significato biologico della 5-idrossitriptamina (enteramina, serotonina). Medicina (Parma) 5, 1—34 (1955a).
— Le système entérochromaffine et la 5-hydroxytryptamine entéramine, sérotonine). Triangle (Basel) 11, 129—138 (1955b).
— Fenilalchil- e fenilalcanolamine nell'organismo vivente. Farmaco, Ed. sci. 13, 842—855 (1958).
— Isolamento della leptodactylina (m-idrossifenil-etil-trimetilammonio) dagli estratti di pelle di Leptodactylus. Ric. Sci. 28, 2065—2069 (1958a).
— Isolation of leptodactyline (m-hydroxyphenylethyltrimethyl-ammonium) from extracts of Leptodactylus skin. Arch. Biochem. Biophys. 82, 431—438 (1959).
— The biological significance of 5-hydroxytryptamine. Present status of the problem. XXI. Congr. Internat. de Ciencias Fisiologicas, Buenos Aires 1959. Lectures p. 216—222.
— Recent research in the field of 5-hydroxytryptamine and related indolealkylamines. Progress Drug Research 3, 151—367 (1961).
— Pharmacologically active substances of mammalian origin. Ann. Rev. Pharmacol. 1, 175—218 (1961a).
— 5-Hydroxytryptamine. In: U. S. v. EULER and H. HELLER, Comparative Endocrinology, vol. 2, p. 159—181. New York and London: Academic Press 1963.
—, and A. ANASTASI: Structure and pharmacological actions of eleidosin, the active endecapeptide of the posterior salivary glands of Eledone. Experientia (Basel) 18, 58—59 (1962).
—, e F. DORDONI: Sulla murexina, nuovo derivato colinico degli estratti di organo ipobranchiale di Murex trunculus, Murex brandaris e Tritonalia erinacea. Ric. Sci. e Ricostruz. 16, 1114—1116 (1946).

ERSPAMER, V., e F. DORDONI: Ricerche chimiche e farmacologiche sugli estratti di ghiandola ipobranchiale di Murex trunculus, Murex brandaris e Tritonalia erinacea. III. Presenza negli estratti di un nuovo derivato della colina o di una; colina omologica: la murexina. Arch. int. Pharmacodyn. **74**, 263—285 (1947).
—, and A. TESTINI: Observations on the release and turnover rate of 5-hydroxytryptamine in the gastrointestinal tract. J. Pharm. Pharmacol. **11**, 618—623 (1959).
—, and M. VIALLI: Presence of enteramine in the skin of Amphibia. Nature (Lond.) **167**, 1033 (1951).
— — Ricerche preliminari sulle indolalchilamine e sulle fenilalchilamine degli estratti di pelle di Anfibio. Ric. Sci. e Ricostruz. **22**, 1420—1425 (1952).
FÄNGE, R.: The salivary gland of *Neptunea antiqua*. Ann. N.Y. Acad. Sci. **90**, 689—694 (1960).
FALCK, B.: Observations on the possibilities of the cellular localization of monoamines by a fluorescence method. Acta physiol. scand. **56**, Suppl. 197, 6—25 (1962).
—, and N.-Å. HILLARP: A note on the chromaffin reaction. J. Histochem. Cytochem. **7**, 149 (1959).
— — and A. TORP: Some observations on the histology and histochemistry of the chromaffin cells probably storing dopamine. J. Histochem. Cytochem. **7**, 323—328 (1959).
— — — A new type of chromaffin cells, probably storing dopamine. Nature (Lond.) **183**, 267—268 (1959a).
—, and A. TORP: A fluorescence method for histochemical demonstration of noradrenalin in the adrenal medulla. Med. exp. **5**, 429—432 (1961).
— — New evidence for the localization of noradrenalin in the adrenergic nerve terminals. Med. exp. **6**, 169—172 (1962).
FARAGGIANA, R.: Sulla presenza di due tipi di ghiandole granulose nella pelle di Bombinator pachypus Fitz. Monit. zool. ital. **48**, 13—16 (1937).
— Ricerche istologiche sulle ghiandole cutanee granulose degli Anfibi anuri. I. Bufo vulgaris e Bufo viridis. Arch. ital. Anat. Embriol. **39**, 327—376 (1937a).
— La struttura sinciziale e il meccanismo di secrezione delle ghiandole cutanee granulose di Anfibi anuri. Monit. zool. ital. **49**, 105—107 (1938).
— Ricerche istologiche sulle ghiandole cutanee granulose degli Anfibi. II. Rana esculenta, Rana agilis e Bombinator pachypus. Arch. ital. Anat. Embriol. **41**, 390—410 (1939).
FEARON, W. R., and W. A. BOGGUST: Pigments derived from tryptophan: (1) Urorosein, (2) Tryptochrome. Biochem. J. **46**, 62—67 (1950).
FERNER, H.: Über die Entwicklung der Langerhansschen Inseln nach Geburt und die Bedeutung der versilberbaren Zellen im Pankreas des Menschen. Z. mikr.-anat. Forsch. **44**, 451—488 (1938).
— Weitere Untersuchungen über die Bedeutung der Silberzellen in den Langerhansschen Inseln des Menschen. Anat. Anz. (Jena) **88**, Erg.-H. 104—112 (1939).
— Das Inselsystem des Pankreas. Stuttgart: Georg Thieme 1952.
FEYRTER, F.: Carcinoid und Carcinom. Ergebn. allg. Path. path. Anat. **29**, 305—489 (1934).
— Über diffuse endokrine epitheliale Organe. Leipzig: Johann Ambrosius Barth 1938.
— Über die argyrophilen Epithelzellen des Menschen. Verh. dtsch. Ges. Path. **33**. Tagg, 155—160 (1949).
— Über die peripheren endokrinen (parakrinen) Drüsen des Menschen. Wien-Düsseldorf: Maudrich 1953.
FIORENTINI, A.: Sulla distribuzione delle cellule enterocromaffini nel tubo gastroenterico di Rana esculenta. Riv. Istochim. norm. pat. **5**, 544 (1959).
— Observations histochimiques sur les glandes salivaires postérieures de Eledone moschata. 1st Internat. Congr. Histochem. and Cytochem., Abstracts, p. 142, Paris 1960.
— Osservazioni istochimiche sulle ghiandole salivari posteriori di *Eledone moschata*. Ann. Histochim. **9**, 195—200 (1964).
—, e E. MIRA: Presenza di cellule enterocromaffini tipiche nelle vie aeree di Anfibi anuri. Riv. Istochim. norm. pat. **9**, 193—194 (1963).
FODDEN, J. H.: The enterochromaffin and pancreatic alpha cells: a comparison. Amer. J. clin. Path. **23**, 994—997 (1953).
FRIEDLÄNDER, P.: Über die Farbstoffe aus Purpura aperta und Purpura lapillus. Ber. dtsch. chem. Ges. **55**, 1655—1658 (1922).
FRIEDMANN, I.: Ein Beitrag zur Kenntnis der basalgekörnten, gelben Zellen des Darmtraktes beim Menschen. Z. mikr.-anat. Forsch. **36**, 99—136 (1934).
FROUTIN, G. H.: Contribution a l'étude du tissu conjonctif des mollusques et plus particulièrement des Lamellibranches et des Gastéropodes. Arch. Morph. gén. exp. **30**, 7—162 (1937).
GARDOSI, D.: Le cellule del sistema enterocromaffine nel pancreas degli Anfibi. Z. Anat. Entwickl.-Gesch. **109**, 60—74 (1938).

GASKELL, E. J.: The cromaffine system of annelids and the relation of this system to the contractile vascular system in the Leech Hirudo medicinalis. Phil. Trans. B. **205**, 153–211 (1914).

GERARD, P., R. CORDIER et L. LISON: Sur la nature de la réaction chromaffine. Bull. Histol. appl. **7**, 133—139 (1930).

GEREBTZOFF, M. A., et A. DRESSE: Contribution à la recherche des catécholamines au microscope de fluorescence. Ann. Histochim. **6**, 125—130 (1961).

GERNGROSS, O., K. VOSS u. H. HERFELD: Über eine hochempfindliche, streng tyrosinspezifische Farbreaktion auf para-substituierte Phenole. Der Tyrosin-Gehalt verschiedener Proteine, insbesondere von Kollagen und Gelatine. Ber. dtsch. chem. Ges. **66**, 435—442 (1933).

GERSH, I., J. VERGARA and G. L. ROSSI: Use of anhydrous vapors in post-fixation and in staining of reactive groups of proteins in frozen-dried specimens for electron microscopic studies. Anat. Rec. **138**, 445—459 (1960).

GERZELI, G.: Ricerche istochimiche sulla ovogenesi nei Policladi. Rend. Ist. Lombardo Sci. Cl. Sci. (B) **94**, 195—204 (1960).

— Presence of enterochromaffin cells in the gut of Amphioxus. Nature (Lond.) **189**, 237—238 (1961).

— Ricerche quantitative sugli ovociti in corso di sviluppo di Thysanozoon Brocchii Grube: II. L'accumulo delle granulazioni specifiche. Z. mikr.-anat. Forsch. **69**, 31—41 (1962).

— Istochimica delle cellule follicolari e delle cellule testali in diverse Ascidiacee. Rend. Ist. Lombardo Sci. Cl. Sci. (B) **96**, 165—178 (1962a).

— Le cellule enterocromaffini nei tunicati. Pubbl. Staz. zool. Napoli **33**, 117—124 (1963).

— Osservazioni interferometriche sulle cellule enterocromaffini. Ann. Histochim. **9**, 169—179 (1964).

—, e F. GHIRINGHELLI: Valutazione quantitativa di reazioni istochimiche in elementi microscopici non omogenei attraverso la misurazione di assorbimenti complessi per "annerimento" o per "colore". Mikroskopie **16**, 274—282 (1961).

— — e E. MIRA: Dati di istochimica enzimatica della mucosa gastrica come premessa per uno studio istofunzionale. Med. clin. sper. **12**, 329—347 (1962).

GESSNER, O.: Tierische Gifte. In: HEFFTER, Handbuch der experimentellen Pharmakologie, Suppl. 6, S. .1—83. Berlin: Springer 1938.

GHIDINI, G. M.: Ricerche embriologiche e sperimentali sulle cellule enterocromaffini nel pollo. Anat. Anz. **89**, 197—204 (1940).

GHIRETTI, F.: Cephalotoxin: the crab-paralysing agent of the posterior salivary glands of Cephalopods. Nature (Lond.) **183**, 1192—1193 (1959).

GHIRINGHELLI, F.: Sulla presenza di cellule enterocromaffini nella prostata e nella uretra prostatica del cane. Riv. Istochim. norm. pat. **2**, 235—238 (1956).

— Contribution à l'étude des cellules entérochromaffines selon la technique de congélation-dessication. 1st Internat. Congr. Histochem. and Cytochem., Abstracts, p. 7, Paris 1960.

— L'uso del microdensitometro integratore secondo Deeley per la valutazione quantitativa della carica granulare delle cellule enterocromaffini poste in evidenza con la reazione di MASSON-HAMPERL. Biochim. Biol. sper. No 2, 187—192 (1961).

— Le cellule enterocromaffini in ratti ipofisectomizzati. Arch. Sci. biol. (Bologna) **45**, 127—133 (1961a).

— Ricerche istochimiche sul sistema cellulare enterocromaffine. Nota V. Osservazioni su alcune reazioni presentate dalle cellule enterocromaffini. Riv. Istochim. norm. pat. **7**, 185—196 (1961b).

— Contributo allo studio delle cellule enterocromaffini con la tecnica del freezing-drying. Ann. Histochim. **9**, 181—186 (1964).

—, e G. BERTACCINI: Le cellule enterocromaffini, la 5-idrossitriptamina e l'acido 5-idrossindolilacetico nel ratto trattato con colchicina. Rend. Ist. Lombardo Sci. Cl. Sci. (B) **95**, 156—166 (1961).

—, e D. BOTTINO: Ricerche istochimiche sul sistema cellulare enterocromaffine. Nota II. Esame comparativo del colore delle cellule enterocromaffini e mucipare dopo reazione di Hotchkiss mediante metodo spettrofotometrico e "tristimulus". Mikroskopie **14**, 161—165 (1959).

— — Ricerche istochimiche sul sistema cellulare enterocromaffine. Nota IV. Su una presunta componente lipidica nelle cellule enterocromaffini tipiche di Cavia. Acta histochem. (Jena) **10**, 265—270 (1960).

—, e E. MIRA: Per una migliore valutazione dell'effetto della reserpina sulle cellule enterocromaffini. Riv. Istochim. norm. pat. **5**, 563 (1959).

— — Azione della reserpina sulle cellule enterocromaffini del ratto e sua valutazione quali- e quantitativa. Arch. Biol. (Liège) **70**, 875—900 (1959a).

— — Le cellule enterocromaffini nell'intestino di ratto tenuto a dieta di banane. Rend. Ist. Lombardo Sci. Cl. Sci. (B) **94**, 31—42 (1960).

GHIRINGHELLI, F., E. MIRA e G. BERTACCINI: Le cellule enterocromaffini e la 5-idrossitriptamina dell'intestino di ratti ipofisectomizzati e trattati con ormone somatotropo. Arch. Biol. (Liège) **72**, 485—499 (1961).
— — — Le cellule enterocromaffini e la 5-idrossitriptamina dell'intestino del ratto surrenectomizzato. Folia endocr. (Roma) **14**, 571—580 (1961a).
— — — Il comportamento delle cellule enterocromaffini nell'intestino di ratto dopo resezione del crasso. Riv. Istochim. norm. pat. **7**, 77—88 (1961b).
GIBBS, H. D.: Phenol tests. I. A classification of the tests and a review of the literature. Chem. Rev. **3**, 291—319 (1927).
— Phenol tests. III. The indophenol test. J. biol. Chem. **72**, 649—664 (1927a).
GILLMAN, J.: The structure of the basal granular cell (argentaffine) in the human (Bantu) alimentary canal with special reference to the anti-anaemic factor. S. Afr. J. med. Sci. **7**, 144—159 (1942).
GIROUD, A., et C. P. LEBLOND: L'acide ascorbique dans les tissus et sa détection. Paris: Hermann 1936.
— — Histological study of renal elimination of ascorbic acid. Anat. Rec. **68**, 113—126 (1937).
GLENNER, G. G., and R. D. LILLIE: Pepsin release of guinea pig enterochromaffin substance. J. Histochem. Cytochem. **7**, 204 (1959).
GLICK, D., S. L. BONTING and D. DEN BOER: Histochemistry. XLIV. Use of density gradient for isolation of mast cells. Proc. Soc. exp. Biol. (N.Y.) **92**, 357—359 (1956).
GOMORI, G.: Chemical character of the enterochromaffin cells. Arch. Path. **45**, 48—55 (1948).
— Pitfalls in histochemistry. Ann. N.Y. Acad. Sci. **50**, 968—981 (1950).
— Microscopic histochemistry. Chicago: Chicago University Press 1952.
— Histochemistry of the enterochromaffin substance. J. Histochem. Cytochem. **1**, 50—53 (1954).
GRÜTZNER, P., u. H. MENZEL: Über Bildung und Ausscheidung von Fermenten. Pflügers Arch. ges. Physiol. **20**, 395—419 (1879).
GRYNFELTT, E.: De quelques réactions chimiques et histochimiques de la glandé à pourpre de "Murex trunculus" comparées à celles de la substance médullo surrénale des vertébrés. Nouv. Montpellier Med. **29**, 127—132 (1909).
— Glande hypobranchiale et organe de la pourpre chez quelques Murex indigènes de côtes du Languedoc. Bull. Acad. Sci. Lett. Montpellier **5**, 21—30 (1913).
— Sur la genèse des boules picriphiles dans la glande hypobranchiale de "Murex trunculus". Bull. Acad. Sci. Lett. Montpellier **5**, 119—127 (1913a).
GURR, E.: Encyclopaedia of microscopic stains. London: Leonard Hill (Books) Limited 1960.
HAMPERL, H.: Über die „gelben (chromaffinen)" Zellen im Epithel des Verdauungstraktes. Z. mikr.-anat. Forsch. **2**, 506—535 (1925).
— Über die „gelben (chromaffinen)" Zellen im gesunden und kranken Magendarmschlauch. Virchows Arch. path. Anat. **266**, 509—548 (1927).
— Was sind argentaffine Zellen? Virchows Arch. path. Anat. **286**, 811—833 (1932).
— Über argyrophile Zellen. Virchows Arch. path. Anat. **321**, 482—507 (1952).
HARTROFT, W. S., G. A. WRENSHALL and W. D. WILSON: Absence of degenerative changes in argentaffin cells of intestinal mucosa of cobalt-injected guinea-pigs. Amer. J. Path. **30**, 621—622 (1954).
HEIDENHAIN, A.: Untersuchungen über den Bau der Labdrüsen. Arch. mikr. Anat. **6**, 368—406 (1870).
HELANDER, H. F.: A preliminary note on the ultrastructure of the argyrophile cells of the mouse gastric mucosa. J. Ultrastruct. Res. **5**, 257—262 (1961).
— Ultrastructure of fundus glands of the mouse gastric mucosa. J. Ultrastruct. Res., Suppl. **4**, 5—123 (1962).
HELLERSTRÖM, C., and B. HELLMAN: Some aspects of silver impregnation of the islets of Langerhans in the rat. Acta endocr. (Kbh.) **35**, 518—532 (1960).
HELLMAN, B., U. ROTHMAN and C. HELLERSTRÖM: Identification of a specific type of α-cell located in the central part of the pancreatic islets of the horse. Gen. comp. Endocr. **2**, 558—564 (1962).
HELLWEG, G.: Über Vorkommen und gegenseitiges Verhalten der argentaffinen und argyrophilen Zellen im menschlichen Magen-Darmtrakt. Z. Zellforsch. **36**, 546—551 (1952).
HENZE, M.: p-Oxyphenyläthylamin, das Speicheldrüsengift der Cephalopoden. Hoppe-Seylers Z. physiol. Chem. **87**, 51—58 (1913).
HILLARP, N.-Å., and B. HÖKFELT: Histochemical demonstration of noradrenalin and adrenalin in the adrenal medulla. J. Histochem. Cytochem. **3**, 1—5 (1955).
HOESCHEN, T.: Über Menge und Verteilung der basalgekörnten Zellen im Darm des Meerschweinchens. Z. Zellforsch. **27**, 711—719 (1938).
HOFMANN, H.: Gelbe (basalgekörnte) Zellen in der Schleimhaut einer ekstrophierten Harnblase. Virchows Arch. path. Anat. **300**, 466—472 (1937).

HOLCENBERG, J., and E. BENDITT A reaction for indoleethylamines. J. Histochem. Cytochem. **7**, 303—304 (1959).
— — A new color reaction for tryptamine derivatives. Histochemical application to enterochromaffin cells. Lab. Invest. **10**, 144—158 (1961).
ITO, S., and R. J. WINCHESTER: The fine structure of the gastric mucosa in the bat. J. Cell Biol. **16**, 541—577 (1963).
JACOBSON, W.: The argentaffine cells and pernicious anaemia. J. Path. Bact. **49**, 1—19 (1939).
— The yellow pigment of the argentaffine cells of the mammalian gastro-intestinal tract. Ciba Foundation Symposium on Chemistry and Biology of Pteridines 1954, pp. 314—327.
—, and P. M. GOOD: The argentaffine cells and the nature of the anti pernicious anaemia factor. Exp. Cell Res., Suppl. **1**, 300—303 (1949).
—, and D. M. SIMPSON: The fluorescence spectra of pterins and their possible use in the elucidation of the antipernicious anaemia factor. Part 1. Biochem. J. **40**, 3—9 (1946).
— — The fluorescence spectra of pterins and their possible use in the elucidation of the antipernicious anaemia factor. Part 2. Biochem. J. **40**, 9—14 (1946a).
KAUFMANN-WOLF, M.: Kurze Notiz über Belegzellen, Panetsche Zellen und basalgekörnte Zellen im Darm des Menschen. Anat. Anz. **39**, 670—672 (1911).
KIRBERGER, E., u. L. BRAUN: Über das Vorkommen von 5-Hydroxytryptamin in der Walnuß (Juglans regia). Biochim. biophys. Acta (Amst.) **49**, 391—393 (1961).
KOHN, A. J.: Piscivorous gastropods of the genus *Conus*. Proc. nat. Acad. Sci. (Wash.) **42**, 168—171 (1956).
— P. R. SAUNDERS, and S. WIENER: Preliminary studies on the venom of the marine snail *Conus*. Ann. N.Y. Acad. Sci. **90**, 706—725 (1960).
KOJECKY, Z., L. BENÝŠEK, R. KODOUŠEK, and J. MALINSKÝ: The diagnostic value of enterobiopsies. Vnitřni Lék. **9**, 564—567 (1963).
— et R. KODOUŠEK: Etudes histo-enzymatiques de la muqueuse intestinale dans les carcinoides malins. Arch. Mal. Appar. dig. **50**, 1194—1196 (1961).
KULL, H.: Die basalgekörnten Zellen des Dünndarmepithels. Arch. mikr. Anat. **81**, 185—195 (1913).
— Die chromaffinen Zellen des Verdauungstraktes. Z. mikr.-anat. Forsch. **2**, 163—200 (1925).
KUROSUMI, K., S. SHIBASAKI, G. UCHIDA and Y. TANAKA: Electron microscope studies on the gastric mucosa of normal rats. Arch. hist. jap. **15**, 587—624 (1958).
LACY, P. E.: Electron microscopic identification of different cell types in the islets of Langerhans of the guinea pig, rat, rabbit and dog. Anat. Rec. **128**, 255—267 (1957).
— Electron microscopy of normal islets of Langerhans; studies in dog, rabbit, guinea pig and rat. Diabetes **6**, 498—507 (1957a).
LAGUNOFF, D., M. PHILLIPS and E. P. BENDITT: The histochemical demonstration of histamine in mast cells. J. Histochem. Cytochem. **9**, 534—541 (1961).
LANERI, A. V.: Risposte delle cellule enterocromaffini alla reazione di MASSON-HAMPERL di varia durata. Riv. Istochim. norm. pat. **7**, 500 (1961).
— Unpublished observations.
LEBLOND, C. P., and B. MESSIER: Renewal of chief cells and goblet cells in the small intestine as shown by radioautography after injection of thymidine-H^3 into mice. Anat. Rec. **132**, 247—259 (1958).
LEMBECK, F., u. W. KLEMENTSCHITZ: Papierchromatographische Untersuchungen über die Reaktionsprodukte des Oxytryptamins mit Formaldehyd. Naunyn-Schmiedeberg's Arch. exp. Path. Pharmak. **225**, 129 (1955).
LEWIS, G. P.: 5-Hydroxytryptamine. London: Pergamon Press 1958.
— Histochemistry in biology. View points in Biology **1**, 50—89 (1962).
LIEBECQ-HUTTER, S., and Z. M. BACQ: Disparition de la 5-hydroxytryptamine dans les granulations des glandes de la peau de Discoglossus pictus et de Rana temporaria après injection de réserpine. Experientia (Basel) **14**, 180—181 (1958).
— J. F. RENSON and P. FISCHER: Action de la réserpine sur la teneur de 5-hydroxytryptamine des tissus de Discoglossus pictus. Arch. int. Physiol. Biochem. **67**, 144—147 (1959).
LILLIE, R. D.: Histopathologic technic and practical histochemistry. New York: Blakiston Co., Inc. 1954.
— The p-Dimethylaminobenzaldehyde reaction for pyrroles in histochemistry: Melanins, enterochromaffin, zymogen granules, lens. J. Histochem. Cytochem. **4**, 118—129 (1956).
— The xanthydrol reaction for pyrroles and indoles in histochemistry: Zymogen, Granules Lens, Enterochromaffin and Melanins. J. Histochem. Cytochem. **5**, 188—195 (1957).
— Adaptation of the Morel-Sisley protein diazotization procedure to the histochemical demonstration of protein bound tyrosine. J. Histochem. Cytochem. **5**, 528—532 (1957a).

LILLIE, R. D.: Acetylation and nitrosation of tissue amines in histochemistry. J. Histochem. Cytochem. 6, 352—362 (1958).
— Preferred common names, formulae, colour index references and synonyms of stable diazonium salts used in histochemistry. J. Histochem. Cytochem. 7, 281—284 (1959).
— Investigations on the structure of the enterochromaffin substances. J. Histochem. Cytochem. 9, 184—189 (1961).
—, and H. J. BURTNER: The ferricyanide reduction test in histochemistry. J. Histochem. Cytochem. 1, 87—92 (1953).
— — and J. P. GRECO HENSON: Diazosafranin for staining enterochromaffin cells. Histochem. Cytochem. 1, 154—159 (1953).
—, and G. G. GLENNER: Histochemical reactions in carcinoid tumors of the human gastrointestinal tract. Amer. J. Path. 36, 623—651 (1960).
—, H. WEISSBACH and G. G. GLENNER: On the experimental discharge of the gastric and intestinal argentaffin cells. J. Histochem. Cytochem. 7, 23—26 (1959).
LISON, L.: Etudes histochimiques sur les phénols et leurs dérivés. Arch. Biol. (Liège) 41, 343—436 (1931).
— Chromaffinité et pseudo-chromaffinité. (Etudes histochimiques sur la glande à pourpre des Muricidés. I.) Arch. Soc. Sci. méd. et biol. Montpellier 9, 542—553 (1932).
— Composés phénoliques dans la glande a venin des Crapauds. C. R. Soc. Biol. (Paris) 111, 657—658 (1932a).
— Etudes histochimiques sur la glande a pourpre des Murex. Composés indoliques. J. Physiol. Path. gén. 31, 82—99 (1933).
— La cellule a polyphénols du tube digestif des Ascidies, homologue de la cellule de KULTSCHITZKY des vertébrés. C. R. Soc. Biol. (Paris) 112, 1237—1239 (1933a).
— Histochimie et Cytochimie Animales Principes et Méthodes, III. edit. Paris: Gauthier-Villars 1960.
LOJDA, Z., and P. FRIČ: Enzymes of the jejunal enterochromaffine cells in man. Histochemie 3, 455—461 (1964).
— B. VEČEREK and H. PELICHOVĂ: Some remarks concerning the histochemical detection of acid phosphatase by azo-coupling reactions. Histochemie 3, 428—454 (1964).
LUSE, S. A., and P. E. LACY: Electron microscopy of a malignant argentaffin tumor. Cancer (Philad.) 13, 334—346 (1960).
MARCHE MARCHAD, I., H. GIONO, A. MAZER et R. LEMAIRE: Effets pharmacodynamiques d'extraits de glande de Leiblen de *Cymbium patulum*. C. R. Soc. Biol. (Paris) 155, 873—875 (1961).
MARCOLI, C. G.: Il metodo al protargolo di Bodian applicato allo studio delle cellule enterocromaffini e preenterocromaffini. Studia Ghisleriana (Milano) Ser. III 1, 169—171 (1949).
MARKS, B. H., R. W. SORGEN and E. R. HAYES: Effects of reserpine and chlorpromazine upon enterochromaffin cells of the rat. Proc. Soc. exp. Biol. (N.Y.) 97, 413—415 (1958).
MARTOJA, M.: Données histologiques sur l'appareil venimeux de *Conus mediterraneus* Brug. Ann. Sci. nat. Zool., Sér. XII 2, 513 (1960).
MASSON, P.: La glande endocrine de l'intestin chez l'homme. C. R. Acad. Sci. (Paris) 158, 59—61 (1914).
— Anciennes et nouvelles méthodes de détection des cellules chromo-argentaffines de l'intestin. Trans. roy. Soc. Can., Sect. V, 45 (1932).
MATHIAS, A. P., D. M. ROSS and M. SCHACHTER: Identification and distribution of 5-hydroxytryptamine in a sea anemone. Nature (Lond.) 180, 658 (1957).
MIRA, E.: Action de l'hormone somatotrope préhypophysaire sur les cellules entérochromaffines de rat. 1st Internat. Congr. Histochem. Cytochem., Abstracts, pp. 147—148, Paris 1960.
— Comportamento del sistema cellulare enterocromaffine dopo trattamento con ormone somatotropo. Rend. Ist. Lombardo Sci. e Lett., Cl. Sci. (B) 97, 300—314 (1963).
— Azione dell'ormone somatotropo preipofisario sulle cellule enterocromaffini di ratto. Ann. Histochim. 9, 217—225 (1964).
—, e A. FIORENTINI: Presenza di cellule enterocromaffini nel sacco laringotracheale degli anfibi anuri e possibili rapporti istogenetici con i carcinoidi bronchiali. Boll. Mal. Orecch. 81, 45—55 (1963).
MONESI, V.: L'epoca di comparsa delle cellule argentofile e delle cellule argentaffini nell'in testino di embrione di pollo. Boll. Zool., 26, 537—544 (1959).
— The appearance of enterochromaffin cells in the intestine of the chick embryo. Acta anat. (Basel) 41, 97—114 (1960).
— La differenziazione delle cellule enterocromaffini nell'intestino di embrione di pollo coltivato in vitro. Monit. zool. ital., Suppl. 68, 393—402 (1960a).
— Differentiation of argyrophil and argentaffin cells in organotypic cultures of embryonic chick intestine. J. Embryol. exp. Morph. 8, 302—313 (1960b).

MOSCA, L.: Istofisiologia delle isole pancreatiche. Milano: Fondazione D. Ganassini, Ed. del Premio Ganassini 1958.
MÜNCH, H.: Über Menge und Verteilung der basalgekörnten Zellen im Darm der weißen Ratte. Z. mikr.-anat. Forsch. **45**, 244—254 (1939).
NICOLAS, A.: Recherches sur l'épithélium de l'intestin grêle. Internat. Monatss. Anat. Physiol. **8**, 1—62 (1891).
NUSSBAUM, M.: Über den Bau und die Thätigkeit der Drüsen. III. Mittheilung. Die Fermentbildung in den Drüsen. Arch. mikr. Anat. **16**, 532—544 (1879).
PAASONEN, M. K.: 5-hydroxytryptamine in mammalian thyroid gland. Experientia (Basel) **14**, 95—96 (1958).
PAGE, I. H.: Serotonin (5-hydroxytryptamine); the last four years. Physiol. Rev. **38**, 277—335 (1958).
PAGÈS, A.: Essai sur le système des "cellules claires" de FEYRTER. Montpellier: P. Dèhan 1955.
PAGÈS, P., et A. PAGÈS: Etudes sur l'intégration biologique. Le rôle du "système des cellules claires". Causse Graille Castelnau Imprimeurs, Montpellier 1957.
PARAT, M.: Contribution à l'histophysiologie des organes digestifs de l'embryon. L'apparition corrélative de la cellule de KULTSCHITZKY et de la sécrétine chez l'embryon. C. R. Soc. Biol. (Paris) **90**, 1023—1024 (1924).
— Contribution à l'histophysiologie des organes digestifs de l'embryon. L'apparition des glandes de BRUNNER, des cellules de KULTSCHITZKY, des plaques de PEYER chez l'embryon humaine. C. R. Ass. Anat. **19**, 232—236 (1924a).
PATZELT, V.: Die gelben oder basalgekörnten Zellen. In: W. v. MÖLLENDORFFs Handbuch der mikroskopischen Anatomie des Menschen, Bd. V/3, S. 137—152. Berlin: Springer 1936.
— Die feinere Ausbildung des menschlichen Darmes von der fünften Woche bis zur Geburt. Z. mikr.-anat. Forsch. **27**, 269—518 (1931).
PAULETTA, G.: Contributo alla conoscenza istochimica delle cellule testacee e follicolari nelle Ascidie. Arch. ital. Anat. Embriol. **47**, 659—672 (1942).
PEARSE, A. G. E.: Application of the alkaline tetrazolium reaction to the study of reducing groups in tissue sections. J. Path. Bact. **67**, 129—136 (1954).
— A contribution to the chemistry of mammalian enterochromaffin cells. Riv. Istochim. norm. pat. **2**, 103—110 (1956).
— Histochemistry theoretical and applied, second edit. London: J. & A. Churchill Ltd. 1960.
—, and W. J. A. PEPLER: A probable peptidase in carcinoid tumours. Nature (Lond.) **179**, 589 (1957).
PELLEGRINO DE IRALDI, A., and E. DE ROBERTIS: Action of reserpine on the submicroscopic morphology of the pineal gland. Experientia (Basel) **17**, 122—124 (1961).
PERRONE, O., y W. ACOSTA FERREIRA: Sobre la existencia de células argentafines en el timo del pollo y del nandù. Arch. Soc. Biol. Montevideo **15**, 120—122 (1948—1949).
— — Sobre la presencia de células argentafines en la bolsa de Fabricio. Arch. Soc. Biol. Montevideo **17**, 58—67 (1950).
PETERSSON, B., C. HELLERSTRÖM, and B. HELLMAN: Some characteristics of the two types of A-cells in the islets of Langerhans of guinea-pigs. Z. Zellforsch. **57**, 559—566 (1962).
PHILIPPS, J. H.: Isolation of active nematocysts of Metridium senile and their chemical composition. Nature (Lond.) **178**, 932 (1956).
PICCINELLI, D.: Azione della reserpina su alcune localizzazioni di indolalchilamine e fenilalchilamine in vertebrati inferiori e molluschi. Arch. int. Pharmacodyn. **117**, 452—459 (1958).
PLENK, L.: Der Magen. In: W. v. MÖLLENDORFFs, Handbuch der mikroskopischen Anatomie des Menschen, Bd. 5/2, S. 1—234. Berlin: Springer 1932.
PLETSCHER, A.: Topographical difference of the behaviour of 5-hydroxytryptamine in the gastric mucosa after reserpine administration. In: G. P. LEWIS, 5-Hydroxytryptamine, pp. 84—85. London: Pergamon Press 1957.
POLL, H., u. A. SOMMER: Über phaeochrome Zellen im Centralnervensystem des Blutegels. Arch. Anat. z. Physiol., Physiol. Abt. 549—550 (1903).
PRETL, K.: Zur Frage der Endokrinie der menschlichen Vorsteherdrüse. Virchows Arch. path. Anat. **312**, 392—404 (1944).
PRUSOFF, W. H.: The distribution of 5-hydroxytryptamine and adenosinetriphosphate in cytoplasmic particles of the dog's small intestine. Brit. J. Pharmacol. Chemoth., **15**, 520—524 (1960).
— Effect of reserpine on the 5-hydroxytryptamine and adenosinetriphosphate of the dog intestinal mucosa. Brit. J. Pharmacol. **17**, 87—91 (1961).
QUARONI, E.: Presenza di cellule preenterocromaffini argentofile nel timo di pollo. Riv. Istochim. norm. pat. **2**, 185—187 (1956).

RATZENHOFER, M.: Zur Histochemie der Carcinoide. Acta histochem. (Jena) **1**, 53—54 (1954).
REGGIANI, M.: Ricerche sulle cellule enterocromaffini. I. Azione della formalina sulla fluorescenza. Boll. Soc. ital. Biol. sper. **20**, 584—585 (1945).
— Contributo alla conoscenza delle cellule cromaffini del timo nel pollo. Boll. Soc. ital. Biol. sper. **22**, 108—109 (1946).
RICE, W. G., and J. W. MITCHENER: Histochemical evidence of 5-hydroxytryptamine in a dog mast cell tumour. Nature (Lond.) **189**, 767—768 (1961).
RILEY, J. F.: Fluorescent mast cells in precancerous mouse skin. Experientia (Basel) **14**, 141 (1958).
ROAF, H. E.: The situation in the mantle of Purpura lapillus of the cells which yield a pressor substance. Quart. J. exp. Physiol. **4**, 89—92 (1911).
—, and M. NIERENSTEIN: The physiological action of the extract of the hypobranchial gland of "Purpura lapillus". J. Physiol. (Lond.) **36**, V—VIII (1907).
ROMANINI, M. G.: Contributo alla conoscenza istochimica delle ghiandole salivari posteriori di Eledone cirrosa. Boll. Soc. ital. Biol. sper. **28**, 1116—1117 (1952).
SCARLATO, G., B. MANZINI e N. CANAL: 5-idrossitriptamina e sistema nervoso. Dati biologici. Spunti patogenetici e clinici. Riv. sper. Freniat. **83**, 1087—1193 (1959).
SCHAUER, A., and E. WERLE: Zur histochemischen Darstellung des Histamins der Mastzellen. Z. ges. exp. Med. **131**, 100—104 (1959).
SCHOFIELD, G.: The argentaffin and mucous cells of the human intestine. Acta anat. (Basel) **18**, 256—272 (1953).
SIMARD, L. C.: Sur les relations des cellules argentaffines de l'intestin avec les nerfs. C. R. Soc. Biol. (Paris) **111**, 766 (1932).
— Sur la presence de cellules argentaffines dans les nerfs de l'intestin du phoque. Trans. roy. Soc. Can., Sect. V, 97—98 (1933).
— Sur les relations des cellules argentaffines de l'intestin avec les nerfs chez l'embryon de veau. Arch. Anat. micr. Morph. exp. **30**, 235—248 (1934).
—, and E. VAN CAMPENHOUT: The embryonic development of argentaffin cells in the chick intestine. Anat. Rec. **53**, 141—152 (1932).
SINGH, I.: A note on enterochromaffin cells in islets of ectopic intestinal mucosa in the human stomach. J. anat. Soc. India **11**, 57—59 (1962).
— The staining of enterochromaffin cells by the Bodian silver impregnation method. Acta anat. (Basel) **51**, 292—297 (1962a).
— The prenatal development of enterochromaffin cells in the human gastro-intestinal tract. J. Anat. (Lond.) **97**, 377—387 (1963).
— On the alleged presence of non argyrophile argentaffin cells in the human gastro-intestinal tract. Z. Zellforsch. **59**, 615—624 (1963a).
— Further observations on the alleged presence of non-argyrophile argentaffin cells in the human gastro-intestinal tract. Z. Zellforsch. **62**, 121—124 (1964).
SOLCIA, E.: Studio del pancreas endocrino di alcuni vertebrati mediante osservazione in campo oscuro di sezioni fresche. Boll. Soc. ital. Biol. sper. **38**, 1192—1194 (1962).
SUTHERLAND, E. W., and CH. DE DUVE: Origin and distribution of the hyperglycemic-glycogenolytic factor of the pancreas. J. biol. Chem. **175** (2), 663—674 (1948).
TAYLOR, J., and E. R. HAYES: An electron microscopic study of the ultrastructure of the argentaffin cell. J. appl. Physics **30**, 2033 (1959).
TRAVERSO, G., e M. VIALLI: Aspetti chimici ed istochimici della diazoreazione di alcune sostanze indoliche. Riv. Istochim. norm. pat. **6**, 129—140 (1960).
TRIER, J. S.: Studies on small intestinal crypt epithelium. I. The fine structure of the crypt epithelium of the proximal small intestine of fasting humans. J. Cell Biol. **18**, 599—620 (1963).
TWAROG, B. M.: Response of a molluscan smooth muscle to acetylcholine and 5-hydroxytryptamine. J. cell. comp. Physiol. **44**, 141—163 (1954).
UGGERI, B.: Ricerche sulle cellule enterocromaffini e sulle cellule argentofile dei pesci. Z. Zellforsch. **28**, 648—673 (1938).
VALCURONE, M.: Ricerche istochimiche sui granuli vitellini dei policladi. Arch. Zool. ital. **38**, 245—267 (1953).
VERNE, M. J.: La réaction chromaffine en histologie et sa signification. Bull. Soc. Chim. biol. (Paris) **5**, 227—235 (1923).
VETTER, J.: Über das Verhalten der basalgekörnten Zellen bei hungernden Tieren (Meerschweinchen, weiße Ratten und weiße Mäuse). Z. mikr.-anat. Forsch. **43**, 623—632 (1938).
— Über die Frage der Beteiligung der basalgekörnten Zellen an den Resorptions- und Sekretionsvorgängen des Darmes. Z. mikr.-anat. Forsch. **47**, 33—48 (1939).
VIALLI, M.: Ricerche sull'intestino dei rettili. IV. L'Epitelio intestinale. Arch. Biol. (Liège) **39**, 527—581 (1929).

VIALLI, M.: Ricerche istochimiche sui vitellogeni dei platelminti. (Nota preventiva). Boll. Zool. **4**, 135—138 (1933).
— Ricerche istochimiche sul veleno cutaneo degli Anfibi. Boll. Soc. ital. Biol. sper. **8**, 1740—1741 (1933a).
— Ricerche istochimiche sui granuli vitellini dei policladi. Boll. Zool. **5**, 21—23 (1934).
— Sulle caratteristiche istochimiche della ghiandola della porpora in Murex trunculus. Boll. Soc. ital. Biol. sper. **9**, 203—206 (1934a).
— Ricerche istochimiche sul veleno cutaneo degli Anfibi. Nota II. Boll. Soc. med.-chir. Pavia **48**, 600—605 (1934b).
— Le cellule cromaffini dei gangli nervosi degli irudinei. Atti Soc. ital. Sci. nat. **73**, 57—73 (1934c).
— La reazione cromaffine e alcune presunte localizzazioni adrenaliniche. Boll. Zool. **6**, 147—151 (1935).
— Il veleno granuloso degli Anfibi studiato al microscopio a fluorescenza. Monit. zool. ital. **48**, 237—243 (1937).
— Considerazioni sul significato istochimico della cromaffinità nel veleno cutaneo di rospo. Boll. Zool. **11**, 119—127 (1940).
— La reazione metacromatica nelle ghiandole granulose cutanee dei Bufonidi. Monit. zool. ital. **51**, 275—281 (1940a).
— Su alcuni caratteri di fissabilità dei granuli del veleno nelle ghiandole granulose cutanee di Rana esculenta. Boll. Soc. ital. Biol. sper. **21**, 307 (1946).
— Contributo alla conoscenza istochimica delle ghiandole salivari posteriori di Eledone moschata e di Octopus macropus. Boll. Soc. ital. Biol. sper. **22**, 107—108 (1946a).
— Su alcune reazioni istochimiche dei granuli del veleno nelle ghiandole granulose cutanee di Rana esculenta. Boll. Soc. ital. Biol. sper. **21**, 308 (1946b).
— Il ciclo di maturazione del veleno granuloso di Rana esculenta. Boll. Soc. ital. Biol. sper. **21**, 190—191 (1946c).
— Considerazioni morfologiche e biologiche sulle localizzazioni di enteramina. Rend. Ist. Lombardo Sci. Cl. Sci. **87**, 61—85 (1954).
— Contributo alla conoscenza delle ghiandole cutanee e dello strato cribroso di Bufo kisoloensis. Rend. Ist. Lombardo Sci. Cl. Sci. **88**, 243—249 (1955).
— Phénols, indols et le système cellulaire entèrochromaffine. 1st Internat. Congr. of Histochem. and Cytochem., Abstracts, p. 134, Paris 1960.
— Presenza di cellule enterocromaffini in Latimeria chalumnae. Riv. Istochim. norm. pat. **7**, 499—500 (1961).
— L'istochimica e i problemi biologici riguardanti la 5-idrossitriptamina (enteramina-serotonina). Riv. Anat. pat. **21**, 392—438 (1962).
— Classificazione delle tecniche istochimiche. Acta histochem. (Jena) **13**, 123—128 (1962a).
— Presenza di cellule enterocromaffini in Latimeria chalumnae. Monit. zool. ital. **70—71**, 313—319 (1962—1963).
— Phénols et indols et le système entèrochromaffine. In: R. WEGMANN, Hystochemistry and Cytochemistry, pp. 63—137. Oxford: Pergamon Press 1963.
— Considerazioni su alcuni problemi ancora aperti nello studio delle cellule enterocromaffini. Rend. Ist. Lombardo Sci. e Lett., Cl. Sci. (B), **97**, 267—290 (1963a).
— Histochemistry: Its general problems and its relationships to the other biological sciences. In: Handbuch der Histochemie (1964) (to be published).
—, e L. BOLOGNANI: Prime osservazioni sulla presenza di ATP nel veleno di rospo. Boll. Soc. ital. Biol. sper. **39**, 1291—1292 (1963).
—, e C. CASATI: La localizzazione istochimica della enteramina in Calliactis parasitica. Rend. Ist. Lombardo Sci. Cl. Sci. **92**, 329—335 (1958).
—, e G. CERIOTTI: Sulla presenza di cellule enterocromaffini nell'apparato urogenitale di "Lacerta muralis". Nota preventiva. Anat. Anz. 88, 387—392 (1939).
— — Sulla presenza di cellule enterocromaffini nell'epitelio vescicale di Rana esculenta. Monit. zool. ital. **51**, 29—36 (1939a).
—, e V. ERSPAMER: Cellule enterocromaffini e cellule basigranulose acidofile nei vertebrati (Ricerche istochimiche). Z. Zellforsch. **19**, 743—773 (1933).
— — Contributo alla conoscenza istochimica delle cellule enterocromaffini. Arch. ital. Anat. Embriol. **37**, 411—436 (1936).
— — Ricerche sul secreto delle cellule enterocromaffini. Nota I. Estratti alcoolici di mucosa gastrica e loro reazioni. Boll. Soc. med.-chir. Pavia **51**, 357—363 (1937).
— — Ricerche sul secreto delle cellule enterocromaffini. Nota II. Prove di controllo su estratti gastrici varii. Boll. Soc. med.-chir. Pavia **51**, 365—370 (1937a).
— — Ricerche sul secreto delle cellule enterocromaffini Nota. III. Comportamento della sostanza specifica delle enterocromaffini di fronte ad alcuni agenti precipitanti. Boll. Soc. med.-chir. Pavia **51**, 371—376 (1937b).

VIALLI, M., e V. ERSPAMER: Ricerche sul secreto delle cellule enterocromaffini. Nota IV. La sostanza specifica delle cellule enterocromaffini non può essere adrenalina. Boll. Soc. med.-chir. Pavia **51**, 377—383 (1937c).
— — Ricerche sul secreto delle cellule enterocromaffini. Nota V. Comportamento della sostanza specifica delle enterocromaffini di fronte ai solventi organici. Boll. Soc. med.-chir. Pavia **51**, 431—441 (1937d).
— — Ricerche sul secreto delle cellule enterocromaffini. Nota VI. Sulla azione biologica di estratti bruti di mucosa gastrica di coniglio. Boll. Soc. med.-chir. Pavia **51**, 443—450 (1937e).
— — Ricerche sul secreto delle cellule enterocromaffini. Nota VII. Osservazioni critiche su alcuni problemi inerenti alla istochimica delle enterocromaffini. Z. Zellforsch. **27**, 81—99 (1937f).
— — Ricerche sul secreto delle cellule enterocromaffini. Nota IX. Intorno alla natura chimica della sostanza specifica. Boll. Soc. med.-chir. Pavia **51**, 1111—1116 (1937g).
— — Ricerche sul secreto delle cellule enterocromaffini. Nota X. Nuovi dati sugli estratti gastrici di coniglio. Boll. Soc. med.-chir. Pavia **52**, 1167—1173 (1938).
— — Ricerche istochimiche sulla ghiandola salivare posteriore di "Octopus vulgaris". Mikrochemie **24**, 253—261 (1938a).
— — Ricerche sulla diazoreazione. Nota I. Introduzione, diazoreazione in ambiente acido, in ambiente alcalino e in ambiente alcalino con successiva acidificazione. Arch. Fisiol. **39**, 1—19 (1939).
— — Considerazioni sul sistema enterocromaffine (A proposito di una recente monografia di FEYRTER.) Z. Zellforsch. **29**, 487—501 (1939a).
— — Ricerche di caratterizzazione chimica delle sostanze fenoliche presenti negli estratti acetonici di ghiandole salivari posteriori di Octopus vulgaris. Arch. Fisiol. **40**, 293—312 (1940).
— — Sulle reazioni chimiche colorate dell'enteramina. I. Ricerche su estratti acetonici di mucosa gastro-intestinale. Arch. Sci. biol. (Bologna) **28**, 101—121 (1942).
—, e G. GERZELI: Primo contributo alle ricerche di microscopia interferenziale. Riv. Istochim. norm. pat. **1**, 503—518 (1955).
—, e F. GHIRINGHELLI: L'azione della benzochinolizina sulle cellule del sistema enterocromaffine. Riv. Istochim. norm. pat. **4**, 343 (1958).
— — Riduzione numerica delle cellule enterocromaffin nell'intestino di ratto per azione della benzochinolizina. Rend. Ist. Lombardo Sci., Cl. Sci. **92**, 511—514 (1958a).
— — Osservazioni sulle cellule enterocromaffini nell'intestino di ratti colchicinizzati. Arch. int. Pharmacodyn. **129**, 438—454 (1960).
—, e E. QUARONI: Osservazioni su una recente reazione proposta da Pearse per la enteramina. Riv. Istochim. norm. pat. **2**, 213—220 (1956).
— — Azione della reserpina sulle cellule enterocromaffini nel pollo. (Nota preventiva.) Riv. Istochim. norm. pat. **2**, 111—116 (1956a).
— — Azione della reserpina sulle cellule del sistema enterocromaffine in alcune specie di anfibi. Quad. Anat. Prat., Ser. XII, No 1—4, 153—158 (1957).
—, e G. TRAVERSO: Aspetti chimici della fissazione formolica e della reazione iodaffine nella istochimica di alcune sostanze indoliche. Rend. Ist. Lombardo Sci. e Lett. Cl. Sci. **94**, 167—184 (1960).
— — Applicazione in istochimica del blocco degli OH fenolici con diazometano. Riv. Istochim. norm. pat. **6**, 397—400 (1960a).
VOSS, H.: Beobachtungen über die Henlesche Chromreaktion an der Körnerdrüse des Frosches. Z. Anat. Entwickl.-Gesch. **89**, 445—452 (1929).
WALASZEK, E. J., and L. G. ABOOD: Fixation of 5-hydroxytryptamine by brain mitochondria. Fed. Proc. **16**, 133 (1957).
WELSH, J. H.: Hydroxytryptamine: a neurohormone in the invertebrates. Fed. Proc. **13**, 162—163 (1954).
— Papers in marine biology and oceanography. Deep-Sea Research **3**, Suppl., 287 (1955).
— Evidence for 5-HT granules in molluscan ganglia. Anat. Rec. **132**, 516 (1958).
—, and M. MOORHEAD: The quantitative distribution of 5-hydroxytriptamine in the invertebrates, especially in their nervous system. J. Neurochem. **6**, 146—169 (1960).
WIELAND, H., W. KONZ u. H. MITTASCH: Die Konstitution von Bufotenin und Bufotenidin. Über Kröten-Giftstoffe. VII. Justus Liebigs Ann. Chem. **513**, 1—25 (1934).
—, u. TH. WIELAND: Zur Kenntnis der Krötengiftstoffe. X. Die Konstitution des Bufothionins. Justus Liebigs Ann. Chem. **528**, 234—246 (1937).
WETZSTEIN, R., and W. DOERFLER: Elektronenmikroskopie enterochromaffiner Zellen. Anat. Anz., Erg.-Heft, **111**, 113—120 (1962).
— — u. A. SCHWINK: Die Feinstruktur der enterochromaffinen Zellen und ihrer spezifischen Granula. Protoplasma (Wien) **55**, 303—312 (1962).

WETZSTEIN, R., W. DOERFLER and A. SCHWINK: Electron-microscopy of enterochromaffin cells after release of 5-hydroxytryptamine by reserpine. German med. Res. **2**, 2 (1964).

YAMASAKI, M.: Mikroskopische Untersuchung über die tageszeitlichen Veränderungen am enterochromaffinen System der weißen Ratte. Arb. anat. Inst. Sendai **23**, 123—131 (1940).

ZANOTTI, L.: Applicazione di un istofotometro universale per assunzione di curve di fluorescenza e di assorbimento. Ann. Histochim., Suppl. **2**, 155—164 (1962).

ZBINDEN, G.: Biochemische, funktionelle und morphologische Organveränderungen durch Beeinflussung des 5-Hydroxytryptamin-Stoffwechsels. Ergebn. allg. Path. path. Anat. **39**, 225—259 (1960).

— A. PLETSCHER u. A. STUDER: Regionäre Unterschiede der Reserpinwirkung auf enterochromaffine Zellen und 5-Hydroxytryptamin-Gehalt im Magendarmtrakt. Schweiz. med. Wschr. **87**, 15—19 (1957).

— — — Hemmung der Reserpin-bedingten 5-Hydroxytryptamin-Freisetzung im enterochromaffinen System durch Isopropyl-Isonicotinsäurehydrazid. Klin. Wschr. **35**, 565—567 (1957a).

ZORZOLI, G. C., e R. D. LILLIE: Ricerche istochimiche sulle cellule enterocromaffini. Riv. Istochim. norm. pat. **2**, 283—294 (1956).

Chapter 2

Chemical analysis of indolealkylamines and related compounds

By

Arne Hanson

With 11 figures

Introduction

A close parallel between methodology and understanding has been recognized throughout modern scientific research, and is germane to the topics of indolealkylamines and related compounds. Although 5-hydroxytryptamine was first isolated from biological material by Erspamer in 1937, further developments in this field were sparse until the early 1950's, when more advanced analytical techniques were employed. Within the past ten years, isolation, identification, and quantitation of indole compounds has rapidly proliferated, and the metabolic pathways, physiological rôles, and pharmacological effects of these compounds have been increasingly understood. Of crucial importance to this progress has been the application of three analytical techniques: paper chromatography, spectrophotometry, and spectrophotofluorometry.

Indolealkylamines often have marked biological activity. Hence, determination of tissue concentration and excretion may involve measurements in the microgram range. The high sensitivity and narrow specificity of present methods permits examination of indole compounds under physiological circumstances, and recognition of derangements in indole metabolism.

In this review, physical and chemical methods, pertinent to analysis of indolealkylamines and related compounds in biological material will be presented. For practical reasons, emphasis is given to methods which have gained wide usage, or which are judged to have a potentially broad application.

Reviews which cover different aspects of indole analysis have been published by Erspamer (1954), Dalgliesh (1958), Udenfriend et al. (1958), Jepson (1960), Udenfriend (1962), Sandler (1963) and Udenfriend and Weissbach (1963).

A. Isolation and fractionation from biological material

If solid compounds are to be examined no problems of isolation arise; the material is dissolved in a suitable solvent and appropriate identification procedures started (see below). However, biochemical and pharmacological work on indoles mostly concern their occurrence, distribution or fate in animal tissues. Hence, they have to be isolated from tissue before any identification or assay studies can be made. Further, very often the compounds studied occur in tissues in such minute amounts that a concentration procedure must be included in the initial stages of investigation.

In the following section general procedures for the isolation and separation of indoles from biological material will be briefly described. For a thorough discussion of separation techniques, the reader is referred to MORRIS and MORRIS (1963).

I. Extraction procedures

1. Acetone extraction

Acetone has been the classical extraction solvent for indole analysis since it was introduced in 1940 by ERSPAMER for the extraction of 5-HT from tissues (see ERSPAMER 1954, ERSPAMER and BERTACCINI 1962). In the early investigations which led to the isolation of 5-HT as enteramine from mammalian gastrointestinal mucosa and salivary glands of octopods by ERSPAMER and coworkers in 1937 (see ERSPAMER 1954) and as serotonin from serum by RAPPORT and coworkers in 1948 (RAPPORT et al. 1948) acetone was extensively used in the extraction procedures.

Acetone extraction is carried out as follows (ERSPAMER 1955, 1956; ERSPAMER and BERTACCINI 1962):

Tissues. — Tissues are minced with scissors and extracted with 80 per cent aqueous acetone (4 ml of acetone per gram fresh tissues) for 24 hours. After decanting acetone, the tissues are reextracted with the same volume of acetone for another 24 hours. The combined acetone extracts, which can be kept indefinitely at low temperature, are evaporated in vacuo, or, if small volumes are used, by rapid evaporation in a boiling water bath under an air stream. The residue is then dissolved in water or other suitable solvent.

It has been found that 80 per cent acetone assures a complete extraction not only of 5-HT but also of 5-HTP and 5-HIAA (ERSPAMER and BERTACCINI 1962).

It should be stressed that homogenization of the tissues before extraction does not offer any advantages; on the contrary, it may be harmful to 5-HT when tissues rich in monoamine oxidase are analyzed.

Plasma and serum. Samples are treated with 4 volumes of acetone, left standing in a refrigerator overnight and then filtered or centrifuged. The precipitate is washed once with acetone, and the combined acetone extracts evaporated in vacuo and treated as above.

Urine. Urine is concentrated in vacuo, at 40—50^0, to a 1/20 of the original volume. 1 volume of 95 per cent ethanol and 4 volumes of acetone are then added with stirring. After standing in a refrigerator for 8—24 hours the precipitate formed is filtered off and the filtrate evaporated in vacuo. The residue is taken up in a mixture of 1 ml water + 3 ml ethanol + 25 ml acetone for every 100 ml of initial urine volume. The solution thus obtained is repeatedly evaporated to dryness, after being successively redissolved in the following solvents: a) 0.5 ml ethanol + 10 ml acetone; b) 0.25 ml ethanol + 20 ml acetone; c) 0.25 ml ethanol + 2—3 ml acetone + 5—10 ml ether. In each instance, the residue which is not soluble is discarded. Finally, the solute is dissolved in a mixture of ethanol and acetone, in which it is stable, in the cold, for months, and used for chromatographic separation of component indoles.

Recovery of most indolic acids is 95 per cent in the final filtrate. If ether insoluble compounds are anticipated in the starting material, ether should be omitted from the final precipitation mixture.

BUMPUS and PAGE (1955) also used acetone for the preparation of extracts of urine containing 5-HT, N-methyl-5-HT and bufotenine.

2. Butanol extraction

Butanol saturated with 0.1 N HCl is a useful solvent for the extraction of most indolic acids from biological material. Extraction may be performed using the original aqueous solution (e.g. urine or tissue homogenates), as the butanol is immiscible with water. However, it is necessary to adjust the solution to 0.1 N with respect to HCl before extraction with the acid butanol.

5-HT can also be extracted by acid butanol if salt is present in the solution (MEAD and FINGER 1961).

However, for the isolation of 5-HT the method of choice is the alkaline butanol extraction procedure introduced by UDENFRIEND et al. (1955b). Although this method has been somewhat modified in details in successive publications (Bogdanski et al. 1956, Udenfriend et al. 1958) in brief it is as follows: after acid homogenization of the tissues, followed by adjustment to pH 10, the 5-HT is extracted into n-butanol from a salt-saturated solution buffered with borate to pH 10. Saturation with salt facilitates the extraction of 5-HT into butanol. Washing of the butanol extract with salt-saturated borate buffer removes 5-HTP, TP and normally occurring blank impurities. The addition of heptane to the butanol lowers the polarity, so that 5-HT can be reextracted into dilute acid in which it can be assayed.

This method can, of course, also be used for other indolealkylamines. Bufotenine, which is much more soluble in organic solvents than 5-HT, can be completely extracted into butanol from an alkaline aqueous solution without salt saturation (Udenfriend et al. 1958).

A detailed description of the alkaline butanol extraction procedure is given on p. 99.

Quay (1962) has studied the differential extractions of diverse 5-hydroxy- and 5-methoxyindoles from tissues. By combination of alkaline butanol extraction and p-cymene and ether extractions 5-HT, N-acetyl-5-HT, 5-HTP, 5-HIAA, 5-methoxy IAA, and melatonin can be each selectively extracted.

3. Other solvent extractions

When indolic acids present in biological material (e.g. urine) are studied by paper chromatography they are preferably first isolated by extraction. As most of these acids are soluble in ether or ethyl acetate, a simple extraction with one of these solvents is made. Such an extract eliminates amino compounds and other non-ether soluble compounds which may subsequently interfere with analysis. Moreover, such an extract can be evaporated, yielding a solution ten to twenty times more concentrated and may thus reveal minor components as well as reduce the volume of solution to be applied to the chromatogram.

Armstrong et al. (1958), who studied the indolic acids of human urine, prepared an ethyl acetate extract of the urine preliminary to paper chromatography.

II. Chromatographic procedures

1. Adsorption chromatography

Adsorption chromatography on alumina has been used by several workers for the partial purification and separation of indole derivatives from biological material.

Bumpus and Page (1955) used a 2.3×21 cm alumina column (aluminium oxide, Merck, for chromatography) for the separation of 5-HT, N-methyl-5-HT and bufotenine from human urine. The column was initially prepared in benzene, then washed with benzene diluted with increasing quantities of methanol until a final washing was made with 100 ml of absolute methanol. Urine extracts prepared with acetone (see above) were then added to the column in 5 ml portions of methanol solution and eluted with methanol diluted with increasing amounts of water as follows:

95 ml of absolute methanol,
100 ml of 80% methanol,
100 ml of 60% methanol,
25 ml of 40% methanol,
25 ml of 20% methanol and
50 ml of water.

The eluates were collected in 5 ml fractions. After removal of the methanol at reduced pressure (50°) the indolealkylamines were identified and determined by chromatography and biological assay. Fig. 1 shows the distribution of the three indolealkylamines in such a fractionation.

A similar column was also used by McIsaac and Page (1959) for partial fractionation of metabolites of 5-HT in rats and rabbits.

The same adsorbent has been used by Erspamer and Bertaccini (1962) for a partial purification and separation of 5-HTP metabolites in rat urine. The urine was concentrated in vacuo (50°) to 5 ml and 100 ml of 96 per cent ethanol added. The turbid liquid was transferred to a 3.3×21 cm alumina column (alkaline alumina, Merck, for chromatography) and passed through it. Elution was carried out first with decreasing concentrations of ethanol, then with distilled water, and finally with 10 per cent acetic acid. The eluates were collected in single fractions of 100 ml each, and samples of the different fractions were examined by paper chromatography after suitable concentration.

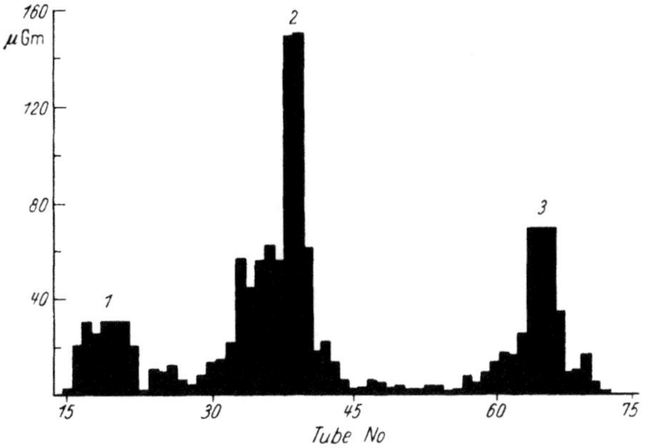

Fig. 1. Aluminium oxide chromatography of bufotenine (peak 1), N-methyl-5-HT (peak 2) and 5-HT (peak 3). From Bumpus and Page (1955).

2. Ion exchange chromatography

Ion exchange chromatography can greatly facilitate both isolation and fractionation of indoles occurring in biological material at extremely low concentrations.

Generally, indolealkylamines are taken up by a weak acid exchanger (e.g. Amberlite IRC-50 or Zeo-Karb 226) at pH 6—8, under which conditions the amines exist as cations. The amines are eluted either with acid, which suppresses the ionization of the exchanger, or with alkali, which suppresses the ionization of the amine.

In Table 1 are given some of the ion exchange resins which have been used for the isolation of indolealkylamines.

Table 1. *Some ion exchange resins used for the separation of indolealkylamines and related compounds*

Exchange resin	Indoles studied	Reference
Amberlite IRC-50 . .	5-HT	Dengler (1959), Oates (1961)
Amberlite XE-97 . .	5-HT	Gluckman and Abrams (1959)
Amberlite CG-50 . . .	5-HT and T	Davis and Awapara (1960), Cooper and Melcer (1962), McIlwain and Rodnight (1962)
Zeo-Karb 226	Indolealkylamines	Rodnight (1956), Blau (1961)
Dowex 1	5-HT and 5-HTP	Schanberg (1962)
Dowex 50	Phenolic amines (incl. 5-HT)	Kakimoto and Armstrong (1962)
Permutit	5-HT	Lovenberg et al. (1962)

RODNIGHT (1956) used columns containing 4 g of Zeo-Karb 226 (H form, 90—120 mesh). After repeated regeneration with 1 N H_2SO_4 and 1 N NaOH and washing with water, the resin was buffered with 0.5 M Na_2HPO_4-HCl buffer pH 6. A 75—120 ml sample of urine, adjusted to pH 6 and diluted to 250 ml with water was then run through the column. The resin was then washed with 125 ml de-gassed water, followed by 125 ml de-gassed 50 per cent ethanol. The indolealkylamines were then eluted with 350 ml of 0.02 N acetic acid in 75 per cent ethanol.

BLAU (1961) has used the same ion exchange resin for the separation of amines (including indolealkylamines) from biological material. However, here the resin was buffered at pH 7.3 and the amines were eluted with buffer pH 5.

MCILWAIN and RODNIGHT (1962) have described a similar method for the isolation of 5-HT and T from urine but use Amberlite CG-50 buffered at pH 6 with 0.5 M Na_2HPO_4—HCl. Columns (1 cm diameter) are loaded with 2 g (dry weight) of the resin which is regenerated with acid and buffered as described by RODNIGHT (1956) for Zeo-Karb 226, except that the alkaline washing is omitted. The diluted urine is allowed to run through the column at about 100 ml/hr. and the effluents discarded. The column is washed with 40 ml of water. The amines are eluted with 30 ml of 2 N H_2SO_4 after running through and discarding 4 ml of 2 N H_2SO_4. The flow rates for both stages of elution should not exceed 1 ml/min. The eluates are collected in centrifuge bottles and are made alkaline (pH 10—11) by gradual addition of 6 g of anhydrous Na_2CO_3. 60 mg of ascorbic acid and 60 ml of n-butanol-benzene (1:1) are added and the bottles are shaken and centrifuged. Of the upper phases 50 ml are transferred to bottles containing 30 ml of heptane and 5 ml of 2 N formic acid. The mixtures are shaken for a few minutes and centrifuged. The whole of the aqueous layer is removed and taken to dryness by freeze-drying or in vacuo evaporation. The residues are then dissolved in 80 per cent methanol and used for paper chromatography.

Another carboxylic acid resin suitable for the isolation of 5-HT and other indolealkylamines is Amberlite IRC-50. This resin was used by OATES (1961) for the determination of 5-HT in urine. A description of his method is given on p. 102.

DENGLER (1959) also used Amberlite IRC-50 for the isolation and separation of 5-HT and 5-HIAA from carcinoid tumour tissues. The tumour tissues are homogenized with 5 per cent perchloric acid. The homogenate centrifuged and the supernatant adjusted to pH 6 with KOH. The precipitate of perchlorate is removed by filtration and the filtrate run through an Amberlite IRC-50 column equilibrated with 1 M acetate buffer pH 6.5. 5-HIAA passes through the column and is determined in the effluent. 5-HT is eluted with dilute H_2SO_4.

The carboxylic acid resins may be most useful in the separation of substrate and reaction product in studies involving the 5-HTP decarboxylase. 5-HTP and 5-HT present in the incubation mixtures can be easily separated on resins such as Amberlite CG-50 (DAVIS and AWAPARA 1960).

Indolealkylamines like 5-HT and T can also be separated from their corresponding amino acids by cation exchange absorption on Permutit. LOVENBERG et al. (1962) in their studies on the L-amino acid decarboxylase applied a Permutis method originally described by DIETRICH (1953). Aliquots of the incubateq (pH 9) were diluted to 5 ml with water. After centrifugation the supernatant solution was passed through a 0.5×3 cm Permutit column. The column was washed with 20 ml of boiling water to remove the amino acid, and the amine was then eluted with 3 ml of 20 per cent NaCl. The recovery of added amine in the salt eluate ranged between 90 to 100 per cent.

In the concentration and purification of phenolic amines of human urine, KAKIMOTO and ARMSTRONG (1962) used the strong acid cation exchanger Dowex 50.

3. Paper chromatography

Paper chromatography, which will be discussed here primarily as a method of identification, may, however, be most useful as a method for isolation and separation of small amounts of indole compounds.

Chromatograms employed primarily for identification may be contrasted with those used to achieve isolation of a given substance. In the former, minute volumes are applied as a small, discreet spot; in the latter, thick papers, heavily overloaded with starting material are used.

For isolation one-way chromatograms are frequently used and the solution is applied as a large streak parallel to the origin line. When thick papers, such as Whatman 31 or 3 MM, are used, up to 0.2 ml of solution may be applied and after drying the paper, application of the same volume may be repeated several times prior to the chromatographic run. Thus, relatively large volumes may be conveniently chromatographed. The papers are then chromatographed in the usual way and the components separate in horizontal bands. After drying, the indole compounds are located using suitable reagents. Physical methods (e.g. ultraviolet fluorescence) are preferable but a guide-strip (1—2 cm wide) may also be cut from one side of the paper, in the direction of the solvent flow, and treated with the location reagent to find the position of the compound. This strip is then realigned with the untreated paper. The material is eluted from the paper by cutting it into small pieces and extracting with solvent.

With the above technique it may be possible to isolate indole compounds in amounts up to the milligram level. For further technical details, the reader is referred to BLOCK et al. (1958), HAIS and MACEK (1958), LINSKENS (1959) and SMITH (1960).

Larger amounts of material can be isolated by use of column procedures. It is often found that columns of cellulose powders will allow separations similar to those obtained on paper if the same solvents are employed. A preliminary paper chromatographic analysis may thus be useful to guide a later large scale separation on a cellulose powder column.

ERSPAMER and NOBILI (1962a) have isolated metabolites of 4-HTP on a cellulose powder column. Eluates from an alumina column (see p. 69) were concentrated and chromatographed on a column of Whatman 1 cellulose powder using the ascending technique and a solvent of n-butanol-acetic acid-water (4:1:5). The column was prepared in a glass tube formed by two adherent hemi-cylinders which could be opened longitudinally. The tube was positioned upright, exactly as if it were a paper sheet and placed into a chromatographic cabinet with the solvent at the bottom. After a convenient run, the tube was taken out. To locate the desired compounds, the column was opened longitudinally, paper strips were pressed gently on to the column surface, and then removed and sprayed with NNCD reagent (see p. 87). From the location of the coloured spots on the paper, the column segment containing the desired material could be accurately identified and subsequently eluted. This technique exactly parallels the "guide-strip" method as described above.

4. Molecular sieving (gel filtration)

Cross-linked dextran gels have recently been developed for molecular sieving. Solutes vary greatly in their ability to penetrate the pores of such gels and the extent of their penetration reflects primarily the molecular size of the solute.

Different grades of dextran gels (designated Sephadex G-25, G-50, G-75, G-100 and G-200) are commercially available. Sephadex G-25 will completely exclude neutral compounds with a molecular weights greater than 3500—4500. The process of separating molecules of different size by passage through a column of a dextran gel is termed *gel filtration* (for technical details, see FLODIN and PORATH 1961, BOARDMAN 1962, MORRIS and MORRIS 1963). The chromatographic behaviour of small molecules on Sephadex G-25 has been thoroughly investigated by GELOTTE (1960) and his paper should be consulated for details. Substances of similar size may also show a difference in migration rates, because dextran gels are not completely devoid of sorption and ion exchange effects.

Table 2. *Separation of indole compounds on Sephadex G-25.* (SCHLOSSBERGER et al. 1963)

Compound	Fraction number
Urea	16—26
Citrulline	18—24
Indican	26—30
Tryptophan	28—39
Tryptamine	34—50
Indoleacetic acid	40—45
5-Hydroxytryptophan	39—48
5-Hydroxytryptamine	46—66
5-Hydroxyindoleacetic acid	42—60
5,6-Dihydroxytryptophan	36—46
5,6-Dihydroxytryptamine	44—52
5,6-Dihydroxyindoleacetic acid	44—50

SCHLOSSBERGER et al. (1963) have used gel filtration with Sephadex G-25 for the separation of indole derivatives from urine. A 10 ml sample of the urine is first concentrated to 2 ml by evaporation. An 0.8 ml aliquot of the centrifuged concentrate is applied to a 1.4×20 cm Sephadex G-25 column which has been equilibrated with 0.5 per cent ascorbic acid solution to prevent oxidation of the unstable 5,6-dihydroxyindoles. The elution of the indoles is also made with 0.5 per cent ascorbic acid solution and the eluates collected in 1 ml fractions. The indoles are then identified in the eluates by means of thin layer chromatography (adsorbent: cellulose powder; solvent: butanol-acetic acid-water, 12:3:5; spray reagent: p-dimethylaminocinnam aldehyde).

Table 2 shows the distribution of a number of indole derivatives on Sephadex G-25.

III. Paper electrophoresis

Paper electrophoresis will be discussed here mainly as an identification method. However, it may be used as an isolation and separation procedure in the same way as described above for paper chromatography. Most paper electrophoretic techniques lend themselves to the separation of quantities up to a few hundred milligrams, by employing either a stack of filter paper or a single thick paper strip. For further details, see LEDERER (1955).

B. Identification

I. Ultraviolet absorbancy

The absorption spectra of 5-hydroxyindoles in neutral and acid solution show a maximum in the ultraviolet at 275 mμ with a subsidiary peak at 295 mμ. In alkali, the subsidiary peak is shifted to 325 mμ (Fig. 2). The molecular extinction of 5-HT in acid at 275 mμ is 5.3×10^3 (UDENFRIEND et al. 1958).

The introduction of a second hydroxy group at position 6 of the indole ring results in a reversal of the magnitude of the peaks described above. For 5,6-dihydroxytryptophan in neutral solution, the larger peak is at 295 mμ, while the subsidiary peak is at 265—270 mμ (SCHLOSSBERGER and KUCH 1963, see Fig. 3).

Simple indoles which are not substituted in the ring show an absorption maximum at 280 mμ with a small subsidiary peak at 288 mμ in both acid and alkaline solutions (Fig. 4). This lack of acid-base shift of ultraviolet absorption maxima seen in simple indoles is also found in compounds which have their ring hydroxyls blocked by methylation (e.g. melatonin and 5-methoxy-IAA), see Fig. 5.

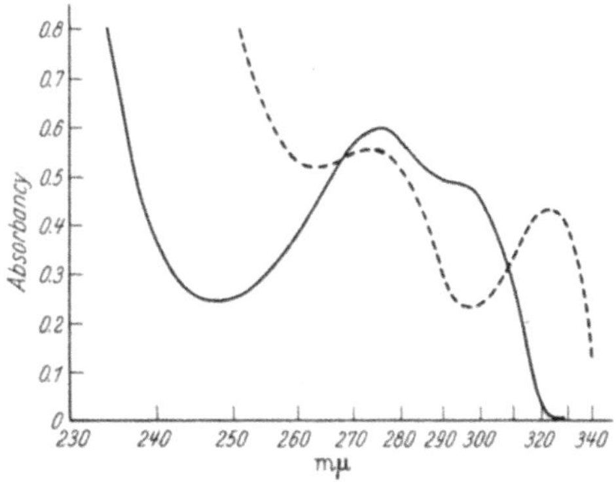

Fig. 2

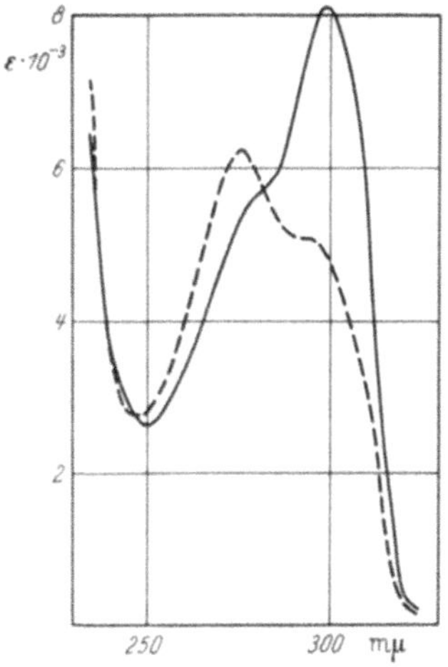

Fig. 3

Fig. 2. Spectral absorbancy curves of 5-HT (0.1 μM per ml) in 0.1 N HCl (———) and in 0.1 N NaOH (— — — —)

Fig. 3. Ultraviolet absorption spectra of DL-5-HTP (— — — —) and DL-5,6-dihydroxy-TP (———) in water (SCHLOSSBERGER and KUCH, 1963)

Measurement of absorption in acid at 275—280 mμ is the simplest procedure for the determination of indoles. However, the low sensitivity and lack of specificity make it inapplicable to studies of endogenous indoles in biological samples.

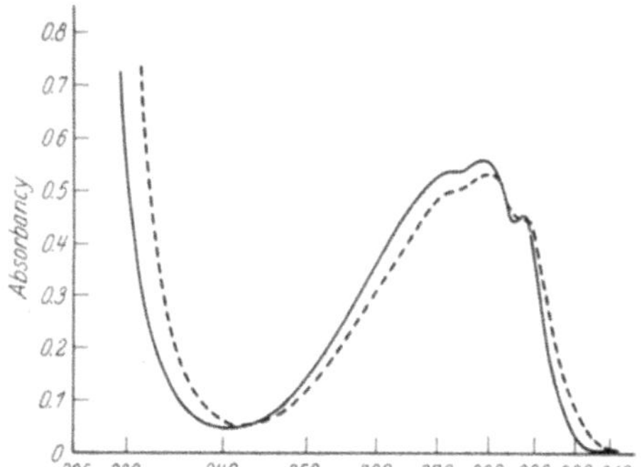

Fig. 4

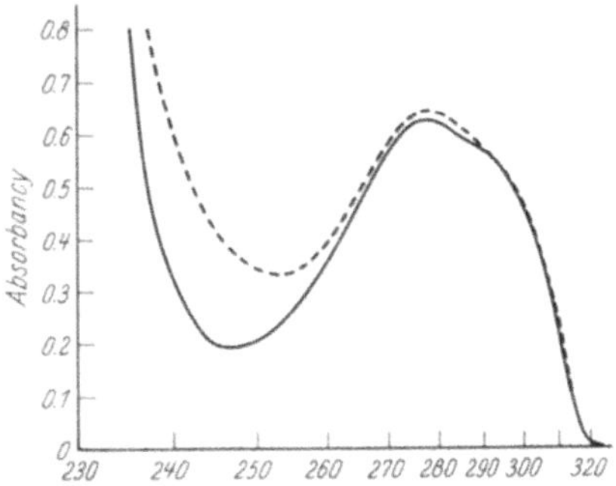

Fig. 5

Fig. 4. Spectral absorbancy curves of T (0.1 μM per ml) in 0.1 N HCl (———) and in 0.1 N NaOH (— — — —)

Fig. 5. Spectral absorbancy curves of melatonin (0.1 μM per ml) in 0.1 N HCl (———) and in 0.1 N NaOH (— — — —)

It has been successfully applied, however, to the measurement of enzymatic formation and destruction of 5-HT in tissue preparations (UDENFRIEND et al. 1955b, DAVIS and AWAPARA 1960). The amount of 5-HT in such experiments is large and the blank is minimal, because a comparatively small amount of tissue is taken through the extraction procedure.

II. Fluorescence

Many of the biologically occurring indoles exhibit a very intense fluorescence which make them readily detectable in minute amounts in extracts and on chromatograms.

Indoles which are not substituted in the ring (e.g. TP, T and IAA) fluoresce in weak acid or neutral solutions at 350 mμ, when activated at 275 mμ, and 5-hydroxyindoles (5-HTP, 5-HT and 5-HIAA) emit a maximum fluorescence at 350 mμ, when activated at 295 mμ (Bowman et al. 1955).

In strong acid (3 N HCl) 5-hydroxy- and 5-methoxyindoles fluoresce at 550 mμ and this fluorescence is also maximally activated at 295 mμ. This shift of fluorescence, from the ultraviolet to the visible, with increasing acidity, is completely reversible and is not accompanied by a noticable change in the absorption spectrum. No corresponding shift in fluorescence is observed with the simple indoles. In fact, these compounds loose their fluorescence in 3 N HCl. The fluorescence shift in strong acid is a function of the phenolic group and distinguishes 5-hydroxy- and 5-methoxy-indoles from other indoles (Udenfriend et al. 1955a, Quay 1963).

Fluorescence assay permits better discrimination among indole compounds than do spectrophotometric and colorimetric methods. All 5-hydroxyindoles have exactly the same colour with several reagents, e.g. 1-nitroso-2-naphtol. In neutral or weak acid solutions they are all activated to fluoresce by ultraviolet light of the same wavelength (295 mμ) and emit the same fluorescence at 350 mμ. However, each compound has its own optimal pH for maximal fluorescence. Thus, it becomes possible to distinguish between various 5-hydroxyindole derivatives by selecting the proper pH in which to make the fluorescence measurements.

In addition to their native fluorescence, several indole compounds give highly fluorescent reaction products when treated with certain reagents. Indoleethylamine derivatives (e.g. T) condense with formaldehyde to the nonfluorescent tetrahydronorharman which on dehydrogenation with hydrogen peroxide forms the highly fluorescent norharman, 3-carboline (Hess and Udenfriend 1959).

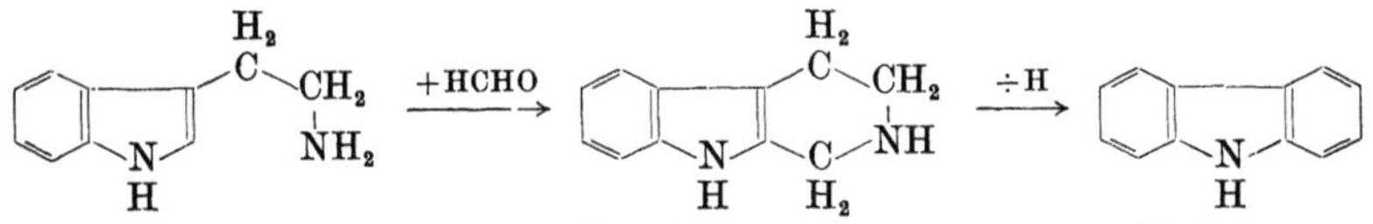

This reaction is used in a very sensitive method for the determination of T in tissues (see p. 95).

Another reaction also based on the formation of a carboline derivative is that described by Jepson and Stevens (1953) for the detection of certain tryptamines on paper chromatograms. When 5-HT and other primary indole-alkylamines are treated on paper chromatograms with ninhydrin in acetic acid they yield 3,4-dihydro-3-carbolines (Jepson 1960). These derivatives show an intense greenish-blue fluorescence in ultraviolet light, detectable at levels as low as 0.01 μg per cm^2 paper. However, here the fluorescence only occurs when the 3,4-dihydro-3-carbolines are adsorbed on paper (see p. 88).

Procházka (1953) has developed a fluorescence reaction for the detection of indole compounds on paper chromatograms . When the latter are sprayed with a mixture of formaldehyde and hydrochloric acid most indoles substituted at position 3 show orange to brown colours with characteristic yellow or orange fluorescence (see p. 88). The substituted group must be separated from the ring system by a methylene group.

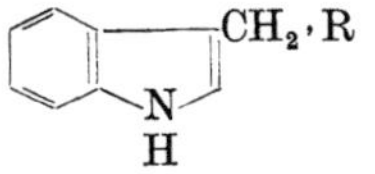

However, derivatives where R is a OH-, indolyl- or dimethylamine group only show red to violet colours.

A similar reaction has been described by SHEPHERD et al. (1953) who use formaldehyde and potassium dichromate. When treated on chromatograms with this reagent, 5-HT, bufotenin and bufotenidin produce a golden-yellow fluorescence in amounts as small as 0.2 μg (see p. 89).

Although histochemical methods will not be treated in this review, mention must be made here of the highly sensitive fluorescence methods for histochemical detection of catecholamines and 5-HT at the cellular level, as developed by FALCK and coworkers (see FALCK 1962). The technique used in these methods is briefly as follows: Pieces of the tissues to be studied are frozen in propane cooled by liquid nitrogen and dried in vacuo at —35°. After thorough drying the pieces are treated with formaldehyde gas at +80° in a closed glass vessel containing paraformaldehyde. During this treatment 5-HT condenses with formaldehyde yielding a product with intense yellow fluorescence, which is not extracted with hot paraffin or xylene. The preparations are then inbedded in vacuo with paraffin and sectioned. The sections (8—10 μ) are placed on nonfluorescent slides and mounted. The details of the technique and the equipment used for fluorescence microscopy are described by FALCK (1962). Results obtained with this technique have shown that it has a sensitivity much greater than that of hitherto available histochemical methods for 5-HT. This is well illustrated by the following findings: The 5-HT in normal rat mast cells, which has hitherto been beyond the reach of histochemical detection, gives a very strong fluorescence, and single granules from disrupted cells are readily seen. Further, the 5-HT in blood platelets shows a distinct fluorescence when the content exceeds about 100 μg per ml.

TP and T form the highly fluorescent tryptochrome when oxidized in acetic acid with iodate (FEARON and BOGGUST 1950):

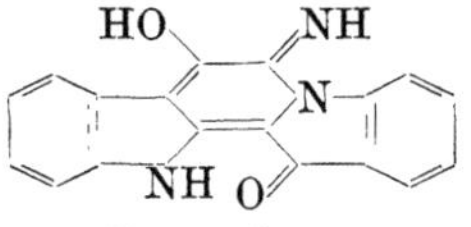

Tryptochrome

As a fluorescent test for TP and T the sensitivity of the tryptochrome reaction is about 1 in 10^6. EGELHAAF (1957) has reported a very sensitive chromatographic method for TP in which the tryptochrome is measured fluorometrically.

HOLMSTEDT and LUNDGREN (1964) have found that solutions of psilocin (N,N-dimethyl-4-hydroxytryptamine) turn yellow at pH 12 and fluoresce at 500 mμ, when activated at 370 mμ. Psilocybin (N,N-dimethyl-4-phosphoryltryptamine) does not show any fluorescence at this pH.

The development of spectrophotofluorometers capable of delivering high-intensity monochromatic activation at all wave lengths from 240 to 800 mμ, and concomitant availability of automatic spectral analysis of resulting fluorescence throughout the same range have brought extreme sensitivity into fluorometric methodology (UDENFRIEND 1962). In many cases these methods, which allow the detection of indoles in amounts far below the microgram level, offer distinct advantages over other physical and chemical methods.

Table 3. *Fluorescence characteristics of some biologically important indoles*

Compound	Medium	Activation mμ	Fluorescence mμ	Reference
Tryptophan derivatives:				
Tryptophan	pH 2—11	275	360	1, 3
Tryptophan	as norharman	365	440	5
Tryptamine	pH 2—11	275	360	1, 3
Tryptamine	as norharman	365	440	5
Indoleacetic acid	pH 2—11	275	360	1, 3
4-Hydroxytryptophan derivatives:				
4-Hydroxytryptamine	pH 7	none	none	13
4-Hydroxytryptamine	3 N HCl	none	none	13
N,N-Dimethyl-4-hydroxytryptamine (psilocin)	pH 12	370	500	14
N,N-Dimethyl-4-phosphoryltryptamine (psilocybin)	pH 12	none	none	14
5-Hydroxytryptophan derivatives:				
5-Hydroxytryptophan	pH 2—11	295	330	1, 3
5-Hydroxytryptophan	3 N HCl	295	550	2
5-Hydroxytryptamine	pH 2—11	295	330	1, 3
5-Hydroxytryptamine	3 N HCl	295	550	2
N,N-Dimethyl-5-hydroxytryptamine (bufotenine)	3 N HCl	295	550	4
N-Acetyl-5-hydroxytryptamine	3 N HCl	295	550	4
5-Methoxytryptamine	3 N HCl	295	550	4
N-Acetyl-5-methoxytryptamine (melatonin)	pH 7	290	360	6
N-Acetyl-5-methoxytryptamine (melatonin)		304	333, 338	12
N-Acetyl-5-methoxytryptamine (melatonin)	3 N HCl	300	540	4,6
5-Hydroxyindoleacetic acid	pH 2—11	295	330	1.3
5-Hydroxyindoleacetic acid	3 N HCl	295	550	2
5-Methoxyindoleacetic acid	3 N HCl	295	550	4
5-Methoxyindoleacetic acid		304	338	11
6-Hydroxytryptophan derivatives:				
6-Hydroxytryptamine	pH 7	290	365	13
6-Hydroxytryptamine	3 N HCl	none	none	13
6-Hydroxyindoleacetic acid	pH 7	290	365	13
7-Hydroxytryptophan derivatives:				
7-Hydroxytryptamine	pH 7	none	none	13
7-Hydroxytryptamine	3 N HCl	none	none	13
7-Hydroxyindoleacetic acid	pH 7	none	none	13
Other indole compounds:				
Indole	pH 2—11	275	360	1, 3
5-Hydroxyindole	pH 1	290	355	7
Lysergic acid diethylamide (LSD)	pH 7	325	465	8, 9
Lysergic acid diethylamide (LSD)	pH 9	315	440	1
2-Brom-lysergic acid diethylamide (Brom-LSD)	pH 1	315	460	7, 8
Harmine	pH 1	330, 365	400	7, 8
Reserpine	pH 1	300	375	7, 8
Reserpine	selenious acid oxid.	365	420	10

References to Table 3. [1] BOWMAN et al. (1955). — [2] UDENFRIEND et al. (1955). — [3] SPRINCE et al. (1957). — [4] QUAY (1963). — [5] HESS and UDENFRIEND (1959). — [6] AXELROD and WEISSBACH (1961). — [7] Data sheet to Aminco bulletin, No. 2278. — [8] UDENFRIEND et al. (1957). — [9] AXELROD et al. (1957). — [10] HESS et al (1956). — [11] LERNER et al. (1959a). — [12] LERNER et al. (1959b). — [13] JEPSON et al. (1962). — [14] HOLMSTEDT and LUNDGREN (1964).

Fluorescence characteristics of biologically important indoles and some other related compounds are given in Table 3. For the instrumentation and general principles of spectrophotofluorometric analysis the reader is referred to the monograph of UDENFRIEND (1962).

III. Colour reactions

The literature pertinent to colour reactions of indole compounds is voluminous, and will not be extensively reviewed here. Only methods which confer particular advantage in terms of either specificity or sensitivity will be described.

1. Aldehyde reactions

Most indoles condense with aromatic aldehydes to form coloured derivatives. The oldest reaction of this type — introduced by Ehrlich already in 1901 — is that involving p-dimethylaminobenzaldehyde.

The aldehydes react with the indoles at the free 2- or 3-position. As most biologically important indoles are already substituted at their 3-position the condensation consequently takes place at the 2-position, i.e.

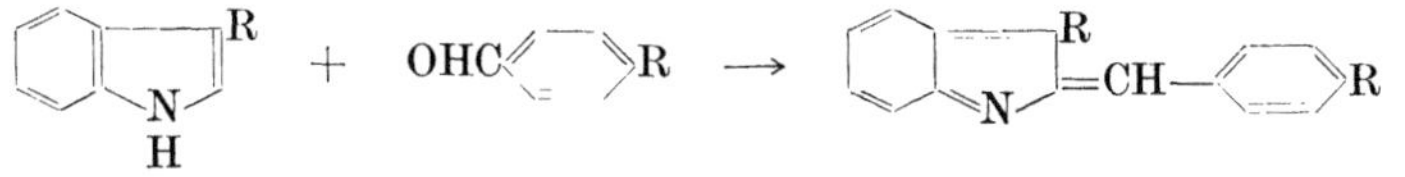

Indole Derivative Aromatic Aldehyde Coloured Reaction Product

Other aldehydes often used for the detection and quantitative determination of biologically important indole compounds are p-dimethylaminocinnamaldehyde and cinnamaldehyde.

a) p-Dimethylaminobenzaldehyde

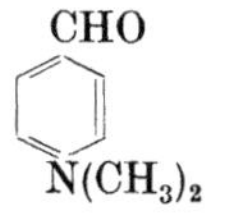

p-Dimethylaminobenzaldehyde in acid solution — often called Ehrlich's reagent — is the most useful of the general tests for indoles and has been widely used for both the detection and quantitation of biologically important indole compounds. It reacts with a wide range of indoles, and shows significant variations in colour development which are useful in the identification of a specific compound concerned.

Simple compounds like TP and its derivatives (e.g. T and IAA) show some shade of purple. Substitution of OH- or OR- at position 5 shifts the colour towards blue. Substitution at position 6 changes it to blue-green.

The p-dimethylaminobenzaldehyde reaction is not absolutely specific for the indole nucleus, but a blue colour developing rapidly in the cold is a very good indication of an indole. Purple colours are, however, more dubious and cannot *per se* be attributed to indoles as certain non-indoles give similar colours. Among such naturally occurring compounds should be mentioned simple pyrroles like porphobilinogen, pyrrol-2-carboxylic acid (from mucoproteins) and 2-methyl-pyrrol (from hexosamine).

b) p-Dimethylaminocinnamaldehyde

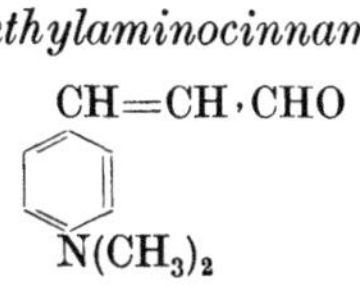

Strell and Kalojanoff (1954) suggested the use of vinyl homologues of p-dimethylaminobenzaldehyde for the detection of pyrroles. These compounds also react with indoles to form intensively coloured products.

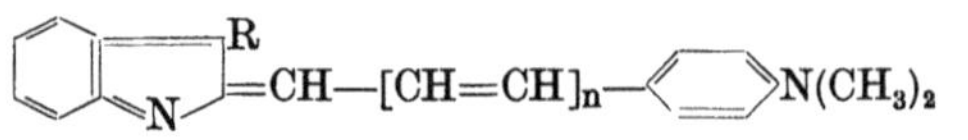

p-Dimethylaminocinnamaldehyde was used by HARLEY-MASON and ARCHER (1958) for the detection of indoles and reported to be preferable to p-dimethylaminobenzaldehyde in paper chromatography. It is, in fact, in most cases about ten times more sensitive than the p-dimethylaminobenzaldehyde reagent. Its selectivity is, however, low and the background colour may be troublesome (JEPSON 1960). Certain indoles which do not react with p-dimethylaminobenzaldehyde (e.g. β:β-dimethyltryptamine) can, however, be detected with this reagent.

c) Cinnamaldehyde

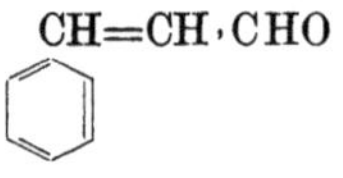

Cinnamaldehyde reacts in acid solution with indoles in the same way as the other aromatic aldehydes already described. However, the reaction products formed are differently coloured. While the products formed with p-dimethylaminobenzaldehyde and its vinylogue are mostly purple or blue, those formed with cinnamaldehyde are red to brown.

The cinnamaldehyde reaction has been used most frequently for the detection of indoles in paper chromatography and paper electrophoresis (MÜLLER 1953).

2. Xanthydrol reaction

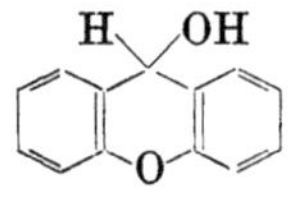

Indole compounds react with xanthydrol in acid solution to form highly coloured acid-stable products (DICKMAN and WESCOTT 1954; DICKMAN and CROCKETT 1956). In the presence of excess xanthydrol the formation of xanthydrylindoles is directly related to the concentration of indole compound in the solution.

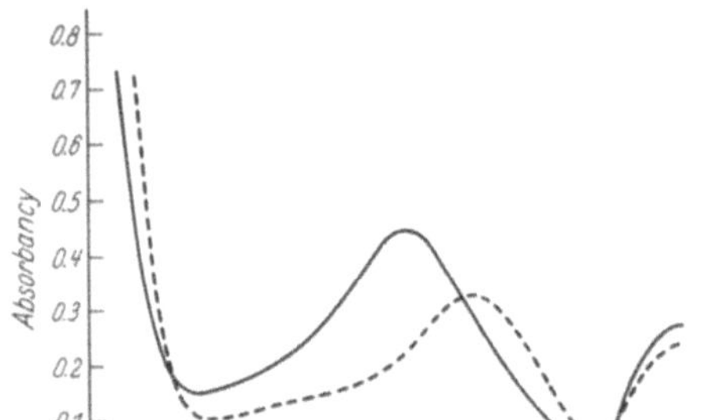

Fig. 6. Spectral absorbancy curves of xanthydryl-T (———) and xanthydryl-5-HT (— — — —). 0.5 μM of the compound in 5 ml of water was treated with 1 mg of xanthydrol in 5 ml of 6N HCl for 15 minutes at 100° and the solution extracted twice with benzene before absorbancy was measured

The xanthydryls formed with simple indoles such as TP, T and IAA show an absorption peak at 510 mμ. A hydroxy group in position 5 shifts this peak to 557 mμ (Fig. 6).

Briefly, a sample to be analyzed should contain 0.1 to 0.5 μM of the indole compound in a maximal volume of 5 ml; it is added to a mixture of 1 ml of xanthydrol (1 mg per ml) in concentrated HCl and 4 ml of concentrated HCl. This solution is then diluted to 10 ml with H_2O and the tube heated in a boiling water bath for 15 minutes. After cooling it is extracted three times with wet benzene, and the excess benzene is evaporated from the aqueous phase with a stream of air. The solution is finally diluted to volume with 6 N HCl. The content of indole compound can be calculated from the absorbancy of the solution at 510 mμ form a calibration curve.

Detailed procedures for the quantitative determination of TP and 5-HT have been reported by DICKMAN and CROCKETT (1956).

3. 1-Nitroso-2-naphtol reaction

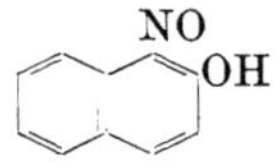

This reagent, which was originally introduced by GERNGROSS et al. (1933) for the detection of p-substituted phenols (tyrosin and tyramine) reacts almost exclusively with 5-hydroxyindoles to form coloured derivatives under certain conditions (UDENFRIEND et al. 1955b).

In dilute HCl or H_2SO_4, containing traces of nitrite, 5-hydroxyindoles react to give a violet-purple chromophore, the structure of which is as yet unknown. Tyramine and tyrosin react with 1-nitroso-2-naphtol only in the presence of strong nitric acid. TP, T, 7-HTP and 7-HT do not react at all, and of twenty phenolic compounds reported by UDENFRIEND et al. (1955b) only p-hydroxy-acetanilide gave a positive colour reaction. However, recently other compounds — mostly urinary metabolites of ingested drugs — have been found to give a colour similar to that given by 5-hydroxyindoles (see p. 105).

Colorimetric methods based on the 1-nitroso-2-naphtol reaction have been used for analyses of the following indoles: 5-HIAA acid in urine; 5-HT in carcinoid tumours; enzymatic experiments involving 5-HTP and 5-HT. These methods have about the same sensitivity as the ultraviolet absorption technique, but are preferable when tissue extracts contain large amounts of ultraviolet-absorbing material.

The following procedure can be employed for the detection and determination of all the 5-hydroxyindoles after they have been separately isolated (UDENFRIEND and WEISSBACH 1963).

To 2 ml of an acid extract containing 0.03 to 0.8 uM of 5-hydroxyindole in a glass-stoppered shaking tube are added 1 ml of 1-nitroso-2-naphtol reagent (0.1% in 95% ethanol). After thorough mixing, 1 ml of nitrous acid reagent (freshly prepared mixture of 5 ml 2 N H_2SO_4 or HCl and 0.2 ml 2.5% $NaNO_2$) is added. The tube is stoppered, shaken again, and allowed to stand at room temperature for 10 minutes. 10 ml of ethylene dichloride are then added, and the tube is shaken for a sufficient time to extract all excess 1-nitroso-2-naphtol. After low speed centrifugation the aqueous layer is transferred to a cuvette, and the optical density of the stable purple chromophore measured at 540 mμ in a spectrophotometer.

4. Diazo reactions

Phenolic compounds, including 4-, 5- and 6-hydroxyindoles, react with diazonium salts (diazo coupling) to give azo dyes which are strongly coloured. These reactions are very sensitive and often allow the detection of hydroxyindoles below the microgram level. In non-hydroxylated, and in such compounds where the phenolic group is blocked by ether or ester formation little colour occurs with simple diazonium salts. However, certain complex diazonium salts give colours with indole acids and indolealkylamines and these salts may be useful for identification.

The diazonium compounds which give the most satisfactory results in indole analysis are the following:

a) Benzenesulphonic acid diazonium chloride, diazotized sulphanilic acid, VAN DEN BERGH'S or PAULY'S reagent

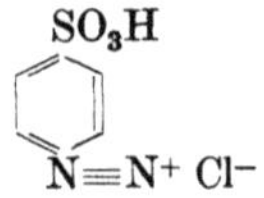

b) p-Nitrobenzenediazonium chloride, diazotized p-nitroaniline

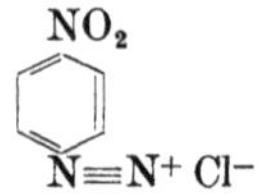

c) p-Nitrobenzenediazonium tetrafluoroborate

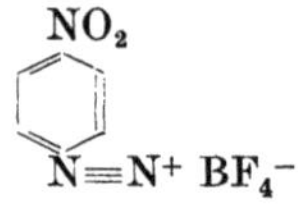

d) 2-Chloro-4-nitrobenzenediazonium naphtalene-2-sulphonate, NNCD reagent

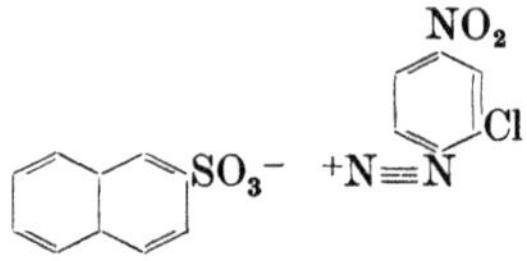

Unfortunately, most solid diazonium salts are explosive. Even small quantities of these compounds may explode violently on mechanical shock and cause accidents; hence they are rarely prepared in the dry state. The first two of the diazonium salts mentioned above are such compounds and are therefore mostly prepared in aquoeus solutions. These solutions are not stable and must be prepared fresh before use.

Diazonium salts form complexes with many metallic salts, of which one of the most important is the fluoroborate, $(Ar \cdot N_2)^+BF_4^-$. These complex salts can be prepared in the dry state and handled with relative safety. They are also stable in solution and hence offer a means of stabilizing a diazonium salt solution. One such compound is p-nitrobenzediazonium tetrafluoroborate. Aqueous solutions of this compound are stable even at room temperature. The solid reagent is easily prepared (CHERONIS and ENTRIKIN 1957) and is also commercially available[1]. It is a very effective reagent for the detection of certain indoles and may be useful in the differentiation of hydroxylated and non-hydroxylated compounds (see p. 87).

Another stabilized and safe diazonium compound is 2-chloro-4-nitrobenzenediazonium naphtalene-2-sulphonate (NNCD reagent), which is also commercially available in solid form[2]. This compound was introduced by HEINRICH and SCHULER (1948) for the determination of dihydroxyphenols and has been extensively used for the detection of indoles in paper chromatography (ERSPAMER and BORETTI 1951, ERSPAMER 1954, 1955; see p. 87). Not only phenolic indoles, but also IAA and T react with this reagent.

With phenolic compounds, diazo coupling is best performed in slightly alkaline solution (alkaline coupling). However, with certain diazonium salts, a coupling occurs also in acid solution (acid coupling). The extent of coupling and the resulting colour vary considerably — as a function of pH. When diazo reactions are used for analytical purposes both acid and alkaline coupling should be used, as the colours obtained very often show marked differences which may be characteristic of a given compound.

[1] Eastman Organic Chemicals, Rochester, U.S.A.
[2] Hopkin & Williams Ltd. Chadwell Heath, Essex, England.

In indole analysis the diazo reactions are almost exclusively used after separation by paper chromatography. Chromatograms are first sprayed with the acid diazonium salt, and examined for the appearance of colour. Then, an alkaline pH is obtained by spraying with sodium carbonate, and again the appearance of colours is noted (see p. 87).

6-Hydroxy- and 6-alkoxyindoles with a free 2-position react immediately with diazotized sulphanic acid or p-nitroaniline in strong acid to give brillant red colours (JEPSON et al. 1962). Indoles hydroxylated at positions 4, 5 or 7 only give slowly forming brownish-purple or yellow colours. The sensitivity of the reaction with diazotized sulphanilic acid in strong acid is several times as great for 6-hydroxyindoles as for 7-hydroxyindoles. The absorption spectra of the coloured products from 6-HT and 6-HIAA have peaks at 525 mμ and 510 mμ, respectively. The colour obtained with 7-HT and 7-HIAA show a broader maximum at 555 mμ, with an absorbancy only 0.3 that of 6-HT at their respective maxima. JEPSON et al. (1962) have used this reaction with diazotized sulphanilic acid for the quantitative determination of 6-hydroxyindoles.

IV. Countercurrent distribution

Countercurrent distribution is a separation process, based directly on the principle that a pure solute, when shaken with two immiscible solvents in which it is soluble, will distribute itself between the two liquid layers according to a certain characteristic preference. The preference at a given concentration level and temperature is a constant determined by the Nernst distribution law.

Countercurrent distribution is used mostly for the separation of organic substances, and offers certain advantages in the isolation of biological products: it avoids extremes of temperature; it is applicable both on a preparative scale and at micro levels. Several excellent reviews of countercurrent distribution are available, e.g. HECKER (1955), CRAIG and CRAIG (1956), TITUS (1960) and CRAIG (1961).

The pattern of distribution of a substance in the countercurrent distribution system can be predicted from its partition coefficient by very simple mathematical procedures which greatly facilitate the analytical uses of this process. One common application is to measure small amounts of impurities by means of the discrepancies between observed and theoretical distribution patterns.

The partition coefficient of a substance in a carefully defined two-phase system can also serve as an identifying physical constant, a fact which has been successfully exploited by UDENFRIEND and his collaborators in establishing the specificity of analytical procedures for several indole compounds.

BOGDANSKI et al. (1956) identified 5-HT in brain of rat and rabbit by means of countercurrent distribution, which was carried out in glass-stoppered centrifuge tubes using the solvents n-butanol and 0.55 M pyrophosphate buffer pH 9.4; each solvent was previously saturated with respect to the other. After distribution, the partition coefficient of 5-HT in each tube was determined by measurement of its concentration in each phase. Analysis of the butanol phase was made after extracting the 5-HT into 0.1 N HCl, following the addition of two volumes of heptane (see p. 99). The 5-HT in the buffer phase and in the 0.1 N HCl was determined from its fluorescence at 550 mμ, after the solution had been made 3 N with respect to HCl. Countercurrent distribution curves obtained for the apparent 5-HT extracted from rabbit brain are shown in Fig. 7. The location of the peaks and the shape of the curves were found to be almost identical; both curves were almost the same as that calculated from the measured partition coefficient of authentic 5-HT. It was also apparent that no bufotenine occurs in the brain. To obtain additional evidence that the 450 mμ fluorescence represented 5-HT, the distribution of the apparent 5-HT between the two phases was measured in each tube. Except in a few of the last tubes the ratio of the amount of material in the butanol phase to the total amount in both phases was constant, and almost identical with that found for authentic 5-HT measured at the same time. A small amount of non-5-HT material was found in a few of the last tubes. The theoretical amount of 5-HT that should be present in these tubes was calculated from the measured partition coefficient of 5-HT by application of the binomial expansion in the manner described by WILLIAMSON and CRAIG (1947) and was found to be about 9 per cent. However, the same tubes had been found by analysis to contain a total of about 16 per cent of the total apparent 5-HT. Therefore, non-5-HT material represented about 7 per cent of the material measured in brain as 5-HT.

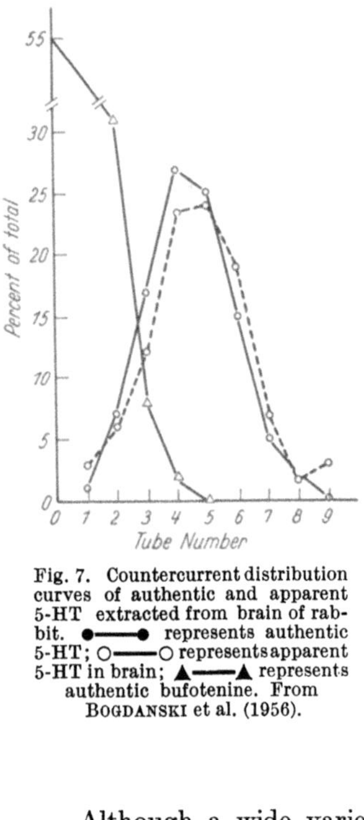

Fig. 7. Countercurrent distribution curves of authentic and apparent 5-HT extracted from brain of rabbit. ●——● represents authentic 5-HT; ○——○ represents apparent 5-HT in brain; ▲——▲ represents authentic bufotenine. From BOGDANSKI et al. (1956).

The above countercurrent distribution technique was also used by SJOERDSMA et al. (1959) to identify T isolated from human urine (see p. 94). Countercurrent distribution was carried out with benzene and 0.25 M borate buffer, pH 9.4 as solvents. After distribution, the partition coefficient of T was determined by measurement of its concentration in each phase. The organic phas was assayed after extraction of the T into 0.1 N HCl. The T from both phases was determined by spectrophotofluorometry after readjusting to pH 9—10. From the countercurrent distribution curves obtained and corresponding theoretical calculations, it was found that only 5 per cent of the material measured as T consisted of non-T substances. Further, N-methyl analogues of T, such as N-methyl-5-HT and bufotenine, could be excluded as urinary metabolites, since their countercurrent distribution curves were clearly different from that of T.

V. Paper chromatography

Although a wide variety of analytical methods are presently available for indole analysis, paper chromatography still retains a unique position in this field. Historically, it has been the most widely used method for separation and identification of indoles. Practically, it requires minute amounts of starting material, and is simple to perform without elaborate equipment.

Paper chromatography of indole compounds has been discussed by several workers, e.g. ERSPAMER (1954), DALGLIESH (1955, 1956), PROCHÁZKA (1958), ARMSTRONG et al. (1958), JEPSON (1960) and SANDLER (1963).

For the principles and practice of paper chromatography the reader is referred to the many excellent monographs available, e.g. HAIS and MACEK (1958), BLOCK et al. (1958), LINSKENS (1959), SMITH (1960), MACEK (1961) and CONSDEN (1961).

1. Chromatography paper

A large variety of chromatography papers has been used in indole analysis. However, the literature indicates that Whatman No. 1 and No. 4 have been used more than any other kind for qualitative work. The former is a "medium rate" paper; the latter is "fast", about two times that of No. 1. In recent years Whatman No. 1 has in some countries been replaced by Schleicher & Schüll 2043 b, which is a standard filter paper which is usable in practically all types of chromatographic separations. Whatman No. 5 and No. 42 are "slow" papers. For isolation purposes a thick paper may be required, e.g. Whatman No. 3 or 3 MM (see p.71).

2. Solvent systems

A large number of solvent systems are used, far too many to list in this discussion. Here, only some of the most widely used systems will be given:

a) Butanol-acetic acid-water (4:1:5)

This is a good general solvent for indole compounds and has been used by many workers (e.g. ERSPAMER 1955, DALGLIESH 1956, ARMSTRONG et al. 1958, McISAAC and PAGE 1959, ERSPAMER and NOBILI 1962a, b). In this solvent chromatograms are usually run overnight.

b) Isopropanol-ammonia-water (8:1:1)

This is an excellent solvent for indoles by virtue of its high resolution power. It is remarkably little affected by the presence of inorganic ions, and solutions so chromatographed need no prior desalting.

The R_f values obtained with this solvent are rather dependent on the ammonia concentration and this must be carefully controoled.

This solvent system has been used by ARMSTRONG et al. (1958), McISAAC and PAGE (1959), ERSPAMER and NOBILI (1962a, b) and others. Chromatograms are usually run overnight.

c) Potassium chloride

Potassium chloride, 20 per cent water solution.

This solvent, which was applied to indole analysis by DALGLIESH (1956), allows rather rapid separation of many indole compounds; a run usually requires only 3—4 hours. Compact spots are usually obtained, and the R_f values are remarkably constant.

This solvent has ben used by several other workers, e.g. ARMSTRONG et al. (1958) and ERSPAMER and NOBILI (1962a, b).

d) Benzene-propionic acid-water (100:70:5)

This solvent, which was introduced by ARMSTRONG et al. (1958), is particularly useful for the separation of indole acids.

The four above systems have been chosen for mention here because they give the best chromatograms in general indole investigations and screening operations. Furthermore, a larger number of indole compounds have been run with these solvents than with any other systems. A large number of other solvent systems have been described for smaller groups of indole compounds; some of these are given in Table 4.

For two-dimensional chromatography of indole compounds several combinations of solvent systems have been recommended. Generally, a basic solvent and a neutral or acidic solvent will give the best separations. JEPSON (1955) recommends isopropanol-ammonia-water (20:1:2) in the first dimension, followed by butanol-acetic acid-water (12:3:5) in the second dimension. This combination

Table 4 a. *R_f values of indolealkylamines and related compounds*

Compound	Solvent system								
	a	b	c	d	e	f	g	h	i
Indolealkylamines:									
Tryptamine	0.70	0.72	0.48		0.94	0.76	0.90	0.44	
1-Methyltryptamine	0.70	0.84				0.75			
2-Methyltryptamine	0.75	0.87				0.80			
α-Methyltryptamine	0.78	0.88				0.82			
N-Methyltryptamine	0.73	0.88				0.76		0.48	
N-Ethyltryptamine	0.83	0.93	0.60			0.79			
α-Ethyltryptamine	0.84	0.92	0.52			0.86			
N,N-Dimethyltryptamine	0.74	0.92	0.60			0.82		0.48	
α,α-Dimethyltryptamine	0.82	0.90	0.60			0.87			
β,β-Dimethyltryptamine	0.81	0.92	0.58			0.79			
N,N-Diethyltryptamine	0.85	0.98	0.62			0.83			
4-Hydroxytryptamine	0.60	0.66	0.36			0.75			
4-Hydroxytryptamine glucuronide	0.18	0.05	0.65						
N,N-Dimethyl-4-hydroxytryptamine (Psilocin)	0.74								
5-Hydroxytryptamine	0.48	0.69	0.37		0.86	0.70	0.62	0.20	
5-Hydroxytryptamine glucuronide	0.14	0.09	0.66						
5-Methoxytryptamine	0.64	0.76	0.30			0.72	0.80	0.34	
N-Methyl-5-hydroxytryptamine	0.49	0.73			0.83	0.72			
Bufotenine	0.62	0.92			0.91	0.79			
Bufotenidine	0.59	0.20			0.15				
Bufothionine	0.51	0.24	0.43		0.34	0.72			
Dehydrobufotenine	0.76	0.46			0.09				
N-Acetyl-5-hydroxytryptamine	0.81	0.75			0.86				
Melatonin	0.90	0.83							
N-Acetyl-5-methoxy-6-hydroxy-tryptamine	0.67								
N-Acetyl-5-methoxy-6-hydroxy-tryptamine glucuronide		0.22							
N-Acetyl-5-methoxy-6-hydroxy-tryptamine sulphate		0.55							
6-Hydroxytryptamine	0.44	0.53	0.33			0.72			
6-Methoxytryptamine	0.65	0.75	0.30			0.72			
7-Hydroxytryptamine	0.53	0.46				0.76			
5,6-Dimethoxytryptamine	0.50	0.65	0.24			0.62			
Indole amino acids:									
Tryptophan	0.37	0.34	0.54	0.07	0.08	0.56			0.77
N-Acetyltryptophan	0.83	0.53	0.74	0.42		0.70			0.80
N-Methyltryptophan	0.60	0.37				0.65			0.95
4-Hydroxytryptophan	0.29	0.30	0.67						
4-Hydroxytryptophan glucuronide	0.08								
5-Hydroxytryptophan	0.22	0.27	0.43		0.03	0.40			0.46
5-Hydroxytryptophan glucuronide	0.08		0.70						
N-Acetyl-5-hydroxytryptophan	0.75		0.66				0.23		
N-Acetyl-5-hydroxytryptophan glucuronide	0.23		0.70						
N-Acetyl-5-acetoxytryptophan	0.81		0.75				0.21		
5-Methoxytryptophan	0.27	0.32	0.36	0.06		0.52			0.76
Indole carboxylic acids:									
Indole-3-									
carboxylic acid	0.83	0.35	0.36	0.71		0.93			0.60
glyoxylic acid	0.67	0.48	0.42	0.11		0.72			0.60
glyoxylamide	0.76	0.85	0.11	0.49					
glycolic acid	0.82	0.39	0.74	0.18		0.56			0.50
acetic acid	0.85	0.47	0.63	0.72	0.12	0.84	0.52	0.84	0.75
acetamide	0.77	0.85	0.51	0.67		0.90			0.95

Table 4a (continued)

Compound	Solvent system								
	a	b	c	d	e	f	g	h	i
Indoleaceturic acid	0.76	0.48	0.65	0.29		0.65	0.46	0.58	0.82
N-(Indole-3-acetyl)-									
α-alanine	0.84	0.60	0.71	0.47					
β-alanine	0.82	0.51	0.70	0.46					
β-aminoisobutyric acid	0.86	0.60	0.71	0.66					
γ-aminobutyric acid	0.84	0.52	0.67	0.56					
aspartic acid	0.72	0.11	0.78	0.14		0.55			0.48
asparagine	0.59	0.33	0.72	0.17		0.60			0.78
glutamic acid	0.78	0.12	0.78	0.19		0.43			0.51
glutamine	0.65	0.37	0.70	0.19		0.58			0.82
β-(Indole-3)-									
pyruvic acid	0.80			0.41					
lactic acid	0.78	0.48	0.61	0.29		0.71			0.63
propionic acid	0.86	0.53	0.44	0.80	0.19	0.89			0.78
acrylic acid	0.83	0.45	0.15	0.73		0.94			0.70
4-Hydroxyindoleacetic acid	0.87	0.55	0.42						
4-Hydroxyindoleacetic acid glucuronide	0.24								
5-Hydroxyindole-									
2-carboxylic acid	0.72	0.29	0.24	0.17					
3-carboxylic acid	0.70	0.19	0.30	0.13					
3-acetic acid	0.72	0.27	0.51	0.14	0.03	0.61	0.16	0.60	0.46
3-acetic acid-5-sulphate ester	0.28	0.05	0.70						
3-acetic acid glucuronide	0.24								
5-Hydroxyindoleaceturic acid	0.84	0.23							
β-(5-Hydroxyindole-3)-lactic acid	0.53	0.29	0.50	0.03					
5-Methoxyindole-									
2-carboxylic acid	0.82	0.45	0.20	0.76					
3-carboxylic acid	0.82	0.32	0.29	0.71					
3-acetic acid	0.83	0.39	0.49	0.66		0.82	0.44	0.78	0.78
β-(5-Methoxyindole-3)-lactic acid	0.70	0.44	0.50	0.27					
6-Hydroxyindoleacetic acid	0.76	0.14				0.58			
7-Hydroxyindoleacetic acid	0.84	0.13				0.68			

Table 4b. Solvent Systems

System	Composition	R_f values given by:
a	Butanol-acetic acid-water (4:1:5), see p. 83	ARMSTRONG et al. (1958), JEPSON (1960), McISAAC and PAGE (1959), JEPSON et al. (1962), ERSPAMER and BERTACCINI (1962), ERSPAMER and NOBILI (1962).
b	Isopropanol-ammonia-water (8:1:1), see p. 83	
c	Potassium chloride, 20% water sol., see p. 83	ARMSTRONG et al. (1958), JEPSON (1960), ERSPAMER and BERTACCINI (1962), ERSPAMER and NOBILI (1962).
d	Benzene-propionic acid-water (100:70:5), see p. 83	ARMSTRONG et al. (1958).
e	Methyl ethyl ketone-2 N NH_3 (2:1)	McISAAC and PAGE (1959).
f	Butanol-pyridine-water (1:1:1)	JEPSON (1960).
g	Butanol-methylamin 25% (8:3)	ERSPAMER (1955), ERSPAMER and NOBILI (1962b)
h	Butanol, saturated with 1 N HCl	ERSPAMER (1955).
i	Phenol-ammonia	JEPSON (1960).

gives excellent separation of most indoles and is sepecially useful in the analyses of urine or tissue extracts. For a detailed description of this system, the reader is referred to JEPSON (1960).

DALGLIESH (1956) recommends the organic layer of butanol-acetic acid-water (4:1:5) for the first dimension and 20 per cent KCl for the second dimension.

3. Location of spots

a) Colour reactions

All the colour reactions mentioned above (p. 77) are useful in paper chromatography.

α) Aldehyde reagents (see. p. 77). p-Dimethylaminobenzaldehyde in dilute HCl (EHRLICH's reagent) is by far the most important of these reagents. As a spray reagent it is usually employed in an acid alcohol solution (2 g of p-dimethylaminobenzaldehyde dissolved in a mixture of 80 ml of 95 per cent ethanol and 20 ml of 6 N HCl). It can also be made up with acetone and used as a dip reagent. JEPSON (1960) prefers the latter and uses a mixture of 1 volume of 10 per cent p-dimethylaminobenzaldehyde in conc. HCl and 4 volumes of acetone. This mixture is prepared just before use.

Spots appearing with p-dimethylaminobenzaldehyde range in colour from blue-green through blue to bright pink. The rate of development of these colours varies considerably with different indole compounds; some compounds may develop maximal colour within 5 minutes while others may require more than 24 hours (see ARMSTRONG et al. 1958). When working with this reagent it is very important to note the *initial* colours, *changes* in colour, and the *permanance* of the colours. The sequence of colours in the development of the spots may be quite characteristic, and is therefore useful in the identification of a given indole compound. Sometimes a spot may appear strongly, fade almost to disappearance and reappear later with an enhanced or different colour. 5-HIAA may be taken as an example: its colour sequence is a rapid blue spot, changing to faint grey, and later to stable blue over a 30 minute period. Hence, as pointed out it is advisable to inspect the chromatograms at intervals over the first hour and again the next day.

p-Dimethylaminocinnamaldehyde, which was used by HARLEY-MASON and ARCHER (1958), is prepared for spraying by dissolving 2 g of the aldehyde in a mixture of 100 ml of 6 N HCl and 100 ml of 95 per cent ethanol. For dipping, a 1 per cent solution of the aldehyde in conc. HCl is diluted with 4 volumes of acetone just before use. Most 5-hydroxyindoles react with this reagent to give blue colours. 4-Hydroxyindoles only give grey, 6-hydroxyindoles a grey-blue and 7-hydroxyindoles a green colour.

Cinnamaldehyde is usually sprayed as a 1 per cent solution in methanol. The chromatograms are then exposed to HCl vapours in a glass container until the spots are clearly developed (MÜLLER 1953).

β) Xanthydrol reagent (see. p. 78). A 0.1 per cent solution of xanthydrol in 95 per cent ethanol containing 5 per cent conc. HCl is used as a spray reagent. The solution is prepared fresh on the day of use. Colour appears on drying the paper at room temperature. The paper may also be sprayed with an alcoholic xanthydrol solution, and after drying placed over conc. HCl in a sealed container.

For quantitative work, the coloured material can be eluted from the paper with methanol, the latter evaporated, and the residue taken up in 6 N HCl and the absorbancy determined (DICKMAN and CROCKETT 1956).

γ) 1-Nitroso-2-naphtol reagent (see p. 79). The paper is first sprayed with a 0.1 per cent 1-nitroso-2-naphtol solution in 95 per cent ethanol. After drying the paper is sprayed with a freshly prepared mixture of 25 ml of 2 N HCl and 1 ml of 2.5 per cent $NaNO_2$. The 5-hydroxyindoles appear as violet spots on a faint yellow background. At least 5 to 10 μg of compound are needed with this reagent (UDENFRIEND and WEISSBACH 1963).

4-Hydroxyindoles give a weak yellow and 6- and 7-hydroxyindoles a weak brown colour with this reagent (JEPSON et al. 1962).

δ) Diazo reagents (see p. 79). Diazotized sulphanilic acid is used in both acid (van den Bergh reaction) and in sodium carbonate (PAULY's reaction). The *acid* reagent is made up as follows:

a) Sulphanilic acid, 9 g, conc. HCl 90 ml, water 900 ml	10 vol.
b) Sodium nitrite, 5 per cent in water	1 vol.

The two solutions are mixed and immediately placed in an ice-bath for 5 minutes. Then the remaining nitrous acid is destroyed with solid ammonium sulphamate. When sprayed with this reagent 6-hydroxy- and 6-methoxyindoles react *immediately* and specifically to give brilliant red colours. 4-, 5- and 7-Hydroxyindoles yield yellow-brown to purple colours which develop rather slowly.

Diazotized sulphanilic acid in *alkaline* solution is prepared as follows:

a) Sulphanilic acid, see above	1 vol.
b) Sodium nitrite, see above	1 vol.
c) Sodium carbonate, 10 per cent in water	2 vol.

When required the stock solutions of a and b are mixed and allowed to stand for 5 minutes at room temperature. Solution c is then added carefully as the mixture vigorously effervesces. The reagent is used immediately and is usually sprayed on the chromatograms. 4-Hydroxyindoles are coloured brown-violet, 5-hydroxyindoles red-brown, 6-hydroxyindoles purple, and 7-hydroxyindoles grey-brown (JEPSON et al. 1962).

Diazotized p-nitroaniline may be used in the same way as diazotized sulphanilic acid. A suitable reagent is made up as follows:

a) p-Nitroaniline, 0.1 per cent in 1 N HCl	1 vol.
b) Sodium nitrite, 0.2 per cent in water	1 vol.
c) Potassium carbonate, 10 per cent in water	2.5 vol.

The separate reagents are kept in stock solutions at 5°. For the *acid* reagent a and b are mixed and kept cool for a further 5 minutes and then sprayed on the paper. When the *alkaline* reagent is required, an additional spray is made with solution c. If an alkaline reagent is to be used directly, c is added to the cooled mixture of a and b and the paper sprayed at once. This spray reagent must be prepared fresh and used immediately as it deteriorates rapidly. A volume of 10 ml is sufficient for one 25×25 cm chromatogram.

Diazotized p-nitroaniline in *acid* also gives an immediate intense red colour with 6-hydroxyindoles. 4-, 5- and 7-Hydroxyindoles react more slowly yielding colours which vary from yellow to red-brown. In the *alkaline* version 6-hydroxyindoles give purple colours, 4-hydroxyindoles grey-blue, 5-hydroxyindoles pink, and 7-hydroxyindoles green-blue colours.

p-Nitrobenzenediazoniumtetrafluoroborate is used as a 0.5 per cent aqueous solution, which is stable at room temperature. 5-Hydroxyindoles give red to brown-red colours. Simple indoles, such as TP, T and IAA, show yellow to orange colours. A further differentiation may be obtained by subsequently spraying with a 10 per cent sodium carbonate solution.

2-Chloro-4-nitrobenzenediazonium naphtalene-2-sulphonate (NNCD reagent) is usually employed as a freshly prepared 0.1—0.3% solution in 0.1 N HCl. After spraying, the chromatograms are allowed to dry in air. Simple indoles, e.g. T, IAA, N-methyl-T and N,N-dimethyl-T react to give orange colours. 4- and 5-Hydroxyindoles result in red colours (ERSPAMER 1955, ERSPAMER and NOBILI 1962a).

ε) Other colour reactions. Several other colour reactions have been used for the location of indole compounds on chromatograms: descriptions of these are to be found in the monographs by JEPSON (1960) and CLOTTEN and CLOTTEN (1962) and in the publications of DALGLIESH (1955, 1956).

b) Fluorescence reactions

Although most indoles *adsorbed on paper* do not fluoresce, it is always advisable to examine the untreated chromatogram in ultraviolet light, and again after each colour reagent has been applied. After reacting with a reagent, ultraviolet light can sometimes provide a more sensitive means for examining weak spots on chromatograms than visible light.

However, when sprayed with a number of reagents indole compounds show fluorescence (see p. 74) and may thus be detected on developed chromatograms.

α) HCl-fluorescence. When sprayed with 0.1 N HCl and examined under an ultraviolet lamp 5-HT and other 5-hydroxyindoles emit a pink fluorescence. This fluorescence is fairly specific, but not very sensitive (5—10 μg required per spot). However, it may be useful as a location method when chromatography or electrophoresis on paper are used as isolation procedures (see p. 71).

β) Ninhydrin-acetic acid fluorescence (see. p. 74). The chromatograms are dipped in or sprayed with a freshly prepared reagent of the following composition:

Ninhydrin, 0.1 per cent in acetone	9 vol.
Acetic acid, conc.	1 vol.

After drying the paper, it is heated at 110° for 2 minutes. Susceptible tryptamines show an intense greenish-blue fluorescence in ultraviolet light which is detectable at concentrations as low as 0.01 μg per cm^2 paper. This test, which is specific for certain tryptamines, depends upon the formation of 3,4-dihydro-3-carboline (JEPSON 1960). A strongly positive reaction specifically indicates a compound with a tryptamine structure not more substituted than the following:

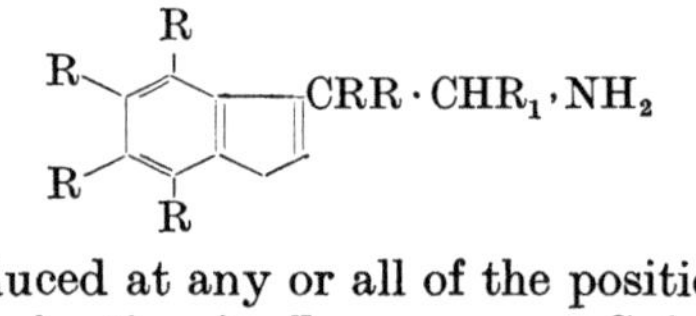

Alkyl groups can be introduced at any or all of the positions shown in the above structure, without any diminution in fluorescence. Substitution of any of the hydrogen atoms shown in the structure abolishes fluorescence. R_1 cannot be —COOH (tryptophan), but may well be —CH_2OH (tryptophanol). With tryptamines bearing a substitutent at position 6 the fluorescence colour is yellowish.

Tryptamines, N-alkyltryptamines and N,N-dialkyltryptamines, which react similarly with p-dimethylaminobenzaldehyde reagent, can be distinguished by their response to the ninhydrin-acetic acid reagent. Tryptamines-(NH_2) give strong visible colour and strong fluorescence, N-alkyltryptamines-(NHR) strong visible colour but little fluorescence, and N,N-dialkyltryptamines-(NRR) no visible colour and no fluorescence.

γ) Formaldehyde-HCl-fluorescence (see p. 74). The chromatograms are sprayed with the following mixture:

Formaldehyde (35—40 per cent)	1 vol.
HCl, conc.	1 vol.
Water	2 vol.

and then dried at 90°. Most indoles substituted at the 3-position show orange to brown visible colours with characteristic yellow or orange fluorescence (PRO-

CHAZKA 1953). For structural requirements of the molecules for this reaction, see p. 75.

δ) Formaldehyde-K_2Cr0_7-fluorescence (see. p. 75). SHEPHERD et al. (1953) have described a similar fluorescence reaction but use potassium dichromate instead of hydrochloric acid. Their reagent is the following:

Potassium dichromate, 0.1 per cent in water	9 vol.
Formaldehyde (35—40 per cent)	1 vol.

After spraying, the chromatograms are heated at 100—110° for 5 minutes. When examined in ultraviolet light 5-HT shows a golden-yellow fluorescence immediately after heating, and this persists for days; amounts as small as 0.2 μg of 5-HT can be detected. The behaviour of bufotenine and bufotenidine is quite similar to that of 5-HT. T gives a bright yellow fluorescence if more than 2.5 μg are present, but this develops slowly. TP likewise gives a yellowish fluorescence if 2.5 μg are present, while 5-methoxy-T gives yellow-orange fluorescence if similar amounts are present.

ε) Iodate-acetic acid-fluorescence (see p. 75). When chromatograms are sprayed with a saturated solution of potassium iodate in 50 per acetic acid (about 2.5 per 100 ml) and then heated at 60° for 5 minutes, TP and T form tryptochrome which shows a brown-red visible colour with intense orange fluorescence (EGELHAAF 1957). 0.1 μg of TP may be detected.

4. R_f values of indolealkylamines and related compounds

In Table 4 R_f values are given for a number of biologically important indolealkylamines and related compounds in different solvents.

5. Quantitative paper chromatography

Although paper chromatography cannot, by its very nature, be more than semi-quantitative, it may be necessary to use it when no other quantitative procedure exists.

GOBLE et al. (1955) used the fluorescence reaction of JEPSON and STEVENS (1953) for 5-HT measurements, comparing the unknown spots with standards. RODNIGHT (1956) used a similar procedure with p-dimethylaminobenzaldehyde spots for the determination of urinary 5-HT and T. However, these spots are not ideal for this purpose, as colours may change and the speed at which they appear may vary depending on whether the indoles are present together with urine or in pure solution (see p. 86).

SCHREIER and GAEDTKE (1956) measured 5-HT and IAA in pure solutions by spraying the chromatograms with a mixture of equal parts of 10 per cent xanthydrol in methanol and acetic acid. The spots were then cut out, eluted with a mixture of acetic acid and methanol (2:1) and the colour read at 580 mμ. GAEDTKE and SCHREIER (1956) used the same technique for determination of 5-HT in urine, but acetylated the 5-HT before chromatography.

CORREALE (1955) used paper chromatography for the determination of 5-HIAA. The spots were eluted with water and the 5-HIAA determined in the eluates by using the p-dimethylaminobenzaldehyde reaction.

CARCASONA et al. (1959b) separated 5-HTP, 5-HT and 5-HIAA by paper chromatography, sprayed the papers with p-dimethylaminobenzaldehyde, 1-nitroso-2-naphtol or diazotized sulphanilic acid. The papers were then made transparent with a mixture of α-bromonaphtalene and paraffin oil and the spots scanned densitometrically.

VI. Thin layer chromatography

Whereas paper chromatography has proven an effective and useful tool for separation of indole compounds, an alternative method — thin layer chromatography — providing equivalent resolution has been recently developed.

The principles and techniques of thin layer chromatography will not be treated here. Excellent reviews have been published by WOLLISH et al. (1961) and DEMOLE (1959), and the various techniques are comprehensively reviewed in the books by STAHL (1962), RANDERATH (1962), TRUTER (1963) and BOBBITT (1963).

Table 5. *R_f values of indole compounds on silica gel G layers*

Compound	R_f values in		References
	Solvent 1	Solvent 2	
Indole	0.84	0.73	1
3-Hydroxymethylindole	0.84	0.45	1
Indoleacetic acid	0.31	0.28	1
Indolepropionic acid	0.38	0.34	1
Indolebutyric acid	0.40	0.38	1
Indoleacrylic acid	0.33	0.29	1
5-Hydroxyindoleacetic acid	0.19	0.04	1
Tryptamine	0.77	0	1
5-Methoxytryptamine	0.62	0	2
5-Hydroxytryptamine	0.65	0	1, 2
Melatonin	0.89	0.26	2
N-Acetyl-5-hydroxytryptamine	0.90	0.08	2
Tryptophan	0.23	0	1
5-Methoxytryptophan	0.28	0	1
5-Hydroxytryptophan	0.14	0	1
Bufotenine	0.90	0	2
N-Acetyltryptophan	0.56	0.07	2

Solvent 1: Methyl acetate-isopropanol-25% ammonia (9:7:4). Solvent 2: Chloroform-96% acetic acid (19:1).

References to Table 5. [1] STAHL and KALDEWEY (1961). [2] HANSON (1964).

Thin layer chromatography, a technique essentially complementary to paper chromatography, may offer such advantages as:

1. Small, sharply defined spots, frequently better than those which can be obtained with the same compounds by paper chromatography.

2. Extraordinary rapid development.

3. The results can be readily applied to large-scale preparative separations on columns.

4. There are no limitations on the reagents which can be used for localization of the spots.

The method can frequently be used with amounts ten to hundred times less than those needed for paper chromatography.

These advantages are all well illustrated by the results obtained with indole compounds. Thin layer chromatography here is about one hundred times as sensitive as paper chromatography, a feature which is very important in studies of biological materials.

STAHL and KALDEWEY (1961) and HANSON (1964) have used neutral, unbuffered silica gel *G* (Merck) as an adsorbent, and this material gives a good separation with many indole compounds. The chromatoplates are of the size 20×20 cm and each development is carried to a distance of about 10 cm. Methyl acetate-isopropanol-25% ammonia (9:7:4) and chloroform-96% acetic acid (19:1) were used as solvent systems, either singly, or combined for two-dimensional chromatography. In these systems the development usually takes about 30 minutes. The indoles are located with either of the following reactions (STAHL and KALDEWEY 1961):

Van Urk reaction. Reagent: 1 g of p-dimethylaminobenzaldehyde is dissolved in a mixture of 50 ml of 25% HCl and 50 ml of 96% ethanol. Each 20×20 cm chromatoplate is sprayed with about 10 ml of the reagent. Ammonia from the developing solvent should be removed by first warming the chromatoplate to 50° for 5 minutes. After the sprayed chromatoplate has been warmed to 50° for 20 minutes it is exposed to the vapours from aqua regia. Indole compounds then appear as blue, violet or red spots. This reaction, which was found to be the most specific, allows a detection of 0.05 to 0.1 μg of most indole components.

Prochazka fluorescence reaction. Reagent: 10 ml of 35% formaldehyde is mixed with 10 ml of 25% HCl and 20 ml of 96% ethanol. Again the chromatoplate is sprayed with 10 ml of the reagent and after about 5 minutes heated to 100°. Indole compounds form yellowish brown visible spots which have an intense orange fluorescence in ultraviolet light (see p. 74). Exposure of the sprayed plate to the vapours of aqua regia, or simple storage in air for 24 hours results in an intensification of the fluorescence. This reaction, which was found by STAHL and KALDEWEY (1961) to be the most sensitive, allows a detection of 0.005 to 0.01 μg of most indole compounds.

Instead of the above van Urk reagent, the p-dimethylaminobenzaldehyde reagent with acetone (described in the above section on paper chromatography, p. 86) is equally satisfactory for thin layer chromatography.

HANSON (1964) has used thin layer chromatography for the rapid analysis of carcinoid urines. A small volume (2—3 ml) of acidified urine is extracted with ether or ethyl acetate. The extract is dried with anhydrous sodium sulphate and evaporated. The residue is taken up in 0.1—0.2 ml of ethanol and 5 μl of the extract is spotted on a chromatoplate. After development in the above described methyl acetate-isopropanol-ammonia system, the plate is sprayed with p-dimethylaminobenzaldehyde-acetone reagent and dried. It is then inspected for the presence of 5-HIAA and other indole compounds. In this way the chromatographic analysis of a urine sample can be completed in about 1 hour.

Table 5 summarizes R_f values for some biologically important indole compounds, as resolved on neutral silica gel.

VII. Gas chromatography

The failure to apply gas-liquid chromatography to indole analysis apears to be based on technical features presently inherent in the instrumentation involved. For current gas chromatography columns, only a very small volume may be applied (1—10 μl); hence, very high indole concentrations must be achieved

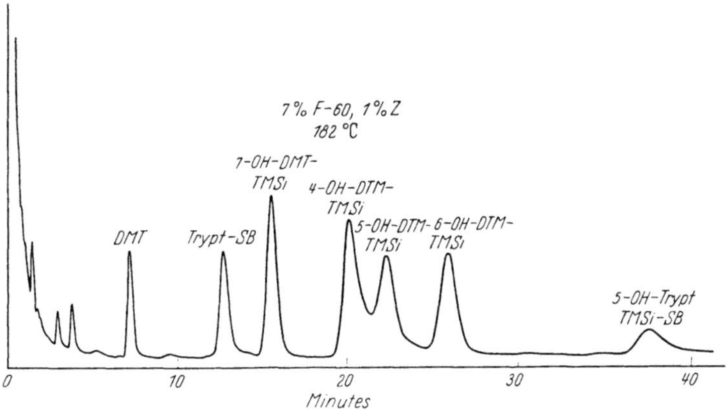

Fig. 8. Gas chromatographic separation of a mixture of closely related T derivatives. The compounds are N,N-dimethyl-T (DMT). The acetone condensation product (Schiff base) of T (TRYPT-SB); 7-trimethylsilyloxy-N,N-dimethyl-T (7-OH-DMT-TMSi); 4-trimethyl-silyloxy-N,N-dimethyl-T (4-OH-DMT-TMSi); 5-trimethylsilyloxy-N,N-dimethyl-T (5-OH-DMT-TMSi); 6-trimethylsilyloxy-N,N-dimethyl-T (6-OH-DMT-TMSi); acetone condensation product of 5-trimethylsilyloxy-T (5-OH-TRYPT-TMSi-SB). From HOLMSTEDT et al. (1964)

for suitable detection. This is in contrast to spectrophotofluorometrical techniques whereby indoles may be detected at the 0.1 μg level in 1 ml of fluid. However, in situations where high concentrations can be obtained, gas-liquid chromatography permits not only qualitative resolution, but quantitative estimation as well. A final outstanding feature well documented for gas-liquid chromatography is the ability to resolve closely related indoles.

The principles and practice of gas-liquid chromatography will not be discussed here; for this the reader is referred to the many manuals available (e.g. KEULEMANS 1959, BURCHFIELD and STORRS 1962).

SWEELEY and WILLIAMS (1961) have used gas-liquid chromatography to separate and quantitatively estimate aromatic acids-including IAA and 5-HIAA — from human urine after conversion of the acids to their methyl esters.

FALES and PISANO (1962) were able to separate microgram quantities of a number of biogenic amines including T, dimethyl-T, 5-methoxy-T, 5-HT, N-acetyl-T and melatonin.

HOLMSTEDT et al. (1964) have studied the separation and identification of a number of tryptamine related indole bases by gas-liquid chromatography. The indoles studied were N,N-dimethyl-T, N,N-diethyl-T, T, 5-methoxy-T, 5-methoxy-N,N-dimethyl-T, 5-HT, 4-hydroxy-N,N-dimethyl-T, 5-hydroxy-N,N-dimethyl-T, 6-hydroxy-N,N-dimethyl-T and 7-hydroxy-N,N-dimethyl-T. These compounds were chromatographed both directly and as the trimethylsilyl ethers. The latter derivatives provided a satisfactory separation of the positional isomers 4-, 5-, 6- and 7-hydroxy-N,N-dimethyl-T (see Fig. 8).

By means of their gas-liquid chromatographic technique the latter workers were able to identify 5-methoxy-N,N-dimethyl-T as the major indole base of *epená*, a South American snuff with reported hallucinogenic properties.

VIII. Paper electrophoresis

Electrophoresis on filter paper offers another method, complementary to paper chromatography, for the separation and identification of minute quantities of closely related indole compounds.

According to the potential gradient used distinction is made between low and high voltage electrophoresis. *Low voltage electrophoresis* is carried out at voltages not exceeding 300—400 volts or a potential gradient of not more than 10 volts per cm in the direction of the migration. In *high voltage electrophoresis*, which is the most important recent development in zonal electrophoresis, much higher voltages (1000 to 10,000 volts) and potential gradients (20 to 200 volts per cm) are employed.

The theory and practice of paper electrophoresis will not be treated here; for this the reader is referred to the books by LEDERER (1955), BLOCK et al. (1958), RIBEIRO et al. (1961) and MORRIS and MORRIS (1963) for techniques of low voltage electrophoresis, and to EFRON (1960) and CLOTTEN and CLOTTEN (1962) for comprehensive reviews of high voltage electrophoresis.

A number of low voltage electrophoretic systems have been described for the analysis of indole compounds. Plant extracts were analyzed for indoles by DENFFER et al. (1952), who used a phosphate buffer of pH 7 and a potential of 110 volts for 8 hours. TP and IAA separated without difficulty in this system. MÜLLER (1953) also studied these compounds by paper electrophoresis.

LANGEMANN and KÄGI (1956) used low voltage electrophoresis for the separation of 5-HT and 5-HIAA in a case of carcinoid. The electrophoresis was run for 6 to 10 hours in 0.2 M acetate buffer pH 4.8 or 0.067 M barbital buffer pH 8.6 at a voltage of 220 volts.

ROBERTSON and ANDREWS (1961) used low electrophoresis in the detection and estimation of 5-HT in human plasma. A 0.1 ml plasma sample was applied to the paper strip which was run in a citrate buffer pH 3.8 at a potential gradient of 10 volts per cm for 6 hours. After elution of the appropriate area with Tyrode solution 5-HT was determined by biological assay.

Carcasona et al. (1960) separated 5-HTP, 5-HT and 5-HIAA by using barbital buffer pH 8.6, phosphate buffer pH 7.0 or acetate buffer pH 5.05 and a potential gradient of 3.5 volts per cm. In these systems 5-HT migrates towards the cathode and 5-HIAA towards the anode, while 5-HTP migrates very little. The time necessary for optimal separation was 8 to 12 hours. The paper strips were sprayed with p-dimethylaminobenzaldehyde reagent and, after drying, made transparent with a mixture of α-bromonaphtalene and paraffin oil. The colour intensity of the spots was then determined by densitometry.

The time necessary for separation of small molecules by low voltage electrophoresis is usually long and during this time substances not only migrate according to their electrical charge but also diffuse into the surrounding media. This often results in large, faint, overlapping spots and consequently poor resolution. For this reason is often proves advantageous to use a high voltage gradient to complete the process of migration rapidly. The resulting heat which is generated requires special arrangements for cooling, which somewhat complicates the equipment, but the definition of the spots and the degree of resolution is unequalled by any alternative methods.

It is thus apparent that there are two major advantages of high voltage electrophoresis for the separation of small molecules: The separation is rapid, and diffusion is minimized. To these can further be added that specimens usually need not be desalted. Urine and plasma samples can be applied directly to the paper strips without any prior preparation.

A large number of high voltage electrophoretic systems have been described for the analysis of indole compounds (see Clotten and Clotten 1962).

Some of the most useful buffers for the separation of indole compounds commonly encountered in biological specimens are the following:

1. Borate buffer pH 10 (Efron 1960).
2. Pyridine-acetate buffer pH 6.1 (Efron 1960).
3. Citrate buffer pH 3.8 (Robertson and Andrews 1961).
4. Pyridine-acetate buffer pH 3.6 (Zylka and Köhler 1957, Sturm 1961).
5. Pyridine-acetate buffer pH 2.3 (Gayer 1956).
6. Formate-acetate buffer pH 1.9 (Nöller and Stelgens 1957).

The two first are the most effective for the separation of indolic acids from other indole compounds. The migration of most compounds is towards the anode in these systems. However, exceptions are 5-HT and other tryptamines which migrate towards the cathode. For separation of the amines the more acid buffers usually give better results.

With a high voltage applied, a very rapid separation of the compounds can be effected; e.g. a potential of 6000 volts often gives adequate separation in 30 minutes.

Following the electrophoretic separation the indole compounds may be located by any of the reagents described in the section on paper chromatography (p. 86).

After location of the individual indole compounds, their determination can be made either directly by densitometry or, after elution, by colorimetry, ultraviolet absorbancy, spectrophotofluorometry or biological assay.

If there is a large number of similarly charged compounds present in a specimen, overlapping of the spots often occurs. In such cases a separation in a second dimension may be very effective. This can be done by high voltage electrophoresis in one direction followed by chromatography performed in a perpendicular direction on the same paper. When such a two-way separation is made, electrophoresis should always be used for the first separation for three reasons: it automatically desalts the specimen, it effectively separate the compounds from deproteinizing agents if such have been used, and it avoids leaving chromatographic solvents on the paper, as these may interfere with electrophoretic separation. For details on this combination of high voltage electrophoresis and chromatography, see EFRON (1960).

Specific high voltage electrophoretic methods for the determination of 5-HT in biological material have been described by NÖLLER and STELGENS (1957), ZYLKA and KÖHLER (1957) and STURM (1961) and for that of 5-HIAA by STURM (1962).

GAYER (1956) has been used a special technique for the detection of certain biogenic amines, including T and 5-HT. These amines are first converted to their tetraphenyl borates and are then separated by high voltage electrophoresis.

DEAVER et al. (1958) also applied a somewhat variant electrophoretic technique for the fractionation of mixtures containing indoles. Here use was made of the phenomenon of ionophoretic mobility equilibria as first described by DURRUM (see BLOCK et al. 1958).

C. Quantitative determination of specific compounds

In the following section a number of different methods for the quantitative determination of T and 5-HT, their precursors TP and 5-HTP and major metabolites IAA and 5-HIAA will be described.

I. Simple indoles

1. Tryptamine

T can be isolated from biological material by alkaline extraction into benzene, returned to an acid aqueous phase, and here determined either colorimetrically or fluorometrically.

a) Colorimetric determination

T forms a coloured product with xanthydrol which is very similar in optical characteristics to xanthydryltryptophan, i.e. showing an absorption maximum at 510 mμ (DICKMAN and WESCOTT 1954) and can thus be determined by the xanthydrol methods described for TP (p. 96) and IAA (p. 98).

b) Spectrophotofluorometric determination

Native fluorescence of T (SJOERDSMA et al. 1959). The following method is based on the fluorescence at 360 mμ shown by T when activated at 285 mμ and it is well suited for the determination of T in human urine:

A urine sample of 15 ml in a 50 ml glass-stoppered centrifuge tube is alkalinized to pH 11—14 by dropwise addition of 10 N NaOH. 30 ml of benzene are added, the tube is shaken for 20 minutes on a shaking machine and then centrifuged. If an emulsion occurs at the solvent interface, it is dispersed with a stirring rod and the tube is recentrifuged. The benzene layer is transferred to a similar tube and washed twice by shaking with 5 ml of 0.1 N NaOH. After centrifugation, a 25 ml aliquot of the benzene layer is transferred to a 35 ml tapered glass-stoppered centrifuge tube containing 0.7 ml of 0.1 N HCl. The tube is shaken for 15 minutes and centrifuged, following which the benzene layer is aspirated and discarded. A 0.5 ml aliquot of the acid solution is transferred to a test tube containing 1 ml of 0.13 M borate buffer pH 10. T in this buffered solution is then determined in the spectrophotofluorometer, using 285 mμ for activation and 360 mμ for fluorescence.

A T standard (about 2 μg) and a reagent blank are carried through the entire procedure. The T content of the unknown sample is calculated from the readings obtained with the standard and blank. As little as 0.1 μg of T in 15 ml of urine may be measured by the method. Fluorescence is proportional to T concentrations of 0.1 to 8 μg.

As some drugs may produce extractable fluorescent material which interferes with the determination it is advisable to examine both the activation and fluorescence spectra of the sample (see Fig. 9) when assaying T. The average T excretion in man is about 75 μg per day, with values ranging from 25 to 130 μg.

Norharman fluorescence (Hess and Udenfriend 1959, Hess 1961).

The method based on the native fluorescence of T works well with human urine, but is not sensitive and specific enough for the assay of T in tissues or urine of some laboratory animals. A method involving extraction of the T, its condensation with formaldehyde and dehydrogenation to a highly fluorescent product, apparently norharman (see p. 74), exhibits such a great sensitivity as to allow the determination of T present in tissues in concentrations higher than 0.1 μg per gram. Since norharman formation only occurs with indoleethylamine derivatives compounds such as IAA and 5-HIAA do not interfere in the determination of T (Fig. 10). However TP gives a comparable fluorophor when treated with formaldehyde and H_2O_2 but it is not extracted by the benzene and therefore does not interfere in the method.

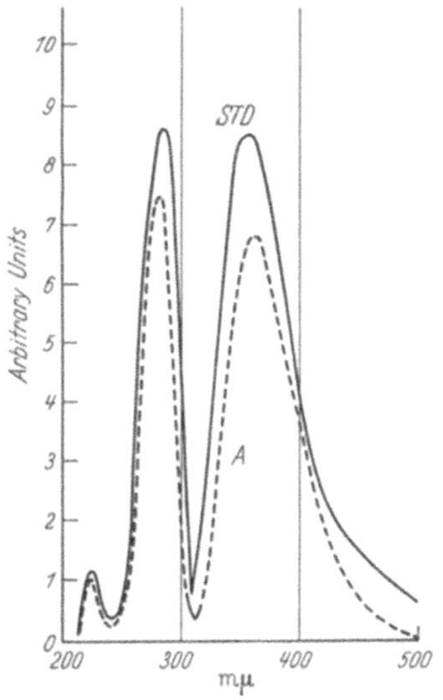

Fig. 9

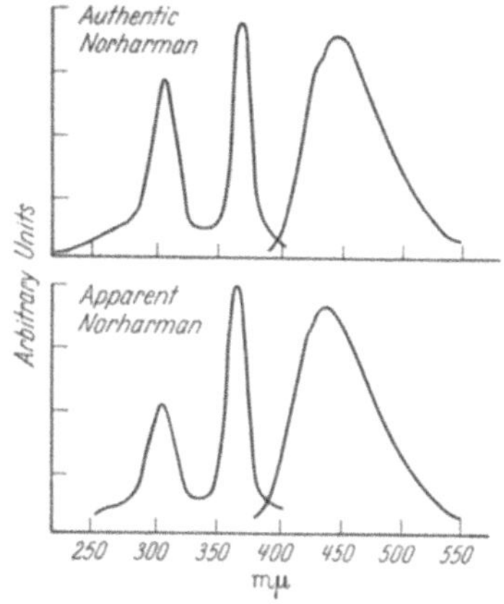

Fig. 10

Fig. 9. Activation and fluorescence spectra of authentic T (STD) and apparent T (A) from urine (Sjoerdsma et al. 1959)

Fig. 10. Activation and fluorescence spectra of authentic and apparent norharman. The apparent norharman was prepared from T extracted from the liver of a guinea pig treated with TP and monoamine oxidase inhibitor (iproniazid). From Hess and Udenfriend (1959)

The procedure for tissues is as follows: To 3 ml of tissue homogenate (1 g tissue + 2 ml 0.1 N HCl), or urine containing 0.1 to 5 μg of T, in a glass-stoppered centrifuge tube are added 0.3 ml of 10 N NaOH to bring the pH to about 11. 20 ml of benzene are then added and the tube is shaken for 15 minutes on a shaking machine. The tube is then centrifuged and as much of the benzene as possible is transferred to another tube containing 5 ml of 0.1 N NaOH. The tube is shaken for 5 minutes, centrifuged, and 15 ml of the benzene are transferred to another tube containing 4 ml of 0.1 N H_2SO_4. This tube is also shaken for 5 minutes, centrifuged, and 3 ml of the acid layer transferred to a test tube containing 0.1 ml of 18 per cent formaldehyde. The tube is covered with a glass-marble and placed in a boiling water bath for 20 minutes following which 0.1 ml of 5 per cent aqueous H_2O_2 is added and the heating is continued for another 20 minutes. After cooling to room temperature fluorescence is measured in a spectrophotofluorometer at 440 mμ when activated at 365 mμ.

The distribution of T between the various solvents used in this procedure is such that about 70 to 80 per cent appears in the final extract. Accordingly, standards are prepared by carrying known amounts of T through the entire procedure. Fluorescence is proportional to T concentration over the entire range. T added to tissues is recovered in 90 to 100 per cent, based on extracted standards.

When the reagents themselves are carried through the entire extraction procedure and compared to 0.1 N H_2SO_4 the resulting fluorescence is equivalent to about 0.2 to 0.3 μg of T. This blank fluorescence limits the sensitivity of the method. The amounts of T normally present in the tissues of several laboratory animals are too small (0.05 to 0.1 μg per gram) to give values significantly above the reagent blank range. The normal values are presumably less than 0.08 μg per gram. However, following the administration of L-TP or of monoamine oxidase inhibitors, the concentration of T in tissues rises to values between 1 and 2 μg per gram (HESS et al. 1959).

c) Other methods for the determination of tryptamine

RODNIGHT (1956) has described a method for the isolation and determination of urinary 5-HT and T. The method, which involves ion-exchange and paper chromatography, is rather time-consuming and not very precise.

Thin-layer chromatography has been applied quantitatively for the assay of T in plasma by EBLE and BROOKER (1962).

2. Tryptophan

a) Colorimetric determination

p-Dimethylaminobenzaldehyde method (UDENFRIEND and PETERSON 1957).

This method, wich is an adaptation of the procedure of GRAHAM et al. (1947) can be used to determine TP in tissues and biological extracts:

Transfer 0.5 ml of the deproteinized sample containing 0.05 to 0.5 μM of TP to a tube containing 2.5 ml of reagent (p-dimethylaminobenzaldehyde, 0.5% in 12 N HCl) and allow to stand for 30 minutes at room temperature, preferably in the dark. Then add 2.5 ml of absolute ethanol and 2 to 3 drops of 0.2% sodium nitrite, and let stand at room temperature for another 30 minutes. The optical density of the resulting blue chromophore is measured at 620 mμ. Standards are prepared at exactly the same time by adding known amounts of TP dissolved in 0.50 ml of solution to 0.5 ml of deproteinized tissue blank and developing the colour described.

In a Beckman spectrophotometer with a 1 cm light path an optical density of about 0.275 is obtained for 0.1 μM of TP. A linear relation between optical density and concentration is obtained up to 0.5 μM of TP.

The sample can be deproteinized by either trichloroacetic acid or zinc acetate and NaOH.

As the p-dimethylaminobenzaldehyde method is not specific for TP the above procedure is not applicable to studies involving the conversion of TP to other indole derivatives (e.g. T or 5-HTP) unless these compounds are first removed.

Xanthydrol method (DICKMAN and CROCKETT 1956).

This method has been elaborated for the determination of TP in plasma and serum but may, with slight modifications, be applicable to other tissues as well:

To 1 ml of plasma in a centrifuge tube are added 5 ml of 1% picric acid and 370 mg of ammonium sulphate. After thorough mixing, the sample is centrifuged for 15 minutes, and the supernatant solution is filtered through a small cotton plug. A 4 ml aliquot is added to a mixture composed of 4 ml of 12 N HCl, 1 ml of glacial acetic acid, and 1 ml of xanthydrol (1 mg per ml in 12 N HCl) in a glass-stoppered tube. The tube is placed in boling water bath for 15 minutes, then cooled in an ice bath. Saturated NaOH is added until the solution reaches pH 3.5 where it becomes colourless. Excess alkali must be avoided or false low results will be obtained. The solution is then extracted with 10 ml of isoamyl acetate and the upper phase is removed. 1.4 ml of 6 N HCl are added to the organic phase and the mixture is shaken in a glass-stoppered test-tube. The aquerous phase is removed and its absorbancy is measured at 510 mμ in a spectrophotometer. The TP content is calculated from a standard curve made up under the same conditions from TP samples of 10 to 80 μg per ml.

b) Spectrophotofluorometric determination

Native fluorescence of TP (DUGGAN and UDENFRIEND 1956).

This method, which is based on the native fluorescence of TP at 360 mμ, when activated at 280 mμ, has been applied to plasma from various laboratory animals and man. TP is the only substance normally present in plasma in concentrations high enough to show a measurable fluorescence under the conditions employed; in man the fasting level is about 10 μg per ml. The method is, however, less suited for other tissues, since they usually contain interfering substances and here TP has to be isolated before its determination can be made.

A 1 ml sample of plasma is diluted with 4 volumes of water and acidified with 0.5 ml of 0.6 N H_2SO_4. Protein is precipitated by the addition of 0.5 ml of 10% sodium tungstate ($Na_2WO_4 \cdot 2H_2O$) with constant stirring and is removed by centrifugation. Tungstate ions, which have a slight quenching effect on TP fluorescence, are precipitated by the addition of 1 ml of 0.25 Mbarium chloride to a 3 ml aliquot of the clear tungstic acid filtrate. The precipitate of barium sulphate and barium tungstate is removed by centrifugation. A 2 ml aliquot of the solution is treated with 0.5 ml of 2 M sodium carbonate to precipitate excess barium ions and bring the pH of the sample to the optimal value for TP fluorescence (pH 11). The barium carbonate precipitate is removed by centrifugation for 10 minutes at 3000 r.p.m. A small portion (1 to 1.5 ml) of the supernatant fluid, which should be clear and colourless, is withdrawn and its fluorescence measured at 360 mμ when activated at 280 mμ in a spectrophotofluorometer. Standards prepared by appropriate dilutions of TP in 0.3 M sodium carbonate as well as internal standards (TP added to plasma) are run together with the unknown samples. A reagent blank in which pure water is substituted for plasma is carried through the entire procedure to serve as a fluorescence blank.

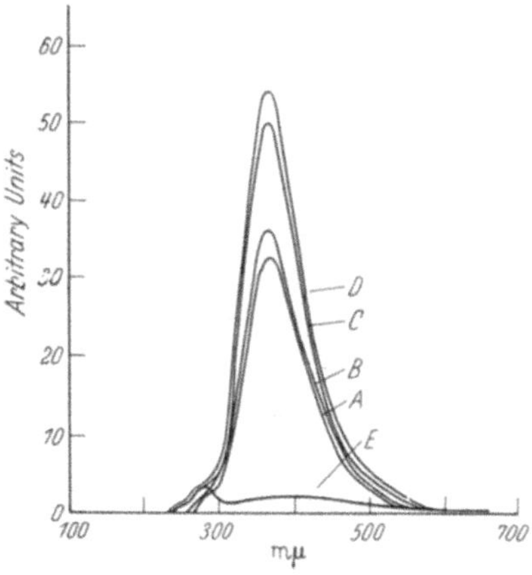

Fig. 11. Fluorescence spectra of TP standards (curves *A* and *C*), plasma TP (curve *B*), plasma plus added TP (curve *D*) and reagent blank (curve *E*). From DUGGAN and UDENFRIEND (1956).

The fluorescence spectra of sample, internal and absolute standards, and blank in a TP determination with the above method is shown in Fig. 11.

Norharman fluorescence (HESS and UDENFRIEND 1959).

When treated with formaldehyde and hydrogen peroxide TP yields — like T — norharman, which is highly fluorescent. This reaction can be applied to trichloroacetic acid filtrates of both plasma and tissue, and offers an extremely specific method for the determination of TP. The sensitivity has been reported to be so great as to allow the assay of TP in fingertip blood. The details of this reaction are given on p. 95, in regard to T.

c) Other methods for the determination of tryptophan

The methods described above are those usually employed in biochemical and pharmacological studies. They are not strictly specific for TP and, of course, do not distinguish between D- and L-TP. The only available procedures which are strictly specific for the L-isomer of TP are those involving microbiological or enzymatic assay. Microbiological assay procedures for L-TP have been published by DUNN et al. (1945) and by SCHWEIGERT et al. (1946). These procedures are, however, rather time-consuming.

SCOTT (1961) has described an enzymatic method for the estimation of L-TP in biological material in the range of 1 to 60 μg. L-TP is converted quantitativly into indole by the enzyme tryptophanase (prepared from acetone dried powder of Escherichia coli), and the indole measured colorimetrically after extraction with light petroleum, with either p-dimethylaminobenzaldehyde or p-dimethylaminocinnamaldehyde reagents.

3. Indoleacetic acid

IAA can be extracted from acidified solutions into non-polar solvents and then returned to aqueous alkali. This separates IAA from related indoles and other interfering substances and it can then be determined by fluorometric or colorimetric methods.

a) Spectrophotofluorometric determination
(WEISSBACH et al. 1959)

A very sensitive procedure for the determination of IAA is based on its fluorescence at 365 mμ when activated at 285 mμ. The procedure is as follows:

An aliquot of deproteinized sample containing 1 to 10 μg of IAA is transferred to a 40 ml glass-stoppered centrifuge tube and acidified by the addition of 0.3 ml of 6 N HCl. 15 ml of chloroform are added and the tube shaken for 1 to 2 minutes. After centrifugation the aqueous layer is removed and discarded. The chloroform phase is washed by shaking with 10 ml of 0.1 N HCl, thus removing any tryptophan that may have been extracted into the chloroform. 10 ml of the chloroform are then transferred to another 40 ml glass-stoppered shaking tube containing 1.5 ml of 0.5 M phosphate buffer pH 7. After thorough shaking and centrifugation, the chloroform layer is discarded. The aqueous phase is transferred to a cuvette and fluorescence determined in a spectrophotofluorometer (e.g. AMINCO-BOWMAN) at 365 mμ when activated at 285 mμ. Standards and reagent blanks are all treated in the same manner.

b) Colorimetric determination
(WEISSBACH et al. 1959).

This method which is based on the xanthydrol reaction of DICKMAN and CROCKETT (1956) is not as sensitive as the fluorometric procedure but may be used on materials where IAA is present in larger amounts, e.g. in human urine. The procedure is as follows:

4 ml of urine in a 40 ml glass-stoppered centrifuge tube are acidified by the addition of 0.36 ml of 12 N HCl. 10 ml of chloroform are added and the tube shaken for 5 minutes. After centrifugation 9 ml of the chloroform are transferred to another 40 ml glass-stoppered tube containing 0.6 ml of 0.5 M phosphate buffer pH 7. The tube is shaken for 5 minutes and the chloroform layer is aspirated and discarded. An aliquot (0.4 ml) of the buffer extract is transferred to a test tube containing 0.4 ml of 12 N HCl; 1 ml of 0.1% xanthydrol in glacial acetic acid (freshly prepared) is added, followed 5 minutes later by 0.5 ml of 5% sodium bisulfite. The solution is mixed and the pink colour measured within 5 to 10 minutes at 520 mμ in a spectrophotometer. Standards and reagent blanks are treated in the same manner. As little as 8 μg of IAA can be detected by this procedure. Optical density is proportional to IAA concentration over the range from 8 to 200 μg. 20 μg IAA carried through the entire method gives an optical density of 0.130.

IAA is usually excreted in the urine in conjugated form and unless a hydrolysis step is included in the procedure, low values — representing only free IAA — will be obtained. The tubes containing the 4 ml urine sample and 0.36 ml of 12 N HCl (see above) are placed in a boiling water bath for 15 minutes. After cooling, the urine is assayed as described above. The normal urinary excretion of indoleacetic acid in man is 3 to 8 mg (as free IAA) and 5 to 14 mg (as total IAA after acid hydrolysis) per 24 hours.

II. 5-Hydroxyindoles

In pharmacology and biochemistry most studies of the 5-hydroxyindoles concern the active 5-HT, its precursor 5-HTP or its main metabolite 5-HIAA.

In the following section different methods for the quantitative determination of these compounds will be described. Reviews of the detection and estimation of 5-hydroxyindoles and related compounds have been published by UDENFRIEND et al. (1958), DALGLIESH (1958), UDENFRIEND and WEISSBACH (1963) and SANDLER (1963).

Determination of total 5-hydroxyindoles

All 5-hydroxyindoles show the same fluorescence characteristics and in tissues where their total content is greater than 1 μg per gram they may be determined directly after precipitation of the proteins with zinc hydroxide (WEISSBACH et al. 1958, UDENFRIEND and WEISSBACH 1963). The following procedure is recommended:

Tissues are homogenized in at least 2 volumes of 0.1 N HCl, and an aliquot of the homogenate corresponding to no more than 2 grams is made up to 8 ml with water. The proteins are then precipitated by the addition of 1 ml of 10 % zinc sulphate followed by 0.5 ml of 1 N NaOH. After thorough shaking the precipitated protein is removed by centrifugation for 15 minutes at 10.000×g. Then 1 ml of the supernatant fluid is transferred to a test tube containing 0.3 ml of 12 N HCl and the fluorescence measured in a spectrophotofluorometer at 550 mμ, using an activation of 295 mμ. Standards (e.g. of 5-HT) and a reagent blank, in which the tissue aliquot is replaced by water, are treated in the same manner.

1. 5-Hydroxytryptamine

The method from which most others for 5-HT assay derive to a greater or lesser extent, is that of UDENFRIEND et al. (1955b), the principle of which was described above in the discussion of extraction procedures (see p. 67).

5-Hydroxytryptamine in tissues

The extraction method which will be described below can be used for most tissues, e.g. brain, lung, gastric and intestinal mucosa, spleen, skin and tumour material (carcinoids). However, for blood and plasma of most animal species this method is not sufficiently sensitive and alternate methods must be employed (see p. 101).

Reagents. Borate Buffer. To 94.2 g of boric acid in 3 liters of water are added 165 ml of 10 N NaOH. The buffer solution is then saturated with purified n-butanol and NaCl by adding these substances in excess and shaking. Excess n-butanol is removed by aspiration and excess salt permitted to settle. The final pH should be approximately 10.

n-Butanol. Reagent grade n-butanol is purified by shaking first whith an equal volume of 0.1 N NaOH, then with an equal volume of 0.1 N HCl, and finally twice with distilled water.

Heptane. Practical grade of heptane is treated in the same manner as the n-butanol.

Procedure. The tissues are homogenized in 2 parts of 0.1 N HCl. A 3 ml aliquot of the homogenate is transferred to a 60 ml glass-stoppered bottle and adjusted to pH 10 by the addition of anhydrous sodium carbonate. After addition of 5 ml of borate buffer pH 10 the solution is diluted with water to a volume of 15 ml and 5 g of NaCl and 15 ml of n-butanol are added. The bottle is shaken for 10 minutes, then centrifuged and the fluid decanted from the solid material into a glass-stoppered centrifuge tube. After centrifugation the aqueous layer is removed by aspiration and the butanol phase washed by shaking with an equal volume of borate buffer. After centrifugation 10 ml of the butanol phase is transferred to another tube containing 20 ml of heptane and 1.5 ml of 0.1 N HCl. After shaking and centrifugation of the tube the supernatant solvent is removed. The aqueous phase containing the extracted 5-HT is then assayed by one of the three following methods:

α) Assay by ultraviolet absorption. The absorption of 5-HT at 275 mμ can be used for the assay when the amine is present in amounts of 0.08 to 0.8 μM per gram of tissue (see p. 73). The method can be applied to studies of the activities of 5-HTP decarboxylase and monoamine oxidase in tissue preparations. The amounts of 5-HT involved in such studies are usually large and the extraction procedure also effectively separates it from either precursor (5-HTP) or end-product (5-HIAA). In experiments where 5-HT is present in tissues, the butanol extract should be washed three times with borate buffer instead of once.

β) Colorimetric assay. The 1-nitroso-2-naphtol method (see p. 79 for procedure) has about the same sensitivity as the ultraviolet absorption technique. However, it is the method of choice when tissue extracts contain large amounts of ultraviolet-absorbing material.

γ) Spectrophotofluorometric assay. The extreme sensitivity of the spectrophotofluorometric assay offers a distinct advantage over both the ultraviolet absorption and the colorimetric method. Depending on the nature of the material to be studied, two methods of measuring the fluorescence may be used:

a) Fluorescence at 330 mμ. In weakly acid solutions (pH 2—4) 5-HT shows a maximal fluorescence at 330 mμ when activated at 295 mμ. This is the most sensitive method available for 5-HT assay. In pure solutions 0.01 μg per ml may be detected.

When this technique is used the final acid solution in the extraction procedure should be adjusted to pH 2—4 — or the 0.1 N HCl replaced by a 0.5 M formate buffer of pH 4 — to obtain maximal fluorescence.

b) Fluorescence at 550 mμ. Extracts of certain tissue (e.g. brain) normally contain materials that fluoresce near 330 mμ and therefore make analysis by the above technique difficult. In such cases the fluorescence at 550 mμ shown by 5-HT in strong acid (3 N HCl), when activated at 295 mμ, is the method of choice. Under these conditions very little interference from other physiological substances occurs. The fluorescence at 550 mμ, although less sensitive than the 335 mμ fluorescence at pH 2—4, is thus more specific for 5-HT and is now the method of assay generally employed in studies of biological material. As little as 0.1 μg of 5-HT can be measured by this technique.

When using the 550 mμ fluorescence for assay, 1 ml of the final HCl extract is added to 0.3 ml of concentrated HCl in a quartz cuvette and the fluorescence determined in a spectrophotofluorometer with activation at 295 mμ (for further details see p. 74).

Specificity of the extraction method

The specificity of the technique described above for the assay of 5-HT has been thoroughly discussed by Bogdanski et al. (1956) and Udenfriend et al. (1958). The material extracted from brain exhibit the same activation and fluorescence spectra as 5-HT. In a counter-current extraction system the 550 mμ fluorescing material was distributed almost identically with 5-HT (see p. 81), and also had the same pharmacological activity on the *Venus mercenaria* heart. Material isolated from rabbit stomach and intestine also proved to be chromatographically identical with 5-HT.

Nevertheless, the technique is not absolutely specific for 5-HT since N-methyl-5-HT and N,N-dimethyl-5-HT, (bufotenine) are also extracted to a minor degree. Fortunately, these compounds are not normally present in mammalian tissues. 5-Methoxy-T, which has the same fluorescence spectrum as 5-HT, also interferes with the procedure. However, 5-methoxyindoles seem thus far to be limited in occurrence to the pineal gland in mammalia, and here occur in rather minute amounts.

Sensitivity and recovery

5-HT added to brain was recovered to the extent of 92—102%. Approximately 0.1 μg of 5-HT can be detected in the procedure but at least 0.3 μg are needed for accurate assay (Bogdanski et al. 1956).

Modifications of the extraction method

A number of modifications of the Udenfriend extraction method have been reported. However most of these concern minor details and seem to have resulted in little improvement of the original technique. Accordingly only a few of these modifications will be mentioned.

Dalgliesh and Dutton (1957) have reported that better recoveries are obtained with a borate buffer of pH 9.5—9.8 than with of pH 10. Crawford and Rudd (1962) confirmed this observation. In the method of Dalgliesh and Dutton the final extraction of 5-HT is further made into 3 N HCl instead of dilute HCl and its fluorescence measured in a filter fluorometer. The method is reported to be satisfactory to a concentration of 0.02 μg per ml of 5-HT.

In the method of Crawford and Rudd (1962) proteins are precipitated with trichloroacetic acid, which is then removed by ether extraction. The rest of their method differs only in the use of isooctane instead of heptane, presumably used because pure isooctane is available commercially.

Cais (1961) deproteinizes sample with perchloric acid and extracts with butanol at pH 11; he replaces heptane with petroleum ether.

5-Hydroxytryptamine in blood

α) Direct assay after protein precipitation. In some animals (e.g. rabbits and chickens) as well as in patients with carcinoid tumours, 5-HT occurs in blood in sufficiently high concentrations (i.e. above 1 μg per ml) to permit an assay by fluorescence techniques made directly on the deproteinized blood filtrate. The procedure, which is that of Weissbach et al. (1958), is as follows:

The blood to be assayed is collected in a siliconized vessel containing anticoagulant (heparin). 1 ml of blood is diluted with 6 ml of water, deproteinized with zinc sulphate and sodium hydroxide and then further treated as described above for the determination of total 5-hydroxyindoles (p. 99).

5-HT concentrations exceeding 0.5—1 μg per ml of blood can be measured by this method . The recovery of 5-HT added to blood is from 85 to 95%.

It must be kept in mind that this is a method for *total 5-hydroxyindoles* measuring not only 5-HT but all other indoles hydroxylated in the 5 position which may be present in the blood. In rabbits and chickens, 5-HT is the only 5-hydroxyindole present, and here the method may be considered specific for this compound.

However, in patients which carcinoid tumours, 5-HIAA is occasionally found in the blood in concentrations as high as 0.5 to 1 μg per ml. In such cases 5-HT must be separated from this compound, and possibly from other 5-hydroxyindoles by extraction of the deproteinized blood with butanol (see below).

β) Assay after protein precipitation and butanol extraction. The 5-HT concentration in blood of many species (e.g. man, dog, guinea-pig, rat and mouse) is so low (less than 0.5 μg per ml) that the above direct method cannot be used for its assay. A combined protein precipitation and butanol extraction procedure has proved satisfactory, however. Such a procedure not only results in specificity, but also increases the sensitivity of the method, since a large volume of deproteinized blood filtrate can be extracted, and since the 5-HT is returned to a small volume of dilute acid.

Waalkes (1959) has described a sensitive fluorometric method for 5-HT in human blood and plasma which is based on the above combination of protein precipitation and butanol extraction. A 3 ml sample of whole blood or plasma collected with EDTA as anticoagulant, is deproteinized with zinc hydroxide. After salt saturation of the blood filtrate, the 5-HT is isolated and concentrated by two alternative methods; either the ordinary butanolheptane method or the ethyl acetate extraction followed by cotton acid succinate as an ion exchange medium. In both methods the 5-HT is obtained in an acid solution, and it is determined by its fluorescence at 550 mμ when activated at 295 mμ.

The range of values for the 5-HT in human blood was found by this method to be 0.09 to 0.18 μg per ml.

5-Hydroxytryptamine in blood platelets

Virtually all the circulating 5-HT found in blood is contained in the platelets.

The method of DILLARD et al. (1951) has been recommended for the isolation of platelets (WEISSBACH et al. 1958, UDENFRIEND et al. 1958, UDENFRIEND and WEISSBACH 1963). The platelets obtained by this method from a 10 ml blood sample are suspended in a measured volume (about 3.5 ml) of saline. An aliquot is taken for protein determination and the remainder used for spectrophotofluorometric 5-HT assay, either using the direct method (see p. 99) or the butanol extraction method (see p. 99). The results are expressed as μg of 5-HT per mg of platelet protein.

5-HT seems to be the only 5-hydroxyindole present in platelets. The direct method of determination is therefore well suited for platelet studies provided the 5-HT concentration is not too low for detection.

5-Hydroxytryptamine in urine

Only small amounts of unchanged 5-HT are normally excreted in the urine (e.g. in humans 50 to 100 μg per day). However, its determination may be indicated on various occasions; in studies of amino acid decarboxylase inhibitors when 5-HTP has been administered or in patients with the carcinoid syndrome. In the latter the 5-HT excretion may increase to 1—2 mg per day.

5-HT in urine may be determined by the method of UDENFRIEND et al. (1955b), described above, but a more recent method of OATES (1961) is the one of choice because of its sensitivity, high recovery and comparative simplicity. The procedure, which employs a carboxylic acid ion exchange resin to separate 5-HT from the urine and a spectrophotofluorometric assay of the latter in the eluate, is as follows:

Amberlite IRC-50 resin (H^+ form) is converted to the NH^+ form by washing twice with approximately 3 volumes of 3 N NH_4OH. The resin is then washed three times with 3 volumes of water and stored in 0.2 N ammonium acetate at pH 7.5.

In a 20 cm long ion exchange column is placed a 50 × 5 mm layer of Amberlite IRC-50 prepared as above. The resin is washed on the column with 5 ml of 0.2 N ammonium acetate pH 7.5 A 1 to 5 ml sample (the volume depending on the expected 5-HT concentration) of the filtered urine is diluted to 6 ml with water. The sample is then adjusted to pH 7.5 with 0.2 N NaOH and applied to the column. After the sample has passed through, the column is carefully washed, first with 10 ml and then 5 ml of 0.02 N ammonium acetate pH 7.5. The 5-HT is then eluted from the column with 5.5 ml of 1 N HCl and the eluate is collected in a graduated tube and made up to 6 ml with 0.1 N HCl. A 1 ml aliquot of the eluate is transferred to a small tube containing 0.3 ml of 12 N HCl and the fluorescence at 540 mμ measured in a spectrophotofluorometer when activated at 290 mμ. Standards which contain 10 μg of 5-HT in 6 ml water, and a water blank, are carried through the procedure together with the unknown sample. The fluorescence is proportional to the 5-HT concentration up to 20 μg in the sample.

Recovery of 5-HT added to urine is 95±5 %. The lower limit of sensitivity of the method is approximately 125 μg of 5-HT per liter of urine when a 5 ml sample is applied to the column.

Urine for 5-HT assay should be kept refrigerated during the collection period and frozen if not analyzed immediately.

Other Methods for the assay of 5-hydroxytryptamine

MEAD and FINGER (1961) have used the catecholamine extraction method of SHORE and OLIN (1958) and found that 5-HT passes into acid butanol as long as salt is present. This renders possible a determination of both the catecholamines and 5-HT on the same tissue homogenate . The acid extraction method is not satisfactory if 5-HTP is present. However, WIEGAND and SCHERFLING (1962) overcame this problem by passing the acid extract from heptane thorough a cation exchange resin with separate elution of 5-HTP, followed by 5-HT.

Several methods employing only ion exchange columns for the separation of 5-HT have been reported. DAVIS and AWAPARA (1960) in their studies of amino acid decarboxylases separated 5-HT from 5-HTP by using a weak cation exchange resin, Amberlite CG-50-H^+. The amino acid passes through the column and the 5-HT is retained, and subsequently eluted with a weak acid.

GLUCKMAN and ABRAMS (1959) employed two columns, and their method is briefly as follows: Tissue homogenates are made with two parts of 0.5 perchloric acid. Following centrifugation, the precipitate is washed twice by rehomogenization with 0.5 M perchloric acid. The combined supernatants are passed through a Dowex 1-OH^- column to remove the perchlorate ions. The eluate is neutralized to pH 7 and its volume reduced to half in a flash evaporator. This material is passed through an Amberlite XE-97-NH_4^+ column. The column is washed with an equal volume of 0.03 M ammonium acetate buffer pH 7 and the 5-HT finally eluted with 1 M formic acid and determined spectrophotofluorometrically (fluorescence 540 mμ and activation 295 mμ).

Several workers have used paper chromatographic and paper electrophoretic procedures for the assay of 5-HT. Some of these methods have been reviewed in the above section on paper chromatography and electrophoresis (see p. 89 and 94). However, most of them are rather laborious, not very accurate and derive from an earlier period of indole biochemistry and pharmacology.

2. 5-Hydroxytryptophan

The amounts of 5-HTP normally present in animal tissues are too small to be detected by any of the methods presently available. However, in experimental work where this amino acid is administered to animals, large amounts (5 μg per gram tissue) are found in the tissues and may be determined spectrophotofluorometrically (UDENFRIEND et al. 1957a). The following procedure is recommended for this type of work.

Spectrophotofluorometric determination (UDENFRIEND et al. 1957a).

To determine 5-HTP the tissues are homogenized in 2 volumes of 0.1 N HCl. 1 ml of this homogenate is diluted with 2 ml of water, and is deproteinized by the addition of 1 ml of 40% trichloroacetic acid. After centrifugation, a 3 ml portion of the supernatant solution is extracted twice with ether to remove trichloroacetic acid and any 5-HIAA present. After the addition of 0.5 ml of 20% Na_2CO_3 to the aqueous phase, it is extracted with 15 ml of n-butanol to remove 5-HT. To 1 ml of the residual aquous solution is added 0.6 ml of 12 N HCl and the fluorescence at 550 mμ measured in a spectrophotofluorometer, using 295 mμ as activation wavelength. Standards of known amounts of 5-HTP are carried through the entire precipitation and the extraction procedure. Reagent blanks are run in the same manner, water being substituted for tissue homogenate.

Tissues from normal animals contain no detectable amounts of 5-HTP. However, they do contain small amounts of some material showing a nonspecific fluorescence at 550 mμ. This fluorescence should be substracted from the values obtained after 5-HTP administration.

When the above method is used it is always advisable to check its specificity by paper chromatography of the residual aqueos extract.

Other methods for 5-hydroxytryptophan

SANDLER and SNOW (1958) have described a small group of carcinoid patients having certain atypical chemical features. In these patients, the urine contains not only 5-HIAA but also relatively large quantities of both 5-HTP and 5-HT. It has been suggested that in these cases the main tumour product is not 5-HT but 5-HTP some of which is then decarboxylated to 5-HT elsewhere in the body (SANDLER et al. 1961).

After Sandlers report the determination of this amino acid in urine of carcinoid patients has assumed increasing importance. SJOERDSMA et al. (1960) have elaborated a method for the determination of 5-HTP in urine which may also be used successfully on tissue extracts. After adjusting to pH 8.4 diluted urine is passed through an Amberlite IRC 50 column which removes any 5-HT present. The column effluent is incubated with a guinea-pig decarboxylase preparation, made from animals which have been pretreated with a monoamine oxidase-inhibitor so that 5-HT formed during incubation is not further metabolized. The incubation mixture is then passed through another IRC 50 column, from which the 5-HT is eluted and measured spectrophotofluorometrically.

3. 5-Hydroxyindoleacetic acid

5-Hydroxyindoleacetic acid in urine

The greater part of 5-HT formed in the body is excreted as 5-HIAA which is a normal constituent of mammalian urine (TITUS and UDENFRIEND 1954, ERSPAMER 1955). Measurement of the urinary excretion of 5-HIAA can, therefore, be used as an indication of the production and metabolism of 5-HT in the body.

Either ultraviolet absorption or fluorescence can be used for determining 5-HIAA, just as for 5-HT as has been already described. However, these methods are less readily applicable to urine than in the case of 5-HT, as extracts containing 5-HIAA essentially free of interfering substances are less readily obtained from urine than are extracts containing 5-HT.

Colorimetric determination.

Colorimetric procedures which are less influenced by other substances in the urine extracts are usually applied for the determination of 5-HIAA. Most procedures described are based either on the 1-nitroso-2-naphtol or the p-dimethylaminobenzaldehyde reaction (see p. 79 and 77).

1-Nitroso-2-naphtol methods

The most popular procedure seems to be a 1-nitroso-2-naphtod methol introduced by UDENFRIEND et al. (1955c). The method depends on the ability to extract 5-HIAA from a salt-saturated aqueous solution into ether. Keto acids, which interfere with the colour reaction, are removed from the urine by treatment with 2,4-dinitrophenylhydrazine and IAA which gives a slight colour with nitrous acid, is extraced with chloroform.

Reagents. *1-Nitroso-2-naphtol,* 0.1% solution in ethanol.

Nitrous acid reagent. To 5 ml of 2 N H_2SO_4 is added 0.2 ml of 2.5% $NaNO_2$. This reagent should be prepared fresh daily.

Ethyl ether. Reagent grade washed once with a dilute solution of ferrous sulphate and twice with water, to remove peroxides.

2,4-Dinitrophenylhadrazine, 0.5% in 2 N HCl.

Phosphate buffer. 0.5 M, pH 7.

Procedure. To 6 ml of urine are added 6 ml of 2,4-dinitrophenylhydrazine solution. After 30 minutes, 25 ml of chloroform are added and the mixture shaken for a few minutes and then centrifuged. The organic layer is removed, replaced with a fresh 25 ml portion of chloroform and the extraction repeated. After centrifugation, a 10 ml aliquot of the aqueous layer is transferred to a glass-stoppered centrifuge tube containing about 4 g of NaCl and 25 ml of ether. The mixture is shaken for 5 minutes. After centrifugation, a 20 ml aliquot of the ether is transferred to another glass-stoppered centrifuge tube containing 1.5 ml of phosphate buffer. The tube is shaken for 5 minutes, centrifuged, and the ether layer is removed by aspiration. 1 ml of the aqueous phase is transferred to a small glass-stoppered centrifuge tube containing 0.5 ml of 1-nitroso-2-naphtol reagent. Following this, 0.5 ml of nitrous acid reagent is added. The sample is then mixed well and warmed at 37° for 5 minutes. Unreacted 1-nitroso-2-naphtol is removed by extraction of the sample with two 5 ml portions of ethyl acetate. The optical density of the final coloured aqueous layer is measured at 540 mμ. Standards of 10 to 200 μg of 5-HIAA per 6 ml and a reagent blank of 6 ml water are treated in the same manner as the unknown sample.

The recovery of 5-HIAA added to urine is about 85%.

The range of urinary 5-HIAA excretion in normal man was found by this method to be 2.0 to 8.2 mg per 24 hours; in dogs, 1.4 to 2.7 mg; and in rabbits, 0.3 to 0.6 mg per 24 hours.

Other methods based on the 1-nitroso-2-naphtol reaction

The above method of Udenfriend et al. (1955c) is rather laborious and low recoveries have been reported by several workers. Modifications have therefore been made. Rivalling it in popularity is the method of Macfarlane et al. (1956; see also Dalgliesh 1958). This method is shorter; requiring about one half the time when compared with the original method. The 2,4-dinitrophenylhydrazine step is omitted, as urines containing significant amounts of keto acids are considered, *a priori*, to be rare. The chloroform step is also omitted, as the interfering pink colour with IAA is quantitatively extracted at the ethyl acetate step of the colour reaction. As all extractions are done in acid solution in which 5-HIAA is relatively stable, it is unneccessary to use peroxide-free ether to prevent destruction of 5-HIAA. The procedure is as follows:

To 5 ml of urine, adjusted to pH 3 with acetic acid, are added 2 g of NaCl and 25 ml of ether. The mixture is shaken for 1 minute and the two phases are then separated by centrifugation. 20 ml of the ether layer is transferred to a flask in which the ether is rapidly removed under reduced pressure. The residue is taken up in 4 ml of water and a measured volume (up to 3 ml, the volume depending on the 5-HIAA content) is transferred to a test tube. 1 ml each of 1-nitroso-2-naphtol reagent and nitrite reagents (see above) are added, and the tubes warmed at 55° for 5 minutes. The solution is then extracted with 10 ml of ethyl acetate, which removes both excess 1-nitroso-2-naphtol and the interfering colour given by IAA. The optical density of the lower layer is read at 540 mμ, preferably after half an hour. The results are obtained from a standard curve prepared at the same time with pure 5-HIAA in amounts of 0 to 90 μg. Recoveries are essentially quantitative, and the standard curve can be made without putting the pure 5-HIAA through the entire procedure. A standard curve may also be prepared using equivalent amounts (on a 5-hydroxyindole basis) of the more stable 5-HT.

The mean excretion of 5-HIAA of man was found to be 7 mg per 24 hours with a range of 3.2 to 13.7 mg.

Schön et al. (1960) obtained very low recoveries (25 to 56%) when 5-HIAA was added to urine and determined by the original method of Udenfriend et al. (1955c). They postulated that this was due to losses incurred at the chloroform extraction step due to formation of emulsions during prolonged shaking. They therefore omitted the chloroform step and passed a dried ethyl acetate extract through an alumina column before taking it back into buffer for the colour reaction with 1-nitroso-2-naphtol.

Drugs interfering with the 1-nitroso-2-naphtol reaction

A source of error in the determination of 5-HIAA in urine arises from the ingestion of certain drugs. After ingestion of phenacetin and related drugs, p-hydroxyacetanilide occurs in the urine and gives a colour reaction (UDENFRIEND et al. 1955b). Ingestion of mephenesin, 3-ortho-toloxy-1,2-propanediol (CURZON 1955, HORNET et al. 1959) and methocarbamol, 3-(o-methoxyphenoxy)-1,2-propanediol monoacarbamate (HORNET et al. 1959) results in metabolites which give an unspecific colour reaction of the urine with 1-nitroso-2-naphtol in the chemical carcinoid screening test of SJOERDSMA et al. (1955). Glyceryl ether of guaiacol, which is widely used as expectorant, also produces urinary metabolites which interfere with the 1-nitroso-2-naphtol reaction — not only in the screening test (SJOERDSMA 1958) but also in the quantitative method of UDENFRIEND et al. (1955c). After ingestion of therapeutic doses of this drug the determination shows falsely high values for 5-HIAA, as high as those usually encountered in malignant carcinoid (PITKÄNEN et al. 1962). Some metabolic product of glyceryl guaiacol ether seems to be the cause of the reaction, as the drug does not react in vitro.

Various derivatives of phenothiazine (e.g. chlorpromazine) have been found to cause a quenching of the colour in the 1-nitroso-2-naphtol reaction (SJOERDSMA et al. 1957, Ross et al. 1958). CHADWICK and WILKINSON (1960) have made a careful study of this quenching effect and found that although these drugs markedly interfere with the screening test of SJOERDSMA et al. (1955), their effect can be minimized by using the more specific extraction method of UDENFRIEND et al. (1955c) before the colour reaction.

p-Dimethylaminobenzaldehyde methods

The p-dimethylaminobenzaldehyde reaction (see p. 77) has been used by several workers for the determination of 5-HIAA in urine.

HANSON and SERIN (1955) used the following procedure for studies of the 5-HIAA excretion in patients with malignant carcinoid:

A 2 ml aliquot of the filtered urine is acidified with one or two drops of 10% HCl and twice extracted with 25 ml of ether. The pooled ether extracts are then filtered, dehydrated with about 3 g anhydrous sodium sulphate, and evaporated to dryness at 50°. The residue is dissolved in 1 ml of 0.1 N HCl, and to 0.2 ml of this solution in a test tube is added 5 ml of p-dimethylaminobenzaldehyde reagent (2% solution in 20% HCl). The solution, and a blank consisting of 0.2 ml of 0.1 N NCl and 5 ml of reagent, are then heated for 2 hours in a water bath at 45—50°. The solutions are next removed from the water bath and immediately diluted with cold 50% ethanol to a volume of 10 ml and the optical density measured in a spectrophotometer at 590 mμ. The results are read from a standard curve made up from known amounts of 5-HIAA. This method permits a determination of 5 μg of 5-HIAA (i.e. 12.5 mg per 1000 ml of urine). The method is not specific for 5-HIAA (see p. 77). However, in cases of malignant carcinoid the 5-HIAA is always the predominating indole and the method is satisfactory for routine clinical work.

ERSPAMER (1956) has used the p-dimethylaminobenzaldehyde reaction after paper chromatographic separation. Concentrated urine is repeatedly precipitated with alcohol-acetone and acetone-ethyl ether (ERPSAMER 1955, see also p. 67) and then chromatographed on paper using the n-butanol-acetic acid-water mixture (4:1:5) as solvent and p-dimethylaminobenzaldehyde reagent as locating reagent. The 5-HIAA spots are then visually compared with respect to area and density of colour with spots obtained with known amounts of pure 5-HIAA.

Another, more precise paper chromatographic method is based on the elution of the spots with water and colorimetric determination of 5-HIAA in the eluate with p-dimethylaminobenzaldehyde reagent (ERSPAMER 1955). To 2 volumes of the eluate is added 1 volume of freshly prepared 2% solution of p-dimethylaminobenzaldehyde in concentrated HCl. The solution is then placed in a water bath at 56—58° for 10—12 hours. The coloured solution is then read in a spectrophotometer at 600 mμ (CORREALE 1955).

In experiments in which 5-HIAA was added to fresh human and dog urine recovery was between 90 and 100% with these paper chromatographic methods.

Storage of urine for 5-hydroxyindoleacetic acid assay

In animal experiments, as well as in clinical work, urine samples for 5-HIAA assay often have to be stored for later analysis. A consensus seems to be that the most satisfactory way to obtain minimal destruction is to bring the urine immediately to pH 2—3 with HCl (DEGKWITZ et al. 1962, FUCHS and FUCHS 1960). When stored for longer periods the acidified samples should be kept frozen.

Fruit diet and 5-hydroxyindoleacetic acid assay

A number of varieties of fruit have been found to contain relatively large amounts of 5-HT. Walnuts may contain as much as 170—340 μg per gram (KIRBERGER and BRAUN 1961), banana peels 50—150 μg per gram and banana pulp 20—30 μg per gram (ANDERSON et al. 1958, UDENFRIEND et al. 1959), grape fruit 10—20 μg per gram (BRUCE 1960, WEST 1960) and tomatoes 5—6 μg per gram (WEST 1958). After ingestion of these fruits 5-HT is metabolized to and excreted as 5-HIAA which may result in falsely high values when endogenous excretion is determined. Ingestion of walnuts and bananas may even increase 5-HIAA excretion enough to falsely suggest a diagnosis of malignant carcinoid (see e.g. CROUT and SJOERDSMA 1959, KIRBERGER 1962).

In experimental studies on 5-hydroxyindole metabolism, as well as in clinical work, it is therefore absolutely mandatory to omit these fruits from the diet before specimens of urine are collected for assay.

5-Hydroxyindoleacetic acid in tissues

The amounts of 5-HIAA normally found in tissues are too small to be determined. However, when 5-HT is added to crude tissue preparations which contain monoamine oxidase and aldehyde dehydrogenase it is oxidized to 5-HIAA via 5-hydroxyindoleacetaldehyde. In studies of this reaction 5-HIAA can be determined spectrophotofluorometrically by the following procedure (UDENFRIEND and WEISSBACH 1963):

An aliquot of the incubation mixture (containing about 2 μg of 5-HIAA is transferred to a glass-stoppered tube, acidified with 1 ml of 1 N HCl, and diluted to 4 ml. The aqueous phase is saturated with solid NaCl, and extracted with 15 ml of peroxide-free ether. After centrifugation, 10 ml of the ether layer are transferred to another tube containing 1.5 ml of 0.5 M phosphate buffer pH 7. After shaking and centrifuging the buffer layer is assayed spectrophotofluorometrically at 340 mμ, when activated at 295 mμ. Standards and reagent blanks are treated in the same manner.

References

ANDERSON, J. A., M. R. ZIEGLER, and D. DOEDEN: Banana feeding and urinary excretion of 5-hydroxyindoleacetic acid. Science **127**, 236—238 (1958).

ARMSTRONG, M. D., K. N. F. SHAW, M. J. GORTATOWSKI, and H. SINGER: The indole acids of human urine. Paper chromatography of indole acids. J. biol. Chem. **232**, 17—30 (1958).

— — and P. E. WALL: The phenolic acids of human urine. J. biol. Chem. **218**, 293—303 (1956).

AXELROD, J., R. O. BRADY, B. WITKOP, and E. V. EVARTS: The distribution and metabolism of lysergic acid diethylamide. Ann. N.Y. Acad. Sci. **66**, 444—435 (1957).

—, and H. WEISSBACH: Purification and properties of hydroxyindole-O-methyl transferase. J. biol. Chem. **236**, 211—213 (1961).

BLAU, K.: Chromatographic methods for the study of amines from biological material. Biochem. J. **80**, 193—200 (1961).
BLOCK, R. J., E. L. DURRUM, and G. ZWEIG: A manual of paper chromatography and paper electrophoresis. New York 1958.
BOARDMAN, N. K.: Molecular sieving other than dialysis. In: H. F. LINSKENS and M. V. TRACEY (eds.), Modern methods of plant analysis, vol. 5, p. 205—213. Berlin-Göttingen-Heidelberg: Springer 1962.
BOBBIT, J. M.: Thin-layer chromatography. New York 1963.
BOGDANSKI, D. F., A. PLETSCHER, B. B. BRODIE, and S. UDENFRIEND: Identification and assay of serotonin in brain. J. Pharmacol. exp. Ther. **117**, 82—88 (1956).
BOWMAN, R. L., P. A. CAULFIELD, and S. UDENFRIEND: Spectrophotofluorometric assay in the visible and ultraviolet. Science **122**, 32—33 (1955).
BRUCE, D. W.: Serotonin in pineapple. Nature (Lond.) **188**, 147 (1960).
BUMPUS, F. M., and I. H. PAGE: Serotonin and its methylated derivatives in human urine. J. biol. Chem. **212**, 111—116 (1955).
BURCHFIELD, H. P., and E. E. STORRS: Biochemical applications of gas chromatography. New York 1962.
CAIS, M.: The spectrofluorometric assay of serotonin and histamine in tissues following a common extraction procedure. Med. exp. (Basel) **5**, 73—76 (1961).
CARCASONA, A., J. CERVOS-NAVARRO u. F. UNTERHARNSCHEIDT: Untersuchungen zur quantitativen Bestimmung von 5-Hydroxytryptamin und 5-Hydroxyindolessigsäure mit dem Spektralphotometer. Klin. Wschr. **37**, 253—254 (1959a).
— F. UNTERHARNSCHEIDT u. J. CERVOS-NAVARRO: Die quantitative Bestimmung von 5-Hydroxytryptophan, 5-Hydroxytryptamin und 5-Hydroxyindolessigsäure mit der Papierchromatographie. Klin. Wschr. **37**, 761—763 (1959b).
— — — u. W. GELLER: Untersuchungen zur quantitativen Bestimmung von 5-Hydroxytryptophan, 5-Hydroxytryptamin und 5-Hydroxyindolessigsäure mit Hilfe der Papierelektrophorese. Klin. Wschr. **38**, 457—460 (1960).
CHADWICK, B. T., and J. H. WILKINSON: The effects of phenothiazine drugs on the determination of urinary 5-hydroxyindolylacetic acid. Clin. chim. Acta **5**, 879—886 (1960).
CHERONIS, N. D., and J. B. ENTRIKIN: Semimicro qualitative organic analysis, p. 730. New York 1957.
CLOTTEN, R., u. A. CLOTTEN: Hochspannungs-Elektrophorese. Stuttgart 1962.
CONSDEN, R.: Paper chromatography. In C. LONG (ed.), Biochemists' Handbook, p. 127—160. London 1961.
COOPER, J. R., and I. MELCER: The enzymic oxidation of tryptophan to 5-hydroxytryptophan in the biosynthesis of serotonin. J. Pharmacol. exp. Ther. **132**, 265—268 (1961).
CORREALE, P.: Colorimetric and spectrophotometric titration of 5-hydroxyindoleacetic acid. Experientia (Basel) **11**, 315 (1955).
CRAIG, L. C.: Countercurrent distribution. In: C. LONG (ed.), Biochemists' Handbook, p. 98—105. London 1961.
—, and D. CRAIG: Extraction and distribution. In: A. WEISSBERGER (ed.), Technique of organic chemistry, vol. 3, p. 171—311. New York 1956.
CRAWFORD, N., and B. T. RUDD: A spectrophotofluorometric method for the determination of serotonin (5-hydroxytryptamine) in plasma. Clin. chim. Acta **7**, 114—121 (1962).
CROUT, J. R., and A. SJOERDSMA: The clinical and laboratory significance of serotonin and catecholamines in bananas. New Engl. J. Med. **261**, 23—26 (1959).
CURZON, G.: A rapid chromatographic test for high urinary 5-hydroxy-indole-acetic acid and 5-hydroxytryptamine. Lancet **1955 II**, 1361—1362.
DALGLIESH, C. E.: Isolation and examination of urinary metabolites containing an aromatic system. J. clin. Path. **8**, 73—78 (1955).
— Two-dimensional paper chromatography of urinary indoles and related substances. Biochem. J. **64**, 481—485 (1956).
— The 5-hydroxyindoles. Advance. clin. Chem. **1**, 193—235 (1958).
—, and R. W. DUTTON: Biogenesis of 5-hydroxytryptophan. Brit. J. Cancer **11**, 296—309 (1957).
DAVIS, V. E., and J. AWAPARA: A method for the determination of some amino acid decarboxylases. J. biol. Chem. **235**, 124—127 (1960).
DEAVER, G. L., W. E. CRISP, and W. J. FRAJOLA: Use of ionophoretic mobility equilibria in fractionation of mixtures containing indoles. Proc. Soc. exp. Biol. (N.Y.) **98**, 632—635 (1958).
DEGKWITZ, R., R. FROWEIN, E. KIRBERGER, C. KULENKAMPFF u. U. MOHS: Über Normalwerte der stündlichen 5-HIES-Ausscheidung im Urin beim Menschen und die Messungen störende Faktoren. Klin. Wschr. **40**, 285—289 (1962).
DEMOLE, E.: Chromatostrips and chromatoplates. Chromatogr. Rev. **1**, 1—10 (1959).

DENFFER, D. VON, M. BEHRENS u. A. FISCHER: Papierelektrophoretische Trennung von Indolderivaten aus Pflanzenextrakten. Naturwissenschaften **39**, 258—259 (1952).

DENGLER, H.: Atypisches Carcinoidsyndrom mit vermehrter Ausscheidung von 5-Hydroxyindolessigsäure bei Pankreascarcinom. Klin. Wschr. **37**, 1245—1248 (1959).

DICKMAN, S. R., and A. L. CROCKETT: Reactions of xanthydrol. IV. Determination of tryptophan in blood plasma and in proteins. J. biol. Chem. **220**, 957—965 (1956).

—, and W. L. WESCOTT: Reactions of xanthydrol. I. Amino acids. J. biol. Chem. **210**, 481—489 (1954).

DIETRICH, L. S.: A rapid method for the determination of dihydroxyphenylalanine decarboxylase in animal tissues. J. biol. Chem. **204**, 587—591 (1953).

DILLARD, G. H. P., G. BRECHER, and E. P. CRONKITE: Separation, concentration, and transfusion of platelets. Proc. Soc. exp. Biol. (N.Y.) **78**, 796—799 (1951).

DUGGAN, D. E., and S. UDENFRIEND: The spectrophotofluorometric determination of tryptophan in plasma and of tryptophan and tyrosine in protein hydrolysates. J. biol. Chem. **223**, 313—319 (1956).

DUNN, M. S., H. F. SCHOTT, W. FRANKL, and L. B. ROCKLAND: Investigations of amino acids, peptides, and proteins: determination of apparent free tryptophan in blood by microbiological method. J. biol. Chem. **157**, 387—394 (1945).

EBLE, J. N., and R. M. BROOKER: A novel quantitative application of thin layer chromatography: Assay of tryptamine. Experientia (Basel) **18**, 524 (1962).

EFRON, M.: High voltage paper electrophoresis. In: I. SMITH (ed.), Chromatographic and electrophoretic techniques, p. 158—189. London 1960.

EGELHAAF, A.: Der Gehalt an freiem Tryptophan und Kynurenin bei den Genotypen a^+ und a von Ephestia kühniella während der Entwicklung. Z. Naturforsch. **12**b, 465—472 (1957).

ERSPAMER, V.: The enterochromaffin cell system and enteramin (5-hydroxytryptamin). R. C. sci. Farmitalia **1**, 1—193 (1954).

— Observations on the fate of indolalkylamines in the organism. J. Physiol. (Lond.) **127**, 118—133 (1955).

— Some observations on the fate of exogeneous 5-hydroxytryptamine (enteramine) in the rat. J. Physiol. (Lond.) **133**, 1—9 (1956).

—, and G. BERTACCINI: Observations on the antidiuretic action and the fate of 5-hydroxy-DL-tryptophan in the rat organism. Arch. int. Pharmacodyn. **137**, 6—23 (1962).

—, and G. BORETTI: Identification and characterization, by paper chromatography, of enteramine, octopamine, tyramine, histamine and allied substances in extracts of posterior salivary glands of octopoda and in other tissue extracts of vertebrates and invertebrates. Arch. int. Pharmacodyn. **88**, 296—332 (1951).

—, and M. B. NOBILI: Observations on the fate of 4-hydroxy-DL-tryptophan in the organism of the rat and man. Arch. int. Pharmacodyn. **137**, 24—38 (1962a).

— — Observations on the fate of DL-5-hydroxy-N-acetyltryptophan and DL-5-acetoxy-N-acetyltryptophan in the rat organism. Arch. int. Pharmacodyn. **139**, 433—446 (1962b).

FALCK, B.: Observations on the possibilities of the cellular localization of monoamines by a fluorescence method. Acta physiol. scand. **56**, Suppl. 197 (1962).

FALES, H. M., and J. J. PISANO: Gas chromatography of biologically important amines. Analyt. Biochem. **3**, 337—342 (1962).

FEARON, W. R., and W. A. BOGGUST: Pigments derived from tryptophan: (1) Urorosein, (2) Tryptochrome. Biochem. J. **46**, 62—67 (1950).

FLODIN, P., and J. PORATH: Molecular sieve processes. In: E. HEFTMANN (ed.), Chromatography, p. 328—343. New York 1961.

FUCHS, A. R., and F. FUCHS: Urinary excretion of 5-hydroxyindoleacetic acid during the menstrual cycle. Dan. med. Bull. **9**, 39—45 (1960).

GAEDTKE, K., u. K. SCHREIER: Eine Methode zur Serotoninbestimmung im Urin. Clin. Chim. Acta **1**, 475—477 (1956).

GAYER, J.: Zum Nachweis biogener Amine. Biochem. Z. **328**, 39—43 (1956).

GELOTTE, B.: Gel filtration. Sorption properties of the bed material sephadex. J. Chromatog. **3**, 330—342 (1960).

GERNGROSS, O., K. VOSS u. H. HERFELD: Über eine hochempfindliche, streng tyrosinspezifische Farbreaktion auf para-substituierte Phenole. Ber. dtsch. chem. Ges. **66**, 435—442 (1933).

GLUCKMAN, M. I., and R. ABRAMS: A method for serotonin determination. Fed. Proc. **18**, 395 (1959).

GOBLE, A. J., D. R. HAY, and M. SANDLER: 5-Hydroxytryptamine metabolism in acquired heart-disease associated with argentaffin carcinoma. Lancet **1955 II**, 1016—1017.

GRAHAM, C. E., E. P. SMITH, S. W. HIER, and D. KLEIN: An improved method for the determination of tryptophane with p-dimethylaminobenzaldehyde. J. biol. Chem. **168**, 711—716 (1947).

HAIS, I. M., u. K. MACEK: Handbuch der Papierchromatographie, Bd. 1. Jena 1958.

HANSON, A.: Unpublished results 1964.

—, and F. SERIN: Determination of 5-hydroxyindoleacetic acid in urine and its excretion in patients with malignant carcinoids. Lancet **1955 II**, 1359—1361.

HARLEY-MASON, J., and A. A. P. G. ARCHER: Use of p-dimethylaminocinnamaldehyde as a spray reagent for indole derivatives on paper chromatograms. Biochem. J. **69**, 60 P (1958).

HECKER, E.: Verteilungsverfahren im Laboratorium. Weinheim 1955.

HEINRICH, P., u. W. SCHULER: Stabilisierte Diazoniumsalze als Reagenzien zur Bestimmung von Dioxybenzolderivaten. II. Über eine kolorimetrische Bestimmungsmethode des 1,2-Dioxybenzols, des Methylaminomethyl-[3,4-dioxy-phenyl]-carbinols und der α-Amino-β-[3,4-dioxyphenyl]-propionsäure. Helv. chim. Acta **31**, 320—330 (1948).

HESS, S. M.: Chemical estimation of tryptamine. In: J. H. QUASTEL (ed.), Methods in Medical Research, vol. 9, p. 175—177. Chicago 1961.

— B. G. REDFIELD, and S. UDENRFIEND: The effect of monoamine oxidase inhibitor and tryptophan on the tryptamine content of animal tissues and urine. J. Pharmacol. exp. Ther. **127**, 178—181 (1959).

— P. A. SHORE, and B. B. BRODIE: Persistence of reserpine action after the disappearance of drug from brain: effect of serotonin. J. Pharmacol. exp. Ther. **118**, 85—89 (1956).

—, and S. UDENFRIEND: A fluorometric procedure for the measurement of tryptamine in tissues . J. Pharmacol. exp. Ther. **127**, 175—177 (1959).

HOLMSTEDT, B., and G. LUNDGREN: Unpublished results 1964.

— V. J. A. VANDENHEUVEL, W. L. GARDINER, and E. C. HORNING: The separation and identification of tryptamine-related indole bases by gas chromatographic methods. Analyt. Biochem. **8**, 151—157 (1964).

HORNET, J. C., T. V. CASEY, and J. W. RUNYAN: False-positive urinary test for 5-hydroxyindoleacetic acid due to methocarbamol and mephenesin carbamate. New Engl. J. Med. **261**, 188—190 (1959).

JEPSON, J. B.: Paper chromatography of urinary indoles. Lancet **1955 II**, 1009—1011.

— Indoles and related Ehrlich reactors. In: I. SMITH (ed.), Chromatographic and electrophoretic techniques, vol. 1, p. 183—211. London 1960.

—, and B. J. STEVENS: A fluorescence test for serotonin and other tryptamines. Nature (Lond.) **172**, 772 (1953).

— P. ZALTZMAN, and S. UDENFRIEND: Microsomal hydroxylation of tryptamine, indoleacetic acid and related compounds, to 6-hydroxy derivatives. Biochim. biophys. Acta (Amst.) **62**, 91—102 (1962).

KAKIMOTO, Y., and M. D. ARMSTRONG: The phenolic amines of human urine. J. biol. Chem. **237**, 208—214 (1962).

KEULEMANS, A. I. M.: Gas chromatography, 2 ed. New York 1959.

KIRBERGER, E.: Differentialdiagnostische Überlegungen bei vermehrter 5-Hydroxyindolessigsäure-Ausscheidung im Harn. Dtsch. med. Wschr. **87**, 829—834 (1962).

—, u. L. BRAUN: Über das Vorkommen von 5-Hydroxytryptamin in der Walnuß. Biochim. biophys. Acta (Amst.) **49**, 391 (1961).

LANGEMANN, H., u. J. KÄGI: Oxytryptamin- und Oxyindolessigsäurebestimmungen bei einem Fall von Carcinoidsyndrom, nebst einigen anderen Untersuchungen über Oxytryptamin. Klin. Wschr. **34**, 237—241 (1956).

LEDERER, M.: A introduction to paper electrophoresis and related methods. Amsterdam 1955.

LERNER, A. B., J. D. CASE, K. BIEMANN, R. V. HEINZELMAN, J. J. SZMUSZKOVICZ, W. C. ANTHONY, and A. KRIVIS: Isolation of 5-methoxyindole-3-acetic acid from bovine pineal glands. J. Amer. chem. Soc. **81**, 5264 (1959a).

— — and R. V. HEINZELMAN: Structure of melatonin. J. Amer. chem. Soc. **81**, 6084 (1959b).

LINSKENS, H. F.: Papierchromatographie in der Botanik. Berlin-Göttingen-Heidelberg 1959.

LOVENBERG, W., H. WEISSBACH, and S. UDENFRIEND: Aromatic L-amino acid decarboxylase. J. biol. Chem. **237**, 89—94 (1962).

MACEK, K.: Techniques of liquid-liquid partition chromatography. In: E. HEFTMANN (ed.), Chromatography, p. 112—163. New York 1961.

MACFARLANE, P. S., C. E. DALGLIESH, R. W. DUTTON, B. LENNOX, L. M. NYHUS, and A. N. SMITH: Endocrine aspects of argentaffinoma, with special reference to the use of the urinary 5-hydroxyindoleacetic acid estimations in diagnosis. Scot. med. J. **1**, 148—155 (1956).

MCILWAIN, H., and R. RODNIGHT: Practical neurochemistry. London 1962.

MCISAAC, W. M., and I. H. PAGE: The metabolism of serotonin (5-hydroxytryptamine). J. biol. Chem. **234**, 858—864 (1959).

MEAD, J. A., and K. F. FINGER: A simple extraction method for the determination of both norepinephrine and serotonin in brain. Biochem. Pharmacol. **6**, 52—53 (1961).

MOHLER, D. N.: Evaluation of the urine test for serotonin metabolites. J. Amer. med. Ass. **163**, 1138 (1957).
MORRIS, C. J. O. R., and P. MORRIS: Separation Methods in Biochemistry. London 1963.
MÜLLER, R.: Zur quantitativen Bestimmung von Indolylessigsäure mittels Papierchromatographie und Papierelektrophorese. Beitr. Biol. Pflanzen **30**, 1—32 (1953).
NÖLLER, H. G., u. P. STELGENS: Die hochspannungselektrophoretische Abtrennung des Serotonins von den übrigen xanthydrolpositiven Substanzen. Clin. chim. Acta **2**, 304—306 (1957).
OATES, J. A.: Measurement of urinary tryptamine, tyramine, and serotonin. In: J. H. QUASTEL (ed.), Methods in medical research, vol. 9, p. 169—174. Chicago 1961.
PITKÄNEN, E., M. M. AIRAKSINEN, O. O. MUSTALA, and J. PALOHEIMO: Observations on the specificity of the urinary 5-hydroxyindoleacetic acid determination with 1-nitroso-2-naphtol. Scand. J. clin. Lab. Invest. **14**, 571—577 (1962).
PROCHÁZKA, Z., 1953: Cited after PROCHAZKA (1958).
— Indolderivate. In: I. M. HAIS u. K. MACEK (eds.), Handbuch der Papierchromatographie, vol. 1, p. 585—592. Jena 1958.
QUAY, W. B.: Differential extractions for the spectrophotofluorometric measurement of diverse 5-hydroxy- and 5-methoxyindoles. Analyt. Biochem. **5**, 51—59 (1963).
RANDERATH, K.: Dünnschicht-Chromatographie. Weinheim 1962.
RAPPORT, M. M., A. A. GREEN, and I. H. PAGE: Serum vasoconstrictor (serotonin). IV. Isolation and characterization. J. biol. Chem. **176**, 1243—1251 (1948).
RIBEIRO, L. P., E. MITIDIERI, and O. R. AFFONSO: Paper Electrophoresis. Amsterdam 1961.
ROBERTSON, J. I. S., and T. M. ANDREWS: Free serotonin in human plasma. Qualitative and quantitative estimation. Lancet **1961 I**, 578—580.
RODNIGHT, R.: Separation and characterization of urinary indoles resembling 5-hydroxytryptamine and tryptamine. Biochem. J. **64**, 621—626 (1956).
ROSS, G., I. B. WEINSTEIN, and B. KABAKOW: The influence of phenothiazine and some of its derivatives on the determination of 5-hydroxyindoleacetic acid in urine. Clin. Chem. **4**, 65—76 (1958).
SANDLER, M.: The determination of hydroxyindoles in biological materials. In: H. VARLEY and A. H. GOWENLOCK (eds.), The clinical chemistry of monoamines, p. 116—130. Amsterdam 1963.
— P. J. SCHEUER, and P. J. WATT: 5-Hydroxytryptophan-secreting bronchial carcinoid tumour. Lancet **1961 II**, 1067—1069.
—, and P. J. D. SNOW: An atypical carcinoid tumour secreting 5-hydroxy-tryptophan. Lancet **1958 I**, 137—139.
SCHANBERG, S. M.: A study of the transport of 5-hydroxytryptophan and 5-hydroxytryptamin (serotonin) into brain. J. Pharmacol. exp. Ther. **139**, 191—200 (1963).
SCHLOSSBERGER, H. G., u. H. KUCH: Synthese von 5,6-Dihydroxytryptophan und verwandten Verbindungen. Justus Liebigs Ann. Chem. **662**, 132—138 (1963).
— — u. I. BUHROW: Abtrennung von Indol-Derivaten aus Urin mittels Sephadex G 25. Hoppe-Seylers Z. physiol. Chem. **333**, 152—153 (1963).
SCHÖN, H., W. ORDNUNG u. E. SCHMID: Zum Nachweis der 5-Hydroxyindolessigsäure im Harn. Klin. Wschr. **38**, 405—406 (1960).
SCHREIER, K., u. K. GAEDTKE: Über die papierchromatographische Bestimmung von Serotonin und anderen Indolkörpern. Naturwissenschaften **43**, 130 (1956).
SCHWEIGERT, B. S., H. E. SAUBERLICH, C. A. ELVEHJEM, and C. A. BAUMANN: Free tryptophan in blood and urine. J. biol. Chem. **164**, 213—221 (1946).
SCOTT, T. A.: An enzymic method for the estimation of L-tryptophan. Biochem. J. **80**, 462—464 (1961).
SHEPHERD, D. M., G. B. WEST, and V. ERSPAMER: Detection of 5-hydroxytryptamine by paper chromatography. Nature (Lond.) **172**, 357 (1953).
SHORE, P. A., and J. S. OLIN: Identification and chemical assay of norepinephrine in brain and other tissues. J. Pharmacol. exp. Ther. **122**, 295—300 (1958).
SJOERDSMA, A.: Clinical and laboratory features of malignant carcinoid. Arch. intern. Med. **102**, 938—940 (1958).
— J. A. OATES, P. ZALTZMAN, and S. UDENFRIEND: Identification and assay of urinary tryptamine; application as an index of monoamine oxidase inhibition in man. J. Pharmacol. exp. Ther. **126**, 217—222 (1959).
— — — — Serotonin synthesis in carcinoid patients. Its inhibition by α-methyl-DOPA, with measurement of associated increases in urinary 5-hydroxytryptophan. New Engl. J. Med. **263**, 585—588 (1960).
— L. L. TERRY, and S. UDENFRIEND: Malignant carcrnoid, a new metabolic disorder. Arch. intern. med. **99**, 1009—1012 (1957).
— H. WEISSBACH, and S. UDENFRIEND: Simple test for diagnosis of α-metastatic carcinoid (argentaffinoma). J. Amer. med. Ass. **159**. 397 (1955).

SMITH, I. (ed.): Chromatographic and electrophoretic techniques. London 1960.
SPRINCE, H., G. R. ROWLEY, and D. JAMESON: Spectrofluorometric studies of 5-hydroxyindoles and related compounds. Science **125**, 442—443 (1957).
STAHL, E. (ed.): Dünnschicht-Chromatographie. Berlin-Göttingen-Heidelberg: Springer 1962.
—, u. H. KALDEWEY: Spurenanalyse physiologisch aktiver einfacher Indolderivate. Hoppe-Seylers Z. physiol. Chem. **323**, 182—191 (1961).
STRELL, M., u. A. KALOJANOFF: Polymethinfarbstoffe. V. Mitt. Eine Erweiterung der Ehrlichschen Reaktion. Chem. Ber. **87**, 1025—1032 (1954).
STURM, A.: Die Bestimmung des Serotonins in Serum mit Hilfe der Hochspannungselektrophorese. Klin. Wschr. **39**, 365—367 (1961).
— Die Bestimmung der 5-Hydroxyindolessigsäure mit Hilfe der Hochspannungselektrophorese. Clin. chim. Acta **7**, 714—721 (1962).
SWEELEY, C. C., and C. M. WILLIAMS: Microanalytical determination of urinary aromatic acids by gas chromatography. Analyt. Biochem. **2**, 83—86 (1961).
TITUS, E. O.: Countercurrent distribution. In: C. D. STEWART, and A. STOLMAN (eds.), Toxicology, vol. 1, p. 392—422. New York 1960.
—, and S. UDENFRIEND: Metabolism of 5-hydroxytryptamine (serotonin). Fed. Proc. **13**, 411 (1954).
TRUTER, E. V.: Thin film chromatography. London 1963.
UDENFRIEND, S.: Fluorescence assay in biology and medicine. New York 1962.
— D. F. BOGDANSKI, and H. WEISSBACH: Fluorescence characteristics of 5-hydroxytryptamine (serotonin). Science **122**, 972—973 (1955a).
— D. E. DUGGAN, B. M. VASTA, and B. B. BRODIE: A spectrophotofluorometric study of organic compounds of pharmacological interest. J. Pharmacol. exp. Ther. **120**, 26—32 (1957b).
— W. LOVENBERG, and A. SJOERDSMA: Physiologically active amines in common fruits and vegetables. Arch. Biochem. **85**, 487—490 (1959).
—, and R. E. PETERSON: Assay of aromatic amino acids. III. Tryptophan. In: S. P. COLOWICK and N. O. KAPLAN (eds.), Methods in enzymology, vol. 3, p. 613—614. New York 1957.
— E. TITUS, and H. WEISSBACH: The identification of 5-hydroxy-3-indoleacetic acid in normal urine and a method for its assay. J. biol. Chem. **216**, 499—505 (1955c).
—, and H. WEISSBACH: 5-Hydroxytryptophan and derivatives. In: S. P. COLOWIGK, and N. O. KAPLAN (eds.), Method in enzymology, vol. 6, p. 598—605. New York 1963.
— — and D. F. BOGDANSKI: Increase in tissue serotonin following administration of its precursor 5-hydroxytryptophan. J. biol. Chem. **224**, 803—810 (1957a).
— — and B. B. BRODIE: Assay of serotonin and related metabolites, enzymes, and drugs. In: D. GLICK (ed.), Methods of Biochemical Analysis, vol. 6, p. 95—130. New York 1958.
— — and C. T. CLARK: The estimation of 5-hydroxytryptamine (serotonin) in biological tissues. J. biol. Chem. **215**, 337—344 (1955b).
WAALKES, T. P.: The determination of serotonin (5-hydroxytryptamine) in human blood. J. Lab. clin. Med. **53**, 824—829 (1959).
— A. SJOERDSMA, C. R. CREVELING, H. WEISSBACH, and S. UDENFRIEND: Serotonin, norepinephrine and related compounds in banana. Science **127**, 648—650 (1958).
WEISSBACH, H., W. KING, A. SJOERDSMA, and S. UDENFRIEND: Formation of indole-3-acetic acid and tryptamine in animals. A method for estimation of indole-3-acetic acid in tissues. J. biol. Chem. **234**, 81—86 (1959).
— T. P. WAALKES, and S. UDENFRIEND: A simplified method for measuring serotonin in tissues; simultaneous assay of serotonin and histamine. J. biol. Chem. **230**, 865—871 (1958).
WEST, G. B.: Tryptamines in edible fruits. J. Pharm. Pharmacol. **10**, 589 (1958).
— Carcinoid tumours and pineapples. J. Pharm. Pharmacol. **12**, 768 (1960).
WIEGAND, R. G., and E. SCHERFLING: Determination of 5-hydroxytryptophan and serotonin. J. Neurochem. **9**, 113—118 (1962).
WOLLISH, E. G., M. SCHMALL, and M. HAMRYLYSHYN: Thin-layer chromatography. Recent development in equipment and applications. Analyt. Chem. **33**, 1138—1142 (1961).
ZYLKA, W., u. T. KÖHLER: Anwendung verschiedener Methoden zum quantitativen Nachweis von 5-Hydroxytryptamin und 5-Hydroxyindolessigsäure bei einem Fall von metastasierendem Dünndarmcarcinoid. Klin. Wschr. **35**, 622—626 (1957).

Chapter 3

Bioassay of indolealkylamines*

By

VITTORIO ERSPAMER

With 5 Figures

I. Extraction of 5-HT and related indolealkylamines from tissues and organic fluids

For a satisfactory extraction of 5-HT from tissues it is sufficient that they be carefully cleaned, minced finely with scissors and then treated with 4 parts (w/v) of pure acetone, to give a final concentration of acetone of approximately 80%.

The completeness and accuracy of this extremely simple procedure, first suggested by ERSPAMER (1940), has been generally confirmed (FELDBERG and TOH 1953, AMIN et al. 1954). However, BONNYCASTLE et al. (1957) claim that simple mincing of the tissues with scissors before extraction with acetone allows only an incomplete extraction and that better results may be obtained if tissues are first minced with scissors and then homogenized before extraction.

On the other hand, AMIN et al. (1954) affirm that 80% acetone extracts from tissues not only 5-HT but also other substances, such as substance *P*, which are capable of interfering with the bioassay of 5-HT especially when using the rat uterus preparation. To eliminate the disturbing polypeptide they recommend extraction of the tissues with 19 parts of acetone, instead of with 4 parts, to give a final concentration of 95% acetone. This suggestion was widely accepted but it soon appeared that 95% acetone, while eliminating to a large extent the interference of substance *P*, failed to produce a satisfactory extraction of 5-HT (CORREALE 1957, BENDITT and WONG 1957).

Table 1 shows the results of unpublished experiments which have been carried out on the ox spleen and the rabbit small intestine in order to determine the suitability of the different procedures which have been suggested for the extraction of 5-HT from tissues.

The extraction procedures used were as follows:

1. the tissue was simply minced with scissors and then extracted with 4 parts of acetone (1a) or 19 parts of acetone (1b);

2. the tissue was passed through a meat grinder and then extracted with 4 parts of acetone (2a), 19 parts of acetone (2b), 4 parts of absolute ethanol (2c), 4 parts of absolute methanol (2d), or boiled for 20 min with 2 parts of distilled water and then treated with 4 parts of acetone (2e);

3. the tissue was homogenized with an equal volume of isotonic saline (homogenizer flask cooled with ice!) and the resulting homogenate extracted with either 4 parts (3a) or 19 parts of acetone (3b);

* The work done in the reviewer's laboratory which is described in this chapter and in chapters 4, 7 and 8 was supported by research grants from the Consiglio Nazionale delle Ricerche, Roma, and the Rockefeller Foundation, New York.

4. the tissue was homogenized directly with 4 parts of acetone (4a) or 19 parts of acetone (4b);

5. the tissue was homogenized with 2 parts of 0.1 N HCl and, after neutralization with Na OH, the homogenate was treated with 4 parts of acetone.

Table 1. *Extraction of 5-HT from ox spleen and rabbit intestine by different solvents and extraction procedures* (explanation in the text)

Extraction procedure	Ox spleen		Rabbit intestine	
	Absolute extraction (μg 5-HT/g tissue)	Percent extraction[1]	Absolute extraction (μg 5-HT/g tissue)	Percent extraction[1]
1a	9.7	100	3.6	100
1b	3.7	38	2.1	57
2a	9.5	97	—	—
2b	4.1	42	—	—
2c	5.2	53	—	—
2d	7.3	75	—	—
2e	10.2	105	—	—
3a	9.5	97	2.6	72
3b	7.1	73	1.1	30
4a	8.1	83	3.6	100
4b	5.6	57	0.9	25
5	7.7	79	3.9	108

[1] Extraction obtained with procedure 1a is considered = 100.

The first extraction lasted 24 hr, then the material was re-extracted for another 24 hr with 3—4 parts of the same solvent, having the same final concentration.

All the extracts were assayed on the rat uterus preparation.

Recovery of 5-HT added to ox spleen homogenates, obtained with either isotonic saline or 0.1 N HCl, before addition of 4 parts of acetone, was 90—107%.

The results of some additional experiments carried out on rat tissues and on the posterior salivary glands of *Eledone moschata* are shown in Table 2.

Ox spleen and posterior salivary glands minced with scissors and then extracted twice with 95% acetone, were re-extracted with 60% acetone and then boiled with distilled water. Only a fraction of the 5-HT retained in the tissues following treatment with 95% acetone was recovered in this way.

Unlike tissue 5-HT, serum 5-HT can be extracted with 19 vol of acetone as completely as with 4 vol. Eighty per cent or, still better, 70% acetone affords a complete extraction of the indolealkylamines and phenylalkylamines contained in dry amphibian skin. It is, however, advisable to prolong extraction for 7—14 days (Erspamer, unpublished observations).

Table 2. *Extraction of 5-HT from rat tissues and posterior salivary glands of Eledone moschata by different procedures* (explanation in the text)

Tissue	Yield of 5-HT (μg/g) after extraction procedure					
	1a	1b	3a	3b	4a	4b
Rat brain . . .	0.7	0.27	0.55	0.25	—	—
intestine .	4.3	2.4	3.4	2.1	—	—
spleen . .	3.2	1.2	3.6	2.0	—	—
Eledone moschata posterior salivary glands .	450	140	420	180	430	160

Fenster and Towne (1963) and Towne and Kalayil (1964) have called attention to the possibility that lipids extracted from tissues by acetone produce a solubilization of 5-HT in lipid solvents such as petroleum ether, which is sometimes used to remove fats. This solubilization might represent a remarkable source of error in the bioassay of 5-HT.

Generally treatment of acetone extracts with petroleum ether is completely superfluous. If necessary, the eventual passage of 5-HT into ether should be checked.

The above results demonstrate that treatment with 80% acetone, preceded by mincing of the tissues with scissors, represents the most simple and convenient procedure for a complete extraction of 5-HT from the tissues of both vertebrates and invertebrates. 95% acetone, as recommended by several investigators, can be used only for serum and possibly for other organic liquids. For tissues it is incapable of assuring a satisfactory extraction of 5-HT. In fact, only 30 to 50% of tissue 5-HT can be found in 95% acetone and the aliquot of the amine which does not pass into 95% acetone is tenaciously retained in the tissue, from which, subsequently, it cannot be completely recovered with any solvent, not even boiling water. In no instance and under no conditions do homogenized tissues give higher yields of 5-HT than tissues simply chopped up with scissors before extraction. On the contrary, especially when tissues are homogenized with saline, remarkable losses in 5-HT recovery may frequently be observed. They are probably to be ascribed to the monoamineoxidase made disposable in active form during homogenization.

Homogenization of tissues with 0.1 N HCl, as usually carried out in the spectrofluorometric estimation of 5-HT, does not produce any better extraction of the amine than 80% acetone. Besides, acid extracts cannot be stored as easily as acetone extracts.

II. Smooth muscle preparations used in the bioassay of indolealkylamines

1. Rat uterus

a) Erspamer's original method

The isolated rat uterus has been proposed by Erspamer for the quantitative estimation of 5-HT since 1940 (see also 1948, 1954, 1955).

Preparation of the uterus. Young rats, weighing 120—160 g, are ovariectomized and then, after a recovery period of at least a week, injected subcutaneously, on two successive days, with single doses of 100—200 μg of oestradiol dipropionate. The uterus is removed 3—5 days after the first injection and suspended in an aerated 10 ml. bath of Tyrode solution containing atropine (10^{-6}) at 29—31° C. The gimbal lever magnification is generally 4 to 6 and the tension 1 g. The composition of the Tyrode solution is as follows: sodium chloride, 8 g; potassium chloride, 0.2 g; calcium chloride, 0.2 g; magnesium chloride, 0.1 g; sodium bicarbonate, 1 g; sodium dihydrogen phosphate, 0.05 g/l. The response of the uterus preparation is recorded for 3—4 min, and doses are repeated at intervals of 6 to 7 min.

Response of the uterus. The response of the uterus usually consists of a number of contractions between which partial relaxation occurs, so that the full response consists of waves of contraction superimposed on a more or less sustained tonic contraction. Although all aspects of the uterus response must be considered during the assay, particular emphasis is laid on sustained contraction, not only on the height of this contraction but also how well it is maintained. As shown in Fig. 1 the rise in sustained contraction is satisfactorily proportional to the dose of 5-HT. Washing with fresh nutrient liquid produces immediate relaxation and prompt return to the base-line. There is no sign of tachyphylaxis or sensitization.

A good uterine preparation always responds to 5 ng 5-HT/ml and often the sensitivity increases up to 1 ng/ml (Erspamer 1954, Schwartz 1955, Leitsch et al. 1958). Uterine horns which do not react to 10—20 ng/ml 5-HT should be rejected. Satisfactory result are obtained in 70—80% of the experiments. According to Supek and Milković (1956) the average limit of error of the method ($P = 0.05$) is 10.5%, but in the writer's opinion it may be consistently less in good preparations.

Outside the oestrus-period the uterus is considerably less sensitive to 5-HT and unsuitable for the bioassay of the amine (ERSPAMER 1954, ROBSON et al. 1954, BUSCH 1956).

Specificity of the method. The stimulant action of *acetylcholine* may be completely blocked by atropine (10^{-6}—10^{-7}). *Histamine* inhibits the rat uterus, but this inhibitory effect seems to be of no practical importance, since as much as 10 μg histamine is required to reduce by 20% the stimulant action of 0.04 μg 5-HT.

Tyramine, octopamine, dopamine, noradrenaline and *adrenaline* all inhibit the uterus preparation but practically only adrenaline deserves consideration. In fact, 0.1—0.2 μg adrenaline is sufficient to halve the response to 0.2 μg 5-HT Noradrenaline, which is certainly the catecholamine most likely to occur in tissue

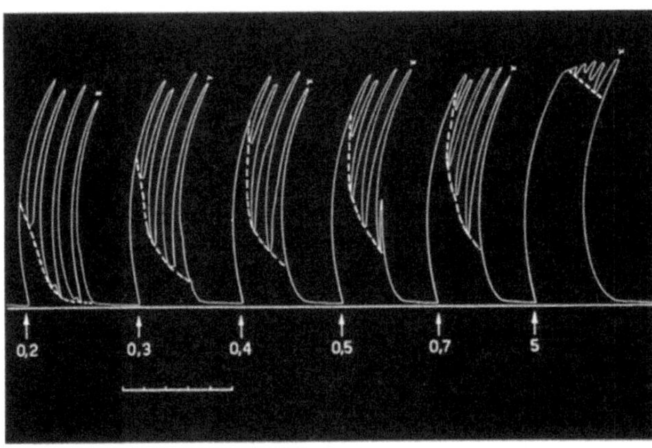

Fig. 1. The response of the rat oestrus-uterus to doses of 5-HT picrate in μg. Bioassay is based not so much on the amplitude of single contractions as on the maintenance of diastolic tone (see area between broken line and base line). A 10 ml bath containing Tyrode solution was used. Time in min. *x* wash. [From Fig. 23, ERSPAMER, V., Rend. sci. Farmitalia 1, 122 (1954).]

extracts together with 5-HT, displays an inhibitory effect which is 50—100 times less intense. If catecholamines, especially adrenaline, are suspected of being present in an extract, they can be differentially destroyed by a procedure such as that used by GARVEN (1956).

Adenosine and *adenosine triphosphate* possess a stimulant action which is at least 2000—5000 times less than that of 5-HT.

Polypeptides probably represent the most important potential source of error in the bioassay of 5-HT by the rat uterus method. However, whereas the uterus is extremely sensitive to some polypeptides, it is rather insensitive to others.

Among the biogenic polypeptides which potently stimulate the uterus are angiotensin, oxytocin and the kinins, the respective threshold concentrations being approximately 1—2 ng, 0.01—0.05 milliunits, and 0.01—0.1 ng/ml (synthetic bradykinin).

A relevant example of the heavy interference of bradykinin-like polypeptides in the bioassay of 5-HT and related indolealkylamines is given by some extracts of amphibian skin which may contain amounts of kinins equiactive to 500—10.000 μg 5-HT per g tissue (ERSPAMER and co-workers, unpublished observations).

The current opinion that substance *P* may consistently disturb the assay of 5-HT in brain or intestinal extracts seems to be hardly tenable after the recent demonstration that pure substance *P* has a very poor stimulant action on the rat uterus (HAEFELI and HÜRLIMANN 1962, CLEUGH and GADDUM 1963).

Eledoisin, physalaemin and other polypeptides behave like substance *P* (ERSPAMER and FALCONIERI ERSPAMER 1962, ERSPAMER and co-workers, unpublished observations).

Fortunately, incubation with chymotrypsin at pH 7.5—8 offers the possibility of destroying the activity of all disturbing polypeptides leaving unaffected that of 5-HT and related indolealkylamines.

As research progresses the number of active compounds which are found in tissues and which are capable of interfering with the bioassay of 5-HT by the rat uterus method is increasing. It is therefore advisable to check the reliability and specificity of the method not only in the case of extracts of different biological materials but even in the case of extracts of the same material obtained from different species.

Obviously, this statement is valid not only for the rat uterus but also for all other smooth muscle preparations used in the bioassay of indolealkylamines.

b) Gaddum's technique

According to GADDUM and HAMEED (1954) and to AMIN et al. (1954) ovariectomy does not appear to be essential. Stilbestrol (0.1 mg/kg in arachis oil) is injected subcutaneously into a virgin rat weighing 160—200 g and the next day the uterus is removed and the middle 2 cm of one horn is suspended in an aerated 2 ml bath of JALON's solution containing atropine (10^{-6}) at 30°. The composition of the JALON's solution is as follows: sodium chloride, 9; potassium chloride, 0.4; calcium chloride, 0.06; sodium bicarbonate, 0.15; glucose, 1 g/l.

The lever magnification is about 10 and the tension 1 g weight. The time interval between doses is usually 4 min and the drug is left in the bath for 40 to 60 sec, the contact being interrupted as soon as the first contraction of the muscle has attained its maximum.

It clearly appears that the criteria adopted by the writer and by GADDUM in evaluating the uterine response are somewhat divergent.

If a higher sensitivity is required from the rat uterus then it may well be worth while trying the technique of superfusion described by GADDUM (1953).

In order to eliminate in the bioassay of 5-HT the interference of disturbing substances, SUPEK and RANDIĆ (1961) suggest enriching tissue extracts, especially brain extracts, with a known amount of exogenous 5-HT (e.g. 2 μg/g fresh tissue). By adding 5-HT artificially, the enriched extract can then be diluted to such an extent that all interfering substances are present in biologically inactive concentrations. According to SUPEK and RANDIĆ the limit of error ($P=0.05$) of assays of this type is relatively high (20%).

Instead of JALON's solution, PUT and HOGENHUIS (1962) recommend a nutrient liquid of the following composition: sodium chloride, 8.1; potassium chloride, 0.246; calcium chloride, 0.139; magnesium chloride $+6\,H_2O$, 0.243; sodium bicarbonate, 1.76; sodium dihydrogen phosphate $+\,H_2O$, 0.066; urea, 0.132; glucose, 0.611; and atropine sulphate, 0.001 g/l. Bath temperature 30°.

2. Rat fundus strip

Preparation of the fundus strip. The stomach is dissected free from the abdomen and dropped into the bathing solution. The pyloric antrum is removed, except for a small band, and the fundal content washed away. The fundus, which appears as a translucent balloon-like tissue, is then cut into a strip by opening the fundus along the lesser curvature and cutting to preserve the longitudinal musculature. The resultant strip is then hung in a small bath and the movements recorded by an isotonic lever. It is convenient to leave a small band of pyloric tissue still attached to the fundus, to act as a marker, and so prevent cutting in the wrong direction after the fundus has been opened into a flat plate (Fig. 2).

After the strip has been suspended it is important for it to be allowed to recover and relax for 15 to 60 min before starting stimulation. During this period the bathing solution is either allowed to perfuse through the organ bath at a rate of about 1 ml/min or is changed by overflow at about 6-min intervals.

Bath and bathing solutions. Generally a bath 15 cm long holding 5 to 10 ml of fluid is used. Of the various bathing solutions which have been tried the most

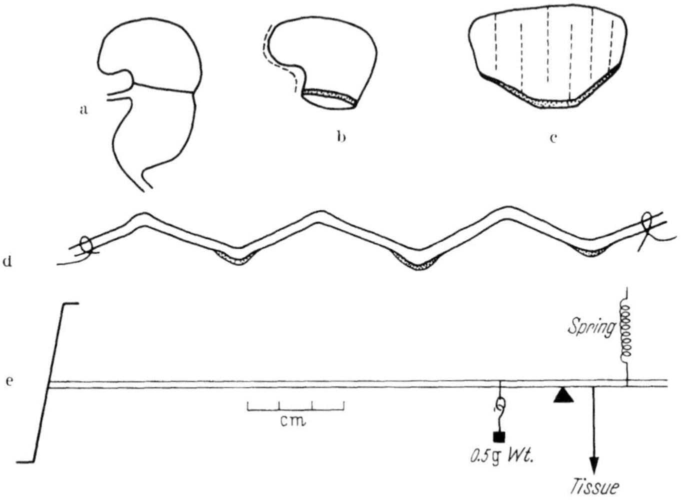

Fig. 2a—e. Diagram showing the method of cutting the rat fundal strip and the arrangement of the lever. (a) The whole stomach. (b) The fundus, left with a thin band of pyloric tissue and cut along the dotted line. (c) The fundus opened into a plate of tissue and cut along the dotted lines. (d) The strip pulled out by cotton tied to each end, so that protrusions of bits of pyloric tissue can be cut off. (e) The lever, showing the relative positions of the load, the tissue and the spring. Without any of these, the lever should come to rest horizontally. The scale refers to the lever only. [From Fig. 1, VANE, J. R., Brit. J. Pharmacol. 12, 345 (1957).]

suitable seem to be the two following, recommended by VANE (1957) and UUSPÄÄ and UUSPÄÄ (1962), respectively:

a) rat uterus Ringer: sodium chloride, 9; potassium chloride, 0.4; calcium chloride, 0.06; sodium bicarbonate, 0.15; glucose, 1 g/l.

b) sodium chloride, 8; potassium chloride, 0.4; calcium chloride, 0.17; sodium bicarbonate, 0.3; glucose, 0.3 g/l.

In both Krebs and Tyrode solutions the muscle is slightly more sensitive to 5-HT, but the spontaneous movements are greater than in rat uterus Ringer solution.

The bathing solution is actively aerated with oxygen at 37°. Lower temperatures make the muscle less sensitive, while higher temperatures elicit greater spontaneous movements. Washing of the preparation is always by overflow.

Lever. A balsa wood lever with a frontal writing point, completed with a light spring and a vibrator was originally used by VANE (1957), but later on abandoned in favour of a simple Palmer lever with an all-metal frontal writing point and PATON's pendulum. Magnification is about 15-fold and the load on the preparation varies between 1 and 3 g (VANE 1958, UUSPÄA and UUSPÄÄ 1962).

Assay cycle. 5-HT is added to the bath and the contraction is allowed to develop for 90—120 sec. The bath is then washed out and a weight added to the lever so that it comes to rest immediately on a bar fixed at a predetermined level.

After a constant time (15 to 30 sec depending on the individual muscles) the extra weight is removed. The tissue rapidly regains its basal length and after a further 2 min the next dose is added. Stretching the muscle to a fixed length is necessary owing to excessive slowness of spontaneous relaxation.

It also seems possible, when the writing point does not fall to the base line spontaneously, to drop the lever by gently knocking against the working table (Uuspää and Uuspää 1962).

The greatest difficulties in using the fundus strip arise from the already mentioned slowness of relaxation after a dose of 5-HT and from changes in the resting length of the muscle. However, when very high sensitivity is not needed and, hence, it is not required to use only the bottom part of the dose/response

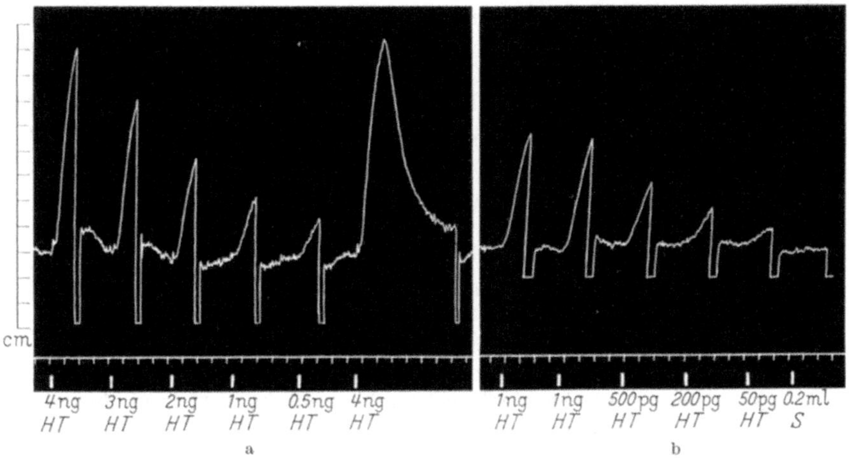

Fig. 3a and b. (a) The response of the rat fundal strip to doses of 5-HT in nanograms (ng). The drum was left running continuously to illustrate the cycle. The second dose of 4 ng 5-HT shows the slowness of relaxation if the tissue is not stretched. (b) A more sensitive preparation showing responses down to 50 picagrams (pg) 5-HT, with an injection of 0.2 ml saline (*S*) at the end. A 5 ml bath containing rat uterus Ringer at 37° was used. The vertical scale is in cm. Time in min. [From Fig. 2, Vane, J. R., Brit. J. Pharmacol. **12**, 346 (1957).]

curve, then it is not necessary to maintain a stable baseline during the assay and, consequently, the preparation becomes easier to handle.

Sensitivity to 5-HT. The most sensitive preparations may give a measurable response even to 0.01 ng 5-HT/ml; tissues with average sensitivity respond to 0.02—0.06 ng 5-HT/ml (Vane 1957) (Fig. 3).

Specificity of the method. According to Vane the following doses of other biogenic compounds are required to produce a contraction similar to that given by 1 ng 5-HT: acetylcholine, 10 ng; histamine, more than 1 μg; adenosine triphosphate, 20 μg; pitressin, 0.4 units; potassium chloride, 2 mg; tryptamine hydrochloride 0.25 μg; 4-hydroxytryptamine 1.8 ng; 5-methoxytryptamine, 20 ng. In their turn Erspamer and Falconieri Erspamer (1962) found that 1 ng 5-HT was equivalent to approximately 25—50 ng eledoisin, 250—1000 ng bradykinin and 3—6 units substance *P*.

Sympathomimetic amines relax the fundal strip and reduce the response to 5-HT. For example, 25—30 ng of either adrenaline or noradrenaline are sufficient to halve the effect of 5 ng 5-HT. In order to render the muscle insensitive to acetylcholine, hyoscine hydrobromide or atropine sulphate (10^{-7}) is added to the bathing fluid. The interference of polypeptides and catecholamines may be excluded in the manner previously described.

Assay precision. According to UUSPÄÄ and UUSPÄÄ the limit of error of the method corresponding to 5% level of significance is 8.8%.

Advantages and disadvantages of the fundus strip in comparison with the uterus. The main advantages of the fundus strip over the rat uterus are, according to VANE (1957), that it does not need pretreatment of the donor rat, that it will work in several bathing solutions, and that it can always be relied upon to respond to 0.2 ng and very often to 0.02 ng 5-HT per ml bathing fluid.

Actually, the only important advantage is that of the greater sensitivity of the fundus strip. This preparation is decidedly to be preferred whenever 5-HT is present in low concentrations and the interference of disturbing substances may be excluded. The other advantages are either inconsistent or largely neutralized by the tedious cutting of the fundal strip, and the difficulty of relaxation of the preparation, requiring stretching and removing of extra weights from the lever. It should be added that the choice between stomach fundus and uterus is not only a matter of sensitivity, but also of specificity. The rat stomach, for example, is relaxed by noradrenaline and contracted by substance *P*, eledoisin and eledoisin-like polypeptides much more potently than the rat uterus and this, conversely, is more sensitive to bradykinin-like polypeptides and to oxytocin than the fundus strip.

3. Rat colon

This preparation was first recommended for the assay of 5-HT by DALGLIESH et al. (1953).

The part of the rat colon nearest the caecum is suspended in 5—20 ml of a Ringer solution of the following composition: sodium chloride, 9; potassium chloride, 0.4; calcium chloride, 0.03; sodium bicarbonate, 0.15; and glucose, 1 g/l. The temperature of the bath is 22—24°. Test substances are added to the bath at 4—5 min intervals and kept in the bath for 1.25—1.5 min.

According to SUPEK and MILKOVIĆ (1956) the average concentration of 5-HT producing a suitable response by the colon preparation is 20—30 ng/ml. It may be seen that this concentration is higher than that required to elicit a similar response by the rat uterus.

The atropinized rat colon is practically insensitive not only to acetylcholine but also to histamine, while giving moderate responses to the usual biogenic polypeptides.

SUPEK and MILKOVIĆ found that the average limit of error ($P = 0.05$) of this method is 8.8%, and they affirm that the colon is to be preferred to the uterus in the assay of 5-HT. This opinion, however, is not shared by GADDUM and HAMEED (1954) nor by the writer.

4. Guinea-pig ileum

Preparation of the ileum. The lowest piece of the gut next the colon is found especially sensitive and animals which have fasted for 18 hr provide the best preparations. The gut is suspended in a 2—10 ml bath containing Tyrode or Krebs solution maintained at 30—37° and the movements of the longitudinal muscle are recorded with a common gimbal lever or with a lever with a frontal writing point. During assays the drug is left in the bath for 40 sec and doses are repeated at intervals of 4—5 min (AMIN et al. 1954, GADDUM and HAMEED 1954, BARLOW and KAHN 1959).

Sensitivity and specificity of response. Not only is the sensitivity of this preparation at least 10 times less than that of the rat uterus but, what is more important, the specificity of the response is unsatisfactory. It is difficult to find another smooth muscle preparation which is contracted by such a variety of active tissue constituents as the guinea-pig ileum is. To remain in the field of polypeptides, the preparation is stimulated by vasopressin, angiotensin, bradykinin-like polypeptides, substance *P*, eledoisin, physalaemin etc. In addition the guinea-pig ileum may be extremely sensitive to lipid-soluble organic acids such as prostaglandin, vesiglandin, darmstoff, irin, slow-reacting substance *A* etc., with the disadvantage that these compounds cannot be inactivated by proteolytic enzymes.

On the whole it may be stated that the guinea-pig ileum is unsuitable not only for the quantitative estimation of 5-HT but even for the qualitative detection of the amine in crude biological materials.

5. Isolated rabbit ear

The isolated rabbit ear is perfused at room temperature through a cannula in the central artery. A special injection device is interposed between the reservoir

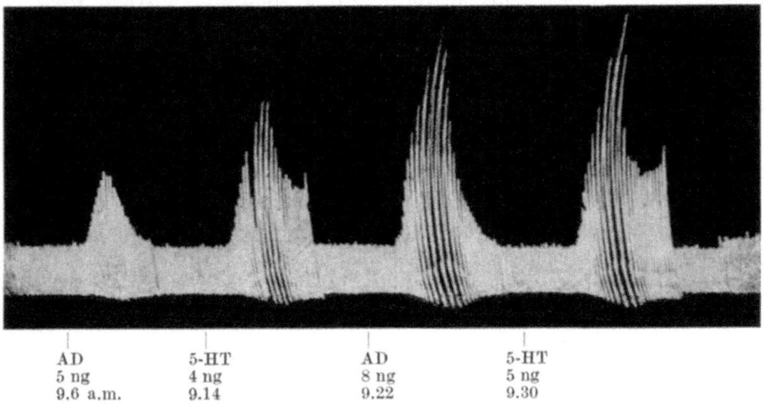

Fig. 4. The response of the perfused rabbit's ear to doses of 5-HT and adrenaline (AD) in nanograms (ng). Height of record shows interval between drops. It may be noted that the vasoconstrictor effect of 5-HT is more potent than that of adrenaline. [From Fig. 5, Gaddum, J. H., and K. A. Hameed, Brit. J. Pharmacol. **9**, 244 (1954).]

containing the perfusion fluid and the arterial cannula. The ear is placed on a draining plate and the perfusate from the cut surface is led to a drop counter system.

The most highly recommended perfusion fluid is that used by Page and Green (1948) for the study of serum vasoconstrictor. It has the following composition: sodium chloride, 8.2; potassium chloride, 0.84; calcium chloride + 2 H_2O, 0.04; magnesium chloride + 6 H_2O, 0.06; sodium bicarbonate, 0.4; and glucose, 1 g/l. To each litre is added 10 ml of phosphate buffer containing 4 parts of 1 *M* K_2HPO_4 to 1 part of 1 *M* KH_2PO_4.

When this solution is used the ear is much more sensitive to vasoconstrictor substances than when Locke's solution is used. The ear is always more sensitive the day after being kept overnight in the refrigerator.

The sensitivity of the preparation to 5-HT is of the order of 1 ng or even less (Gaddum and Hameed 1954, Bertaccini and Zamboni 1961) (Fig. 4).

However, the rabbit ear, while presenting possibilities of advantageous use in the assessment of the relative potencies of pure 5-HT-like substances and in the study of anti-5-HT drugs, does not seem to be suitable for the quantitative estimation of 5-HT or other indolealkylamines in crude tissue extracts.

The preparation is, in fact, tremendously sensitive to catecholamines and remarkably sensitive to other biogenic amines as well as to vasoactive polypeptides and, as a consequence, its response is by no means specific for 5-HT.

6. Molluscan heart

a) *Venus mercenaria*

The isolated heart of *Venus mercenaria* was first recommended by WELSH and TAUB in 1955, and since then it has become the molluscan heart most frequently used in the bioassay of 5-HT.

Method for preparing the heart. Specimens of *Venus mercenaria* with a shell length of 8 to 12 cm have been found to be the most convenient size. After removal from the sea they may be stored for one or two weeks in shallow tanks of aerated sea water, at 15—18°, or kept dry at 5—10°.

The heart is exposed by breaking and removing the dorsal portion of the shells (umbos and hinge) and then cutting away the mantle and pericardium dorsal to the heart. The heart consists of a single median ventricle with laterally disposed, thin-walled atria. Anterior and posterior blood vessels leave the heart in close association with the intestine which passes through the heart. Threads for attaching it to a support in the bath and to a writing lever may be passed under the atria and tied close to the ventricle in order to include some of the thicker-walled ventricular muscle. Cutting the atria distal to the threads and cutting the bloods vessels and the intestine isolate the ventricle, which may then be placed in an appropriate heart bath. A bath holding 10 ml when filled has been found appropriate. The heart lever should be counterweighted to give a pull of 200 to 300 mg.

According to MCINTYRE et al. (1960), for best results the heart should be suspended so that the contiguous segment of gut lies transversely and not parallel with the contraction axis of the heart.

Sea water thermostatically maintained at 15—18° is an adequate perfusion fluid for the isolated heart. Another fluid found satisfactory has the following composition: sodium chloride, 30; potassium chloride, 0.9; calcium chloride, 1.1; magnesium sulphate $+3\ H_2O$, 3.5 g/l; with a phosphate or bicarbonate buffer (pH 7—7.5). Oxygen may be supplied by air or a mixture of 95% O_2 and 5% CO_2 passed through the bath (WELSH and TAUB 1955).

Response of the heart. The response of the *Venus* heart to 5-HT has three components: an increase in amplitude, an increase in frequency, and an increase in the resting tone of the muscle. The relative importance of these components varies with the concentration. Between threshold concentration (about 10^{-10}) and moderately high doses (about 10^{-7}) the response of the *Venus* heart to 5-HT is mainly an increase in the amplitude of beat. There is also an increase in frequency which, however, does not seem to be dependable. Above 10^{-7} 5-HT the relative increase of the tone becomes larger, and at 10^{-6} the effect is almost all increase in tone while rhythmical excursions of the heart are very small (Fig. 5).

The bioassay of 5-HT is mainly based on the difference between the amplitude of beat before and after the addition of the drug. Thus, the most reliable results are obtained with concentrations of 5-HT varying between 1 and 10—20 ng/ml. With these concentrations the heart amplitude varies linearly with the log concentration (WELSH and TAUB 1955, WELSH 1957, GREENBERG 1960a, 1960b, MCINTIRE et al. 1960).

Specificity. There are, on the whole, meagre data on the specificity of the response of the *Venus* heart to 5-HT. However, it should be emphasized that:

(a) acetylcholine displays on the *Venus* heart a powerful inhibitory action, the threshold concentration being 10^{-10} to 10^{-11}. If present, the disturbing action of acetylcholine may be eliminated either by benzoquinonium chloride (10 μg/ml) or by enzymatic hydrolysis.

(b) the *Venus* heart is 5- to 30-fold more sensitive to bufotenine and twice as sensitive to N-methyl-5-HT as to 5-HT itself (Bumpus and Page 1955, Greenberg 1960b). Thus, bioassay of 5-HT is impossible in the presence of these N-methylated derivatives. This statement is valid also when the *Helix* heart is used instead of the *Venus* heart (Bertaccini and Zamboni 1961).

(c) both invertebrate and vertebrate tissues and fluids may contain unknown substances capable of stimulating the *Venus* heart or of increasing its sensitivity to 5-HT and hence of invalidating any attempt at quantitative estimation of the amine (Welsh 1956, Bowers 1962).

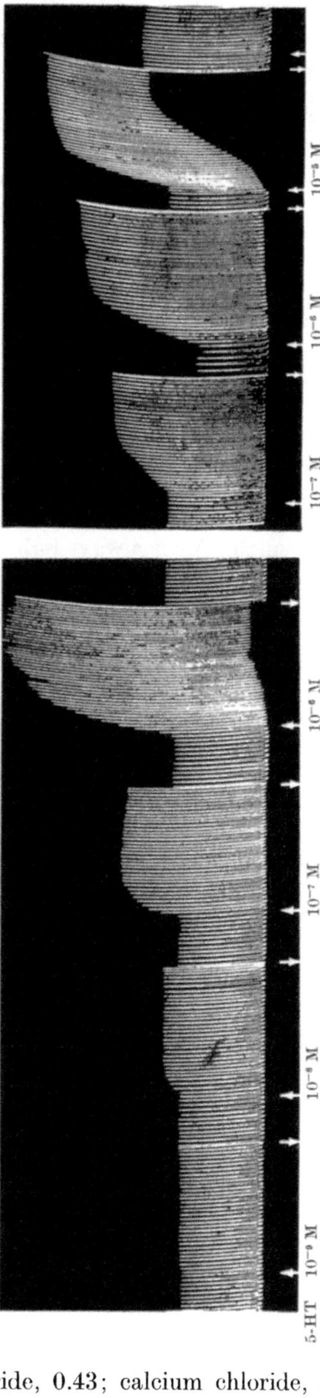

Fig. 5. The action of different concentrations of 5-HT on two preparations of *Venus mercenaria* heart. At each ↓, drum was stopped and bath flushed with sea-water for 5 min. Note the effect of increasing concentrations of 5-HT: at first increase in amplitude and frequency of beat may be seen, then increase in diastolic tone. [From Figs. 3 and 6, Wright, A. M. et al., Brit. J. Pharmacol. **18**, 444, 448 (1962).]

b) Helix (several species)

The ventricles of *Helix aspersa*, *Helix pomatia* and *Helix luconum* are tied by ligatures in the ventriculo-aortic and auriculo-ventricular grooves to the light lever and a fixed support; a small piece of the auricle is retained because this seems to produce a more regular beat. The heart is suspended at room temperature in a 2—3 ml bath, bubbled through with air.

Several perfusion fluids have been recommended. The composition of three of them is as follows:

α) sodium chloride, 6.5; potassium chloride, 0.2; calcium chloride, 0.2; magnesium chloride, 0.1; sodium dihydrogen phosphate, 0.05; sodium bicarbonate 1 g/l (Zetler and Schlosser 1954).

β) sodium chloride, 5; potassium chloride, 0.2; calcium chloride, 0.2; magnesium sulphate $+7\ H_2O$, 0.3; sodium dihydrogen phosphate, 0.1; sodium bicarbonate, 0.1 g/l (Bertaccini and Zamboni 1961).

γ) sodium chloride, 3.45; potassium chloride, 0.43; calcium chloride, 1.17; magnesium chloride $6\ H_2O$, 3.31; sodium bicarbonate 1.1 g/l (Kerkut and Cottrell 1963).

Change of the solution is by overflow.

The threshold concentration of 5-HT causing increase in amplitude and frequency of beat is normally about 1 ng/ml but at times the snail heart can be sensitive even to 0.01 ng/ml 5-HT (KERKUT and COTTRELL 1963). The maximum reaction is reached in about 20 sec and graded responses may be obtained.

Adrenaline and histamine are without effect, but acetylcholine inhibits the heart in about the same doses as 5-HT stimulates it. This effect is not blocked either by atropine or benzoquinonium (10 μg/ml) (GADDUM and PAASONEN 1955, ERSPAMER and GHIRETTI 1951, BERTACCINI and ZAMBONI 1961).

c) *Spisula (Mactra) solida*

The heart of this bivalve mollusc has been especially recommended in the bioassay of 5-HT by GADDUM and PAASONEN (1955).

The *Spisula* specimens are opened by cutting both adductor muscles with a thin scalpel, and then dissecting by the technique of WELSH and TAUB (1948). Threads are tied near the auriculo-ventricular junctions and a small piece of ventricle is included in the ligature because of the fragility of the auricles.

The heart is then suspended at room temperature (13—21°) in a 2 ml bath, the contents of which can be changed by overflow so that the mechanical disturbance is small. Air is always bubbled through the fluid and the movements of the heart are recorded on a smoked drum with a light lever.

The nutrient solution has the following composition: sodium chloride, 23; sodium sulphate, 4; potassium chloride, 0.65; calcium chloride, 1.1; magnesium chloride · 6 H_2O, 10; sodium carbonate, 0.2 g/l. Sometimes the heart gives a better beat when the concentration of Mg is reduced by 2—5 times.

The heart of *Spisula* starts to beat in 5—60 min after dissection at a rate of 12—25 beats per minute. 5-HT increases the amplitude of beat in concentrations as low as 0.1—0.5 ng/ml. Maximal response is reached within 45 to 60 sec and relaxation is rapid. Graded responses are obtained within large dose limits and for the maximum effect the concentration of 5-HT is 1 μg/ml.

Acetylcholine usually inhibits the *Spisula* heart in threshold concentrations of 1—100 ng/ml, the only efficient antagonist of this action being benzoquinonium (1—10 μg/ml). Adrenaline and noradrenaline stimulate the heart in concentrations of 1 μg/ml or more. Histamine is ineffective at this dose level. Adenosine, adenosine-5-phosphate and adenosine diphosphate display a very small stimulant action only in concentrations of 1 mg/ml. Crude preparations of substance *P* and bradykinin are inactive.

d) *Anodonta cygnea*

The isolated ventricle containing a short piece of intestine is suspended in a 10 ml bath bubbled through with air. The nutrient liquid consists of a mixture of 96 parts of distilled water and 4 parts of sea water buffered by $M/400$ sodium bicarbonate.

The *Anodonta* ventricle, either immediately or after an initial standstill of varying duration, begins to beat with a slow even rhythm. Generally the isolated ventricles are able to continue beating for more than 48 h.

The threshold concentration of 5-HT causing increase in amplitude and frequency of beat is about 1 ng/ml, and graded responses are obtained with concentrations up to about 1 μg/ml.

Adrenaline, noradrenaline, tyramine, dopamine, substance *P*, histamine and acetylcholine are either ineffective or produce negligible responses at high concentrations (FÄNGE 1955, MARCZYNSKY 1959).

e) Other molluscs

Hearts of other bivalve molluscs which may be used in the bioassay of 5-HT are those of *Cyprina islandica* (threshold concentration of 5-HT 1 ng/ml), *Mya arenaria* (0.5—50 ng/ml) and *Cardium edule* (0.1—1 ng/ml) but, on the whole, for one reason or another, they do not seem to be as convenient as hearts of *Spisula* or *Venus*. The same dissection technique as described for the *Spisula* heart in used.

No satisfactorily beating hearts have been obtained from *Barnea candida*, *Mactra corallina*, *Mytilus edulis* or *Paphia saxatilis* (GADDUM and PAASONEN 1955).

Hearts of *Buccinum undatum* and of *Octopus* or *Eledone* are employed more rarely in the bioassay of 5-HT. The heart of *Buccinum* is cannulated with a Straub cannula through the aorta and the auricle is tied off (GADDUM and PAASONEN 1955); the heart of *Octopus* is cannulated with a similar cannula which is introduced through one of the atria, all the vessels which open into the ventricle having been ligatured first (ERSPAMER and GHIRETTI 1951).

7. Miscellaneous preparations

Guinea-pig uterus. According to McGOVERN et al. (1961) uterine muscles from guinea-pigs in natural oestrus may serve excellently for the qualitative and quantitative bioassay of 5-HT. 0.5 μg/ml 5-HT gives maximal response.

Perfused pig ear. 5-HT, adrenaline and noradrenaline, in doses from 0.01 to 0.1 μg, produce vasoconstriction proportional to the dose and suitable for recording (GRETTE 1957).

Carotid artery rings or strips. They have been widely used in the past, and more recently by WOOLLEY and SHAW (1953), but have now been completely abandoned owing to the difficulty of obtaining repeatable results, and their poor sensitivity and specificity.

Anterior retractor muscle of the byssus. The superfused isolated anterior retractor muscle of the byssus of *Mytilus edulis* may be used for the identification of 5-HT owing to the capacity of the amine (1—100 ng/ml) to provoke a relaxation of the contraction produced either by electrical stimulation or by acetylcholine (CAMBRIDGE and HOLGATE 1955).

Dorsal muscle of the leech. It has been found by POLONI (1951) that 5-HT causes relaxation of the isolated leech muscle and that this effect can be utilized for its assay in concentrations as low as 0.01 ng/ml. The relaxing effect of 5-HT on the leech muscle has been confirmed by SCHAIN (1961), but it has not been found suitable as a basis for the assay or identification of the amine, mainly because of the difficulty in establishing a stable base line for comparison of relaxations and because of the lack of specificity of the response.

Isolated stomach of Helix pomatia. The isolated stomach of *Helix pomatia* is potently stimulated by 5-HT at exceptionally low concentrations (threshold 5×10^{-8} to 1×10^{-7} μg/ml) and the response is fairly proportional to the dose of 5-HT. Acetylcholine, adrenaline, noradrenaline, histamine, vasopressin and oxytocin all cause similar contraction of the snail stomach but their action is at least 10,000 times less intense than that of 5-HT. In view of these facts, grounds exist, according to GRYGLEWSKI and SUPNIEWSKI (1963) for undertaking the elaboration of a method for bioassay of 5-HT in body fluids and tissues using the above preparation.

III. The relative potency of natural and synthetic indolealkylamines

As a direct consequence of the enormous interest raised by 5-HT and the other naturally occurring indolealkylamines, numerous related indole derivatives have been synthesized and studied.

Detailed results of these studies will be reported in due course in chapter 7. Here we wish only to summarize in Tables 3 and 4 the relative activities of the most important indolealkylamines and indazolealkylamines, as assessed on some of the smooth muscle preparations most commonly used in the bioassay of 5-HT.

The following indole aminoacids and acids have proved to be inactive or at least 10,000 times less active than 5-HT on the smooth muscle preparations employed: L-tryptophan, 5-HTP, 4-HTP, 6-HTP, 7-HTP, 2-HTP, 5-hydroxy-N-acetyl-TP, 5-acetoxy-N-acetyl-TP, 5-hydroxy-N,N-dimethyl-TP, 5-hydroxy-2-methyl-TP, 5-amino-TP, 5-nitro-TP, IAA, 5-HIAA, 4-HIAA, 7-HIAA, 6-HIAA and 5-methoxy-IAA.

It may easily be seen from the tabulated data that no general conclusion is possible in regard to the relationship between chemical constitution and pharmacological activity. Therefore discussion will be limited to some of the data collected on the rat uterus and rat stomach preparations, which behave in a fairly similar manner:

a) Shifting of the phenolic-OH group from position 5 to other positions regularly produces a decay of biological activity, which is moderate when the transposition is to position 4, but tremendous when the transposition is to position 6 or 7.

b) Substitution on the indole nucleus of groups other than —OH groups regularly reduces biological activity. The reduction is moderate in the case of amino- and methoxy-groups, but considerable in the case of halo-groups and benzyloxy-groups.

c) Etherification of the phenolic —OH with glucuronic or sulphuric acid practically abolishes biological activity.

d) Lack of any phenolic —OH group, as in tryptamine, is accompanied by a strong reduction in biological activity which, however, is much less than that observed following transposition of the —OH group from position 5 to position 6 or 7 of the indole nucleus.

e) Shifting of the side chain from position 3 to position 2 produces a complete loss of biological activity.

f) The effect of alkyl substitution on the amino nitrogen is variable; in general both an increase in number and size of the alkyl group produces a reduction of biological activity.

g) Substitution of a methyl group on the α-carbon of the side chain, i.e. introduction of a third carbon atom into the side chain, produces either a moderate decay of activity or an increase in activity, depending upon other substituents in the molecule. Substitution of two methyl groups or of one ethyl group is considerably more deleterious.

h) In sharp contrast to what usually happens with phenylalkylamines, substitution of an —OH group on the β-carbon of the side chain produces the practical disappearance of any activity on the rat uterus preparation.

i) Indolealkylamines with a single carbon atom side chain (gramine derivatives) show negligible activity on all preparations tested.

k) Indazolealkylamines show remarkable 5-HT-like activity, which is particularly evident with the first member of the series, more strictly related to 5-HT from a chemical point of view.

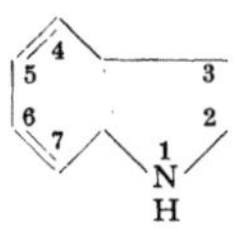

Table 3. *Equipotent molar ratios of indolealkylamines estimated on five isolated smooth muscle preparations.* 5-HT taken as unity.

Ring substituent	Side chain	Stimulant action: Rat uterus[1,2]	Rat stomach[1,3]	Molluscan heart[2,4]	Rabbit ear[2]	Guinea-pig ileum[2]
5—OH	3—CH_2—CH_2—NH_2 (5-Hydroxytryptamine)	1	1	1	1	1
5—OH	3—CH_2—CH_2—$NHCH_3$	1	6.3	=	1.4	7
5—OH	3—CH_2—CH_2—$N(CH_3)_2$ (Bufotenine)	4	10	0.3 (0.028)	11	4
5—OH	3—CH_2—CH_2—$N(C_2H_5)_2$	9	18; 20	=	=	=
5—OH	3—CH_2—CH_2—$N(C_3H_7$ iso$)_2$	16	4.5	=	=	=
5—OH	3—CH_2—CH_2—$N(C_3H_7)_2$	39	16; 4	=	=	=
5—OH	3—CH_2—CH_2—$N(C_4H_9)_2$	540; 1100	151	0	0	450
5—OH	3—CH_2—CH_2—$N(CH_3)_3$ (Bufotenidine)	$>$1000[5]	=	=	=	=
5—OH	3—CH_2—$CH(CH_3)$—NH_2	1.3; 2	1.4; 1.7	8.2 (6)	3.3	8
5—OH	3—CH_2—$C(CH_3)_2$—NH_2	310	=	170	0	24
5—OH	3—CH_2—$CH(C_2H_5)$—NH_2	50	7	50	40	44
5—OH	3—CH_2—CH_2—$NHCOCH_3$	+—[6]	=	=	=	=
5—OH	3—CHOH—CH_2—$N(CH_3)_2$	0	=	0	0	0
5—OH	3—CH_2—C(N)—NH_2	0	=	=	108	=
5—OH, 2,3-dihydro	3—CH_2—CH_2—NH_2	10[7]	=	=	=	=
5—OH	2—CH_2—CH_2—NH_2	0	=	0	0	190
5—OCH_3	3—CH_2—CH_2—NH_2 (5-Methoxytryptamine)	9.6; 8	20; 39	0.5	5.4	9
5—OCH_3	3—CH_2—CH_2—$NHCH_3$	150	=	=	=	=
5—OCH_3	3—CH_2—CH_2—$N(CH_3)_2$	150	=	=	=	=
5—OCH_3	3—CH_2—CH_2—$N(C_4H_9)_2$	0	=	540	0	0
5—OCH_3	3—CH_2—$CH(CH_3)$—NH_2	1.5; 4.3	2.9; 1.4	4.6	1.5	43
5—OCH_3	3—CH_2—CH_2—$NHCOCH_3$ (Melatonin)	0	=	=	345	0
5—$OCOCH_3$	3—CH_2—CH_2—NH_2	=	=	(+)[8]	=	=
5—CH_3	3—CH_2—CH_2—NH_2	173	184; 620	=	=	=
5—CH_3	3—CH_2—$CH(CH_3)$—NH_2	1300; 240	14; 22	190	340	0
5—Cl	3—CH_2—CH_2—NH_2	=	100	=	=	=
5—NH_2	3—CH_2—CH_2—NH_2	11	=	1.3	23	22
5—OC_7H_7	3—CH_2—CH_2—$N(CH_3)_2$	20000	625	=	=	=
5—OC_7H_7	3—CH_2—CH_2—$N(C_2H_5)_2$	10000	470	=	=	=
5—OC_7H_7	3—CH_2—CH_2—$N(C_3H_7)_2$	20000	614	=	=	=
5—OC_7H_7	3—CH_2—CH_2—$N(C_4H_9)_2$	20000	20000	=	=	=
5—OC_7H_7	3—CH_2—$CH(CH_3)$—NH_2	20000	63	=	=	=
5—O-sulphate	3—CH_2—CH_2—$N(CH_3)_2$ (Bufoviridine)	500	=	=	0	1000
5—O-glucuronide	3—CH_2—CH_2—NH_2	0	=	0	=	0
5—O-glucuronide	3—CH_2—CH_2—$N(CH_3)_2$	0	=	0	=	0
5—OH, 2—CH_3	3—CH_2—CH_2—NH_2	=	=	(31.4)	=	=
5—OCH_3, 2—CH_3	3—CH_2—CH_2—NH_2	=	=	(43.8)	=	=
5—OCH_3, 2—CH_3, 1—C_7H_7 (BAS)	3—CH_2—CH_2—NH_2	=	=	(30)[9]	=	=
5—OH, 2—CH_3, 1—C_7H_7 (BAS-phenol)	3—CH_2—CH_2—NH_2	=	=	(300)[9]	=	=
5,6—$(OH)_2$	3—CH_2—CH_2—NH_2	=	~1[10]	=	=	=
5,6—$(OCH_3)_2$	3—CH_2—CH_2—NH_2	58	300	4	140	300
5,6,7—$(OCH_3)_3$	3—CH_2—CH_2—NH_2	110	=	130	560	145
6—OH	3—CH_2—CH_2—NH_2	0	460	47	155	0
6—OCH_3	3—CH_2—CH_2—NH_2	0	1520	174	480	400
4—OH	3—CH_2—CH_2—NH_2	11	1.8	15	22	26

Table 3. (cont.)

Ring substituent	Side chain	Stimulant action: Rat uterus[1,2]	Rat stomach[1,3]	Molluscan heart[2,4]	Rabbit ear[2]	Guinea-pig ileum[2]
4—OH	3—CH_2—CH_2—$N(CH_3)_2$ (Psilocin)	10—20[11]	0[11]	=	=	=
4—O-phosphate	3—CH_2—CH_2—$N(CH_3)_2$ (Psilocybin)	330; 50—100[11]	3—1000[11]	18	0	760
7—OH	3—CH_2—CH_2—NH_2	0	=	0	1300	0
2—CH_3	3—CH_2—CH_2—$N(CH_3)_2$	20000	1200;6600	=	=	=
2—CH_3	3—CH_2—CH_2—$N(C_2H_5)_2$	1000	280	=	=	=
2—CH_3	3—CH_2—CH_2—$N(C_3H_7)_2$	630	70	=	=	=
1—CH_3	3—CH_2—CH_2—NH_2	142	=	0	330	520
1—CH_3	3—CH_2—$CH(CH_3)$—NH_2	1350	69	=	=	=
	3—CH_2—CH_2—NH_2 (Tryptamine)	176; 210	408; 933	22 (9.9)	20	280
	3—CH_2—CH_2—$NHCH_3$	128; 2000	1120;2400	(3.7)	17	48
	3—CH_2—CH_2—NHC_2H_5	2000	250; 350	(9.1)	=	=
	3—CH_2—CH_2—NHC_3H_7	0; 2000	330; 490	0	0	0
	3—CH_2—CH_2—$N(CH_3)_2$	200;1000	196; 350	107 (10.7)	35	58
	3—CH_2—CH_2—$N(C_2H_5)_2$	160; 500	83; 112	650 (7.9)	0	0
	3—CH_2—CH_2—$N(C_3H_7)_2$	95; 200	34; 40	59	0	0
	3—CH_2—CH_2—$N(C_3H_7\ iso)_2$	520	53	=	=	=
	3—CH_2—CH_2—$N(C_4H_9)_2$	720; 500	244	810	0	870
	3—CH_2—$CH(CH_3)$—NH_2	0; 800	31; 60	0 (8.6)	0	0
	3—CH_2—$CH(C_2H_5)$—NH_2	20000	4600	=	=	=
	3—CH_2—$C(CH_3)_2$—NH_2	=	1400	=	=	=
	3—CH_2—CH_2—$NHCOCH_3$	0	=	=	=	=
	3—CHOH—CH_2—$NHCH_3$	0	=	23	370	0
	3—CH_2—C(N)—NH_2	0	=	=	120	=
	3—CH_2—CH_2—CH_2—NH_2	=	1920	=	=	=
	3—CH_2—CH_2—CH_2—$N(CH_3)_2$	=	=	(2000)	=	=
	3—CH_2—NH_2	=	29000	=	=	=
	3—CH_2—$N(CH_3)_2$ (Gramine)	0	=	0 (0)	0	400

Values in parentheses have been obtained on the heart of *Venus mercenaria* (Greenberg 1960b), the others on the heart of *Helix luconum* (Bertaccini and Zamboni 1961).

References to Table 3. [1] Barlow and Kahn (1959a, 1959b). — [2] Bertaccini and Zamboni (1961). — [3] Vane (1959). — [4] Greenberg (1960b). — [5] Erspamer (1954). — [6] McIsaac and Page (1958). — [7] Fellman et al. (1962). — [8] Osborne et al. (1962). — [9] Woolley (1959). [10] Colhoun (1963). — [11] Woolley and Campbell (1962).

The aldehydes corresponding to 5-HT and tryptamine, generated *in vitro* by purified oxidative deaminase preparations and isolated free of amines, do not show any activity on the rat uterus and the guinea-pig ileum at concentrations several hundred times higher than the parent amines nor do they possess any inhibitory or potentiating effect on the activity of the amines. Since the aldehydes are taken up and metabolized by the smooth muscle preparations, their inactivity is not due to impermeability (Renson et al. 1964).

Vane (1959) has observed that the relative potency of many of the examined indolealkylamines changes considerably following introduction of a MAO inhibitor into the nutrient bath of the isolated rat stomach. He suggests that MAO block increases the potency of those compounds which more easily enter the cells where MAO is active.

The tabulated data show that the molluscan heart frequently gives results which differ strikingly from those obtained with the rat uterus or stomach preparations. This fact should not be overlooked when submitting to bioassay crude extracts from vegetable or animal tissues. The presence, for example, of N-alkylated indolealkylamines would greatly impair the accuracy of estimation of 5-HT.

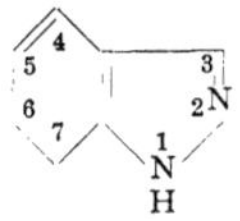

Table 4. *Equipotent molar ratios of indazolealkylamines estimated on four isolated smooth muscle preparations* (BERTACCINI and ZAMBONI 1961). 5-HT taken as unity.

Ring substituent	Side-chain	Stimulant action			
		Rat uterus	*Helix* heart	Rabbit ear	Guinea-pig ileum
5—OH	3—CH_2—CH_2—NH_2	4.3—5[1]	3.9	27	5.3
5—OH	3—CH_2—CH_2—$NHCH(CH_3)_2$	227	172	0	0
5—OC_7H_7	3—CH_2—CH_2—NH_2	0	0	0	0
5—OC_7H_7	3—CH_2—CH_2—$N(CH_3)_2$	0	0	0	0
5—OC_7H_7	3—CH_2—CH_2—$NHCH(CH_3)_2$	0	0	0	0
	3—CH_2—CH_2—NH_2	360	335	134	0
	3—CH_2—CH_2—$N(CH_3)_2$	39	7.2	85	20
	3—CH_2—CH_2—$NHCH(CH_3)_2$	0	0	0	0
	2—CH_2—CH_2—NH_2	0	0	700	570
	1—CH_2—CH_2—NH_2	870	0	66	185

[1] AINSWORTH 1958.

SCHÖTENSACK et al. (1963) have carried out comparative studies on the pharmacological actions of some indolealkylamines and their oxa-analogues. On the blood pressure of rats pretreated with tetraethylammonium, tryptamine and 5-HT were 3 and 500 times, respectively, more potent than the corresponding benzofuranalkylamines; on the rat uterus 10 and 10000 times more active, and on the rat fundus strip 100 and 1000 times more active.

References

AINSWORTH, C.: Substituted β-aminoethylindazoles. J. Amer. chem. Soc. **80**, 965—967 (1958).

AMIN, A. H., T. B. B. CRAWFORD and J. H. GADDUM: The distribution of substance *P* and 5-hydroxytryptamine in the central nervous system of the dog. J. Physiol. (Lond.) **126**, 596—618 (1954).

BARLOW, R. B., and I. KAHN: Actions of some analogues of tryptamine on the isolated rat uterus and on the isolated rat fundus strip preparations. Brit. J. Pharmacol. **14**, 99—107 (1959a).

— — Actions of some analogues of 5-hydroxytryptamine on the isolated rat uterus and the rat fundus strip preparations. Brit. J. Pharmacol. **14**, 265—272 (1959b).

— — The use of the guinea-pig ileum preparation for testing the activity of substances which imitate or antagonize the actions of 5-hydroxytryptamine and tryptamine. Brit. J. Pharmacol. **14**, 553—558 (1959c).

BENDITT, E. P., and R. L. WONG: On the concentration of 5-hydroxytryptamine in mammalian enterochromaffin cells and its release by reserpine. J. exp. Med. **105**, 509—519 (1957).

BERTACCINI, G., and P. ZAMBONI: The relative potency of 5-hydroxytryptamine-like substances. Arch. int. Pharmacodyn. **133**, 138—156 (1961).

BONNYCASTLE, D. D., N. J. GIARMAN, and M. K. PAASONEN: Anticonvulsant compounds and 5-hydroxytryptamine in rat brain. Brit. J. Pharmacol. **12**, 228—231 (1957).

BOWERS jr., M. B.: Stimulation and sensitization of isolated Venus heart by cerebrospinal fluid. Brit. J. Pharmacol. **19**, 295—298 (1962).

BUMPUS, F. M., and I. H. PAGE: Serotonin and its methylated derivatives in human urine. J. biol. Chem. **212**, 111—116 (1955).

BURDON, K. L., K. OZKARAGOZ, H. S. KAUFMAN, and J. P. MCGOVERN: The effect of estrus on the response of the excised mouse uterus to serotonin, acetylcholine and specific antigen; Schultz-Dale tests with the physiograph. Ann. Allergy **18**, 972—979 (1960).

BURN, J. H.: Practical Pharmacology, p. 17. Oxford: Blackwell Sci. Publ. 1953.
BUSCH, E.: Über die Erregbarkeit des Rattenuterus im Cyclus. Naunyn-Schmiedebergs Arch. exp. Path. Pharmakol. **228**, 153—154 (1956).
CAMBRIDGE, G. W., and J. A. HOLGATE: A method for identification of 5-hydroxytryptamine. J. Physiol. (Lond.) **130**, 22P (1955).
CLEUGH, J., and J. H. GADDUM: The stability of purified preparations of substance *P*. Experientia (Basel) **19**, 72—73 (1963).
COLHOUN, E. H.: Synthesis of 5-hydroxytryptamine in the American cockroach. Experientia (Basel) **19**, 9—10 (1963).
CORREALE, P.: The biological estimation of 5-hydroxytryptamine (enteramine) in the presence of substance *P*. J. Neurochem. **2**, 201—208 (1958).
DALGLIESH, C. E., C. C. TOH, and T. S. WORK: Fractionation of the smooth muscle stimulants present in extracts of the gastrointestinal tract. Identification of 5-hydroxytryptamine and its distinction from substance *P*. J. Physiol. (Lond.) **120**, 298—310 (1953).
ERSPAMER, V.: Pharmakologische Studien über Enteramin. I. Über die Wirkung von Acetonextrakten der Kaninchenmagenschleimhaut auf den Blutdruck und auf isolierte überlebende Organe. Naunyn-Schmiedebergs Arch. exp. Path. Pharmakol. **196**, 343—365 (1940).
— Active substances in the posterior salivary glands of octopoda. I. Enteramine-like substance. Acta pharmacol. (Kbh.) **4**, 213—223 (1948).
— Il sistema cellulare enterocromaffine e l'enteramina (5-idrossitriptamina). Rend. sci. Farmitalia **1**, 1—193 (1954).
— Observations of the fate of indolalkylamines in the organism. J. Physiol. (Lond.) **127**, 118—133 (1955).
— and G. FALCONIERI ERSPAMER: Pharmacological actions of eledoisin on extravascular smooth muscle. Brit. J. Pharmacol. **19**, 337—354 (1962).
—, and F. GHIRETTI: The action of enteramine on the heart of molluscs. J. Physiol. (Lond.) **115**, 470—481 (1951).
FÄNGE, R.: Use of the isolated heart of a freshwater mussel (*Anodonta cygnea* L.) for biological estimation of 5-hydroxytryptamine. Experientia (Basel) **11**, 156 (1955).
FELDBERG, W., and C. C. TOH: Distribution of 5-hydroxytryptamine (serotonin, enteramine) in the wall of the digestive tract. J. Physiol. (Lond.) **119**, 352—362 (1953).
FELLMAN, J. H., T. S. FUJITA, and C. J. BELBER: 2,3-Dihydro-5-hydroxytryptamine. Biochem. Pharmacol. **11**, 557—561 (1962).
FENSTER, E., and J. C. TOWNE: Solubilization of serotonin by rat brain extracts in lipid solvents. Fed. Proc. **22**, 624 (1963).
GADDUM, J. H.: The technique of superfusion. Brit. J. Pharmacol. **8**, 321—326 (1953).
—, and K. A. HAMEED: Drugs which antagonize 5-hydroxytryptamine. Brit. J. Pharmacol. **9**, 240—248 (1954).
—, and M. K. PAASONEN: The use of some molluscan hearts for the estimation of 5-hydroxytryptamine. Brit. J. Pharmacol. **10**, 474—483 (1955).
GARVEN, J. D.: The estimation of 5-hydroxytryptamine in the presence of adrenaline. Brit. J. Pharmacol. **11**, 66—70 (1956).
GREENBERG, M. J.: The response of the *Venus* heart to catechol amines and high concentrations of 5-hydroxytryptamine. Brit. J. Pharmacol. **15**, 365—374 (1960a).
— Structure-activity relationship of tryptamine analogues on the heart of *Venus mercenaria*. Brit. J. Pharmacol. **15**, 375—388 (1960b).
GRETTE, K.: Determination of 5-hydroxytryptamine with the isolated, perfused pig ear. Acta pharmacol. (Kbh.) **13**, 177—183 (1957).
GRYGLEWSKI, R., and J. SUPNIEWSKI: Influence of 5-hydroxytryptamine and other biologically active substances on the movements of the isolated stomach of *Helix pomatia* Bull. Acad. pol. Sci., Ser. Sci. Biol. **11**, 53—56 (1963).
HAEFELI, W., and A. HÜRLIMANN: Substance *P*, a highly active naturally occurring polypeptide. Experientia (Basel) **18**, 297—303 (1962).
KERKUT, G. A., and G. A. COTTRELL: Acetylcholine and 5-hydroxytryptamine in the snail brain. Comp. Biochem. Physiol. **8**, 53—63 (1963).
LEITSCH, J. L., D. MARYN and J. B. MOORE: Note on sensitivity of the isolated perfused rat uterus to serotonin. J. Amer. pharm. Ass. (Sci. Ed.) **47**, 535 (1958).
MARCZYNSKI, T.: Preliminary investigations of the pharmacological properties of 5-methoxy-N-methyltryptamine. The freshwater crustacean *Anodonta cygnea* L. as a test for serotonin and related compounds. Diss. pharm. (Kraków) **11**, 297—313 (1959).
McGOVERN, J. P., K. OZKARAGOZ, A.E, HENSEL, and K.L. BURDON: Qualitative and quantitative studies with 5-hydroxytryptamine (serotonin) in the Schultz-Dale apparatus. J. Allergy **32**, 321—326 (1961).

McIntyre, A. D., D. E. Williams, and F. L. Humoller: Bioassay of 5-hydroxytryptamine on heart of Venus mercenaria. Fed. Proc. **19**, 283 (1960).
McIsaac, W. M., and I. H. Page: New metabolites of serotonin in carcinoid urine. Science **128**, 537 (1958).
Osborne, M., R. Detar, and L. Gabel: Comparison between the autonomic pharmacology of 5-hydroxytryptamine and 5-acetyltryptamine (5 AT). Fed. Proc. **21**, 324 (1962).
Page, I. H., and A. A. Green: Perfusion of rabbit's ear for study of vasoconstrictor substances. Meth. med. Res. **1**, 123—129 (1948).
Poloni, A.: Il muscolo dorsale di sanguisuga quale test biologico per l'evidenziamento dell'attività serotoninica nei liquidi organici. Cervello **31**, 472—476 (1955).
Put, T. R., and L. A. H. Hogenhuis: Brain serotonin and thyroid function. Acta physiol. pharmacol. neerl. **10**, 343—352 (1962).
Ravenna, F.: Sintesi e attività biologica del 5-ammino-triptofano. Experientia (Basel) **14**, 273—274 (1958).
Renson, J., H. Weissbach, and S. Udenfriend: Studies on the biological activities of the aldehydes derived from norepinephrine, serotonin, tryptamine and histamine. J. Pharmacol. exp. Ther. **143**, 326—331 (1964).
Robson, J. M., Trounce, and K. A. H. Didcock: Factors affecting the response of the uterus to serotonin. J. Endocr. **10**, 129—132 (1954).
Schain, R. J.: Effects of 5-hydroxytryptamine on the dorsal muscle of the leech (Hirudo medicinalis). Brit. J. Pharmacol. **16**, 257—261 (1961).
Schötensack, W., P. Bischler u. G. Richarz: Vergleich pharmakologischer Wirkungen von Indol- und Benzofuran-alkylaminen. Naunyn-Schmiedebergs Arch. exp. Path. Pharmakol. **245**, 120—121 (1963).
Schwartz, I. L.: Assay of serotonin with antimetabolites. Amer. J. Physiol. **183**, 659—660 (1955).
Supek, Z., and S. Milković: Quantitative biological determination of 5-hydroxytryptamine. Experientia (Basel) **12**, 71—72 (1956).
—, and M. Randić: An improved method for biological determination of 5-hydroxytryptamine in acetone brain extracts in the presence of interfering substances. Biochem. Pharmacol. **8**, 79 (1961).
Towne, J. C., and Ph. K. Kalayil: Lipid solvent-amine interaction. Fed. Proc. **23**, 492 (1964).
Uuspää, V. J., and V. I. Uuspää: Vane's rat fundus strip method in determination of 5-hydroxytryptamine. Ann. Acad. Sci. fenn. A IV, **60**, 1—17 (1962).
Vane, J. R.: A sensitive method for the assay of 5-hydroxytryptamine. Brit. J. Pharmacol. **12**, 344—349 (1957).
— The relative activities of some tryptamine analogues on the isolated rat stomach strip preparation. Brit. J. Pharmacol. **14**, 87—98 (1959).
Welsh, J. H.: Neurohormones of invertebrates. I. Cardio-regulators of *Cyprina* and *Buccinum*. J. Mar. Biol. Ass. U. Kingd. **35**, 193—201 (1956).
— Serotonin as a possible neurohumoral agent: evidence obtained in lower animals. Ann. N. Y. Acad. Sci. **66**, 618—630 (1957).
—, and R. Taub: The action of choline and related compounds on the heart of *Venus mercenaria*. Biol. Bull. **95**, 346—353 (1948).
Woolley, D. W.: Highly potent antimetabolites of serotonin with little serotonin-like action. Biochem. Pharmacol. **1**, 51—59 (1959).
—, and N. K. Campbell: Serotonin-like and antiserotonin properties of psilocybin and psilocin. Science **136**, 777—779 (1962).
Zetler, G., u. L. Schlosser: Über das Vorkommen von 5-Hydroxytryptamin (Enteramin oder Serotonin) im Gehirn von Säugetieren. Naunyn-Schmiedebergs Arch. exp. Path. Pharmakol. **222**, 345—351 (1954).

Chapter 4

Occurrence of indolealkylamines in nature

By

Vittorio Erspamer

With one Figure

I. Introduction

Quantitative data on the occurrence of 5-HT and related indolealkylamines in nature are presented in Tables 1—23 of this chapter and in Tables 1—6 of chapter 13. The interest of these data is obvious, especially for the interpretation of the physiological significance of indolealkylamines in their different localizations. However, it seems opportune to call attention at once to a few points.

The occurrence of 5-HT or another indolealkylamine in a tissue does not of necessity imply that the amine has particular importance in this tissue. In fact, it is obvious that one is authorized to surmise that a given localization of an indolealkylamine has a general biological significance only if this localization occurs in all or in a great number of species.

Quantitative data on the concentration of indolealkylamines in a tissue reflect only a static situation, and they give no indication of the rapidity of synthesis and metabolism of the amines. There is no doubt that knowledge of the turnover rate of the amines in a tissue is considerably more important, from every point of view, than knowledge of the content of the amines at a given moment.

To give only one example, it is probable that the amount of 5-HT synthetized and destroyed in a 24-hour period in the rat brain is considerably larger than that metabolized in the skin of *Bombina variegata pachypus* or *Discoglossus pictus*. Yet, it will be seen that the first tissue contains as little as 0.4—0.6 μg/g 5-HT, the second 200—450 μg/g. Obviously, the functional significance of 5-HT in these two localizations cannot be the same.

II. Vertebrates

1. Gastro-intestinal tract

Found for the first time in extracts of rabbit's gastric mucosa (Vialli and Erspamer 1937, Erspamer 1940b), 5-HT has since been recognized in extracts of the gastrointestinal mucosa of all examined vertebrates, as well as of ascidians (Erspamer 1946, 1953b, 1954a, 1954b, Feldberg and Toh 1953, Dalgliesh et al. 1953). At variance with previous negative results, small amounts of 5-HT could be detected also in gastrointestinal extracts of *Telostei* (Erspamer unpublished observations).

The general occurrence of 5-HT within the gastrointestinal mucosa of all vertebrates represents the most convincing proof of the general biological significance of the 5-HT of enterochromaffin origin. It has been conclusively demonstrated that, with a few exceptions, the alimentary canal is the only source of the 5-HT found in blood of vertebrates.

Table 1. *The 5-HT content of rat extracerebral tissues*

Tissue	5-HT content (in µg/ml or µg/g)
Blood	
Whole blood	0.31[1]; 0.43[2]; 0.87 ± 0.07[3]; 0.73 ± 0.06[4]; 1.04[5]
Serum	0.57—1.72[6]; 0.65[7]; 0.53—0.82[8]; 0.4—0.6[9]; 0.3—0.54[10]
Platelet protein (1 mg)	1.0—2.0[11]
Plasma (platelet free) .	0.008[32]
Spleen	2.8[6]; 2.15[7]; 1.9—3.0[8]; 2.5[12]; 2.99 ± 0.16[4]; 0.8 ± 0.1[13]; 1.8—2.2[5]; 4.43 ± 0.44[31]; 3.2—9.2[34]
Gastrointestinal tract . .	2.1[7]; 1.87—2.45[20]
Stomach	1.4[6]; 1.45 ± 0,07[14]; 1.8F, 2.1P[15]; 5.6[16]; 3.9P[18], 1.9P[17]; 9.31 ± 0.7P[31]; 0.68 ± 0.09F, 0.80 ± 0.19 P[35]
Small intestine	1.2[6]; 4.18[5]; 6.5[16]; 2.8 ± 0.6[17]; 1.06—1.35[10]; 5.04 ± 0.23[4]; 2.9[19]; 1.1—4.0[21]; 3.48 ± 0.25[38]
cranial third	5.6[15]; 2.9[18]; 2.3 ± 0.13[20]; 6.26 ± 0.48[31]; 3.28 ± 0.52[35]
medium third . . .	3.2[15]; 1.6[18] } 2.57 ± 0.16[20]
caudal third	5.5[15]; 3.3[18] } 2.57 ± 0.16[20]
Large intestine	3.8[15]; 4.75—6.0[18]; 5.9 ± 1.4[17]; 5.76[19]; 6.32 ± 0.5[20]
Liver	0.14[15]; 0.27—0.45[8]; 0.18[7]; 0.65 ± 0.08[31]; 0.48—0.68[36]
Lung	1.16[12]; 1.0[1]; 0.55 ± 0.16[22]; 3.9[15]; 2.7—3.5[21]; 1.9—3.3[8]; 1.3[7]; 2.43 ± 0.25[31]
Heart	0.15[7]; 0.58[19]; 0.7—0.8[30]
Uterus	0.15 ± 0.05[13]
Testicles	0.05[7]
Kidney	0.08[7]
Thyroid gland	2.5—5.0[23]; 3.55[37]
Salivary glands	0.56 (parotid), 0.25 (submaxill.), 0.8 (sublingual)[23]
Uvea and retina	2.70—5.20[33]
Lid	1.53[33]
Skin	
ear	1.0[24]; 3.20 (base), 1.40 (margin)[25]; 1.9[15]; 0.32—0.67[8]; 0.55[7]
groin	1.5[24]; 4.36[25]
throat	4.26[25]
abdomen	1.3[24]; 1.9[15]; 0.66—1.56[26]; 0.8—1.1[27]
tail	0.33[24]; 0.9[25]
feet	0.7[24]; 1.5[15]; 1.5—4.0[28]; 0.75[29]
Paws	0.34[7]; 0.15—0.44[8]
Adipose tissue	
interscapular brown fat	1.04 ± 0.054[38]
epididymal white fat .	0.154 ± 0.018[38]

P = pyloric or glandular stomach; F = fundic stomach.

References to Table 1. [1] Skillen et al. (1961a). — [2] Gordon (1961). — [3] Ershoff and Gal (1961). — [4] Ershoff et al. (1962). — [5] Gal and Drewes (1961). — [6] Erspamer (1954a, 1954b). — [7] Erspamer and Bertaccini (1962). — [8] Bertaccini (1960). — [9] Schmidt et al. (1960). — [10] Cass and Marshall (1962). — [11] Shore et al. (1956). — [12] Parratt and West (1957a). — [13] Boréus and Westerholm (1962). — [14] Nikodijević and Trajkov (1963). — [15] Telford and West (1960). — [16] Toh (1960). — [17] Resnick et al. (1961). — [18] Nobili, unpublished data. — [19] Schone and Lindner (1960). — [20] Bertaccini and Erspamer (1962). [21] Weissbach et al. (1958). — [22] Kindwall et al. (1962). — [23] Paasonen (1958). — [24] Parratt and West (1956a). — [25] Parratt and West (1958). — [26] Brocklehurst et al. (1960). — [27] Johansson (1960). — [28] Mörsdorf (1959, 1961). — [29] Supek et al. (1961). — [30] Skillen et al. (1962). — [31] Uuspää and Uuspää (1962). — [32] Kärki and Paasonen (1960). — [33] Levene (1962). — [34] Varagić et al. (1963). — [35] Moran and Westerholm (1963). — [36] Boggs et al. (1963). — [37] Magus et al. (1964). — [38] Stock and Westermann (1963a, 1963b).

In the mucosa of the digestive tract 5-HT is localized, to a great extent at least, in the enterochromaffin cells, which the writer considers to constitute a "diffuse endocrine organ", in the sense of Feyrter (1953), designed for the production and storage of 5-HT. The abundant evidence definitely supporting this view has been discussed elsewhere (see pages 138, 140 and 203).

From the enterochromaffin cells 5-HT is released into the circulatory stream, where most of it is taken up by the platelets (Toh 1954, Erspamer and Testini 1959, Adams 1960, Bertaccini 1960, Kärki et al. 1960a).

It has been claimed that elevation of the intraluminal pressure and/or motility of an isolated or *in situ* loop of the guinea-pig intestine causes the appearance in the intestinal lumen of detectable amounts of 5-HT (Bülbring and Crema 1959a, 1959b) and similarly that a fraction of the 5-HT released by HCl from the wall of an obstructed loop of the rat intestine can be recovered intraluminally (Resnick and Gray 1962). Although an external secretion by the enterochromaffin

Table 2. *The 5-HT content of dog and cat extracerebral tissues*

Tissue	5-HT content (in μg/ml or μg/g)	
	Dog	Cat
Blood		
Whole blood	0.2—0.8[1]	0.9—4.5[1]; 1.8[2]
Serum	0.08—0.57[3]; 0.2—0.6[1]; 0.55[4] 0.28[5]; 0.2—0.6[6]	1.2—7.4[3]; 0.3—5.7[1]; 4.3[2]
Plasma (platelet free)	0.002—0.005[5]; <0.006[7]	
Spleen	0.61—2.5[3]; 4.6[9]	5.7—10.5[3]; 8.5[9]
Gastrointestinal tract		
Stomach	5.2[3]; 1.6—2.3[8]	0.45[3]; 0.52[8]
Small intestine		
cranial half	2.0[8]; 3.7[3]	1.4[8]; 0.9[3]
caudal half	1.7[8]; 4.3[3]	1.0[8]; 0.5[3]
Large intestine	1.5[8]; 2.8[3]	1.7[8]; 1.2[3]
Lung	0.1[1]; 0.26[9]	0.2[1]; 0.62[9]
Liver	0.54[9]	0.56[9]
Heart	0.02—0.26[12]	=
Skin	<0.03[9]	0.08—0.13[9]
Salivary glands		
parotid	0.017[10]	=
submaxillary	0.012[10]; 0.35—1.4[11]	=
Thyroid gland	0.025[10]	

References to Table 2. [1] Sanders et al. (1959). — [2] Smith and Smith (1955). — [3] Erspamer (1954a, 1954b). — [4] Rosenberg et al. (1960). — [5] Cambridge and Holgate (1958). — [6] Erspamer and Testini (1959). — [7] Toh (1956). — [8] Nobili, unpublished data. — [9] Parratt and West (1957a). — [10] Paasonen (1958). — [11] Iachello et al. (1962). — [12] Bhatt et al. (1963).

cells cannot be excluded (the chromaffin cells of the posterior salivary glands of octopods, for example, possess both an internal and an external secretion) there is as yet no decisive evidence that the enterochromaffin cells discharge, under strict physiological conditions, part of their 5-HT into the intestinal lumen.

Evidently, the problem is whether the delicate intestinal epithelium may be considered completely normal in isolated or obstructed intestinal loops. Moreover, it should not be forgotten that the typical normal enterochromaffin cells of the pancreatic islets of some mammals and of the thymus of some birds lack the anatomical possibility of an external secretion.

Administration of a diet of meat or liver or of a diet containing added tryptophan to rats or mice produces an increase in the 5-HT content of the small intestine (Stacey and Sullivan 1957, Eber and Lembeck 1958, Sullivan 1960). The opposite can be observed in rabbits, guinea-pigs, rats and mice on feeding a low-tryptophan diet (Eber and Lembeck 1958, Zbinden et al. 1958, Gal and Drewes 1962). This observation points to the decisive role of tryptophan in the biosynthesis of 5-HT.

Of interest is the finding of BEAVER and WOSTMANN (1962) that the 5-HT content of the intestines may vary conspicuously (up to 100%) in different mouse strains kept on the same diet.

5-HT levels in the intestinal wall of conventional animals having a normal intestinal flora are lower than those found in the intestinal wall of germ-free

Table 3. *The 5-HT content of guinea-pig and rabbit extracerebral tissues*

Tissue	5-HT content (in μg/ml or μg/g)	
	Guinea-pig	Rabbit
Blood		
Whole blood	0.2[1]	3.2—6[1]; 4—6[2]; 3.5[3]; 2.52 ± 0.3[4]
Serum	0.07—0.27[5]; 0.15—0.7[6]	1.8—5.6[5]; 4.4[6]; 2.0[7]; 3.3—10[8]
Platelets	0.3—0.5 μg/mg platelet protein[9]	2.7 per 10^8 platelets[10]
Plasma (platelet free)	=	0.01—0.07[11]
Spleen	0.25—1.6[5]; 1.1[12]; 3.7 ± 0.5[13]	16.4—22.5[5]; 11.7[14]; 24.3[12]
Gastrointestinal tract		
Stomach	1.4[5]; 3.9[15]; 1.15[16]	0.85P, 4.9F[5]; 0.9P, 5.7F[16]; 6.2[14]
Duodenum	7.2[15]; 3.3[16]	3.2[16]
Jejunum	5.0[5]; 6.2[15]; 2.0[16]	3,3[5]; 1.8[16]
Ileum	3.4[5]; 4.5[15]; 2.0[16]; 3.6[13]	3.7[5]; 1.5[16]
Caecum	0.8[15]; 0.9[16]	0.7[16]
Large intestine	0.7[5]; 0.8[15]; 0.45[16]	2.7[5]; 2.2[16]; 3.5[14]
Intestine (?)		10—17[2]; 17[1]; 5.9[17]
Liver	< 0.02[12]	0.55[12]; 2.3[1]; 0.27[14]; 0.6[17]
Lung	0.06[12]; 0.2—0.3[2]; 0.2[1]; 0.21[22]	1.6[12]; 1.2—4,7[1]; 5—5.5[2]; 0.13[14]; 0.1[17]; 1.7—7.1[18]
Uterus	< 0.003[13]	=
Heart	=	0.4[1]; < 0.1[17]; 0.02[14]
Kidney	=	< 0.1[17]; 0.09[14]
Thyroid gland	=	0.09—0.29[20]; 0.09[14]
Salivary glands	=	0.13—0.16[20]; 0.07[14]
Skin	< 0.02—0.18[12]; < 0.01[13]	< 0.04—0.11[12]; < 0.04[19]
Thymus, pancreas, bladder, skeletal muscle	=	< 0.1[14]
Uvea and retina	1.5—2.1[21]	0.45—1.3[21]
Lid	0.92[21]	0.24[21]
Adipose tissue	0.015—0.03[23]	=

P = pyloric stomach; F = fundic or glandular stomach.

References to Table 3. [1] WAALKES and COBURN (1959, 1960a, 1960b). — [2] WEISSBACH et al. (1957, 1958). — [3] SHORE et al. (1956). — [4] CERHOVÁ (1962). — [5] ERSPAMER (1954a, 1954b). [6] MACHAFFIE et al. (1960). — [7] VANE (1958). — [8] DAVIS et al. (1961). — [9] HAVERBACK et al. (1957). — [10] WOOLLEY and EDELMAN (1958). — [11] KÄRKI et al. (1960a). — [12] PARRATT and WEST (1957a). — [13] BORÉUS and WESTERHOLM (1962). — [14] HAGMÜLLER et al. (1961). — [15] GARVEN (1956). — [16] NOBILI, unpublished data. — [17] KAKIMOTO and ARMSTRONG (1962). — [18] SANYAL and WEST (1958). — [19] WAALKES and COBURN (1960b). — [20] PAASONEN (1958). — [21] LEVENE (1962). — [22] ROBILLARD and ALARIE (1963). — [23] STOCK and WESTERMANN (1963b).

animals. BEAVER and WOSTMANN (1962) have observed 20—40% differences in rats, and 30—90% differences in mice, PHILLIPS et al. (1961) 10—55% differences in chickens. Oral administration of antibiotics causes a significant increase in intestinal 5-HT in mice, whereas in rats the increase is not considered to be significant. Sterilization of the gut acts probably by preventing bacterial metabolism of dietary tryptophan (STACEY and SULLIVAN 1957, SULLIVAN 1961). With the exception of neomycin, antibiotics only affect the 5-HT content of the intestine in mice.

The 5-HT content of the stomach and the duodenum of the hedgehog shows no statistically significant differences during activity and hibernation (UUSPÄÄ 1963).

The small intestine of thiamine-deficient rats presents, like blood and spleen, reduced levels of 5-HT; that of starved rats normal levels (GAL and DREWES 1961). Pyridoxine-deficiency causes in chickens a fall in the 5-HT content of the intestine from 5.0 to 1.2 μg/g, possibly owing to lessened activity of dopadecarboxylase (UDENFRIEND et al. 1957). Chronic administration of ethanol to mice and guinea-pigs, up to 3—7 months, does not produce significant changes either in the number of enterochromaffin cells or in the 5-HT content of the gastrointestinal tract (HAGMÜLLER et al. 1961).

Table 4. *The 5-HT content of hamster and mouse extracerebral tissues*

Tissue	5-HT content (in μg/ml or μg/g)	
	Hamster	Mouse
Blood		
Whole blood	=	1.8—4.6[1]
Serum	0.37[2]	1.48[2]
Spleen	20.5[3,12]	1.8[2]; 2.7[3]; 5.9[4]; 3.5[5]
Gastrointestinal tract		
Stomach	1.7—3.7[6]; 0.85[12]	25P, 2.15F[6]; 8.85[2]; 5.2[7]; 1.1[12]
Small intestine		1.6[2]; 3.5—4.5[1]; 3.1[4]; 2.8—3.7[9]
cranial third	0.95[6]	2.5[6]; 2.8[7]
medium third	0.95[6]	1.7[6]
caudal third	0.85[6]	0.7[6]; 2.6[7]
Caecum	0.73[6]	2.1[6]; 2.2[7]
Colon	1.3[6]	4,5[6]; 8.7[7]; 3.1[2]
Liver	0.22[3]	0.6—1.1[1]; 0.24[5]
Lung	2.75[3]	1.4—6[1]; 2.7[4]; 2.59 ± 0.37[10]; 1.9[8]
Kidney	=	1.3[4]
Skin	0.08[3,12]; < 0.08[13]	0.37 (abdomen), 1.12 (ears)[3]
Adipose tissue	=	0.12 (interscapular), 0.025 (epididymal)[14]
Placenta	=	0.14—0.52[15]
Whole body	=	1.5[11]

P = pyloric stomach; F = fundic stomach.

References to Table 4. [1] WAALKES and COBURN (1959, 1960a). — [2] ERSPAMER (1954a, 1954b). — [3] PARRATT and WEST (1957b). — [4] DONALDSON et al. (1960). — [5] MELCHING et al. (1960). — [6] NOBILI, unpublished data. — [7] HAGMÜLLER et al. (1961). — [8] WEISSBACH et al. (1957). — [9] SMITH (1960). — [10] KIND et al. (1961). — [11] SJOERDSMA et al. (1957). — [12] WEST (1958b). — [13] CHIECO BIANCHI et al. (1963). — [14] STOCK and WESTERMANN (1963b). — [15] ROBSON and SENIOR.

Table 5. *The 5-HT content of the gastrointestinal tract of some large domestic mammals* (FAUSTINI 1955)

	5-HT content (in μg base per g fresh tissue)							
	Stomach				Intestine			
	Rumen	Reticulum	Omasum	Abomasum	Small intest. proximal	Small intest. distal	Large intest. proximal	Large intest. distal
Ox	0	0	0	1.6	5.1	1.6	1.2	4.9
Calf	0	0	?	1.2	3.6	3.0	3.7	4.5
Goat	0	0	?	3.2	4.1	2.0	2.5	2.9
Hog	0.5				4.0	0.5	0.3	0.5
Horse	?				0.7	0.3	0.5	1.0

Table 6. *The 5-HT content of the gastrointestinal tract of other vertebrate species* (in μg 5-HT base per g fresh tissue)

Animal species	Stomach	Small intestine proximal	Small intestine medium	Small intestine distal	Large intestine	Reference
Monkey *(Papio hamadryas)*	1.2—1.5	2.1	1.65	1.4	1.8—2.5	1
Marmot	0.2	1.1	0.6	0.9	1.1—2	2
Hedgehog	6.3		2.8		3.9	3
Bat *(Rhinolophus ferrum equinum)*			1.6			3
Chicken	0—0.65	2.0	3.4	1.0	1.3—1.9	1
	1.4	4.9		4.5	4.1	3
		8.3 ± 1.3		6.1 ± 0.8		4
Pigeon	0.3—0.7	0.7	0.8	1.0	1.3—1.9	1
Duck	=	3.1		4.1	3.6	3
Tortoise			3.2			3
Rana pipiens	3.0		5.4, 1.4—2.0		=	6,7
Hyla cinerea	3.6		4.8		=	6
Hyla radiana			0.9			5
Hyla faber			0.6			5
Pleurodema tucumana			0.8			5
Calyptocephallela gayi			0.3			5
Phyllomedusa sauvagi			0.8			5
Leptodactylus ocellatus			1.4			5
Leptodactylus chaquensis			1.5			5
Leptodactylus bufonius			0.7			5
Leptodactylus pentadactylus labyrinthicus			1.0; 4.9			1
Leptodactylus laticeps			1.7			5
Bufo bufo bufo	2.2		1.6			3
Bufo americanus	2.6		5.1		=	6
Bufo marinus	2.7		7.1		=	6
Bufo marinus			0.4, 0.77			5,7
Bufo arenarum			1.5			1
Bufo spinulosus			0.7			5
Bufo granulosus major			2.0			5
Odontophrynus americanus			3.0			5
Bombina variegata pachypus	1.0		0.75			3
Desmognatus fuscus	3.0		5.0		=	6
Ambystoma tigrinum	1.1		2.1		=	6
Necturus maculosus	1.8, 0.28		1.4, 0.26		=	6,7
Scyliorhinus canicula	0.6		2.6			3
Scyliorhinus stellaris	0.3		2.3			3
Torpedo marmorata	1.35		2.5			3
Acipenser naccarii	0.3		0.34			3
Acipenser sturio			0.38			3
Ameiurus catus, Anguilla anguilla, Tinca tinca			<0.2—0.4 (?)			3
Carassius auratus	1.1		1.1		=	6
Amia calva	1.6		1.2		=	6
Ameiurus nebulosus	(mucosa) 0.15—0.36		0.4—0.74		=	7
Petromyzon planeri			0.2			3

References to Table 6. [1] Nobili, unpublished data. — [2] Bertaccini, unpublished data. — [3] Erspamer (1954a, 1954b). — [4] Phillips et al. (1961). — [5] Roseghini, unpublished data. — [6] Bogdanski et al. (1963), Brodie et al. (1964). — [7] Welsh (1964).

Quantitative data on the occurrence of 5-HT in foetal tissues have been collected in bovine foetuses by Faustini (1955) and by Bertaccini et al. (unpublished observations). They are shown in Table 7.

It clearly appears from the tabulated data that small amounts of 5-HT are detectable very early in the intestinal tract of bovine foetuses, at the time of the first appearance of the enterochromaffin cells in the mucosa and, similarly, that spleen tissue contains considerable amounts of 5-HT from the time of its first differentiation.

Table 7. *Occurrence of 5-HT in some tissues during foetal life (bovine foetuses)* (FAUSTINI 1955, BERTACCINI et al. to be published)

Gestation time	Content of 5-HT base (in μg per g fresh tissue)		
	Gastrointestinal tract*	Spleen	Brain
up to 30 days	non detectable	=	=
30—60 days	trace amounts	=	=
60—90 days	0.35—0.7	3—3.3	=
90—120 days	0.65—0.7	3.1—3.3	=
120—150 days	0.7	3.4	=
	A 0.9—2; S 0.6—1.6; L 0.9—2	1.7—2.7	0.2—0.4
150—180 days	A 1.6—1.7; S 2.6—3.4; L 2.7—3.5	2.2—5.0	0.15—0.25
180—210 days	A 2.7; S 2.4; L 2.2	6.0	0.16
240 days	A 1.6; S 1.6; L 2.0	5.8	0.12

* A = abomasus, S = small intestine, L = large intestine.

In guinea-pigs, 5-HT first appears in the small intestine in measurable amounts after 30—40 days of intrauterine life, i.e. only half way through the gestation period. Thereafter the concentration in the gut rises rapidly till at birth it reaches a level about 60% of the adult. The rise in concentration of the 5-HT in the platelets follows the rise in the intestine, a result which supports the view that platelet 5-HT is derived from the intestine (STACEY and YOUNG 1964).

Data on the subcellular localization of 5-HT in the enterochromaffin cells and on the turnover rate of 5-HT in the gastrointestinal tract are presented in Chapter 5.

2. Blood

As early as 1912, O'CONNOR, as a result of his careful experimental observations, supposed that the serum vasoconstrictor did not pre-exist in the circulating plasma, but was released, during coagulation or defibrination of the blood, from the blood cells or, more probably, from the platelets. The hypothesis of the thrombocytic origin of the serum vasoconstrictor was later supported, with ever more convincing evidence, by ZUCKER and STEWART (1913), JANEWAY et al. (1918), HIROSE (1918), FREUND (1920a, 1920b), SIMON (1938, 1939), ZUCKER (1944, 1947, 1951), BRACCO and CURTI (1953, 1954), BRACCO et al. (1956) and finally by RAND and REID (1951, 1952) and by ZUCKER and RAPPORT (1954) and ZUCKER et al. (1954). By fractional centrifugation of ox blood rendered non-coagulable with sodium citrate, RAND and REID succeeded in establishing definitively that the presence of platelets at the time of clotting was a necessary condition for the appearance of 5-HT in the serum. ZUCKER and co-workers, in their turn, found that the content of 5-HT in bovine platelets was more than sufficient to account for all the 5-HT present in bovine serum. No other indolic or phenolic substances were found in the platelet extracts.

It is evident that the thrombocytes contain substances or active groups capable of anchoring 5-HT with especial selectivity and tenacity. This anchoring is very important in that, amongst other things, it provides a defence for 5-HT against amine oxidase and other enzymes, to which the substance would otherwise inevitably be exposed.

HUMPHREY and TOH (1954) first demonstrated that washed dog platelets possess the capacity of absorbing 5-HT from their suspending medium and these results have since then been confirmed, both *in vitro* and *in vivo*, by a number of research workers. From all the studies on this topic it clearly emerged on the one hand that there exists for every animal species a definite limit to the capacity of the thrombocytes to take up 5-HT and, on the other hand, that the absorption capacity of 5-HT by the thrombocytes is by no means saturated under normal conditions.

In fact, the maximum uptake of 5-HT observed by BORN and GILLSON (1959) for human platelets was 1.08 μg per 10^8 platelets, the normal content being 0.025—0.038 μg.

In fractioning experiments, carried out on suspensions of destroyed human thrombocytes, 95% of the platelet 5-HT was found by SCHULTZ et al. (1964) in the hyalomer fraction and only 5% in the granulomer fraction.

5-Hydroxy-α-methyltryptamine is taken up by ox platelets in the same way as 5-HT and the uptake is inhibited competitively by α-methyltryptamine (LONG 1962). Tryptamine is taken up by the platelets by a different mechanism and in the presence of tryptamine the uptake of 5-HT is depressed. Tryptophan, 5-HTP and DOPA do not affect 5-HT uptake by the platelets (STACEY 1961).

Specific hetero-antibodies (anti-human-platelet serum prepared in the rabbit) and iso-antibodies (serum from patients who have received multiple blood transfusions) strongly inhibit the *in vitro* uptake of 5-HT by platelets (BRIDGES et al. 1963).

When thrombocytes disintegrate, in the spleen, in other tissues or in the blood itself, 5-HT is of necessity set free either into the plasma or inside the macrophages. The further fate of the substance may then be very different inasmuch as, according to the circumstances, it may either be taken up by other thrombocytes, or undergo enzymatic inactivation, or finally act on the effector structures to provoke its peculiar biological actions.

There is at present no doubt that platelet 5-HT is of intestinal origin, with the possible partial exception of the few animal species containing 5-HT in their mast cells. Mature platelet is, in fact, not capable of forming 5-HT from its precursor 5-HTP (GADDUM and GIARMAN 1956).

Through the use of radioactive tryptophan it has been calculated that the half-life of platelet 5-HT is 24 to 73 hours, i.e. that the platelets lose their 5-HT only when disintegrating (UDENFRIEND and WEISSBACH 1958; MELMON and SJOERDSMA 1963).

Assuming in man a daily production of 5—20 mg 5-HT — as inferred from the urinary excretion of 5-HIAA (ERSPAMER and TESTINI 1959) — and a total 5-HT content in the platelets of 0.5—1 mg 5-HT (TODRICK et al. 1958), it should be concluded either that the turnover rate of 5-HT in the platelets is considerably faster than that calculated or that barely 2.5—20% of the 5-HT produced by the enterochromaffin cells is absorbed by the platelets.

Recent studies have concordantly shown that platelet 5-HT exchanges with other body depots of the amine and that it may be re-utilized after release from the platelets (PARKER-WILLIAMS et al. 1963; JACKSON et al. 1963, ZUCKER et al. 1964).

If we allow that thrombocytic 5-HT has its origin in the enterochromaffin cells of the gastrointestinal mucosa, then it must of necessity be admitted that a part of the 5-HT, though perhaps a very small part, does exist and circulates free in the plasma. In fact, the exchange of 5-HT between thrombocytes and enterochromaffin cells can take place only through the mediation of plasma, and the substance released following damage or lysis of the platelets must obviously penetrate, at least in part, into the plasma. The well-known extreme fragility of thrombocytes accounts for the circumstance that unambiguous quantitative data on plasma 5-HT are very difficult to collect.

HUMPHREY and JAQUES (1954b) indicate for dog, rabbit, and human plasmas a possible 5-HT content of 2 to 5 ng/ml, ARMIN and GRANT (1957a) a content in dog plasma of less than 0.1 ng/ml. It may be inferred that normal plasma 5-HT values exceeding 10 ng/ml are to be considered erroneous.

Table 8. *The 5-HT content of the serum (or whole blood) and spleen of other vertebrates* (in μg 5-HT base per g fresh tissue or ml serum)

Animal species	Serum (whole blood *)	Spleen	Reference
Ox	1.48	7.8	1
Goat	2.2	4.8	1
Sheep	0.85	3.8	1
Horse	0.4	1.75	1
Ass	0.4	3.1	1
Hog	0.26; 0.4*	1.2	1, 2
Hedgehog	1.8	1.8	1
Bat *(Rhinolophus ferrum equinum)*	3.6	19	1
Chicken	2.8; 2—3*	12.5	1, 3
Guinea-hen	2.7	=	1
Turkey	0.1	=	1
Duck	1.15	4.1	1
Goose	350 μg/g platelets	=	4
Pigeon	0.33	=	1
Sea gull	0.7	=	1
Stork	0.03	=	1
Tropidonotus natrix	0.4	0.16	1
Testudo graeca	0.01	0.01	1
Rana esculenta	0.18	0.08	1
Bufo bufo bufo	0.02	=	1
Scyliorhinus canicula	<0.02	<0.06	1
Scyliorhinus stellaris	<0.04	<0.06	1
Torpedo marmorata	<0.02	<0.06	1
Acipenser naccarii	0.01	0.03	1
Acipenser sturio	0.025	0.03	1
Anguilla anguilla	<0.05	<0.05	1
Tinca tinca	<0.04	<0.05	1
Ameiurus catus	<0.05	=	1
Petromyzon planeri	<0.05	=	1
Petromyzon marinus	<0.03	=	1

References to Table 8. [1] ERSPAMER (1954a, 1954b). — [2] GRETTE (1957). — [3] WEISSBACH et al. (1958). — [4] BRACCO and CURTI (1954).

For a better understanding of the data shown in the Tables 1—4 and 8 it should be emphasized that blood serum contains only part (43—59%) of the 5-HT present in the blood. The remainder is lost during the separation of serum owing to irreversible absorption by red cells or to enzyme attack (see page 746).

Blood 5-HT is reduced in thiamine-deficient rats (from 1.04 to 0.7 μg/ml) and in tryptophan-deficient rats (from 0.86 to 0.12 μg/ml), but not in starved rats (GAL and DREWES 1961, 1962). Similarly, there is a very conspicuous reduction of the 5-HT level in blood of pyridine-deficient chickens (from 5.5 to 0.4 μg/ml) (UDENFRIEND 1957).

Removal of the large intestine in rats does not cause any change in serum 5-HT levels, in spite of reduced biosynthesis of 5-HT. On the contrary, total removal of the gastrointestinal tract produces a conspicuous decrease in the serum 5-HT content. Decrease is of 50% after 24 hr, and of 85% after 3 days (BERTACCINI 1960). A similar 90% decrease of platelet 5-HT has been described by HAVERBACK and DAVIDSON (1958) in a patient with resection of large and small intestine.

This demonstrates unequivocally that the enterochromaffin cells of the gastrointestinal mucosa represent both in man and in the rat the main, if not the only, source of blood 5-HT.

Data on the content of 5-HT in foetal blood are scanty, but it may be supposed that, as in spleen tissue, 5-HT in blood makes its appearance rather early.

Pepeu and Giarman (1962) observed that whereas in the goat foetal blood contains more 5-HT than maternal blood (1.83—8 μg/ml as compared with 0.27 to 4.2 μg/ml) in the rabbit the level of 5-HT in maternal blood is almost twice as high as that found in foetal blood (1.2—2.5 μg/ml as compared with 0.53 to 2 μg/ml).

3. Spleen

5-HT is regularly present, in considerable amounts, in spleen tissue. The substance is contained to the greatest extent in the thrombocytes and thrombocyte fragments caught in the spleen. Mast-cell 5-HT contributes scarcely, even in rats and mice, to the total spleen 5-HT (Parratt and West 1957b). Generally, the amine is particularly abundant in the spleen tissue of animal species whose blood is rich in 5-HT (Erspamer 1940b, 1954b, c).

Faustini (1955) has been able to establish that 5-HT appears in the spleen from the earliest stages of its embryonic development (cf. Table 7).

4. Mast cells

The occurrence of 5-HT in mast cells was first demonstrated by Benditt et al. in 1955 (b). Since then, considerable work has been dedicated to the study of this peculiar localization of 5-HT in the mammalian organism and some fundamental facts may now be considered as firmly established:

a) Only rat and mouse mast cells contain important amounts of 5-HT. The amine is not detectable in the mast cells of other mammalian species, either under normal or pathological conditions (Bhattacharya and Lewis 1956, Parratt and West 1957a, Adams-Ray et al. 1964). The consequence of this statement is that, from a general biological point of view, 5-HT in the mast cells of the above rodents is little more than a biochemical rarity, and exactly the same may be said of the occurrence of 5-HT in the hypobranchial body of some molluscs or in the coelenteron tissue of some coelenterates.

It is obvious that those animal species which contain 5-HT in their mast cells display considerable 5-HT levels in nearly all their parenchymatous tissues (cf. Tables 1 and 4). However, a correlation between mast-cell population and 5-HT concentration is not always evident, i.e. mast cells do not necessarily contain the same quantity of 5-HT in the different rat tissues, nor is the 5-HT/histamine ratio everywhere the same (Bhattacharya and Lewis 1956). Parratt and West (1957a), for example, maintain that the abundant 5-HT which is found in the outer layer of the rat skin is not held in mast cells, at least in the typical metachromasia-yielding mast cells. This opinion is shared by Smith and Lewis (1961) on the basis of results obtained in rats treated with an anti-mast-cell serum, which caused no fall of skin 5-HT at the time when histamine and mast cells in the skin were very low. Similarly, mast-cell origin is doubtful in the case of the 5-HT found in the rat thyroid gland.

Green et al. (1960a, 1960b) found that heparin from rat tissues and from a mouse mastocytoma yielded, on fractionation, an unusual heparin fraction. They suggest that the anomalous occurrence of 5-HT in the mast cells of rats and mice may be explained by the presence of this unique heparin.

b) In the mouse 5-HT is present not only in normal mast cells, but also in neoplastic mast cells, namely in those of mastocytoma and of mast cell leukaemia.

Moreover, during chemical skin carcinogenesis in the mouse the 5-HT content of the skin at different stages of papilloma formation rises from 0.3 to 4.5 μg/g. 5-HT is apparently contained in cells giving a golden-yellow fluorescence with no or very little metachromasia (RILEY 1958, COUPLAND and RILEY 1960, FIORE-DONATI et al. 1962).

On the contrary, animals lacking 5-HT in their normal mast cells do not show any detectable 5-HT either in tissues abnormally rich in mast cells (mastocytosis) or in mastocytomas (Table 9).

Table 9. *The 5-HT content of mast cells*

Animal species and mast cell type	Content of 5-HT base	Reference
Rat Normal mast cells		
peritoneal cavity . . .	630—700 μg/ml cells	BENDITT et al. (1955b)
peritoneal cavity . . .	0.35—0.46 μg/10^6 cells	KELLER (1957)
peritoneal cavity . . .	1.02—1.59 μg/10^6 cells	MORAN et al. (1962, 1963)
feet, areolar tissue . . .	760 μg/ml cells	BENDITT (1957)
feet, dermis	780 μg/ml cells	BENDITT (1957)
back, areolar tissue . . .	800 μg/ml cells	BENDITT (1957)
back, dermis	1150 μg/ml cells	BENDITT (1957)
Mouse Mastocytoma		
tumoral tissue	6—714 μg/g tissue	FURTH et al. (1957) SJOERDSMA et al. (1957a) ONO et al. (1959)
tumoral cells in culture .	0.06—1.5 μg/10^6 cells	SCHINDLER et al. (1959) GREEN and DAY (1960b)
Mast cell leukemia . . .	7.74 μg/ml blood	ONO et al. (1959)
Dog Mastocytoma		
tumoral tissue	<0.2 μg/g fresh tissue	SJOERDSMA et al. (1957a) PARRATT and WEST (1957a)
tumoral tissue	0.32—0.83 μg/g lyophilized tissue	MEIER (1959)
Cow Mastocytoma		
tumoral tissue	no detectable 5-HT	PARRATT and WEST (1957a)
Man Mastocytoma	no detectable 5-HT	PARRATT and WEST (1957a)
Urticaria pigmentosa . .	<0.25 μg/g skin	PARRATT and WEST (1957a) SJOERDSMA et al. (1957a)
Spleen mastocytosis . .	no increase in 5-HT level	ENDE and CHERNISS (1958)
Liver mastocytosis . . .	no 5-HT detectable	GARDNER and TYCE (1958)
Cutaneous mastocytosis	<0.05 μg/g skin or ml blister content	STURM and STÜTTGEN (1962)

RICE and MITCHENER (1961) claim to have obtained histochemical evidence of the occurrence of 5-HT in a dog mast cell tumour. Unfortunately, the investigators were unable to support their not completely persuasive histochemical data (variable silver reaction!) with any biochemical or biological evidence.

ENERBACK (1963) in his turn affirms that mast cells occurring in human carcinoid tumours exhibit histochemical reactions suggesting that they contain 5-HT and that a large number of mast cells with positive enterochromaffin reactions may occur even in so-called anargentaffin carcinoids.

Apart from the fact that it is difficult to accept, in the case of a neoplastic tissue, the statement of ENERBACK that a cell which contains metachromatic granules *must* be a mast cell (why not an enterochromaffin cell with abnormal content in metachromatic granules?) the above finding demonstrates only that under conditions of enhanced 5-HT secretion, human mast cells are capable of "storing" 5-HT. Biosynthesis of 5-HT has never been demonstrated in human mast cells.

Similarly, the possible occurrence of 5-HTP in extracts of human skin affected by mastocytosis, as described by STURM and STÜTTGEN (1962) in a single clinical case, awaits confirmation. Perplexity seems justified not only by the meagre direct evidence, but even more by the lack of detectable 5-HT in the extracts.

It should be stressed at this point that, in a study by MEIER (1959), eight canine mastocytomas revealed only negligible quantities of 5-HT (?), averaging 0.49 μg per g dry lyophilized tumour material, although histochemically large amounts of indole compounds could be demonstrated, and that FIORE-DONATI et al. (1963) were unable to find any increase of 5-HT during chemical skin carcinogenesis in the hamster.

c) 5-HT in the mast cells is probably of completely autochthonal origin, i.e. it may be synthesized from L-tryptophan within the mast cells themselves. This has been shown by SCHINDLER et al. (1959) and by DAY and GREEN (1959) and GREEN and DAY (1960b), who found that neoplastic mast cells obtained from a mouse mastocytoma after many generations in culture maintained, or even increased, their high intracellular level of 5-HT. Of necessity, 5-HT is formed at the expense of the L-tryptophan in the cultural medium.

The above statement does not exclude the possibility that exogenous 5-HT may contribute to the store in mast cells. In fact, mast cells from the peritoneal fluid of the rat are capable of taking up 5-HT and histamine (not dopamine and noradrenaline) both in vitro and in vivo. The distribution ratios of 5-HT and histamine between cells and medium are 78 and 9.2, respectively (FURANO and GREEN 1964).

d) The turnover rate of mast-cell 5-HT is not known. Indirect evidence supports the view that under normal conditions it is probably rather slow, but that in the case of mastocytoma it may become more rapid. In fact, BERTACCINI (1960) has shown that removal of the entire gastrointestinal tract in rats causes the practical disappearance of 5-HIAA in urine, while leaving largely unaffected the mast-cell 5-HT in the skin, which accounts for more than 50% of the total 5-HT in the body. On the other hand, SJOERDSMA et al. (1957) have found that mouse mastocytoma provokes not only a huge increase in the 5-HT content of the mouse body (from 1.5 to 20 μg/g) but also a similar increase in the urinary 5-HIAA (from 6 to 70 μg/ml).

STOLK (1963) has described in the lizard a mast cell reaction during chemical skin carcinogenesis identical, in every detail, to that seen in the mouse by FIORE-DONATI et al. (1962). This raises the problem of the occurrence of 5-HT in mast cells of vertebrates other than mammals.

LEWIS (1957) considers each mast cell of rats and mice to be a minute pharmacological armamentarium destined not only to serve as outer defence in the body defence mechanism against tissue injury, but also as a store-house of vasoactive substances which may well be released physiologically to control the vasculature of the connective tissue. This view has recently been strengthened by the observation that mast cells may contain not only histamine and 5-HT but, at least in ungulates, dopamine also (COUPLAND and HEATH 1961).

5. Other extracerebral tissues of mammals

Concerning unusual localizations of 5-HT in animal species not containing 5-HT in their mast cells, two seem of particular interest: that in the rabbit lung and that in the sheep thyroid gland.

The 5-HT in the rabbit lung clearly originates from blood platelets, as shown by the fact that during anaphylactic shock, in which circulating platelets are caught in the lung, lung 5-HT may increase by 5 to 10 times (WAALKES and COBURN 1959).

The origins of the 5-HT contained in the sheep thyroid gland (2.4—7.5 μg/g fresh tissue) and the rat thyroid gland (2.4—5 μg/g) are unknown. The rabbit thyroid contains 0.09—0.29 μg/g 5-HT, the dog thyroid only 0.025 μg/g PAASONEN 1958). FALCK (1962) has recently shown that in the rat thyroid gland 5-HT may be localized in peculiar fluorescent cells. It would seem advisable to extend the search for typical enterochromaffin cells or fluorescent 5-HT-containing cells to the thyroid gland of the sheep and other animal species.

No significant changes in the 5-HT content of the rat thyroid gland are seen following single doses of methimazole or potassium thiocyanate. Repeated administration of methimazole, however, produces a significant increase of the total 5-HT in the gland (PAASONEN and PELTOLA 1960). As expected, the 5-HT level in the rat thyroid gland is raised also by administration of iproniazid and 5-HTP (PAASONEN et al. 1961).

Table 10. *The 5-HT content of miscellaneous vertebrate tissues*

Tissue		Content of 5-HT base (μg/g fresh tissue)	Reference
Man	Placenta	0.13 ± 0.04	KURIAKI and INOUE (1956)
	Lung	0.1	SANDERS et al. (1959)
	Skin	0.03	PARRATT and WEST (1957a)
			JOHANSSON (1960)
Monkey	Uvea and retina	0.15—0.97	LEVENE (1962)
	Lid	0.25	LEVENE (1962)
Goat	Placenta	0.25—0.27	PEPEU and GIARMAN (1962)
	Lung	0.8—2.2	PEPEU and GIARMAN (1962)
Sow	Urinary tract	0.13 (mucosa) 0.02 (muscular layer)	KOCH and ENGELHARDT (1959)
Hedgehog	Liver	1.46—2.79	UUSPÄÄ (1963)
	Lung (perfused)	0.71—0.94	UUSPÄÄ (1963)
	Kidney	0.21—0.59	UUSPÄÄ (1963)
Pigeon	Liver	0.22—0.48	APRISON et al. (1962)
	Heart	0.11—0.30	APRISON et al. (1962)
	Lung	0.08—0.26	APRISON et al. (1962)
Ameiurus nebulosus (fish)	Skin	< 0.02	WELSH (1964)

Minute amounts of 5-HT have been described in a variety of tissue extracts (see Tables 2, 3 and 10) but very often one cannot avoid the impression that this 5-HT may be referred to the blood contained in the tissues (GARVEN 1956), or that colour reactions, fluorescence reaction or pharmacological effects considered specific for 5-HT may in reality depend on substances other than 5-HT. It is hoped that the histochemical fluorescence method of FALCK (1962) will be of decisive importance, owing to its extreme sensitivity and high specificity, in solving many of the present doubts.

The 5-HT content of nearly all rat tissues shows a progressive increase during postnatal development. For example, the lung, liver and gastrointestinal tract of male rats weighing 36 g contains 0.52, 0.03 and 1.45 μg/g 5-HT, respectively; the same organs of rats weighing 300 g 2.02, 0.14 and 2.8 μg/kg, respectively (BERTACCINI 1958).

It is interesting to note that two days after weaning, the 5-HT and histamine values for ears, abdominal skin and skin of feet are about double those found in the unweaned rats of the same age. No detectable difference has been found in the 5-HT content of tissues secured from male and female rats of similar age (PARRATT and WEST 1956b).

Several parenchymatous tissues (lung, liver, kidney) contain apparently small amounts (0.05—0.2 μg/g) of tryptamine (HESS and UDENFRIEND 1959, HESS et al. 1959). This is all we know at present about the occurrence and distribution of this amine in the mammalian organism.

6. Central and peripheral nervous system

The occurrence of 5-HT in the CNS was first demonstrated by AMIN et al. (1954) and by TWAROG and PAGE (1953) and was soon confirmed by numerous other research workers. It may be seen from Tables 11 and 12 that all vertebrate species examined contain 5-HT in the brain. This fact represents again, as in the case of gastrointestinal mucosa, strong evidence that 5-HT in the brain has a general biological significance.

Table 11. *The 5-HT content of the central nervous system of the rat*

	The 5-HT content (in μg per g fresh tissue) as estimated by	
	Bioassay	Spectrofluorometric method
Whole brain	Rat uterus: 0.23—0.38[1]; 0.26—0.50[2]; 0.25—0.52[3]; 0.41—0.48[4]; 0.2—0.25[40] Rat stomach: 0.35[5]; 0.346 ± 0.01[6]; 0.286 ± 0.05[7] Venus heart: 0.34—0.42[8]; 0.21—0.45[9]; *0.36[10]; *0.36 ± 0.007[11]; *0.38 ± 0.02[12]	0.4[13]; 0.54[14]; 0.48—0.53[15]; 0.41—0.77[16]; 0.4—0.45[17]; 0.6 ± 0.1[18]; 0.63 ± 0.14[19]; 0.58 ± 0.014[20]; 0.78 ± 0.1[21]; 0.53[22]; 0.47[23]; 0.41[24]; 0.5—0.8[25]; 0.474[26]; 0.371 ± 0.048[27]; 0.81 ± 0.05[28]; 0.54 ± 0.08[29]; 0.57[32]; 0.49—0.62[33]; 0.58 ± 0.033[34]; 0.78—0.80[39] *0.54—0.59[10]; *0.43—0.52[11]; *0.52 ± 0.02[12] °0.62 (r.h.)—0.60 (l.h.)[42]
Frontal cortex		0.162 ± 0.014[31]
Cerebellum		0.029 ± 0.002[31]; 0.31[25]
Hippocampal gyrus		0.328 ± 0.07[31]
Hypothalamus		0.429 ± 0.123[31]
Anterior hypothalamus		3.8 ± 1.4[30]
Midbrain + stem		0.94[25]
Pons + mesencephalon + diencephalon		1.07—1.34[39]
Whole brain bound 5-HT		60—75%[35]; 85%[36]; 70%[37]; 82%[38]; 55%[41]
free 5-HT		25—40%; 15%; 30%; 18%; 39%

° r.h. = right hemibrain; l.h. = left hemibrain.

* Comparative assays with the Venus heart method and the spectrofluorometric method.

References to Table 11. [1] BERTACCINI (1959). — [2] BERTACCINI (1960). — [3] ERSPAMER and BERTACCINI (1962). — [4] BERTACCINI and ERSPAMER (1962). — [5] PAASONEN and KÄRKI (1959). [6] KIVALO et al. (1961). — [7] GÖRÖG and SZPORNI (1962). — [8] BONNYCASTLE et al. (1957). — [9] PAASONEN and GIARMAN (1958). — [10] FREEDMAN (1961). — [11] BONNYCASTLE et al. (1962). — [12] ANDERSON et al. (1962). — [13] BOGDANSKI et al. (1956). — [14] PLETSCHER (1956), PLETSCHER et al. (1956). — [15] MAAS and NIMMO (1959). — [16] TABACHNICK and RUBIN (1959). — [17] UDENFRIEND et al. (1958). — [18] RESNICK et al. (1961). — [19] SKILLEN et al. (1961). — [20] YUWILER and LOUTTIT (1961). — [21] SCHWABE et al. (1961). — [22] MOORE and BRODY (1961). — [23] EHRINGER et al. (1961). — [24] GAL and DREWES (1961). — [25] HESS and DOEPFNER (1961). — [26] GREEN et al. (1962). — [27] MAYNERT et al. (1962). — [28] ERSHOFF and GAL (1961). — [29] ERSHOFF et al. (1962). — [30] QUAY and HALEVY (1962). — [31] JOYCE (1962). — [32] SCHONE and LINDNER (1960). — [33] PUT and HOGENHUIS (1962). — [34] TOWNE et al. (1962). — [35] WHITTAKER (1959). — [36] GLUCKMAN (1960). — [37] SCHANBERG and GIARMAN (1962). — [38] GREEN and SAWYER (1962). — [39] MAAS (1963). — [40] WALASZEK and ABOOD (1959). — [41] CARLINI and GREEN (1963). — [42] HARVEY et al. (1963).

Table 12. *The 5-HT content of the whole brain in representatives of different vertebrate classes*

Animal species	5-HT content (in μg per g fresh tissue)
Rhesus monkey	0.43—0.53[22]
Rabbit	0.57 ± 0.08[1]; 0.46 ± 0.03[2]; 0.45—0.67[3]; 0.35 ± 0.014[4]
Guinea-pig	0.46 ± 0.05[2]; 0.6[5]; 0.44 ± 19[6]; 0.428[7]; 0.68—0.72[21] 0.56 ± 0.23[27]; 0.49 ± 0.24[28]
Mouse	0.85—1.0[8]; 0.48—0.62[9]; 0.66 ± 0.01[10]; 0.82 ± 0.02[11]; 0.59 ± 0.04[12]; 0.52 ± 0.05[13]; 0.78—0.93[14]; 0.53 ± 0.03[4]; 0.32[15]
Marmot	0.13[16]
Hedgehog	0.56—0.96[24]
Goat	0.08—0.12 parietal and frontal lobes, 0.11—0.12 hippocampus and basal ganglia[17]
Chicken	1.13[18]; 1.0[23]; 0.88 ± 0.08 hemispheres, 0.70 ± 0.10 midbrain, 0.51 ± 0.96 pons-medulla, 0.16 ± 0.05 cerebellum[26]
Pigeon	0.7[23]; 0.78—1.24 telencephalon, 0.6—1.2 diencephalon + optic lobes, 0.12—0.44 cerebellum, 0.93—1.5 pons-medulla[20]
Turkey	0.4[19]
Water snake	0.2[19]
Sceloporus cyanogenys	3.1[23]
Alligator mississipiensis	0.21—0.68 telencephalon, 0.46—1.56 diencephalon, 0.34—0.69 rhombencephalon, 0.5 cerebellum, 0.51—0.87 optic lobes[30]
Rana esculenta	0.25—0.35[29]
Rana pipiens	3.7[23]; 0.23—0.62 telencephalon, 0.75—1.6 diencephalon; 0.32—0.71 rhombencephalon, 1.1—1.6 optic lobes[30]
Rana catesbiana	0.36—0.7 telencephalon, 1.29—1.8 diencephalon, 0.36—1.0 rhombencephalon[30]
Hyla cinerea	2.0[23]
Bufo americanus	9.1[23]
Bufo marinus	1.5[23]
Bufo arenarum	0.8—1.3[25]
Bufo paracnemis	0.8[25]
Leptodactylus chaquensis	0.6—1.0[25]
Telmatobius hauthali	0.57[25]
Desmognatus fuscus	2.8[23]
Ambystoma tigrinum	2.9[23]
Necturus maculosus	1.1[23]
Scyliorhinus canicula	0.2[19]
Carassius auratus	0.15[23]
Amia calva	0.48[23]

References to Table 12. [1] Brodie et al. (1956); Shore and Brodie (1957). — [2] Bogdanski et al. (1956). — [3] Gursey et al. (1959), Gursey and Olson (1960). — [4] Haggendal et al. (1957). — [5] Pletscher (1956a). — [6] Whittaker (1962). — [7] Ryall (1962). — [8] Pletscher (1956)b. — [9] Bartlet (1960). — [10] Dubnick et al. (1960, 1962). — [11] Wiegand and Perry (1961). — [12] Wiegand and Scherfling (1962). — [13] Leroy (1962). — [14] Albrecht et al. (1956). — [15] Melching et al. (1960). — [16] Bertaccini, unpublished observations. — [17] Pepeu and Giarman (1962). — [18] Udenfriend et al. (1957). — [19] Correale (1956). — [20] Aprison et al. (1962). — [21] Haverback et al. (1957). — [22] Weissman and Finger (1962). — [23] Bogdanski et al. (1963), Brodie et al. (1954). — [24] Uuspää (1963). — [25] Nobili, unpublished observations. — [26] Pscheidt and Himwich (1963); Pscheidt (1964). — [27] Hsia et al. (1963). — [28] Michaelson and Whittaker (1963). — [29] de Caro and Roseghini, to be published. — [30] Welsh (1964).

Tables 13 and 14 of this chapter and Table 4 of chapter 13 show that, at least in mammals, 5-HT is preferentially contained in specific areas of the brain (brain stem structures, rhinencephalic structures, neostriatum) some of which are part of, or are functionally connected with, the autonomic system or the reticular activating system.

Although the problem of the origin of cerebral 5-HT is not solved, indirect evidence seems to support the view that brain 5-HT may originate locally from

L-tryptophan. We refer to the experiments of BERTACCINI (1960) showing that 5-HT is present, in nearly normal amounts, in the brain of rats deprived operatively of the whole gastrointestinal tract, and to the occurrence of considerable quantities of 5-HT in ganglia and peripheral nerves of molluscs containing only traces of the amine in all other tissues.

Table 13. *Regional distribution of 5-HT in the brain of the dog, cat and rabbit*

	5-HT content in μg base per g fresh tissue		
	Dog	Cat	Rabbit
Brain stem	0.75[1]; 0.43 ± 0.10[3]; 1.28[16]	0.79[1]	0.65[1]; 0.58—0.7[2]; 0.425 ± 0.05[3]
Spinal cord cervical	0.26 ± 0.013 (above Th2)[14]	0.24[4]	
sacral	0.25 ± 0.02 (below Th2)[14]	0.82[4]	
Medulla	0.55—0.62[5]	0.55—1.2[5]	
Area postrema	0.26[7]		
Floor 4th ventricle	0.17—0.37[7]		
Medulla-pons	0.56[15]	0.88[15]	0.63[9]
Pons	0.42—0.38[5]	0.33[6]; 0.7[5]	
Pontile reticular formation		0,89[6]	
Cerebellum	0.07—0.09[5]; 0.11 ± 0.04[16]	0.3—0.27[5]	0.12[9]
Cerebellar cortex	0.007—0.012[7]		
Inferior colliculus		0.76[6]	
Midbrain	0.97—1.0[5]	1.23—1.7[5]	0.83[9]
Midbrain reticular formation		2.6[6]	
Midbrain-hypothalamus	1.31[15]	0.5 ± 0.08[10]; 1.45[15]	
Hypothalamus	1.75[5]; 0.37[8]; 1.28[16]	1.78—2.0[5]	0.43 ± 0.12[11]
anterior		2.4[6]	
posterior		2.5[6]	
Thalamus	0.65[5]; 0.48[15]	0.78[5]; 0.43[6]; 0.91[15]	
Basal thalamic area		0.88[6]	
Caudate nucleus	0.27[8]; 0.72[5]; 0.48—0.63[12]; 0.61[15]; 0.51[16]	1.6[6,5]; 0.84[15]	
Intralaminar and midline nuclei		0.56[6]	
Olfactory bulb	0.38[5]; 0.04[7]; 0.08[8]		
Septal region	0.46[8]	2.0[6]	
Brain gyri	0.17[5]	0.24[5]	
White matter	0.07—0.13[5]; 0.02[8]	0.13[5]	
Cortical grey matter	0.27—0.34[5]	0.68[5]	
Central grey matter		1.6[6]	
Amygdala	2.1[5]; 0.48[8]	1.6[6]	
Hippocampus	0.64[5]; 0.25[8]; 0.46[15]	0.71[15]	0.33 ± 0.07[11]
Putamen	0.11[8]		
Hypnogenic zone of HESS		1.8[6]	
Neocortex		0.69[6]	
Frontal cortex			0.055 ± 0.002[11]
Auditory cortex		0.41[6]	
Pyriform cortex	0.94[5]; 0.18—0.48[8]	1.4[6]	
Posterior pituitary	0[7]		
Sympathetic ganglia	0[7]	0.2[13]	

References to Table 13. [1] BRODIE et al. (1959). — [2] SPECTOR et al. (1960). — [3] MAYNERT et al. (1962). — [4] ANDERSON and CUDIA (1962). — [5] BOGDANSKI and UDENFRIEND (1956), BOGDANSKI et al. (1957). — [6] KUNTZMAN et al. (1961). — [7] PAASONEN and VOGT (1956). — [8] PAASONEN et al. (1957). — [9] COSTA and APRISON 1958). — [10] ANTONELLI et al. (1961). — [11] JOYCE (1962). — [12] ASHCROFT and SHARMAN (1962). — [13] GERTNER et al. (1959). — [14] CARLSSON et al. (1963). — [15] PSCHEIDT et al. (1964). — [16] TYCE et al. (1964).

Quite recently direct evidence that brain tissue is capable of hydroxylating L-tryptophan has been furnished by several groups of research workers [e.g. GREEN, H., and J. L. SAWYER, Fed. Proc. 24, 604 (1965)].

Concerning the problem of the distribution of 5-HT at cellular and subcellular levels within the brain tissue, there is still considerable uncertainty and perplexity. Three main possibilities should be kept in mind, namely that:

a) 5-HT is contained, at least in some areas, in glia cells instead of in true nervous cells. This possibility is supported, α) by the finding that in autoradiographs of brain tissue obtained after injection of radioactive 5-HTP, the 5-HT appears to be distributed fairly evenly throughout the brain with no relation to nervous elements (LEWIS 1958), β) by the observation that in the dog whole CNS the highest concentrations of 5-HT are found in the area postrema which consists of highly vascular neuroglia tissue and only some nervous cells (STACEY 1959), γ) by the observation that in mount rabbit brain cortex cultures and subtransplants some glial elements and fibers contain yellow fluorescent monoamines (5-HT ?) (GEIGER et al. 1964), and finally, γ) by the stimulating experimental results of UTLEY (1963), who found that removal in the cat of cortical areas known as A I, A II, Ep, S II, temporal and insular (which results in retrograde degeneration and gliosis in all portions of the principal division of the medial geniculate body, with a 45% decrease in weight) produced a 70% increase of 5-HT in the residual atrophic tissue (from 1.2 to 2.05 μg/g). This 5-HT concentration persisted even after successive lesions of the brachium of the inferior colliculus.

Table 14. *Regional distribution of 5-HT in the brain of the monkey (Macacus rhesus)* (PSCHEIDT and HIMWICH 1963)

	5-HT content, in μg base per g fresh tissue *
Pons-medulla	0.49 ± 0.11
Midbrain (hypothalamus)	0.77 ± 0.16
Caudate	0.36 ± 0.06
Thalamus	0.56 ± 0.15
Hippocampus (amigdala)	0.29 ± 0.08
Various cortical structures	0.17 ± 0.04
Temporal pole	0.20—0.24
Lenticular thalamic mass	0.29—0.35

* Spectrofluorometric method.

JOYCE (1963) has recently shown that glioma tissue contains less 5-HT than normal surrounding cerebral tissue. However, in the writer's opinion this observation, while certainly not in favour of the theory that 5-HT is localized in glia cells, does not disprove this theory. In fact, data obtained in neoplastic cells can hardly be transferred to normal cells.

b) 5-HT is present in the body of the nervous cell. This is the opinion shared, tacitly or expressly, by the majority of research workers. According to WALASZEK and ABOOD (1959) most of the 5-HT present in rat brain is bound to the mitochondria, but other investigators (GLUCKMAN 1960, GIARMAN and SCHANBERG 1959, INOUYE et al. 1962, KATAOKA 1962, CARLINI and GREEN 1963) while confirming that 60—80% of the brain 5-HT resides in granules, eschew a more precise definition of the nature of these granules.

c) 5-HT is contained in the nerve endings, more precisely in the synaptic vesicles or in particles quite similar to them. This theory, which has been advanced by WHITTAKER (1959, 1961, 1962) and MICHAELSON and WHITTAKER (1962, 1963) is at present the most satisfactory and attractive. WHITTAKER suggests that, like acetylcholine, 5-HT also may be bound to the particles partly in a highly labile state and partly in a more stable state. Subcellular particles containing 5-HT are distinct from those storing acetylcholine (cf. also RYALL 1963, 1964).

CARLSSON et al. (1963) have recently shown that a week after transection of the rabbit spinal cord at the 2nd thoracic segment the 5-HT in the portion below the section was only about 15% of that found in the cervical portion (0.04 ± 0.015 as compared to 0.32 ± 0.02 μg/g). According to the Swedish investigators this fact may be interpreted to mean that 5-HT in the cord is mostly localized, like noradrenaline, in the fibres descending from more centrally sited cell bodies. The interpretation is not in contrast with the WHITTAKER's theory.

The turnover rate of 5-HT in the CNS is high. With the aid of powerful, promptly-acting monoamineoxidase inhibitors it has been demonstrated that the half-life of cerebral 5-HT is not longer than 10 to 20 min (UDENFRIEND et al. 1958), and according to 5-HT estimates in brains of rats anaesthetized with pentobarbital sodium it is even shorter (2 minutes) (ANDERSON and BONNYCASTLE 1960).

ALBRECHT et al. (1956) found that the brain 5-HT level is slightly higher in female mice than in male adult mice (0.93 and 0.78 μg/g, respectively) and that a small but significant decrease in 5-HT concentration of brain pools is noted prior to the usual time of arousal. On the average the concentration of 5-HT in brain is higher before and around noon than at or after 4.30 p.m. (difference 0.12 μg/g).

MAAS (1963) has recently called attention to the possible existence of neurochemical differences among different strains of mice. He found that whereas the 5-HT in total brain did not differ significantly in the two examined strains (0.807 and 0.783 μg/g), the 5-HT in pons + mesencephalon + diencephalon was 1.34 ± 0.046 μg/g in strain BABL/CJ and 1.07 ± 0.037 μg/g in strain C57BL/10J.

Data on the appearance of brain 5-HT during embryonic life are still incomplete and in part contrasting.

NACHMIAS (1960) found that 5-HT is present in the brain of newborn rats at about a third of the concentration in adult brain and increases in a linear fashion thereafter; KÄRKI et al. (1960, 1962) observed that three days before birth rat brain 5-HT is about 25% (norepinephrine 15%), at birth 50% (norepinephrine 20%), and two weeks later 70% (norepinephrine 40%) of normal, with values of the mature animals (0.47 ± 0.02 μg/g) being approached in seven weeks; finally WANG et al. (1962) noted, in full confirmation of the above results, that in rat brain 5-HT increases gradually from birth, attaining 0.45 ± 0.02 μg/g at 20 days of age and 0.77 ± 0.03 μg/g at 39 days of age.

Rabbits behave like rats (brain 5-HT levels in newborn and adult rabbits = 0.33 ± 0.05 and 0.60 ± 0.02 μg, respectively), whereas in guinea-pigs the amount of 5-HT stored in the brain of newborn animals approaches the adult figure (0.26 ± 0.01 μg/g, as compared to 0.33 ± 0.01 μg/g) (KÄRKI et al. 1962, SMITH et al. 1961, PEPEU and GIARMAN 1960, 1962).

It has been suggested that the above biochemical differences should be correlated with differences in the functional development or degree of maturity of the various species at birth. However, this hypothesis does not seem to have a general value since in goat foetuses, late in gestation, the 5-HT content of different brain areas is considerably larger than that of the corresponding maternal brain areas (foetus and mother, respectively: parietal lobe 0.36 and 0.10, occipital lobe 0.29 and 0.09, hippocampus 0.25 and 0.15, basal ganglia 0.27 and 0.17 μg/g) (PEPEU and GIARMAN 1960, 1962).

The observations on the influence of the diet on brain 5-HT levels in rats are of considerable interest.

Young rats maintained for 1 to 7 weeks on a diet supplemented with 2—7% phenylalanine regularly present a marked decrease (20—35%) in the brain 5-HT level. This decrease is even greater (70%) in animals kept on a tryptophan-free diet. On the contrary, rats kept on a high-tryptophan diet show a consistent increase (30—35%) in 5-HT levels. Finally, rats kept on a diet supplemented with both phenylalanine and tryptophan present, depending on the ratio between the two aminoacids, increased, unchanged or decreased 5-HT concentrations in the brain (WANG et al. 1961, 1962; YUWILER and LOUTTIT 1961; GAL et al. 1961; SCHANBERG et al. 1962; GREEN et al. 1962; GAL and DREWES 1962; CULLEY et al. 1963). The depressive effect of a low-tryptophan diet on brain 5-HT has been confirmed by ZBINDEN et al. (1958) in the guinea-pig and in the mouse, that of a high-phenylalanine diet by HSIA et al. (1963) in the guinea-pig.

Excess dietary tyrosine (7%) causes little or no change in brain 5-HT, excess valine (6—9%) a 17% decrease of the amine, phenylacetic acid (5%) a 22% increase (BOGGS et al. 1963).

The mode of action of tryptophan excess or deficiency is obvious; phenylalanine is believed to act as a depressor of dopadecarboxylase via its metabolites.

Table 15. *The 5-HT content (in μg/g) of the hedgehog brain during activity and hibernation* (UUSPÄÄ 1963)

	Summer active state	Cold season	
		active state	hibernating
Whole brain	0.56 ± 0.026	0.85 ± 0.056	0.96 ± 0.045
Cerebellum	0.05 ± 0.004	0.07 ± 0.02	0.06 ± 0.02
Medulla and pons	0.78 ± 0.02	1.00 ± 0.07	1.21 ± 0.08
Mesencephalon	1.37 ± 0.04	1.76 ± 0.07	1.79 ± 0.08
Diencephalon	1.00 ± 0.05	1.25 ± 0.08	1.22 ± 0.06
Cerebral hemispheres	0.37 ± 0.04	0.75 ± 0.08	0.89 ± 0.06
Olfactory bulbs	0.27 ± 0.08	0.41 ± 0.04	0.47 ± 0.04

UUSPÄÄ (1963) has carried out a comparative study on the 5-HT content of the hedgehog brain during activity and hibernation. Results are shown in Table 15.

It may be seen that whereas an increase in the 5-HT content occurs during the cold season, this increase seems to be independent of the activity of the animal. In fact, no significant differences are found in brain 5-HT levels between hibernating hedgehogs and animals kept at room temperature during the cold season.

Neither starvation nor thiamine deficiency produces any change in the brain 5-HT levels of rats (GAL and DREWES 1961). Pyridoxine-deficiency causes only a small decrease in the 5-HT concentration of the rat brain (YEH et al. 1959), but a conspicuous decrease in the brain 5-HT level of chickens (UDENFRIEND et al. 1957).

TOH (1960) observed that the 5-HT content of the brain of rats exposed to extreme heat or cold was lower (0.20 and 0.24 μg/g) than that of control rats (0.38 μg/g).

BARCHAS and FREEDMAN (1963) noted that swimming to exhaustion produced a 13—15% increase in brain 5-HT levels and wheel a 10% increase, whereas a number of other stressors (exposure to cold, electroshock, 72 hours of food and water deprivation, anoxia in a nitrogen chamber, adrenalectomy) failed to evoke significant changes.

TYCE et al. (1962) could not find any change in the brain 5-HT levels of dogs submitted to hepatectomy or of Eck-fistula dogs.

Results obtained in the rat were at variance. In fact, TYCE et al. (1963) observed that in this species 24 hr after hepatectomy the concentration of 5-HT in the brain showed a twofold, and that of 5-HIAA a 3-fold increase, indicating a rapid turnover of 5-HT. Tryptophan showed a 4- to 5-fold increase.

Not only 5-HT but also tryptamine must be considered a normal constituent of brain tissue. The brain content of this amine seems, however, to be rather low (HESS et al. 1959, HESS and DOEPFNER 1961) and information about regional differences in its distribution is lacking.

Among the metabolites of 5-HT the only one so far detected in brain tissue is 5-HIAA, but there is the possibility that other acidic or basic 5-hydroxyindole compounds are present (ASHCROFT and SHARMAN 1962).

According to PLETSCHER et al. (1963) rat brains contain 0.37 ± 0.01 μg 5-HIAA per g tissue, as compared to the 0.57 ± 0.02 μg/g 5-HT found in the same brains.

Among the areas of the CNS, the pineal gland occupies a unique position since, in addition to large amounts of 5-HT and 5-HIAA, it contains two unusual 5-hydroxyindole derivatives: melatonin and its metabolite 5-methoxyindoleacetic acid (LERNER and CASE 1960). Table 16 shows that the 5-HT levels in the pineal gland are the highest ever reported in any neuronal structure of all species examined. However, it should be stressed that only part and less than half of the material that is measured in the rat pineal by the fluorescence method is 5-HT (QUAI and HALEVY 1962).

Table 16. *Indole derivatives in the pineal gland*

	Content in μg per g fresh tissue				Reference
	5-HT	5-HIAA	Melatonin	5-Methoxy IAA	
Steer . . .	0.2—0.63	2	0.2	2	1, 2, 3, 4
Monkey .	1.2—10.1				3
Man . . .	0.36—22.8				3
Rat . . .	11; 10—90;	4—18	1—3	1	5, 8
	56.9—72.6				7
Goat . . .	1.2—7				6

References to Table 16. [1] GIARMAN and DAY (1958). — [2] GIARMAN et al. (1959). — [3] GIARMAN and FREEDMAN (1960). — [4] LERNER et al. (1959b), LERNER et al. (1960). — [5] QUAY (1963c, 1964). — [6] PEPEU and GIARMAN (1962). — [7] OWMAN (1963). — [8] DE IRALDI et al. (1963).

The content of 5-HT and related indole amines in the rat pineal gland nearly doubles during the second postnatal week and attains nearly adult levels. Continuous artificial light for either $4^1/_2$ or $21^1/_2$ weeks significantly reduces the amine content (from 89 to 45.3 μg/g and from 120.7 to 71.7 μg/g, respectively). A similar reduction is produced by transection of the optical tracts $4^1/_2$ weeks before removal of the pineals for analysis (QUAI and HALEVY 1962).

DE IRALDI and DE ROBERTIS (1961) suggest that 5-HT is contained, together with other amines, in the secretory processes of the pinealocyte, and more precisely in the heterogeneous vesicles of these processes. This suggestion is supported by the disappearance of the heterogeneous vesicles following reserpine administration.

However, fluorescence microscopy seems to indicate that in the rat, mouse, guinea-pig and dog pineal gland indolealkylamines may be contained also in pineal nerves, more precisely in the network of nerve fibres enclosing the vessels. In cat and rabbit pineals, on the contrary, the fluorescence reaction in the nerves indicates the presence of a primary catecholamine. In the rat, an intense tryptamine-fluorescence also develops in the parenchymal cells.

After bilateral cervical sympathectomy and after single reserpine injections no fluorescence occurs in the nerves and the 5-HT of the rat pineal gland is decreased to 50% (OWMAN 1963).

The decrease in the pineal 5-HT content following bilateral gangliectomy has been confirmed by DE IRALDI et al. (1963), who similarly suggest, continuing their previous studies, that there are probably two different pools of 5-HT in the rat pineal gland, one located in the parenchymal cells and the other in the sympathetic nerve fibres and endings.

Of considerable importance are the recent observations of QUAY (1963c, 1964) on the existance of a daily cycle or circadian rhythm of surprising amplitude for the 5-HT, 5-HIAA and melatonin contained in the pineal body of the rat.

Pineal 5-HT rises from a nocturnal minimum of 10 ng/pineal to a midday maximum of over 90 ng/pineal and falls rapidly at the start of darkness (Fig. 1). If the start of darkness is delayed, the nocturnal drop of pineal 5-HT is reduced or even abolished. The time at which the lights turn on in the morning has much less effect on 5-HT levels.

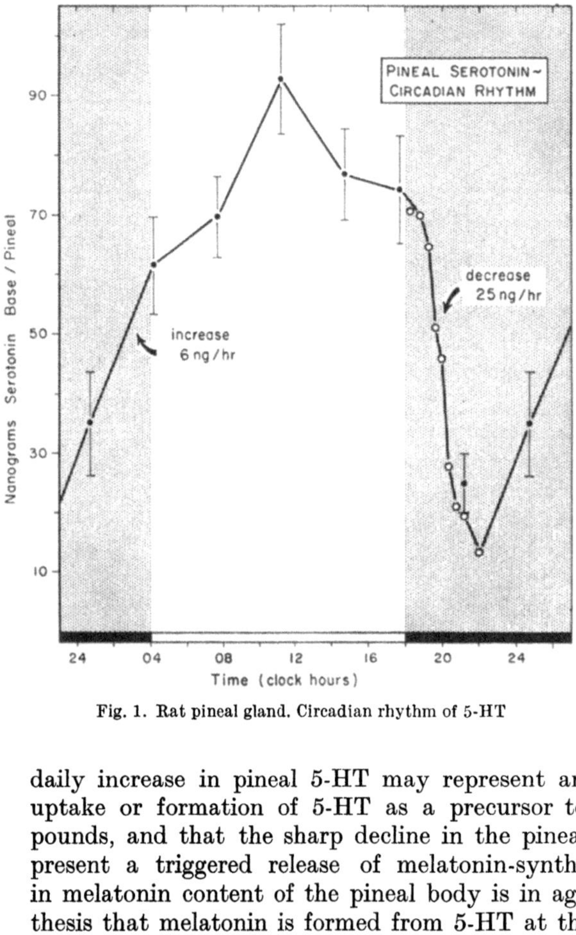

Fig. 1. Rat pineal gland. Circadian rhythm of 5-HT

Pineal 5-HIAA similarly rises from a nocturnal basal level of about 4 ng/pineal to an early afternoon maximum of about 18 ng/pineal and again falls sharply at the start of darkness. However, the time of maximum 5-HIAA content of the pineal is significantly later than the time of maximum 5-HT content. In sharp con, trast to 5-HT and 5-HIAA-pineal melatonin rises on the start of darkness, from 1 to 3 ng/pineal. 5-Methoxyindoleacetic acid, averaging 0.98 ng/pineal, shows no circadian change.

The physiological meaning of the circadian rhythm in pineal 5-HT is not clear. QUAY suggests that the slow daily increase in pineal 5-HT may represent an intrinsic rate of continuous uptake or formation of 5-HT as a precursor to melatonin and related compounds, and that the sharp decline in the pineal 5-HT in the evening may represent a triggered release of melatonin-synthesizing activity. The rhythm in melatonin content of the pineal body is in agreement with the above hypothesis that melatonin is formed from 5-HT at the start of darkness.

The 5-HT, 5-HIAA and melatonin content of the rat pineal is, to a slight but significant degree, modified by, or shows fluctuations correlated with, the estrous cycle. Early morning pineal 5-HT, for example, shows a trend of increasing during the estrous period, and evening 5-HT a trend in reduction. The behaviour of melatonin is similar, the behaviour of 5-HIAA opposite to that of 5-HT (QUAY 1964).

Feeding a high-tryptophan diet leads to a 250% increase in pineal 5-HT levels, feeding a high-phenylalanine diet to a 30% reduction (QUAY 1963b).

Other very important studies on melatonin in the pineal gland were carried out by AXELROD and co-workers. The main results so far obtained are summarized below, but research on this topic is still in progress.

Exposure to light reduces the ability of the rat pineal gland to synthesize melatonin (from 5 to 2 ng/hr/pineal) and decreases the weight of the gland (from 1.2 to 0.95 mg in female rats weighing 160—180 g). When the sympathetic nerves to the pineal are cut, light no longer has an effect on melatonin synthesis or pineal weight. The response of the gland does not require that the gonads or the pituitary gland be present (WURTMAN et al. 1964).

In surprising contrast with the rat pineal gland, the hen pineal gland shows a highly significant decrease in the activity of the melatonin-forming enzyme when the animals are kept in darkness for 5 days. The activity of hydroxyindole-O-methyl transferase per mg of pineals in hens is at least 200 times that of the rat (AXELROD et al. 1964).

The 5-HT content in the vertebrate eye which is, in part, derived from the central nervous system, has been thoroughly investigated by WELSH (1964). He found that 5-HT was present in the retina and pigment epithelium-choroid complex of several representative vertebrates, in amounts ranging from 2—2.5 μg/g (*Pomolabrus pseudoharengus*, a fish) to < 0.05 μg/g (retina of *Bos taurus*). Where the retina could be cleanly separated from pigmented tissue, the values for the two layers were about the same. Other values of 5-HT in the retina and pigment epithelium-choroid complex were as follows: *Rana pipiens* 0.7—0.8 μg/g, *Rana catesbiana* 0.2—0.4 μg/g, *Bufo marinus* 0.4—0.6 μg/g, *Alligator mississipiensis* 0.25—0.41 μg/g, *Rattus norvegicus* 0.22—0.27 μg/g, *Lepus cuniculus* 0.1—0.2 μg/g.

The problem of whether the autonomic ganglia of mammals contain 5-HT or are capable of synthesizing the substance cannot be considered solved by the partially positive results of GERTNER et al. (1959), which contrast with the negative results of AMIN et al. (1954). At any rate no measurable 5-HT appears in the perfusate from the functioning superior cervical ganglion of the cat *in situ* unless iproniazid is added to the perfusion liquid. But even in this case there is a delay of 2 hr before 5-HT appears in the effluent (GERTNER et al. 1959).

Peripheral nerves apparently do not contain 5-HT (AMIN et al. 1954, GARVEN 1956). However, a melatonin-like substance has been described in some of them (LERNER et al. 1959).

The occurrence of 5-HT in normal cerebrospinal fluid has never been demonstrated with certainty either in man or in the dog. In fact, the values given by the different investigators (2—20 ng/ml) are beyond the practical limits of sensitivity of the available biological and fluorometric methods (AMIN et al. 1954; FELDMAN et al. 1957; TURNER and MAUSS 1959; ASHCROFT and SHARMAN 1960, 1961; DERRY et al. 1961; BOWERS 1962; PERRY et al. 1964). This statement is more relevant when one considers that cerebrospinal fluid may contain substances disturbing both bioassay (BOWERS 1962) and spectrofluorometric estimation of 5-HT (ASHCROFT and SHARMAN 1962).

5-HT is not detectable in cerebrospinal fluid even after MAO inhibitors (BOWERS 1962, PERRY et al. 1961) or after intravenous infusion of large amounts of 5-HT (SOUTHERN 1960). The same significance has the lack of 5-HT in the cerebrospinal fluid of carcinoid patients (SJOERDSMA et al. 1957b).

According to ASHCROFT and SHARMAN (1960, 1961) and ROOS (1963) the cerebrospinal fluid contains acidic 5-hydroxyindole derivatives, among which the most important is 5-HIAA (0.03—0.04 μg/ml).

The occurrence of tryptamine in pooled human cerebrospinal fluid, at a concentration of about 0.02 μg/ml has been reported by JENSEN (1962), but not confirmed by PERRY et al. (1964).

7. Venom of reptiles

Zarafonetis and Kalas (1960) have described the presence of minute amounts of 5-HT in the venom of certain reptiles: *Heloderma horridum*, 2,2 μg 5-HT base/ml venom; *Crotalus atrox*, 0.15—0.3 μg/ml; *Crotalus adamanteus*, 0.1 μg/ml; *Agkistrodon piscivorus*, 0.35 μg/ml. 5-HT is accompanied by other known (tryptamine, 5-HIAA, IAA) and unknown indole compounds.

It seems futile to ascribe to these unimportant amounts of indolealkylamines any significance in the complex action of the snake venom.

8. Amphibian skin

Amphibian skin represents one of the most conspicuous localizations of indolealkylamines in the living organism. No tissue can compete with the parotoid glands of some toads as regards the absolute values of indolealkylamines, and in no tissue is there such a variety of indolealkylamines. It is therefore conceivable that comparative studies of the skin of adult and larval amphibians may contribute substantially to a better understanding of the metabolic possibilities of these substances in the living organism.

Table 17 shows the indolealkylamine content of the skin of a number of amphibians studied in the writer's laboratory since 1957.

In the skin of the following species of amphibians, none of the tabulated indole derivatives could be found in detectable amounts: *Euproctes rusconi*, *Pleurodeles waltlii*, *Triton cristatus*, *Ambystoma tigrinum* (Axolotl), *Leptodactylus chaquensis*, *Leptodactylus ocellatus*, *Leptodactylus bolivianus*, *Leptodactylus prognatus*, *Leptodactylus bufonius*, *Physalaemus fuscumaculatus*, *Physalaemus centralis*, *Pleurodema tucumana*, *Pleurodema cinerea*, *Pleurodema bibroni*, *Ceratophrys ornata*, *Cycloramphus fuliginosus*, *Eleutherodactylus ranoides*, *Corythomantis brunoi*, *Trachycephalus nigromaculatus*, *Gastrotheca boliviana*, *Batracophrynus macrostomum*, *Sphoenorhyncus aurantiacus*, *Thoropa petropolitana*, *Telmatobius hauthali*, *Elosia aspera*, *Elosia lateristrigata*, *Phyllomedusa sauvagi*, *Phyllomedusa annae*, *Phyllomedusa hypochondrialis*, *Phyllomedusa burmeisteri*, *Hyla lanciformis*, *Hyla faber*, *Hyla radiana*, *Hyla trachytorax*, *Hyla nasica*, *Hyla raniceps*, *Hyla semiguttata*, *Hyla albomarginata*, *Hyla ansper*, *Rana megapoda*, *Rana limnocharis*, *Hynobius nebulosus*, *Triturus pyrrhogaster*, *Polypedates buergeri*, *Dicroglossus occipitalis*, *Racophorus madagascariensis*, *Rana fuscigola*, *Chiromantis rufescens*, *Phyctimantis verrucosus*, *Ptychadena mascariniensis*, *Leptopelis karissimbensis*, *Arthroleptis adolphi-friederici*, *Callixalus* sp., *Chrysobatrachus* sp. *Hyla spegazzini*, *Hyla multilinea*, *Telmatobius montanus*, *Lepidobathracus hanensis*, *Lepidobathracus salinicola*, *Eleutherodactylus bufoniformis*, *Leptodactylus sibilatrix*, *Eupsophus roseus*, *Eupsophus nodosus*, *Pseudis paradoxa*, *Physalaemus bresslaui*.

It may be seen that nearly all indolealkylamines so far found in the animal kingdom are present also in the amphibian skin, and it is certain that other indolealkylamines will be discovered in the systematic screening of skin extracts from new amphibian species.

In all probability indolealkylamines in this localization are of completely autochthonal origin, i.e. they are fully independent, in regard to biosynthesis, of gastrointestinal mucosa. In fact, whereas the 5-HT content of the gastrointestinal mucosa is practically the same in the different amphibian species (0.5—3 μg/g), that of the skin may vary within extremely wide limits (O to 1000 μg/g).

Indolealkylamines in the skin of amphibians are destined exclusively for external secretion and their biosynthesis is therefore strictly connected with the

Table 17. *The content of indolealkylamines in the amphibian skin*[1]
(in μg per g dry or fresh$^+$ tissue)

Amphibian species	5-HT	N-Methyl-5-HT	Bufotenine	Bufotenidine	Dehydrobufotenine	Bufothionine	Tryptamine
Bufo bufo bufo$^+$	20	10	450	50	130	260	0
Bufo viridis$^+$	5—10	20—30	350—630	30	0	0	(Bufoviridine 450—520)
Bufo calamita$^+$	6—8	13—15	95—110	30—40	0	0	(Bufoviridine 220—230)
Bufo arenarum	40—250	40—200	800—2600	40—130	250—700	150—450	0
Bufo paracnemis							
whole skin	25—70	10—200	2.8—4.3 mg	180—220	120—180	110—290	0
a) parotoid glands	100—150	=	13—20 mg	650—1600	500—700	220—350	0
b) coxal glands	150	=	16—20 mg	500—1000	300—400	120	0
c) remaining skin	20—70	=	0.4—0.5 mg	30—50	30—100	100—270	0
Bufo marinus	30—140	40—130	<2—4	0	2200—6000	30—375	0
Bufo marinus poeppigi	160	100—140	0	0	270—1100	210—240	0
Bufo ictericus	5—70	<4—50	<2—15	0	1800—4500	35—375	0
Bufo granulosus major	60—250	25—130	140—200	0	<10—1000	300—750	0
Bufo granulosus fernandezae	60—750	300—650	80—150	0	1200—2400	900—1500	0
Bufo spinulosus spinulosus	5—50	0	15—230	<3—80	180—4000	360—3600	0
Bufo spinulosus trifolium	0	0	550	100	0	0	0
Bufo terrestris	0	0	0	80	0	0	0
Bufo boreas	0	3—10	230—300	20—50	0	250—360	0
Bufo valliceps	1600	traces	0	0	0	0	0
Bufo alvarius	4—6	30—40	250—1500	0	0	0	15—30 mg 5-Methoxy-N,N-dimethyl-tryptamine
Bufo cognatus	600	20	0	0	20	0	0
Bufo speciosus	600—4500	80—450	0	0	50—300	0	0
Bufo canaliferus	3000	120—130	0	80	0	200	0
Bufo debilis$^+$	24—30	30	0	15 (?)	750	450	0
Bufo horribilis	500—520	300	30	25—30	3000	? (<30)	0
Bufo typhonius	5—10		0	0	450	630	0
Bufo variegatus	0	0	8500	750	0	0	0
Bufo woodhousei	500—800	40	0	950—1200	150—200	0	0
Bufo punctatus	0	0	20	0	125—1000	100—750	0
Bufo haematiticus	2100	0	0	0	9000	0	0
Bufo americanus	++	+	++	++		+	0
Bufo fowleri	++	+	++	++		+	0
Bufo mauretanicus	150—300	0	0	0	0	0	0
Bufo funereus	180	0	0	0	0	0	0
Bufo regularis	550—2500	0	0	0	0	0	0
Bufo berghei	150	0	0	0	0	0	0
Bufo kisoloensis	600	0	0	0	0	0	0
Bufo formosus	80—100	60	150	130—150	15—30	300	0
Bufo gargarizans Chan Su	++	+	?	++			0
Bufo melanostictus	125	0	15	1250	8—9	0	0
Pseudobufo subasper	8—10	0	0	0	0	0	0
Leptodactylus laticeps	570	0	0	0	0	0	0
Leptodactylus pentadactylus pentadactylus	130—150	0	0	0	0	0	0
Leptodactylus pentadactylus labyrinthicus	100—1800	0	0	0	0	0	0
Leptodactylus pentadactylus dengleri	40—65	0	0	500—700	3	0	0

Table 17. (Continued)

Amphibian species	5-HT	N-Methyl-5-HT	Bufotenine	Bufotenidine	Dehydrobufotenine	Bufothionine	Tryptamine
Leptodactylus podicipinus podicipinus	640	0	0	15—20	0	0	0
Leptodactylus podicipinus petersi	1—1.5	0	0	2.5—3	0	0	0
Leptodactylus rubido cope	7	0	0	40—45	0	0	0
Leptodactylus melanonotus	35	10	0	25	0	0	0
Odontophrynus americanus	300—1700	0	0	0	0	0	0
Odontophrynus occidentalis	500	0	0	0	0	0	0
Scaphiopus hammondi .	550—600	0	0	70	0	0	0
Scaphiopus couchi . . .	320	0	0	0	0	0	0
Xenopus laevis+	100—200	0	0	600—1800	0	0	0
Melanophryniscus moreirae	40—70	0	2400—3000	30	0	0	0
Thoropa miliaris . . .	2—10	0	0	0	0	0	0
Osteocephalus taurinus .	2—3	0	0	0	0	0	0
Bombina variegata pachypus+	400—450	0	0	0	0	0	0
Bombina bombina . . .	++	0	0	0	0	0	0
Discoglossus pictus+ . .	200—350	0	0	0	0	0	0
Rana esculenta+	20—40	0	0	0	0	0	0
Rana temporaria+ . . .	20—200	3—10	7—100	0—22	0	0	0
Rana latastei+	4—16	2—10	12—95	10—15	0	0	0
Rana dalmatina	100	?	1900	200	0	0	0
Rana japonica	60—70	0	0	0	0	0	0
Rana nigromaculata . .	70—80	0	0	0	0	0	0
Rana rugosa.	750	0	0	0	0	0	0
Rana palmipes	4—60	0	0	0	0	0	0
Rana pipiens	3—60	0	0	0	0	0	0
Rana clamitans	?	0	0	0	0	0	0
Rana palustris	+	0	0	0	0	0	0
Rana madagascariensis .	+	0	0	0	0	0	0
Rana labrosa	+	0	0	0	0	0	0
Pleurodema bufonina							
coxal glands	230—250	0	0	0	0	0	0
remaining skin . . .	0	0	0	0	0	0	0
Phyllomedusa rohdei . .	0	0	7—25	0	0	0	0
Hyla caerulea	200	0	0	0	0	0	0
Hyla infrafrenata . . .	500	0	0	0	0	0	0
Hyla arborea (europea)+	10—100	0	0	0	0	0	0
Hyla arborea (japonica) .	10	0	0	0	0	0	0
Hyla fuscovaria	10—15	0	0	0	0	0	0
Hyla peroni	250	12	15	0	0	0	0
Lepidobathracus asper .	5	0	0	0	0	0	0
Salamandra salamandra+	10	0	0	0	0	0	45
Salamandra atra+ . . .	10	0	0	0	0	0	2.5

0 = not detectable (<2—3 μg/g).
[1] Erspamer (1954a, 1954b), Erspamer, Cei and co-workers (to be published).

biosynthesis of the other constituents of the "cutaneous venom". This suggests that, in spite of all appearances, the turnover rate of the amines in the skin must be very slow.

The biological significance of the indolealkylamines in the amphibian skin is largely obscure. It may be that they play some part in the defence of the animal, but it is also possible that they simply constitute metabolic end products.

Before concluding it should be emphasized that amphibian skin may represent a formidable store-house not only of indolealkylamines, but also of phenylalkylamines, imidazolealkylamines and highly active polypeptides (Erspamer 1958; Erspamer et al. 1962a, 1962b, 1963).

9. Fish tissues and venoms

Male reproductive tract of the dogfish. The undiluted secretion of clasper siphons of sexually mature specimens of *Squalus acanthias* (250 mg of fluid per pair of clasper siphons) contains, according to Mann (1960), the tremendous amount of 25—34 mg 5-HT base per g secretion; the siphon tissue itself (2.8—3.6 g per kg body weight) 1.2 mg 5-HT per g wet tissue. This would correspond to not less than 10 mg 5-HT per animal weighing 1 kg. 5-HT is absent or present only in traces in the sperm removed directly from the seminal ducts and in the so-called seminal vesicles. Clasper siphons of immature males, weighing 100 mg, contain only 0.07—0.2 mg 5-HT per g tissue.

It has been suggested that the 5-HT present in a secretion which represents an integral part of semen might play a part in the reproductive process, either by affecting the mechanism of copulation and ejaculation in the male, or by eliciting contractions of the female reproductive tract, thus influencing passage of sperm and fertilization.

Fish venoms. The dried venom obtained from the dorsal spines of the lesser weever-fish, *Trachinus vipera,* contains about 1—20 μg 5-HT per mg. According to Carlisle (1962) the 5-HT appears to be responsible for the immediate pain about wounds inflicted by this fish.

10. Urine

Table 18 summarizes the most important available data on the occurrence of indolealkylamines and indole acids in normal urine.

The origin of the 5-HT found in normal human urine is obscure. A first possibility is that urinary 5-HT originates from plasma 5-HT either by glomerular filtration or tubular excretion; a second possibility that at least part of the 5-HT in urine is contributed directly by kidney metabolism (Rodnight 1956, Airaksinen and Uupää 1961). This would, however, require the presence of 5-HTP in the blood or in kidney tissue.

In the chicken, exogenous 5-HT is excreted by tubular excretion. In fact, 80 μg of 5-HT base given to normal chicken or to chicken pre-treated with a MAO inhibitor by unilateral leg vein infusion produces an ipsilateral excess of excretion of 5-HT of such magnitude that it proves a tubular excretion of the compound (Sanner and Wortman 1962).

Apparently 5-HT is transported in the chicken tubule by the ordinary organic base system (Sanner 1963).

According to Despopoulos (1956, 1957) 5-HIAA is excreted by the kidney both by glomerular filtration and by tubular excretion, and this opinion is shared by Barac (1961). In fact, the intravenous administration of 2 g of probenecid to patients with a high rate of excretion of 5-HIAA is followed by a decrease in the rate of excretion of 5-HIAA and an increase in its concentration in plasma.

Neither in man nor in the rat is there any significant change in the excretion rate of 5-HIAA with varying urinary pH. The mean excretion rate in human acid urine (pH 5.5—6.5) is 240 μg/hr, and in alkaline urine (pH above 7.8) 280 μg/hr (Milne et al. 1960, Degkwitz et al. 1962).

Data on the diurnal rhythm in the excretion of urinary 5-HIAA are at variance. According to Johnsen et al. (1958) and Sochor and Lakatua (1964) the peak in the daily 5-HIAA excretion occurs in the 3-hour period on either side of

Table 18. *Indolealkylamines and indole acids in urine*

	Indolealkylamines		Indole acids	
	5-HT	Tryptamine	5-HIAA	Other acids
Man	20—100[1], 45—120 μg/24 hr[2]; 0.01—0.7[3], 0.23 μg/ml[4]	20—100[1], 45—120[2], 25—250[35] 30—120[5], 30—126 μg/24 hr[6]	2—9[7]; 3.2—13.7[8], 1.3—5.6[9]; 2—7[10]; 5.7 ± 1.4[11]; 4.77 ± 0.32[12]; 3.54 ± 0.18[13] mg per day 229[14]; 203[15]; 240—280[16]; 238[17]; 206 ± 53 μg per hour[18] 3.9 mg per g creatinine[19]	indoleacetic, indolelactic, indoleacetylglutamic, indole-3-carboxylic, indoleacrylic, indoleglycolic acids; indoleacetylglutamine; acetyltryptophan[20]; indoleacetamide[20, 21]
Rat		4.4—8.2 μg per 10 mg creatinine[28]	146[22]; 145—200[23]; 113—133[24]; 110—140[25]; 130[26]; 250—280[27] μg/kg/24 hr	166 μg IAA per 100 mg creatinine[28]
Guinea-pig		0.6 mg/24 hr/animal[29]	60--150 μg/day/animal[34]	
Mouse			6 μg/ml[32]; 130—157 μg/kg/16 hr[33]	
Monkey			1.6—19.4 μg/hr[31]	
Dog			40—120 μg/kg/24 hr[30]	
Cow			3.34 ± 0.24 μg/ml[36]	

References to Table 18. [1] Davies et al. (1954). — [2] Rodnight (1956). — [3] Lembeck and Neuhold (1955). — [4] Kuriaki and Inoue (1956). — [5] Sjoerdsma et al. (1959, 1960). — [6] Brune and Himwich (1961). — [7] Udenfriend et al. (1955), Sjoerdsma et al. (1956). — [8] Macfarlane et al. (1956). — [9] Nikkila (1958). — [10] Peltola and Leppänen (1960). — [11] Olson et al. (1960). — [12] Barbeau and Jasmin (1961). — [13] Schwemmle et al. (1961). — [14] Kopin (1959). — [15] Feldstein et al. (1959). — [16] Milne et al. (1960). — [17] Perman (1961). — [18] Degkwitz et al. (1962). — [19] Pare et al. (1960). — [20] Armstrong et al. (1958). — [21] Sprince et al. (1961). — [22] Ferrari et al. (1957). — [23] Bertaccini (1960). — [24] Bertaccini and Nobili (1961). — [25] Bertaccini and Erspamer (1962). — [26] Kivalo et al. (1961). — [27] Cass and Marshall (1962). — [28] Donaldson (1962), Donaldson et al. (1961). — [29] Hess et al. (1959). — [30] Erspamer and Testini (1959). — [31] Anderson et al. (1958). — [32] Sjoerdsma et al. (1957). — [33] Bartlet (1963). — [34] Krüger and Smith (1960b). — [35] Gottfries and Magnusson (1962). — [36] Bertaccini and Cheli (1963).

noon, according to Peltlola and Leppänen (1960) between 5 p.m. and 9 p.m., according to Bettendorf et al. (1962) between 1 p.m. and 4 p.m.

Peltola and Leppänen (1960) found that on the average one half of the daily amount of 5-HIAA is excreted during the night, Schwemmle et al. (1961) and Degwitz et al. (1962, 1964) that nocturnal excretion of 5-HIAA is approximately 15% less than diurnal, finally Bettendorf et al. (1962) that 50% of the total 5-HIAA is excreted between 10 p.m. and 7 a.m.

Administration of tap water by stomach tube or of isotonic NaCl solution orally or subcutaneously produces a conspicuous increase in the urinary excretion of 5-HIAA in the rat. The same increase can be observed after administration of water plus posterior-pituitary antidiuretic hormone. Tap water is less effective than physiological saline; the latter, in its turn, is more effective by the subcutaneous route than by mouth. Increase of 5-HIAA may be, for short periods, as high as 3 times normal. The minimum oral dose of tap water causing a significant increase in urinary 5-HIAA is 2 ml/kg, that of physiological saline 1 ml/kg. Generally excess 5-HIAA coincides with excess urine elimination, but there is no obligatory correlation of the intensity of the two phenomena (Bertaccini and Erspamer 1962). The above observation have been essentially confirmed in man (Bertaccini and co-workers, unpublished observations; Degkwitz et al. 1962), but the mechanism of action of water or saline remains still to be elucidated.

Removal of large segments of the intestine is followed both in the experimental animal and in man by a more or less conspicuous reduction in the urinary excretion of 5-HIAA. This is a direct consequence of the removal of an important part of the 5-HT secreting tissue (BERTACCINI 1960, HAVERBACK and DAVIDSON 1958, BERTACCINI and CHIEPPA 1960).

Administration of excess dietary tryptophan or of a tryptophan load is followed by a conspicuous increase in the urinary excretion of 5-HIAA, in all probability depending on accelerated biosynthesis of 5-HT. In the rat the minimum oral dose of L-tryptophan producing a significant increase in urinary 5-HIAA is 100 mg/kg; 200 mg/kg may cause a 300% increase for a 4-hour period (BERTACCINI and NOBILI 1961).

Conversely, in the rat the absence of tryptophan from the diet is reflected in a 50% fall of urinary 5-HIAA, within 3 days (TOWSEND et al. 1958).

Neither nicotinic acid deficiency in the dog, nor pyridoxine or riboflavine deficiency in the rat causes any significant change in the urinary excretion of 5-HIAA (FERRARI et al. 1957, HARDING-GAUDIN 1961, EDELSTEIN et al. 1962).

The statement of PIGEAUD et al. (1958) that 5-HIAA excretion increases during pregnancy was not confirmed by SCHWEMMLE et al. (1961).

The urinary excretion of 5-HIAA in the rat is increased from 157 to 250—265 μg/kg/24 hr after 2—3 weeks of exposure of the animal to cold (6^0), and this increase persists as long as exposure is continued, up to 12 months. According to LEBLANC (1963) the changed excretion of 5-HIAA may not be specific to cold and may parallel the increased metabolic activity.

In the presence of a localized area of intestinal stasis produced in rats surgically by the creation of midintestinal diverticula, the excretion in the urine of 5-HT, tryptamine and 5-HIAA is not altered, whereas that of indican and IAA, free and conjugated, is significantly increased (DONALDSON et al. 1961, DONALDSON 1962).

11. Biological fluids and liquids other than urine

Mammalian semen. The statement by KATSH (1959) that human seminal plasma contains as much as 135 μg/ml 5-HT has not been confirmed. HAWKER et al. (1960) and ELIASSON (1961) could not find any 5-HT either in human or in ram semen and MANN et al. (1961) assessed by spectrofluorometric estimation the following "5-HT equivalents" in the semen of mammals: man 0.15 μg, bull 1 μg, ram 0.5 μg, boar 0.05 μg, dog 0.15 μg/ml.

Amniotic fluid. The amniotic liquid of the goat and the rabbit contains, if any, only traces of 5-HT: 0.006—0.03 and < 0.05 μg/ml, respectively (PEPEU and GIARMAN 1962, BERTACCINI unpublished data).

In human amniotic liquid the 5-HT content was found by KOREN et al. (1961) to vary between 0 and 0.38 μg/ml. However, the credibility of these values is impaired by the apparent unsuitability of the chemical assay procedure employed (1-nitroso-2-naphtol reagent).

Allantoid fluid. According to PEPEU and GIARMAN (1962) the 5-HT concentration in the allantoid fluid of the goat ranges between 0.12 and 0.4 μg/ml.

III. Invertebrates

So far 5-HT has been detected in particularly large amounts in some venom apparatuses of molluscs, scorpions, insects and coelenterates (Table 19) and in much less conspicuous but important amounts in the nervous tissue of molluscs (Table 20).

Table 19. *Occurrence of 5-HT and related indole derivatives in invertebrate tissues other than nervous tissue*

Animal species and tissue	5-HT	Other indole derivatives	Reference
Molluscs			
Posterior salivary glands			
Octopus vulgaris (Bari)	300—500 μg		1
Octopus vulgaris (Bermudas)	68—72 μg		2
Octopus macropus	—0.5 μg		1
Octopus bimaculata	present		3
Eledone moschata	280—750 μg		1
Median salivary glands			
Loligo pealii	0.38 μg		2
Anterior salivary glands			
Octopus vulgaris (Bermudas)	0.48—2.4 μg		2
Hypobranchial body			
Murex trunculus	80—290 μg		4
Murex brandaris	present		4
Gills			
Mytilus edulis	0.1—1.0 μg	5-HTP	5
	1.45 μg	0.05—0.5 μg	6
Modiolus demissus	0.3 μg		6
Tissues from different molluscan species			2
Intestine	0.6—0.7 μg		
Heart	0.2—0.5 μg		
Kidney	0.3—2.0 μg		
Musculature	0.08—1.0 μg		
Connectives	2.2 μg		
Skin	0.04 μg		
Crustaceans			
Green glands	0.06—1.0 μg		2
Pericardial organ	17 μg	5,6-dihydroxy-tryptamine	2,7
Heart		6-HT	17, 19
Insects			
Acanthoscurria atrox	0.058 μg per mg dry venom		18
Acanthoscurria sternalis	0.14 μg per mg dry venom		
Pterinopelma vellutinum	0.033 μg per mg dry venom		
Lycosa erythrognatha	0.014 μg per mg venom gland		
Phoneutria fera	0.52—2.65 μg per mg dry venom		
Polybia occidentalis	0.28 μg per abdomen		
Polistes versicolor	1.04—1.2 μg per sting apparatus		
Polistes versicolor vulgatus	1.94 μg per sting apparatus		
Polistes gallica	0.7—0.8 μg per venom apparatus		10
Vespa vulgaris	0.32 μg per mg dry venom		8
Vespa crabro	7.5—19 μg per mg dry venom sac		9
Vespa maculata	1.29 μg per sting apparatus		18
Synoeca surinama	0.97—2.74 μg per sting apparatus		18
Apis mellifera	5 ng; 0.03 μg per venom apparatus		2,8,10
Luciola italica	1 μg per head, 2 μg per thorax, 1 μg per abdomen, 2 μg per pair of wings		20
Periplaneta americana			
♂ utriculi majores	?	o-dihydroxy-indolealkyl-amine	11

Table 19. (Continued)

Animal species and tissue	5-HT	Other indole derivatives	Reference
corpora cardiaca glands . . .	present		11
Scorpions			
Leiurus quinquestriatus	2—4 μg per mg dry venom		12
Buthotus minax	0.03—0.04 μg per mg dry venom		12
Vejovis sp.	58—138 μg per sting segment		2
Hadrurus arizonensis	0.55 μg per sting segment		2
Parabuthus hunteri	present		12
Worms			
Dugesia tigrina whole	2 μg		2
Dugesia dorotocephala whole . .	1.5—3.4 μg		
Lineus ruber whole	0.18—0.43 μg		
Cerebratulus lacteus whole . . .	0.08—2.9 μg		
Arenicola marina body wall . .	2.3 μg		
Amphitrite ornata gills	0.26 μg 0.19 μg		
Fasciola hepatica	0.06—0.07 μg		13
Coelenterates			
Hydra oligactis whole	1.5 ng per animal		2,14
Sagartia luciae whole	50—100 ng per animal		2,14
Calliactis parasitica			
coelenteric tissue	500—660 μg per g freeze-dried tissue		15
column	13—36 μg per g freeze-dried tissue		
tentacles	6—12 μg per g freeze-dried tissue		
Metridium senile			
whole animal.	0.04—0.05 μg		2,14,16
body wall	0.02—0.09 μg		
oral disk and tentacles . . .	0.08—0.17 μg		
tentacles	0.24—0.47 μg	bufotenine,	
acontia	0.60—1.3 μg	5-HTP	
Anemonia sulcata	non detectable		15
Actinia equina	non detectable		15
Physalia	non detectable		15

Unless otherwise stated the above values are per g fresh tissue.

References to Table 19. [1] ERSPAMER (1948b, 1954b, 1954c), ERSPAMER and BORETTI (1951), ANASTASI and ERSPAMER (1962). — [2] WELSH and MOORHEAD (1959, 1960). — [3] CLARK (1960), HARTMAN et al. (1960). — [4] ERSPAMER (1948a, 1954b, 1954c). — [5] AIELLO (1962). — [6] GOSSELIN et al. (1962). — [7] CARLISLE (1956), CARLISLE and KNOWLES (1959), CARLISLE (1964), MAYNARD and WELSH (1959). — [8] JAQUES and SCHACHTER (1954). — [9] BHOOLA et al. (1960, 1961). — [10] ERSPAMER (1954c). — [11] DAVEY (1960), COLHOUN (1963, 1964), — [12] ADAM and WEISS (1956, 1959). — [13] MANSOUR et al. (1957). — [14] WELSH (1960). — [15] MATHIAS et al. (1957, 1958, 1960). — [16] PHILIPPS (1956). — [17] KERKUT and PRICE (1963). — [18] WELSH and BATTY (1963). — [19] KERKUT and PRICE (1964). — [20] BERTACCINI et al. (to be published).

It is certain that numerous other examples of indolealkylamines will be discovered in invertebrates.

Quite recently, for example, an unexpected localization of 5-HT has been described by MANN (1963) in the octopus. MANN found that the glandular portion of the spermatogenic sac of the octopus contained 120 μg 5-HT per g fresh tissue in the smallest specimens and as much as 1690 μg/g in the largest specimens. The weight of the glandular portion was 2.5—3 g per kg octopus. It is suggested that this 5-HT may play a part in the ejaculatory process. This might perhaps be envisaged as an induction of either the discharge of the spermatophores from the spermatophoric sac, or a stimulation of contractions within the male or female reproductive tract, assisting the passage of spermatozoa to the site of fertilization.

Table 20. *Occurrence of 5-HT in nervous tissue of invertebrates*

Animal species	Tissue	5-HT content (in µg base per g wet tissue)	Reference
Molluscs			
Venus mercenaria	pooled ganglia	30—40	1
Pecten magellanicus	visceral ganglia	36	
Mytilus edulis	ganglia	10—15	
Artica islandica	ganglia	20	
Spisula solidissima	ganglia	8—14.3	
Ensis directus	ganglia	21—39	
Mya arenaria	ganglia	22	
Buccinum undatum	ganglia	7.7	
Busycon canaliculatum	ganglia	8.4—9.7	
	nerves	2—2.5	
Fasciolaria tulipa	ganglia and nerves	7.6—9.4	
Polinices heros	ganglia	10.6	7
Crepidula fornicata	ganglia	5.0	
Melongena corona	ganglia	4.5	
Viviparus japonicus	ganglia	1.2	
Helix pomatia	ganglia	2—3; <1	2,3
	nerve cords	non detectable	3
Astacus leptodactylus	nerve cords	non detectable	3
Astacus fluviatilis	nerve cords	non detectable	3
Loligo pealii	"brain"	0.7	1
	optic ganglia	1.15	1
Octopus briareus	pooled ganglia	1.6	1
Octopus vulgaris	"brain"	0.8; 0.25	1,4
	optic ganglia	2.3; 2.3	1,4
	stellate ganglia	0.72	4
	nerves	1.5	4
Eledone moschata	optic ganglia	2—4	5
	nerves	1.5—2	5
Crustaceans			
Cancer irroratus, Cancer borealis, Carcinus moenas, Homarus americanus, Panulirus argus, Orconectes virilis, Palinurus vulgaris, Gecarcinus lateralis	nerve cords, ventral ganglia, leg nerves, "brain"	< 0.1	1,4
Worms			
Lumbricus terrestris	nerve cords	10.4	1
Hirudo medicinalis	nerve cords	6.9	1
	nerve cords	0.2	4
Amphitrite ornata	nerve cords	5.4	1
Arenicola marina	nerve cords	3.1	1
Glycera dibranchiata	nerve cords	4.6	1
Insects			
Blaberus gigantea	nerve cords	< 0.02	1
Locusta migratoria	ganglia	< 0.2	4
Periplaneta americana	"brain"	present	6
	ventral nerve cord	present	6
Holothurians			
Thyone briareus	region of nerve ring	0.03—0.05	1

References to Table 20. [1] WELSH and MOORHEAD (1959, 1960). — [2] MENG (1958). — [3] JULLIEN et al. (1961), CARDOT et al. (1962, 1963). — [4] ERSPAMER, unpublished data. — [5] BERTACCINI (1961). — [6] COLHOUN (1963). — [7] MIROLLI and WELSH (1964).

The resemblance of this localization with that found in the male reproductive tract of the dogfish (MANN 1960) is evident. It would be instructive to carry out comparative studies on different octopod or cephalopod species to see whether the occurrence of 5-HT in the spermatogenic sac is a constant finding.

The 5-HT in the venom glands does not seem to have any particular significance but that of a facultative constituent of the venom. In fact, the venom of strictly related species may present, for completely unknown reasons, striking differences in 5-HT content. This is true of the posterior salivary glands and the hypobranchial body of molluscs, the venom apparatus of *Hymenoptera*, the venom apparatus of scorpions, etc. The opinion cannot be rejected that here, as in the case of amphibian skin, 5-HT may merely be a metabolite destined for external secretion.

Things are completely different with the 5-HT present in molluscan nervous tissue. All the investigators found that molluscan ganglia and peripheral nerves contain important amounts of 5-HT and that this 5-HT behaves, towards different drugs, exactly like the 5-HT occurring in the brain of mammals. Moreover, it has been demonstrated that the turnover rate of 5-HT in the ganglia of molluscs is very high, the half-life of the amine being not longer than 15 to 20 minutes (Bertaccini 1961).

From this it may reasonably be inferred that, in sharp contrast to other localizations of 5-HT in the molluscan body, neuronal 5-HT must have a general biological significance, probably in the transmission of nervous impulses. Appropriate procedure indicates that 5-HT is stored in granules in the molluscan ganglia (Welsh 1958).

It is conceivable that a thorough study of the 5-HT in the nervous tissue of molluscs may offer a key to a better understanding of the function of the amine in the brain of vertebrates.

According to Cardot (1963) the nerve cords of *Helix pomatia* also contain trace amounts of tryptamine.

IV. Plants

The data reported in Table 21 are intended merely to be an exemplification of the wide distribution of indolealkylamines in the vegetable kingdom. It may be anticipated that these compounds will be met with in numerous other plant tissues.

Tables 22 and 23 show the content of tryptamines and other amines in the different parts of some edible fruits and their appearance during the ripening process.

There appears to be more 5-HT in unripe pineapples (50—60 μg/g) than in the ripe fruit (19 μg/g). A trace of the amine is also detectable in the stalk (0.2 μg/g), but none in the leaves of the crown or in the base (Foy and Parratt 1961).

It is very interesting to note that not only 5-hydroxyindoles but also 4-hydroxyindoles and 2-hydroxyindoles have been found in the vegetable kingdom. We refer to psilocin and psilocybin (see Table 21) and to 2-hydroxyindoleacetic acid, which has been detected in the shooting seeds of *Brassica rapa* and the red gooseberry as well as in the caryopsides of Indian corn (Klambt 1959). This means that the vegetable cells contain enzymes capable of hydroxylating the indole nucleus at the 4- and 2-positions also.

The significance of indolealkylamines in plants is not very well understood. It may be that in some cases they act as growth factors or as precursors of auxines and that in other cases they intervene in the synthesis of pigments. But a third, likely possibility is that, as in the animal kingdom, some examples of indolealkylamines in plants are to be considered mere metabolic end products possessing no particular significance.

Table 21. *Occurrence of 5-HT and related indole derivatives in the vegetable kingdom*

Species	5-HT	Other indole derivatives	Reference
Neurospora crassa		β-hydroxy-pseudo-tryptophan	1
Panaeolus campanulatus	80 μg/g	other indole derivatives	2, 25
Panaeolus foenesecii	240 μg/g		25
Panaeolus sphinctrinus	present	psilocybin 1.9 μg/g, 5-HTP	3, 28
Psilocybe (several species)		psilocybin 0.1—6 μg/g psilocin 0—2.5 μg/g	4
Stropharia cubensis		psilocybin 0.1—5 μg/g psilocin 0—2.5 μg/g	3
Amanita mappa		bufotenine	5
Piptadenia peregrina (seeds)		bufotenine 9.4 μg/, 5-HIAA	6
Piptadenia peregrina (bark)		N-methyltryptamine, 5-methoxy-N-methyltryptamine, 5-methoxy-N,N-dimethyltryptamine	7
Piptadenia colubrina (seeds)		bufotenine	8
Piptadenia macrocarpa (seeds and pods)		bufotenine, bufotenine oxide, N,N-dimethyltryptamine, N,N-dimethyltryptamine oxide	9
Gossypium hirsutum (fruit)	present		10
Symplocarpus foetidus (leaves)	present		10
Citrullus vulgaris	present		11
Dictyoloma incanescens (bark)		5-methoxy-N,N-dimethyltryptamine	8
Mimosa hostilis (roots)		N,N-dimethyltryptamine	8
Urtica dioica (stings)	3—5 ng/sting		12
Laportea moroides (hairs)	1 ng/hair		13
Mucuna pruriens (trichomes)	150 μg per g trichomes		14
Prestonia amazonica (leaves)		N,N-dimethyltryptamine	15
Acacia fluribunda (tops)		tryptamine	16
Phalaris arundinacea		5-methoxy-N-methyltryptamine	17
Acer saccharinum		gramine	8
Acer rubrum (fruit)		gramine	18
Hippophae rhamnoides	present		19
Arundo donax		gramine	20
Barley		gramine, N-methyltryptamine	21
Girgensohnia diptera		N-methyltryptamine	26
Girardinia heterophylla	present		29
Maize (chopped green)	13.7 μg/g dry matter		27
Ananas comosus			
unripe fruit	50—60 μg/g		22
ripe fruit	19 μg/g		
fresh juice	12—22 μg/ml		
canned juice	1.3—25 μg/ml		
Carica papaya (fruit)	1.1—2.1 μg/g		23
Passiflora foetida (fruit)	1.4—3.5 μg/g		23
Juglans regia (nut)	170—340 μg per g kernel		24
Eggplant (fruit)	2 μg/g	tryptamine 0.5—3 μg/g	25
Avocado	10 μg/g		25
Red plum	10 μg/g	tryptamine 0.2 μg/g	25
Blue-red plum	8 μg/g	tryptamine 2 μg/g	25
Banana	see Tables 22 and 23		
Plantain	see Tables 22 and 23		
Tomatoes	see Tables 22 and 23		

References to Table 21. [1] Sherwood (1957). — [2] Tyler (1958). — [3] Delay et al. (1959), Cerletti (1960), Marmo (1960). — [4] Hofmann et al. (1958, 1963), Hofmann and Troxler (1959). — [5] Wieland and Motzel (1953). — [6] Stromberg (1954), Fish et al. (1955). — [7] Legler and Tschesche (1963). — [8] Pachter et al. (1959). — [9] Fish et al. (1955, 1956). — [10] Bulard and Leopold (1958). — [11] Dannenbourg and Liverman (1957). — [12] Collier and Chesher (1956). — [13] Robertson et al. (1957). — [14] Bowden et al. (1954). — [15] Hochstein and Paradies (1957). — [16] White (1944). — [17] Wilkinson (1958). — [18] Pachter (1959). — [19] Purkhalskaia and Menshikov (1960). — [20] Orchoff and Norkina (1935). — [21] Brandt et al. (1935), v. Euler et al. (1936), Kirkwood and Marion (1950). — [22] Bruce (1960, 1961), West (1960), Foy and Parratt (1961). — [23] Foy and Parratt (1960). — [24] Kirberger and Braun (1961). — [25] Wier and Tyler (1963). — [26] Yurashewskii (1941). — [27] Neumark (1964). — [28] Tyler and Groger (1964). — [29] Saxena et al. (1964).

Numerous research workers (WAALKES et al. 1958, WEST 1960, KIRBERGER and BRAUN 1961) have called attention to the possibility that ingestion of edible fruits, especially bananas, containing large amounts of 5-HT and catecholamines

Table 22. *Indolealkylamines and phenylalkylamines in bananas (μg/g wet tissue)*

	5-HT	Tryptamine	Tyramine	Dopamine	Noradrenaline
a) Banana					
Hard green					
outer peel	0.1[2]; 74[1]				
inner peel	0.2; 13	=	=	=	=
pulp . . .	25; 24				
Ripe					
outer peel	52; 96	0[1]	65[1]	700[1]	122[1]
inner peel	40; 38				
pulp . . .	19; 36	0	7	8	2
Over-ripe					
outer peel	39; 161				
inner peel	30; 170	=	=	=	=
pulp . . .	22; 35				
b) Plantain					
Unripe					
skin . . .	13[3]; 1[4]	0[4]	=	=	5[3]; 1.8[4]
pulp . . .	50; 16	0	=	=	2.0[4]
Ripe					
skin . . .	41[3]	=	=	=	6.2[3]
pulp . . .	57; 45[1]	=	=	=	2.5
Over-ripe .					
skin . . .	6[3]	=	=	=	15[3]
pulp . . .	12	=	=	=	10

References to Table 22. [1] WAALKES et al. (1958), UDENFRIEND et al. (1959). — [2] WEST (1958). — [3] FOY and PARRATT (1960). — [4] MARSHALL (1959).

may lead to erroneous chemical diagnosis of carcinoid tumour or pheocromocytoma. In this regard the observation by FOY and PARRATT (1962) seems relevant that whereas there is no significant difference between the urinary 5-HIAA of Nigerians not on a plantain diet and Europeans living in Nigeria (5.3 and 4.5 mg/24 hr),

Table 23. *Tryptamines in tomatoes (μg/g wet tissue)* (WEST 1959a, 1959b)

	5-HT	Tryptamine	Tryptophan		5-HT	Tryptamine	Tryptophan
Young plant				Fruit			
main stems .	0	0	2.5	unripe pulp .	0.2	1.0	0.2
leaf stems .	0.3	0	2.5	ripe skin . .	1.5	1.8	0.2
leaves . . .	0.5	0	2.0	ripe pulp . .	3.4	4.0	0.8
				ripe pips . .	1.0	4.8	0.4

5-HTP and 5-HIAA are not present in detectable amounts.

Nigerian subjects on two main plantain meals present a urinary excretion of 5-HIAA as high as 28 mg/24 hr.

The possibility that 5-HT in edible fruits may constitute a contributory factor in intestinal disorders (MARSHALL 1959) has been minimized by UDENFRIEND et al. (1959) and by CROUT and SJOERDSMA (1959).

References

Adam, K. R., and C. Weiss: 5-Hydroxytryptamine in scorpion venom. Nature (Lond.) **178**, 421—422 (1956).

— — Distribution of 5-hydroxytryptamine in scorpion venoms. Nature (Lond.) **183**, 1398—1399 (1959).

Adams, B. G.: Serum 5-hydroxytryptamine levels following experimental increase in gastrointestinal activity in man. Lancet **1960 I**, 207—208.

Adams-Ray, J., A. Dahlström, K. Fuxe, and N.-Å. Hillarp: Mast cells and monoamines. Experientia (Basel) **20**, 80—82 (1964).

Aiello, E. L.: Identification of the cilioexcitatory substance present in the gill of the mussel *Mytilus edulis*. J. cell. comp. Physiol. **60**, 17—21 (1962).

Airaksinen, M. M., and V. J. Uuspää: Is urinary 5-hydroxytryptamine formed in the kidney? Biochem. Pharmacol. **8**, 46 (1961).

Albrecht, P., M. B. Visscher, J. J. Bittner and F. Halberg: Daily changes in 5-hydroxytryptamine concentration in mouse brain. Proc. Soc. exp. Biol. (N.Y.) **92**, 703—706 (1956).

Amin, A. H., T. B. B. Crawford and J. H. Gaddum: The distribution of substance P and 5-hydroxytryptamine in the central nervous system of the dog. J. Physiol. (Lond.) **126**, 596—618 (1954).

Anastasi, A., and V. Erspamer: Occurrence and some properties of eledoisin in extracts of posterior salivary glands of eledone. Brit. J. Pharmacol. **19**, 326—336 (1962).

Anderson, E. G., and D. D. Bonnycastle: A study of the central depressant action of pentobarbital, phenobarbital and diethyl ether in relationship to increases in brain 5-hydroxytryptamine. J. Pharmacol. exp. Ther. **130**, 138—143 (1960).

—, and J. Cudia: The anatomical localization of norepinephrine and 5-hydroxytryptamine in cat spinal cord. Fed. Proc. **21**, 341 (1962).

— S. D. Markowitz and D. D. Bonnycastle: Brain 5-hydroxytryptamine and anticonvulsant activity. J. Pharmacol. exp. Ther. **136**, 179—182 (1962).

Anderson, J. A., M. R. Ziegler and D. Doeden: Banana feeding and urinary excretion of 5-hydroxyindoleacetic acid. Science **127**, 236—238 (1958).

Antonelli, A. R., G. Bertaccini and P. Mantegazzini: Relationship between mesencephalic and hypothalamic concentration of 5-hydroxytryptamine and cortical electrical activity of cats. J. Neurochem. **8**, 157—158 (1961).

Aprison, M. H., M. A. Wolf, G. L. Poulos and T. L. Folkerth: Neurochemical correlates of behavior. III. Variation of serotonin content in several brain areas and peripheral tissues of the pigeon following 5-hydroxytryptophan administration. J. Neurochem. **9**, 575—584 (1962).

Armin, J., and R. T. Grant: Further observations on vasoconstrictor substances in blood of rabbit and man. J. Physiol. (Lond.) **138**, 401—416 (1957).

Armstrong, M. D., K. N. F. Shaw, M. J. Gortawski and H. Singer: The indole acids of human urine. Paper chromatography of indole acids. J. biol. Chem. **232**, 17—30 (1958).

Ashcroft, G. W., and D. F. Sharman: 5-Hydroxyindoles in human cerebrospinal fluid. Nature (Lond.) **186**, 1050—1051 (1960).

— — The effect of reserpine on the concentration of 5-OR indolyl compounds in the caudate nucleus and the cerebrospinal fluid of the dog. J. Physiol. (Lond.) **158**, 32—33 P (1961).

— — Drug-induced changes in the concentration of 5-OR indolyl compounds in cerebrospinal fluid and caudate nucleus. Brit. J. Pharmacol. **19**, 153—160 (1962).

Axelrod, J., R. J. Wurtman, and Ch. M. Winget: Melatonin synthesis in the hen pineal gland and its control by light. Nature (Lond.) **201**, 1134 (1964).

Barac, G.: Elimination rénale de l'acide 5-hydroxyindoleacétique chez le Chien. C. R. Soc. Biol. (Paris) **155**, 1732—1734 (1961).

Barbeau, A., et G. Jasmin: Dosage de l'acide 5-hydroxyindoleacétique urinaire dans la maladie de Parkinson. Rev. canad. Biol. **20**, 837—838 (1961).

Barchas, J. D., and D. X. Freedman: Brain amines: response to physiological stress. Biochem. Pharmacol. **12**, 1232—1235 (1963).

—, and A. B. Lerner: Localization of melatonin in the nervous system. J. Neurochem. **11**, 489—491 (1964).

Bartlet, A. L.: The 5-hydroxytryptamine content of mouse brain and whole mice after treatment with some drugs affecting the central nervous system. Brit. J. Pharmacol. **15**, 140—146 (1960).

— The influence of chlorpromazine on the excretion of 5-hydroxyindoleacetic acid from mice. J. Physiol. (Lond.) **165**, 25—26 P (1963).

Beaver, M. H., and B. S. Wostmann: Histamine and 5-hydroxytryptamine in the intestinal tract of germ-free animals, animals harbouring one microbial species and conventional animals. Brit. J. Pharmacol. **19**, 385—393 (1962).

BENDITT, E. P.: 5-Hydroxytryptamine and 5-hydroxytryptophan decarboxylase in rat mast cells. In: G. P. LEWIS (Ed.), 5-Hydroxytryptamine, p. 31—34. London: Pergamon Press 1957.
— S. BADER and K. B. LAM: Studies of the mechanisms of acute vascular reactions to injury. Arch. Path. **60**, 104—115 (1955a).
— J. HOLCENBERG, and D. LAGUNOFF: The role of serotonin (5-hydroxytryptamine) in mast cells. Ann. N.Y. Acad. Sci. **103** (3), 179—184 (1963).
— R. L. WONG, M. ARASE and E. ROEPER: 5-Hydroxytryptamine in mast cells. Proc. Soc. exp. Biol. (N.Y.) **90**, 303—304 (1955b).
BERTACCINI, G.: Osservazioni sul contenuto in 5-idrossitriptamina di vari tessuti del ratto durante lo sviluppo postnatale. Ric. Sci. **28**, 2261—2263 (1958).
— Effect of convulsant treatment on the 5-hydroxytryptamine content of brain and other tissues of the rat. J. Neurochem. **4**, 217—222 (1959).
— Tissue 5-hydroxytryptamine and urinary 5-hydroxyindoleacetic acid after partial or total removal of the gastro-intestinal tract in the rat. J. Physiol. (Lond.) **153**, 239—249 (1960).
— Discussion. In: S. S. KETY and J. ELKES (Eds.), Regional Neurochemistry, p. 305—306. London: Pergamon Press 1961.
—, e R. CHELI: Considerazioni sulla eliminazione urinaria di acido 5-idrossiindolilacetico nel bovino. Arch. Sci. biol. (Bologna) **47**, 336—338 (1964).
—, and S. CHIEPPA: Urinary excretion of 5-hydroxyindoleacetic acid after removal of the large intestine in man. Lancet **1960 I**, 881.
—, and V. ERSPAMER: The effect of the administration of water or isotonic NaCl solution on the urinary excretion of 5-hydroxyindoleacetic acid in the rat. J. Pharm. Pharmacol. **14**, 687—697 (1962).
—, and M. B. NOBILI: Effect of L-tryptophan on diuresis and 5-hydroxyindoleacetic acid excretion in the rat. Brit. J. Pharmacol. **17**, 519—525 (1961).
BETTENDORF, G., A. P. MOJE u. H.-J. SCHMERMUND: Der Einfluß der Strahlenbehandlung auf die 5-Hydroxy-Indol-Essigsäure-Ausscheidung. Strahlentherapie **117**, 370—376 (1962).
BHATT, K. G. S., H. R. K. ARORA, H. L. DHAR and R. K. SANYAL: Changes in serotonin content in the heart following acute myocardial infarction in the dog. Med. exp. **9**, 46—48 (1963).
BHATTACHARYA, B. K., and G. P. LEWIS: The release of 5-hydroxytryptamine by histamine liberators. Brit. J. Pharmacol. **11**, 202—208 (1956).
BHOOLA, K. D., J. D. CALLE and M. SCHACHTER: The identification of acetylcholine, 5-hydroxytryptamine and other substances in hornet venom. J. Physiol. (Lond.) **151**, 35—36P (1960).
— — — Identification of acetylcholine, 5-hydroxytryptamine, histamine, and a new kinin in hornet venom *(V. crabro)*. J. Physiol. (Lond.) **159**, 167—182 (1961).
BOGDANSKI, D. F., L. BONOMI and B. B. BRODIE: Occurrence of serotonin and catecholamines in brain and peripheral organs of various vertebrate classes. Life Sciences No 1, 80—84 (1963).
— A. PLETSCHER, B. B. BRODIE and S. UDENFRIEND: Identification and assay of serotonin in brain. J. Pharmacol. exp. Ther. **117**, 82—88 (1956).
—, and S. UDENFRIEND: Serotonin and monoamine oxidase in brain. J. Pharmacol. exp. Ther. **116**, 7—8 (1956).
— H. WEISSBACH and S. UDENFRIEND: The distribution of serotonin, 5-hydroxytryptophan decarboxylase, and monoamine oxidase in brain. J. Neurochem. **1**, 272—278 (1957).
BOGGS, D. E., R. ROSENBERG and H. A. WAISMAN: Effects of phenylalanine, phenylacetic acid, tyrosine and valine on brain and liver serotonin in rats. Proc. Soc. exp. Biol. (N.Y.) **114**, 356—358 (1963).
BONNYCASTLE, D. D., M. F. BONNYCASTLE and E. G. ANDERSON: The effect of a number of central depressant drugs upon brain 5-hydroxytryptamine levels in the rat. J. Pharmacol. exp. Ther. **135**, 17—20 (1962).
— N. J. GIARMAN and M. K. PAASONEN: Anticonvulsant compounds and 5-hydroxytryptamine in rat brain. Brit. J. Pharmacol. **12**, 228—231 (1957).
BORÉUS, L. O., and B. WESTERHOLM: 5-Hydroxytryptamine in the Schultz-Dale reaction. Acta physiol. scand. **56**, 17—25 (1962).
BORGERT, H., u. K. KEITEL: Über die vasokonstriktorischen Substanzen im Blutserum. Biochem. Z. **175**, 1—7 (1962).
BORN, G. V. R., and R. E. GILLSON: Studies on the uptake of 5-hydroxytryptamine by blood platelets. J. Physiol. (Lond.) **146**, 472—491 (1959).
BOWDEN, K., B. G. BROWN and J. E. BATTY: 5-Hydroxytryptamine: its occurrence in cowhage. Nature (Lond.) **174**, 925—926 (1954).

BOWERS jr., M. B.: Stimulation and sensitization of the isolated Venus heart by cerebrospinal fluid. Brit. J. Pharmacol. **19**, 295—298 (1962).

BRACCO, M., e P. C. CURTI: Ricerche sulla natura del fattore vasocostrittore delle piastrine. Haematologica **37**, 721—736 (1953).

— — The vasoconstrictor factor of platelets. Experientia (Basel) **10**, 71—72 (1954).

— — e V. GIULIANO: Identificazione della 5-OH-triptamina nei trombociti degli uccelli. Experientia (Basel) **12**, 31—33 (1956).

BRANDT, K., H. v. EULER, H. HELLSTRÖM u. N. LOFGREN: Gramin und zwei Begleiter desselben in Laubblättern von Gerstensorten. Hoppe-Seylers Z. physiol. Chem. **235**, 37—42 (1935).

BRIDGES, J. M., M. BALDINI, C. FICHERA and W. DAMESHEK: Effect of antiplatelet antibodies on the *in vitro* uptake of 5-hydroxytryptamine by blood platelets. Nature (Lond.) **197**, 364—366 (1963).

BROCKLEHURST, W. E., J. H. HUMPHREY and W. L. M. PERRY: Cutaneous antigen-antibody reactions in the rat. J. Physiol. (Lond.) **150**, 489—500 (1960).

BRODIE, B. A., P. A. SHORE and A. PLETSCHER: Serotonin-releasing activity limited to Rauwolfia alkaloids with tranquilizing action. Science **123**, 992—993 (1956).

BRODIE, B. B., D. F. BOGDANSKI, and L. BONOMI: Formation, storage and metabolism of serotonin (5-hydroxytryptamine) and catecholamines in lower vertebrates. In: D. RICHTER Ed., Comparative Neurochemistry, pp. 367—377. Oxford: Pergamon Press 1964.

—, S. SPECTOR and P. A. SHORE: Interaction of monoamine oxidase inhibitors with physiological and biochemical mechanisms in brain. Ann. N.Y. Acad. Sci. **30** (3), 609—616 (1959).

BRUCE, D. W.: Serotonin in pineapple. Nature (Lond.) **188**, 147 (1960).

— Carcinoid tumours and pineapples. J. Pharm. Pharmacol. **13**, 256 (1961).

BRUNE, G., and H. E. HIMWICH: Effects of reserpine on urinary tryptamine and indole-3-acetic acid excretion in mental deficiency, schizophrenia and phenylpyruvic oligophrenia. In: G. TONINI (Ed.), Techniques for the study of psychotropic drugs, p. 176—184. Modena: Soc. Tip. Modenese 1961.

BÜLBRING, E., and A. CREMA: The release of 5-hydroxytryptamine in relation to pressure exerted on the intestinal mucosa. J. Physiol. (Lond.) **146**, 18—28 (1959a).

— — The action of 5-hydroxytryptamine, 5-hydroxytryptophan and reserpine on peristalsis in anaesthetized guinea-pigs. J. Physiol. (Lond.) **146**, 29—53 (1959b).

BULARD, C., and A. C. LEOPOLD: 5-Hydroxytryptamine chez les plantes supérieures. C. R. Acad. Sci. (Paris) **247**, 1282—1284 (1958).

CAMBRIDGE, G. W., and J. A. HOLGATE: 5-HT in plasma. J. Physiol. (Lond.) **142**, 53—54P (1958).

CARDOT, J.: Mise en évidence de la tryptamine dans les extraits nerveux du Mollusque *Helix pomatia*. C. R. Soc. Biol. (Paris) **157**, 853—854 (1963).

—, et J. RIPPLINGER: Recherches sur les amines indoliques cardio-actives présentes dans le tissue nerveux du mollusque *Helix pomatia*. J. Physiol. (Paris) **55**, 217—218 (1963).

— — et M. LONCHAMPT: Sur la non spécificité tissulaire des acides aminés basiques et des amines chez l'Escargot (*Helix pomatia* L.) C. R. Soc. Biol. (Paris) **156**, 1433—1435 (1962).

CARLINI, E. A., and J. P. GREEN: The subcellular distribution of histamine, slow-reacting substance and 5-hydroxytryptamine in the brain of the rat. Brit. J. Pharmacol. **20**, 264—277 (1963).

CARLISLE, D. B.: An indole-alkylamine regulating heart-beat in Crustacea. Biochem. J. **63**, 32—33P (1956).

— On the venom of the lesser weeverfish, Trachinus vipera. J. mar. biol. Ass. U. Kingd. **42**, 155 (1962).

— The neurohumoral control of heart rate in crustaceans. In: D. RICHTER Ed., Comparative Neurochemistry, pp. 323—328. Oxford: Pergamon Press 1964.

—, and F. KNOWLES: Endocrine control in Crustacea, p. 72. Cambridge: Cambridge University Press 1959.

CARLSSON, A., T. MAGNUSSON and E. ROSENGREN: 5-Hydroxytryptamine of the spinal cord normally and after transection. Experientia (Basel) **19**, 359 (1963).

CASS, R., and P. B. MARSHALL: Effect of adrenocortical hormones on tissue histamine and 5-hydroxytryptamine in the rat. Arch. int. Pharmacodyn. **136**, 311—332 (1962).

CERHOVÁ, M., A. ŠIDLOVA and A. ZELENÝ: The effect of skin inflammation on blood content of serotonin and histamine. Physiol. bohemoslov. **11**, 136—141 (1962).

CERLETTI, A.: Über Vorkommen und Bedeutung der Indolstruktur in der Medizin und Biologie. Progr. Drug Res. **2**, 227—249 (1960).

CHIECO BIANCHI, L., L. FIORE DONATI, N. PENNELLI and G. BERTACCINI: Mast cell reaction and 5-hydroxytryptamine content in the skin of syrian golden hamsters painted with 9:10-dimethyl-1:2-benzanthracene. Nature (Lond.) **199**, 293—294 (1963).

CLARK, W. G.: Amine content and biosynthesis in mastocytomas and Octopus salivary glands. Fed. Proc. **19**, 9 (1960).
COLHOUN, E. H.: Synthesis of 5-hydroxytryptamine in the American cockroach. Experientia (Basel) **19**, 9—10 (1963).
— Aspects of biologically active substances in insects with particular reference to the cockroach, *Periplaneta americana*. In: D. RICHTER Ed., Comparative Neurochemistry, pp. 333—339. Oxford: Pergamon Press 1964.
CORREALE, P.: The occurrence and distribution of 5-hydroxytryptamine (enteramine) in the central nervous system of vertebrates. J. Neurochem. **1**, 22—31 (1956).
COSTA, E., and M. H. APRISON: Distribution of intracarotidly injected serotonin in the brain. Amer. J. Physiol. **192**, 95—100 (1958).
COUPLAND, R. E., and I. D. HEATH: Chromaffin cells, mast cells and melanin. II. The chromaffin cells of the liver capsule and gut in ungulates. J. Endocr. **22**, 71—76 (1961).
—, and J. F. RILEY: Mast cells and 5-hydroxytryptamine in precancerous mouse skin. Nature (Lond.) **187**, 1128—1129 (1960).
CRAWFORD, N.: Plasma free serotonin (5-hydroxytryptamine). Clin. chim. Acta **8**, 39—45 (1963).
CROUT, J. R., and A. SJOERDSMA: The clinical and laboratory significance of serotonin and catechol amines in bananas. New Engl. J. Med. **261**, 23—26 (1959).
CULLEY, W. J., R. N. SAUNDERS, E. T. MERTZ and D. H. JOLLY: Plasma tryptophan and brain serotonin levels of rats fed a tryptophan deficient diet. Fed. Proc. **22**, 203 (1963); — Proc. Soc. exp. Biol. (N.Y.) **113**, 645—648 (1963).
DALGLIESH, C. E., C. C. TOH and T. S. WORK: Fractionation of the smooth muscle stimulants present in extracts of the gastrointestinal tract. Identification of 5-hydroxytryptamine and its distinction from substance P. J. Physiol. (Lond.) **120**, 298—310 (1953).
DANNENBOURG, W. N., and J. L. LIVERMAN: Conversion of tryptophan-2-C^{14} to indoleacetic acid by watermelon tissue slices. Plant Physiol. **32**, 263—269 (1957).
DAVEY, K. G.: A pharmacologically active agent in the reproductive system of insects. Canad. J. Zool. **38**, 39—45 (1960).
DAVIES, D. F., K. M. WOLFE and H. M. PERRY: Studies on primary amines. II. Their natural occurrence in urine of normotensive and hypertensive patients. J. Lab. clin. Med. **43**, 620—632 (1954).
DAVIS, R. B., W. R. MEEKER jr. and W. L. BAILEY: Serotonin release by bacterial endotoxin. Proc. Soc. exp. Biol. (N.Y.) **108**, 774—776 (1961).
DAY, S., and J. P. GREEN: Levels of heparin, histamine and 5-hydroxytryptamine in neoplastic mast cells in vivo. Fed. Proc. **18**, 381 (1959).
DEGKWITZ, R., R. FROWEIN, E. KIRBERGER, C. KULENKAMPFF u. U. MOHS: Über Normalwerte der stündlichen 5-HIES-Ausscheidung im Urin beim Menschen und die Messungen störender Faktoren. Klin. Wschr. **40**, 285—289 (1962).
— O. SCHULENBURG u. H. SIEROSLAWSKI: Die 5-HIES-Ausscheidung im Urin beim Schlafen und Wachen. Klin. Wschr. **42**, 102—103 (1964).
DE IRALDI, A. P., and E. DE ROBERTIS: Action of reserpine on the submicroscopic morphology of the pineal gland. Experientia (Basel) **17**, 122—124 (1961).
— L. M. ZIEHER and E. DE ROBERTIS: The 5-hydroxytryptamine content and synthesis of normal and denervated pineal gland. Life Sci. **9**, 691—696 (1963).
DELAY, J., P. PICHON et T. LAMPERIÈRE: La psilocybine (Historique-Pharmacophysiologie-Clinique). Presse méd. **67**, 1731—1733 (1959).
DESPOPOULOS, A.: Renal metabolism of 5-hydroxyindole acetic acid. Fed. Proc. **15**, 48 (1956); — Amer. J. Physiol. **189**, 548—550 (1957).
DEULEFEU, V., and B. BERINZAGHI: Picrolonates of bufotenine, bufotenidine and dehydrobufotenine. J. Amer. chem. Soc. **68**, 1665—1666 (1946).
DONALDSON jr., R. M.: Excretion of tryptamine and indole-3-acetic acid in urine of rats with intestinal diverticula. Amer. J. Physiol. **202**, 289—292 (1962).
— H. A. DOLCINI and S. J. GRAY: Urinary excretion of indolic compounds in rats with intestinal pouches. Amer. J. Physiol. **200**, 794—796 (1961).
— S. MALKIEL and S. J. GRAY: Serotonin studies on mouse tissues. Proc. Soc. exper. Biol. (N.Y.) **103**, 261—263 (1960).
DUBNICK, B., G. A. LEESON, M. CHESSIN and CH. C. SCOTT: Accumulation of serotonin in the brain of reserpine-treated mice after inhibition of monoamine oxidase: effect of body temperature. Arch. int. Pharmacodyn., **126**, 194—202 (1960).
— — and G. E. PHILLIPS: An effect of monoamine-oxidase inhibitors on brain serotonin of mice in addition to that resulting from inhibition of monoamine oxidase. J. Neurochem. **9**, 299—306 (1962).
EBER, O., u. F. LEMBECK: Hydroxytryptamingehalt des Rattendarmes bei verschiedenem Tryptophangehalt der Nahrung. Pflügers Arch. ges. Physiol. **265**, 563—566 (1958).

EDELSTEIN, E. L., Y. PFEIFER, J. E. STEINER and F. G. SULMAN: Excretion of urinary 5-HIAA in dog pellagra. Proc. Soc. exp. Biol. (N.Y.) **110**, 13—16 (1962).
EHRINGER, H., O. HORNYKIEWICZ u. K. LECHNER: Die Wirkung von Methylenblau auf die Monoaminoxydase und den Katecholamin- und 5-Hydroxytryptaminstoffwechsel des Gehirnes. Naunyn-Schmiedeberg's Arch. exp. Path. Pharmak. **241**, 568—582 (1961).
ELIASSON, R.: Critical evaluation of the occurrence of 5-hydroxytryptamine in human semen. J. Urol. **86**, 676—678 (1961).
ENDE, N., and E. I. CHERNISS: Mast cells, histamine and serotonin. Amer. J. clin. Path. **30**, 35—36 (1958).
ENERBACK, L.: Serotonin in human mast cells. Nature (Lond.) **197**, 611 (1963).
ERSHOFF, B. H., and E. M. GAL: Effects of radiation on tissue serotonin levels in the rat. Proc. Soc. exp. Biol. (N.Y.) **108**, 160—162 (1961).
— R. HELLMERS and A. F. WELLS: Effects of a radioprotective agent on tissue serotonin levels in the X-irradiated rat. Proc. Soc. exp. Biol. (N.Y.) **110**, 536—538 (1962).
ERSPAMER, V.: Pharmakologische Studien über Enteramin. I. Über die Wirkung von Acetonextrakten der Kaninchenmagenschleimhaut auf den Blutdruck und auf isolierte überlebende Organe. Naunyn-Schmiedeberg's Arch. exp. Path. Pharmak. **196**, 343—365 (1940a).
— Pharmakologische Studien über Enteramin. III. Über das Vorhandensein eines enteraminähnlichen Stoffes in Milzextrakten. Naunyn-Schmiedeberg's Arch. exp. Path. Pharmak. **196**, 391—407 (1940b).
— Presenza di enteramina o di una sostanza enteraminosimile negli estratti gastrointestinali e splenici dei pesci e negli estratti gastroenterici delle ascidie. Experientia (Basel) **2**, 369—371 (1946).
— Ricerche chimiche e farmacologiche sugli estratti di ghiandola ipobranchiale di Murex. IV. Presenza negli estratti di enteramina o di una sostanza enteraminosimile. Arch. int. Pharmacodyn. **76**, 308—326 (1948a).
— Active substances in the posterior salivary glands of octopoda. I. Enteramine-like substance. Acta pharmacol. (Kbh.) **4**, 213—223 (1948b).
— Über den 5-Hydroxytryptamin-(Enteramin-)Gehalt des Magen-Darmtraktes bei den Wirbeltieren. Naturwissenschaften **40**, 318—319 (1953).
— Il sistema cellulare enterocromaffine e l'enteramina (5-idrossitriptamina). Rend. sci. Farmitalia **1**, 1—193 (1954a).
— Pharmacology of indolealkylamines. Pharmacol. Rev. **6**, 425—487 (1954b).
— Quantitative estimation of 5-hydroxytryptamine in gastrointestinal tract, spleen and blood of vertebrates. Ciba Foundation, Symposium on Hypertension, p. 78—84. London: Churchill 1954 c.
— Isolation of bufoviridine from the skin of *Bufo viridis* and its identification as dihydrobufothionine. Biochem. Pharmacol. **2**, 270—275 (1959a).
— Isolation of leptodactyline (*m*-hydroxyphenylethyltrimethylammonium) from extracts of *Leptodactylus* skin. Arch. Biochem. Biophys. **82**, 431—438 (1959b).
—, and B. ASERO: Isolation of enteramine from extracts of posterior salivary glands of *Octopus vulgaris* and *Discoglossus pictus* skin. J. biol. Chem. **200**, 311—318 (1953).
—, G. BERTACCINI and J. M. CEI: Occurrence of an eleidosin-like polypeptide (physalaemin) in skin extracts of *Physalaemus fuscumaculatus*. Experientia (Basel) **18**, 562—563 (1962a).
— — — Occurrence of bradykinin-like substances in the amphibian skin. Experientia (Basel) **18**, 563—564 (1962b).
—, and G. BORETTI: Identification and characterization, by paper chromatography, of enteramine, octopamine, tyramine, histamine and allied substances in extracts of posterior salivary glands of octopoda and in other tissue extracts of vertebrates and invertebrates. Arch. int. Pharmacodyn. **88**, 296—332 (1951).
—, u. R. FAUSTINI: Über den 5-Hydroxytryptamin-(Enteramin-, Serotonin-)Gehalt des Serums und des Milzgewebes bei Wirbeltieren sowie der Hämolymphe bei Octopoden. Naturwissenschaften **40**, 317—318 (1953).
—, and A. TESTINI: Observations on the release and turnover rate of 5-hydroxytryptamine in the gastrointestinal tract. J. Pharm. Pharmacol. **11**, 618—623 (1959).
—, and M. VIALLI: Presence of enteramine in the skin of amphibia. Nature (Lond.) **167**, 1033 (1951).
— — Ricerche preliminari sulle indolalchilamine e fenilalchilamine degli estratti di pelle di anfibio. Ric. sci. **22**, 1420—1425 (1952).
— T. VITALI, M. L. ROSEGHINI and J. M. CEI: Occurrence of new imidazolealkylamines (spinaceamine and 6-methylspinaceamine) in skin extracts of *Leptodactylus pentadactylus labyrinthicus*. Experientia (Basel) **19**, 346—347 (1963).
EULER, H. v., H. ERDTMAN u. H. HELLSTRÖM: Über das Alkaloid Gramin. Ber. dtsch. chem. Ges. **69**, 743—747 (1936).

FALCK, B.: Observations on the possibilities of the cellular localization of monoamines by a fluorescence method. Acta physiol. scand. **56**, Suppl. 197, 1—25 (1962).
FAUSTINI, R.: The enteric distribution of 5-hydroxytryptamine (enteramine, serotonin) in some large domestic mammals and the appearance of 5-hydroxytryptamine and the enterochromaffin cell system in the embryonic calf. Amer. J. vet. Res. **16**, 397—400 (1955).
FELDBERG, W., and C. C. TOH: Distribution of 5-hydroxytryptamine (serotonin, enteramine) in the wall of the digestive tract. J. Physiol. (Lond.) **119**, 352—362 (1953).
FELDMAN, S., G. IZAK and D. NELKEN: Blood coagulation studies and serotonin determinations in serum and cerebrospinal fluid in multiple sclerosis. Acta psychiat. scand. **32**, 37—49 (1957).
FELDSTEIN, A., H. HOAGLAND and H. FREEMAN: Blood and urinary serotonin and 5-hydroxyindole acetic acid levels in schizophrenic patients and normal subjects. J. nerv. ment. Dis. **129**, 62—68 (1959).
FERRARI, V., E. GINOULHIAC e L. T. TENCONI: Osservazioni sperimentali sui derivati 5-idrossiindolici nella carenza da piridossina. Boll. Soc. ital. Biol. sper. **33**, 1418—1421 (1957).
FEYRTER, F.: Über die peripheren endokrinen (parakrinen) Drüsen des Menschen. Wien u. Düsseldorf: Maudrich 1953.
FIORE-DONATI, L., G. DE BENEDICTIS, L. CHIECO-BIANCHI and G. BERTACCINI: Development of mast cell reaction during chemical skin carcinogenesis of mouse. Nature (Lond.) **193**, 287—288 (1962).
FISCHER, E., F. A. VAZQUES, T. A. FERNÁNDEZ and L. LISKOWSKI: Bufotenin in human urine. Lancet **1961 I**, 890—891.
FISH, M. S., and E. C. HORNING: Studies on hallucinogenetic snuffs. J. nerv. ment. Dis. **124**, 33—37 (1956).
—, N. M. JOHNSON and E. C. HORNING: Piptadenia alkaloids. Indole bases of P. peregrina (L.) Benth. and related species. J. Amer. chem. Soc. **77**, 5892—5895 (1955).
FOY, J. M., and J. R. PARRATT: A note on the presence of noradrenaline and 5-hydroxytryptamine in plantain *(Nusa sapientum* var., *paradisiaca)*. J. Pharm. Pharmacol. **12**, 360—364 (1960).
— — 5-Hydroxytryptamine in pinneaples. J. Pharm. Pharmacol. **13**, 382—383 (1961).
— — Urinary excretion of 5-hydroxyindoleacetic acid in West Africans. Lancet **1962 I**, 942—943.
FRANKLAND, M., F. KENDRICKS and M. GREIPEL: Serotonin concentration in the spleen. Amer. J. dig. Dis. **7**, 347—355 (1962).
FREEDMAN, D. X.: Effects of LSD-25 on brain serotonin. J. Pharmacol. exp. Ther. **134**, 160—166 (1961).
FREUND, H.: Über die pharmakologischen Wirkungen des defibrinierten Blutes. Naunyn-Schmiedeberg's Arch. exp. Path. Pharmak. **86**, 266—280 (1920).
FRYDMAN, B., and V. DEULOFEU: Isolation of 5-hydroxytryptamine from the skin of the toad Bufo arenarum Hensel. Experientia (Basel) **17**, 545—546 (1961).
FURANO, A. V., and J. P. GREEN: The uptake of biogenic amines by mast cells of the rat. J. Physiol. (Lond.) **170**, 263—271 (1964).
FURTH, J., P. HAGEN and E. I. HIRSCH: Transplantable mastocytoma in the mouse containing histamine, heparin and 5-hydroxytryptamine. Proc. Soc. exp. Biol. (N.Y.) **95**, 824—828 (1957).
GADDUM, J. H., and N. J. GIARMAN: Preliminary studies on the biosynthesis of 5-hydroxytryptamine. Brit. J. Pharmacol. **11**, 88—92 (1956).
GAL, E. M., and P. A. DREWES: Levels of serotonin during convulsion and the effect of reserpine. Nature (Lond.) **189**, 234 (1961a).
— — Studies on the metabolism of 5-hydroxytryptamine (serotonin). I. Effect of starvation and thiamine deficiency. Proc. Soc. exp. Biol. (N.Y.) **106**, 295—297 (1961b).
— — Studies on the metabolism of 5-hydroxytryptamine (serotonin). II. Effect of tryptophan deficiency in rats. Proc. Soc. exp. Biol. (N.Y.) **110**, 368—371 (1962).
— — and C. A. BARRACLOUGH: Effect of reserpine and the metabolism of serotonin in tryptophan deficient rats. Biochem. Pharmacol. 8, 32 (1961).
GARDNER, L. I., and A. A. TYCE: Histamine and related compounds in urticaria pigmentosa: analyses of tissues having mast-cell infiltration. Pediatrics **21**, 805—812 (1958).
GARVEN, J. D.: The estimation of 5-hydroxytryptamine in the presence of adrenaline. Brit. J. Pharmacol. **11**, 66—70 (1956).
GEIGER, R. S., N. CANTOR and F. A. GIBBS: Localization of monoamines and action of hallucinogens on them in adult mammalian brain cells in long term culture. Fed. Proc. **23**, 351 (1964).
GERSCH, M., F. FISCHER, H. UNGER u. W. KABITZER: Vorkommen von Serotonin im Nervensystem von *Periplaneta americana* L. *(Insecta)*. Z. Naturforsch. B **16**, 351—352 (1961).

GERTNER, S. B., M. K. PAASONEN and N. J. GIARMAN: Studies concerning the presence of 5-hydroxytryptamine (serotonin) in the perfusate from the superior cervical ganglion. J. Pharmacol. exp. Ther. **127**, 268—275 (1959).
GIARMAN, N. J., and M. DAY: Presence of biogenic amines in the bovine pineal body. Biochem. Pharmacol. **1**, 235 (1958).
— — and G. PEPEU: Presence of neuro-humors in bovine pineal glands. Fed. Proc. **18**, 394 (1959).
—, and D. X. FREEDMAN: Serotonin content of the pineal glands of man and monkeys. Nature (Lond.) **186**, 480—481 (1960).
—, and S. L. M. SCHANBERG: The intracellular distribution of 5-hydroxytryptamine (HT, serotonin) in the rat's brain. Biochem. Pharmacol. **1**, 301—306 (1959).
GIRARD, J.-P.: Le rôle de l'adénosine triphosphorique (ATP) dans la fixation intraplaquettaire de la sérotonine. Schweiz. med. Wschr. **93**, 1456—1459 (1963).
GLUCKMAN, M. I.: Cerebral free and bound serotonin (5HT) after iproniazid (IIH) and reserpine (R). Fed. Proc. **19**, 264 (1960).
GÖRÖG, P., and L. SZPORNY: The depleting effect of vincamin on the cerebral serotonin level. Biochem. Pharmacol. **11**, 165—166 (1962).
GORDON, P.: Changes in blood serotonin during exposure to cold. Nature (Lond.) **191**, 183—184 (1961).
GOSSELIN, R. E., K. E. MOORE and A. S. MILTON: Physiological control of molluscan gill cilia by 5-hydroxytryptamine. J. gen. Physiol. **46**, 277—296 (1962).
GOTTFRIES, C. G., and T. MAGNUSSON: Excretion of tryptamine in man during treatment with MAO inhibitors. Acta psychiat. scand. **38**, 223—226 (1962).
GREEN, H., S. M. GREENBERG, R. W. ERICKSON, J. L. SAWYER and TH. ELLISON: Effect of dietary phenylalanine and tryptophan upon rat brain amine levels. J. Pharmacol. exp. Ther. **136**, 174—178 (1962a).
—, and J. L. SAWYER: Intracellular distribution of serotonin in rat brain. I. Effect of reserpine and the monoamine oxidase inhibitors, tranylcypromine and iproniazid. Arch. int. Pharmacodyn. **135**, 426—441 (1962).
— — R. W. ERICKSON and L. COOK: Effect of repeated oral administration of monoamine oxidase inhibitors on rat brain amines. Proc. Soc. exp. Biol. (N.Y.) **109**, 347—349 (1962b).
GREEN, J. P., and S. M. DAY: Heparin, 5-hydroxytryptamine, and histamine in neoplastic mast cells. Biochem. Pharmacol. **3**, 190—205 (1960b).
—, M. ROBERTS and S. M. DAY: Fractionation of heparin from a mast cell tumour of the mouse. Fed. Proc. **19**, 133 (1960a).
GRETTE, K.: Determination of 5-hydroxytryptamine with the isolated, perfused pig ear. Acta pharmacol. (Kbh.) **13**, 177—183 (1957).
GURSEY, D., and R. E. OLSON: Depression of serotonin and norepinephrine levels in brain stem of rabbit by ethanol. Proc. Soc. exp. Biol. (N.Y.) **104**, 280—281 (1960).
—, J. W. VESTER and R. E. OLSON: Effect of ethanol administration upon serotonin and norepinephrine levels in rabbit brain. J. clin. Invest. **38**, 1008—1009 (1959).
HADDOX jr., CH. H., and M. S. SASLAW: Urinary 5-methoxytryptamine in patients with rheumatic fever. J. clin. Invest. **42**, 435—441 (1963).
HAGGENDAL, J., and M. LINDQUIST: Ineffectiveness of ethanol on noradrenaline, dopamine or 5-hydroxytryptamine levels in brain. Acta pharmacol. (Kbh.) **18**, 278—280 (1961).
HAGMÜLLER, K., L. HAIDER u. H. HELLAUER: Enterochromaffine Zellen, Serotonin und Zink in der Magen-Darm-Wand des Meerschweinchens und der Maus vor und nach chronischer Zufuhr von Aethanol. Wien. klin. Wschr. **73**, 834—836 (1961).
HARDING-GAUDIN, F.: Excrétion urinaire d'acide 5-hydroxyindolylacétique chez le rat albinos carencé ou non en riboflavine. Acta vitamin. (Milano) **15**, 193—196 (1961).
HARTMAN, W. J., W. G. CLARK, S. D. CYR, A. L. JORDAN and R. A. LEIBHOLD: Pharmacologically active amines and their biogenesis in the octopus. Ann. N.Y. Acad. Sci. **90** (3), 637—666 (1960).
HARVEY, J. A., A. HELLER and R. Y. MOORE: The effect of unilateral and bilateral medial forebrain bundle lesions on brain serotonin. J. Pharmacol. exp. Ther. **140**, 103—110 (1963).
HAVERBACK, B. J., and J. D. DAVIDSON: Serotonin and the gastrointestinal tract. Gastroenterology **35**, 570—578 (1958).
— F. T. DUTSCHER, P. A. SHORE, E. G. TOMICH, L. L. TERRY and B. B. BRODIE: Serotonin changes in platelets and brain induced by small daily doses of reserpine. Lack of effect of depletion of platelet serotonin in hemostatic mechanisms. New Engl. J. Med. **256**, 343—345 (1957).
HAWKER, R. W., V. S. ROBERTS and C. F. WALMSLEY: Some properties of an oxytocic substance in extracts of semen. Endocrinology **67**, 187—193 (1960).

HESS, S. M., and W. DOEPFNER: Behavioral effects and brain amine content in rats. Arch. int. Pharmacodyn. **134**, 89—99 (1961).
— B. G. REDFIELD and S. UDENFRIEND: Tryptamine in animal tissues following administration of iproniazid. Fed. Proc. **18**, 402 (1959a).
— — — The effect of monoamine oxidase inhibitors and tryptophan on the tryptamine content of animal tissues and urine. J. Pharmacol. exp. Ther. **127**, 178—181 (1959b).
—, and S. UDENFRIEND: A fluorometric procedure for the measurement of tryptamine in tissues. J. Pharmacol. exp. Ther. **127**, 175—177 (1959).
HIROSE, K.: Relation between the platelet count of human blood and its vasoconstrictor action after clotting. Arch. int. Med. **21**, 604—612 (1918).
HOCHSTEIN, F. A., and A. M. PARADIES: Alkaloids of Banisteria caapi and Prestonia amazonicum. J. Amer. chem. Soc. **79**, 5735—5736 (1957).
HOFMANN, A., A. FREY, H. OTT, TH. PETRZILKA u. F. TROXLER: Konstitutionsaufklärung und Synthese von Psilocybin. Experientia (Basel) **14**, 397—399 (1958).
— R. HEIM et H. TSCHERTER: Présence de la psilocybine dans une espèce européenne d'Agaric, le *Psilocybe semilanceata* Fr. C. R. Acad. Sci. (Paris) **257**, 10—12 (1963).
—, and F. TROXLER: Identifizierung von Psilocin. Experientia (Basel) **15**, 101—102 (1959).
HSIA, D. Y.-Y., K. NISHIMURA and Y. BRENCHLEY: Mechanisms for the decrease of brain serotonin. Nature (Lond.) **200**, 578 (1963).
HUBER, W. G., and R. P. LINK: Relationship of serotonin and reserpine in the chicken. Proc. Soc. exp. Biol. (N.Y.) **109**, 118—120 (1962).
HUMPHREY, J. H., and R. JAQUES: The histamine and serotonin content of the platelets and polymorphonuclear leucocytes of various species. J. Physiol. (Lond.) **124**, 305—310 (1954b).
—, and C. C. TOH: Absorption of serotonin (5-hydroxytryptamine) and histamine by dog platelets. J. Physiol. (Lond.) **124**, 300—304 (1954a).
IACHELLO, R., E. RIVA SANSEVERINO e A. URBANO: Sulla presenza di 5-idrossitriptamina in estratti di ghiandola sottomascellare di cane. Boll. Soc. ital. Biol. sper. **38**, 516—518 (1962).
INOUYE, A., K. KATAOKA and J. SHINAGAWA: 5-Hydroxytryptamine in the subcellular particles of rabbit brain. Nature (Lond.) **194**, 286—287 (1962).
JACKSON, H. R., S. J. WILSON and H. E. HEATH: 5-Hydroxytryptamine-C^{14} platelet survival studies. J. Lab. clin. Med. **62**, 887 (1963).
JANEWAY, T. C., H. B. RICHARDSON and E. A. PARK: Experiments on the vasoconstrictor action of blood serum. Arch. intern. Med. **21**, 565—603 (1918).
JAQUES, R., and M. SCHACHTER: The presence of histamine, 5-hydroxytryptamine and a potent slow contracting substance in wasp venom. Brit. J. Pharmacol. **9**, 53—58 (1954).
JENSEN, H.: Chemical studies on toad poisons. *Bufo arenarum*, *Bufo regularis* and *Xenopus laevis*. J. Amer. chem. Soc. **57**, 1765—1768 (1935).
JENSEN, K.: Paper chromatography determination of indoles in human cerebrospinal fluid. Acta neurol. scand. **38**, 278—284 (1962).
JOHANSSON, S.-A.: 5-Hydroxytryptamine in burns. Acta physiol. scand. **48**, 126—132 (1960).
JOHNSEN jr., H. A., R. E. SMITH and W. SIMON: Diurnal variations in the excretion of urinary 5-hydroxyindoles. Clin. Res. **6**, 268—269 (1958).
JOYCE, D.: Changes in the 5-hydroxytryptamine content of rat, rabbit and human brain after death. Brit. J. Pharmacol. **18**, 370—380 (1962).
— 5-Hydroxytryptamine content of glioma. Experientia (Basel) **19**, 187—188 (1963).
JULLIEN, A., J. CARDOT and J. RIPPLINGER: Observations sur les substances cardioactives d'origine nerveuse chez les Crustacés Décapodes et chez les Mollusques Pulmonés. J. Physiol. (Paris) **53**, 381—382 (1961).
KÄRKI, N. T., R. KUNTZMAN and B. B. BRODIE: Norepinephrine and serotonin brain levels at various stages of ontogenetic development. Fed. Proc. **19**, 282 (1960b).
— — — Storage, synthesis, and metabolism of monoamines in the developing brain. J. Neurochem. **9**, 53—58 (1962).
—, and M. K. PAASONEN: Presence of 5-hydroxytryptamine after raunescine in blood plasma in vivo. Nature (Lond.) **185**, 109 (1960).
— — and P. PELTOLA: Factors influencing the release of 5-hydroxytryptamine from the rabbit intestine into the venous blood. Ann. Med. exp. Fenn. **38**, 231—236 (1960a).
KAKIMOTO, Y., and M. D. ARMSTRONG: On the identification of octopamine in mammals. J. biol. Chem. **237**, 422—427 (1962).
KARZEL, K.: Einfluß des Mastzellentumors P-815 der Maus auf den 5-Hydroxytryptamin-Gehalt ihrer Organe. Med. exp. **10**, 115—118 (1964).
KATAOKA, K.: Subcellular distribution of 5-hydroxytryptamine in the rabbit brain. Jap. J. Physiol. **12**, 623—638 (1962).
KATSH, S.: Serotonin and histamine in human ejaculate. J. Urol. **81**, 570—572 (1959).

KELLER, R.: Histamin und 5-Hydroxytryptamin in den Gewebemastzellen der Albinoratte. Helv. physiol. Acta **15**, 371—375 (1957).

KERKUT, G. A., and G. A. COTTRELL: Acetylcholine and 5-hydroxytryptamine in the snail brain. Comp. Biochem. Physiol. **8**, 53—63 (1963).

—, and M. A. PRICE: 6-HT in crab heart. Life Sciences No 2, 129—130 (1963).

— — Chromatographic separation of cardiaccelerators (6 HT and a mucopeptide) from *Carcinus* heart. Comp. Biochem. Physiol. **11**, 45—52 (1964).

KIND, L. S., A. BURKHALTER and R. SHERINS: Increased lung serotonin and pulmonary edema in mice injected with antiserum to EHRLICH's ascites tumor. Proc. Soc. exp. Biol. (N. Y.) **108**, 735—737 (1961).

KINDWALL, E. P., L. O. BORÉUS and B. WESTERHOLM: Failure to show change in rat tissue histamin and serotonin after rapid decompression. Amer. J. Physiol. **203**, 389—390 (1962).

KIRBERGER, E., u. L. BRAUN: Über das Vorkommen von 5-Hydroxytryptamin in der Walnuß (Juglans regia). Biochim. biophys. Acta (Amst.) **49**, 391—393 (1961).

KIRKWOOD, S., and L. MARION: The biogenesis of alkaloids. I. The isolation of N-methyltryptamine from barley. J. Amer. chem. Soc. **57**, 1765—1768 (1950).

KISS, G., u. H. MICHL: Über das Giftsekret der Gelbbauchunke, *Bombina variegata* L. Toxicon **1**, 33—39 (1962).

KIVALO, E., U. K. RINNE and H. KARINKANTA: The effect of imipramine on the 5-hydroxytryptamine content and monoamine oxidase activity of the rat brain and on the excretion of 5-hydroxyindole acetic acid. J. Neurochem. **8**, 105—108 (1961).

KLAMBT, H.-D.: Die 2-Hydroxy-indol-3-essigsäure, ein pflanzliches Indolderivat. Naturwissenschaften **46**, 649 (1959).

KLEEBERG, J., J. BOXER and E. J. STEINER: Studies on almonds. III. The serotonin content of dried sweet almonds. Arch. int. Pharmacodyn. **144**, 432—436 (1963).

KOCH, G., u. G. ENGELHARDT: Über das argyrophile Helle-Zellen-Organ in der Harnröhrenschleimhaut des Säugetieres. Naunyn-Schmiedeberg's Arch. exp. Path. Pharmak. **236**, 463—473 (1959).

KOPIN, I. J.: Tryptophan loading and excretion of 5-hydroxyindoleacetic acid in normal and schizophrenic subjects. Science **129**, 835—836 (1959).

KOREN, Z., B. ECKSTEIN, A. BRZEZINSKI and F. G. SULMAN: Adrenaline, noradrenaline and serotonin estimations in urine and amniotic fluid during delivery. J. Obstet. Gynaec. Brit. Cwlth **68**, 438—440 (1961).

KUNTZMAN, R., P. A. SHORE, D. BOGDANSKI and B. B. BRODIE: Microanalytical procedures for fluorometric assay of brain DOPA-5-HTP decarboxylase, norepinephrine and serotonin, and a detailed mapping of decarboxylase activity in brain. J. Neurochem. **6**, 226—232 (1961).

KURIAKI, K., et T. INOUE: Teneur en 5-hydroxytryptamine du placenta et des urines gravides et post-partum. C. R. Soc. Biol. (Paris) **150**, 1835—1837 (1956).

LEBLANC, J.: Secretion and activity of histamine and serotonin during cold adaptation. Amer. J. Physiol. **204**, 520—522 (1963).

LEGLER, G., u. R. TSCHESCHE: Isolierung von N-Methyltryptamin, 5-Methoxy-N-methyltryptamin und 5-Methoxy-N,N-dimethyltryptamin aus der Rinde von Piptadenia peregrina Benth. Naturwissenschaften **50**, 94—95 (1963).

LERNER, A. B., and J. D. CASE: Melatonin. Fed. Proc. **19**, 590—592 (1960).

— — K. BIEMANN, R. V. HEINZELMAN, J. SZMUSZKOVICZ, W. C. ANTHONY and A. KRIVIS: Isolation of 5-methoxyindole-3-acetic acid from bovine pineal glands. J. Amer. chem. Soc. **81**, 5264 (1959a).

— — W. MORI and M. R. WRIGHT: Melatonin in peripheral nerves. Nature (Lond.) **183**, 1821 (1959b).

— — and Y. TAKAHASHI: Isolation of melatonin and 5-methoxyindole-3-acetic acid from bovine pineal glands. J. biol. Chem. **235**, 1992—1997 (1960).

LEROY, J. G.: 5-Hydroxytryptamine levels in brain of mice pretreated with α-methyl-dopa. Arch. int. Pharmacodyn. **134**, 492—496 (1961).

LEVENE, R. Z.: Mast cells and amines in normal ocular tissues. Invest Ophthal. **1**, 531—543 (1962).

LEWIS, G. P.: 5-Hydroxytryptamine in the mast cells of the rat. In: G. P. LEWIS, 5-Hydroxytryptamine, p. 26—31. London: Pergamon Press 1957.

— 5-Hydroxytryptamine. J. Pharm. Pharmacol. **10**, 529—540 (1958).

LONG, R. F.: Inhibition of 5-hydroxytryptamine uptake by platelets *in vitro* and *in vivo*. Biochem. J. **82**, 4—5 P (1962).

MAAS, J. W.: Neurochemical differences between two strains of mice. Nature (Lond.) **197**, 255—257 (1963).

MAASS, A. R., and M. J. NIMMO: A new inhibitor of serotonin metabolism. Nature (Lond.) **184**, 547—548 (1959).
MACFARLANE, P. S., C. E. DALGLIESH, R. W. DUTTON, B. LENNOX, L. M. NYHUS and A. N. SMITH: Endocrine aspects of argentaffinoma, with special reference to the use of urinary 5-hydroxyindoleacetic acid estimation in diagnosis. Scot. med. J. **1**, 148—155 (1956).
MÄRKI, F., A. V. ROBERTSON and B. WITKOP: Dehydrobufotenine, a novel type of tryciclic serotonin metabolite from *Bufo marinus*. J. Amer. chem. Soc. **83**, 3341—3342 (1961).
MAGUS, R. D., F. W. KRAUSE and B. E. RIEDEL: Release of thyroidal serotonin by reserpine, methyldopa and guanethidine. Biochem. Pharmacol. **13**, 115—117 (1964).
MANN, T.: Serotonin (5-hydroxytryptamine) in the male reproductive tract of the spiny dogfish. Nature (Lond.) **188**, 941—942 (1960).
— 5-Hydroxytryptamine in the spermatophoric sac of Octopus. Nature (Lond.) **199**, 1066—1067 (1963).
— R. F. SEAMARK and D. F. SHARMAN: On the question of the occurrence and metabolism of 5-hydroxytryptamine and related indole compounds in mammalian semen. Brit. J. Pharmacol. **17**, 208—217 (1961).
MANSOUR, T. E., A. D. LAGO and J. L. HAWKINS: Occurrence and possible role of serotonin in *Fasciola hepatica*. Fed. Proc. **16**, 319 (1957).
MARMO, E.: Psilocibina e psilocina: principi attivi dei funghi allucinogeni messicani. Clin. ter. **18**, 464—490 (1960).
MARSHALL, P. B.: Catechols and tryptamines in the "makote" banana (Musa paradisiaca). J. Pharm. Pharmacol. **11**, 639 (1959).
MATHIAS, A. P., D. M. ROSS and M. SCHACHTER: Identification and distribution of 5-hydroxytryptamine in a sea anemone. Nature (Lond.) **180**, 658—659 (1957).
— — — Distribution of histamine, 5-hydroxytryptamine, tetramethylammonium, and other substances in coelenterates possessing nematocysts. J. Physiol. (Lond.) **142**, 56—57P (1958).
— — — The distribution of 5-hydroxytryptamine, tetramethylammonium, homarine, and other substances in sea anemones. J. Physiol. (Lond.) **151**, 296—311 (1960).
MAYNARD, D. M., and J. H. WELSH: Neurohormones of the pericardial organs of brachyuran crustacea. J. Physiol. (Lond.) **149**, 215—227 (1959).
MAYNERT, E. W., G. I. KLINGMAN and H. K. KAJI: Tolerance to morphine. II. Lack of effects on brain 5-hydroxytryptamine and γ-aminobutyric acid. J. Pharmacol. exp. Ther. **135**, 296—299 (1962).
—, R. LEVI and A. J. D. DE LORENZO: The presence of norepinephrine and 5-hydroxytryptamine in vesicles from disrupted nerve-ending particles. J. Pharmacol. exp. Ther. **144**, 385—392 (1964).
— — and K. KURIYAMA: Vesicles containing norepinephrine (NE) and 5-hydroxytryptamine (5-HT) from disrupted nerve-ending particles. Fed. Proc. **23**, 350 (1964).
MEIER, H.: Serotonin (5-hydroxytryptamine) content of canine mastocytoma. Proc. Soc. exp. Biol. (N.Y.) **100**, 815—817 (1959).
MELCHING, H. J., H. ERNST u. H. RÖSSLER: Untersuchungen über einen biologischen Strahlenschutz. XXXVI. Zum Stoffwechsel des 5-Hydroxytryptamins bei der Ganzkörperbestrahlung weißer Mäuse und Ratten. Strahlentherapie **113**, 394—401 (1960).
MELMON, K., and A. SJOERDSMA: Serotonin in platelets. Lancet **1963 II**, 316—318.
MENG, K.: 5-Hydyroxytrptamin und Acetylcholin als Wirkungsantagonisten beim Helix-Herzen. Naturwissenschaften **45**, 470 (1958).
MENGEL, CH. E., and M. G. KELLY: Biochemical and morphologic changes in a mast-cell neoplasm during treatment with cyclophosphamide. Cancer Res. **21**, 1545—1550 (1961).
MICHAELSON, I. A., and V. P. WHITTAKER: The distribution of 5-hydroxytryptamine in brain fractions. Biochem. Pharmacol. **11**, 505—506 (1962).
— — The subcellular localization of 5-hydroxytryptamine in guinea-pig brain. Biochem. Pharmacol. **12**, 203—211 (1963).
MILNE, M. D., M. A. CRAWFORD, C. B. GIRÃO and L. LOUGHRIDGE: The excretion of indolylacetic acid and related indolic acids in man and the rat. Clin. Sci. **19**, 165—179 (1960).
MIROLLI, M., and J. H. WELSH: The effects of reserpine and LSD on molluscs. In: D. RICHTER Ed., Comparative Neurochemistry, pp. 433—443. Oxford: Pergamon Press 1964.
MÖRSDORF, K.: Spectrofluorometrische Bestimmung des 5-Hydroxytryptamingehaltes der Rattenpfote bei experimentellen „Entzündungen". Med. exp. (Basel) **1**, 87—90 (1959).
— Die serotoninfreisetzende Wirkung einiger zur Auslösung experimenteller „Entzündungen" verwendeter Stoffe in vitro. Med. exp. (Basel) **4**, 293—297 (1961).
MOORE, K. E., and T. M. BRODY: The effect of triethyltin on tissue amines. J. Pharmacol. exp. Ther. **132**, 6—12 (1961).
MORAN, N. C., B. UVNÄS and B. WESTERHOLM: Release of 5-hydroxytryptamine and histamine from rat mast cells. Acta physiol. scand. **56**, 26—41 (1962).

MORAN, N. C., and B. WESTERHOLM: The influence of reserpine on 5-hydroxytryptamine and histamine content of rat mast cells and of some rat tissues. Acta physiol. scand. **58**, 20—29 (1963).

NACHMIAS, V. T.: Amine oxidase and 5-hydroxytryptamine in developing rat brain. J. Neurochem. **6**, 99—104 (1960).

NAERS, K., and S. SCHANCHE: Effect of reserpine on serotonin in rabbit serum. Nature (Lond.) **117**, 1130—1131 (1956).

NEUMARK, H.: Formation of serotonin in chopped green maize. Nature (Lond.) **201**, 527—528 (1964).

NIKKILA, E. A.: Urinary excretion of the serotonin metabolite 5-hydroxyindole acetic acid in neurocirculatory asthenia. Acta med. scand. **162**, 231—235 (1958).

NIKODIJEVIĆ, B., and T. TRAJKOV: Mechanism of ulcerogenic action of 5-hydroxytryptamine in rat's stomach. Arch. int. Pharmacodyn. **143**, 442—445 (1963).

O'CONNOR, J. M.: Über den Adrenalingehalt des Blutes. Naunyn-Schmiedeberg's Arch. exp. Path. Pharmak. **67**, 195—232 (1912).

OLSON, R. E., D. GURSEY and J. W. VESTER: Evidence for a defect in tryptophan metabolism in chronic alcoholism. New Engl. J. Med. **263**, 1169—1174 (1960).

ONO, S., L. ZOMPETTI, P. HAGEN and J. FURTH: Relation of mastocytoma to mast cell leukemia, and of heparin, histamine and serotonin to mast cells. Blood **14**, 770—780 (1959).

ORCHOFF, A. P., u. S. S. NORKINA: Über die Alkaloide von *Arundo donax*. Ber. dtsch. chem. Ges. **68**, 436—437 (1935).

OWMAN, CH.: On the presence of 5-hydroxytryptamine in pineal nerves. Biochem. Pharmacol. **12**, Suppl., 112 (1963).

PAASONEN, M. K.: 5-Hydroxytryptamine in mammalian thyroid gland. Experientia (Basel) **14**, 95—96 (1958).

—, and N. J. GIARMAN: Brain levels of 5-hydroxytryptamine after various agents. Arch. int. Pharmacodyn. **114**, 189—200 (1958).

—, and N. T. KÄRKI: Increase of 5-hydroxytryptamine in the rat brain by raunescine. Brit. J. Pharmacol. **14**, 164—167 (1959).

— — and S. MOLKKA: Influence of iproniazid and 5-hydroxytryptophan on the 5-hydroxytryptamine content in the gastro-intestinal tract and thyroid gland of rats. Ann. Med. exp. Fenn. **39**, 405—410 (1961).

— P. D. MACLEAN and N. J. GIARMAN: 5-Hydroxytryptamine (serotonin, enteramine) content of structures of limbic system. J. Neurochem. **1**, 326—333 (1957).

—, and P. PELTOLA: The effect of methimazole and potassium thiocyanate on the 5-hydroxytryptamine content of the rat thyroid gland. Ann. Med. exp. Fenn. **38**, 228—230 (1960).

—, and M. VOGT: The effect of drugs on the amounts of substance P and 5-hydroxytryptamine in mammalian brain. J. Physiol. (Lond.) **131**, 617—626 (1956).

PACHTER, I., D. E. ZACHARIUS and O. RIBEIRO: Indole alkaloids of *Acer saccharinum* (the silver maple), *Dictyoloma incanescens, Piptadenia colubrina*, and *Mimosa hostilis*. J. organ. Chem. **24**, 1285—1287 (1959).

PACHTER, I. J.: A note on the occurrence of gramine in *Acer rubrum* L. J. Amer. pharm. Ass. (sci. Ed.) **48**, 670 (1959).

PARE, C. M. B., M. SANDLER and R. S. STACEY: 5-Hydroxyindoles in mental deficiency. J. Neurol. Neurosurg. Psychiat. **23**, 341—346 (1960).

PARKER-WILLIAMS, E. J., PH. COHEN, P. WALTROUSE and F. H. GARTNER: Platelet preservation studies using platelets labeled with C^{14}-5-hydroxytryptamine. J. clin. Invest. **42**, 963 (1963).

PARRATT, J. R., and G. B. WEST: Tissue histamine and 5-hydroxytryptamine. J. Physiol. (Lond.) **132**, 40—41 P (1956a).

— — Influence of age on tissue histamine and 5-hydroxytryptamine. J. Physiol. (Lond.) **133**, 71—72 P (1956b).

— — 5-Hydroxytryptamine and tissue mast cells. J. Physiol. (Lond.) **137**, 169—178 (1957a).

— — Release of 5-hydroxytryptamine and histamine from tissues of the rat. J. Physiol. (Lond.) **137**, 179—192 (1957b).

— — The relationship of 5-hydroxytryptamine to capillary permeability in the skin of the rat. J. Physiol. (Lond.) **140**, 105—112 (1958).

PELTOLA, P., and V. LEPPÄNEN: Studies on the excretion of 5-hydroxyindoleacetic acid. Ann. Med. intern. Fenn. **49**, 283—291 (1960).

PEPEU, G., and N. J. GIARMAN: Contrasting findings on serotonin (5-HT) in fetal life. Pharmacologist **2**, 91 (1960).

— — Serotonin in the developing mammal. J. gen. Physiol. **45**, 575—583 (1962).

PERMAN, E. S.: Observations on the effect of ethanol on the urinary excretion of histamine, 5-hydroxyindole acetic acid, catecholamines and 17-hydroxycorticosteroids in man. Acta physiol. scand. **51**, 62—67 (1961).

PERRY, TH. L., S. HANSEN and L. C. JENKINS: Amine content of normal human cerebrospinal fluid. J. Neurochem. **11**, 49—53 (1964).
—, N. F. SHAW and D. WALKER: Apparent absence of amines in cerebrospinal fluid of phenylketonurics. Nature (Lond.) **189**, 926—927 (1961).
PHILIPPS, J. H.: Isolation of active nematocysts of *Metridium senile* and their chemical composition. Nature (Lond.) **178**, 932 (1956).
PHILLIPS, A. W., H. R. NEWCOMB, J. E. SMITH and R. LACHAPELLE: Serotonin in the small intestine of conventional and germ-free chicks. Nature (Lond.) **192**, 380 (1961).
PIGEAUD, H., R. BURTHIAULT, R. BETHOUX et S. NELKEN: Le dosage de l'acide 5-hydroxyindole-acétique au cours de la grossesse normale et dans les suites de couches immédiates. Gynéc. et Ostét. **57**, 415—425 (1958).
PLETSCHER, A.: Beeinflussung des 5-Hydroxytryptaminstoffwechsels im Gehirn durch Isonikotinsäurehydrazide. Experientia (Basel) **12**, 479—480 (1956a).
— Wirkung von Isonicotinsäurehydraziden auf den 5-Hydroxytryptaminstoffwechsel in vivo. Helv. physiol. Acta **14**, C 76—79 (1956b).
— W. P. BURKARD, H. BRUDERER and K. F. GEY: Decrease of cerebral 5-hydroxytryptamine and 5-hydroxyindoleacetic acid by an arylalkylamine. Life Sci. No 11, 827—833 (1963).
— P. A. SHORE and B. B. BRODIE: Serotonin as a mediator of reserpine action in brain. J. Pharmacol. exp. Ther. **116**, 84—89 (1956).
PSCHEIDT, G. R.: Serotonin and norepinephrine in chicken brain: distribution, normal level and effect of reserpine and monoamine oxidase. Fed. Proc. **23**, 305 (1964).
—, and H. E. HIMWICH: Reserpine, monoamine oxidase inhibitors and distribution of biogenic amines in monkey brain. Biochem. Pharmacol. **12**, 65—72 (1963).
— C. MORPURGO and H. E. HIMWICH: Studies on norepinephrine and 5-hydroxytryptamine in various species. In: D. RICHTER Ed., Comparative Neurochemistry, pp. 401—412. Oxford: Pergamon Press 1964.
— — Chicken brain amines, with special reference to cerebellar norepinephrine. Life Sci., No 7, 524—526 (1963).
PURKHALSKAIA, E., and G. P. MENSHIKOV: 5-Hydroxytryptamine from *Hippophae rhamnoides* as antitumoral agent in animal experiments. Biul. eksp. Biol. Med. **50**, 105—110 (1960).
PUT, T. R., and L. A. H. HOGENHUIS: Brain serotonin and thyroid function. Acta physiol. pharmacol. neerl. **10**, 343—352 (1962).
QUAY, W. B.: Cytologic and metabolic parameters of pineal inhibition by continuous light in the rat (*Rattus norvegicus*). Z. Zellforsch. **60**, 479—490 (1963a).
— Effect of dietary phenylalanine and tryptophan on pineal and hypothalamic serotonin levels. Proc. Soc. exp. Biol. (N.Y.) **114**, 718—721 (1963b).
— Circadian rhythm in rat pinael serotonin and its modifications by estrous cycle and photoperiod. Gen. comp. Endocr. **3**, 473—479 (1963c).
— Circadian and estrous rhythms in pineal melatonin and 5-hydroxy-indole-3-acetic acid. Proc. Soc. exp. Biol. (N.Y.) **115**, 710—713 (1964).
—, and A. HALEVY: Experimental modification of the rat pineal's content of serotonin and related indole amines. Physiol. Zool. **35**, 1—7 (1962).
RAND, M., and G. REID: Source of "serotonin" in serum. Nature (Lond.) **168**, 385 (1951).
— — On the presence in rabbit serum of thrombotonin (thrombocytin or serotonin). Aust. J. exp. Biol. med. Sci. **30**, 153—161 (1952).
RESNICK, R. H., and S. J. GRAY: Serotonin release by hydrochloric acid. I. In vivo and in vitro demonstration. J. Lab. clin. Med. **59**, 462—468 (1962).
— G. T. SMITH and S. J. GRAY: Endocrine influences on tissue serotonin content of the rat. Amer. J. Physiol. **201**, 571—573 (1961).
RICE, W. G., and J. MITCHENER: Histochemical evidence of 5-hydroxytryptamine in a dog mast cell tumour. Nature (Lond.) **189**, 767—768 (1961).
RILEY, J. F.: Fluorescent mast cells in precancerous mouse skin. Experientia (Basel) **14**, 141 (1958).
ROBERTSON, P. A., and W. V. MACFARLANE: Pain-producing substances from the stinging bush *Laportea moroides*. Aust. J. exp. Biol. med. Sci. **35**, 381—394 (1957).
ROBILLARD, E., and Y. ALARIE: Mechanical properties and histamine and serotonin content of guinea pig lungs as influenced by microparticles inhalation. Canad. J. Biochem. **41**, 2177—2182 (1963).
ROBINSON, B., G. F. SMITH, A. H. JACKSON, D. SHAW, B. FRYDMAN and V. DEULOFEU: Dehydrobufotenin. Proc. Chem. Soc., August 1961, p. 310—311.
ROBSON, J. M., and J. B. SENIOR: The 5-hydroxytryptamine content of the placenta and foetus during pregnancy in mice. Brit. J. Pharmacol. **22**, 380—391 (1964).
RODNIGHT, R.: Separation and characterization of urinary indoles resembling 5-hydroxytryptamine and tryptamine. Biochem. J. **64**, 621—626 (1956).

Roos, B.-E.: The effect of monoamine oxidase inhibitors on the level of 5-hydroxyindoleacetic acid in human cerebrospinal fluid. Life Sci. No 1, 1—4 (1963).

Rosenberg, J. C., R. C. Lillehei, W. H. Moran and B. Zimmermann: Effect of endotoxin on plasma catechol amines and serum serotonin. Proc. Soc. exp. Biol. (N.Y.) **102**, 335—337 (1960).

Ryall, R. W.: Sub-cellular distribution of pharmacologically active substances in guinea-pig brain. Nature (Lond.) **196**, 680—681 (1962).

— The subcellular distributions of acetylcholine, substance P, 5-hydroxytryptamine, γ-aminobutyric acid and glutamic acid in brain homogenates. J. Neurochem. **11**, 131—145 (1964).

Sanders, R., T. P. Waalkes, J. W. Gilbert jr. and L. L. Terry: Serotonin (5-hydroxytryptamine) and pulmonary thromboembolism. Surg. Gynec. Obstet. **109**, 455—459 (1959).

Sanner, E.: Studies on the excretion mechanism of serotonin (5-hydroxytryptamine) in the chicken kidney. Acta physiol. scand. **58**, 330—341 (1963).

—, and B. Wortman: Tubular excretion of serotonin (5-hydroxytryptamine) in the chicken. Acta physiol. scand. **55**, 319—324 (1962).

Sanyal, R. K., and G. B. West: The relationship of histamine and 5-hydroxytryptamine to anaphylactic shock in different species. J. Physiol. (Lond.) **144**, 525—531 (1958).

Saxena, P. R., K. Kishor, M. C. Pant and K. P. Bhargava: Pharmacologically active constituents of *Girardinia heterophylla*. J. Pharm. Pharmacol. **16**, 361 (1964).

Schanberg, S. M., and N. J. Giarman: Drug-induced alterations in the subcellular distribution of 5-hydroxytryptamine in rat's brain. Biochem. Pharmacol. **11**, 187—194 (1962).

— C. M. McKean and N. J. Giarman: A mechanism of the indole defect in experimental phenylketonuria. Fed. Proc. **21**, 269 (1962).

Schindler, R., M. Day and G. A. Fischer: Culture of neoplastic mast cells and their synthesis of 5-hydroxytryptamine and histamine in vitro. Cancer Res. **19**, 47—51 (1959).

Schone, H.-H., u. E. Lindner: Die Wirkung des N-[3′-Phenyl-propyl-(2′)]-1,1-dipenyl-propyl-(3)-amins auf den Stoffwechsel von Serotonin und Noradrenalin. Arzneimittel-Forsch. **10**, 583—585 (1960).

Schulz, H., H. Strobach u. E. Hiepler: Serotoninbestimmungen an Thrombocyten und an Fraktionen von Thrombocyten. Klin. Wschr. **42**, 232—236 (1964).

Schwabe, U., D. Heyl, H. J. Hildebrandt u. T. Hukuhara: Alkylphosphatvergiftung und 5-Hydroxytryptamin-Stoffwechsel des Zentralnervensystems. Naunyn-Schmiedeberg's Arch. exp. Path. Pharmak. **241**, 254—259 (1961).

Schwemmle, K., E. Schmid, F. Scheiffarth, L. Zicha u. E. Schichor: Zur Frage der gegenseitigen Beziehungen zwischen adrenocorticotropem Hormon bzw. Glucocorticoiden und dem Serotonin-Stoffwechsel. Arzneimittel-Forsch. **11**, 616—619 (1961).

Sherwood W. K.,: Experience with "BGE", a naturally occurring indole compound. J. nerv. ment. Dis. **125**, **490**—491 (1957).

Shore, P. A., and B. B. Brodie: LSD-like effects elicited by reserpine in rabbits pretreated with iproniazid. Proc. Soc. exp. Biol. (N.Y.) **94**, **433**—435 (1957).

— A. Pletscher, E. G. Tomich, R. Kuntzman and B. B. Brodie: Release of blood platelet serotonin by reserpine and lack of effect on bleeding time. J. Pharmacol. exp. Ther. **117**, 232—236 (1956).

Simon, A.: Über die Pharmakologie der gefäßverengernden Stoffe der Blutseren. I. Naunyn-Schmiedeberg's Arch. exp. Path. Pharmak. **190**, 273—279 (1938).

— Über die Pharmakologie der gefäßverengernden Stoffe der Blutseren. II. Naunyn-Schmiedeberg's Arch. exp. Path. Pharmak. **192**, 701—707 (1939).

Simon, S. E., K. D. Cairncross, D. G. Satchell, W. S. Gay and S. Edwards: The toxicity of *Octopus maculosus* Hoyle venom. Arch. int. Pharmacodyn. **149**, 318—329 (1964).

Sjoerdsma, A., J. A. Oates and L. Gillespie jr.: Quantitation of monoamineoxidase inhibition produced with various drugs in man. Proc. Soc. exp. Biol. (N.Y.) **103**, 485—487 (1960).

— — P. Zaltzman and S. Udenfriend: Identification and assay of urinary tryptamine: application as an index of monoamine oxidase inhibition in man. J. Pharmacol. exp. Ther. **126**, 217—222 (1959).

— T. P. Waalkes and H. Weissbach: Serotonin and histamine in mast cells. Science **125**, 1202—1203 (1957 L.).

— H. Weissbach, L. L. Terry and S. Udenfriend: Further observations on patients with malignant carcinoid. Amer. J. Med. **23**, 5—15 (1957 b).

— — and S. Udenfriend: A clinical, physiologic and biochemical study of patients with malignant carcinoid. Amer. J. Med. **20**, 520—532 (1956).

Skillen, R. G., C. H. Thienes, J. Cangelosi and L. Strain: Brain 5-hydroxytryptamine in ozone-exposed rats. Proc. Soc. exp. Biol. (N.Y.) **108**, 121—122 (1961).

SKILLEN, R. G., C. H. THIENES and L. STRAIN: 5-Hydroxytryptamine, 5-hydroxytryptophan decarboxylase and monoamine oxidase in hearts of normal, thyroid fed and propylthiouracil-fed male and female rats. Endocrinology **70**, 743—747 (1962).

SMITH, D. E., and Y. S. LEWIS: Preparation and effects of an anti-mast cell serum. J. exp. Med. **113**, 683—692 (1961).

SMITH, G., and A. N. SMITH: The role of serotonin in experimental pulmonary embolism. Surg. Gynec. Obstet. **101**, 691—700 (1955).

SMITH, S. E.: The pharmacological actions of 3,4-dihydroxyphenyl-α-methylalanine (α-methyldopa), an inhibitor of 5-hydroxytryptophan decarboxylase. Brit. J. Pharmacol. **15**, 319—327 (1960).

— R. S. STACEY and I. M. YOUNG: 5-Hydroxytryptamine and 5-hydroxytryptophan decarboxylase activity in the developing nervous system of rats and guinea-pigs. Biochem. Pharmacol. **8**, 32 (1961).

SNOW, P. J. D., J. E. LENHARD-JONES, G. CURZON and R. S. STACEY: Humoral effects of metastasing carcinoid tumours. Lancet **1955 II**, 1004—1009.

SOCHOR, F., and D. LAKATUA: Daily variations of 5-hydroxyindoleacetic acid urinary excretion. Fed. Proc. **23**, 437 (1964).

SOUTHERN, A. L.: Functioning metastatic bronchial carcinoid with elevated levels of serum and cerebrospinal fluid serotonin and pituitary adenoma. J. clin. Endocr. **20**, 298—305 (1960).

SPECTOR, S., R. KUNTZMAN, P. A. SHORE and B. B. BRODIE: Evidence for release of brain amines by reserpine in presence of monoamine oxidase inhibitors: implication of monoamineoxidase in norepinephrine metabolism in brain. J. Pharmacol. exp. Ther. **130**, 256—261 (1960).

SPRINCE, H., C. M. PARKER, D. JAMESON, J. T. DAWSON jr., M. KNOWLTON and F. C. DOHAN: Detection and isolation of indoleacetamide from human urine: results with schizophrenic and normal subjects. J. Lab. clin. Med. **57**, 763—770 (1961).

STACEY, R. S.: 5-Hydroxytryptamine and other pharmacologically active substances in the central nervous system. Acta physiol. neerl. **8**, 222—239 (1959).

— Uptake of 5-hydroxytryptamine by platelets. Brit. J. Pharmacol. **16**, 284—295 (1961).

—, and T. J. SULLIVAN: Effect of diet and antibiotics on intestinal 5-hydroxytryptamine. J. Physiol. (Lond.) **137**, 63—64 P (1957).

—, and I. M. YOUNG: Concentration of 5-hydroxytryptamine in the small intestine and platelets of the developing guinea pig. Biochem. Pharmacol. **13**, 129—134 (1964).

STOCK, K., u. E. O. WESTERMANN: Biogene Amine im Fettgewebe. Naunyn-Schmiedebergs Arch. exp. Path. Pharmak. **246**, 15—16 (1963).

— — Concentration of norepinephrine, serotonin, and histamine, and of amine-metabolizing enzymes in mammalian adipose tissue. Lipid Res. **4**, 297—304 (1963).

STOLK, A.: Mast cell reaction during chemical skin carcinogenesis of the lizard Lacerta agilis. Experientia (Basel) **19**, 20—21 (1963).

STROMBERG, V. L.: The isolation of bufotenine from *Piptadenia peregrina*. J. Amer. chem. Soc. **76**, 1707 (1954).

STURM jr., A., u. G. STÜTTGEN: Nachweis von 5-Hydroxytryptophan in menschlichen Mastzellen. Klin. Wschr. **40**, 199—201 (1962).

SULLIVAN, T. J.: The effect of diet on the 5-hydroxytryptamine content of the small intestine and of other organs in rats and mice. Brit. J. Pharmacol. **15**, 513—519 (1960).

— Effect of antibiotics on the 5-hydroxytryptamine content of the small intestine and other organs in rats and mice. Brit. J. Pharmacol. **16**, 90—98 (1961).

SUPEK, Z., M. JOVIĆ u. S. KECKES: Der 5-Hydroxytryptamin-Gehalt der Haut der Ratte bei experimenteller Entzündung. Arzneimittel-Forsch. **11**, 132—133 (1961).

TABACHNICK, I. A., and A. A. RUBIN: Some relationships between peripheral monoamine oxidase inhibition and brain 5-hydroxytryptamine levels in brain. Proc. Soc. exp. Biol. (N.Y.) **101**, 435—437 (1959).

TELFORD, J. M., and G. B. WEST: The effects of corticosteroids and related compounds on the histamine and 5-hydroxytryptamine content of rat tissues. Brit. J. Pharmacol. **15**, 532—539 (1960).

TODRICK, A., M. DICK and A. C. TAIT: Effect of reserpine in therapeutic dosage on excretion of 5-hydroxyindoleacetic acid. Brit. med. J. **1958 I**, 496—499.

TOH, C. C.: Release of 5-hydroxytryptamine (serotonin) and histamine from platelets by tissue extracts. J. Physiol. (Lond.) **133**, 402—411 (1956).

— Effect of temperature on the 5-hydroxytryptamine (serotonin) content of tissues. J. Physiol. (Lond.) **151**, 410—415 (1960).

TOWNE, J. C., E. FENSTER, J. O. SHERMAN and T. SCHAEFER: Estimation of serotonin and catechol amines in acetone solution. Fed. Proc. **21**, 420 (1962).

TOWSEND, E. E., J. G. KATIS and T. L. SOURKES: Effect of tryptophan deficiency in rat on liver tryptophan peroxidase-oxidase (TPO) and urinary 5-hydroxy-3-indoleacetic acid (HIAA). Fed. Proc. **17**, 324 (1958).

TURNER, W. J., and E. A. MAUSS: Serotonin (5-hydroxytryptamine) and acetylcholine in human ventricular and spinal fluids. Arch. gen. Psychiat. **1**, 646—650 (1959).

TWAROG, B. M.: Response of a molluscan smooth muscle to acetylcholine and to 5-hydroxytryptamine. J. cell. comp. Physiol. **44**, 141—164 (1954).

—, and I. H. PAGE: Serotonin content of some mammalian tissues and urine. Amer. J. Physiol. **175**, 157—161 (1953).

TYCE, G. M., E. V. FLOCK and CH. A. OWEN: 5-Hydroxindoles in the rat after hepatectomy. Fed. Proc. **22**, 632 (1963).

— G. H. C. STOBIE, E. V. FLOCK and J. L. BOLLMAN: 5-Hydroxytryptamine content of the brain after hepatectomy. Fed. Proc. **21**, 301 (1962).

— — — — 5-Hydroxytryptamine in the gastrointestinal tract after intestinal obstruction and hepatectomy. Proc. Soc. exp. Biol. (N.Y.) **115**, 1068—1072 (1964).

TYLER jr., V. E.: Occurrence of serotonin in a hallucinogenic mushroom. Science **128**, 718 (1958).

—, and D. GROGER: Occurrence of 5-hydroxytryptamine and 5-hydroxytryptophan in *Panaeolus sphinctrinus*. J. pharm. Sci. **53**, 462 (1964).

UDENFRIEND, S., W. LOVENBERG and A. SJOERDSMA: Physiologically active amines in common fruits and vegetables. Arch. Biochem. Biophys. **85**, 487—490 (1959).

— E. TITUS and H. WEISSBACH: The identification of 5-hydroxy-3-indoleacetic acid in normal urine and a method for its assay. J. biol. Chem. **216**, 499—505 (1955).

— H. WEISSBACH and D. F. BOGDANSKI: Biochemical findings relating to the action of serotonin. Ann. N.Y. Acad. Sci. **66** (3), 602—608 (1957).

— B. WITKOP, B. G. REDFIELD and H. WEISSBACH: Studies with reversible inhibitors of monoamine oxidase: harmaline and related compounds. Biochem. Pharmacol. **1**, 160—165 (1958).

UTLEY, J. D.: Gamma aminobutyric acid and 5-hydroxytryptamine concentrations in neurons and glial cells in the medial geniculate body of the cat. Biochem. Pharmacol. **12**, 1228—1230 (1963).

UUSPÄÄ, V. J.: The 5-hydroxytryptamine content of the brain and some other organs of the hedgehog *(Erinaceus europaeus)* during activity and hibernation. Experientia (Basel) **19**, 156—158 (1963).

—, and V. I. UUSPÄÄ: VANE's rat fundus strip method in determination of 5-hydroxytryptamine. Ann. Acad. Sci. fenn. A, IV, **60**, 1—17 (1962).

VARAGIĆ, V., M. KRSTIĆ, S. STEPANOVIĆ and S. HAJDUKOVIĆ: The effect of γ-irradiation on the amount of 5-hydroxytryptamine in the gut and spleen in the early phase after irradiation. Experientia (Basel) **19**, 647—648 (1963).

VIALLI, M., e V. ERSPAMER: Ricerche sul secreto delle cellule enterocromaffini. IX. Intorno alla natura chimica della sostanza specifica. Boll. Soc. med.-chir. Pavia **51**, 1111—1116 (1937).

WAALKES, T. PH., and H. COBURN: The role of platelets and the release of serotonin and histamine during anaphylaxis in the rabbit. J. Allergy **30**, 394—407 (1959).

— — The role of histamine and serotonin during anaphylaxis in the mouse. J. Allergy **31**, 151—161 (1960a).

— — Serotonin, histamine, and the Arthus phenomenon. J. Allergy **31**, 181—184 (1960b).

— — and L. L. TERRY: The effect of reserpine on histamine and serotonin. J. Allergy **30**, 408—414 (1959).

— A. SJOERDSMA, C. R. CREVELING, H. WEISSBACH and S. UDENFRIEND: Serotonin, norepinephrine and related compounds in bananas. Science **127**, 648—650 (1958).

WALASZEK, E. J. and L. G. ABOOD: Fixation of 5-hydroxytryptamine by brain mitochondria. Proc. Soc. exp. Biol. (N.Y.) **101**, 37—40 (1959).

WANG, H. L., V. H. HARWALKER and H. A. WAISMAN: Effect of dietary phenylalanine and triptophan on brain serotonin. Arch. Biochem. Biophys. **96**, 181—184 (1962).

— — —: Influence of dietary phenylalanine and tryptophan on tissue serotonin. Fed. Proc. **20**, 6 (1961).

WEISSBACH, H., T. PH. WAALKES and S. UDENFRIEND: Presence of serotonin in lung and its implication in the anaphylactic reaction. Science **125**, 235—236 (1957).

— — — A simplified method for measuring serotonin in tissues; simultaneous assay of both serotonin and histamine. J. biol. Chem. **230**, 865—871 (1958).

WEISSMAN, A., and K. F. FINGER: Effects of benzquinamide on avoidance behavior and brain amine levels. Biochem. Pharmacol. **11**, 871—880 (1962).

WELSH, J. H.: Neurohormones of invertebrates. I. Cardio-regulators of *Cyprina* and *Buccinum*. J. Mar. biol. Ass. U. Kingd. **35**, 193—201 (1956).

Welsh, J. H.: Serotonin as a possible neurohumoral agent: evidence obtained in lower animals. Ann. N.Y. Acad. Sci. **66** (3), 618—630 (1957).
— Evidence for 5-HT granules in molluscan ganglia. Anat. Rec. **132**, 516 (1958).
— 5-Hydroxytryptamine in coelenterates. Nature (Lond.) **186**, 811—812 (1960).
— The quantitative distribution of 5-hydroxytryptamine in the nervous system, eyes and other organs of some vertebrates. In: D. Richter Ed., Comparative Neurochemistry, pp. 355—366. Oxford: Pergamon Press 1964.
—, and C. S. Batty: 5-Hydroxytryptamine content of some arthropod venoms and venom-containing parts. Toxicon **1**, 165—173 (1963).
—, and M. Moorhead: Identification and assay of 5-hydroxytryptamine in molluscan tissues by fluorescence method. Science **129**, 1491—1492 (1959).
— — The quantitative distribution of 5-hydroxytryptamine in the invertebrates, especially in their nervous system. J. Neurochem. **6**, 146—169 (1960).
West, G. B.: Tryptamines in edible fruits. J. Pharm. Pharmacol. **10**, 589—590 (1958a).
— Comparison of the release of histamine and 5-hydroxytryptamine from tissues of the rat, mouse and hamster. Int. Arch. Allergy **13**, 336—347 (1958b).
— Tryptamine in tomatoes. J. Pharm. Pharmacol. **11**, 319—320 (1959a).
— Indole derivatives in tomatoes. J. Pharm. Pharmacol. **11**, 275—277 T (1959b).
— Carcinoid tumours and pineapples. J. Pharm. Pharmacol. **12**, 768 (1960).
White, E. P.: Alkaloids of the leguminosae. VIII—XIII. N. Z. J. Sci. Technol., Sect. B **25**, 137—162 (1944).
Whittaker, V. P.: The isolation and characterization of acetylcholine-containing particles from brain. Biochem. J. **72**, 694—706 (1959).
— The subcellular localization of transmitter substances in the central nervous system. Biochem. Pharmacol. **5**, 392—398 (1961).
— Sub-cellular distribution of 5-hydroxytryptamine in guinea pig brain. Nature (Lond.) **195**, 1100 (1962).
Wiegand, R. G., and J. E. Perry: Effect of L-Dopa and N-methyl-N-benzyl-2-propynylamine. HCl on dopa, dopamine, norepinephrine, epinephrine and serotonin levels in mouse brain. Biochem. Pharmacol. **7**, 181—186 (1961).
—, and E. Scherfling: Determination of 5-hydroxytryptophan and serotonin. J. Neurochem. **9**, 113—114 (1962).
Wieland, Th., u. W. Motzel: Über das Vorkommen von Bufotenin im gelben Knollenblätterpilz. Justus Liebigs Ann. Chem. **581**, 10—16 (1953).
Wier, J. K., and V. E. Tyler jr.: Quantitative determination of serotonin in Panaeolus species. J. pharm. Sci. **52**, 419—422 (1963).
Wilkinson, S.: 5-Methoxy-N-methyltryptamine: a new indole alkaloid from *Phalaris arundinacea* L. J. chem. Soc. **2**, 2079—2081 (1958).
Wurtman, R. J., J. Axelrod and J. E. Fischer: Melatonin synthesis in the pineal gland: effect of light mediated by the sympathetic nervous system. Science **143**, 1328—1330 (1964).
Yeh, S. D. J., J. D. Solomon and B. F. Chow: Influence of vitamin B 6 on tissue serotonin levels in rats. Fed. Proc. **18**, 357 (1959).
Yurashevskii, M. K.: Alkaloids of *Girgensohnia diptera*, family Chenopodiaceae. J. gen. Chem. (U.S.S.R.) **10**, 1781—1783 (1940).
Yuwiller, A., and R. T. Louttit: Effects of phenylalanine diet on brain serotonin in the rat. Science **134**, 831—832 (1961).
Zarafonetis, C. J. D., and J. P. Kalas: Serotonin, catecholamines and amine oxidase activity in the venom of certain reptiles. Amer. J. med. Sci. **240**, 764—768 (1960).
Zbinden, G., A. Pletscher u. A. Studer: Alimentäre Beeinflussung der enterochromaffinen Zellen und des 5-Hydroxytryptamin-Gehaltes von Gehirn und Darm. Z. ges. exp. Med. **129**, 615—620 (1958).
Zieher, L. M., and E. de Robertis: Subcellular localization of 5-hydroxytryptamine in rat brain. Biochem. Pharmacol. **12**, 596—598 (1963).
Zucker, M. B., B. K. Friedman and M. M. Rapport: Identification and quantitative determination of serotonin (5-hydroxytryptamine) in blood platelets. Proc. Soc. exp. Biol. (N.Y.) **85**, 282—285 (1954).
— L. Hellman and B. Zumoff: Rapid disappearance of C^{14}-labeled serotonin from platelets in patients with carcinoid syndrome. J. Lab. clin. Med. **63**, 137—146 (1964).
—, and M. M. Rapport: Identification and quantitative determination of serotonin (5-hydroxytryptamine) in platelets, the source of serum serotonin. Fed. Proc. **13**, 170—171 (1954).

Chapter 5

Biosynthesis of indolealkylamines. Physiological release and transport of 5-hydroxytryptamine

By

PAUL B. HAGEN and LEONARD H. COHEN

With 3 Figures

I. Introduction

During the past fifty years research on pharmacologically active bases normally present in mammalian tissues has provided considerable insight into the metabolism and physiological functions of acetylcholine, noradrenaline and adrenaline in peripheral nervous tissue and into the role of histamine in hypersensitivity. When, about ten years ago, attention was drawn to the presence in animal tissues of comparable amounts of yet another chemically related base, 5-hydroxytryptamine (RAPPORT 1948; RAND and REID 1951; ERSPAMER and ASERO 1952), which also had pharmacological activity, it was natural that interest should develop in its biosynthesis and metabolism. It is probable that work on the biochemistry of indolealkylamines was considerably stimulated by the expectation that 5-hydroxytryptamine might be particularly important in mental activity and might, in fact, function as a chemical transmitter in the central nervous system much as acetylcholine or noradrenaline were known to function in neuromuscular and autonomic nervous transmission. This suggestion was based, firstly, on the presence in the central nervous system of trace amounts of 5-hydroxytryptamine (AMIN, CRAWFORD and GADDUM 1954) and on the ability of several compounds which are structurally related to 5-hydroxytryptamine, and which block its effect on smooth muscle (GADDUM 1953b), to influence mental activity (STOLL 1947; GADDUM 1953a and 1953b; WOOLLEY and SHAW 1954) and, secondly, on the ability of tranquilizing drugs to reduce the amounts of this newly discovered amine in cerebral tissue (PLETSCHER, SHORE and BRODIE 1956). It was thought that knowledge of the biochemistry of 5-hydroxytryptamine might facilitate the development of compounds which could inhibit its synthesis or destruction, or which could mimic or block its pharmacological actions or its physiological activity, whatever that might turn out to be.

Probably the first report of the ability of mammalian tissue extracts to catalyze the synthesis of an indolealkylamine was that of WERLE and MENNICKEN (1937). They reported the formation of tryptamine when tryptophan was incubated with an extract of guinea pig kidney, and identified the tryptamine by its pressor effect. Although this report has recently been confirmed with the more sensitive chemical techniques now available (HESS, REDFIELD and UDENFRIEND 1959; LOVENBERG, WEISSBACH and UDENFRIEND 1962), their claim for the presence of tryptophan decarboxylase in mammalian tissue did not gain general acceptance for some time because the amount of tryptamine formed on prolonged incubation was very small, and, although precautions had been taken, the possibility of bacterial contamination could not be altogether excluded. [The formation of tryptamine by putrefactive bacteria has been known for many years (EWINS and LAIDLAW 1910).] Moreover, attempts to demonstrate the decarboxylation of tryptophan in mammalian preparations by manometric measurement of CO_2 production have always been unsuccessful. The low rates of decarboxylation of tryptophan served as the basis for a suggestion by BLASCHKO (1952) that the natural substrate for this reaction might be 5-hydroxytryptophan. "The occurrence of 5-hydroxytryptamine raises the question: how is it formed? The very weak action on tryptophan of the decarboxylase described by WERLE and MENNICKEN might be explained if the natural substrate of this enzyme in the body were not tryptophan but 5-hydroxytryptophan." (BLASCHKO 1952). Presumably the hydroxytryptophan would be formed by the hydroxylation of tryptophan.

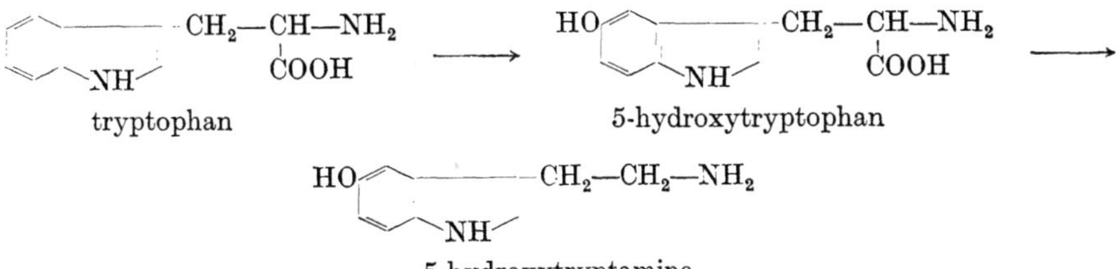

This suggestion received strong support from the discovery by UDENFRIEND, CLARK and TITUS (1953) of an enzyme in mammalian kidney which could decarboxylate synthetic 5-hydroxytryptophan and from their report that the enzyme had no activity on tryptophan, or 7-hydroxytryptophan (CLARK, WEISSBACH and UDENFRIEND 1954). Moreover, there has never been convincing evidence for the hydroxylation of tryptamine in the 5 position (UDENFRIEND, CREVELING, POSNER, REDFIELD, DALY and WITKOP 1959). The validity of the pathway shown above has since been well established. It is interesting that the discovery fourteen years previously of an enzyme that could effect the decarboxylation of another amino acid, dihydroxyphenylalanine (HOLTZ, HEISE and LUDTKE 1938) had likewise led to the proposal of a pathway for adrenaline biosynthesis (BLASCHKO 1939) which was also subsequently confirmed (DEMIS, BLASCHKO and WELCH 1956; HAGEN 1956).

Further evidence that 5-hydroxytryptophan is an intermediate in the synthesis of 5-hydroxytryptamine is the observation that animals given isotopically labelled tryptophan or 5-hydroxytryptophan can convert them to 5-hydroxytryptamine (UDENFRIEND and WEISSBACH 1958). Moreover, the administration of 5-hydroxytryptophan to animals produced an increase in the amounts of 5-hydroxytryptamine in brain and platelets, the appearance of 5-hydroxytryptamine in organs in which it is not normally detected and an increase in the urinary excretion of 5-hydroxyindoleacetic acid (UDENFRIEND, WEISSBACH and BOGDANSKI 1957), a metabolic product of 5-hydroxytryptamine (BLASCHKO 1952; ERSPAMER 1955; TITUS and UDENFRIEND 1954).

It has recently been convincingly demonstrated that 5-hydroxytryptophan decarboxylase and dopa decarboxylase are one and the same enzyme. It has also been possible to demonstrate the conversion of tryptophan to 5-hydroxytryptophan by phenylalanine hydroxylase of mammalian liver (FREEDLAND, WADZINSKI and WAISMAN 1961; RENSON, WEISSBACH and UDENFRIEND 1962). However, there is reason to believe that phenylalanine hydroxylase is of minor importance in this reaction and that the hydroxylation of tryptophan in mammals is probably effected by a different enzyme. The presence of a different tryptophan hydroxylating system has been reported in alimentary mucous membrane (COOPER and MELCER 1961), which may be of importance in the synthesis of most of the body 5-hydroxytryptamine. Unfortunately, the existence of this enzyme has been questioned (RENSON, WEISSBACH and UDENFRIEND 1962) and further experimental work will be necessary to settle its status.

II. The hydroxylation of tryptophan

Despite considerable effort, attempts to demonstrate either the presence of 5-hydroxytryptophan or the hydroxylation of tryptophan in mammalian tissues were for some time not very successful (DALGLIESH and DUTTON 1957a and 1957b). However, evidence for the hydroxylation of tryptophan in nature was provided by UDENFRIEND and his colleagues. They observed the formation of 5-hydroxytryptophan from tryptophan in the venom gland of the toad, *Bufo marinus*, a tissue rich in 5-hydroxyindole compounds (UDENFRIEND, CLARK and TITUS 1952). They fed L-tryptophan-2-C^{14} to toads for five days and were able to isolate from the venom glands a radioactive derivative of 5-hydroxytryptophan (UDENFRIEND, TITUS, WEISSBACH and PETERSON 1956). They also observed the direct conversion of tryptophan to 5-hydroxytryptophan by *Chromobacterium violaceum*, an organism in which conversion to 5-hydroxytryptophan is apparently one of the major metabolic pathways of tryptophan (MITOMA, WEISSBACH and UDENFRIEND 1956). In 1956 for the first time 5-hydroxytryptophan was provisionally identified in urine of a patient with an argentaffinoma (DALGLIESH 1956), a neoplasm of enterochromaffin tissue. The state of our knowledge of the hydroxylation reaction in 1958 was well summarized by UDENFRIEND: "Although conversion of tryptophan to HT [5-hydroxytryptamine] and 5-hydroxyindoleacetic acid (5-HIAA) has been shown in mammalian tissues, 5-HTP [5-hydroxytryptophan] formation has not yet been demonstrated. In fact, it was only recently that this amino acid was detected in mammalian material (DALGLIESH 1956). Tryptophan is not converted to 5-HTP by any of the known aromatic hydroxylating systems, phenylalanine hydroxylase, kynurenine hydroxylase or aniline hydroxylase. Attempts to demonstrate tryptophan hydroxylation in various isolated organ tissues have thus far been unsuccessful." Within the past few years 5-hydroxytryptophan has been isolated from the urine of several patients with metastasizing argentaffinomas. Although patients with this condition have much larger amounts of 5-hydroxytryptamine in their blood and urine than normal persons (SJOERDSMA and UDENFRIEND 1955; WALDENSTROM, PERNOW and SILWER 1956) they usually do not excrete 5-hydroxytryptophan (SMITH, NYHUS, DALGLIESH, DUTTON, LENNOX and MACFARLANE 1957). In one study of seven cases of argentaffinoma, 5-hydroxytryptophan was found in the urine of one patient (SMITH, NYHUS, DALGLIESH, DUTTON, LENNOX and MACFARLANE 1957). In a later study two more argentaffinoma patients were found to have 5-hydroxytryptophan in their urine. When they were given C^{14}-labelled tryptophan by mouth, C^{14}-labelled 5-hydroxytryptophan was recovered in the urine (DONALDSON, GRAY and LETSOU 1959). Thus by 1959 it seemed clear that tryptophan could be converted to 5-hydroxytryptophan in mammalian tissue. However, two important questions remained unanswered. In what organ or organs was the hydroxylation effected and by what kind of enzyme?

Within the past few years a number of remarkable and still unexplained observations have been reported, which may or may not be related to the synthesis of 5-hydroxytryptophan but which none the less have influenced research on the enzymic hydroxylation of tryptophan. The first of these was the report by PARE, SANDLER and STACEY (1957) that the urinary excretion of 5-hydroxyindoleacetic acid and the serum content of 5-hydroxytryptamine are much reduced in the congenital disease phenylketonuria (PARE, SANDLER and STACEY 1957, 1958, 1959). This observation suggested that in this disease the increased concentration of phenylalanine in the body fluids might competitively inhibit the hydroxylation of tryptophan. This concept was supported by the observation (BERENDES, ANDERSON, ZIEGLER and RUTTENBERG 1958; BALDRIDGE, BOROFSKY, BAIRD, REICHLE and BULLOCK 1959) that treatment of phenylketonuria by reduction of the intake of phenylalanine in the diet could restore the urinary excretion of 5-hydroxyindoleacetic acid to normal values. As the basic biochemical defect in phenylketonuria is considered to be a lack of the enzyme phenylalanine hydroxylase (JERVIS 1953), these observations make it seem most unlikely that this enzyme could be involved in the hydroxylation of tryptophan. Nevertheless it was these experiments on phenylketonuria which led to the demonstration that phenylalanine hydroxylase can to a limited extent catalyze the conversion of tryptophan to 5-hydroxytryptophan. In 1960 FREEDLAND, KRAKOWSKI and WAISMAN made the surprising discovery that the phenylalanine hydroxylase activity of rat liver could be decreased by feeding excess phenylalanine or increased by feeding excess tryptophan or tyrosine. The brain 5-hydroxytryptamine content was also decreased by the feeding of supplementary phenylalanine (YUWILER and LOUTTIT 1961). These observations suggested that phenylalanine hydroxylase was involved in the synthesis of 5-hydroxytryptamine. FREEDLAND, WADZINSKI and WAISMAN (1961) then demonstrated a small but definite hydroxylation of tryptophan by an enzyme system in rat liver. UDENFRIEND and his colleagues (RENSON, GOODWIN, WEISSBACH and UDENFRIEND 1961) confirmed this observation. They found the enzyme activity in the 78,000 $\times$ g supernatant fraction of rat liver and showed that the hydroxylation required two enzymes which were similar to the two enzymes of the previously described phenylalanine hydroxylating system (UDENFRIEND, WEISSBACH and CLARK 1955; MITOMA 1956; KAUFMAN 1959; KAUFMAN and LOVENBERG 1959) and that, as in the case of the hydroxylation of phenylalanine, a pteridine coenzyme was required. One enzyme effects the hydroxylation while the other enzyme keeps the coenzyme in an active form (KAUFMAN 1959). By analogy with the reactions involved in the hydroxylation of phenylalanine, the hydroxylation of tryptophan by this system can probably be represented as follows:

$$\text{tetrahydropteridine} + \text{tryptophan} + O_2 \rightarrow \text{5-HTP} + \text{dihydropteridine}$$
$$\text{dihydropteridine} + \text{TPNH} + H^+ \rightarrow \text{tetrahydropteridine} + \text{TPN}^+$$

Evidence that the same enzyme is involved in the hydroxylation of both amino acids was afforded by the demonstration of competition between L-phenylalanine and L-tryptophan for the enzyme system, in that L-phenylalanine competitively inhibited the hydroxylation of L-tryptophan, and by the observation that the relative rates of hydroxylation of both phenylalanine and tryptophan remained constant throughout different stages of the enzyme purification procedure. Tryptophan was hydroxylated at one-thirtieth the rate of phenylalanine. The enzyme had a much higher Michaelis constant (K_M) for tryptophan than for phenylalanine. The K_M for tryptophan was 3×10^{-3} M (RENSON, GOODWIN, WEISSBACH and UDENFRIEND 1961) or 6.8×10^{-3} M (RENSON, WEISSBACH and UDENFRIEND 1962), the K_M for phenylalanine was 1×10^{-5} M (RENSON, GOODWIN, WEISSBACH and UDENFRIEND 1961) or 2×10^{-6} M (MITOMA 1956).

There can be little doubt that phenylalanine hydroxylase can catalyze the hydroxylation of tryptophan. However, there are several reasons why it is unlikely that this enzyme plays more than a minor role, if any, in the conversion of tryptophan to 5-hydroxytryptophan in the body.

Firstly, phenylalanine hydroxylase is not found in any other organs than the liver (UDENFRIEND and COOPER 1952), whereas almost all the body 5-hydroxytryptamine is synthesized in the enterochromaffin tissue of the alimentary mucous membrane (ERSPAMER and TESTINI 1959). Available evidence indicates that this tissue synthesizes its 5-hydroxytryptamine from 5-hydroxytryptophan it has made itself. It is unlikely that the 5-hydroxytryptophan reaches it from the liver since careful experiments have failed to detect any release of 5-hydroxytryptophan from the liver into the circulation (DALGLIESH and DUTTON 1957a and 1957b) and observations by SANDLER and SNOW (1958) and OATES and SJOERDSMA (1962,) indicate that certain types of metastatic argentaffinoma, neoplastic enterochromaffin tissue, actually secrete 5-hydroxytryptophan into the circulation. Were this 5-hydroxytryptophan originally derived from liver, at least the same amount would also have to be secreted into the circulation by the liver. Moreover, were 5-hydroxytryptophan formed in the liver and distributed throughout the body in the circulation, 5-hydroxytryptamine might be formed in any tissue which contains dopa decarboxylase (5-hydroxytryptophan decarboxylase). As already mentioned the injection into animals of 5-hydroxytryptophan has led to the appearance of 5-hydroxytryptamine in tissues in which it is not normally found (UDENFRIEND, WEISSBACH and BOGDANSKI 1957), even including the chromaffin granules of adrenal medulla (BERTLER, ROSENGREN and ROSENGREN 1960). If 5-hydroxytryptophan were secreted by the liver one would expect to find 5-hydroxytryptamine normally in these tissues.

Secondly, it has been shown (RENSON, WEISSBACH and UDENFRIEND 1962) that, although the feeding of large amounts of phenylalanine to rats can reduce the amount of 5-hydroxytryptamine in the brain to about half its original level within two hours, the amount of 5-hydroxytryptamine in the gut or the excretion of 5-hydroxyindoleacetic acid in the urine are not reduced. Thus, even under conditions where the liver phenylalanine hydroxylase activity would be expected to be considerably reduced (FREEDLAND, KRAKOWSKI and WAISMAN 1960), 5-hydroxyindoleacetic acid excretion, indicative of 5-hydroxytryptamine and therefore of 5-hydroxytryptophan synthesis, remained unchanged.

Finally, the lack of phenylalanine hydroxylase in phenylketonuria (JERVIS 1953) strongly suggests that in this condition the hydroxylation of tryptophan must be effected by a different enzyme and that the increase in the urinary 5-hydroxyindoleacetic acid which follows the reduction in the dietary phenylalanine (BERENDES, ANDERSON, ZIEGLER and RUTTENBERG 1958; BALDRIDGE, BOROFSKY, BAIRD, REICHLE and BULLOCK 1959) must be due to an effect on some enzyme other than phenylalanine hydroxylase. On the other hand it is possible that the genetic lesion in phenylketonuria may not be an actual lack of the phenylalanine hydroxylase as is generally accepted, but perhaps rather a modification of the structure of the enzyme such that its affinity for phenylalanine is greatly reduced while its affinity for tryptophan remains unchanged. This type of modification of an enzyme has been described in mutations in Neurospora (DEMOSS and BONNER 1959).

An entirely different enzyme system which can catalyze the hydroxylation of tryptophan has recently been reported (COOPER and MELCER 1961). It is located in a particulate fraction obtained from rat intestinal mucous membrane. This system requires ascorbic acid and cupric ions but does not require oxygen or a pyridine nucleotide coenzyme. Presumably the enzyme is in the enterochromaffin cells of the intestine. Unfortunately, RENSON, WEISSBACH and UDENFRIEND (1962) claim that they are unable to demonstrate a hydroxylation of tryptophan in this system. This is an important discrepancy and further information on this system will be eagerly awaited. It is possible that more light might be thrown on the hydroxylation of tryptophan by the identification of the enzyme which carries out the reaction in mouse mastocytoma, a tissue which can effect the net synthesis of 5-hydroxytryptophan from tryptophan in tissue culture (SCHINDLER 1958; SCHINDLER, DAY and FISCHER 1959). It would be interesting to know whether mouse mastocytoma tissue possesses a phenylalanine hydroxylase.

Despite attempts to demonstrate it, there is at present no evidence for the hydroxylation of tryptophan at other than the 5 position in mammalian tissues. However, in view of the difficulties in demonstrating the hydroxylation at the 5 position, the possibility of hydroxylation at other positions should not be altogether dismissed at the present time, especially since certain fungi *(Psilocybe)* are known to synthesize a 4 hydroxylated indolealkylamine (HOFMANN 1960). Tryptamine, on the other hand, can be hydroxylated at the 6 position by a microsomal preparation from rat or rabbit liver (JEPSON, UDENFRIEND and ZALTMAN 1959; UDENFRIEND, CREVELING, POSNER, REDFIELD, DALY and WITKOP 1959). An earlier report suggesting that liver extracts convert tryptamine to the 5 and 7 hydroxylated derivatives (ICHIHARA, SAKAMOTO, INAMORI and SAKAMOTO 1957) is now believed to have been incorrect (JEPSON, ZALTZMAN and UDENFRIEND 1962). The significance of this hydroxylation reaction is unknown. However, the very limited formation of tryptamine in the body makes unlikely any extensive synthesis of hydroxylated tryptamines from tryptamine.

III. The decarboxylation of 5-hydroxytryptophan

In contrast to the lack of precise information about the enzymic hydroxylation of tryptophan, a vast amount of information is available concerning the decarboxylation of 5-hydroxytryptophan. About ten years ago the discovery of 5-hydroxytryptophan decarboxylase (UDENFRIEND, CLARK and TITUS 1953) made highly probable the steps of the presently accepted pathway for the synthesis of 5-hydroxytryptamine from tryptophan. Soon after its discovery the enzyme was greatly purified by fractional ammonium sulfate precipitation and adsorption on silica gel (CLARK, WEISSBACH and UDENFRIEND 1954). Over the last eight years cogent evidence has accumulated that this enzyme is identical with the enzyme dopa decarboxylase which was first found in guinea pig kidney by HOLTZ, HEISE and LÜDTKE in 1938 and subsequently extensively studied by BLASCHKO (1950a and 1950b) and his coworkers, and which catalyses an important step in the biosynthesis of adrenaline and noradrenaline (BLASCHKO 1939; HAGEN and WELCH 1956; DEMIS, BLASCHKO and WELCH 1956).

1. The identity of 5-hydroxytryptophan decarboxylase with dopa decarboxylase

In 1956 LANGEMANN and KÄGI drew attention to the occurrence of both enzyme activities together in a carcinoid tumor, and used the unspecific term "amino acid decarboxylase" to describe the enzyme. Both activities were also found together in mouse mastocytoma (HAGEN and LEE 1958) and in brain and other tissues (WESTERMANN, BALZER and KNELL 1958). In a survey of several tissues WESTERMANN, BALZER and KNELL found 5-hydroxytryptophan decarboxylase activity confined to tissues possessing dopa decarboxylase activity. Homogenates and partially purified preparations of the enzyme decarboxylate both L-5-hydroxytryptophan and L-Dopa (WESTERMANN, BALZER and KNELL 1958; FELLMAN 1959; WERLE and AURES 1959; YUWILER, GELLER and EIDUSON 1959; ROSENGREN 1960; UDENFRIEND, LOVENBERG and WEISSBACH 1960; KUNTZMAN, SHORE, BOGDANSKI and BRODIE 1961; HAGEN 1962; LOVENBERG, WEISSBACH and UDENFRIEND 1962). LOVENBERG, WEISSBACH and UDENFRIEND (1962) found that the ratio of the rates of decarboxylation of 5-hydroxytryptophan and dopa remained constant throughout the different stages of preparation of the enzyme up to 50 or 100 fold purification.

Further evidence for the identity of the dopa and 5-hydroxytryptophan decarboxylating enzymes was obtained by competition experiments in which dopa and 5-hydroxytryptophan were incubated together or separately with preparations of the enzyme, and the rate of decarboxylation with both substrates

Table 1. *Comparison of the distribution of 5-hydroxytryptophan decarboxylase activity throughout different tissues in several mammals with the amounts of 5-hydroxytryptamine naturally present.* (Modified from GADDUM and GIARMAN 1956)

5-hydroxytryptamine (μg/g tissue) naturally present and formed from added substrate (4×10^{-4} M).

[No. of observations in parentheses. G and E indicate data of GARVIN (1956) and ERSPAMER (1954) respectively.]

Tissue	Formed				Naturally present			
	Guinea-pig	Rat	Rabbit	Man	Guinea-pig	Rat	Rabbit	Man
Kidney	200 (9)	120 (3)	45 (3)	—	—	—	0.03 G	—
Liver	25 (3)	20	15	—	—	—	0.4 G	—
Stomach	33 (4)	—	—	—	1.40 E	1.40 E	4.9 E	3.35 E
Spleen	3.3	1.02	4.65	—	1.06 E	2.8 E	19.6 E	0.83 E
Serum	—	—	—	—	0.21 E	0.55 E	3.53 E	0.12 E
Plasma with platelets	0	—	0	0	—	—	—	—
Bone marrow	0	—	0.65	—	—	—	0.33 G	—

Guinea-pig tissue	Formed	Naturally present (ERSPAMER)
Stomach, whole	33.0	1.4
Stomach, fundus	88.8	—
Stomach, body	50.3	—
Stomach, pylorus	112.5	—
Duodenum	127.5	5.0
Ileum	88.4	3.4
Caecum	110.0	—
Colon	15.0	0.7

Neural tissue	Formed			Naturally present		
	Dog	Ox	Hog	Dog	Ox	Hog
Sympathetic ganglia*	16.6	44.7	—	0	0	—
Peduncles	—	6.7	—	0	—	—
Pons	—	2.6	—	—	—	—
Medulla (whole)	4.7	2.6	—	0.03	—	—
Caudate nucleus	—	0.6	12.7	0.12	0.2	0.32
Hypothalamus	—	0.45	1.72	0.37	—	—
Floor 4th ventricle	—	—	1.5	0.1	—	—
Cerebellar cortex	0	—	—	0.01	—	—
Motor and premotor areas	0	—	—	0.02	—	—
Area postrema	—	0	0	0.21	—	—

* Combined stellate and superior cervical ganglia of dogs; stellate ganglia only of oxen.

together was found to be intermediate between the rates of reaction with either substrate alone (BERTLER and ROSENGREN 1959; FELLMAN 1959; WERLE and AURES 1959; YUWILER, GELLER and EIDUSON 1959; HAGEN 1962). Moreover, α-methyl dopa, a competitive inhibitor of dopa decarboxylation (SOURKES 1954), also blocks the decarboxylation of 5-hydroxytryptophan by tissue extracts (WESTERMANN, BALZER and KNELL 1958).

2. Distribution of 5-hydroxytryptophan decarboxylase (dopa decarboxylase) within the body

Although considerable information had been obtained about dopa decarboxylase long before it was known to act on 5-hydroxytryptophan, the first systematic

Table 2. *Activities of DOPA and 5-hydroxytryptophan decarboxylase and levels of noradrenaline and 5-hydroxytryptamine in various regions of cat brain.* (From KUNTZMAN, SHORE, BOGDANSKI and BRODIE 1961)

Area	Concentration (μg/g)		Decarboxylase activity*	
	NE	5-HT	DOPA	5-HTP
Anterior hypothalamus	3.6	2.4	750	185
Posterior hypothalamus	2.0	2.5	896	175
Septum	1.5	2.0	420	—
Midbrain reticular formation	1.4	2.6	810	85
Central grey matter	1.2	1.6	519	—
Olfactory tubercle	0.95	2.0	930	264
Pontile reticular formation	0.97	0.89	383	85
Medial geniculate	0.50	—	129	30
Neocortex	0.49	0.69	39	—
Hypnogenic zone of HESS	0.45	1.8	261	45
Amygdala	0.30	1.6	291	35
Caudate nucleus	0.36	1.6	1260	300
Pyriform cortex	0.35	1.4	159	20
Auditory cortex	0.35	0.41	51	—
Cochlear nucleus	0.32	—	90	20
Inferior colliculus	0.26	0.76	201	40
Thalamus (whole)	0.17	0.43	231	50
Pons	0.25	0.33	300	40
Intralaminar and midline nuclei	0.40	0.56	400	80
Basal thalamic area	1.00	0.88	660	135
Cingulate cortex	0.35	0.41	51	—

Each value represents the mean obtained from 2—6 cats.

* Units for DOPA decarboxylase: μg dopamine formed/g per 3 hr. Units for 5-HTP decarboxylase: μg 5-HT formed/g per hr. Abbreviations above are NE, noradrenaline; 5-HT, 5-hydroxytryptamine; 5-HTP, 5-hydroxytryptophan.

study of its distribution throughout the body was made when GADDUM and GIARMAN in 1956 investigated the formation of 5-hydroxytryptamine from 5-hydroxytryptophan by extracts of various tissues. They paid particular attention to the distribution of the enzyme throughout the brain. The three tables from their paper (Table 1) indicate the distribution of 5-hydroxytryptophan decarboxylase in various organs and brain regions of several species of mammals. The amounts of 5-hydroxytryptamine present in these tissues are also shown.

They found highest activity in the kidney. Considerable activity was also found in liver and alimentary canal. There was no significant activity in platelets or bone marrow. In nervous tissue the greatest activity was found in sympathetic ganglia.

In addition to the tissues studied by these workers high dopa decarboxylase (5-hydroxytryptophan decarboxylase) activity has been found in adrenal medulla

(LANGEMANN 1951; BLASCHKO, HAGEN and WELCH 1955), pheochromocytoma (BURGER and LANGMANN 1956; HAGEN 1962), neoplastic enterochromaffin tissue (LANGEMANN 1958, HAGEN 1962) and normal and neoplastic mouse mast cell tissue (LAGUNOFF, LAM, ROEPER and BENDITT 1957; HAGEN and LEE 1958; HAGEN, WEINER, ONO and LEE 1960).

A more detailed study of the distribution of dopa decarboxylase throughout the brain of the cat was made by KUNTZMAN, SHORE, BOGDANSKI and BRODIE (1961) and is indicated in table 2.

Their results show that there is throughout brain a fairly constant relationship between dopa decarboxylase and 5-hydroxytryptophan decarboxylase activities.

Although comparisons of activities reported by different workers who studied different tissues are not altogether satisfactory it seems justifiable to conclude that very high activity is found in kidney, liver, adrenal medulla, sympathetic ganglia and intestine (presumably enterochromaffin tissue) and in the mast cells of rodents. Bone marrow, platelets and lung seem to be devoid of activity and no information is available for skeletal muscle. There does not, however, seem to be a parallel between the 5-hydroxytryptamine content of a tissue and its 5-hydroxytryptophan decarboxylase activity (PAASONEN, MACLEAN and GIARMAN 1957).

3. Intracellular distribution of 5-hydroxytryptophan decarboxylase (dopa decarboxylase)

In 1955 BLASCHKO, HAGEN and WELCH reported that in adrenal medulla the dopa decarboxylase activity was in the fluid (nonparticulate) cytoplasm. Subsequently it has been shown to be restricted to the fluid cytoplasm of mouse mastocytoma cells (HAGEN, WEINER, ONO and LEE 1960) and has been prepared in high yield from the fluid cytoplasm of ox adrenal medulla, human argentaffinoma, human pheochromocytoma (HAGEN 1962) and guinea pig kidney (LOVENBERG, WEISSBACH and UDENFRIEND 1962).

4. Pyridoxal phosphate as a coenzyme of 5-hydroxytryptophan decarboxylase (dopa decarboxylase)

In 1945 GREEN, LELOIR and NOCITO demonstrated that the addition of pyridoxal phosphate could increase the activity of dialysed dopa decarboxylase prepared from pig kidney. Subsequently a number of investigators reported low activities of dopa decarboxylase and 5-hydroxytryptophan decarboxylase in tissues from pyridoxine deficient animals (BLASCHKO, CARTER, O'BRIEN and SLOANE-STANLEY 1948; BUXTON and SINCLAIR 1956; BUZARD and NYTCH 1959; WEISSBACH, BOGDANSKI, REDFIELD and UDENFRIEND 1957). Both activities could be restored by addition of the cofactor, provided the state of deficiency were not excessively prolonged (BLASCHKO, CARTER, O'BRIEN and SLOANE-STANLEY 1948; BUZARD and NYTCH 1959). Apparently, prolonged deficiency of the coenzyme can lead to a decline in the amount of apoenzyme.

Even in the absence of vitamin deficiency an increase in decarboxylase activity on the addition of pyridoxal phosphate to homogenates of ox adrenal medulla (BLASCHKO, HAGEN and WELCH 1955), rat brain (HOLTZ and WESTERMANN 1956) and rat kidneys (BUZARD and NYTCH 1957) has been reported. Presumably the coenzyme was diluted to suboptimal concentration in the course of homogenization. However, no increase in activity has been observed on the addition of pyridoxal phosphate to homogenates of mouse brain or liver (BLASCHKO and CRUŚCIEL 1960). In the mouse tissues the pyridoxal phosphate is apparently either present in larger amounts or else is so firmly bound that dilution of the coenzyme during the homogenization has little effect.

5. Substrate specificity of 5-hydroxytryptophan decarboxylase (dopa decarboxylase)

Failure to recognize the identity of dopa decarboxylase and 5-hydroxytryptophan decarboxylase has led to a confusing situation in the literature with regard to substrate specificity. There are three main groups of studies, early studies of dopa decarboxylase with phenylalanine analogues, later studies of 5-hydroxytryptophan decarboxylase with tryptophan analogues and the more recent studies with both phenylalanine and tryptophan analogues, which have had the additional advantage of more sensitive methods of enzyme measurement. These three phases will be discussed in sequence. It will become apparent that a few of the earlier observations are at variance with more recent findings. This is probably due to differences in enzyme source, enzyme purity and methods of assay.

The early studies of BLASCHKO and his colleagues (BLASCHKO 1949; BLASCHKO and HOLTON 1950; BLASCHKO, HOLTON and SLOANE-STANLEY 1949; BLASCHKO and SLOANE-STANLEY 1948) showed that the substrate specificities of mammalian dopa decarboxylase were different from those of the bacterial enzyme (tyrosine decarboxylase) and permitted the formulation of some general rules about the substrate specificity of dopa decarboxylase (BLASCHKO 1950b). Of the various phenylalanine derivatives tested, the mammalian enzyme acted only on those possessing a hydroxyl group at either the 2 or 3 position of the ring, preferably at the 3 (meta) position. The importance of the free meta hydroxyl group was emphasized by SOURKES, HENEAGE and TRANO (1952), who showed that if it were replaced by a methoxy group the resulting compound was not a substrate. Changes in the side chain also modify activity. The early work of BLASCHKO and his colleagues established that the α-carbon must be of the L configuration and the amino group unsubstituted. In addition, the introduction of a methyl radical at the α-carbon atom converted dopa into an inhibitor of the enzyme (α-methyl dopa) (SOURKES 1954). The introduction of a hydroxyl group at the β-carbon atom of dopa made the compound (3,4 dihydroxyphenylserine) a poor substrate; of the two diasteroisomers only one was decarboxylated at a substantial rate (BLASCHKO, BURN and LANGEMANN 1950), later shown to be the threo form (HARTMAN, POGRUND, DRELL and CLARK 1955). Among tryptophan derivatives the enzyme decarboxylates 5-hydroxytryptophan (UDENFRIEND, CLARK and TITUS 1953) and 4-hydroxytryptophan (ERSPAMER, GLÄSSER, PASINI and STOPPANI 1961) at about the same rate but does not act on 7-hydroxytryptophan (UDENFRIEND, CLARK and TITUS 1953). FRETER, WEISSBACH, UDENFRIEND and WITKOP (1957) resolved the L and D isomers and showed that only the L isomer was decarboxylated *in vitro*. Until the last few years it was thought that 5-hydroxytryptophan decarboxylase could not decarboxylate tryptophan, phenylalanine or tyrosine (CLARK, WEISSBACH and UDENFRIEND 1954). However, the development of very sensitive techniques for the measurement of small amounts of the corresponding amines (see UDENFRIEND 1962) has made possible the detection of some activity towards all naturally occurring aromatic L-amino acids. The relative rates of decarboxylation of a number of aromatic L-amino acids are shown in table 3.

The finding that o-tyrosine is decarboxylated more rapidly than m-tyrosine by the guinea pig kidney enzyme does not apply to all tissues. The reverse is the case with enzymes from several sources (BLASCHKO 1949; HAGEN 1962). The rate of decarboxylation of 3,4-dihydroxyphenylserine or 3-hydroxyphenylserine was shown by WERLE and AURES (1959) to be slightly faster than the rate of decarboxylation of 5-hydroxytryptophan. In addition these workers reported competition experiments with greatly purified enzyme indicating that a single enzyme effected the decarboxylation of 5-hydroxytryptophan, dopa and the phenylserines. The table also shows tryptophan to be decarboxylated at an appreciable rate. There is evidence that tryptophan is also decarboxylated *in vivo* (HESS, REDFIELD and UDENFRIEND 1959).

Recently there has been considerable discussion as to whether histidine decarboxylase is identical with dopa decarboxylase. The existence of a separate enzyme specific for histidine has been assumed for many years and was supported by the demonstration of the decarboxylation of histidine in human urticaria pigmentosa tissue (BIRT, HAGEN and ZEBROWSKI 1961) and in rat hepatoma (MACKAY, RILEY and SHEPHERD 1961) both of which tissues lack a dopa decarboxylase. Likewise, the inability to demonstrate activity by dopa decarboxylase of ox adrenla medulla, mouse mastocytoma or human argentaffinoma tissue towards histidine, p-tyrosine, or tryptophan (HAGEN 1962) has suggested that the dopa decarboxylase from these specific amine storing tissues might be somewhat different from that of the guinea pig kidney enzyme. Recently there have been reports (GANROT, ROSENGREN and ROSENGREN 1961; WEISSBACH, LOVENBERG and UDENFRIEND 1961) that although kidney dopa (5-hydroxytryptophan) decarboxylase can decarboxylate histidine, mast cells possess a specific histidine decarboxylase which lacks dopa decarboxylase activity; 5-hydroxytryptophan and histidine do not compete with each other for the latter enzyme. On the other hand WERLE and AURES (1959) have produced evidence that histidine decarboxylase and dopa decarboxylase of guinea pig kidney are different enzymes. Only further experiments can settle this question.

Table 3. *Substrate specificity of guinea pig kidney enzyme.* (Modified from LOVENBERG, WEISSBACH and UDENFRIEND 1962)

Substrate	Relative specific activity*
Dopa	6400
o-Tyrosine	4750
m-Tyrosine	2000
5-Hydroxytryptophan	1000
Tryptophan	220**
Phenylalanine	104**
p-Tyrosine	34**
α-Methyl-dopa	32
α-Methyl-5-hydroxytryptophan	13
Histidine	10**
α-Methyltryptophan	5
α-Methyl-m-tyrosine	4
Kynurenine	1—2
5-Methyltryptophan	<0.1
6-Methyltryptophan	<0.1
5-Methoxytryptophan	<0.1

* An enzyme which had been purified from guinea pig kidney about 10-fold was used in this study.
** Estimated V_{max} from Lineweaver-Burk plots.

6. Inhibitors of 5-hydroxytryptophan decarboxylase (dopa decarboxylase)

Although a separate chapter of this volume is devoted to inhibitors of dopa decarboxylase (PLETSCHER, Chapter XII) a brief mention of some inhibitors is included here in so far as it is pertinent to the understanding of the decarboxylase reaction.

The interpretation of the effects of inhibitors may be hampered by the fact that any compounds which can prevent pyridoxal phosphate from functioning as a coenzyme in the decarboxylation reaction will inhibit the enzyme. It is interesting that several compounds which are structural analogues of the substrates and some which are themselves substrates will react with the carbonyl group of pyridoxal phosphate although they are not ordinarily considered to be carbonyl reagents. This type of inhibition can be no more specific than inhibition by carbonyl reagents such as hydrazine and semicarbazide. The first example of this type of inhibition, which at the time was unexplained, was the inhibition of histidine decarboxylase by D-dopa (WERLE 1942). Subsequently SCHOTT and CLARK (1952) showed that dopa and a number of related compounds react with pyridoxal phosphate to form a product lacking coenzyme activity. The most reactive compounds were phenylethylamines or aromatic amino acids which possessed a ring hydroxyl group at the meta position and lacked substituents on the amino group. In addition histamine seemed to be quite reactive despite the lack of a ring hydroxyl. They did not study the condensation of 5-hydroxytryptophan or 5-hydroxytryptamine with pyridoxal phosphate. However, as tryptophan did react slowly it is possible that 5-hydroxytryptophan and 5-hydroxytryptamine would condense quite readily. Several of the compounds studied were substrates of the enzyme and they showed that under certain conditions dopa inhibits dopa decarboxylase by this mechanism. It seems likely that many of the more recently studied compounds may owe part of their inhibitory action to this phenomenon. The contribution by this type of inhibition would be least when initial rates were used in the enzyme assay and would be greatest if the enzyme were preincubated with the inhibitor.

The first study of the inhibitory effects of a number of analogues of dopa was made by SOURKES (1954). Unfortunately it was not realized at the time that 5-hydroxytryptophan was decarboxylated by the same enzyme and no tryptophan derivatives were included in the study. SOURKES found that 2,3-dihydroxy-α-methyl-phenylalanine (α-methyl dopa) could cause 98% inhibition at a concentration of 5×10^{-4} M with a substrate concentration (dopa) of 2×10^{-3} M. In fact, because of lack of resolution of D and L isomers it is probable that the concentration of active inhibitor was only 2.5×10^{-4} M. Dialysis could reverse the inhibition. SOURKES demonstrated that this inhibition was not due to complexing of the pyridoxal phosphate. The importance of the meta hydroxyl group was again illustrated by the observation that methyl substitution at that site to form the 3-methoxy-4-hydroxy-α-methylphenylalanine reduced the inhibitory activity of the compound under the conditions of the study from 95% to 18%. As previously mentioned α-methyl dopa has recently been shown to be very slowly decarboxylated by the enzyme (UDENFRIEND, LOVENBERG and WEISSBACH 1960; CARLSSON and LINDQVIST 1962; LOVENBERG, WEISSBACH and UDENFRIEND 1962). α-methyl-5-hydroxytryptophan, α-methyl-meta-tyrosine, α-methyl-2,5-dopa have also recently been shown to inhibit the enzyme (MURPHY and SOURKES 1961).

Extensive studies of the inhibitory activity of a large number of phenylethylamine derivatives and other compounds were made by HARTMAN, AKAWIE and CLARK (1955) and YUWILER, GELLER and EIDUSON (1960). They found the most potent inhibitor to be 5(3,4-dihydroxycinnamoyl)salicylic acid. This inhibitor was competitive and produced 87% inhibition at a concentration onethousandth that of the substrate (dopa).

Inhibition of the decarboxylation of dopa by phenylpyruvic, phenyllactic and phenylacetic acids (FELLMAN 1956) and of the decarboxylation of 5-hydroxytryptophan by phenylacetic and phenyllactic acids (DAVISON and SANDLER 1958) has been reported. It would be interesting to know whether 5-hydroxyindoleacetic acid and dihydroxyphenylacetic acid, the products of 5-hydroxytryptamine and dopamine oxidation, are also inhibitors. If this should be the case this inhibition may represent a mechanism for feedback control of the biosynthesis of these amines.

Although many compounds have been studied which are inhibitors or substrates or both, knowledge of the factors which affect affinity as contrasted to those which influence turnover (V_{max}) is still rudimentary. Such information would be highly desirable for a better understanding of the enzyme mechanism and also in order to design compounds with greater potency and specificity. Our present information about this is limited to data concerning the K_M[1] for various substrates from the studies of SOURKES (1954) and LOVENBERG, WEISSBACH and UDENFRIEND (1962). From the data of SOURKES mentioned above it would appear that methylation of the α-carbon of dopa reduces both K_M and V_{max}

Table 4. *Effect of α-methylamino acids on decarboxylation of aromatic amino acids.* (Modified from LOVENBERG, WEISSBACH and UDENFRIEND 1962)

Substrate	Concentration of inhibitor for 50% inhibition			
	α-Methyl-DPA	α-Methyl-HTP	α-Methyl-m-tyrosine	α-Methyl-tryptophan
Dopa (10^{-3} M)	1×10^{-3}			
5-Hydroxytryptophan (1.5×10^{-3} M)	2×10^{-4}	3×10^{-4}	3×10^{-4}	$>10^{-3}$
Tryptophan (6.7×10^{-3} M)	2×10^{-6}	8×10^{-6}	1×10^{-5}	1×10^{-3}
Phenylalanine (1.6×10^{-2} M)	1×10^{-6}			

A similar effect was obtained with α-methylation of tryptophan and 5-hydroxytryptophan (LOVENBERG, WEISSBACH and UDENFRIEND 1962). This can be seen from the data shown in Tables 4 and 5.

With 1.5×10^{-3} M 5-hydroxytryptophan as substrate the concentration of α-methyl 5-hydroxytryptophan required to give 50% inhibition is only 3×10^{-4} M indicating approximately one fifth the K_M. Similarly α-methyl tryptophan inhibits the decarboxylation of tryptophan by 50% at a concentration of about one-seventh that of 5-hydroxytryptophan. Surprisingly, methyl dopa had about the same K_M as dopa in disagreement with SOURKES' report. In all cases decarboxylation of the methylated compound was considerably slower than that of the unmethylated compound. These effects are remarkably similar to those of methylation of the corresponding carbon of substrates of amine oxidase (BLASCHKO 1952).

Table 5. *K_M of various substrates for aromatic L-amino acid decarboxylase.* (Modified from LOVENBERG, WEISSBACH and UDENFRIEND 1962)

Substrate	$K_M\times10^5$	V_{max}
Dopa	40	6400
5-Hydroxytryptophan	2	1000
Tryptophan	300	220
p-Tyrosine	1300	34
Phenylalanine	2000	104
Histidine	2200	10
α-Methyl-dopa	54	32

An apparent anomaly in the data shown above can be seen in the effects of α-methyl dopa on the decarboxylation of dopa and of 5-hydroxytryptophan. One would expect that a higher concentration of inhibitor would be required to produce 50% inhibition when 5-hydroxytryptophan was the substrate than when dopa was the substrate since the K_M for 5-hydroxytryptophan is much lower. The data indicated (LOVENBERG, WEISSBACH and UDENFRIEND 1962) show the opposite.

7. Studies on 5-hydroxytryptophan decarboxylase (dopa decarboxylase) in vivo

The first deliberate *in vivo* studies on this enzyme showed that the feeding of 5-hydroxytryptophan caused an increase in the amount of 5-hydroxytryptamine in the brain and in tissues in which it cannot normally be detected (UDENFRIEND, BOGDANSKI and WEISSBACH 1956). The injection of an equivalent amount of

[1] It should be emphasized that affinity between enzyme and substrate is not the same as $1/K_M$, although it is one factor influencing K_M.

5-hydroxytryptamine did not cause this effect (UDENFRIEND, WEISSBACH and BOGDANSKI 1957). Thus it would appear that each tissue in which 5-hydroxytryptamine accumulates following the injection of 5-hydroxytryptophan contains the decarboxylase. ERSPAMER (1961) has obtained chromatographic evidence for the presence in brain not only of 5-hydroxytryptophan, but also of 4-hydroxytryptophan, 6-hydroxytryptophan and 7-hydroxytryptophan after the administration of these amino acids to animals; and SCHANBERG and GIARMAN (1960) have reported *in vitro* studies suggesting the participation of an active transport system in the uptake of 5-hydroxyryptophan by brain tissue. Clear evidence that the decarboxylation actually takes place *in situ* has been provided by PLETSCHER and GEY (1961). They found that the intraperitoneal injection of 5-hydroxytryptophan into rats shortly before death caused considerable accumulation of 5-hydroxytryptamine in brains *post mortem* and showed that decarboxylation of 5-hydroxytryptophan continues in the brain for several hours after decapitation. It is remarkable that even chromaffin granules of adrenal medulla, which normally store only dopamine and its derivatives adrenaline and noradrenaline, can accumulate 5-hydroxytryptamine following the injection of 5-hydroxytryptophan (BERTLER, ROSENGREN and ROSENGREN 1960). It is clear that the nature of the amine stored depends upon which substrate of the decarboxylase is available, which normally is determined by the nature of the hydroxylating enzyme present in the tissue. Indeed, it is possible to promote the accumulation of abnormal amines in tissues by providing substrates not normally available to them.

The injection of 4-hydroxytryptophan in rats has been shown to cause the appearance of 4-hydroxytryptamine and 4-hydroxyindoleacetic acid in the brain and other tissues (ERSPAMER, GLÄSSER, NOBILI and PASINI 1960; ERSPAMER and NOBILI 1962). This compound can also be decarboxylated in man, as evidenced by the excretion of 4-hydroxyindoleacetic acid in urine following its oral administration (ERSPAMER and NOBILI 1961). HESS, REDFIELD and UDENFRIEND (1959) observed an increase in the amount of tryptamine in tissues following the administration of tryptophan and iproniazid, the latter to prevent the destruction by amine oxidase of any tryptamine formed. The tryptamine content of brain and liver, normally less than 0.03 μg/g, was increased to 1 to 2 μg/g following the administration of iproniazid (100 mg/kg) and L-tryptophan (800 mg/kg). The possibility that this tryptamine might have been formed by bacterial tryptophan decarboxylase in the alimentary canal and absorbed when its oxidation was prevented by the inhibitor was excluded by the demonstration that the feeding of tryptamine even in large amounts after the administration of amine oxidase inhibitors did not increase the urinary excretion of tryptamine. On the other hand, the feeding of small amounts of tryptophan caused an increase in the urinary tryptamine (SJOERDSMA, OATES, ZALTZMAN and UDENFRIEND 1959). The decarboxylation of dopa (CARLSSON, LINDQVIST, MAGNUSSON and WALDECK 1958), of α-methyl dopa and of α-methyl m-tyrosine has also been demonstrated *in vivo* (CARLSSON and LINDQVIST 1962). The amounts of various amines that have been found in several tissues following the administration of the corresponding amino acids are indicated in Table 6.

An inhibition of dopa decarboxylase *in vivo* by α-methyl dopa has been suggested by the demonstration that this compound can largely prevent the pharmacological effects of injected dopa (DENGLER and REICHEL 1958) or 5-hydroxytryptophan (WESTERMAN, BALZER and KNELL 1958) and can lower the concentration of dopamine and noradrenaline in brain (MURPHY and SOURKES 1959). However, the effect on amine content may be due, in part at least, to a release of amines from the tissue (SOURKES, MURPHY, CHAVEZ and ZIELINSKA 1961).

Table 6. *Amounts of several amines found in tissues following the administration of the corresponding amino acids*

Tissue	Amino acid and mode of administration	Content of amine in μg/g wet weight of tissue		
		before	after	time
Rat brain	5-hydroxytryptophan 150 mg/kg I.P.	0.4	2.4	3 hr.
	5-hydroxytryptophan 100 mg/kg S.C.	0.25	0.56	1 hr.
	5-hydroxytryptophan 100 mg/kg I.P.	0.25	0.85	$^1/_2$ hr.
Dog brain				
hypothalamus .	5-hydroxytryptophan 60 mg/kg I.P.	1.5	13.3	$1^1/_2$ hr.
cortex	5-hydroxytryptophan 60 mg/kg I.P.	0.2	2.4	$1^1/_2$ hr.
cerebellum . . .	5-hydroxytryptophan 75 mg/kg I.V.	0.11	0.29	2 hr.
Guinea pig brain .	tryptophan 800 mg/kg oral	0.1	1.4	2 hr.
Rat brain	4-hydroxytryptophan 100 mg/kg I.P.	—	1.5	1 hr.
Dog liver.	5-hydroxytryptophan 60 mg/kg I.P.	0	6.2	$1^1/_2$ hr.
Rat liver	5-hydroxytryptophan 100 mg/kg I.P.	0	6.0	3 hr.
Rat liver	5-hydroxytryptophan 100 mg/kg I.P.	0.18	0.64	$^1/_2$ hr.
Rat uterus	5-hydroxytryptophan 100 mg/kg I.P.	0	2.5	3 hr.
Rat kidney	5-hydroxytryptophan 100 mg/kg I.P.	0.15	12	1 hr.
Rat heart	5-hydroxytryptophan 100 mg/kg I.P.	0	3.1	9 hr.

The values given in the table are from the following sources: COSTA and RINALDI (1958), ERSPAMER and NOBILI (1962), ERSPAMER and BERTACCINI (1962), UDENFRIEND, WEISSBACH and BOGDANSKI (1957). Abbreviations: I.P., intraperitoneal; I.V., intravenously; S.C., subcutanously.

Further evidence for such an action has been produced by PORTER, TOTARO and LEIBY (1961). They found that the 5-hydroxytryptamine content of brain was decreased by the administration of 3-hydroxy, 2,3-dihydroxy and 3,4-dihydroxy derivatives of DL-α-methylphenylalanine. However, a similar effect was obtained with α-methyl-metatyramine, which is not an inhibitor of the decarboxylase. Thus it is quite possible that the effects of the α-methylated amino acids on the tissue amine stores involves their prior conversion to the corresponding amines which act as releasers (CARLSSON and LINDQVIST 1962). Indeed, such amines have been found in brain after the administration of α-methyl dopa and α-methyl m-tyrosine (CARLSON and LINDQVIST 1962). The evidence also suggests that catecholamines are released to a greater extent than 5-hydroxytryptamine by these α-methyl amines. Recently, inhibition of the enzyme in brain and intestine by α-methyl dopa *in vivo* has been demonstrated by SMITH (1960). Figure 1 shows the onset of and recovery from inhibition of 5-hydroxytryptophan decarboxylase of mouse brain homogenates after pretreatment of the mice with α-methyl dopa. A similar effect of α-methyl-meta-tyrosine has been observed with other tissues (HESS, CONNAMACHER, OZAKI and UDENFRIEND 1961).

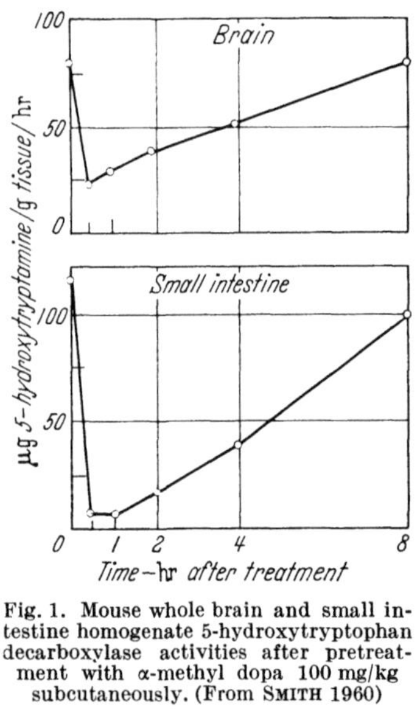

Fig. 1. Mouse whole brain and small intestine homogenate 5-hydroxytryptophan decarboxylase activities after pretreatment with α-methyl dopa 100 mg/kg subcutaneously. (From SMITH 1960)

8. Mechanism of the Decarboxylase reaction

Virtually nothing is known concerning the chemical structure of the apodecarboxylase. There is evidence that a reduced sulfhydryl group is necessary for activity.

FELLMAN (1959) found that N-ethyl maleimide and mercuric ions can inactivate the enzyme. Likewise LOVENBERG, WEISSBACH and UDENFRIEND (1962) found that the enzyme was inhibited by 10^{-5} M p-chloromercuribenzoate, but that no stimulation of activity was obtained by the addition of sulfhydryl compounds. On the other hand, BUZARD and NYTCH (1957) could find no evidence that thiol groups were necessary for activity. Further experiments will be necessary to settle this question.

From his studies on the substrate specificity of dopa decarboxylase BLASCHKO (1950a and 1950b) was able to present a rough picture of the spatial relationships of the reactive groups of the enzyme. Some extension of this picture is now possible in the light of more recent studies, especially that of LOVENBERG, WEISSBACH and UDENFRIEND (1962).

The ability of the enzyme to decarboxylate only L-isomers of amino acids indicates attachment between enzyme and substrate at three or more points. The preference of the enzyme for compounds possessing an aromatic hydroxyl group suggests that this hydroxyl group is one point of attachment. The carboxyl group and the amino group are apparently other points of attachment because the D-isomer does not combine with the enzyme, as evidenced by its failure to inhibit. These three sites of the enzyme might for convenience be referred to as an "aromatic site", a "carboxyl site" and an "amino site". The part of the enzyme which accomodates the aromatic hydroxyl group must be fairly strictly localized, in view of the great preference for phenylalanine derivatives with the hydroxyl group at position 2 or 3 of the ring or the indolaleanine derivative with the hydroxyl group at the 4 or 5 position. The data of LOVENBERG, WEISSBACH and UDENFRIEND (1962) (Tables 3, 4 and 5) mentioned previously show that both affinity and turnover rate are markedly increased by the presence of these hydroxyl groups. The actual site of attachment of the amino group is generally considered to be the coenzyme, pyridoxal phosphate. During the past fifteen years the efforts of a number of investigators (see BRAUNSTEIN 1960) have indicated an interaction between the aldehyde group of pyridoxal phosphate and the amino group of amino acids and evidence has been obtained that such an interaction is involved in the action of all types of enzymes which use pyridoxal phosphate as a coenzyme.

In 1951 WERLE proposed a mechanism for the decarboxylation of α-amino acids. This involved the formation of a Schiffs base between the aldehyde radical of pyridoxal phosphate and the amine radical of the amino acid; then followed a shifting of the double bond to a position between the nitrogen and the α-carbon of the substrate to form an imino carboxylic acid with loss of the hydrogen attached to the α-carbon of the substrate. This proposal required modification when at WESTHEIMER'S suggestion MANDELES, KOPPELMAN and HANKE (1954) studied the decarboxylation of tyrosine by bacterial tyrosine decarboxylase in a deuterium oxide medium and showed that the hydrogen atom initially attached to the α-carbon remained attached throughout the decarboxylation reaction. The course of the reaction which they pro posed is depicted below (Fig. 2).

Although this reaction was studied with bacterial tyrosine decarboxylase and not with mammalian dopa decarboxylase (5-hydroxytryptophan decarboxylase), it would be most unlikely that the mechanism of the decarboxylation would be different. Differences might be expected in the steric fit of the enzyme and the amino acid at the "aromatic site" but the actual mechanics of the reaction with the amino and carboxyl groups would not be expected to differ. The drastic reduction in the rate of decarboxylation brought about by the introduction of a methyl group at the α-carbon of the substrate might

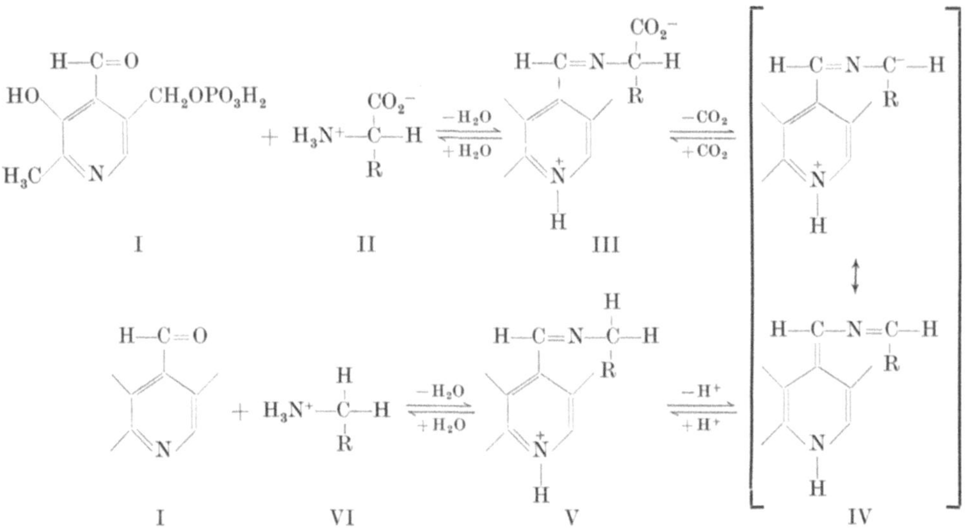

Fig. 2. WESTHEIMER'S proposal for decarboxylation. I, pyridoxal phosphate; II, amino acid; III, pyridoxylidene amino acid; IV, resonance hybrid of the pyridoxylidene amine; V, ionic form of the pyridoxylidene amine; VI, amine. (From MANDELES, KOPPELMAN and HANKE 1954.)

be due to an increase in the electron density at the α-carbon atom or to a change in the relation of the amino acid to a catalytic group of the enzyme. Present knowledge about the mode of attachment of the substrate is illustrated in the following diagram.

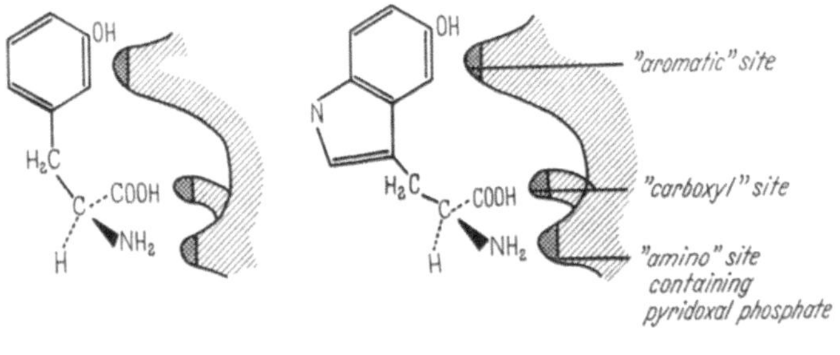

9. Differences in 5-hydroxytryptophan decarboxylase activity with age

HUANG, TANNENBAUM and HSIA (1960) have shown that in rats 5-hydroxytryptophan decarboxylase activity in the kidney first appears at about two to five days after birth and approaches adult activity after about twenty to thirty days (Table 7).

Table 7. *Kidney 5-hydroxytryptophan decarboxylase activity in rats of different ages.* (From HUANG, TANNENBAUM and HSIA 1960)

Age	No. of exp.	No. of animals	5-Hydroxy-tryptophan decarboxylase activity *	Age	No. of exp.	No. of animals	5-Hydroxy-tryptophan decarboxylase activity *
Foetal** . . .	3	45	0	21—23 days .	7	21	0.66 ± 0.13
1 day	3	23	0	33 days . . .	4	8	1.19 ± 0.47
2— 5 days .	4	24	0.21 ± 0.21	Adults	14	14	1.34 ± 0.58
7—12 days .	5	26	0.38 ± 0.10				

* Mean values expressed as μmoles 5-hydroxytryptamine formed per 100 mgm of dry weight of kidneys per hr. ** 1—3 days before term.

IV. Biosynthesis of melatonin

Another indolealkylamine, melatonin, has recently been isolated from pineal gland (LERNER, CASE, TAKAHASHI, LEE and MORI 1958) and found in peripheral nervous tissue (LERNER, CASE, MORI and WRIGHT 1959). It is N-acetyl-5-methoxytryptamine (LERNER, CASE and HEINZELMAN 1959).

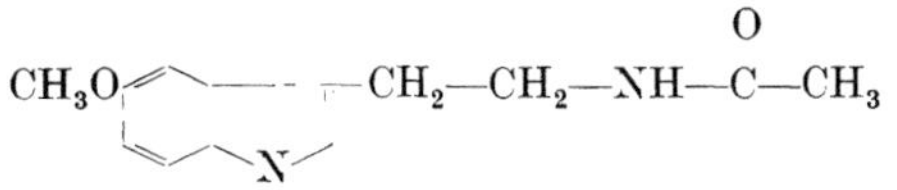

Melatonin (N-acetyl-5-methoxytryptamine)

Melatonin causes lightening of frog skin and blocks the darkening effect of the melanocyte stimulating hormone of the pituitary. Its lightening effect is exerted by exceedingly minute doses.

Melatonin is synthesized from 5-hydroxytryptamine. The 5-hydroxytryptamine is first acetylated to form N-acetyl-5-hydroxytryptamine, which is then methylated.

Table 8. *Substrate specificity of the amine-acetylating enzyme*

Substrate	Acetylamine formed (mμmoles)
Serotonin	4.2
Tryptamine . . .	4.9
Histamine	5.1
Phenylethylamine .	2.2
Tyramine	3.7
Octopamine . . .	0.7
Normetanephrine .	1.1

Amount of acetylamine formed when the same amount of rat liver preparation was incubated with the different substrates in the presence of an acetyl coenzyme A regenerating system. (From WEISSBACH, REDFIELD and AXELROD 1961).

5-hydroxytryptamine + acetyl coenzyme A → N-acetylhydroxytryptamine
N-acetylhydroxytryptamine + S-adenosylmethionine → melatonin

The enzyme which effects the acetylation has been found in nonparticulate cytoplasm of rat liver, rat brain and of beef pineal glands (WEISSBACH, REDFIELD and AXELROD 1960). This enzyme is not specific for 5-hydroxytryptamine but can also acetylate other amines. Table 8 indicates the relative rates of acetylation of a number of different amines by this enzyme in the presence of an acetyl coenzyme A regenerating system (WEISSBACH, REDFIELD and AXELROD 1961).

The enzyme hydroxyindolemethyl transferase, which catalyzes the reaction of N-acetyl-5-hydroxytryptamine with S-adenosylmethionine has been found only in the nonparticulate cytoplasm of ox and monkey pineal tissue. It catalyzes the methylation of 5-hydroxytryptamine at only one-tenth the rate at which it catalyzes the methylation of N-acetyl-5-hydroxytryptamine. This preference for N-acetyl-5-hydroxytryptamine suggests that the first step in the conversion of 5-hydroxytryptamine is acetylation and that the methylation of the N-acetyl-5-hydroxytryptamine occurs subsequently. Further aspects of the substrate specificity are shown in Table 9.

Table 9. *Substrate specificity*

Substrate	Relative activity %
N-Acetylserotonin	100
Bufotenine	14
5-Hydroxyindoleacetic acid * .	12
N-Methylserotonin	9
Serotonin *	7
4-Hydroxy-N-acetyltryptamine	8
4-Hydroxydimethyltryptamine	< 5
2-Hydroxytryptamine	< 5
6-Hydroxydiethyltryptamine .	< 5

* The methoxy derivatives formed were identified chromatographically.

The relative rates of methylation of a number of tryptamine derivatives on incubation with a fixed amount of pineal 0-methyl transferase. The rates were measured at pH 8. (Modified from AXELROD and WEISSBACH 1961).

It has recently been shown that a further hydroxylation of melatonin at the 6 position can be catalyzed by a relatively nonspecific oxidizing system previously described by UDENFRIEND, CLARK, AXELROD and BRODIE (1954), which is also known to hydroxylate tryptamine at the 6 position (KOPIN, PARE, AXELROD and WEISSBACH 1960). C^{14}-N-acetyl-5-methoxy-6-hydroxytryptamine has been recovered from the urine of rats injected with C^{14} melatonin (KOPIN, PARE, AXERLOD and WEISSBACH 1960). Thus 6 hydroxylation may be involved in the metabolism of melatonin *in vivo*.

V. Storage of 5-hydroxytryptamine

5-hydroxytryptamine is stored principally in the enterochromaffin cells of the alimentary mucous membrane (ERSPAMER and ASERO 1952), the blood platelets (RAND and REID 1951), and the spleen (ERSPAMER 1954). That which is in spleen may be localized in platelets. 5-hydroxytryptamine is also found in mast cells of rodents (BENDITT, WONG, ARASE and ROEPER 1955; FURTH, HAGEN and HIRSCH 1957) but not of other species (PARRATT and WEST 1957; STURM and STÜTTGEN 1962). ERSPAMER (1955) has estimated that a 10 kilogram dog "contains altogether 1.58 mg 5-hydroxytryptamine, of which as much as 1.42 is in the gastrointestinal mucosa, 0.086 in the spleen and only 0.073 in the blood". Although the amounts in other tissues are insignificant by comparison they may be very important, and the 5-hydroxytryptamine in the brain has been intensively studied because it has been regarded by many workers as important for cerebral activity.

In those tissues which contain the greatest amounts of 5-hydroxytryptamine, namely, enterochromaffin cells, platelets and, in mice, mast cells, the compound appears to be stored in granules. By centrifugation of homogenates of dog alimentary mucous membrane in sucrose density gradients BAKER (1958 and 1959) obtained evidence that the 5-hydroxytryptamine storage granules are distinct from mitochondria and have a higher specific gravity. PRUSOFF (1960) extended these observations and showed that isolated preparations of enterochromaffin granules were rich in ATP (adenosine triphosphate) as well as 5-hydroxytryptamine. BARER et al. (1964) made electron micrographs of sections of dog alimentary mucous membranes and demonstrated the presence of enterochromaffin granules in the intact enterochromaffin cell. The isolated granules appear densely and uniformly osmiophilic as they do in electron micrographs of intact cells (see Fig. 3).

In platelets, also, 5-hydroxytryptamine is stored together with ATP within granules of high specific gravity, which can be isolated by centrifugation procedures (BAKER, BLASCHKO and BORN 1959). In electron micrographs of platelets, densely osmiophilic granules, similar to those within the enterochromaffin cells, are clustered in the chromomere region (LOW and FREEMAN 1958). Likewise, in rodent mastocytoma cells the 5-hydroxytryptamine is held within similar dense granules, which can be isolated and separated from mitochondria by centrifugation procedures (HAGEN, BARRNETT and LEE 1959). In this case the granule fraction containing 5-hydroxytryptamine also contains the histamine and heparin. Although this fraction appears to be homogeneous, the possibility cannot be excluded that there may be specific granules for each compound. The localization of pharmacologically active amines in special granules in those tissues in which they are stored would seem to be of general occurrence. Thus, in adrenal medulla the adrenaline and noradrenaline are stored within specific chromaffin granules (BLASCHKO and WELCH 1953) which are biochemically and morphologically distinct from mitochondria (HAGEN and BARRNETT 1960) and which, like enterochromaffin granules, are highly osmiophilic and of a higher specific gravity than mitochondria. A function of the storage granules may be to protect the amines from enzymes which could destroy them. The alimentary canal is especially rich in amine oxidase, which may be in the enterochromaffin tissue.

In the case of brain, it is not certain whether 5-hydroxytryptamine is localized in granules. By centrifugation of homogenates the 5-hydroxytryptamine can be sedimented together with acetyl choline in particles of lower specific gravity than mitochondria (WHITTAKER 1958). On electron microscopy, however, these particles have been shown to consist of fragments of damaged nerve fibres (GRAY and WHITTAKER 1962). These fragments contain many very small vesicles, which may be the normal storage site of 5-hydroxytryptamine. Noradrenaline, too, has been found in particles of low density isolated from homogenates of brain tissue (CRUŚCIEL 1960).

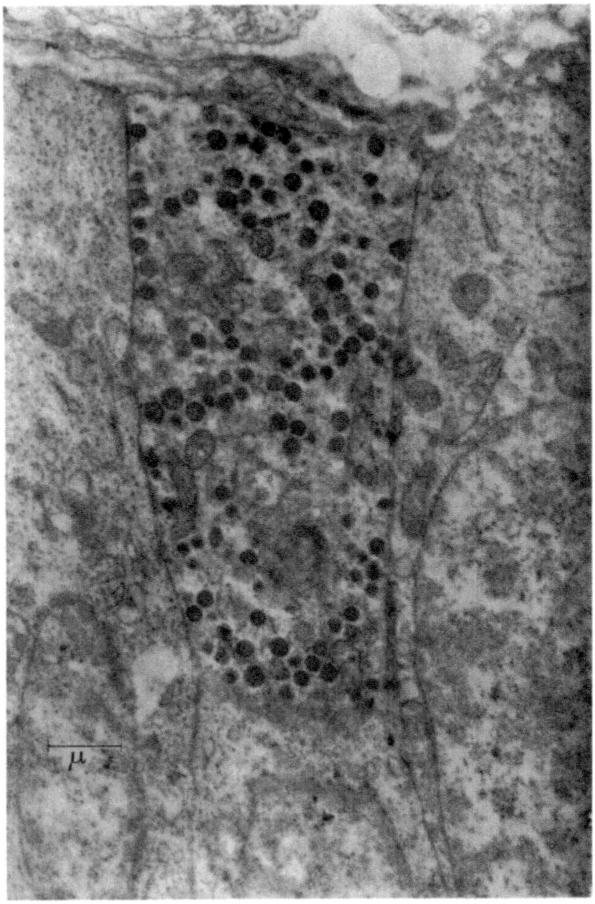

Fig. 3. Electron micrograph of an enterochromaffin cell of the alimentary mucous membrane of the dog. (The authors are grateful to Drs. R. BARER, H. BLASCHKO, G. A. MEEK and W. H. PRUSOFF for this illustration.)

The remarkably high content of ATP in platelets (BORN 1958; SCHMITZ, SCHLEIPEN and GROSS 1962) and in enterochromaffin granules (PRUSOFF 1960 and 1961) has suggested that this nucleotide is probably involved in the binding of 5-hydroxytryptamine within the granules. It is probably more than coincidence that a similar high concentration of ATP is found within the adrenal medulla chromaffin granules (BLASCHKO, BORN, D'IORIO and EADE 1956), which store adrenaline and noradrenaline.

The intracellular localization of 5-hydroxytryptamine within storage granules might suggest that the granules are the sites of its synthesis. However, such does not appear to be the case. In human carcinoid tumor (HAGEN 1962), mouse mastocytoma (HAGEN, WEINER, ONO and LEE 1960) and guinea pig intestine (LOVENBERG, WEISSBACH and UDENFRIEND 1962) the 5-hydroxytryptophan decarboxylase has been found in the nonparticulate cytoplasm. The results with carcinoid tissue suggest that in normal enterochromaffin tissue too, the 5-hydroxytryptophan is decarboxylated in the fluid cytoplasm (HAGEN 1962). In tissues which do not store 5-hydroxytryptamine but contain 5-hydroxytryptophan decarboxylase (dopa decarboxylase), i.e., ox adrenal medulla (BLASCHKO, HAGEN and Welch 1955) and human pheochromocytoma (Hagen 1962), the enzyme is also found in the nonparticulate cytoplasm. Moreover, platelets, which lack 5-hydroxytryptophan decarboxylase (Udenfriend and Weissbach 1954), store their 5-hydroxytryptamine in granules (Baker, Blaschko and Born 1959). From the above data it seems highly probable that the 5-hydroxytryptamine is formed by the decarboxylation of 5-hydroxytryptophan in the fluid cytoplasm and then enters the storage granules. In the case of platelets the 5-hydroxytryptamine must be taken up from the plasma. As will be discussed later, platelets can take up large amounts of 5-hydroxytryptamine both *in vivo* and *in vitro*.

VI. Turnover of 5-hydroxytryptamine

A number of studies on the rate of turnover of 5-hydroxytryptamine in dog and man have been reported. Erspamer (1954 and 1955) and Erspamer and Testini (1959) reported that in humans the daily excretion of 5-hydroxyindoleacetic acid, the only appreciable metabolic product of 5-hydroxytryptamine known, varied between 1.13 and 3.5 mg. They assumed that this represented only about 30% of the amount of 5-hydroxytryptamine metabolized. This assumption was based on the finding that, when large doses of 5-hydroxytryptamine were injected, approximately 30% could be accounted for by the increase in urinary 5-hydroxyindoleacetic acid. They therefore concluded that the total daily metabolism of 5-hydroxytryptamine in man was between 3.39 and 10.5 mg. From the mean value of 7.3 mg they calculated that an amount equal to the 5-hydroxytryptamine content of the alimentary canal was metabolized every 14 to 24 hours. However, the assumption that the endogenous 5-hydroxytryptamine is metabolized at the same rate as administered 5-hydroxytryptamine is not necessarily correct and it is possible that a much larger fraction than 30% may be excreted as 5-hydroxyindoleacetic acid. Thus, up to 3 days might be required to metabolize an amount equivalent to that contained in the alimentary canal. However, their value is not greatly different from that arrived at by Udenfriend and Weissbach (1958) on the basis of isotopic data. Udenfriend and Weissbach labelled the body 5-hydroxytryptamine by repeated injections of C^{14}-tryptophan or C^{14}-5-hydroxytryptophan into rabbits. Then, after they had stopped giving the labels, they measured the rate of decline of radioactivity of platelets, spleen, stomach and intestine. In this way they estimated the half life of 5-hydroxytryptamine in stomach to be 17 hours, in intestine, 11 hours and in platelets and spleen, 33—48 hours. One of the assumptions inherent in the isotope experiments is that the 5-hydroxytryptamine in each tissue behaves as a homogeneous pool. However, there might well be several compartments with different rates of turnover, especially since the 5-hydroxytryptamine is stored in particles.

Despite the difficulties in determining turnover accurately the results of the two laboratories do indicate that 5-hydroxytryptamine is rapidly metabolized. It is most unlikely that more than a very small fraction of the 5-hydroxytryptamine formed and excredet each day ever enters the platelets. Even if the replacement time of 5-hydroxytryptamine were two or three days instead of one, the amount synthesized per day would certainly exceed the total 5-hydroxytryptamine content of all the body platelets. Since the average life span of human platelets is estimated to be 8—11 days (see Wintrobe 1961), it is clear, as pointed out by Erspamer (1955), that the 5-hydroxytryptamine liberated during destruction of platelets represents only a small fraction of the 5-hydroxytryptamine metabolized. Nor is there extensive turnover of 5-hydroxytryptamine during the life of the platelets, for the half life of platelet 5-hydroxytryptamine (UDENFRIEND and WEISSBACH 1958; WEISSBACH, BOGDANSKI and UDENFRIEND 1958; BERTACCINI 1960) is of the same order of magnitude as that reported for platelets themselves (ODELL, GAMBLE and FURTH 1953; ADELSON, RHEINGOLD and CROSBY 1957). Thus, most of the 5-hydroxytryptamine is metabolized without ever having been taken up by the platelets. The main site of this metabolism is probably the liver, but the alimentary canal cannot be excluded. If it is liver, then free 5-hydroxytryptamine should be present in the plasma of the portal vein. Although 5-hydroxytryptamine has not been detected free, i.e., outside platelets, in portal plasma (TOH 1954), concentrations that would be sufficient to account for all of the 5-hydroxyindoleacetic acid excreted would be difficult to detect, especially since the time required for collection of the plasma might permit further uptake of 5-hydroxytryptamine by the platelets.

There is considerable evidence that the 5-hydroxytryptamine found in the platelets is derived from the enterochromaffin tissue of the alimentary mucous membrane. In 1954 TOH reported that perfusates of the dog stomach contain 5-hydroxytryptamine and that portal blood contains about three times as much 5-hydroxytryptamine as systemic arterial blood. Since it had been demonstrated that platelets take up 5-hydroxytryptamine *in vitro* (HUMPHREY and TOH 1954), TOH suggested that 5-hydroxytryptamine is released from the enterochromaffin tissue into the portal blood, where it is picked up by the platelets. Uptake of 5-hydroxytryptamine by platelets *in vivo* has also been demonstrated (ERSPAMER 1956; WEISSBACH, BOGDANSKI and UDENFRIEND 1958). The evidence for the release of 5-hydroxytryptamine from the alimentary canal and its uptake by platelets is amply supported by the observations that the platelet 5-hydroxytryptamine content falls after removal of alimentary canal in humans and in animals (HAVERBACK 1958; ROSENBERG, DAVIS, MORAN and ZIMMERMANN 1959; BERTACCINI and CHIEPPA 1960; BERTACCINI 1960; and ERSPAMER and TESTINI 1959). That this 5-hydroxytryptamine originates from the enterochromaffin cells is indicated by the large amounts present in these cells (ERSPAMER 1954) and by the elevation of blood 5-hydroxytryptamine in patients with carcinoid tumors (SJOERDSMA and UDENFRIEND 1955).

TOH suggested in 1954 that the uptake of 5-hydroxytryptamine by platelets protects it during passage through the liver. Indeed the blood from the hepatic vein does contain more 5-hydroxytryptamine than systemic venous blood (ERSPAMER and TESTINI 1959), indicating that at least part of the 5-hydroxytryptamine released by the gut survives passage through the liver. However, the liver can remove some 5-hydroxytryptamine from the blood, as indicated by the observation that the injection of a higher dose of 5-hydroxytryptamine into the portal vein is required to produce the same quantitative response on the cat's nictitating membrane as a given dose injected into the jugular vein (INNES 1963). This is not surprising in view of the known capacity of the liver to remove other amines from the circulation (DAWES 1946). The uptake of 5-hydroxytryptamine by liver probably prevents free 5-hydroxytryptamine from enteiing the systemic circulation. Another obstacle is the lung, which has been shown to remove 5-hydroxytryptamine from perfusing fluids (GADDUM, HEBB, SILVER and SWAN 1953). Further evidence that platelets protect 5-hydroxytryptamine is the very slow turnover of the amine in platelets compared with that of the bulk of the body 5-hydroxytryptamine. This apparent protection suggests that the compound may have a physiological role (but none has yet been established). The most likely sites of such a role would be the sites of platelet destruction, namely sites of clot formation and the reticulo-endothelial system (principally the spleen). The possibility of release of 5-hydroxytryptamine from platelets under physiological or pathological circumstances other than blood coagulation is suggested by the observation of TOH (1956) that alkaline extracts of kidney or of gastric mucous membrane of several animal species (dog, rabbit or sheep) could release 5-hydroxytryptamine from platelets. Alkaline extracts of rat brain are also very active in releasing 5-hydroxytryptamine (GIARMAN and POTTER 1958). The only evidence so far concerning a physiological role of platelet 5-hydroxytryptamine is negative, namely the observation that depletion of platelets of their 5-hydroxytryptamine by administration of reserpine does not influence bleeding time (SHORE, PLETSCHER, TOMICH, KUNTZMANN and BRODIE 1956).

A number of studies of the uptake of 5-hydroxytryptamine by platelets *in vitro* have been reported (BORN and GILLSON 1959; BORN, INGRAM and STACEY 1958; HARDISTY and STACEY 1955; HUMPHREY and TOH 1954; WEISSBACH, BOGDANSKI and UDENFRIEND 1958; ZUCKER and BORELLI 1956). Large amounts are taken up when platelets are incubated in various media containing very low concentrations of 5-hydroxytryptamine even when the concentration in the platelets greatly exceeds that in the medium. Once taken up, 5-hydroxytryptamine does not seem to be readily released from the platelets. Only a small amount is removed by washing with plasma or saline, and this loss may well be due to damage to platelets. An extensive study of factors affecting the rate and extent of uptake of 5-hydroxytryptamine by platelets has recently been reported by BORN and GILLSON (1959). The maximum amount that could be taken up was five to ten times the amount found in freshly prepared platelets. The 5-hydroxytryptamine taken up could exchange rapidly with 5-hydroxytryptamine of the medium. Since earlier evidence suggested that the uptake capacity depended upon the ATP content of the platelets (BORN, INGRAM and STACEY 1958) they suggested that the ATP probably behaved like a cation exchange resin. It was interesting that the initial rate of uptake varied with the concentration of 5-hydroxytryptamine in such a way as to indicate the involvement of a catalyst or carrier. The uptake was essentially unaffected by cyanide or iodoacetate.

BÜLBRING and LIN (1958) have shown that small amounts of 5-hydroxytryptamine can be released from isolated intestine when it contracts in response to an increase in intraluminal pressure. The 5-hydroxytryptamine is released into the lumen. Whether 5-hydroxytryptamine is normally released into the lumen of the intestine in the living animal is still unknown.

Nothing definite is known about the turnover of 5-hydroxytryptamine in brain. Measurements of turnover by isotopic tracer methods have indicated a half life of about ten hours (SJOERDSMA, WEISSBACH, TERRY and UDENFRIEND 1957). However, the investigators believed that for technical reasons this value was misleading. On the basis of experiments in which the 5-hydroxytryptamine content of rat brain was found to rise sharply after the administration of amine oxidase inhibitors to prevent its destruction they have since suggested that the turnover is many times faster than their original estimate (UDENFRIEND and WEISSBACH 1958).

The foregoing discussion should make it clear that our knowledge of the turnover of 5-hydroxytryptamine is still far from satisfactory. It appears that most of the body 5-hydroxytryptamine is in the enterochromaffin tissue, which is the principal site of its synthesis. Of the large amount synthesized each day the greater part is metabolized and excreted in the urine as 5-hydroxyindoleacetic acid. A small fraction is taken up by platelets and most or all of it held there until the death of the platelets. The platelet 5-hydroxytryptamine accounts for virtually all that is found in the blood.

References

ADELSON, E., J. J. RHEINGOLD and W. H. CROSBY: Studies of platelet survival *in vivo* with P^{32}. J. Lab. clin. Med. **50**, 570—576 (1957).

AMIN, A. H., T. B. B. CRAWFORD and J. H. GADDUM: The distribution of substrates P and 5-hydroxytryptamine in the central nervous system of the dog. J. Physiol. (Lond.) **126**, 596—618 (1954).

AXELROD, J., and H. WEISSBACH: Purification and properties of hydroxyindole-0-methyl transferase. J. biol. Chem. **236**, 211—213 (1961).

BAKER, R. V.: Observations on the localization of 5-hydroxytryptamine. J. Physiol. (Lond.) **142**, 563—570 (1958).

— Mitochondria and storage granules for 5-hydroxytryptamine. J. Physiol. (Lond.) **145**, 473—481 (1959).

— H. BLASCHKO and G. V. R. BORN: The isolation from blood platelets of particles containing 5-hydroxytryptamine and adenosine triphosphate. J. Physiol. (Lond.) **149**, 55P—56P (1959).

BALDRIDGE, R. C., L. BOROFSKY, H. BAIRD III, F. REICHLE and D. BULLOCK: Relationship of serum phenylalanine levels and ability of phenylketonurics to hydroxylate tryptophan. Proc. Soc. exp. Biol. (N.Y.) **100**, 529—531 (1959).

BARER, R., H. BLASCHKO, G. A. MEEK and W. H. PRUSOFF: Personal communication (1964).

BENDITT, E. P., R. L. WONG, M. ARASE and E. ROEPER: 5-hydroxytryptamine in mast cells. Proc. Soc. exp. Biol. (N.Y.) **90**, 303—304 (1955).

BERENDES, H., J. A. ANDERSON, M. A. ZIEGLER and D. RUTTENBERG: Disturbance of tryptophane metabolism in phenylketonuria. Amer. J. Dis. Child. **96**, 430 (1958).

BERTACCINI, G.: Tissue 5-hydroxytryptamine and urinary 5-hydroxyindoleacetic acid after partial or total removal of the gastro-intestinal tract in the rat. J. Physiol. (Lond.) **153**, 239—249 (1960).

—, and S. CHIEPPA: Urinary excretion of 5-hydroxyindoleacetic acid after removal of the large intestine in man. Lancet **1960 I**, 881

BERTLER, A., A. M. ROSENGREN and E. ROSENGREN: *In vivo* uptake of dopamine and 5-hydroxytraptamine by adrenal medullary granules. Experientia (Basel) **16**, 418—419 (1960).

—, and E. ROSENGREN: Distribution of monoamines and enzymes responsible for their formation in brain. Experientia (Basel) **15**, 382—384 (1958).

BIRT, A. R., P. HAGEN and E. ZEBROWSKI: Amino acid decarboxylase of urticaria pigmentosa mast cells. J. invest. Derm. **37**, 273—276 (1961).

BLASCHKO, H.: The specific action of L-dopa decarboxylase. J. Physiol. (Lond.) **96**, 50P—51P (1939).

— The decarboxylation of o-hydroxyphenylalanine. Biochem. J. **44**, 268—270 (1949).

— Remarks on chemical specificity. Proc. roy. Soc. B **137**, 307—311 (1950a).

— Substrate specificity of amino acid decarboxylases. Biochim. biophys. Acta (Amst.) **4**, 130—137 (1950b).

— Amine oxidase and amine metabolism. Pharmacol. Rev. **4**, 415—458 (1952).

— Enzymatic oxidation of 5-hydroxytryptamine in mammalian and cephalopod tissue. Biochem. J. **52**, X (1952).

— G. V. R. BORN, A. D'IORIO and N. R. EADE: Sedimentation of adrenal medullary granules in hypertonic sucrose. J. Physiol. (Lond.) **132**, 44P (1956).

— J. H. BURN and H. LANGEMANN: The formation of noradrenaline from dihydroxyphenylserine. Brit. J. Pharmacol. **5**, 431—437 (1950).

— C. W. CARTER, J. R. P. O'BRIEN and G. H. SLOANE-STANLEY: Pyridoxin in relation to amine formation in the mammalian liver. J. Physiol. (Lond.) **107**, 18P—19P (1948).

—, and T. L. CHRUŚCIEL: The decarboxylation of amino acids related to tyrosine and their awakening action in reserpine-treated mice. J. Physiol. (Lond.) **151**, 272—284 (1960).

— P. HAGEN and A. D. WELCH: Observations on the intracellular granules of the adrenal medulla. J. Physiol. (Lond.) **129**, 27—49 (1955).

—, and P. HOLTON: Enzymic formation of ortho-tyramine (o-hydroxyphenylethylamine). J. Physiol. (Lond.) **110**, 482—487 (1950).

— — and G. H. SLOANE-STANLEY: Enzymic formation of pressor amines. J. Physiol. (Lond.) **108**, 427—439 (1949).

—, and G. H. SLOANE-STANLEY: Decarboxylation of tyrosine and its derivatives by mammalian and bacterial enzymes. Biochem. J. **42**, iii—iv (1948).

—, and A. D. WELCH: Localization of adrenaline in cytoplasmic particles of the bovine adrenal medulla. Naunyn-Schmiedeberg's Arch. exp. Path. Pharmak. **219**, 17—22 (1953).

BORN, G. V. R.: Changes in the distribution of phosphorus in platelet rich plasma during clotting. Biochem. J. **68**, 695—704 (1958).

Botn, G. V. R., and R. E. Gillson: Studies on the uptake of 5-hydroxytryptamine by blood platelets. J. Physiol. (Lond.) **146**, 472—491 (1959).
— G. I. C. Ingram and R. S. Stacey: The relationship between 5-hydroxytryptamine and adenosine triphosphate in blood platelets. Brit. J. Pharmacol. **13**, 62—64 (1958).
Braunstein, A. E.: Pyridoxal phosphate. In: P. D. Boyer, H. Lardy and K. Myrback, The enzymes, vol. 2, part A. New York: Academic Press 1960.
Bülbring, E., and R. C. Y. Lin: The effect of intraluminal application of 5-hydroxytryptamine and 5-hydroxytryptophan on peristalsis: The local production of 5-HT and its release in relation to intraluminal pressure and propulsive activity. J. Physiol. (Lond.) **140**, 381—407 (1958).
Burger, M., u. H. Langemann: Bestimmungen von Adrenalin und Noradrenalin sowie von Decarboxylase- und Aminoxydase-Aktivitäten in Zellfraktionen von Phaochromocytomen. Klin. Wschr. **34**, 941—944 (1956).
Buxton, J., and H. M. Sinclair: Pyridoxal phosphate as a coenzyme of 5-hydroxytryptophan decarboxylase. Biochem. J. **62**, 27 P (1956).
Buzard, J. A., and P. D. Nytch: Some characteristics of rat kidney 5-hydroxytryptophan decarboxylase. J. biol. Chem. **227**, 225—230 (1957).
— — The relation of dietary pyridoxine to the 5-hydroxytryptophan decarboxylase activity of rat kidney. J. biol. Chem. **229**, 409—413 (1959).
Carlsson, A., and M. Lindqvist: In vivo decarboxylation of α-methyl DOPA and α-methyl metatyrosine. Acta physiol. scand. **54**, 87—94 (1962).
— — T. Magnusson and B. Waldeck: On the presence of 3-hydroxytyramine in brain. Science **127**, 471 (1958).
Chruściel, T. L.: Observations on the localization of noradrenaline in homogenates of dog's hypothalamus. Ciba Foundation Symposium on Adrenergic Mechanisms, p. 539—543. London: Churchill 1960.
Clark, C. T., H. Weissbach and S. Udenfriend: 5-Hydroxytryptophan decarboxylase: preparation and properties. J. biol. Chem. **210**, 139—148 (1954).
Cooper, J. R., and I. Melcer: The enzymic oxidation of tryptophan to 5-hydroxytryptophan in the biosynthesis of serotonin. J. Pharmacol. exp. Ther. **132**, 265—268 (1961).
Costa, E., and F. Rinaldi: Biochemical and electroencephalographic changes in the brain of rabbits injected with 5-hydroxytryptophan (Influence of chlorpromazine premedication). Amer. J. Physiol. **194**, 214—220 (1958).
Dalgliesh, C. E.: Two-dimensional paper chromatography ofin urary indoles and related substances. Biochem. J. **64**, 431—485 (1956).
—, and R. W. Dutton: Biogenesis of 5-hydroxytryptophan. Brit. J. Cancer **11**, 296—309 (1957a).
— — On the site of formation of 5-hydroxytryptophan. Biochem. J. **65**, 21 P—22 P (1957b).
Davidson, J., A. Sjoerdsma, L. N. Loomis and S. Udenfriend: Studies with the serotonin precursor, 5-hydroxytryptophan, in experimental animals and man. J. clin. Invest. **36**, 1594—1599 (1957).
Davison, A. N., and M. Sandler: Inhibition of 5-hydroxytryptophan decarboxylase by phenylalanine metabolites. Nature (Lond.) **181**, 186—187 (1958).
Dawes, G. S.: Amidines, guanidines and adrenaline inactivation in the liver. Brit. J. Pharmacol. **1**, 21—37 (1946).
Demis, D. J., H. Blaschko and A. D. Welch: The conversion of dihydroxyphenylalanine-2-C^{14} (Dopa) to norepinephrine by bovine adrenal medullary homogenates. J. Pharmacol. exp. Ther. **117**, 208—212 (1956).
DeMoss, J. A., and D. M. Bonner: Normal and genetically altered tryptophan synthetase from neurospora crassa. Proc. nat. Acad. Sci. (Wash.) **45**, 1405—1412 (1959).
Dengler, H., u. G. Reichel: Hemmung der Dopadecarboxylase durch α-Methyldopa *in vivo*. Naunyn-Schmiedeberg's Arch. exp. Path. Pharmak. **234**, 275—281 (1958).
Donaldson jr., R. M., S. J. Gray and V. C. Letsou: 5-hydroxytryptophan as an intermediate of serotonin biosyntheses in malignant carcinoidosis. Lancet **1959 II**, 1002—1003.
Erspamer, V.: Quantitative estimation of 5-hydroxytryptamine in gastrointestinal mucosa, spleen and blood of vertebrates. Ciba Foundation Symposium on Hypertension, p. 78—85. London: Churchill 1954.
— Pharmacology of indolealkylamines. Pharmacol. Rev. **6**, 425—487 (1954).
— Observations on the fate of indolealkylamines in the organism. J. Physiol. (Lond.) **127**, 118—133 (1955).
— Some observations on the fate of exogenous 5-hydroxytryptamine (enteramine) in the rat. J. Physiol. (Lond.) **133**, 1—9 (1956).
— Recent research in the field of 5-hydroxytryptamine and related indolealkylamines. Fortschr. Arzneimittelforsch. **3**, 151—367 (1961).

ERSPAMER, V., and B. ASERO: Identification of enteramine, the specific hormone of the enterochromaffin cell system, as 5-hydroxytryptamine. Nature (Lond.) **169**, 800—801 (1952).
—, and G. BERTACCINI: Observations on the antidiuretic action and the fate of 5-hydroxy-DL-Tryptophan in the rat organism. Arch. int. Pharmacodyn. **137**, 6—23 (1962).
— A. GLÄSSER, B. M. NOBILI and C. PASINI: The fate of 4-hydroxytryptophan in the rat organism. Experientia (Basel) **16**, 506—507 (1960).
— — — The fate of 5-hydroxy-N-acetyltryptophan and 5-acetoxy-N-acetyl-tryptophan in the rat organism. Arch. Biochem. **93**, 673—674 (1961).
— — C. PASINI and G. STOPPANI: In vitro decarboxylation of tryptophans by mammalian decarboxylase. Nature (Lond.) **189**, 483 (1961).
—, and M. B. NOBILI: Observations on the fate of oral 4-hydroxytryptophan in man. Experientia (Basel) **17**, 351—352 (1961).
— — Observations on the fate of 4-hydroxy-DL-tryptophan in the Organism of the rat and man. Arch. int. Pharmacodyn. **137**, 24—38 (1962).
—, and A. TESTINI: Observations on the release and turnover rate of 5-hydroxytryptamine in the gastrointestinal tract. J. Pharm. Pharmacol. **11**, 618—623 (1959).
EWINS, A. J., and P. P. LAIDLAW: The syntheses of 3-β-aminoethylindole and its formation from tryptophan. Proc. chem. Soc. **26**, 343 (1910).
FELLMAN, J. H.: Inhibition of DOPA decarboxylase by aromatic acids associated with phenylpyruvic oligophrenia. Proc. Soc. exp. Biol. (N.Y.) **93**, 413—414 (1956).
— Purification and properties of adrenal L-dopa decarboxylase. Enzymologia **20**, 366—376 (1959).
FREEDLAND, R. A., M. C. KRAKOWSKI and H. A. WAISMAN: Influence of dietary aromatic amino acids on phenylalanine hydroxylase activity. Fed. Proc. **19**, 7 (1960).
— I. M. WADZINSKI and H. A. WAISMAN: The enzymatic hydroxylation of tryptophan. Biochem. biophys. Res. Commun. **5**, 94—98 (1961).
FRETER, K., H. WEISSBACH, S. UDENFRIEND and B. WITKOP: Biochemical and pharmacological studies with D- and L-5-hydroxytryptophan. Proc. Soc. exp. Biol. (N.Y.) **94**, 725—728 (1957).
FURTH, J., P. HAGEN and E. I. HIRSCH: Transplantable mastocytoma in the mouse containing histamine, heparin, 5-hydroxytryptamine. Proc. Soc. exp. Biol. (N.Y.) **95**, 824—828 (1957).
GADDUM, J. H.: Antagonism between lysergic acid diethylamide and 5-hydroxytryptamine. J. Physiol. (Lond.) **121**, 15P (1953a).
— Drugs antagonistic to 5-hydroxytryptamine. Ciba Foundation on Hypertension 75—77 (1953b).
—, and N. J. GIARMAN: Preliminary studies on the biosynthesis of 5-hydroxytryptamine. Brit. J. Pharmacol. **11**, 88—92 (1956).
— C. O. HEBB, A. SILVER and A. A. B. SWAN: 5-hydroxytryptamine. Pharmacological action and destruction in perfused lungs. Quart. J. exp. Physiol. **38**, 255—262 (1953).
GANROT, P. O., A. M. ROSENGREN and E. ROSENGREN: On the presence of different histidine decarboxylating enzymes in mammalian tissues. Experientia (Basel) **17**, 263—264 (1961).
GIARMAN, N. J., and L. T. POTTER: Release of serotonin by extracts of mammalian tissues. Fed. Proc. **17**, 371 (1958).
GRAY, E. G., and V. P. WHITTAKER: The isolation of nerve endings from brain: An electron-microscopic study of cell fragments derived by homogenization and centrifugation. J. Anat. (Lond.) **96**, 79—88 (1962).
GREEN, D. E., L. P. LELOIR and V. NOCITO: Transaminases. J. biol. Chem. **161**, 559—582 (1945).
HAGEN, P.: Biosynthesis of norepinephrine from 3,4-dihydroxyphenylethylamine (Dopamine). J. Pharmacol. exp. Ther. **116**, 26 (1956).
— Observations on the substrate specificity of dopa decarboxylase from ox adrenal medulla, human phacochromocytoma and human argentaffinoma. Brit. J. Pharmacol. **18**, 175—182 (1962).
— and R. J. BARRNETT: The storage of amines in the chromaffin cell. Ciba Foundation Symposium on Adrenergic Mechanisms, p. 83—99 (1960).
— — and F. L. LEE: Biochemical and electron microscopic study of particles isolated from mastocytoma cells. J. Pharmacol. exp. Ther. **126**, 91—108 (1959).
—, and F. L. LEE: Amino acid decarboxylases of mouse mast cells. J. Physiol. (Lond.) **143**, 7B—8B (1958).
— N. WEINER, S. ONO and F. L. LEE: Amino acid decarboxylases of mouse mastocytoma tissue. J. Pharmacol. exp. Ther. **130**, 9—12 (1960).
—, and A. D. WELCH: The adrenal medulla and the biosynthesis of pressor amines. Recent Progr. Hormone Res. **12**, 27—44 (1956).

HARDISTY, R. M., and R. S. STACEY: 5-hydroxytryptamine in normal human platelets. J. Physiol. (Lond.) **130**, 711—720 (1955).

HARTMANN, W. J., R. I. AKAWIE and W. G. CLARK: Competitive inhibition of 3,4-dihydroxy phenylalanine (Dopa) decarboxylase *in vitro*. J. biol. Chem. **216**, 507—529 (1955).

— R. S. POGRUND, W. DRELL and W. G. CLARK: Studies on the biosynthesis of arterenol, enzymatic decarboxylation of diastereoisomers of hydroxyphenylserines. J. Amer. chem. Soc. **77**, 816—817 (1955).

HAVERBACK, B. J.: Serotonin and the gastrointestinal tract. Clin. Res. **6**, 57 (1958).

HESS, S. M., R. H. CONNAMACHER, M. OZAKI and S. UDENFRIEND: The effects of α-methyl-dopa and α-methyl-meta-tyrosine on the metabolism of norepinephrine and serotonin *in vivo*. J. Pharmacol. exp. Ther. **134**, 129—138 (1961).

— B. G. REDFIELD and S. UDENFRIEND: The effect of monoamine oxidase inhibitors and tryptophan on the tryptamine content of animal tissues and Urine. J. Pharmacol. exp. Ther. **127**, 178—181 (1959a).

HOFMANN, A. v.: Die psychotropen Wirkstoffe der mexikanischen Zauberpilze. Separatabdruck aus Chimia **14**, 309—318 (1960).

HOLTZ, P., R. HEISE u. K. LÜDTKE: Fermentativer Abbau von 1-Dioxyphenylalanin (Dopa) durch Niere. Naunyn-Schmiedeberg's Arch. exp. Path. Pharmak. **191**, 87—118 (1938).

—, and E. WESTERMANN: Dopa (α-(3,4-dihydroxyphenyl)alanine) decarboxylase and histidine decarboxylase in nerve tissue. Naunyn-Schmiedeberg's Arch. exp. Path. Pharmak. **227**, 538—546 (1956).

HUANG, I., S. TANNENBAUM and D. Y.-Y. HSIA: Development of 5-hydroxytryptophan decarboxylase activity in rat kidney. Nature (Lond.) **186**, 717—718 (1960).

HUMPHREY, J. H., and C. C. TOH: Absorption of serotonin (5-hydroxytryptamine) and histamine by dog platelets. J. Physiol. (Lond.) **124**, 300—304 (1954).

ICHIHARA, K., A. SAKAMOTO, K. INAMORI and Y. SAKAMOTO: Studies on the acid diazo-reaction and 5- or 7-hydroxyindole derivatives. J. Biochem. (Tokyo) **44**, 649—659 (1957).

INNES, I. R.: Uptake of 5-hydroxyhyptamine and adrenaline by the liver. Brit. J. Pharmacol. **21**, 202—207 (1963).

JEPSON, J. B., S. UDENFRIEND and P. ZALTZMAN: The enzymic conversion of tryptamine to 6-hydroxytryptamine. Fed. Proc. **18**, 254 (1959).

— P. ZALTZMAN and S. UDENFRIEND: Microsomal hydroxylation of tryptamine, indole-acetic acid and related compounds, to 6-hydroxy derivatives. Biochim. biophys. Acta (Amst.) **62**, 91—102 (1962).

JERVIS, G. A.: Phenylpyruvic oligophrenia deficiency of phenylalanine-oxidizing system. Proc. Soc. exp. Biol. (N.Y.) **82**, 514—515 (1953).

KAUFMAN, S.: Studies on the mechanism of the enzymatic conversion of phenylalanine to tyrosine. J. biol. Chem. **234**, 2677—2682 (1959).

—, and B. LOVENBERG: Further studies on the phenylalanine-hydroxylation cofactor. J. biol. Chem. **234**, 2683—2688 (1959).

KOPIN, I. J., C. M. B. PARE, J. AXELROD and H. WEISSBACH: 6-hydroxylation, the major metabolic pathway for melatonin. Biochim. biophys. Acta (Amst.) **40**, 377—378 (1960).

KUNTZMAN, R., P. A. SHORE, D. BOGDANSKI and B. B. BRODIE: Microanalytical procedures for fluorometric assay of brain DOPA-5HTP decarboxylase, norepinephrine and serotonin, and a detailed mapping of decarboxylase activity in brain. J. Neurochem. **6**, 226—232 (1961).

LAGUNOFF, D., K. B. LAM, E. ROEPER and E. P. BENDITT: 5-hydroxytryptamine formation from 5-hydroxytryptophan by mast cells. Fed. Proc. **16**, 363 (1957).

LANGEMANN, H.: Enzymes and their substrates in the adrenal gland of the ox. Brit. J. Pharmacol. **6**, 318—324 (1951).

— 5-hydroxytryptamine (ed. G. B. LEWIS), p. 153—157. London: Pergamon Press 1958.

—, u. J. KÄGI: Oxytryptamin- und Oxyindolessigsäurebestimmungen bei einem Fall von Carcinoidsyndrom, nebst einigen anderen Untersuchungen über Oxytryptamin. Klin. Wschr. **34**, 237—241 (1956).

LERNER, A. B., J. D. CASE and R. V. HEINZELMAN: Structure of melatonin. J. Amer. chem. Soc. **81**, 6084—6085 (1959).

— — W. MORI and M. R. WRIGHT: Melatonin in peripheral nerve. Nature (Lond.) **183**, 1821 (1959).

— — Y. TAKAHASHI, T. H. LEE and W. MORI: Isolation of melatonin, the pineal gland factor that lightens melanocytes. J. Amer. chem. Soc. **80**, 2587 (1958).

LOVENBERG, W., H. WEISSBACH and S. UDENFRIEND: Aromatic L-amino acid decarboxylase. J. biol. Chem. **237**, 89—93 (1962).

LOW, F. N., and J. A. FREEMAN: Electronmicroscopic atlas of normal and leukemic human blood. New York: McGraw-Hill 1958.

MACKAY, D., J. F. RILEY and D. M. SHEPHERD: Amino acid decarboxylase activities in rat hepatoma. J. Pharm. Pharmacol. **13**, 257—261 (1961).
MANDELES, S., R. KOPPELMAN and M. E. HANKE: Deuterium studies on the mechanism of enzymatic amino acid decarboxylation. J. biol. Chem. **209**, 327—336 (1954).
MITOMA, C.: Studies on partially purified phenylalanine hydroxylase. Arch. Biochem. **60**, 476—484 (1956).
— H. WEISSBACH and S. UDENFRIEND: 5-hydroxytryptophan formation and tryptophan metabolism in chromobacterium violaceum. Arch. Biochem. **63**, 122—130 (1956).
MURPHY, G. F., and T. L. SOURKES: Effect of catecholamino acids on the catecholamine content of rat organs. Rev. canad. Biol. **18**, 379—388 (1959).
— — The action of antidecarboxylases on the conversion of 3,4-dihydroxyphenylalanine to dopamine *in vivo*. Arch. Biochem. **93**, 338—343 (1961).
OATES, J. A., and A. SJOERDSMA: A unique syndrome associated with secretion of 5-hydroxytryptophan by metastatic gastric carcinoids. Amer. J. Med. **32**, 333—342 (1962).
ODELL, T. T., F. N. GAMBLE and J. FURTH: Life span of naturally labelled platelets of rats. Fed. Proc. **12**, 398—399 (1953).
PAASONEN, M. K., P. D. MACLEAN and N. J. GIARMAN: 5-hydroxytryptamine (serotonin, enteramine) content of structures of the limbic system. J. Neurochem. **1**, 326—333 (1957).
PARE, C. M. B., M. SANDLER and R. S. STACEY: 5-hydroxytryptamine deficiency in phenylketonuria. Lancet **1957 I**, 551—553.
— — — Decreased 5-hydroxytryptophan decarboxylase activity in phenylketonuria. Lancet **1958 II**, 1099—1101.
— — — The relationship between decreased 5-hydroxyindole metabolism and mental defect in phenylketonuria. Arch. Dis. Childh. **34**, 422—425 (1959).
PARRATT, R. J., and G. B. WEST: 5-hydroxytryptamine and tissue mast cells. J. Physiol. (Lond.) **137**, 169—178 (1957).
PLETSCHER, A., and K. F. GEY: Assay of 5-hydroxytryptophan decarboxylation in intact brain. Nature (Lond.) **190**, 918—919 (1961).
— P. A. SHORE and B. B. BRODIE: Serotonin as a mediator of reserpine action in brain. J. Pharmacol. exp. Ther. **116**, 84—89 (1956).
PORTER, C. C., J. A. TOTARO and C. M. LEIBY: Some biochemical effects of α-methyl-3,4-dihydroxyphenylalanine and related compounds in mice. J. Pharmacol. exp. Ther. **134**, 139—145 (1961).
PRUSOFF, W. H.: The distribution of 5-hydroxytryptamine and adenosine triphosphate in cytoplasmic particles of the dog's small intestine. Brit. J. Pharmacol. **15**, 520—524 (1960).
— Effect of reserpine on the 5-hydroxytryptamine and adenosine triphosphate of the dog intestinal mucosa. Brit. J. Pharmacol. **17**, 87—91 (1961).
RAND, M., and G. REID: Source of "serotonin" in serum. Nature (Lond.) **168**, 385 (1951).
RAPPORT, M. M.: Serum vasoconstrictor (serotonin) V Presence of creatinine in complex. Proposed structure of vasoconstrictor principle. J. biol. Chem. **180**, 961—969 (1948).
RENSON, J., F. GOODWIN, H. WEISSBACH and S. UDENFRIEND: Conversion of tryptophan to 5-hydroxytryptophan by phenylalanine hydroxylase. Biochem. biophys. Res. Commun. **6**, 20—25 (1961).
— H. WEISSBACH and S. UDENFRIEND: Hydroxylation of tryptophan by phenylalanine hydroxylase. J. biol. Chem. **237**, 2261—2264 (1962).
ROSENBERG, J. C., R. B. DAVIS, W. H. MORAN and B. ZIMMERMANN: Serum serotonin concentration and urinary 5-hydroxyindoleacetic acid excretion following intestinal obstruction and resection. Fed. Proc. **18**, 503 (1959).
ROSENGREN, E.: Are dihydroxyphenylalanine decarboxylase and 5-hydroxytryptophan decarboxylase individual enzymes? Acta physiol. scand. **49**, 364—369 (1960).
SANDLER, M., and P. J. D. SNOW: An atypical carcinoid tumour secreting 5-hydroxytryptophan. Lancet **1958 I**, 137—139.
SCHANBERG, S. M., and N. J. GIARMAN: Uptake of 5-hydroxytryptophan by rat brain. Biochim. biophys. Acta (Amst.) **41**, 556—558 (1960).
SCHINDLER, R.: The conversion of C-labelled tryptophan to 5-hydroxytryptamine by neoplastic mast cells. Biochem. Pharmacol. **1**, 323—327 (1958).
— M. DAY and G. A. FISCHER: Culture of neoplastic mast cells and their synthesis of 5-hydroxytryptamine and histamine *in vitro*. Cancer Res. **19**, 47—51 (1959).
SCHMITZ, H., TH. SCHLEIPEN u. R. GROSS: Freie Nucleotide in normalen menschlichen Blutplättchen. Klin. Wschr. **40**, 13—15 (1962).
SCHOTT, H. F., and W. G. CLARK: Dopa decarboxylase inhibition through the interaction of coenzyme and substrate. J. biol. Chem. **196**, 449—462 (1952).
SHORE, P. A., A. PLETSCHER, E. G. TOMICH, R. KUNTZMAN and B. B. BRODIE: Release of blood platelet serotonin by reserpine and lack of effect on bleeding time. J. Pharmacol. exp. Ther. **117**, 232—236 (1956).

SJOERDSMA, A., J. A. OATES, P. ZALTZMAN and S. UDENFRIEND: Identification and assay of urinary tryptamine: Application as an index of MAO inhibition in man. J. Pharmacol. exp. Ther. **126**, 217—222 (1959).

—, and S. UDENFRIEND: Studies on indole metabolism in patients with malignant carcinoid (argentaffinoma). J. clin. Invest. **34**, 914—915 (1955).

— H. WEISSBACH, L. L. TERRY and S. UDENFRIEND: Further observations on patients with malignant carcinoid. Amer. J. Med. **23**, 5—15 (1957).

SMITH, A. N., L. M. NYHUS, C. E. DALGLIESH, R. W. DUTTON, B. LENNOX and P. S. MACFARLANE: Further observations on the endocrine aspects of argentaffinoma. Scot. med. J. **2**, 24—38 (1957).

SMITH, S. E.: The pharmacological actions of 3,4-dihydroxyphenyl-α-methylalanine (α-methyldopa), an inhibitor of 5-hydroxytryptophan decarboxylase. Brit. J. Pharmacol. **15**, 319—327 (1960).

SOURKES, T. L.: Inhibition of dihydroxyphenylalanine decarboxylase by derivatives of phenylalanine. Arch. Biochem. **51**, 444—456 (1954).

— P. HENEAGE and Y. TRANO: Enzymatic decarboxylation of isomers and derivatives of dihydroxyphenylalanine. Arch. Biochem. **40**, 185—193 (1952).

— G. F. MURPHY, B. CHAVEZ and M. ZIELINSKA: The action of some α-methyl and other amino acids on cerebral catacholamines. J. Neurochem. 8, 109—115 (1961).

STOLL, W. A.: Lysergsäure-diäthylamid, ein Phantastikum aus der Mutterkorngruppe. Schweiz. Arch. Neurol. Psychiat. **68**, 279—323 (1947).

STURM, A., u. G. STÜTTGEN: Nachweis von 5-Hydroxytryptamin in menschlichen Mastzellen. Klin. Wschr. **40**, 199—201 (1962).

TITUS, E. O., and S. UDENFRIEND: Metabolism of 5-hydroxytryptamine (serotonin). Fed. Proc. **13**, 411 (1954).

TOH, C. C.: Release of 5-hydroxytryptamine (serotonin) from the dog's gastro-intestinal tract. J. Physiol. (Lond.) **126**, 248—254 (1954).

— Release of 5-hydroxytryptamine (serotonin) and histamine from platelets by tissue extracts. J. Physiol. (Lond.) **133**, 402—411 (1956).

UDENFRIEND, S.: Metabolism of 5-hydroxytryptamine. 5-hydroxytryptamine. (Ed. G. P. LEWIS). London: Pergamon Press 1958.

— D. F. BOGDANSKI and H. WEISSBACH: Increase in tissue serotonin by administration of its precursor, 5-hydroxytryptophan. Fed. Proc. **15**, 493 (1956).

— C. T. CLARK, J. AXELROD and B. B. BRODIE: Ascorbic acid in aromatic hydroxylation. J. biol. Chem. **208**, 731—739 (1954).

— — and E. TITUS: The presence of 5-hydroxytryptamine in the venom of Bufo marinus. Experientia (Basel) 8, 379—380 (1952).

— — — 5-hydroxytryptophan decarboxylase: a new route of metabolism of tryptophan. J. Amer. chem. Soc. **75**, 501—502 (1953).

—, and J. R. COOPER: The enzymatic conversion of phenylalanine to tyrosine. J. biol. Chem. **194**, 503—511 (1952).

— C. R. CREVELING, H. POSNER, B. G. REDFIELD, J. DALY and B. WITKOP: On the inability of tryptamine to serve as a precursor of serotonin. Arch. Biochem. **83**, 501—506 (1959).

— W. M. LOVENBERG and H. WEISSBACH: L-amino acid decarboxylase activity in mammalian tissues and its inhibition by α-methyl DOPA. Fed. Proc. **19**, 7 (1960).

— E. TITUS, H. WEISSBACH and R. PETERSON: Biogenesis and metabolism of 5-hydroxyindole compounds. J. biol. Chem. **219**, 335—344 (1956).

—, and H. WEISSBACH: Studies on serotonin (5-hydroxytryptamine) in platelets. Fed. Proc. **13**, 412—413 (1954).

— — Turnover of 5-hydroxytryptamine (serotonin) in tissues. Proc. Soc. exp. Biol. (N.Y.) **97**, 748—751 (1958).

— — and D. F. BOGDANSKI: Increase in tissue serotonin following administration of its precursor 5-hydroxytryptophan. J. biol. Chem. **224**, 803—810 (1957).

— — and C. T. CLARK: The estimation of 5-hydroxytryptamine (serotonin) in biological tissues. J. biol. Chem. **215**, 337—344 (1955).

WALDENSTRÖM, J., B. PERNOW and H. SILWER: Case of metastasizing carcinoma (argentaffinoma?) of unknown origin showing peculiar red flushing and increased amounts of histamine and 5-hydroxytryptamine in blood and urine. Acta med. scand. **156**, 73—83 (1956).

WEISSBACH, H., D. F. BOGDANSKI, B. G. REDFIELD and S. UDENFRIEND: Studies on the effect of vitamin B_6 on 5-hydroxytryptamine (serotonin) formation. J. biol. Chem. **227**, 617—624 (1957).

— F. BOGDANSKI and S. UDENFRIEND: Binding of serotonin and other amines by blood platelets. Arch. Biochem. **73**, 492—499 (1958).

WEISSBACH, H., W. LOVENBERG and S. UDENFRIEND: Characteristics of mammalian histidine decarboxylating enzymes. Biochim. Biophys. Acta (Amst.) **50**, 177—179 (1961).
— B. G. REDFIELD and J. AXELROD: Biosynthesis of melatonin: Enzymic conversion of serotonin to N-acetylserotonin. Biochim. biophys. Acta (Amst.) **43**, 352—353 (1960).
— — — The enzymic acetylation of serotonin and other naturally occurring amines. Biochim. biophys. Acta (Amst.) **54**, 190—192 (1961).
WERLE, E.: Amino acid decarboxylases and histaminases. Biochem. Z. **311**, 270—286 (1942).
— Aminosäure-Decarboxylasen. Angew. Chem. **63**, 550—555 (1951).
—, and D. AURES: Purification and specificity of 3,4-dihydroxyphenylalanine (dopa) decarboxylase. Hoppe-Seylers Z. physiol. Chem. **316**, 45—60 (1959).
—, u. G. MENNICKEN: Über die Bildung von Tryptamin aus Tryptophan und von Tyramin aus Tyrosin durch tierisches Gewebe. Biochem. Z. **291**, 325—327 (1937).
WESTERMANN, E., H. BALZER u. J. KNELL: Hemmung der Serotoninbildung durch α-Methyl-Dopa. Naunyn-Schmiedeberg's Arch. exp. Path. Pharmak. **234**, 194—205 (1958).
WHITTAKER, V. P.: A comparison of the distribution of lysosome enzymes and 5-hydroxytryptamine with that of acetylcholine in subcellular fractions of Guinea pig brain. Biochem. Pharmacol. **1**, 351—352 (1958).
WINTROBE, M. M.: Clinical hematology, p. 280. Philadelphia: Lea & Febiger 1961.
YUWILER, A., E. GELLER and S. EIDUSON: Studies on 5-hydroxytryptophan decarboxylase. I. In vitro inhibition and substrate interaction. Arch. Biochem. **80**, 162—173 (1959).
— — — Studies on 5-hydroxytryptophan decarboxylase. II. Additional inhibition studies and suggestions on the nature of the enzymic site. Arch. Biochem. **89**, 143—147 (1960).
—, and R. T. LOUTTIT: Effects of phenylalanine diet on brain serotonin in the rat. Science **134**, 831—832 (1961).
ZUCKER, M. B., and J. BORRELLI: Absorption of serotonin (5-hydroxytryptamine) by canine and human platelets. Amer. J. Physiol. **186**, 105—110 (1956).

Chapter 6

Metabolism of indolealkylamines

By

HERMANN BLASCHKO and WALTER G. LEVINE

With 3 Figures

A. Introduction

Biological inactivation by enzymes has been of interest to the pharmacologist for a long time. The classical study by OTTO LOEWI of the mechanism of action of eserine has led to the recognition that at many, if not all, cholinergic nerve endings destruction of the mediator by enzymic hydrolysis determines the time course of the response of the effector organ. More recently, ARUNLAKSHANA, MONGAR and SCHILD (1954) have found that inhibitors of the enzyme histaminase enhance the response of the excitable tissue to histamine (see also BLASCHKO and KURZEPA 1962).

However, there are also many suggestions that the time course of the response of the effector cell may be determined by other factors. OGSTON (1955) has pointed out that *diffusion* alone may rapidly lower the effective concentration of a compound locally released, e.g., of a mediator at a nerve ending. Such a lowering of the effective concentration by diffusion may be facilitated if the compound passes readily through cell membranes and enters the effector cell (see BLASCHKO 1954, 1956, 1958); this is somewhat analogous to the mechanism proposed by BROWN and GILLESPIE (1957) for the removal of the mediator at adrenergic nerve endings. For this substance it has also been made likely that, once released, it can again be taken up and stored by the nerve ending (BURN and RAND 1958; HERTTING, AXELROD, KOPIN and WHITBY 1961). Similar mechanisms may have to be discussed for the indolealkylamines.

Whatever the fate of the pharmacologically active compound at the effector site, it must, unless it is excreted unchanged, be ultimately destroyed by enzyme action. This may happen at a place far from the site of action. It is known that the blood platelets take up 5-hydroxytryptamine. Thus this amine may be biologically inactivated at or near the site where the blood platelets are destroyed.

B. Enzymes acting on indolealkylamines

I. Amine oxidases

1. The intracellular (and carbonyl-reagent-insensitive) amine oxidase

The enzyme amine oxidase (also called "mono" amine oxidase by some authors) is a general catalyst of the biological inactivation of many amines, including the catechol amines and the indolealkylamines. It was discovered as tyramine oxidase (HARE 1928), but in 1937 a number of observers showed that the enzyme had a much wider spectrum of substrate specificities and also acted on tryptamine (BLASCHKO, RICHTER and SCHLOSSMANN 1937a, b, c; KOHN 1937; PUGH and QUASTEL 1937a, b). This was soon confirmed (see HOLTZ and BÜCHSEL 1942).

At this time, studies of two still unidentified naturally occurring products led to a renewed interest in amine oxidase. These substances were enteramine and serotonin. ERSPAMER, in a series of papers on "*enteraminase*" showed that this catalyst of the biological inactivation of enteramine in mammalian and cephalopod tissues had properties indistinguishable from amine oxidase. Likewise, REID and his colleagues found that serotonin was inactivated by an amine-oxidase-like catalyst. These observations, which have often been reviewed (BLASCHKO 1952b, 1958; ERSPAMER 1954, 1961), were extended to synthetic material soon after this had become available (FREYBURGER, GRAHAM, RAPPORT, SEAY, GOVIER, SWOAP and VANDER BROOK 1952; BLASCHKO 1952a).

Much work has been done on amine oxidase, but there are still important gaps in our knowledge of this enzyme. These gaps, some of which will be discussed in the following pages, are of relevance for our understanding of the biological inactivation of the indolealkylamines.

a) Preparation of amine oxidase

One of the main difficulties that stand in the way of the purification of the enzyme is its extreme insolubility. Lysolecithin, detergents and ultrasonic disintegration have all been used to solubilize the oxidase, but although by these means highly dispersed preparations have been obtained, the enzyme is always again rapidly rendered insoluble. In 1957, WEISSBACH, REDFIELD and UDENFRIEND described a water-soluble preparation of amine oxidase from guinea-pig's liver and this preparation, which proved very similar to the enzyme preparations commonly described, was used for kinetic studies. In particular, it served to establish beyond doubt that the *primary product* in the *oxidation* of *tryptamine* was *indolylacetaldehyde*. However, otherwise little is known about the properties of the preparation, except that the enzymic activity could be precipitated between 25 and 40 per cent saturation with ammonium sulphate; a further purification was achieved by precipitation at pH 5.0—5.1.

Acetone-dried powders of mammalian liver have also been found useful for kinetic studies, but here the activity is present in the insoluble residue.

b) Intracellular localization of amine oxidase

Our ignorance as to the mechanism of electron transport in the amine oxidase reaction is still as complete as it was in 1952 when this subject was last reviewed (BLASCHKO 1952b). The main location of amine oxidase is in the *mitochondria*. This was first shown for *rat liver* (COTZIAS and DOLE 1951; HAWKINS 1952), but has since been confirmed for the *duodenal mucosa of the dog* (BAKER 1959), for the *bovine adrenal medulla* (BLASCHKO, HAGEN and HAGEN 1957) and for *rat brain* (ARNAIZ and DE ROBERTIS 1962).

A tenfold purification of the *mitochondrial amine oxidase* of rat brain has recently been reported (SEIDEN and WESTLEY 1962) in work where the mitochondria were isolated, lysed and sonicated; kynuramine oxidation was used for enzyme assay.

HAWKINS (1952) always found some of the amine oxidase in the microsomal fraction. In 1952, the question as to whether or not this was a truly microsomal location had to be left open, but further analysis by DE DUVE, BEAUFAY, JACQUES, RAHMAN-LI, SELLINGER, WATTIAUX and DE CONINCK (1960) has confirmed that the distribution of the rat liver amine oxidase is truly bimodal.

About 70 per cent of the total enzymic activity was found to be associated with cytochrome oxidase, a further support for the idea that this is really a mitochondrial location, but there was also a microsomal location. This microsomal component appeared to be present in a special structural element, as the activity could be shown not to be associated with any of the other microsomal enzymes.

Too little is known of the *microsomal amine oxidase* to assess its functional significance. Earlier speculations on the function of amine oxidase were based on the mitochondrial location of the enzyme (BLASCHKO 1954); mitochondria are truly intracellular constituents and this portion of the oxidase can act only on amines which have entered the cell. On the other hand, of the microsomal enzyme we cannot say where it is situated in the intact cell. We must remember that the microsomal fraction is defined only by the technique of centrifugation; it may well include fragments of the cell surface. This has been fully discussed elsewhere (HOLTER 1962; BLASCHKO 1962b).

It may be worthwhile to emphasize that the microsomal amine oxidase here discussed is to be distinguished from the microsomal enzymes that have been described by BRODIE (1956) and by AXELROD (1954); enzymes of this group are conveniently discussed later.

However, for the mitochondrial enzyme it remains true that it will probably only act on amine present within the cytoplasmic fluid.

The extracellular amine oxidases are discussed below.

Work on the chromaffin tissue of the adrenal medulla has shown that the enzyme is present in the tissue in which the catechol amines are made and stored (LANGEMANN 1951; BLASCHKO, HAGEN and HAGEN 1957). There is little analogous information for the enterochromaffin cells, generally believed to be the main seat of 5-hydroxytryptamine formation (VIALLI 1962). The cells that form this system are scattered throughout the epithelial lining of the digestive tract, and although homogenates of the intestinal mucous membrane contain amine oxidase, the tissue from which such homogenates are prepared contains many different types of cell.

LANGEMANN and KÄGI (1956) have examined the amine oxidase content of kidney and liver metastases of human enterochromaffinomata, and homogenates from these have been found to have amine oxidase activity. Thus it looks as if the enterochromaffin cell, like the chromaffin cell, contains both amine-forming and amine-destroying catalysts, but it is known that the elementary particle that stores the amines is not the particle that contains the oxidase (see article by HAGEN and COHEN).

HAGEN (1959) has found an *amine oxidase* in *mouse mastocytoma* tissue, but whereas this enzyme acted on dopamine, 5-hydroxytryptamine was not oxidized; mouse mastocytoma tissue is rich in 5-hydroxytryptamine. Similarly, no significant oxidation of 5-hydroxytryptamine was recently found by DAY and GREEN (1962) in *mouse mastocytoma cells in tissue culture.*

Observations on the *intracellular localization* of the oxidase in *invertebrate* tissues is even more incomplete. Some time ago (BLASCHKO, HAGEN and HAGEN, unpublished) homogenates of the "liver" of *Octopus vulgaris* were prepared in 0.7 M sucrose. The bulk of the amine oxidase and of the succinic dehydrogenase were both recovered in the "large granule" fraction; upon ultracentrifugation of this fraction over a sucrose density gradient, similar to that used by BLASCHKO et al. (1957), the two enzymic activities were very similarly distributed in the gradient tube. This result suggests that in cephalopods, as in mammals, the *main location of amine oxidase is mitochondrial.*

c) *Distribution of amine oxidase*

Much of our knowledge on the distribution of the enzyme has been reviewed before (BLASCHKO 1952b, 1958). In all vertebrates tested, amine oxidase has been found. Apart from skeletal muscle, all organs seem to contain the enzyme, but it is not always certain if the enzyme is present in the parenchymatous tissue, or in nervous tissue present in the organ. Until recently *liver* and *kidneys* were considered the richest sources of amine oxidase, with the exception of the rat kidney, which is poor in enzyme. However, a new rich source of amine oxidase has recently been found in the *human salivary glands*, *parotid* and *submaxillary* (STRÖMBLAD 1959). These two organs contain the highest amine oxidase activity yet encountered in mammalian tissue. Using 10^{-2} M tyramine as substrate, the rate of oxygen uptake, expressed in μl O_2/hr/g of fresh tissue, ranged from 700 to 2850. In one experiment with human submaxillary gland extract the rate of oxidation with 5-hydroxytryptamine was 70 p.c., and that with tryptamine 66 p.c., of the rate of oxidation with tyramine. Thus, the rates of oxidation of the two indolealkylamines tested in the human salivary gland preparation were extremely high. It is of interest that in earlier observations by STRÖMBLAD (1956) on the cat's salivary glands, much lower rates of oxidation of tyramine were found; the mean values for the cat's submaxillary glands were 206 μl O_2/hr/g fresh tissue, and for the parotids the corresponding figure was 105. These are activities of the order of magnitude usually found in mammalian liver. Thus, as far as is known, the high concentration of the oxidase in the human salivary glands is unique.

When we consider the wide distribution of *amine oxidase* in many mammalian tissues and in particular the high concentration of enzyme in many glands and in plain muscle, it appears ar first sight surprising that so much attention has been given to the presence of the enzyme in *nervous tissue*, and in particular in the *central nervous system*, where the concentration of enzyme in terms of tissue weight is only moderate. However, this interest is readily understood if we remember that the substrates of amine oxidase, catechol amines and 5-hydroxytryptamine, are present, and that the level of these amines in the brain can be modified by drug action.

Studies of the distribution of amine oxidase in the mammalian central nervous system have been published by many authors. There are differences in the activity of extracts prepared from different parts of the brain. To quote only one series of observations, in which the enzymic activity was measured, using 5-hydroxytryptamine as substrate, in the dog's brain the hypothalamus has the highest enzymic activity (BOGDANSKI, WEISSBACH and UDENFRIEND 1957). However, compared with other enzymes, e.g. L-dopa decarboxylase, the differences between different parts of the brain are not very great.

A comparative study of the development of amine oxidase in the brain has recently been published by KARKI, KUNTZMAN and BRODIE (1962). They have found that the amine oxidase content of guinea-pig brain at birth is almost the same as that of the adult animal, but that in the rat's brain the amine oxidase content of the adult animal is about three times that of the newborn. However, by the use of a histochemical method, SHIMIZU and MORIKAVA (1959) report changes in the amine oxidase of the rat's brain: whereas at birth the region of the pons, the locus caeruleus, the habenula, the periventricular nuclei of the hypothalamus and the nucleus ambiguus showed moderate to strong action at birth, other parts showed activity or increase in activity only after birth.

The occurrence of *amine oxidase in invertebrates* has been known for a long time (BLASCHKO, RICHTER and SCHLOSSMANN 1937c). The phyla in which the presence of the enzyme has been demonstrated, are the *Annelida*, the *Echinodermata*, the *Mollusca* and the *Arthropoda*.

The Mollusca are by far the best studied invertebrate phylum. Amine oxidase has not been found in all the molluscan species studied, but it should be borne in mind that the manometric technique, which has been used in this work, is relatively insensitive. With more sensitive methods of detection, the oxidase may well be found in species in which it has not hitherto been demonstrated.

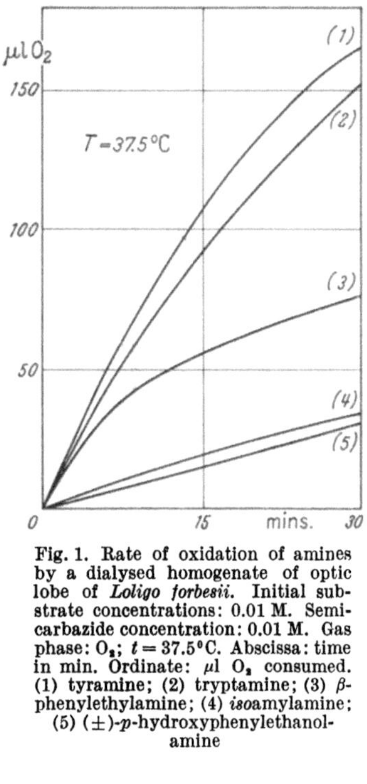

Fig. 1. Rate of oxidation of amines by a dialysed homogenate of optic lobe of *Loligo forbesii*. Initial substrate concentrations: 0.01 M. Semicarbazide concentration: 0.01 M. Gas phase: O_2; $t = 37.5°C$. Abscissa: time in min. Ordinate: µl O_2 consumed. (1) tyramine; (2) tryptamine; (3) β-phenylethylamine; (4) *iso*amylamine; (5) (±)-*p*-hydroxyphenylethanolamine

Eusepia officinalis was the first cephalopod species in which amine oxidase was found to be present in a number of tissues (Blaschko 1941). This was followed by a study of the enzyme in other *Cephalopods* (Erspamer 1948; Blaschko and Hawkins 1952; Blaschko and Himms 1954). All members of this group that have been tested are rich in amine oxidase. With the exception of striated muscle, the enzyme seems to be almost ubiquitous. As in the Vertebrates the tissues of the digestive system are richest in enzyme, followed by excretory organs, and the gonads. The whole of the nervous system is moderately rich in enzyme. In Fig. 1 there is shown an experiment carried out by Blaschko and Himms (1954) on the *optic lobe* of *Loligo forbesii*; it can be seen that the enzymic oxidation of tryptamine was almost as rapid as that of tyramine; in another similar experiment 5-hydroxytryptamine was oxidized almost as rapidly as tryptamine. It may be mentioned here that both tryptamine and 5-hydroxytryptamine are also rapidly oxidized by the tissues of *Octopus vulgaris* (Blaschko 1952a; Blaschko and Philpot 1953). The occurrence of amine oxidase in the Octopods is of interest, because it is known that indolealkylamines occur in some of the tissues. A comparison of the amine oxidase activities of the *posterior salivary glands* of two species of *Octopus* is therefore of interest, *O. vulgaris.* where Erspamer has shown the occurrence of large amounts of 5-hydroxytryptamine in the gland, and *O. macropus*, where 5-hydroxytryptamine is not found in high concentration. The following were the O_2 uptakes (in µl/g fresh tissue/hr) in the two extracts (substrate concentration 1.2×10^{-2} M):

	Substrate			
	Tyramine	β-phenyl-ethyl-amine	Trypt-amine	5-hydr-oxytrypt-amine
O. vulgaris . . .	325	570	215	160
O. macropus . .	120	300	80	47.5

Thus, there were slight differences in the relative rates of oxidation, but all 4 substrates tested were oxidized by both species. One point of interest is the fact that in both the indolethylamine and the β-phenylethylamine series the introduction of a phenolic hydroxyl group lowered the rate of the enzymic reaction. This is different from what was found with the optic lobe extract of *L. for-*

besii. In mammals, tyramine is almost invariably oxidized more rapidly than β-phenylethylamine; the rabbit liver is the only known exception to this rule.

Other molluscan species tested include *Mytilus edulis*. Here no enzymic activity was at first found in the *chief digestive gland* (BLASCHKO and HAWKINS 1952), but after the extreme 5-hydroxytryptamine sensitivity of the anterior retractor muscle of the byssus in Mytilus had been discovered, this question was tackled again. It was now found (BLASCHKO and HOPE 1957) that both the digestive gland and the anterior retractor muscle itself contained small amounts of enzyme. It is interesting that this oxidase differs from enzymes from other sources: no oxygen uptake with *iso*amylamine could be detected. However, both tryptamine and 5-hydroxytryptamine are oxidized. In assessing these results it must be remembered that manometry is not a very sensitive method of amine oxidase assay; there is no doubt that the methods more recently introduced (see OZAKI, WEISSBACH, OZAKI, WITKOP and UDENFRIEND 1960) would readily detect the enzymic activity encountered in these two tissues. This limitation must be borne in mind when it is stated that amine oxidase has not been demonstrated in the gill plates of *Mytilus edulis* (BLASCHKO and HOPE 1957; BLASCHKO and MILTON 1960).

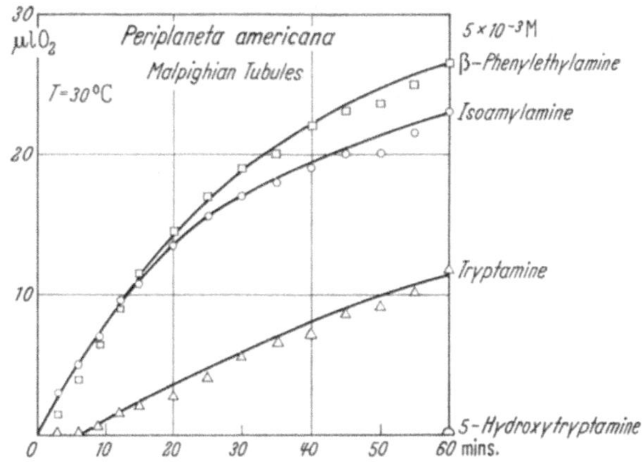

Fig. 2. Oxidation of amines by a homogenate of Malpighian tubules of *Periplaneta americana* (male specimens). Each flask contained the equivalent of about 0.11 gms of tissue

In the study of the amine oxidase of the *earthworm* gut (BLASCHKO and HIMMS 1953) no indolealkylamine was included, but in the polychaete *Annelid*, *Chaetopterus variopedatus*, a homogenate of the gut acted upon tryptamine, at about one-half of the rate of oxidation of β-phenylethylamine.

In the *Echinoderms*, three species of Asteroids, *Luidia ciliaris*, *Asterias rubens* and *Porania pulvillus* readily oxidized tryptamine, the only indolealkylamine tested with these homogenates. It has already been pointed out that nothing is known at present about biogenic amines in this phylum; here is a gap in our present knowledge of this group of substances.

Until recently, nothing was known of the occurence of *amine oxidase* in *Arthropods*. In 1937, no enzymic activity could be detected in the hepatopancreas and the gills of *Cancer pagurus*. At that time, no attention was given to the indolealkylamines. A more systematic attempt to settle the problem of the occurrence of amine oxidase has recently been made. The species selected was the *cockroach Periplaneta americana* (BLASCHKO, COLHOUN and FRONTALI 1961; BLASCHKO and COLHOUN, unpublished). Only one tissue contained enough enzymic activity for a satisfactory quantitative assay of enzymic activity, the *Malpighian tubules*; these are a collection of ducts surrounded by contractile tissue that open into the lumen of the gut at the boundary of mid-gut and hind-gut. They have an excretory function. Fig. 2 gives the result of an experiment with a preparation from the Malpighian tubules. It can be seen that tryptamine was readily oxidized. On the other hand, 5-hydroxytryptamine, tested in a similar experiment, was not attacked.

The Malpighian tubules, although the only tissue that gave extracts with enzymic activity high enough to be studied by manometry, is not the only organ of *P. americana* in which enzymic activity was present. All parts of the gut were enzymically active, but no activity could be detected in homogenates of the nerve cord.

The enzyme in *Periplaneta,* therefore, has two distinctive properties:

1. Absence of any significant action on 5-hydroxytryptamine.
2. Absence of significant enzymic activity in nervous tissue.

The absence of action on 5-hydroxytryptamine with the homogenates of insect tissue is of interest. In a recent study of the distribution of 5-hydroxytryptamine WELSH and MOORHEAD (1960) found a little 5-hydroxytryptamine-like material in some insects; in an extract of the nerve cords of a cockroach, *Blaberus gigantea,* small amounts of 5-hydroxytryptamine were detected. Similarly, COLHOUN (1963) has recently described the presence, in small amounts, of 5-hydroxytryptamine in glands, brain and ventral nerve cord of *P. americana.* He also noted formation of the amine from 5-hydroxytryptophan in *Periplaneta* homogenates; this interesting observation may be an expression of the dopa decarboxylase activity of the tissues (see article by HAGEN and COHEN in this volume).

WELSH and MOORHEAD (1960) did not make a particular study of amine oxidase, but it is of interest that they report that in the *green glands* of *Cancer borealis* and the *coxal glands* of *Limulus polyphemus* they obtained evidence of the presence of amine oxidase. These two glands, like the Malpighian tubules in insects, have an excretory function.

Limulus belongs to another class of the Arthropods, the *Arachnoidea.* Another set of observations on amine oxidase in spiders by WITT, BRETTSCHNEIDER and BORIS (1961) is of interest: these authors, working with homogenates of these three species: *Araneus diadematus, Araneus sericatus* and *Neoscona vertebrata,* have found that the enzymic oxidation of tyramine is inhibited by iproniazid. In these experiments (+)-amphetamine also disappeared when incubated with the homogenates. The mammalian enzyme is known not to act on amphetamine.

d) *Histochemistry of amine oxidase*

All histochemical studies of the distribution of amine oxidase in the tissues are based on the use of tryptamine or 5-hydroxytryptamine as substrates. BLASCHKO and HELLMANN (1953) exploited the observation that both these amines, when oxidized by preparations containing amine oxidase, give rise to pigments. The chemistry of the pigment formation is unknown. It was shown that this simple procedure gave a good picture of the distribution of amine oxidase in *renal tissue.* The main localization of the enzyme was in the proximal convoluted tubules; less was found in the distal convoluted tubules; no enzyme was present in the collecting tubes of the medulla. HELLMANN (1955) also demonstrated amine oxidase in the *apocrine sweat glands* of the horse by the same procedure. ARIOKA and TANIMUKAI (1957) using a similar method, demonstrated the presence of the enzyme in the *brain,* particularly in the peri-vascular spaces. However, it is not certain if these results demonstrate the presence of enzyme at the sites of pigment deposition.

Another procedure, also based upon the oxidation of tryptamine, has been adopted by KOELLE and VALK (1954); here the sections are preincubated with hydrazine, then incubated in presence of both tryptamine and 2-hydroxy-3-naphthoic acid hydrazide; the pigment is then developed with tetrazotized

O-dianisidine. The pictures obtained have confirmed the observations of BLASCHKO and HELLMANN (1953) on the distribution of the enzyme in the kidneys. The method, in the hands of the authors, was unsuitable for use in the central nervous system.

The third method for the histochemical demonstration of amine oxidase is based also on the use of either tryptamine or 5-hydroxytryptamine as substrates (GLENNER, BURTNER and BROWN 1957; GLENNER, WEISSBACH and REDFIELD 1960). It is based on a novel use of tetrazolium salts: the reduction of tetrazolium by indolyl-3-acetaldehyde (or its 5-hydroxylated derivative), to form the corresponding formazan. This method, which is easy in application, gives satisfactory pictures; in the renal tissue they confirm the earlier findings. GLENNER et al. (1957) also give interesting pictures of the localization of the oxidase in the mucosal epithelium of the guinea-pig's duodenum.

SHIMIZU, MORIKAWA and OKADA (1959) have used these methods for the study of the distribution of amine oxidase in the brain of rodents. They could not find any deposition of formazan in the neocortex, but there was a deposition of pigment in the neuropil of the central gray matter. The most conspicuous deposition of formazan was seen in the habenular nuclei and in the midline gray matter of the thalamus; otherwise the thalamic nuclei were negative. Other conspicuously positive areas were: the locus coeruleus, the dorsal nucleus of the vagus nerve, and the area postrema.

Further observations on the distribution of the enzyme in mammalian brain would clearly be desirable (see also SMITH 1963).

e) Indolealkylamines as substrates of amine oxidase

α) Tryptamine and 5-hydroxytryptamine. Both *tryptamine* and *5-hydroxytryptamine* are *oxidized by amine oxidase.* Tryptamine is usually a substrate that is fairly rapidly oxidized in the manometric experiment, but with 5-hydroxytryptamine the rates of oxygen uptake greatly vary from species to species. In mammals, the guinea-pig (liver and kidney) is a species where the two amines are oxidized at relatively rapid rates, the cat (liver and kidney) one in which they are both slowly oxidized in comparison with tyramine. There are other species, e.g. the rabbit, where tryptamine is relatively rapidly oxidized, but where the oxidation of 5-hydroxytryptamine is very slow.

In addition to species differences, differences in the relative rate of oxidation of 5-hydroxytryptamine have been described (HAGEN and WEINER 1959; HOPE and SMITH 1960). For instance, HAGEN and WEINER reported that mouse mastocytoma tissue readily acts on tryptamine and β-phenylethylamine, but has no detectable action on 5-hydroxytryptamine. HOPE and SMITH also studied the rate of enzymic oxidation of tryptamine and 5-hydroxytryptamine in extracts of various mouse tissues. Taking the rate of oxidation of 5-hydroxytryptamine as 100, the rate with *tryptamine* was:

in brain	49
in liver	147
in kidney	47
in spleen	61
in lung	35

In mouse liver, benzylamine was oxidized at approximately the same rate as *5-hydroxytryptamine*; in mouse kidney benzylamine was not oxidized.

These observations raise the question as to the homogeneity of amine oxidase. It is impossible at present to decide whether the observations just described find their explanation in the presence of more than one enzyme in one and the same tissue extract or whether they are due to the presence of a different organ-specific oxidase in each tissue.

β) N-substituted amines. The di-N-methylated derivative of 5-hydroxytryptamine, bufotenine, is oxidized by amine oxidase at a scarcely measurable rate (BLASCHKO and PHILPOT 1953; GOVIER, HOWES and GIBBONS 1953). In the β-phenylethylamine series, there are marked species differences in the rate of oxidation of the N-substituted amines; this is confirmed for the tryptamine derivatives by the study of GOVIER et al. (1953). Using a preparation of guinea-pig's liver these authors found the following rates of oxygen uptake:

with tryptamine	165 μl
with N-methyltryptamine	160 μl
with N-*iso*propyltryptamine	0 μl
with N-dimethyltryptamine	0 μl
with 5-hydroxytryptamine	152 μl
with N-methyl-5-hydroxytryptamine	158 μl
with N-dimethyl-5-hydroxytryptamine (bufotenine) .	28 μl

γ) Other indolealkylamines. ERSPAMER, FERRINI and GLÄSSER (1960) have compared the oxidation of the following compounds by guinea-pig kidney and liver homogenates; the oxygen uptake with 5-hydroxytryptamine was taken as 100:

	With liver	With kidney
4-hydroxytryptamine . .	49	48
6-hydroxytryptamine . .	49	54
7-hydroxytryptamine . .	71	74
5-methoxytryptamine . .	90	94
Iso-5-hydroxytryptamine.	10	26
Tryptamine	118	130
Psilocybine	0	5

VANE (1959) has found that 5-methyltryptamine is readily oxidized by the amine oxidase present in rat gastric fundus, this preparation also acted on tyramine, tryptamine, 5-hydroxytryptamine, but not on 5-hydroxy-α-methyltryptamine.

FELLMAN, FUJITA and BELBER (1962) have recently shown that the 2:3-dihydro-derivative of 5-hydroxytryptamine is also oxidized by amine oxidase; the rate of oxidation is similar to that of 5-hydroxytryptamine but the affinity of the dihydro derivative is much less.

2. Amine oxidases inhibited by carbonyl reagents

It is now known that the classical intracellular amine oxidase is not the only enzyme that removes amino groups from monoamines. The enzyme that has been discussed in the preceding paragraphs is characterized by two properties:

a) Immunity from inhibition by carbonyl reagents, e.g. *semicarbazide*, and by cyanide;

b) Ability to oxidize *secondary* as well as *primary amines* (BLASCHKO 1960).

The amine oxidases to be discussed in what follows differ from the classical enzyme in two points. They all are members of a group characterized by sensitivity to both cyanide and carbonyl reagents, and by their *inability to act on secondary amines.* Enzymes of this group active on indolealkylamines are:

1. The *amine oxidase* of pea seedlings. This enzyme is probably present also in other *plants*.

2. The *benzylamine oxidase* of *mammalian blood plasma*.

Plant amine oxidase was first described by WERLE and v. PECHMANN (1949). It has been purified both in WERLE's laboratory and by KENTEN and MANN (1952) (see also MANN 1955, 1961). KENTEN and MANN (1952) compared the relative rates of oxidation of a variety of substrates; they found the following rates of oxidation: with putrescine 342 $\mu l\ O_2$; with cadaverine 378 $\mu l\ O_2$; with β-phenylethylamine 134 $\mu l\ O_2$; with tryptamine 49 $\mu l\ O_2$. In other words, the rate with tryptamine was much lower than with the two diamines. Other indole derivatives were not tested. WERLE, TRAUTSCHOLD and AURES (1961), using a highly purified preparation of *pea* oxidase, report these relative rates of oxidation:

with cadaverine	1000
with spermidine.	570
with β-phenylethylamine	81
with tryptamine	27
with 5-hydroxytryptamine	8
with 5:6-dihydroxytryptamine . .	1

A comparison of the results of these two groups of workers makes one suspect that there may be a second catalyst present in peas that is responsible for the oxidation of the indolealkylamines; this second catalyst appears to be removed in the progressive purification of the diamine oxidase.

As to the plasma oxidases, there are two of these, spermine oxidase and benzylamine oxidase. It has been shown that spermine oxidase occurs mainly in the blood plasma of ruminants (BLASCHKO 1962a; BLASCHKO and BONNEY 1962). The bovine plasma enzyme has recently been obtained in crystalline form by YAMADA and YASUNOBU (1962); the purified enzyme did not act on tryptamine and 5-hydroxytryptamine. With a crude benzylamine oxidase preparation, consisting of 1.6 ml each of the crude dialysed sera rates of oxidation of benzylamine and tryptamine were (BLASCHKO, FRIEDMAN, HAWES and NILSSON 1959):

Substrate	Serum		
	Horse	*Pig*	*Dog*
Benzylamine . . .	29 $\mu l\ O_2$	47 $\mu l\ O_2$	70 $\mu l\ O_2$
Tryptamine . . .	11 $\mu l\ O_2$	15 $\mu l\ O_2$	24 $\mu l\ O_2$

These experiments show that the rate of oxidation of tryptamine was by no means negligible.

The purification and crystallization of the benzylamine oxydase of pig plasma has been recently achieved by BUFFONI and BLASCHKO (1963).

As far as the oxidation of 5-hydroxytryptamine is concerned, the crude sera all acted on it, although at differing rates. However, it was shown that the slow oxidation of 5-hydroxytryptamine by *pig serum* was not due to the amine oxidase present in the plasma; the ability to act on 5-hydroxytryptamine could be separated from the benzylamine oxidase activity, and it was made likely that the catalyst responsible for the *oxidation* of *5-hydroxytryptamine* was *caeruloplasmin* (BLASCHKO and LEVINE 1960b). Whether the more rapid oxidation of *5-hydroxytryptamine* by *horse serum* is due also to caeruloplasmin or whether it is at least in part due to the benzylamine oxidase has not been investigated.

The presence of the plasma amine oxidases is of interest, because of their variable substrate specificity. It seems quite possible that in those species in which this activity occurs, the blood plasma takes an active part in the biological inactivation of indolealkylamines.

3. Microsomal deaminating enzymes

We owe much of our knowledge of the microsomal "detoxicating" enzymes to the work of B. B. Brodie (1956) and his colleagues. It was Axelrod, who in 1954 showed that (—)-amphetamine was deaminated by a suspension of rabbit liver microsomes. A similar pathway has recently been described for *α-methyltryptamine:* rat liver *microsomes* act on α-methyltryptamine, to give *3-indolylacetone:*

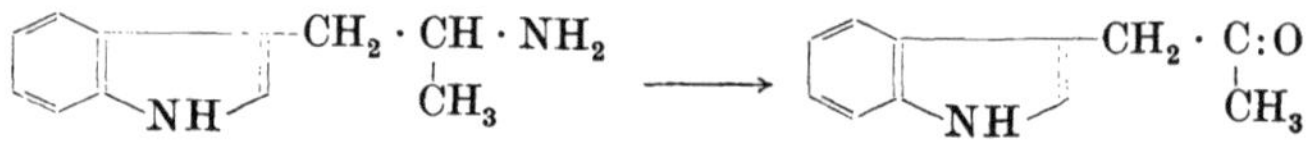

In addition, a 6-hydroxylation occurs (see below); thus 6-hydroxy-3-indolylacetone is also formed (Szara 1961):

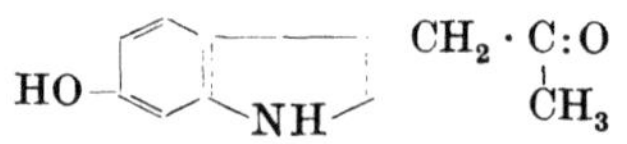

It must remain open whether or not the enzyme described by Axelrod (1954) in the rabbit liver is identical with the rat liver enzyme; however Axelrod found little enzymic activity on amphetamine in the rat liver. Both preparations require the presence of the reduced form of nicotinamide-adenine dinucleotide phosphate.

4. Microsomal demethylating enzymes

These enzymes can also be included under the general heading of "amine oxidases", since the reaction catalysed involves the oxidative fission of a C—N bond; the methyl group gives rise to formaldehyde:

$$R_1CHR_2N \cdot CH_3 + O_2 + H_2O \rightarrow R_1CHR_2NH + HCHO + H_2O_2$$

This was first shown by Axelrod (1953, 1955) for (—)-ephedrine; in these experiments rabbit liver microsomes were used. With rat and dog liver microsomes demethylation of ephedrine was much less, but this may have been due to the presence of an inhibitor, as addition of rat liver microsomes depressed the rate of demethylation of ephedrine by the rabbit liver preparation.

These findings are of interest in view of the observation that the *rabbit liver microsomal* preparation, in the presence of supernatant fraction, nicotinamide-adenine dinucleotide phosphate and semicarbazide, demethylated N,N-dimethyltryptamine, with the formation of N-methyltryptamine and formaldehyde (Szara and Axelrod 1959). Evidence for the formation of dimethyltryptamine-N-oxide was also obtained.

Experiments in rats showed that *N-methyltryptamine* was also formed in this species. These observations are of interest, since they raise the question as to the identity of the demethylating enzymes for ephedrine and the indolealkylamines.

II. Reactions of the phenolic hydroxyl groups

In addition to oxidative deamination of the indolealkylamines, there are enzymic reactions of the phenolic hydroxyl groups which have been studied. The physiological significance of some of these reactions is still unknown.

1. Hydroxyindole oxidases

An oxidation of *5-hydroxytryptamine*, possibly with formation of a quinone-imine, was first discussed by BLASCHKO and PHILPOT (1953), but no experimental evidence in favour of such a reaction was brought forward until PORTER, TITUS, SANDERS and SMITH (1957) reported an oxidation of 5-hydroxytryptamine by *caeruloplasmin*, the *copper*-containing oxidase of mammalian blood plasma. Although GELLER, EIDUSON and YUWILER (1959) were unable to find such an oxidation, the observation by PORTER et al. (1957) has since been confirmed by many authors (NAKAJIMA and THUILLIER 1958; MARTIN, ERIKSEN and BENDITT 1958; SANKAR 1959; ZARAFONETIS and KALAS 1960; LEVINE 1960; BLASCHKO and LEVINE 1960a; CURZON and VALLET 1960).

Another line of enquiry opened up with the finding by BLASCHKO and MILTON (1960), that 5-hydroxytryptamine was oxidized by an extract of the *gill plates* of *Mytilus edulis*. Some purification of the oxidase responsible was achieved later (BLASCHKO and LEVINE 1960a).

Caeruloplasmin is a copper-containing catalyst, and what is known of the *Mytilus* gill plate enzyme, e.g. its *inhibition by cyanide*, is compatible with the view that it also is a copper protein. That iron-containing proteins are also able to attack the phenolic hydroxyl group of 5-hydroxytryptamine, was shown by BLUM and LING (1959), who observed oxidation of the amine, with pigment formation, when it was incubated with denatured oxyhaemoglobin. The authors considered that the oxidation was brought about by a peroxidatic action, a suggestion supported by the observation of RODNIGHT (1958) that carbon monoxide inhibits this type of destruction of 5-hydroxytryptamine. Similarly, HORITA (1962) has demonstrated the oxidation of 5-hydroxytryptamine by the cytochrome-cytochrome oxidase system.

Table 1. *Relative rates of oxidation of different substrates by the hydroxyindole oxidase of Mytilus gill plates and by pig plasma caeruloplasmin* (BLASCHKO and LEVINE 1960a)

Substrate	Hydroxyindole oxidase from *Mytilus* gill plates	Pig plasma caeruloplasmin
4-hydroxytryptamine	520	700
5-hydroxytryptamine	100	100
7-hydroxytryptamine	100	1,100
Psilocine	145	230
Bufotenine	60	44
6-hydroxy analogue of bufotenine	55	170
N-methyl psilocine	120	—
N-methyl bufotenine	78	—
4-hydroxytryptophan	200	0
5-hydroxytryptophan	50	0
7-hydroxytryptophan	100	0
5-hydroxyindoleacetic acid	82	—
5-hydroxyindole	100	0
Paraphenylenediamine	150	6,000

It can thus be stated that both vertebrate and invertebrate enzymes are able to oxidize 5-hydroxytryptamine. It was already shown by BLASCHKO and MILTON (1960) that both *bufotenine* and *5-hydroxytryptophan* were also readily oxidized by the *Mytilus* gill plate enzyme, thus excluding an amine oxidase type of reaction. This led to a systematic study of the substrate specificites of both the *Mytilus* enzyme and pig plasma caeruloplasmin (BLASCHKO and LEVINE 1960a); in the course of this work it was found that indole derivatives substituted with a hydroxyl group in positions 4, 6 or 7 were also attacked. A table showing the rates of oxidation of various substrates, taken from the paper by BLASCHKO and LEVINE (1960a) is appended (Table 1).

The table shows that the substrate specificities are similar, but that there are also some differences. All the hydroxytryptamines tested were oxidized by both preparations, but the mammalian preparation did not act on any of the hydroxytryptophans tested (4-, 5- and 7-hydroxytryptophan), although these were oxidized by the *Mytilus* preparation at rates similar to the rates of oxidation of the corresponding amines.

Thus, we can say that this type of oxidation is widespread in animal preparations. The oxidation reaction, starting from 5-, 6-, or 7-hydroxy compounds, leads to melanin-like pigments. The oxidation product of 5-hydroxytryptamine by caeruloplasmin has been studied by BENDITT and his colleagues (ERIKSEN, MARTIN and BENDITT 1960; MARTIN, BENDITT and ERIKSEN 1960). It was postulated that one of the compounds, probably a precursor of the melanin-like pigment formed, was a dimer formed by dehydrogenative coupling of the benzene ring moieties of two molecules of 5-hydroxytryptamine.

The observations on the enzymic oxidation of the *4-hydroxyindole* compounds are of interest, since these substances do not form melanin-like compounds, but bright-blue substances some of which are water-soluble (BLASCHKO and LEVINE 1960a; HORITA and WEBER 1961; HORITA 1962).

It may be mentioned here that hydroxyindole oxidases may have a wider distribution in Molluscs; one of us has recently found an active enzyme of this type in the *crystalline style of Pinna nobilis*. It is of interest that the crystalline style enzyme will not only act on 5-hydroxytryptamine and on psilocine (on the latter also with the appearance of a blue pigment) but also on catecholamines. In other words, hydroxyindole oxidase activity may be a property of certain phenol oxidases. This agrees with the finding that hydroxyindole oxidase is cyanide-sensitive.

However, the ability to oxidize hydroxyindoles is by no means a property of all phenol oxidases. In Dr. E. BUEDING'S laboratory, MANSOUR (1958) has found that the phenol oxidase of *Fasciola hepatica (the liver fluke)* will readily act on catecholamines and on tyramine, but is without action on *5-hydroxytryptamine*. Yet, the latter is not entirely without effect: in 10^{-2} M concentration, 5-hydroxytryptamine almost completely *inhibits* the oxidation of 5×10^{-3} M tyramine. This inhibition is competitive.

We have confirmed MANSOUR'S statement that the Harding-Passey mouse melanoma oxidase hardly acts on 5-hydroxytryptamine; the preparation is also inactive with psilocine. Here too 5-hydroxytryptamine has an initial inhibitory effect on the oxidation of substrate, (L-dopa), but later the curves of oxygen consumption in the presence and absence of 5-hydroxytryptamine cross, suggesting that in the presence of substrate 5-hydroxytryptamine is oxidized. This is clearly demonstrated in the presence of both substrate (L-dopa) and psilocine; no initial depression of oxygen uptake was seen in the presence of psilocine, but there was an appearance of the typical blue colour, indicative of oxidation of the 4-hydroxyindole derivative (unpublished observation).

The phenol oxidase of fungi is of particular interest in view of the occurrence of 4-hydroxyindoles *(psilocine and psilocybine)* in these plants. We have tested the oxidation of both 5-hydroxytryptamine and psilocine by an extract of an acetone-dried powder of cultivated mushrooms. This preparation did not act on the hydroxyindoles, but the oxygen uptake in the presence of 2×10^{-3} M L-dopa was greatly enhanced when either of the two indolealkylamines was present. In the presence of psilocine, the typical blue colour appeared.

This observation is not without interest for the significance of psilocine in those species of *Psilocybe* in which psilocine or psilocybine occurs. We have, through the courtesy of Dr. A. HOFMANN, of Messrs. SANDOZ, Bâle, tested a dried preparation of *Psilocybe semperviva*. However, this was inactive with both L-dopa and psilocine. Since the condition of the preparation is not known, it must remain an open question whether or not these fungi contain an oxidase that will act on psilocine, either directly or indirectly, in the presence of a catechol substrate. It seems interesting that one of the members of this group is called *Psilocybe caerulescens* (HEIM 1959). One is tempted to speculate if these hydroxyindoles serve as regulators of oxygen uptake in the species in which they occur. Such a view would be in conformity with the theories of certain plant biochemists, who consider the phenolases as "terminal oxidases".

α) 5:6-Dihydroxytryptamine. The possibility that this compound may serve as a hormone in *Arthropods* (CARLISLE 1956) appears to have found confirmation in the work by CARLISLE and TIWARI (1961). This compound, prepared by SCHLOSSBERGER and KUCH (1960), was kindly given to us by Dr. H. G. SCHLOSSBERGER; we have found that it is oxidized by pig plasma caeruloplasmin and the Mytilus gill plate preparation (unpublished observation). In each case there was appearance of a dark colour. In assessing this result, we must remember that the action on 5:6-dihydroxytryptamine is probably a manifestation of the general catechol oxidase activity of these preparations.

2. Conjugases and dephosphorylase

Observations on intact animals, to be discussed below, make it certain that enzymic *conjugations* with *glucuronate* and *sulphate* occur in animals. The presence of *psilocybine* in fungi (discussed in other sections of this volume) also shows that *phosphorylation* reactions do occur. Nothing, however is known about the enzymes responsible for these reactions.

HORITA and WEBER (1961) in their study of the oxidation of psilocine have shown that rat kidney homogenates, by the action of alkaline phosphatase, rapidly convert psilocybine to psilocine. They discuss the possibility that psilocine is the pharmacologically active compound. A study of the enzymic hydrolysis in various animals shows that in the rat and the mouse the kidney was enzymically most active; in guinea-pig and rabbit the small intestine was the most active tissue. Heart and brain tissue also dephosphorylated psilocybine (see also HORITA and WEBER 1962).

3. Hydroxyindole-O-methyl transferase

The elucidation, by LERNER, of the chemical structure of *melatonin* led to a study of the O-methylation mechanism by AXELROD and WEISSBACH (1960, 1961). The method of enzyme assay employed was the study of the enzymic transfer of the methyl group from S-adenosylmethionine, labelled with C14 in the methyl group, to N-acetyl-5-hydroxytryptamine. A preparation from *bovine pineal glands* was prepared, purified by ammonium sulphate precipitation (45 to 68% saturation), followed by adsorption to, and subsequent elution from, alumina gel Cγ, until a final preparation was obtained that was 25 times as active as the crude homogenate. The pineal gland is the only organ in which this enzyme has been found; homogenates of pineal glands of *Macaca mulatta* had more than twice the activity, those of the cat about one-half, of that of the bovine glands. The N-acetyl derivative of 5-hydroxytryptamine was the substrate tested that was most rapidly attacked; if its rate of methylation be taken as 100, the corresponding rates were:

with bufotenine	14
with 5-hydroxyindoleacetic acid	12
with N-methyl-5-hydroxytryptamine	9
with 5-hydroxytryptamine	7
with 4-hydroxy-N-acetyltryptamine	8

No 5-hydroxyindole-O-methyl transferase was found in the "parotid" gland of *Bufo marinus*, the South American toad (MÄRKI, AXELROD and WITKOP 1962).

III. Introduction of the phenolic hydroxyl groups

A very unsatisfactory feature of our knowledge of the formation of 5-hydroxyindole derivatives in the animal body is our ignorance of the enzymic mechanism of the introduction of the phenolic hydroxyl group; this is fully discussed in the contribution of HAGEN and COHEN in this volume.

The introduction of the 4-hydroxyl group, as in psilocine, is also achieved by enzymes hitherto unidentified.

More is known about the mechanism of *6-hydroxylation*. JEPSON, UDENFRIEND and ZALTZMANN (1959) demonstrated the enzymic conversion of *tryptamine* to 6-hydroxytryptamine by rabbit liver microsomes. Other lipid-soluble indoles were also hydroxylated. Similarly, SZARA and AXELROD (1959) described a preparation of rabbit liver microsomes which in the presence of nicotinamide-adenine dinucleotide phosphate, soluble supernatant fraction from liver and semicarbazide, produced a phenolic amine that was, after some initial uncertainty over the exact position of the hydroxyl group, identified as the 6-hydroxy derivative of *dimethyltryptamine*.

In subsequent publications these findings have been extended (SZARA 1961; SZARA and PUTNEY 1961; SZARA, HEARST and PUTNEY 1960): *N,N-diethyltryptamine* was shown to be similarly 6-hydroxylated; rat liver microsomes were shown to convert both α-methyltryptamine and 3-indolylacetone to the corresponding 6-hydroxy compounds (SZARA 1961). Rat liver microsomes incubated with nicotinamide-adenine dinucleotide phosphate and magnesium ions were able to bring about this reaction. SZARA and PUTNEY (1961) found that brain microsomes were not able to catalyse this reaction, but that many lipid-soluble indole derivatives reacted with the rat or rabbit liver microsome system. The hydroxylation could be inhibited by either chlorpromazine or reserpine.

IV. Introduction of N-methyl groups

An *enzyme* capable of *N-methylating 5-hydroxytryptamine* has recently been described by AXELROD (1961, 1962a). This enzyme has a number of remarkable properties. First of all, it occurs in high concentration in *rabbit lungs*; apart from the rabbit it has only been found, and in small amounts, in one human lung, but not in others. No activity has been detected in similar preparations from lungs of rat, mouse, guinea-pig, cat and monkey (*Macaca mulatta* ?). In the rabbit, there was also some activity in these tissues (in decreasing order of activity): adrenal gland, kidney, spleen, heart and liver; there was no activity in extracts of brain, hypothalamus, intestines and salivary gland. Secondly, there is a wide spectrum of substrate specificities; some of the substances tested are shown here:

5-hydroxytryptamine	100	(—)-metanephrine	38
N-methyl-5-hydroxytryptamine	70	Dopamine	16
Tryptamine	81	N-methyldopamine (epinine)	43
4-hydroxytryptamine	22	(—)-noradrenaline	23
6-hydroxytryptamine	65	(—)-adrenaline	13
Tyramine	54	Aniline	85
N-methyltyramine	54	Indole	0
Octopamine	12	Mescaline	37
(±)-ephedrine	21		

Bufotenine appears not to have been investigated as a possible substrate.

The rabbit lung enzyme is a soluble enzyme; it resembles all the other methyl transferases in that it transfers the methyl group of S-adenosylmethionine. The enzyme was inhibited by *p*-chloromercuribenzoic acid, a reagent for sulphydryl groups. Chlorpromazine was a strong inhibitor, causing 45% inhibition in a concentration of 2.5×10^{-5} M. Imipramine, in 10^{-4} M concentration, halved the rate of methylation of 5-hydroxytryptamine.

The enzyme responsible for the N-methylation of noradrenaline, phenylethanolamine-N-methyl transferase, does not act on tryptamine or its 5-hydroxy derivative (AXELROD 1962b). This enzyme, which occurs mainly in the adrenal gland, will not N-methylate some sympathomimetic amines that are substrates of the rabbit lung transferase, e.g., dopamine, amphetamine or tyramine.

The only other source of an "unspecific" *N-methyl transferase* system described occurs in the *South American toad (Bufo marinus)*. The *"parotid"* gland of this animal yields a preparation that will N-methylate 5-hydroxytryptamine, its mono-N-methyl derivative, tryptamine, as well as a number of sympathomimetic amines (MÄRKI et al. 1962).

V. N-acetylase

WEISSBACH, REDFIELD and AXELROD (1960) were able to obtain from homogenates of *rat liver* and of *bovine pineal glands* supernatant fractions that were able to convert 5-hydroxytryptamine to *N-acetyl-5-hydroxytryptamine.* The latter was identified not only by paper chromatography but also enzymically, by demonstrating its conversion to melatonin. The active fractions required the presence of ethylene diamine tetra-acetate and an acetyl-coenzyme-A generating system (coenzyme A and phosphotransacetylase). Rat brain was also active, but the enzyme system appeared more labile.

VI. Oxidative deamination and transamination involving 5-hydroxytryptophan

Reactions involving the formation of 5-hydroxyindolepyruvic acid are of interest because of the possibility that pathways involving this oxo-acid give rise to 5-hydroxyindoleacetic acid (see BLASCHKO and HOPE 1955; UDENFRIEND, TITUS, WEISSBACH and PETERSON 1956).

1. Amino-acid oxidases

BLASCHKO and HOPE (1955, 1956) tested two preparations using DL-5-hydroxytryptophan as substrate; with a preparation from the digestive gland of *Mytilus edulis,* a source of a typical L-amino-acid oxidase, they found these rates of oxygen uptake:

with L-*tryptophan*	60 $\mu l\ O_2$
with DL-*5-hydroxytryptophan* . .	19 $\mu l\ O_2$
with L-phenylalanine	108 $\mu l\ O_2$
with L-tyrosine	110 $\mu l\ O_2$

In another experiment (BLASCHKO and HOPE, unpublished) the L-amino-acid oxidase of *cobra venom* was tested. It may be mentioned that the most active sample used was one collected in India in 1899. Of this sample, 5 mg consumed in the first 15 minutes:

with 10^{-2} M L-tryptophan	195 $\mu l\ O_2$
with 2×10^{-2} M DL-5-hydroxytryptophan .	68 $\mu l\ O_2$

Thus, L-amino-acid oxidase of both vertebrate and invertebrate origin acted on 5-hydroxytryptophan.

2. Transaminases

SANDLER, SPECTOR, RUTHVEN and DAVISON (1960) first demonstrated that *5-hydroxytryptophan* was transaminated in a reaction in which the oxo-acid accepting the amino group was α-oxoglutarate. They suggested that this enzyme, that they found in *rat liver*, was possibly identical with the transaminase for L-*tryptophan*. This was confirmed by SPENCER and ZAMCHEK (1960). There is reason to believe that the rat liver enzyme is less specific than was originally believed: JACOBY and LA DU (1962) have presented evidence that suggests that one and the same enzyme in rat liver acts on tyrosine, phenylalanine and tryptophan.

HAAVALDSEN (1962) has found that liver is not the only tissue that will transaminate 5-hydroxytryptophan; he has described a transaminase for this amino acid in *rat brain* that will use either α-oxoglutarate or pyruvate as acceptors.

C. Metabolism of indolealkylamines

I. Metabolites arising from deamination reactions

1. Metabolites of tryptamine and of its N-methylated derivatives

Although the occurrence of tryptamine derivatives in mammals was securely established only when 5-hydroxytryptamine was identified a little over ten years ago, it had been known for some time that tryptamine is metabolized. In 1913, EWINS and LAIDLAW fed tryptamine to a *dog* and isolated from the *urine* a compound that they identified as *indoleaceturic acid*, the product of condensation of indoleacetic acid and glycine (see also GUGGENHEIM and LÖFFLER 1916):

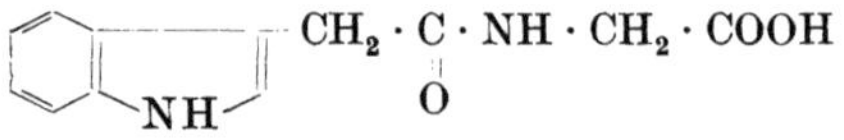

Indoleaceturic acid

WEISSBACH, KING, SJOERDSMA and UDENFRIEND (1959) have since described observations indicating that *indole-3-acetic* acid is a normal metabolite. They estimate that in *normal human urine* about 5—18 mg of the acid are excreted in 24 hrs, but that in certain abnormal conditions the excretion of the acid may rise to as much as ten times this amount. The acid is present partly free, partly in a form from which it is set free by acid hydrolysis. Pathological conditions in which indole-3-acetic acid excretion was high were: *diabetes*, FRIEDREICH'S *ataxia*, *progressive muscular dystrophy, amyotrophic lateral sclerosis and idiopathic sprue*. In a case of *sprue* 53—67 mg of the free acid, and 175—220 mg of total acid, as determined after acid hydrolysis, were excreted in 24 hrs. *Loading* the *diet* with L-*tryptophan* (20 mg per kg of body weight) led to an increase mainly of free *indole-3-acetic acid*. It may be mentioned that there was no concomitant increase in the excretion of 5-hydroxyindoleacetic acid (5-HIAA) in this experiment. The authors believe that both bacterial and mammalian enzymes are involved. Most of the acid is believed to arise, by transamination in the presence of both α-oxoglutarate and pyridoxal-5-phosphate, from indolyl-3-pyruvic acid, bypassing the amine stage. However, WEISSBACH et al. (1959) found that mammalian tissues (kidney and liver) as well as faecal bacteria formed tryptamine from L-tryptophan. Some of the acid, therefore, was probably derived from tryptamine by oxidation. We can summarize these findings by saying that the ultimate source of indole-3-acetic acid is L-tryptophan, but that it remains open how much of this had first been converted to tryptamine.

The work just quoted was preceded by a study of the urinary excretion of metabolites after administration of tryptamine and its N-methylated derivatives in the *rat*. ERSPAMER (1955) identified both *indoleacetic* and *indoleaceturic acids* as metabolites of *tryptamine*, *N-methyltryptamine* and *N,N-dimethyltryptamine*. With increasing methyl substitution the percentage recoveries of the acids decreased: 85 p.c. recovery from tryptamine, 36 p.c. from N-methyltryptamine and 17 p.c. from N,N-dimethyltryptamine. The low recovery of the acid from the tertiary amine is what would be expected from what is known of the metabolic fate of the compound *in vitro*.

This may also be an appropriate place to refer to the work of ARMSTRONG, SHAW, GORTAKOWSKI and SINGER (1958), who have made a careful paper-chromatographic study of over a hundred *normal human urines*. They identified and characterized numerous compounds, all *indole derivatives*. However, the question as to the origin of these substances, listed in Table 2, was left open.

Table 2.
List of some indole derivatives identified in normal human urine (ARMSTRONG et al. 1958)

Indole-3-carboxaldehyde	β-(indole-3)-propionic acid
Indole-3-carboxylic acid	β-(indole-3)-acrylic acid
Indole-3-glyoxylic acid	Tryptophan
Indole-3-glyoxylamide	N-acetyl tryptophan
Indole-3-glycolic acid Na	5-hydroxyindole
Indole-3-acetic acid	5-hydroxyindole-2-carboxylic acid
Indole-3-acetamide	5-hydroxyindole-3-carboxylic acid
Indoleaceturic acid	5-hydroxyindole-3-acetic acid
N-(indole-3-acetyl)-α-alanine	β-(5-hydroxyindole-3)-lactic acid
N-(indole-3-acetyl)-β-alanine	5-hydroxytryptophan
N-(indole-3-acetyl)-β-amino*iso*butyric acid	5-methoxyindole
N-(indole-3-acetyl)-γ-aminobutyric acid	5-methoxyindole-2-carboxylic acid
N-(indole-3-acetyl)-aspartic acid	5-methoxyindole-3-carboxylic acid
N-(indole-3-acetyl)-glutamic acid	5-methoxyindole-3-acetic acid
N-(indole-3-acetyl)-glutamine	β-(5-methoxyindole-3)-lactic acid
β-(indole-3)-pyruvic acid	5-methoxytryptophan
β-(indole-3)-pyruvic acid oxime	2-pyrrolecarboxylic acid
β-(indole-3)-lactic acid	

ARMSTRONG et al. (1958) give these quantitative data on the excretion in *normal human urine*:

Indole-3-acetic acid	1—10 μg per mg of creatinine excreted
Indolelactic acid	0.2—2 μg per mg of creatinine excreted
Indoleacetylglutamine	1—3 μg per mg of creatinine excreted
5-hydroxyindoleacetic acid . .	1—5 μg per mg of creatinine excreted

2. Metabolites of 5-hydroxytryptamine and related amines

a) 5-Hydroxytryptamine

The role of amine oxidase in the catabolism of 5-hydroxytryptamine was independently and almost simultaneously established in work from UDENFRIEND'S and ERSPAMER'S laboratories (TITUS and UDENFRIEND 1954; UDENFRIEND, TITUS and WEISSBACH 1955; UDENFRIEND, TITUS, WEISSBACH and PETERSON 1956; ERSPAMER 1954, 1955, 1956). This work elucidated what is now known to be the main pathway of 5-hydroxytryptamine breakdown, the oxidative deamination of the amine by amine oxidase, followed by a further oxidation of the aldehyde formed, to give the corresponding carboxylic acid, *5-hydroxyindoleacetic acid* (5-HIAA):

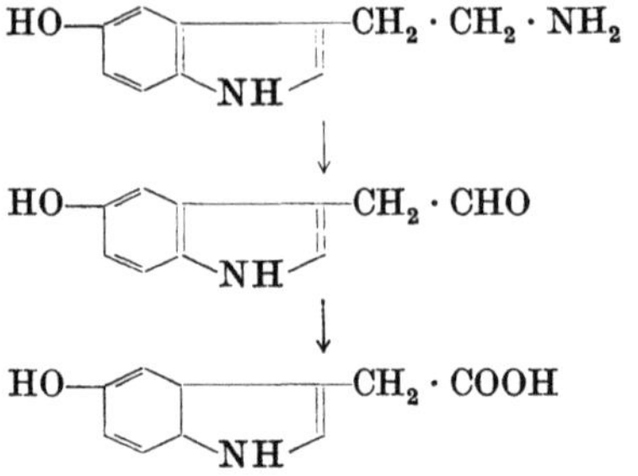

5-Hydroxytryptamine

5-Hydroxyindolylaldehyde

5-HIAA

This is the general pathway of biological inactivation of amines in the animal body (see BLASCHKO 1952b).

The work of UDENFRIEND and of ERSPAMER has given rise to a great volume of observations on the excretion of 5-HIAA in man and in animals. In these observations it has been established that 5-HIAA could be derived both from endogenous and from exogenous 5-hydroxytryptamine (and 5-hydroxytryptophan). To quote only one example of amine from an exogenous source: ANDERSON, ZIEGLER and DOEDEN (1958) discovered the high 5-hydroxytryptamine content of *bananas* in their study of the urinary excretion of 5-HIAA in monkeys and in children. ERSPAMER (1961) gives a number of references to papers in which an increased output of 5-HIAA was reported after administration of the amine in animals and in man; since then, ERSPAMER and BERTACCINI (1962) have published new observations on the fate of *administered* — *orally* and *parenterally* — LD-*5-hydroxytryptophan* in rats. They found that administration of large doses of the racemic amino acid led to an increase in the excretion not only of 5-HIAA but also of its glucuronide.

The discovery by LEMBECK (1953) of *5-hydroxytryptamine* in a *carcinoid* tumour *(enterochromaffinoma)* was followed by that of a great increase in the *urinary* excretion of *5-HIAA* in this condition (PAGE, CORCORAN, UDENFRIEND, SJOERDSMA and WEISSBACH 1955; SJOERDSMA, WEISSBACH and UDENFRIEND 1955; UDENFRIEND, WEISSBACH and SJOERDSMA 1956).

Conversely, after *removal of the large intestine in man* the *urinary* excretion of *5-HIAA* is markedly *reduced* (HAVERBACK and DAVIDSON 1958; BERTACCINI and CHIEPPA 1960). The latter authors report a decrease in the 24 hr interval from 3.04 ± 1.24 mg in normal control subjects to 1.44 ± 0.39 mg in operated subjects (see also BERTACCINI 1958).

The *excretion of 5-HIAA*, its basic value and its increase, due either to an increased turnover of endogenous amine or in response to an increased intake of the amine or its precursor, leave no doubt that the determination of the level of 5-HIAA can serve as a useful index of the metabolism of 5-hydroxytryptamine. The most important clinical application is in the diagnosis of enterochromaffinoma.

However, it is still uncertain to whait extent we are permitted to use the urinary excretion of 5-HIAA as a quant tative indicator of the breakdown of 5-hydroxytryptamine *in vivo*.

The considerations that limit the use of the measurement of the urinary output of 5-HIAA can be conveniently discussed under these headings:

α) 5-HIAA may arise from 5-hydroxytryptophan without the intermediate formation of 5-hydroxytryptamine.

β) Oxidative deamination of the amine may occur, but the aldehyde formed as the first reaction product may not be further oxidized to give 5-HIAA.

γ) Rupture of the indole ring may occur.

δ) 5-Hydroxytryptamine may be metabolized by other routes: N-acetylation, O-methylation or O-conjugation, and

ε) 5-Hydroxytryptamine may be excreted unchanged.

ad α) 5-HIAA may be formed by reactions that bypass the amine, by way of 5-hydroxyindolepyruvic acid, in transamination or oxidative deamination. However, although such reactions are known to occur *in vitro* it is at present not known how important they are in metabolism. One suspects that they are more likely to occur with ingested 5-hydroxytryptophan than when the amino acid is formed *in vivo.*

ad β) The possibility of alternate reactions of the aldehyde was first discussed when the appearance of a dark pigment in the *oxidative deamination of 5-hydroxytryptamine* was described (see BLASCHKO 1958); it was believed that *pigment formation* was due to a condensation reaction of the aldehyde formed in the oxidative deamination catalysed by amine oxidase.

The possibility that the *low* excretion of 5-HIAA in *herbivores* (rabbit and guinea-pig) is due to reactions of the aldehyde other than oxidation to the carboxylic acid is also discussed by NAKAI (1958).

A possibly more important source of error under this heading has recently come to light in the work of KVEDER, ISKRIĆ and KEGLEVIĆ (1962). These authors administered C14-labelled 5-hydroxytryptamine to rats and showed that the *O-glucuronide of 5-hydroxytryptophol* was a major *metabolite;* some of the *O-sulphate* of *5-hydroxytryptophol* was also excreted. These observations indicate the following two pathways of breakdown of 5-hydroxytryptamine, both involving oxidative deamination:

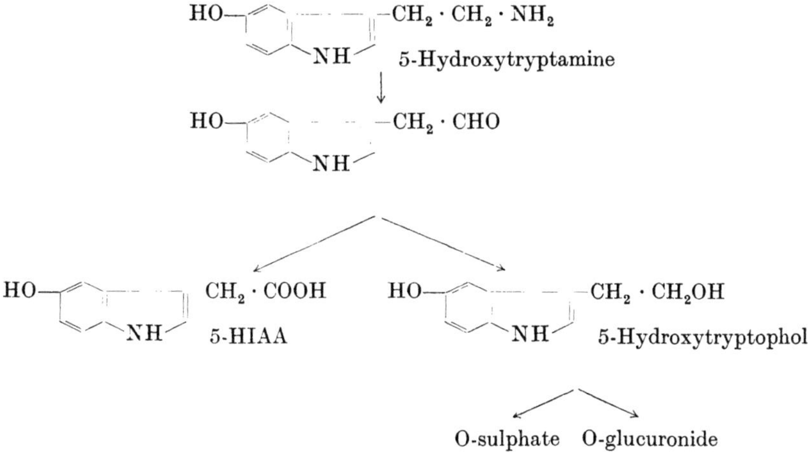

KVEDER et al. (1962) *question* the importance of *N-acetyl-5-hydroxytryptamine* as a major metabolite of 5-hydroxytryptamine (see MCISAAC and PAGE 1959). It may be mentioned here that the *N-acetyl* derivative was found in *rat urine* after the administration of 5-hydroxytryptamine by WEISSBACH, LOVENBERG, REDFIELD and UDENFRIEND (1961), but in amounts smaller than those reported by MCISAAC and PAGE (1959). Both WEISSBACH et al. (1961) and KVEDER et al. (1962) discuss the possibility of an "amine oxidation" insensitive to the known inhibitors of "mono" amine oxidase. The possibility that amine oxidases akin to the mammalian plasma oxidases discussed above may act, must be borne in mind but no evidence for the presence of such enzymes in the tissues of the rat has hitherto been obtained.

It may be mentioned that *5-hydroxytryptophol* as a metabolite of the amine in mammals has its counterpart in the catecholamine series; these are observations that originated with the isolation of what was first described as "substance Z" and eventually identified as ω-hydroxy-acetovanillone (see v. EUW, NEHER, REICHSTEIN, TAIT, TAIT and WETTSTEIN 1959; AXELROD, KOPIN and MANN 1959).

ad γ) There is no positive evidence in favour of the suggestion that hydroxyindole oxidase might be active *in vivo* and initiate a pathway of breakdown that would lead to a rupture of the indole ring. Conditions under which such oxidases might operate in the living animal have been discussed elsewhere (BLASCHKO and LEVINE 1960c); it was pointed out that the situation for 5-hydroxytryptamine is somewhat analogous to that for adrenaline, where the possibility of the formation of adrenochrome has been discussed for a long time, without satisfactory evidence forthcoming so far.

ad δ) There can be no doubt that both O-methylation and N-acetylation of 5-hydroxytryptamine can occur; this has been discussed already. As already mentioned, the work of KVEDER et al. (1962) throws some doubt on the extent of N-acetylation.

ad ε) The *urinary* excretion of *5-hydroxytryptamine*, first suggested by TWAROG and PAGE (1953) and supported by the observations of RODNIGHT (1956) and others (see ERSPAMER 1961), is well-established. However, the contribution of the excretion of the free amine to the total catabolism of the 5-hydroxyindoles is small.

Since ERSPAMER's (1961) review, ERSPAMER and BERTACCINI (1962) have reported observations on rats that had received the racemic form of *5-hydroxytryptophan* by various routes. Whereas after the *administration* of the amine the amounts of free amine excreted in the urine were small, amounting to about 1.5 p.c. or less of the dose administered (see also GESSNER, KHAIRALLAH, McISAAC and PAGE 1960), after the intraperitoneal injection of the amino acid, the amine excreted could amount to as much as one-quarter of the L-form of the amino acid administered.

In man, free 5-hydroxytryptamine was first found in patients with carcinoid tumours (PERNOW and WALDENSTRÖM 1954). For a recent classification of carcinoid tumours excreting both 5-hydroxytryptamine and 5-hydroxytryptophan see WILLIAMS and SANDLER 1963; PEART, PORTER, ROBERTSON, SANDLER and BALDOCK 1963.

Summing up the findings discussed so far we can say that the importance of *amine oxidase* as a major instrument for the *biological inactivation of 5-hydroxytryptamine* is firmly established. In contrast to the urinary indoleacetic acid, which seems mainly, although not exclusively, derived from tryptophan via the oxo-acid, most of the 5-HIAA excreted in the urine appears to have passed through the stage of free 5-hydroxytryptamine, and provided that known exogenous sources of 5-hydroxytryptophan or of 5-hydroxytryptamine are excluded, most of the acid seems to be "endogenous", that is to say, material that has been 5-hydroxylated *in vivo*, probably with the amine contributing the major portion. This still leaves an uncertainty, the fate of much of the 5-hydroxytryptamine that is not excreted as 5-HIAA. ERSPAMER (1955) has given several instances of the recovery of 5-HIAA after administration of 5-hydroxytryptamine. The recovery *varied* from *species* to species; in the guinea-pig it was 0.5—1 p.c., in the rabbit 1—1.5 p.c., in the rat 5.5—33 p.c., in the dog 25 p.c. and in man 20—52 p.c. It is particularly interesting that *5-HIAA* was readily detected in the *urine* of *young ruminants*, but absent from that of *adult* animals. It is known that in newborn ruminants the plasma oxidases are absent or poorly developed (Blaschko and Hawes 1959; Blaschko and Bonney 1962), but it is unknown if these observations can account for the differences in the 5-HIAA excretion. It may be mentioned that caeruloplasmin, a mammalian hydroxyindole oxidase. is also absent from the blood plasma or poorly developed at birth (Elsner, Hornykiewicz, Lindner and Niebauer 1953; Scheinberg and Sternlieb 1960).

b) Other 5-hydroxyindolealkylamines

According to Erspamer (1955), *excretion* of *5-HIAA* after administration to rats of *bufotenidine*, the fully N-methylated quaternary onium compound derived from 5-hydroxytryptamine, was doubtful, but with the tertiary amine, *bufotenine*. *5-HIAA* was definitely identified as a *metabolite*. In addition, unchanged bufotenine was also recovered from the urine. This observation is in keeping with the slow oxidation of bufotenine by amine oxidase; this has already been discussed.

Gessner, Khairallah, McIsaac and Page (1960) have since reported that after subcutaneous or intraperitoneal injection of bufotenine in rats an average of 22 p.c. of unchanged *bufotenine* and of 7 p.c. of *5-HIAA* was found in the urine in the first 48 hrs; conjugation with glucuronic acid was doubtful. The authors suggest that the longlasting effects of the tertiary amines, *bufotenine* and *psilocybine*, are related to their *relative immunity* from the action of *amine oxidase*.

c) Derivatives of 5-hydroxyindoles

Erspamer, Glässer and Nobili (1961) have found that both *5-hydroxy-N-acetyltryptophan* and *5-acetoxy-N-acetyltryptophan*, administered intraperitoneally to rats, are *hydrolysed*, the latter first by removal of the O-acetyl group; then further hydrolysis removes the N-acetyl group. A surprising result was that of the two substances administered a relatively large portion is excreted as free 5-hydroxytryptamine; the authors take this as an indication that the hydrolytic removal of the N-acetyl group occurs mainly in the kidneys; removal of the N-acetyl group is immediately followed by decarboxylation of the 5-hydroxytryptophan, also in the kidneys.

3. 4-Hydroxyindoles

Work on these compounds has been stimulated by the discovery of the two hallucinogenic amines *psilocybine* and *psilocine* and by the elucidation of their chemical constitution (Hofmann, Heim, Brack, Kobel, Frey, Ott, Petrzilka and Troxler 1959). On finding that the L-form of 4-hydroxytryptophan was a substrate of the mammalian decarboxylase (Erspamer, Glässer, Pasini and Stoppani 1961), the metabolic fate of both *4-hydroxytryptophan* and *4-hydroxytryptamine* was investigated (Erspamer, Glässer, Nobili and Pasini 1960; Erspamer and Nobili 1961, 1962). 4-DL-Hydroxytryptophan was administered to rats, orally, subcutaneously or intraperitoneally, and to human subjects by mouth. Six urinary metabolites were definitely identified: *4-hydroxytryptophan*, *4-hydroxytryptamine* and *4-HIAA*, together with their *glucuronides* (the enteric juice of *Helix* served as source of β-glucuronidase for the chromatographic identification). Of these metabolites, the glucuronides were demonstrated only in rat's urine; they were not found in human urine.

In assessing these results, it must be remembered that of the racemic amino acid probably the L-form only is metabolized by decarboxylation. The traces of free amine, therefore, can with a high degree of certainty be considered as derived from the L-form.

It is of interest that in the experiments in *man*, with doses of 200—1000 mg of the DL-amino acid ingested, only about 10—12 p.c. appeared as 4-HIAA in the urine; the amine represented about 3—5 p.c. of the dose given. In the rat, 25—40 p.c. of the dose could be accounted for as the 4-hydroxyindoles and their O-glucuronides, with the latter contributing an important fraction. No evidence of excretion of an O-sulphate or of N-acetyl-4-hydroxytryptamine was obtained. In view of the ease of oxidation of 4-hydroxytryptamine by hydroxyindole oxidases one is wondering if such an oxidation might have contributed to the breakdown of the 4-hydroxyindoles. However, this possibility has not hitherto been explored.

GESSNER et al. (1960) report that in rat urine about 11 p.c. of unchanged psilocybine appears after 48 hrs; there also is some evidence fort he excretion of a glucuronide.

II. N-Acetylated metabolites

Although the work, already quoted (WEISSBACH et al. 1961; ERSPAMER and BERTACCINI 1962; KVEDER et al. 1962) throws some doubt on the quantitative importance of N-acetylation as a metabolic route for the breakdown of 5-hydroxytryptamine, it seems unsafe at present to rule it out altogether. We have to remember the observations, also quoted already, on the occurrence of an N-acetylase acting on 5-hydroxytryptamine in rat and bovine tissues (WEISSBACH, REDFIELD and AXELROD 1960). Although such an enzyme, at least in the pineal gland, is probably mainly concerned with the formation of melatonin, it seems interesting that the rat liver also contains the enzyme. It seems therefore at present advisable to keep the possibility in mind that in some species at least N-acetylation may contribute to the biological inactivation of 5-hydroxytryptamine, although it may be less important than originally believed by McISAAC and PAGE (1959).

III. Excretion of O-sulphates

There is some doubt as to the extent to which O-sulphate formation contributes to the breakdown of 5-hydroxytryptamine. CHADWICK and WILKINSON (1960) incubated rat liver homogenates with the amine, and they isolated a compound that they tentatively identified as the O-sulphate of 5-hydroxytryptamine. They also reported that of the amine administered, about 30 p.c. was excreted as 5-HIAA, and that of this amount again 70 p.c. was excreted as the O-sulphate of 5-HIAA. This statement sill lacks confirmation by other observers. ERSPAMER and BERTACCINI (1962) have tentatively identified one of the substances of which they obtained evidence by paper chromatography as the *O-sulphate* of *5-hydroxytryptamine*, and KVEDER et al. (1962) discuss the possibility that one of the metabolites of 5-hydroxytryptamine is the O-sulphate of 5-hydroxytryptophol.

However, there is good evidence, to be discussed below, that the *O-sulphate* of *6-hydroxymelatonin* is a principal metabolite in the catabolism of melatonin (KOPIN, PARE, AXELROD and WEISSBACH 1961). It is of interest that *etryptamine*, 3-(2-aminobutyl) indole, is reported to be *excreted* as the *O-sulphate* and the *O-glucuronide* (EBERTS and DANIELS 1962).

IV. Excretion of O-glucuronides

There is little doubt that in some species of mammals the *O-glucuronide of 5-hydroxytryptamine* is an important *metabolite* of the amine. This was first studied by WEISSBACH, REDFIELD and UDENFRIEND (1958) and by MCISAAC and PAGE (1959); the latter authors found the O-glucuronide of 5-hydroxytryptamine as a major metabolite in the rabbit.

WEISSBACH et al. (1961) studied the presence of radioactive metabolites in mice after administering C14-labelled 5-hydroxytryptamine. The mice were killed $1\frac{1}{2}$ hrs after receiving 1 mg of the amine. In normal mice 30 p.c. of the total radioactivity was recovered as the O-glucuronide; in mice that had previously received a dose of iproniazid the percentage rose to 70. In *mouse urine*, collected for 12 hrs after giving 250 mg/kg of 5-hydroxytryptamine, 30 p.c. was present as the *O-glucuronide*; this value was 73 p.c. in urine from iproniazid-treated mice. The *O-glucuronide of 5-HIAA* was also present, mainly in the animals not treated with the inhibitor of amine oxidase; in the former it amounted to about 10 p.c. of the total radioactivity recovered. The authors mention that in urine from patients suffering from malignant *carcinoid (enterochromaffinoma)* the *O-glucuronide* was *a minor metabolite*, together with a little N-acetyl-5-hydroxytryptamine.

That the O-glucuronide of 5-hydroxytryptophol is excreted in rat urine after administration of the amine, has already been discussed (KVEDER et al. 1962).

It may be worthwhile to mention that the method of identification of the O-glucuronide employed by WEISSBACH et al. (1961) was an enzymic method, the fluorometric assay of the free amine formed after incubation with bacterial β-glucuronidase.

V. Formation and excretion of phenolic compounds

Experiments on tissue preparations in which hydroxylation reactions occur, have already been described. There is good evidence to show that these reactions also take place in the intact organism. SZARA and AXELROD (1959) demonstrated that N,N-dimethyltryptamine, administered intraperitoneally to rats led to the appearance of these excretion products in the urine: unaltered *dimethyltryptamine, N-methyltryptamine, indole-3-acetic acid, 6-HIAA, tryptamine, the N-oxides* of both dimethyltryptamine and its 6-hydroxy derivative.

Similarly, after the intraperitoneal injection of α-methyltryptamine in *rats* both 6-hydroxy-α-methyltryptamine, its O-glucuronide as well as the *O-glucuronide* of *6-hydroxy-3-indolylacetone* were *excreted*, indicating that not only substances that are substrates of the classical amine oxidase, but also those that are substrates of microsomal deaminating enzymes undergo this type of hydroxylation (SZARA 1961). Incidentally, the excretion of the acetone derivative clearly shows that the microsomal deaminating enzyme also operates *in vivo*.

Similarly EBERTS and DANIELS (1962) have obtained evidence that sulphate or glucuronide conjugates of its 6-hydroxylated derivative are the principal metabolites of *etryptamine*, 3-(2-aminobutyl)-1-indole. Here also evidence for the occurrence of the microsomal type of oxidative deamination was obtained.

In order to understand the biological significance of these 6-hydroxylation reactions, we must remember that there exists one compound that is present in the body and is normally metabolized by 6-hydroxylation; this is melatonin (see below). An enzyme of this kind is therefore operative not exclusively on substances foreign to the body.

Whether indole compounds with a free 5-hydroxyl group are able to be thus hydroxylated in position 6, is unknown. In view of the instability of the

5,6-dihydroxyindole compound that would arise in such a reaction it might be difficult to demonstrate the occurrence of this type of reaction.

VI. Metabolism of melatonin

Our knowledge of the pathway of synthesis of this hormone is due to the work of AXELROD and his colleagues (WEISSBACH, REDFIELD and AXELROD 1960; AXELROD and WEISSBACH 1961). Beginning from 5-hydroxytryptamine, the work suggested that this amine was N-acetylated, and that *N-acetyl-5-hydroxytryptamine* was *O-methylated.* The enzymes involved in these conversions have already been discussed.

The metabolic fate of melatonin was studied by injecting melatonin tritiated in the acetyl group intravenously into rats. After 30 minutes, melatonin itself

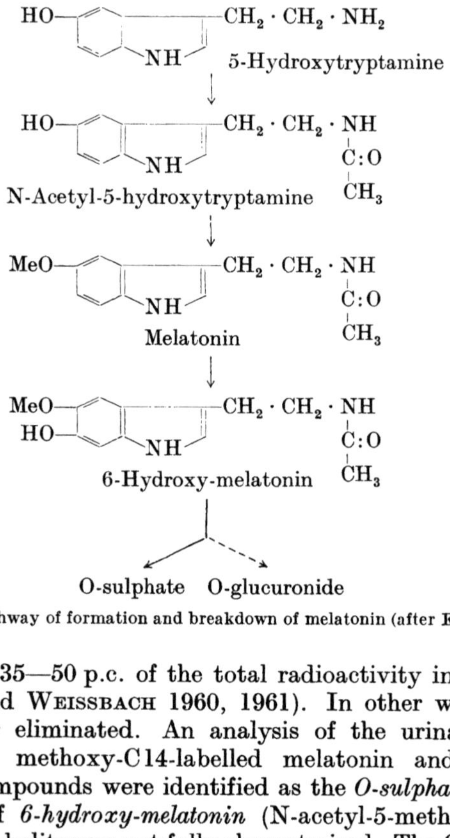

Fig. 3. Main pathway of formation and breakdown of melatonin (after KOPIN et al. 1961)

accounted for only 35—50 p.c. of the total radioactivity in the tissues (KOPIN, PARE, AXELROD and WEISSBACH 1960, 1961). In other words, it was rapidly either destroyed or eliminated. An analysis of the urinary metabolites was carried out, using methoxy-C14-labelled melatonin and acetyl-H3-labelled melatonin. Two compounds were identified as the *O-sulphate* and the *O-glucuronide* respectively of *6-hydroxy-melatonin* (N-acetyl-5-methoxy-6-hydroxytryptamine); a third metabolite was not fully characterized. The O-sulphate accounted for 70—80 p.c. of the total radioactivity of the urine; it thus represented the major metabolite of melatonin. The O-glucuronide accounted for about 5 p.c. of the radioactivity, and the unidentified compound for about 12 p.c.

These experiments have been supplemented by work on *liver microsomes,* suspended with a system that provides reduced nicotinamide-adenine dinucleotide phosphate; under these conditions a substance with the chromatographic properties of *6-hydroxy-melatonin* was formed upon incubation (KOPIN et al. 1961).

From the work just described a sequence of metabolic steps has been proposed which is considered as the main pathway of biosynthesis and breakdown of melatonin, at least in mammals (see Fig. 3). This pathway does not account for the *presence* in the *bovine pineal gland* of *5-methoxyindoleacetic acid* (LERNER and CASE 1960). Several possibilities may account for the presence of this substance: it may represent a stage of the breakdown of that portion of 5-hydroxytryptamine in the gland that is not required for melatonin synthesis, formed either by O-methylation from 5-HIAA, or by oxidative deamination of 5-methoxytryptamine, or it is an indication of an alternative mode of breakdown of melatonin in the bovine pineal gland: hydrolytic removal of the N-acetyl group, followed by oxidative deamination of the 5-methoxytryptamine formed.

That 5-methoxytryptamine is almost quantitatively excreted as 5-methoxyindoleacetic acid, after administration of amine labelled with C14 in the β-carbon atom, has been established by MCISAAC, KVEDER and PAGE (1960). It may be recalled that in the earlier work of ERSPAMER (1955) the recovery of 5-methoxyindoleacetic acid, after the administration of larger amounts of 5-methoxytryptamine, was 40—42 p.c. when the amine was given by mouth, and 71 p.c. after subcutaneous injection.

D. Summary

The study of the breakdown of the indolealkylamines described on the preceding pages is of interest for several reasons. We have already learnt to value the determination of the urinary 5-HIAA as a diagnostic tool. In addition we may hope, as our knowledge of the urinary metabolites of these amines gets more complete, to obtain a reliable estimate of the turnover of the naturally occurring compounds of this group.

For the pharmacologist the fate of a biologically active compound is of interest as an aid for the understanding of the time course of its action. Some of the limitations of this approach have already been discussed in the opening paragraphs of this review.

It has been established in the past decade that the inactivation of the sympathomimetic amines and histamine may proceed by more than one pathway. One of these is always initiated by oxidative deamination, catalysed by one or several of the amine oxidases, but there is also O-methylation with the catechol amines and N-methylation (and, in some species, N-acetylation) with histamine.

For 5-hydroxytryptamine oxidative deamination is also an important pathway. However, there are observations suggesting that amine oxidase is not a factor that determines intensity or time course of the response of the excitable tissue. VANE (1959) has found that the contraction of the plain muscle of the *rat's gastric fundus* preparation in response to a number of *indolealkylamines* is affected by *amine oxidase inhibitors* (iproniazid or phenyl*iso*propylhydrazine). The response of the preparation was potentiated when one of these amines was tested: tryptamine, N-methyltryptamine, 5-methoxytryptamine, 5-chlorotryptamine and 5-methyltryptamine. With these compounds Vane saw a 8.9- to 20-fold *potentiation of the response.* With N'N'-dimethyltryptamine, the response in the presence of an amine oxidase inhibitor was not even doubled; this is in keeping with the feeble action of amine oxidase on tertiary amines. With α-methyltryptamine, a substance not attacked by amine oxidase, there was no potentiation by an amine oxidase inhibitor. These observations can be understood on the assumption that destruction by amine oxidase is a factor that determines the intensity of the response of the excitable tissue, just as histaminase inhibitors modify the response of the guinea-pig's ileum to histamine (ARUNLAKSHANA et al. 1954; BLASCHKO and KURZEPA 1962).

However, when the hydroxytryptamines, 4-hydroxytryptamine, 5-hydroxytryptamine or 6-hydroxytryptamine, were tested on the rat stomach preparation, no similar potentiation was seen. The two compounds carrying hydroxyl groups in position 4 or 5 were the most potent substances tested, but their effects were the same in the presence and in the absence of an inhibitor of amine oxidase. And yet, it is known that both amines are readily oxidized by amine oxidase.

In order to account for this paradox, VANE (1959) suggested that the two hydroxylated compounds were not attacked by amine oxidase, because they could not penetrate the membrane of the muscle cell and thus gain access to the inactivating enzyme, situated in the mitochondria.

This interpretation may be adequate to account for the observations just described, but it presents us with the paradoxical situation that compounds known to be metabolized *in vivo* by oxidative deamination, are not attacked in the isolated rat fundus. We would then have to postulate that the gastric enzyme acts on synthetic amines as would be expected but is without action on the only naturally occurring substance of this group, 5-hydroxytryptamine.

From what has been said before, we are not in doubt that amine oxidase is an important catalyst of the breakdown of 5-hydroxytryptamine in mammals. If we deny to the oxidase in the plain muscle cell a share in the task of biological inactivation of this amine, we have to postulate that in other sites, e.g. in the liver, the *permeability* of the *cell membrane* is such as to allow the intracellular enzyme to act. We also remember that a microsomal localization of liver amine oxidase has been established and that for all we know this fraction of the enzyme may be more closely linked to the cell surface.

Another interpretation of the observations by VANE is implicit in the finding by WEISSBACH et al. (1961), already discussed, which suggests that an amine oxidase inhibitor may not make inactivation impossible, but shift the catabolism of the amine into a different route; this is a possibility that has been discussed for other amines (see DAVISON 1958). We cannot at present assess the importance of such a shift, as the metabolic abilities of the muscle cell, apart from the established presence of amine oxidase, are too imperfectly known.

One fact that has emerged from the study of the metabolism of the indolealkylamines, are the many analogies that exist between the naturally occurring members of this group and the other amines for which GUGGENHEIM has coined the term "biogenic amines". In particular, we find many biochemical relationships between 5-hydroxytryptamine and the catechol amines and we suspect that there exists a cytogenetic counterpart to this relationship, between chromaffin cells and adrenergic neurones on the one side and 5-hydroxytryptamine, enterochromaffin cells and "tryptaminergic" neurones on the other. The enzymic mechanisms that act on the synthetic substances of this group can be seen as instruments of the catabolism of naturally occurring compounds.

Acknowledgments

This article was begun while one of us (W.G.L.) held a Postdoctoral Fellowship (Interdisciplinary Grant) from the National Institute of Mental Health, U.S. Public Health Service. The continued support from the U.S. Air Force, European Office of Aerospace Research, is also gratefully acknowledged.

References

Anderson, J. A., M. R. Ziegler and D. Doeden: Banana feeding and urinary excretion of 5-hydroxyindoleacetic acid. Science **127**, 236 (1958).

Arioka, I., and H. Tanimukai: Histochemical studies of monoamine oxidase in the midbrain of the mouse. J. Neurochem. **1**, 311 (1957).

Armstrong, M. D., K. N. F. Shaw, J. Gortakowski and H. Singer: The indole acids of human urine. Paper chromatography of indole acids. J. biol. Chem. **234**, 17 (1958).

Arnaiz, G. R. de L., and E. de Robertis: Cholinergic and noncholinergic nerve endings in the rat brain. II. Subcellular localization of monoamine oxidase and succinate dehydrogenase. J. Neurochem. **9**, 503 (1962).

Arunlakshana, O., J. L. Mongar and H. O. Schild: Potentiation of pharmacological effects of histamine by histaminase inhibitors. J. Physiol. (Lond.) **123**, 32 (1954).

Axelrod, J.: Studies on sympathomimetic amines. I. The biotransformation and physiological disposition of (—)-ephedrine and (—)-norephedrine. J. Pharmacol. exp. Ther. **109**, 65 (1953).

— An enzyme for the deamination of sympathomimetic amines: properties and distribution. J. Pharmacol. exp. Ther. **110**, 2 (1954).

— The enzymatic deamination of amphetamine (benzedrine). J. biol. Chem. **214**, 753 (1955).

— Enzymatic formation of psychotomimetic metabolites from normally occurring compounds. Science **134**, 343 (1961).

— The enzymatic N-methylation of serotonin and other amines. J. Pharmacol. exp. Ther. **138**, 28 (1962a).

— Purification and properties of phenylethanolamine-N-methyl transferase. J. biol. Chem. **237**, 1657 (1962b).

— I. J. Kopin and J. D. Mann: 3-Methoxy-4-hydroxyphenylglycol sulphate, a new metabolite of epinephrine and norepinephrine. Biochim. biophys. Acta (Amst.) **36**, 576 (1959).

—, and H. Weissbach: Enzymatic O-methylation of N-acetylserotonin to melatonin. Science **131**, 1312 (1960).

— — Purification and properties of hydroxyindole-O-methyl transferase. J. biol. Chem. **236**, 211 (1961).

Baker, R. V.: D. Phil. Thesis, Oxford 1959.

Bertaccini, G.: Effect of removal of large segments of rat intestine on the biosynthesis and metabolism of 5-hydroxytryptamine. Naturwissenschaften **45**, 548 (1958).

—, and S. Chieppa: Urinary excretion of 5-hydroxyindoleacetic acid after removal of the large intestine in man. Lancet **1960 I**, 881.

Blaschko, H.: Amine oxidase in *Sepia officinalis*. J. Physiol. (Lond.) **99**, 364 (1941).

— Enzymic oxidation of 5-hydroxytryptamine in mammalian and cephalopod tissue. Biochem. J. **52**, x (1952a).

— Amine oxidase and amine metabolism. Pharmacol. Rev. **4**, 415 (1952b).

— Metabolism of epinephrine and norepinephrine. Pharmacol. Rev. **6**, 23 (1954).

— Biochemical principles in relation to hypotensive-drug action. In: Hypotensive drugs, p. 21 (Ed. M. Harington). London 1956.

— Biological inactivation of 5-hydroxytryptamine. In: 5-Hydroxytryptamine, p. 50. (Ed. G. P. Lewis). London 1958.

— Primary and secondary amines as substrates of amine oxidases. J. Physiol. (Lond.) **153**, 17P (1960).

— The amine oxidases of mammalian blood plasma. Advanc. comp. Physiol. Biochem. **1**, 68 (1962a).

— In: Enzymes and drug action. Ciba Foundat. Symp., edit. by J. L. Mongar and A. V. S. de Reuck, p. 465ff. London: Churchill 1962b.

—, and R. Bonney: Spermine oxidase and benzylamine oxidase. Distribution, development and substrate specificity. Proc. roy. Soc. B **156**, 268 (1962).

— E. H. Colhoun and N. Frontali: Occurrence of amine oxidase in an insect, *Periplaneta americana* L. J. Physiol. (Lond.) **156**, 28P (1961).

— P. J. Friedman, R. Hawes and K. Nilsson: The amine oxidases of mammalian plasma. J. Physiol. (Lond.) **145**, 384 (1959).

— J. M. Hagen and P. Hagen: Mitochondrial enzymes and chromaffin granules. J. Physiol. Lond. **139**, 316 (1957).

—, and R. Hawes: Observations on spermine oxidase of mammalian plasma. J. Physiol. (Lond.) **145**, 124 (1959).

—, and J. Hawkins: Observations on amine oxidase in cephalopods. J. Physiol. (Lond.) **118**, 88 (1952).

—, and K. Hellmann: Pigment formation from tryptamine and 5-hydroxytryptamine. A contribution to the histochemistry of amine oxidase. J. Physiol. (Lond.) **122**, 419 (1953).

BLASCHKO, H., and J. M. HIMMS: Amine oxidase in the earthworm. J. Physiol. (Lond.) **120**, 445 (1953).

— — Enzymic oxidation of amines in decapods. J. exp. Biol. **31**, 1 (1954).

—, and D. B. HOPE: The oxidation of L-amino-acids in the digestive gland of *Mytilus edulis*. J. Physiol. (Lond.) **128**, 11 P (1955).

— — The oxidation of L-amino acids by *Mytilus edulis*. Biochem. J. **62**, 335 (1956).

— — Observations on the distribution of amine oxidase in invertebrates. Arch. Biochem. **69**, 10 (1957).

—, and S. KURZEPA: Potentiation of the responses to histamine by picolylamines. Brit. J. Pharmacol. **19**, 544 (1962).

—, and W. G. LEVINE: A comparative study of hydroxyindole oxidases. Brit. J. Pharmacol. **15**, 625 (1960a).

— — Enzymic oxidation of 5-hydroxytryptamine by pig serum. J. Physiol. (Lond.) **154**, 599 (1960b).

— — Observations on phenolases. Neuro-Psychopharmacology **2**, 435 (1960c).

—, and A. S. MILTON: Oxidation of 5-hydroxytryptamine and related compounds by Mytilus gill plates. Brit. J. Pharmacol. **15**, 42 (1960).

—, and F. J. PHILPOT: Enzymic oxidation of tryptamine derivatives. J. Physiol. (Lond.) **122**, 403 (1953).

— D. RICHTER and H. SCHLOSSMANN: Inactivation of adrenaline. J. Physiol. (Lond.) **90**, 1 (1937a).

— — — Enzymic oxidation of amines. J. Physiol. (Lond.) **91**, 13 P (1937b).

— — — The oxidation of adrenaline and other amines. Biochem. J. **31**, 2187 (1937c).

BLUM, J. J., and N. S. LING: Oxidation of serotonin and 5-hydroxyindoles during the denaturation of oxyhaemoglobin. Biochem. J. **73**, 530 (1959).

BOGDANSKI, D. F., H. WEISSBACH and S. UDENFRIEND: The distribution of serotonin, 5-hydroxytryptophan decarboxylase, and monoamine oxidase in brain. J. Neurochem. **1**, 272 (1957).

BRODIE, B. B.: Pathways of drug metabolism. J. Pharm. Pharmacol. 8, 1 (1956).

BROWN, G. L., and J. S. GILLESPIE: The output of sympathetic transmitter from the spleen of the cat. J. Physiol. (Lond.) **138**, 81 (1957).

BUFFONI, F., and H. BLASCHKO: Studies of a crystalline preparation of the amine oxidase of pig plasma. Biochem. J. **89**, 111 P (1963). See also: Proc. Roy. Soc. B **161**, 153 (1964).

BURN, J. H., and M. J. RAND: The action of sympathomimetic amines in animals treated with reserpine. J. Physiol. (Lond.) **144**, 314 (1958).

CARLISLE, D. B.: An indole-alkylamine regulating heart beat in Crustacea. Biochem. J. **63**, 32 P (1956).

—, and K. K. TIWARI: In: Report of the council for 1960/61. J. mar. biol. Ass. U. Kingd. **41**, 853 (1961).

CHADWICK, B. T., and J. H. WILKINSON: Some aspects of the metabolism of 5-hydroxytryptamine. Biochem. J. **76**, 102 (1960).

COLHOUN, E. H.: Synthesis of 5-hydroxytryptamine in the American cockroach. Experientia (Basel) **19**, 9 (1963).

COTZIAS, G. C., and V. P. DOLE: Metabolism of amines. II. Mitochondrial localization of monoamine oxidase. Proc. Soc. exp. Biol. (N.Y.) **78**, 157 (1951).

CURZON, G., and L. VALLET: The purification of human caeruloplasmin. Biochem. J. **74**, 279 (1960).

DAVISON, A. N.: The physiological role of monoamine oxidase. Physiol. Rev. **38**, 729 (1958).

DAY, S. M., and J. P. GREEN: The uptake of amino acids and the synthesis of amines by neoplastic mast cells in culture. J. Physiol. (Lond.) **164**, 210 (1962).

DUVE, C. DE, H. BEAUFAY, P. JACQUES, Y. RAHMAN-LI, O. Z. SELLINGER, R. WATTIAUX and S. DE CONINCK: Intracellular localization of catalase and of some oxidases in rat liver. Biochim. biophys. Acta (Amst.) **40**, 186 (1960).

EBERTS jr., F. S., and E. G. DANIELS: Metabolism of 3-(2-aminobutyl-1-C14) indole acetate (etryptamine acetate) in man. Fed. Proc. **21**, 180 (1962).

ELSNER, P., O. HORNYKIEWICZ, A. LINDNER u. G. NIEBAUER: Die Polyphenoloxydaseaktivität im mütterlichen und fötalen Blutserum. Wien. klin. Wschr. **46**, 938 (1953).

ERIKSEN, N., G. M. MARTIN and E. P. BENDITT: Oxidation of the indole nucleus of 5-hydroxytryptamine and the formation of pigments: isolation and partial characterization of a dimer of 5-HT. J. biol. Chem. **235**, 1662 (1960).

ERSPAMER, V.: Active substances in the posterior salivary glands of Octopoda. I. Enteramine-like substances. Acta pharmacol. (Kbh.) **4**, 213 (1948).

— Il sistema cellulare enterocromaffine e l'enteramina. R. C. sci. Farmital. **1**, 5 (1954).

— Observations on the fate of indolealkylamines in the organism. J. Physiol. (Lond.) **127**, 118 (1955).

ERSPAMER, V.: Some observations on the fate of exogenous 5-hydroxytryptamine (enteramine) in the rat. J. Physiol. (Lond.) **133**, 1 (1956).
— Recent research in the field of 5-hydroxytryptamine and related indolealkylamines. Fortschr. Arzneimittelforsch. **3**, 151 (1961).
—, and G. BERTACCINI: Observations on the antidiuretic action and the fate of 5-hydroxy-DL-tryptophan in the rat organism. Arch. int. Pharmacodyn. **137**, 6 (1962).
— R. FERRINI and A. GLÄSSER: A note on the oxidative deamination of 5-hydroxytryptamine and other indolealkylamines. J. Pharm. Pharmacol. **12**, 761 (1960).
— A. GLÄSSER and M. B. NOBILI: The fate of 5-hydroxy-N-acetyltryptophan and 5-acetoxy-N-acetyltryptophan in the rat organism. Arch. Biochem. **93**, 673 (1961).
— — — and C. PASINI: The fate of 4-hydroxytryptophan in the rat organism. Experientia (Basel) **16**, 506 (1960).
— — C. PASINI and G. STOPPANI: *In vitro* decarboxylation of tryptophans by mammalian decarboxylase. Nature (Lond.) **189**, 438 (1961).
—, and M. B. NOBILI: Observations on the fate of oral 4-hydroxytryptophan in man. Experientia (Basel) **17**, 351 (1961).
— — Observations on the fate of 4-hydroxy-DL-tryptophan in the organism of the rat and man. Arch. int. Pharmacodyn. **137**, 24 (1962).
EUW, J. O. v., R. NEHER, T. REICHSTEIN, S. A. S. TAIT, J. F. TAIT and A. WETTSTEIN: "Substanz Z". Helv. chim. Acta **42**, 1817 (1959).
EWINS, A. J., and P. P. LAIDLAW: The fate of indole-ethylamine in the organism. Biochem. J. **7**, 18 (1913).
FELLMAN, J. H., T. S. FUJITA and C. J. BELBER: 2,3-Dihydro-5-hydroxytryptamine. Biochem. Pharmacol. **11**, 557 (1962).
FREYBURGER, W. A., B. E. GRAHAM, M. M. RAPPORT, P. H. SEAY, W. M. GOVIER, O. F. SWOAP and M. J. VAN DER BROOK: The pharmacology of 5-hydroxytryptamine (serotonin). J. Pharmacol. exp. Ther. **105**, 80 (1952).
GELLER, E., S. EIDUSON and A. YUWILER: Oxidation of p-phenylenediamine and adrenaline in enzymatic and copper-catalysed reactions. J. Neurochem. **5**, 73 (1959).
GESSNER, P. K., P. A. KHAIRALLAH, W. M. McISAAC and I. H. PAGE: The relationship between the metabolic fate and pharmacological actions of serotonin, bufotenine and psilocybin. J. Pharmacol. exp. Ther. **130**, 126 (1960).
GLENNER, G. G., H. J. BURTNER and G. W. BROWN: The histochemical demonstration of monoamine oxidase activity by tetrazolium salts. J. Histochem. Cytochem. **5**, 591 (1957).
— H. WEISSBACH and B. G. REDFIELD: The histochemical demonstration of enzymatic activity by a non-enzymatic redox reaction. Reduction of tetrazolium salts by indolyl-3-acetaldehyde. J. Histochem. Cytochem. **8**, 258 (1960).
GOVIER, W. M., B. G. HOWES and A. J. GIBBONS: The oxidative deamination of serotonin and other 3-(beta-aminoethyl)-indoles by monoamine oxidase and the effects of these compounds on the deamination of tyramine. Science **118**, 596 (1953).
GUGGENHEIM, M., u. W. LÖFFLER: Das Schicksal proteinogener Amine im Tierkörper. Biochem. Z. **72**, 325 (1916).
HAAVALDSEN, R.: Transamination of aromatic amino acids in nervous tissue. Nature (Lond.) **196**, 577 (1962).
HAGEN, P.: The substrate specificity of amine oxidase of mouse mastocytoma. Fed. Proc. **18**, 399 (1959).
—, and N. WEINER: Enzymic oxidation of pharmacologically active amines. Fed. Proc. **18**, 1005 (1959).
HARE, M. L. C.: Tyramine oxidase. I. A new enzyme system in liver. Biochem. J. **22**, 968 (1928).
HAVERBACK, B. J., and J. D. DAVIDSON: Serotonin and the gastrointestinal tract. Gastroenterology **35**, 570 (1958).
HAWKINS, J.: The localization of amine oxidase in the liver cell. Biochem. J. **50**, 577 (1952).
HEIM, R.: Les investigations anciennes et récentes propres aux agarics hallucinogènes du Mexique, à leur action et aux substances qui en sont responsables. Actualités pharmacol. **12**, 171 (1959).
HELLMANN, K.: Cholinesterase and amine oxidase in the skin: a histochemical investigation. J. Physiol. (Lond.) **129**, 454 (1955).
HERTTING, G., J. AXELROD, I. J. KOPIN and L. G. WHITBY: Lack of uptake of catecholamines after chronic denervation of sympathetic nerves. Nature (Lond.) **189**, 66 (1961).
HOFMANN, A., R. HEIM, A. BRACK, H. KOBEL, A. FREY, H. OTT, T. PETRZILKA u. F. TROXLER: Psilocybin und Psilocin, zwei psychotrope Wirkstoffe aus mexikanischen Rauschpilzen. Helv. chim. Acta **42**, 1557 (1959).
HOLTER, H.: In: Enzymes and drug action. Ciba Foundat. Symp., edit. by J. L. MONGAR and A. V. S. DE REUCK, p. 467. London: Churchill 1962.

HOLTZ, P., u. H. BÜCHSEL: Über die Substratspezifität und -affinität der d-Aminosäurenoxydase und Aminoxydase. Hoppe-Seylers Z. physiol. Chem. **272**, 201 (1942).
HOPE, D. B., and A. D. SMITH: Distribution and activity of monoamine oxidase in mouse tissues. Biochem. J. **74**, 101 (1960).
HORITA, A.: The influence of pH on serotonin metabolism by rat tissue homogenates. Biochem. Pharmacol. **11**, 147 (1962).
—, and L. J. WEBER: The enzymic dephosphorylation and oxidation of psilocybin and psilocin by mammalian tissue homogenates. Biochem. Pharmacol. **7**, 47 (1961).
— — Dephosphorylation of psilocybin in the intact mouse. Toxicol. appl. Pharmacol. **4**, 730 (1962).
JACOBY, G. A., and B. LA DU: Nonspecificity of tyrosine transaminase: an explanation for the simultaneous induction of tyrosine, phenylalanine and tryptophan transaminase activities in rat liver. Biochem. biophys. Res. Commun. **8**, 352 (1962).
JEPSON, J. B., S. UDENFRIEND and P. ZALTZMAN: The enzymic conversion of tryptamine to 6-hydroxytryptamine. Fed. Proc. **18**, 254 (1959).
KÄRKI, N., R. KUNTZMAN and B. B. BRODIE: Storage, synthesis and metabolism of monoamines in the developing brain. J. Neurochem. **9**, 53 (1962).
KENTEN, R. H., and P. J. G. MANN: The oxidation of amines by extracts of pea seedlings. Biochem. J. **50**, 360 (1952).
KOELLE, G. B., and A. DE T. VALK jr.: Physiological implications of the histochemical localization of amine oxidase. J. Physiol. (Lond.) **126**, 434 (1954).
KOHN, H. I.: Tyramine oxidase. Biochem. J. **31**, 1693 (1937).
KOPIN, I. J., C. M. B. PARE, J. AXELROD and H. WEISSBACH: 6-Hydroxylation the major metabolic pathway for melatonin. Biochim. biophys. Acta (Amst.) **40**, 377 (1960).
— — — — The fate of melatonin in animals. J. biol. Chem. **236**, 3072 (1961).
KVEDER, S., S. ISKRIĆ and D. KEGLEVIĆ: 5-Hydroxytryptophol: a metabolite of 5-hydroxytryptamine in rats. Biochem. J. **85**, 447 (1962).
LANGEMANN, H.: Enzymes and their substrates in the adrenal gland of the ox. Brit. J. Pharmacol. **6**, 318 (1951).
—, u. J. KÄGI: Oxytryptamin- und Oxyindolessigsäurebestimmungen bei einem Fall von Carcinoidsyndrom, nebst einigen anderen Untersuchungen über Oxytryptamine. Klin. Wschr. **34**, 237 (1956).
LEMBECK, F.: 5-Hydroxytryptamine in a carcinoid tumour. Nature (Lond.) **172**, 910 (1953).
LERNER, A. B., and J. D. CASE: Melatonin. Fed. Proc. **19**, 590 (1960).
LEVINE, W. G.: Observations on hydroxyindole oxidases. Biochem. J. **76**, 43 P (1960).
MÄRKI, F., J. AXELROD and B. WITKOP: Catecholamines and methyltransferases in the South American toad *(Bufo marinus)*. Biochim. biophys. Acta (Amst.) **58**, 367 (1962).
MANN, P. J. G.: Purification and properties of the amine oxidase of pea seedlings. Biochem. J. **59**, 609 (1955).
— Further purification and properties of the amine oxidase of pea seedlings. Biochem. J. **79**, 623 (1961).
MANSOUR, T. E.: Effect of serotonin on phenol oxidase from the liver fluke *Fasciola hepatica* and from other sources. Biochim. biophys. Acta (Amst.) **30**, 492 (1958).
MARTIN, G. M., E. P. BENDITT and N. ERIKSEN: Enzymic oxidation of the indole nucleus of 5-hydroxytryptamine: properties of an enzyme in human serum and of the products of oxidation. Arch. Biochem. **90**, 208 (1960).
— N. ERIKSEN and E. P. BENDITT: Oxidation of 5-hydroxytryptamine by human serum and its inhibition by iproniazid. Fed. Proc. **17**, 447 (1958).
MCISAAC, W. M., S. KVEDER and I. H. PAGE: The metabolism of 5-β-^{14}C-methoxy-tryptamine. Biochem. J. **76**, 30 P (1960).
—, and I. H. PAGE: The metabolism of serotonin (5-hydroxytryptamine). J. biol. Chem. **234**, 858 (1959).
NAKAI, K.: Serotonin metabolism in herbivores. Nature (Lond.) **181**, 1734 (1958).
NAKAJIMA, H., et J. THUILLIER: Inactivation de la sérotonine par la ceruloplasmine. C.R. Soc. Biol. (Paris) **152**, 270 (1958).
OGSTON, A. G.: Removal of acetylcholine from a limited volume by diffusion. J. Physiol. (Lond.) **128**, 222 (1955).
OZAKI, M., H. WEISSBACH, A. OZAKI, B. WITKOP and S. UDENFRIEND: Monoamine oxidase inhibitors and procedures for their evaluation *in vivo* and *in vitro*. J. med. pharm. Chem. **2**, 591 (1960).
PAGE, I. H., A. C. CORCORAN, S. UDENFRIEND, A. SJOERDSMA and H. WEISSBACH: Argentaffinoma as endocrine tumour. Lancet **1955 I**, 198.
PEART, W. S., K. A. PORTER, J. I. S. ROBERTSON, M. SANDLER and E. BALDOCK: Carcinoid syndrome due to pancreatic-duct neoplasm secreting 5-hydroxytryptophan and 5-hydroxytryptamine. Lancet **1963 I**, 239.

PERNOW, B., and J. WALDENSTRÖM: Paroxysmal flushing and other symptoms caused by 5-hydroxytryptamine and histamine in patients with malignant tumours. Lancet **1954 II**, 951.
PORTER, C. C., D. C. TITUS, B. E. SANDERS and E. V. C. SMITH: Oxidation of serotonin in the presence of ceruloplasmin. Science **126**, 1014 (1957).
PUGH, C. E. M., and J. H. QUASTEL: Oxidation of aliphatic amines by brain and other tissues. Biochem. J. **31**, 286 (1937a).
— — Oxidation of amines by animal tissues. Biochem. J. **31**, 2306 (1937b).
RODNIGHT, R.: Separation and characterization of urinary indoles resembling 5-hydroxytryptamine and tryptamine. Biochem. J. **64**, 21 (1956).
— Carbon monoxide saturation and the recovery of 5-hydroxytryptamine from whole blood. J. Physiol. (Lond.) **141**, 10P (1958).
SANDLER, M., R. G. SPECTOR, C. R. J. RUTHVEN and A. N. DAVISON: The occurrence and adaptive increase of 5-hydroxytryptophan-α-oxoglutarate transaminase. Biochem. J. **74**, 42P (1960).
SANKAR, D. V. S.: Enzymatic activity of ceruloplasmin. Fed. Proc. **18**, 441 (1959).
SCHEINBERG, I. H., and I. STERNLIEB: Copper metabolism. Pharmacol. Rev. **12**, 355 (1960).
SCHLOSSBERGER, H. G., u. H. KUCH: Synthese des 5,6-Dihydroxy-tryptamins. Chem. Ber. **93**, 1318 (1960).
SEIDEN, L. S., and J. WESTLEY: Partial purification of monoamine oxidase from rat brain. Biochim. biophys. Acta (Amst.) **58**, 363 (1962).
SHIMIZU, N., and N. MORIKAVA: Histochemical study of monoamine oxidase in the developing rat brain. Nature (Lond.) **184**, 650 (1959).
— — and M. OKADA: Histochemical studies of monoamine oxidase of the brain of rodents. Z. Zellforsch. **49**, 389 (1959).
SJOERDSMA, A., H. WEISSBACH and S. UDENFRIEND: Simple test for diagnosis of metastatic carcinoid (argentaffinoma). J. Amer. med. Ass. **159**, 397 (1955).
SMITH, B.: Monoamine oxidase in the pineal gland, neurohypophysis and brain of the albino rat. J. Anat. (Lond.) **97**, 1 (1963).
SPENCER, R. P., and N. ZAMCHEK: Alternate metabolic fate of 5-hydroxytryptophan. Biochem. biophys. Res. Commun. **3**, 386 (1960).
STRÖMBLAD, B. C. R.: Supersensitivity and amine oxidase activity in denervated salivary glands. Acta physiol. scand. **36**, 137 (1956).
— Observations on amine oxidase in human salivary glands. J. Physiol. (Lond.) **147**, 639 (1959).
SZARA, S.: 6-Hydroxylation: an important metabolic route for α-methyltryptamine. Experientia (Basel) **17**, 76 (1961).
—, and J. AXELROD: Hydroxylation and N-demethylation of N,N-dimethyltryptamine. Experientia (Basel) **15**, 216 (1959).
— E. HEARST and F. PUTNEY: Metabolism of hallucinogenic tryptamine derivatives. Fed. Proc. **19**, 23 (1960).
—, and F. PUTNEY: 6-Hydroxylation of tryptamine and derivatives: the enzymatic process. Fed. Proc. **20**, 172 (1961).
TITUS, E. O., and S. UDENFRIEND: Metabolism of 5-hydroxytryptamine (serotonin). Fed. Proc. **13**, 411 (1954).
TWAROG, B. M., and I. H. PAGE: Serotonin content of some mammalian tissues and urine and methods for its determination. Amer. J. Physiol. **175**, 157 (1953).
UDENFRIEND, S., E. TITUS and H. WEISSBACH: Identification of 5-hydroxy-3-indoleacetic acid in normal urine and a method for its assay. J. biol. Chem. **216**, 499 (1955).
— — — and H. E. PETERSON: Biogenisis and metabolism of 5-hydroxyindole compounds. J. biol. Chem. **219**, 335 (1956).
— H. WEISSBACH and A. SJOERDSMA: Studies on tryptophan and serotonin in patients with malignant carcinoids. Science **123**, 669 (1956).
VANE, J. R.: The relative activities of some tryptamine analogues on the isolated rat stomach strip preparation. Brit. J. Pharmacol. **14**, 87 (1959).
VIALLI, M.: L'istochimica e i problemi biologici riguardanti la 5-idrossitriptamina (enteramina-serotonina). Riv. Anat. pat. **21**, 392 (1962).
WEISSBACH, H., W. KING, A. SJOERDSMA and S. UDENFRIEND: Formation of indole-3-acetic acid and tryptamine in animals. J. biol. Chem. **234**, 81 (1959).
— W. LOVENBERG, B. G. REDFIELD and S. UDENFRIEND: *In vivo* metabolism of serotonin and tryptamine: effect of monoamine oxidase inhibition. J. Pharmacol. exp. Ther. **131**, 26 (1961).
— B. G. REDFIELD and J. AXELROD: Biosynthesis of melatonin: enzymic conversion of serotonin to N-acetylserotonin. Biochim. biophys. Acta (Amst.) **43**, 352 (1960).

WEISSBACH, H., B. G. REDFIELD, and S. UDENFRIEND: Soluble monoamine oxidase; its properties and actions on serotonin. J. biol. Chem. **229**, 953 (1957).
— — — Serotonin-O-glucuronide; an alternate route of serotonin metabolism. Fed. Proc. **17**, 418 (1958).
WELSH, J. H., and M. MOORHEAD: The quantitative distribution of 5-hydroxytryptamine in the invertebrates, especially in their nervous system. J. Neurochem. **6**, 146 (1960).
WERLE, E., u. E. v. PECHMANN: Über die Diamin-Oxydase der Pflanzen und ihre adaptive Bildung durch Bakterien. Justus Liebigs Ann. Chem. **562**, 44 (1949).
— I. TRAUTSCHOLD u. D. AURES: Reinigung und Charakterisierung der Diamin-Oxydase aus Erbsen. Hoppe-Seylers Z. physiol. Chem. **326**, 200 (1961).
WILLIAMS, E. D., and M. SANDLER: The classification of carcinoid tumours. Lancet **1963 I**, 238.
WITT, P. N., L. BRETTSCHNEIDER and A. P. BORIS: Sensitivity to d-amphetamine in spiders after iproniazid and imipramine. J. Pharmacol. exp. Ther. **132**, 183 (1961).
YAMADA, H., and K. T. YASUNOBU: Monoamine oxidase. I. Purification, crystallization, and properties of plasma monoamine oxidase. J. biol. Chem. **237**, 1511 (1962).
ZARAFONETIS, C. J. D., and J. P. KALAS: Serotonin degradation by ceruloplasmin and its inhibition by isoniazid and iproniazid. Amer. J. med. Sci. **239**, 203 (1960).

Chapter 7

Peripheral physiological and pharmacological actions of indolealkylamines

By

VITTORIO ERSPAMER

With 16 Figures

I. Acute toxicity of indolealkylamines

5-Hydroxytryptamine base. Mouse, LD 50 by intravenous route: 160 mg/kg (FREYBURGER et al. 1952), 135 mg/kg (HIGGINBOTHAM 1959); by intraperitoneal route: 280 mg/kg (SPENCER and WEST 1961), 340 mg/kg (FISHEL et al. 1962); by subcutaneous route: > 868 mg/kg (FREYBURGER et al. 1952). Rat, LD 50 by intravenous route: 30 mg/kg; by subcutaneous route: approximately 117 mg/kg (FREYBURGER et al. 1952).

Anaesthesia greatly enhances the toxicity of 5-HT. Rats anaesthetized with pentobarbital may die following intravenous doses of the substance as small as 0.1 mg/kg (CORRELL et al. 1952, TAPANI 1963). Similar observations have been made in rabbits, guinea-pigs, hens (CORRELL et al. 1952), dogs (McCAWLEY et al. 1952) and cats (ERSPAMER 1954b). Death is due to respiratory failure.

It is obvious that several drugs when given prior to or at the same time as 5-HT are capable of influencing consistently the acute toxicity of 5-HT itself. To quote a few examples, pretreating of mice with 1 and 1.5 mg/kg of 48/80 increases the 5-HT toxicity 5 and 30 times, respectively (HIGGINBOTHAM 1959), and pretreating of mice with 6 subcutaneous doses of 2 mg/kg thyroxine again raises the toxicity of 5-HT 5 times (SPENCER and WEST 1961).

5-Hydroxy-N,N-dibutyltryptamine HCl. Mouse, LD 50 by intraperitoneal route: 178 mg/kg (HEINZELMAN and SZMUSZKOVICZ 1963).

Bufotenidine. Mouse, LD 50 by intravenous route: 1.3 mg/kg; by subcutaneous route: approximately 90 mg/kg (UEDA et al. 1957).

5-Methoxytryptamine HCl. Mouse, LD 50 by intravenous route: 60 mg/kg; by subcutaneous route: 750 mg/kg. Rat, LD 50 by subcutaneous route: 600 mg/kg (ERSPAMER 1952a).

5-Methoxy-N,N-diethyltryptamine HCl. Mouse, LD 50 by intraperitoneal route: 65 mg/kg (HEINZELMAN and SZMUSZKOVICZ 1963).

Psilocybin. Mouse, LD 50 by intravenous route: > 250 mg/kg (CERLETTI 1959).

Tryptamine. The subcutaneous LD 50 of tryptamine hydrochloride in mice kept at an environmental temperature of 28 to 30° is about 500 mg/kg, death occurring without any marked symptoms of central stimulation (EDERY and SCHATZBERG-PORATH 1960, MAXWELL et al. 1961).

The intravenous administration of sublethal doses of tryptamine HCl (32 to 48 mg/kg) in male mice produces head weave, hind leg spread, arched back and fore-paw clonus (KEASLING et al. 1963). These symptoms are similar to those observed by TEDESCHI et al. (1959) in the rat following intravenous injection of 40 mg/kg tryptamine.

Tryptamine derivatives. Data on the acute toxicity of a series of tryptamine derivatives, reported in a recent review article by HEINZELMAN and SZMUSZKOVICZ (1963) are given below. LD 50 has been determined in the mouse, by intraperitoneal route.

N-methyltryptamine. HCl	200 mg/kg
N-ethyltryptamine. HCl	167 mg/kg
N-propyltryptamine. HCl	77 mg/kg
N-isopropyltryptamine. HCl	205 mg/kg
N-n-butyltryptamine. HCl	65 mg/kg
N-isobutyltryptamine. HCl	167 mg/kg
N-(1'-methyl-)propyltryptamine. HCl	167 mg/kg
N-isopentyltryptamine. HCl	100 mg/kg
N-benzyltryptamine. HCl	200 mg/kg
N-octyltryptamine. HBr	32 mg/kg
N-(2'-ethyl-)tryptamine. HCl	200 mg/kg
N,N-dimethyltryptamine. HCl	167 mg/kg
N,N-diethyltryptamine. HCl	77 mg/kg
N,N-dipropyltryptamine. HCl	56 mg/kg
5-methyltryptamine	200 mg/kg

EDERY and SCHATZBERG-PORATH (1960) found that LD 50 by subcutaneous route in the mouse is 439 mg/kg for *5-fluorotryptamine*, and 320 mg/kg for *5-fluoro-7-methyltryptamine*.

Gramine. Mouse, LD 50 by intravenous route: 44.6$\pm$1.4 mg/kg (POWELL and CHEN 1945), 45.6 mg/kg (AKKERMAN et al. 1951). Rat, LD 50 by intravenous route: 62.9$\pm$2.7 mg/kg (POWELL and CHEN 1945).

Gramine first stimulates the central nervous system (clonic convulsions, hyperpnoea), then depresses it. Death seems to be due to central respiratory failure (SUPNIEWSKI and SERAFINOWNA 1938).

According to SUPNIEWSKI and SERAFIN-GAJEWSKA (1938), *2-methylgramine* is 3 to 4 times more toxic than gramine.

5-Hydroxytryptophan. In the rabbit, intravenous 5-HTP causes lethal hyperpyrexia in doses of 75 mg/kg and more (HORITA and GOGERTY 1958). Rats withstand intraperitoneal doses of 200 mg/kg 5-HTP, repeated every 12 hours for periods up to 12 months, the only toxic effects produced by the amino acid being diarrhoea, failure to gain weight, and persistent cyanotic flush (DAVIDSON et al. 1957a, 1957b).

For other data on the acute toxicity of 5-HT and for data on its chronic toxicity see Chapter 13.

A number of data on the toxicity of a series of indole glyoxamides and indole acetamines are reported by HEINZELMAN and SZMUSZKOVICZ (1963).

II. Action on the systemic blood pressure

Dog. It has been ascertained that the blood pressure response of dogs to parenteral 5-HT depends on a number of known and unknown factors, such as type of anaesthesia, dose, route and rapidity of drug administration, dominant neurogenic vasoconstrictor tone, duration of experiment etc. Only rarely have different research workers obtained exactly superimposable results, and even the same investigator has often failed to elicit identical responses in different dogs, or in the same dog at different stages of an experiment. This justifies the statement by PAGE (1952b) that "the protean character of the response seems to be the most characteristic feature of the action of the tryptamines on arterial pressure."

Rapid intravenous injection or rapid injection into the pulmonary artery (MACCANON and HORVATH 1954) of medium or high doses of 5-HT (10—200 μg/kg) produces either a frank hypertensive response with increase in the systemic vascular resistance, or polyphasic, amphibaric reactions. The rise in pressure is always moderate, rarely exceeding 40—60 mm Hg, and barely correlated with the dose (PAGE 1952a, 1952b, 1954; PAGE and MCCUBBIN 1953a; ERSPAMER 1952a, 1954; HEYMANS and VAN DEN HEUVEL-HEYMANS 1953; DOUGLAS and TOH 1953; SCHNEIDER and YONKMAN 1954; SCHNEIDER et al. 1954; SCARINCI 1955; BINET and BURSTEIN 1955; ABRAHAMS and PICKFORD 1956a; SCHMID et al.

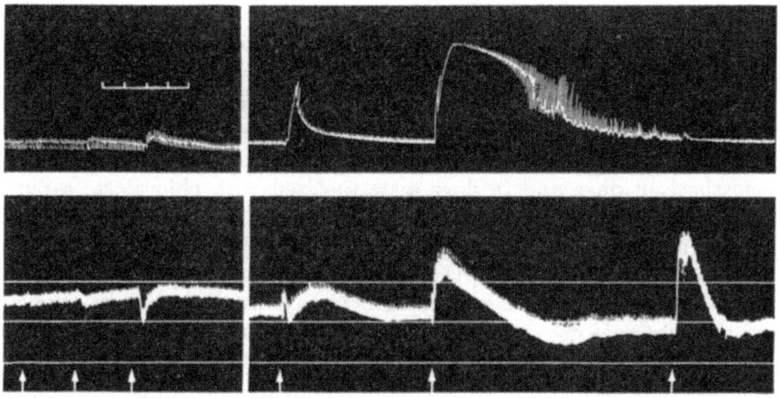

Fig. 1. Dog anaesthetized with pentobarbital. Action of different intravenous doses of 5-HT and of 5 μg/kg adrenaline on carotid blood pressure (lower tracing) and urinary bladder (upper tracing). Time in min. In this experiment low doses of 5-HT produced hypotensive responses, high doses polyphasic or hypertensive responses. Note for the urinary bladder the clear dose/response relationship. [From Fig. 11, ERSPAMER, V., R. C. sci. Farmitalia 1, 40 (1954).]

1956; HOTOVY and ROESCH 1958; JACOB and CUGURRA 1960; BRAUN and STERN 1961; WEIDMANN and CERLETTI 1961; BUÑAG and WALASZEK 1962).

Rapid intravenous injection of small doses of 5-HT (2—8 μg/kg) causes perhaps the most erratic responses: most frequently a slight fall of blood pressure, or biphasic reactions (a fall followed by a slight rise) are seen; more rarely purely hypertensive responses (PAGE 1952b, PAGE and MCCUBBIN 1953a, SCHNEIDER and YONKMAN 1954, ERSPAMER 1954, SCHMID et al. 1956) (Fig. 1).

Finally, slow infusion of 5-HT into the veins or the right atrium constantly produces a drop in mean systolic blood pressure and a decrease in systemic vascular resistance.

At an infusion rate of 8 μg/kg/min of 5-HT base into the right atrium, MAXWELL and co-workers (MAXWELL et al. 1957, 1959; CRUMPTON et al. 1959) obtained an 18% reduction in mean arterial pressure and a 21% reduction in total peripheral resistance; at the same infusion rate into the vein RUDOLPH and PAUL (1957a, 1957b) observed 28% and 55% decreases, respectively; at infusion rates of 60 to 400 μg/kg/min MCGAFF and MILNOR (1962) found decreases of the order of 22% and 38%, respectively.

Following infusion of 5-HT into the left atrium (8 μg/kg/min) the body oxygen consumption does not change, but the arteriovenous difference for oxygen decreases (—17%), while the arterial hematocrit (+4.4%) and hemoglobin (+4.5%) present a slight increase (ROWE et al. 1963).

The hypertensive effect produced by injection of large doses of 5-HT into the femoral vein is reversed to a frank, transient hypotensive response when the amine is injected quickly into the portal vein (BERGAMASCO et al. 1956). When large doses of 5-HT (85 μg/kg of the base) are administered in anaesthetized open-chest dogs into the femoral vein, right heart, pulmonary artery, left heart, ascending aorta or common carotid arteries, it is noted that the latent period before the onset of the pressor response becomes shorter with the shift of the site of the injection towards the ascending aorta. Following injection into the descending aorta a "double-peak" pressor response is obtained (BRAUN and STERN 1961).

Intravenous injections of 5-HT repeated at brief intervals provoke pressor reactions of progressively decreasing intensity (FREYBURGER et al. 1952, ERSPAMER 1954, JACOB and MICHAUD 1962). This tachyphylaxis, however, seems to be of short duration (5—15 min) and this would explain why it was not noted by PAGE (1952b).

Concerning the influence of the type of anaesthesia on the direction of the pressure response to 5-HT, it might be important to confirm the observations of HOTOVY and ROESCH (1958) who found that, in sharp contrast to what happens in unanaesthetized dogs and in dogs anaesthetized with chloralose, rapid intravenous injections of 5-HT in dogs anaesthetized with barbiturates or thiobarbiturates produce a fall of blood pressure and a decrease of peripheral resistances.

In contrast to the intact dog, the spinal dog always responds to intravenous 5-HT with a frank hypertensive reaction which however is barely correlated to the dose and shows some tachyphylaxis (ERSPAMER 1954; PIERRE and CAHN 1956; SCHNEIDER and RINEHART 1956a, 1956b). According to PIERRE and CAHN (1956) the blood pressure of dogs having a pre-medullary brain section does not show any important change following 5-HT administration.

Ganglionic blockade with tetraethylammonium or methonium compounds seems to intensify the hypertensive reaction to 5-HT (PAGE 1952b, PAGE and MCCUBBIN 1953b, SCHNEIDER and YONKMAN 1954). According to PAGE (1952b) the same result might be obtained by transection of the spinal cord at C_6, by atropinization of the animal or by cervical vagotomy. This has not, however, been confirmed (DOUGLAS and TOH 1953, ERSPAMER 1954, FREYBURGER et al. 1952, SCHNEIDER and YONKMAN 1954, BOCK and MEIER 1963). JACOB and CUGURRA (1960) found, on the contrary, that acute vagotomy favoured the appearance of late hypotension.

Nicotine (0.01—2 mg/kg, i.v.) progressively inhibits the 5-HT "spike" (first component of the hypertensive effect). Lower doses of nicotine depress the 5-HT "dome" (second component of the hypertensive effect) and the hypertensive response caused by tryptamine, but higher doses of nicotine enhance them. There is no crossed tachyphylaxis between 5-HT and nicotine (JACOB and MICHAUD 1962).

The hypertensive effect of 5-HT is frequently weakened by sympatholytic agents (piperoxane, priscoline, yohimbine, dibenamine, dibenziline, ergotamine, hydrogenated ergot alkaloids); much more rarely it is abolished or reversed completely (ERSPAMER 1952, 1953; FREYBURGER et al. 1952; PAGE 1952b; PAGE and MCCUBBIN 1953b; SCHNEIDER and YONKMAN 1954; SCARINCI 1955). Procaine (1—10 mg/kg, i.v.) and high doses of cocaine (2—5 mg/kg, i.v.) diminish the blood pressure rise and in most experiments abolish the initial fall (SCHNEIDER and YONKMAN 1954, WEIDMANN and CERLETTI 1961, CERLETTI and WEIDMANN 1962). Low doses of cocaine, however, slightly potentiate the 5-HT effect (WEID-

MANN and CERLETTI 1961, CERLETTI and WEIDMANN 1962). Bilateral adrenalectomy during an acute experiment produced discordant results. Whereas according to SCHNEIDER et al. (1954) it did not seem to alter the cardiovascular or respiratory response to 5-HT, according to SCARINCI (1955) it caused a reduction of the pressor effect of the amine. Bilateral adrenalectomy, followed by administration for several weeks of desoxycorticosterone trimethylacetate, was found even by SCHNEIDER et al. (1954) to decrease the pressor response and to augment the depressor response to 5-HT.

Bilateral nephrectomy selectively augments the pressor actions of 5-HT and tryptamine, though less regularly and less prominently than the actions of angiotonin and renin (McCUBBIN and PAGE 1954). 1-Hydrazinophthalazine does not appear to be a constant and specific inhibitor of 5-HT (ERSPAMER 1954). 2-Methyl-3-ethyl-5-aminoindole and 2,3-dimethyl-5-aminoindole antagonize the circulatory effects of 5-HT inconstantly and partially. If indeed they are occasionally able to attenuate or abolish the hypertensive phase in the reaction to the substance, they never reduce, but sometimes seem rather to accentuate the hypotensive phase. The anti-5-HT action of the nitroindoles given orally is doubtful (PAGE and McCUBBIN 1953b). 2-Methyl-3-ethyl-5-dimethylamino-indole and 1-methyl-2-methyl-3-ethyl-5-dimethylaminoindole, given either orally or subcutaneously, are similarly incapable of protecting normal dogs from the pressor effects of 5-HT (SHAW and WOOLEY 1954).

The pressure rise provoked by 5-HT (30—50 μg/kg) is, on the contrary, potently antagonized by LSD and methysergide (UML) in doses as low as 10 to 20 μg/kg (SCHNEIDER and RINEHART 1956b, FANCHAMPS et al. 1960), and moderately by BAS, given in high doses (4—8 mg/kg) (JACOB and CUGURRA 1960). Surprisingly enough, BOL was found to exhibit weak and inconstant activity towards the cardiovascular responses to 5-HT (SALMOIRAGHI et al. 1957).

The influence of cevadine, veratridine, belladonine, bulbocapnine and harmine on the pressor action of 5-HT in the dog anaesthetized with butallylonal is variable (HOTOVY and ROESCH 1958). According to MILKOVIĆ et al. (1955) both the hypertensive and hypotensive effects of 5-HT in anaesthetized dogs and rabbits are consistently reduced by intravenous infusion of Fe^{++} salts at a rate of 1.3—1.4 mg/kg/min. Dogs premedicated with reserpine respond to infusion of 4 μg/kg/min 5-HT with a gradual additional fall of blood pressure over the reserpine-induced hypotension. Integrity of the vagi is not essential for these results (CRONHEIM and GOURZIS 1956, 1960). The hypertensive effect of 5-HT given by rapid intravenous injection is, on the contrary, either antagonized (SCHNEIDER and RINEHART 1956a, 1956b; RUTLEDGE et al. 1959; WEIDMANN and CERLETTI 1961; CERLETTI and WEIDMANN 1962) or enhanced (SCHNEIDER and RINEHART 1956a, 1956b) by reserpine pretreatment, according to experimental conditions. SCHNEIDER and RINEHART (1956b) suggest that reserpine has a dual effect on the blood pressure response to 5-HT; namely, a peripheral antagonizing effect and a central potentiating effect.

Because the vasoconstrictor effect of 5-HT in dogs anaesthetized with aprobarbital and under ganglionic blockade with chlorisondamine is inhibited by reserpine and since noradrenaline infusion in reserpine-treated animals does not restore the pressor action of 5-HT, unlike that of tyramine, WEIDMANN and CERLETTI (1961, 1962) suggest that 5-HT vasoconstriction has a certain character of its own and that 5-HT acts on a hypothetical synaptic structure at a level intermediate between the site of action of noradrenaline (direct action on the vascular smooth muscle) and tyramine (liberation of noradrenaline-like substances from the depots).

Methylphenidate administered to anaesthetized dogs markedly potentiates the blood pressure response to 5-HT. This potentiating effect, however, disappears after reserpine premedication (RUTLEDGE et al. 1959). Contrary to expectations, pretreatment with MAO-inhibitors (iproniazid, β-phenylisopropylhydrazine, harmine and others) has been found to decrease the cardiovascular effects of 5-HT. According to PAGE and McCUBBIN (1953a, 1953b) the response to 5-HT of dogs with chronic neurogenic hypertension is strikingly different from that seen in normotensive animals. Leaving aside the inconstant appearance of moderate hypertensive peaks, the basic reaction to 5-HT of the hypertensive dog was found to be an unusually conspicuous and prolonged hypotension. In the hypertensive dog even introduction of 5-HT into the perfusion liquid of a hind leg having intact nervous connections but no vascular connections with the body produced evident vasodilatation, in contrast to the usual vasoconstriction. Atropine did not change either the intensity or direction of the pressure reaction; ganglionic blockade, on the contrary, reversed the frankly hypotensive response, making it clearly hypertensive. The above peculiar pressure changes were considerably less conspicuous in dogs with acute neurogenic hypertension, and were lacking in animals made hypertensive by noradrenaline infusion or by increase in endocranic pressure.

On the basis of experiments carried out on normotensive dogs pretreated with ganglion-blocking drugs and in dogs with neurogenic hypertension, as well as in cats and rabbits, both normal and with ganglionic blockade, PAGE and McCUBBIN (1953a, 1953b) and PAGE (1954) consider the pressure response to 5-HT to be the result of various distinct factors: 1) intense direct vasoconstriction; 2) a reflex, possibly in the nature of the Bezold-Jarisch effect, that can be blocked by atropine; 3) transient autonomic ganglion blockade; 4) strong peripheral action that reduces or abolishes neurogenic vasoconstriction; 5) cardiac stimulation. Factors 1) and, to a lesser extent, 5) are believed to be responsible for the hypertension, factors 2) and 3) for the initial transient pressure fall and factor 4) for the more persistent secondary hypotension. PAGE and McCUBBIN are of the opinion that inhibition of neurogenic vasoconstrictor tone is a decidedly more important phenomenon than direct vasoconstriction. They consequently believe that direction and intensity of the pressure response to 5-HT are to a great extent determined by the degree of normal resting vasoconstrictor tone. If this tone is high (dogs with chronic neurogenic hypertension) the predominant response to 5-HT is hypotension, if the tone is low (ganglionic blockade) hypertension has the advantage.

It appears that in the above interpretation of the mechanism of action of 5-HT little, if any, importance is attributed to stimulation of vasal chemoreceptor zones. HEYMANS and VAN DEN HEUVEL-HEYMANS (1953) have carried out careful experiments on this topic. Having ascertained that 5-HT has no stimulant action on the chemoreceptors of the carotid sinus and that its circulatory and respiratory effects do not depend on stimulation of afferent fibres in the carotid sinus nerves or in the cervical vago-aortic nerves, the Belgian investigators maintain that 5-HT hypertension must be due primarily to peripheral vasoconstriction and secondarily to direct stimulation of the vasomotor centers. Only following local bilateral application on the carotid sinuses would large doses of 5-HT (200 μg) cause a depression of the hypertensive reflexes originating from the carotid sinuses, with ensuing reflex hypotension.

However, these essentially negative conclusions have not been entirely accepted by others. JACOB and CUGURRA (1960) found that carotid sinus denervation partly depressed the pressor response to moderate doses of 5-HT (20—40 μg/kg, i.v.) and favoured the appearance of late hypotension. BRAUN and STERN (1961) in their turn, observed that 5-HT (80 μg/kg, i.v.) displayed in the dog a much less pronounced pressor effect after elimination of the carotid and aortic chemoreceptors (bilateral high cervical vagotomy, crushing the carotid bodies and sectioning the carotid sinus nerves), and that shifting of the site of 5-HT injection from the femoral vein towards the ascending aorta shortened the latent period elapsing between amine administration and pressure changes.

It has been previously reported that intravenous infusion of 5-HT constantly produces a sustained pressure fall which differs from the usual amphibaric reaction to single quick injections of the amine. PAGE and MCCUBBIN (1956) suggest that when 5-HT is infused, a release of endogenous histamine may also substantially contribute, together with peripheral inhibition of neurogenic vasoconstriction, to the depressor response. This idea is not new and it has been accepted by other investigators. SCARINCI (1955b, 1955c) noted that 5-HT hypotension was inhibited in dogs, cats and rabbits by antihistaminic drugs, and similarly BUÑAG and WALASZEK (1961a) found that the sustained pressure fall produced by 5-HT in dogs premedicated with BAS-phenol was antagonized by diphenhydramine, an antihistamine agent, but remained unchanged after bilateral vagotomy.

Because 5-HT is apparently capable of eliciting a Bezold-Jarisch reflex, the question has been raised as to whether the reflex seen after veratrine administration could be mediated by 5-HT. The answer was negative (FRAHM et al. 1957).

Responses to 5-methoxytryptamine (ERSPAMER 1952a) and 7-HTP (PAGE 1952a, 1952b) are on the whole similar to those described for 5-HT. Both substances are, however, 3 to 5 times less potent than 5-HT.

4-HT (200—300 μg/kg) elicits a biphasic reaction with the major component depressor (BUÑAG and WALASZEK 1962).

5-Acetyltryptamine consistently produces hypotension both in the "open-chest" and in the "closed-chest" anaesthetized dog (BEN et al. 1962).

Bufotenine, and bufotenidine even more so, differ from 5-HT in being more regularly and potently hypertensive. Injected intravenously in doses of 0.05 to 1 mg/kg they provoke a marked rise in blood pressure, which is potentiated by cocaine and abolished or reversed by yohimbine, and still more by yohimbine plus harmalol (RAYMOND-HAMET 1941, 1942b, 1943a, 1943b, 1944; BUÑAG and WALASZEK 1962c). Sparteine shows no effect (RAYMOND-HAMET 1946). Bufotenine increases the reactivity of the circulatory system to successive injections of adrenaline, but it partly inhibits the pressure rise provoked by carotid occlusion (RAYMOND-HAMET 1942a). On the basis of the above results and of the observation that bufotenine and bufotenidine have only little constrictor effect when applied locally on the vessels, RAYMOND-HAMET (1941, 1942b, 1942c, 1943a) holds the opinion that both substances are to be listed among the nicotine-like drugs, acting on the vessels and on the blood pressure through a discharge of catecholamines.

Small doses of O-methylbufotenine induce tachycardia in dogs and increase blood pressure; large doses have the opposite effect (KANAI et al. 1962).

Concerning the effects on blood pressure of psilocybin and psilocin results are at variance. WEIDMANN et al. (1958) and CERLETTI (1959) found that intravenous administration of 50—100 μg/kg psilocybin produced in the dog a moderate but relatively long-lasting drop in the mean arterial pressure, accompanied by active decrease in kidney volume. MAXWELL et al. (1962) as well as BUÑAG and WALASZEK (1962c), on the contrary, observed that 200—500 μg/kg psilocybin produced a sustained increase in the arterial pressure (17%) and calculated vascular resistances in the body. Psilocin (100—200 μg/kg) had a similarly prolonged pressor effect (BUÑAG and WALASZEK 1962c).

5-HTP given by rapid intravenous injection (30 mg/kg) produces a blood pressure fall both in normal and in reserpinized dogs, but whereas in the former pressure returns toward normal, in the latter it remains low (CRONHEIM 1960).

Tryptamine (0.1—1 mg/kg) causes a rise in systemic arterial pressure which is occasionally preceded or followed by a fall (LAIDLAW 1912, RAYMOND-HAMET 1941a, REID 1952a, PAGE 1952b, BUÑAG and WALASZAK 1962c). These effects can be seen when the vagus nerves are intact or divided. The pressor response is reduced but not completely abolished by yohimbine (2—4 mg/kg) (REID 1952a); it seems, on the contrary, definitely augmented after spinal cord transection, ganglionic blockade and pitressin administration. Piperoxane and priscoline have little or no effect (PAGE 1952b). In sharp contrast to the pressure effects of 5-HT, hypertension elicited by tryptamine is potentiated by prior treatment with MAO-inhibitors or, much more effectively, with MAO-inhibitors plus reserpine (GOLDBERG and SJOERDSMA 1959, BURFORD and WALASZEK 1960).

The response to tryptamine in neurogenic hypertensive dogs is somewhat less than in normal ones (PAGE 1952b).

N,N-dimethyltryptamine (200—500 μg/kg) displays a pressor effect similar to that described for tryptamine (BUÑAG and WALASZEK 1962c).

REID (1952a) ascribes the rise in systemic arterial pressure to direct action on the vascular smooth muscle and, subordinately, to some stimulant action on the heart, the initial pressure fall to pulmonary vasoconstriction and the secondary fall possibly to coronary vasoconstriction; BURFORD and WALASZEK (1960) and WALASZEK and BURFORD (1963) maintain that the pressor effect of tryptamine is produced partly through norepinephrine release and partly through a direct action of its own.

WOOLLEY and SHAW (1957) postulate the existence in the vascular smooth muscle of separate receptors for 5-HT and tryptamine. This is based on the observation that whereas anaesthetized dogs are protected against the pressor response to 5-HT by prior treatment with BAS-phenol, they are not protected against the pressor effects of tryptamine.

The same opinion is substantially shared by VANE et al. (see WOOLEY et al. 1962) on the basis of the observation that the pressor response to tryptamine, unlike that to 5-HT, is (a) prevented by cocaine, (b) abolished by pretreatment of the animal with reserpine, and (c) then restored by an infusion of noradrenaline.

Gramine injected into the dog under chloralose anaesthesia evokes variable responses, depending upon the dose: with 1.25—2.5 mg/kg a moderate hypertension is predominant; with 8—9 mg/kg the transient initial pressure rise is followed by prolonged hypotension. Gramine is to be listed among the minor adrenolytic drugs (RAYMOND-HAMET 1937, 1938).

Serotonamidine (5-hydroxyindoleacetamidine) is 6—7 times more potent than 5-HT as a hypertensive agent in the anaesthetized dog; however, the effect is of shorter duration. Indoleacetamidine displays approximately the same pressor activity as 5-HT. Unlike that of indoleacetamidine, hypertension produced by serotonamidine is blocked by BAS-phenol (WOOLEY and SHAW 1957).

Cat. Hypotension is the predominant pressure response to intravenous 5-HT in the intact cat (Figs. 2 and 14). More rarely, a mixed response (hypotension followed, or interrupted, by a slight pressure increase) or a frank hypertensive reaction can be seen (COMROE 1952; COMROE et al. 1953; ERSPAMER 1952a; FREYBURGER et al. 1952; GINZEL and KOTTEGODA 1954; PAGE and MCCUBBIN 1953a, 1956; REID 1952b; SCHNEIDER and YONKMAN 1953, 1954; POWELL 1955;

KOTTEGODA and MOTT 1955; WEIDMANN and CERLETTI 1955). If present, hypertension is less intense than that provoked by doses of adrenaline or noradrenaline 60 to 100 times smaller (ERSPAMER 1952, FREYBURGER et al. 1952). Simultaneously with the fall in blood pressure an abrupt and marked drop in heart rate is seen, rarely followed by a slight increase in heart rate (SCHNEIDER and YONKMAN 1954).

When correlating preganglionic splancnic outflow with pressor- and chemoreceptor inflow from the carotid sinus and aortic area of the cat, it has been found by DONTAS (1955) that intravenous injection of 4—22 μg 5-HT base produced, at the time of abrupt hypotension and bradycardia, a progressive decrease of pressoreceptor spikes and a simultaneous decrease or abolition of splancnic afferent discharge. During recovery from hypotension the splancnic activity reappeared.

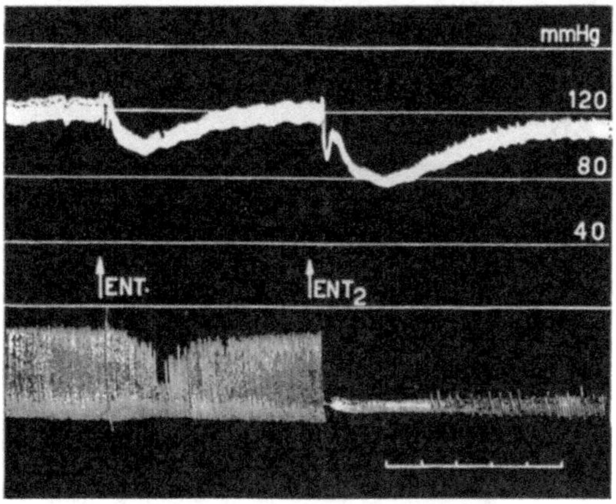

Fig. 2. Cat deeply anaesthetized with secobarbital (35 mg/kg, i.m.). Upper tracing, carotid blood pressure; lower tracing, respiration. Time in min. Blood pressure response to intravenous injection of 4 (ENT_1) and 40 μg/kg 5-HT(ENT_2) was frankly hypotensive. Respiration was strikingly depressed by the drug. [From Fig. 10, ERSPAMER, V., R. C. sci. Farmitalia 1, 39 (1954).]

Cocaine potentiates, as a rule, the pressor response to 5-HT. Purely hypotensive reactions after the alkaloid are rare, hypertension is more sustained and with large doses of 5-HT (20—40 μg/kg) a considerable secondary pressure rise occasionally appears. This has been attributed to stimulation of the suprarenal medulla (FREYBURGER et al. 1952). Procaine 10 mg/kg and nupercaine 0.5 to 0.7 mg/kg antagonize the fall of pressure and bradycardia provoked by large doses of 5-HT (SCHNEIDER and YONKMAN 1953, 1954). Piperoxane and dibenamine generally reduce, but do not suppress, 5-HT hypertension (FREYBURGER et al. 1952). Yohimbine 1—2 mg/kg, on the contrary, does sometimes abolish it completely (PAGE and MCCUBBIN 1954, REID 1952). Cardiovascular responses to 5-HT in the cat are only slightly and irregularly antagonized by BOL and LSD (WEIDMANN and CERLETTI 1957; SALMOIRAGHI, MCCUBBIN and PAGE 1957). Pretreatment with iproniazid (2×50 mg/kg) or reserpine (2 mg/kg) fails to produce pressure changes different from those seen in untreated animals; pretreatment with 2-naphthylguanidine (100—500 μg/kg), on the contrary, causes 5-HT to elicit a rise in blood pressure instead of the usual fall (FASTIER et al. 1959). Whereas it seems well established that ganglionic blockade can abolish the normal depressor action of 5-HT and possibly reverse it to a pressor action (PAGE and MCCUBBIN 1953a, SCHNEIDER and YONKMAN 1954) there exists no agreement concerning the influence of atropine, vagal section and cooling the vagi. The statement of some research workers (COMROE et al. 1953, PAGE 1952b, SCHNEIDER and YONKMAN 1953, KOTTEGODA and MOTT 1955) that the hypotensive effect of 5-HT is largely abolished after atropine, vagotomy or cooling the vagi, and that pressor action increases, has not been confirmed (FREYBURGER et al. 1952, GINZEL and KOTTEGODA 1954, REID 1952b), or confirmed only in part by others (WEIDMANN and CERLETTI 1955).

When given intravenously to the vagotomized cat under dial anaesthesia, 5-HT (0.25—5 mg/kg) reinforces and prolongs the pressor effect of successive doses of adrenaline (5—10 μg/kg). LECOMTE (1953) attributes this sensitization, which disappears after 30 min and cannot be obtained with tryptamine, to the presence of a phenolic hydroxy group in the 5-HT molecule, which retards the oxidation of the adrenaline injected.

In marked contrast to the cat with intact nervous system, the pithed cat and the spinal cat always respond to 5-HT with a frank hypertensive reaction (Fig. 3) which is occasionally enhanced by cocaine, and is always at least 25 to 50 times less than that produced by adrenaline (ERSPAMER 1954, FREYBURGER et al. 1952, PAGE and MCCUBBIN 1953a, SCHNEIDER and YONKMAN 1953, WEIDMANN and CERLETTI 1957). The blood pressure rise produced by 5-HT in spinal cats is due, according to WEIDMANN and CERLETTI (1957) not only to a direct constrictor effect on the vascular smooth muscle, but also to increase in the heart rate and to stimulation of the adrenal medulla. This adrenal effect of 5-HT is enhanced by iproniazid, and cannot be blocked either by hexamethonium or by LSD.

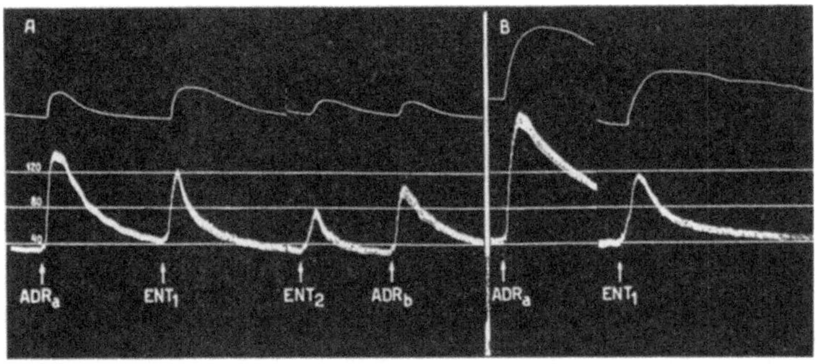

Fig. 3. Spinal cat under artificial respiration. Upper tracing, contraction of the nictitating membrane; lower tracing, carotid blood pressure. Between A and B intravenous injection of 8 mg/kg cocaine hydrochloride. In the spinal cat intravenous 5-HT was, like adrenaline, frankly hypertensive. Cocaine remarkably potentiated all the effects of adrenaline. The effect of 5-HT on the nictitating membrane was clearly reinforced by cocaine, that on the blood pressure remained practically unchanged. [From Fig. 14, ERPSAMER, V., R. C. sci. Farmitalia 1, 47 (1954).]

There is no concordance of opinion in the interpretation of the hypotension caused by 5-HT. REID (1952b) ascribes the short-lived pressure fall that occasionally precedes hypertension to a primary constriction of the pulmonary arterial bed, with ensuing reduction in the volume of blood returning to the left heart; he offers no explanation for the prolonged secondary hypotension. COMROE et al. (1953) believe that the hypotension is largely due to the associated bradycardia. PAGE and MCCUBBIN (1953a) hold that the explanation of pressure changes given for the dog applies equally to the cat. SCHNEIDER and YONKMAN (1954) consider it to be part of a complex cardiopulmonary mechanism. Finally, GINZEL and KOTTEGODA (1954) maintain that the mechanism of the pressure fall may differ depending upon the magnitude of the dose of 5-HT injected. Hypotension which follows the introduction of small doses of 5-HT seems to be due predominantly to baroreceptor stimulation and secondarily to central stimulation; pulmonary vasoconstriction would come into play only with higher doses of the substance. KOTTEGODA and MOTT (1955) are convinced that impulses producing reflex peripheral vasodilatation and reflex bradycardia are carried to the centres by afferent vagal fibres. This idea is based on the previously reported observation that hypotension is reduced or abolished by vagotomy and by cooling the vagi.

Since it is not known in what way 5-HT influences the vessels of the carotid body, the possibility of a constrictor effect giving origin to local anoxaemia cannot be ruled out (GINZEL 1958).

Ginzel and Kottegoda rightly emphasize the ability of 5-HT and tryptamine to produce temporary desensitization to their own actions. It is possible that some contradictory findings with these two substances and with their antagonists can be explained by this self-antagonism.

Cardiovascular responses to 5-HT in the cat are only slightly and irregularly antagonised by BOL and LSD (Salmoiraghi et al. 1957, Weidmann and Cerletti 1957). Pretreatment with iproniazid (2×50 mg/kg) or reserpine (2 mg/kg) fails to produce pressure changes different from those seen in untreated animals; pretreatment with 2-naphthyl-guanidine (100—500 μg/kg), on the contrary, causes 5-HT to elicit a rise in blood pressure instead of the usual fall (Fastier et al. 1959).

Numerous other tryptamine derivatives have been tested on the blood pressure of intact cats, pithed cats or cats with ganglionic blockade. The main results are as follows.

Bufotenine produces in the intact cat depression of arterial pressure or amphibaric responses (Handovsky 1920, Gessner et al. 1961, Buñag and Walaszek 1962c). More rarely, predominant hypertension is seen (Weidmann and Cerletti 1959). The same is true for 5-methoxytryptamine and 5-methylbufotenine. After pithing or blocking, response is frankly hypertensive. 5-Methylbufotenine raises the blood pressure of the pithed cat more potently than bufotenine; 5-methoxytryptamine, on the contrary, is less potent than 5-HT. 5-Methylbufotenine induces tachycardia in small doses but bradycardia in large doses (Kainai et al. 1962). N-acetylation of 5-methoxytryptamine (=melatonin) destroys its activity on blood pressure (Gessner et al. 1961).

Bufotenine O-phosphate displays in the intact cat a hypertensive action which is greater than that produced by bufotenine (Weidmann and Cerletti 1959).

Intravenous administration in the intact cat of 50—100 μg/kg doses of psilocin or psilocybin is followed by a short but distinct rise in pressure, usually accompanied by relative bradycardia. This pressure rise seems more the result of centrally mediated vasoconstriction than of a direct peripheral effect, since the hypertensive response is not enhanced but rather reduced in the spinal cat (Weidmann and Cerletti 1959, Cerletti 1959).

In the intact cat, 4-HT (100 μg/kg, i.v.) produces a rise of blood pressure which is 2 to 6 times less intense but more sustained than that elicited by the same dose of 5-HT. In the spinal cat, 4-HT causes hypertension, like 5-HT, but whereas with 5-HT the pressure rise is proportional to the dose administered, with 4-HT this is not so.

5-HTP, given intravenously in doses of 2.5—5 mg/kg, elicits a moderate fall of blood pressure, which lasts 15—20 min; the same dose of 4-HTP produces a more pronounced rise of blood pressure, lasting 30—50 min (Erspamer et al. 1960).

Both in the intact and in the pithed cat intravenous bufotenidine (20—100 μg/kg) causes a prompt adrenaline-like rise of blood pressure. In the pithed cat it is 5 to 7 times less potent than adrenaline, but 250 times more potent than 5-HT (Powell 1955).

Tryptamine always has the characteristics of a predominantly hypertensive drug, thus giving pressure responses similar to those described in the dog: rise in pressure which is occasionally preceded or followed by a minor fall (Laidlaw 1912, Gyermek 1953, Reid 1952a, Powell 1955, Buñag and Walaszek 1962c). Cocaine does not potentiate tryptamine hypertension; yohimbine, ergotoxine, hydergin and, to a lesser degree, nicotine as well as diphenhydramine and other antihistaminic agents reduce it somewhat; ganglionic blockade, atropine and curare show no remarkable effect (REID 1952, GYERMEK 1953).

Tested on the decerebrated or pithed cat, N-methyltryptamine is less hypertensive than tryptamine, and N,N-dimethyltryptamine still less so (CHEN and CHEN 1933; ERSPAMER 1952a, 1954). The trimethylammonium derivative seems, on the contrary, more active than tryptamine, possessing about $^{1}/_{20}$ of the pressor action of adrenaline (CHEN and CHEN 1933). Gramine causes very moderate hypertensive responses even when given in large doses (5—20 mg/kg) and sometimes hypertension is preceded by a pressure fall (POWELL and CHEN 1945, POWELL 1955).

Finally, several of the substituted β-aminoethylindazoles synthetized by AINSWORTH (1958) prove to be hypotensive in the cat. The most effective members of the series are 5-hydroxy-N,N-dimethylaminoethylindazole, 5-hydroxy-aminoethylindazole and 5-hydroxy-N-isopropylaminoethylindazole. These compounds produce a clear fall of blood pressure at doses of 0.1, 0.5 and 1 mg/kg, respectively.

Man. Single intravenous injections of 5-HT produce both in normotensive and hypertensive subjects variable responses probably dependent, to some extent, on the dose and on the manner of administration of the drug.

SPIES and STONE (1952) found that intravenous injections of 0.5—5 mg 5-HT constantly elicited a rise in both systolic and diastolic pressure independent of the initial pressure level, i.e., in normal as well as in hypotensive and hypertensive patients. After 5 to 10 minutes, the pressure returned to normal. Subsequent injections at intervals of 2 to 3 hours gave identical results.

PAGE and MCCUBBIN (1953a) obtained partly discordant results from continuous pressure recordings in 20 hypertensive patients. They believe that the most common response of hypertensive human beings to small intravenous doses of 5-HT (0.06—0.12 mg) is slight hypotension, with a negligible hypertensive component. Larger doses (0.3—1.8 mg) produce the typical response observed in dogs (brief drop followed by pressure rise and then by a more sustained drop).

The results of HOLLANDER et al. (1956, 1957) in 30 hypertensive patients were again partly at variance. These investigators observed that depressor responses occurred more often after doses of 5-HT smaller than 0.3 mg; biphasic responses (brief fall and then overshoot for 1—5 min) more frequently over 0.3 mg; and pressor responses (increase in both systolic and diastolic pressures for 1 to 6 min, eventually followed by a brief drop) towards 1 mg and more.

Predominant fall of systolic and diastolic blood pressure, sometimes preceded by a short-lived rise, was observed also by other research workers after 0.4—3 mg of intravenous 5-HT (ANNONI et al. 1955, BALDRIGHI and FERRARI 1955, REDISCH et al. 1956, BOCK et al. 1957).

Following infusion of 5-HT into a vein (HOLLANDER et al. 1957, LEMESSURIER et al. 1959) or into the main pulmonary artery (GROVER et al. 1958), at a rate of 10—1000 μg/min, systemic arterial pressure displays only minor and variable variations, while at the highest dosage levels, systemic vascular resistance decreases.

5-HT given intramuscularly in single or repeated doses of 1—4 mg does not appreciably change the systemic blood pressure or only produces unimportant delayed responses (BASSANI and FANTINI 1956, ABBATI et al. 1955, CORREALE 1957).

The blood pressure effects of 5-HT are not prevented by prior administration of hexamethonium, regitine, atropine, antihistamines or reserpine (HOLLANDER et al. 1956, 1957). When 1 mg of 5-HT is injected during pentolinium-induced hypotension, there is a short elevation followed by a marked and sustained drop of both diastolic and systolic pressures exceeding considerably the hypotensive effect of pentolinium alone (REDISCH et al. 1956).

Possible side-effects of intravenous infusion of 5-HT in man are an increase in local venous pressure with occasional reflux of blood into the afferent vessels, burning pain along the course of the vein, which may become prominent, firm and tender; heaviness and tingling in the extremities; pressure in the head and eyes; nausea; cough, shortness of breath; abdominal cramps, and, occasionally, blurred vision, sweating, headache and excessive salivation (HOLLANDER et al. 1957, STEFANINI and MAGALINI 1956, PAGE 1957, LEMESSURIER et al. 1959). Thrombosis of the infused vein is exceptionally frequent (40% and 90%) when 5-HT is infused at a rate of 400 and 800 μg/min (LEMESSURIER et al. 1959).

Intravenous injections into human volunteers of 0.03—0.12 mg/kg bufotenine base over times ranging from 3 to 20 min produce purpling of the skin in the head and neck with slight tendency of blood pressure to increase (FABING et al.

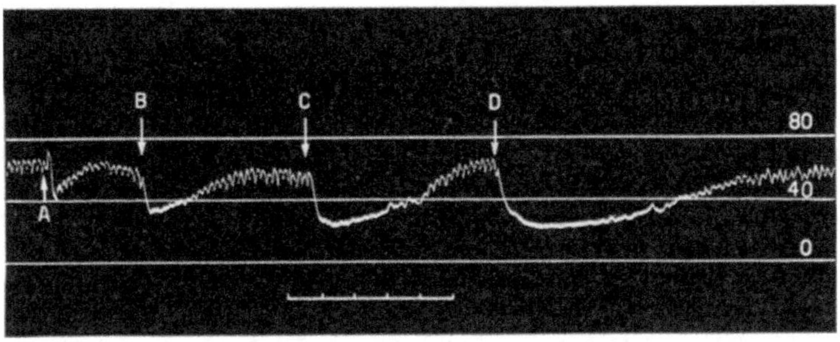

Fig. 4. Rabbit anaesthetized with urethane. Blood pressure response to intravenous injections of 15 (A), 30 (B), 70 (C) and 140 μg/kg (D) 5-HT base. Time in min. 5-HT produced pure hypotension at all dose levels, and decrease of blood pressure was proportional, both in intensity and duration, to the dose of the amine. [From Fig. 15, ERSPAMER, V., R. C. sci. Farmitalia 1, 49 (1954).]

1956). Psilocybin, on the contrary, frequently induces hypotension and bradycardia when given parenterally to normal subjects and to mental patients in doses of 5 to 14 mg (DELAY et al. 1959).

Oral administration of N,N-dimethyltryptamine in a single dose up to 350 mg, or intravenous injection of 5—25 mg of the drug in 3 min does not display obvious cardiovascular effects (TURNER and MERLIS 1959).

Rabbit. The rabbit under urethane or pentobarbital anaesthesia reacts to crude enteramine preparations and to 5-HT with a pure hypotensive response, which is easily repeatable and satisfactorily correlated with the dose (ERSPAMER 1940b, 1940c, 1952a; PAGE and MCCUBBIN 1953a; SCHNEIDER and YONKMAN 1954). Transient slowing of the heart rate associated with cardiac irregularities is also present with uniformity (SCHNEIDER and YONKMAN 1954). Atropine, bilateral section of the vagus nerves and sympatholytic doses of dibenamine show either no effect or only a slight one on the depressor action of 5-HT (ERSPAMER 1940a, 1953a; PAGE and MCCUBBIN 1953a).

This action is, on the contrary, reduced or abolished by large intravenous doses (10—40 mg/kg) of tetrazotized diorthoanisidine (CATO and CAFRUNY 1960).

SCHNEIDER and YONKMAN were not able to confirm the statement by PAGE and MCCUBBIN that ganglionic blockade reverses the action of 5-HT from depressor to pressor.

According to LECOMTE and VAN DE BERG (1957) the blood pressure fall caused in rabbits by 5-HT is to a great extent dependent upon pulmonary vasoconstriction and consequent reduction of cardiac output.

The rabbit is less sensitive to tryptamine than either the dog or the cat. Injections of 0.2—1.8 mg/kg cause a small rise in systemic arterial pressure, which is sometimes preceded by a transient fall and followed by a further fall lasting 2 or 3 min. There is little change in pressure in the right ventricle (REID 1952a). N,N-dimethyltryptamine (125—250 μg/kg, i.v.) produces a more prolonged action than tryptamine (BUÑAG and WALASZEK 1962), whereas with bufotenine (HANDOVSKY 1920, BUÑAG and WALASZEK 1962), bufotenidine (5—100 μg/kg) (UEDA et al. 1957) and large doses of gramine (SUPNIEWSKI and SERAFINOWNA 1938) hypotension is predominant.

Psilocybin (5 mg/kg, i.v.) elicits in the waking rabbit a moderate but sustained elevation of blood pressure, accompanied by transient bradycardia (MONNIER 1959).

Guinea-pig. Intravenous injections of 0.1—0.2 mg/kg 5-HT in animals anaesthetized with pentobarbital usually elicit moderate hypertensive responses. With higher doses (0.4—0.8 mg/kg) hypertension is preceded or followed by a hypotensive phase (ERSPAMER 1952).

Rat. The intact unanaesthetized rat responds to 5-HT given by subcutaneous route in doses of 0.4 mg/kg and more with a regular pressure fall, lasting 90 to 180 min, accompanied by intense dilatation of the cutaneous vessels. Doses of less than 0.4 mg/kg are either ineffective or nearly so. 5-Methoxytryptamine is approximately 4 times less potent than 5-HT (CORREALE 1954, ERSPAMER 1952, ERSPAMER and OTTOLENGHI 1953, TAKÁCS and VAJDA 1963).

The results obtained by SALMOIRAGHI et al. (1956) in anaesthetized rats given rapid intravenous injections of 5-HT were similar. Doses of 5-HT base as low as 4—10 μg/kg produced a small transient fall in arterial pressure (von Bezold-Jarisch-like effect) succeeded by a small pressure rise, followed in turn by marked and prolonged hypotension (25—65 mm Hg for 3—4 min). Vagus section abolished the von Bezold-Jarisch-like effect; neither vagus section nor inactivation of the carotid sinus modified the prolonged depressor response. After ganglionic blockade or pithing, 5-HT elicited only large pressor responses. LSD and BOL in large doses effectively antagonized pressor-depressor responses to 5-HT in rats (SALMOIRAGHI et al. 1957).

Although confirming that the basic effect of intravenous 5-HT in rats is depressor, OUTSCHOORN and JACOB (1960) affirm that the shape of blood pressure response to the amine depends both on the dose (threshold = 0.5—1 μg/kg) and the initial level of blood pressure. The depressor effect is, in fact, less apparent or even absent at low and more pronounced at high pressure levels and the converse applies to the pressor component.

Intravenous infusion of 5-HT causes slight, transient decrease of blood pressure at infusion rates of 0.8—2.5 μg/kg/min, initial larger decrease of pressure with recovery at rates of 3—5 μg/kg/min, and finally biphasic blood pressure curve with initial fall and return to levels higher than control at rates of 5.5—8 μg/kg/min (DEL GRECO and CORCORAN 1956).

The prolonged depressor effect of 5-HT is interpreted by SALMOIRAGHI et al. (1956) as being due partly to depression of neurogenic vasoconstrictor tone and partly to a direct peripheral vasodilator effect of the amine. OUTSCHOORN and JACOB (1960) in their turn suggest that the depressor effect is both of parasympathetic and sympathetic origin, and the pressor effect of sympathetic origin, at least in part.

In contrast to 5-HT, bufotenine and psilocybin produce a pure rise in blood pressure not only in rats with ganglionic blockade but also in normal rats. In addition, the pressor response is considerably more sustained than with 5-HT. BOL is again a good antagonist (GESSNER et al. 1960).

Calf. In calves given a 3-minute intravenous infusion of 0.2 mg/kg/min 5-HT base, carotid blood pressure presents a drop of 28 ± 6.7 mm Hg (KUIDA et al. 1961).

Chicken. 5-HT and tryptamine produce a fall in blood pressure upon intravenous injection in anaesthetized chickens. The minimum effective dose of 5-HT is 1—3 μg/kg and maximal effects are elicited by 100—200 μg/kg. Tryptamine is 3—5 times less active (POWELL 1955; LECOMTE and BEAUMARIAGE 1957; NATOFF and LOCKETT 1957; BUÑAG and WALASZEK 1961b, 1961c; EBLE 1962).

The depressor response is not significantly affected by vagotomy, physostigmine or mecamylamine. It is, on the contrary, reversed in most instances by atropine (0.5—5 mg/kg) and either blocked or altered by antihistaminic drugs, such as parabromdylamine and diphenhydramine (BUÑAG and WALASZEK 1961b, 1961c). Chickens depleted of tissue histamine by repeated injection of 48/80 are found to respond to injections of 5-HT (5—100 μg/kg) or tryptamine (60 to 1000 μg/kg) with a rise in arterial pressure, instead of the usual fall. Moreover, bioassay for histamine done on urine samples taken after injection of 5-HT (50—150 μg/kg) or tryptamine (500—1500 μg/kg) shows significant increments in urine content (BUÑAG and WALASZEK 1962b).

On the basis of these data, BUÑAG and WALASZEK suggest that histamine liberation is the major factor responsible for the depressor response to tryptamine and 5-HT in chickens, and that the latent vasopressor effect of 5-HT, which can be observed in the intact animal only when the normally stronger depressor activity of the drug has been nullified by pretreatment with atropine, antihistaminics or compound 48/80, is mainly produced by a direct peripheral vasoconstriction exerted by the 5-HT molecule *per se.*

Injections of 5-HT (0.01—0.1 μg) into the vessels of the isolated perfused chicken wing cause an intense vasoconstriction, which is directly proportional to the injected dose of the amine.

The above view that histamine release is an important factor in the fall of blood pressure caused by tryptamine is not accepted by EBLE (1962, 1963), who believes that this fall is rather the result of an acute pulmonary hypertension. In fact, systemic hypotension in the chicken is accompanied by a rise in peripheral resistance and in right ventricular pressure. Moreover, the depressive effect of tryptamine (0.1—0.3 mg/kg) is immediate and not delayed, it does not show tachyphylaxis (7 doses within 30 min) or cross tachyphylaxis with 48/80, and is not affected by cholinergic blockade with atropine or methylatropine, nor by adrenergic blockade with tolazoline or dichloroisoproterenol.

The most effective drugs for reversing the hypotensive effect of tryptamine are, according to EBLE, the MAO inhibitors tranylcypromine and β-phenylisopropylhydrazine. The pressor response thus obtained is not blocked either by cocaine or by dibenzyline.

Hypotension produced in the chicken by 5-HT and tryptamine can be blocked by lysergic acid derivatives in the following ascending order of potency: ergotamine, dihydroergotamine, LSD, BOL, ergonovine and UML (BUÑAG and WALASZEK 1962a).

Bufotenine (50—100 μg/kg, i.v.) and 4-HT (50—100 μg/kg), like 5-HT and tryptamine, lower the chicken blood pressure; dimethyltryptamine (300 to 750 μg/kg), psilocin (50—100 μg/kg) and psilocybin (100—200 μg/kg), on the contrary, produce a prolonged pressor response (BUÑAG and WALASZEK 1962c).

Single injections of bufotenidine lower the blood pressure. However, upon repeated injections, the depressor action of bufotenidine is reversed to pressor. Gramine (1 mg/kg) behaves essentially like a hypertensive agent (POWELL 1955).

III. Action on special vascular areas

1. Coronary vascular bed

In dogs anaesthetized with morphine and dial-urethane-nembutal, cardiac output (Fick) and coronary blood flow (NO_2 Fick) were measured before and after the mechanical infusion into the left or the right atrium of 8 μg/kg/min 5-HT base over a period of 25 min. It was found that 5-HT produced a 20 to 169% increase in coronary blood flow, a 27—62.5% decrease in coronary vascular resistance and a 31—107% increase of coronary sinus oxygen content. Thus, the decrease in myocardial oxygen extraction associated with the increase in coronary flow resulted in myocardial oxygen consumption remaining unchanged. Myocardial CO_2 excretion was maintained in a similar manner. Mechanical efficiency of the left ventricle fell by 3%. Coronary blood flow/left ventricle work ratio increased by 65% (MAXWELL et al. 1957, MAXWELL et al. 1959, CRUMPTON et al. 1959, ROWE et al. 1963).

Similar results are obtained following injection of 5-HT (1—30 μg in 1 ml saline) into the left main coronary artery. There is a prompt fall in coronary vascular resistance when the drug reaches the coronary circulation, before a change in heart rate and aortic pressure occurs. The percentage decrease in coronary vascular resistance is related to the dose administered. Myocardial oxygen consumption shows no change from control value (GRIGGS and CASE 1960).

Thus, in confirmation of the previous work of SCHOFIELD and WALKER (1953), 5-HT appears to act in the dog as a potent "benign" coronary dilator increasing the oxygen supply to the myocardium without increasing the ventricular work. These results would seem to exculpate 5-HT as a major factor in the genesis of cardiac infarct (MAXWELL et al. 1959).

In contrast to 5-HT, psilocybin (0.5 mg/kg, i.v.) does not show in the dog any true coronary vasodilator properties, and coronary vascular resistance remains unchanged (MAXWELL, KNEEBONE and ELLIOTT 1962).

In the heart-lung preparation of the rabbit 25 μg 5-HT (0.5—5 μg doses are inactive) causes a 25—60% fall of coronary flow with evident increase in coronary vascular resistance (MAGGI 1960).

Both in the isolated heart of the dog and in that of the cat, 30—300 μg 5-HT introduced into the perfusion fluid produces a clear increase in coronary flow (SCHNEIDER and YONKMAN 1954).

According to KAPILA and ARORA (1962), the intravenous injection of 5-HT (5—20 μg/kg) into dogs subjected, 18 hr previously, to a two-stage ligation of the anterior descending branch of the left coronary artery produces an immediate effect consisting of a short-lasting moderate reduction in ectopic ventricular rate and a slight increase in total heart rate, and a late effect, reaching its peak 20 hr after 5-HT administration, consisting of prolonged reduction in the total heart rate as well as in ectopic ventricular rate.

2. Pulmonary vessels

Owing to the existence of conspicuous species differences in the sensitivity of the pulmonary bed to 5-HT it seems opportune to discuss the response of this vascular area (to the amine) separately in the different animal species, starting with the dog, which has been the object of the most thorough investigation.

Dog. The first study on the haemodynamic effects of 5-HT injected into the pulmonary artery is probably that of MACCANON and HORVATH (1954) who introduced the amine (30—45 μg/kg) directly into the pulmonary artery of dogs anaesthetized with pentobarbital. After a latency of 5—8 seconds a systemic hypertensive response was observed, lasting 2 to 5 min. No alterations in cardiac output or pulmonary blood volume, measured by the tracer dilution technique, were noted at the prehypertensive stage. At the peak of the hypertensive reaction variable responses were obtained.

Apart from these rather ambiguous results, all available evidence concordantly demonstrates that 5-HT is a potent constrictor of the pulmonary vessels in the dog.

Pulmonary vasoconstriction can be elicited by single injections into a vein, into the right atrium or into the pulmonary artery of doses of 5-HT as low as 1—5 μg/kg, or by i.v. infusion of 1—8 μg/kg/min 5-HT (NAHAS 1958, NAHAS and MACDONALD 1959, BORST et al. 1957, RUDOLPH and PAUL 1957, NOBLE and NANSON 1959, DUTEIL and AVIADO 1962).

Single injections of 1 μg/kg 5-HT into the right atrium of an intact dog produce a 37% rise in pulmonary artery-pulmonary vein pressure difference, and this effect remains unchanged after spinal section or vagotomy (NAHAS and MACDONALD 1959). Similarly, single injections of 1.5—8.5 μg 5-HT into the pulmonary artery produce a 53% increase in pulmonary vascular resistance, and injections of 20—47 μg a 62% increase. These results by ROSE and LAZARO (1958) have been confirmed by HARASAWA and RODBARD (1961) who observed that 16 μg/kg 5-HT base injected into the pulmonary artery of anaesthetized, thoracotomized dogs produced an almost immediate elevation of the pulmonary artery pressure, which was maximal (+35%) about 30 seconds after the injection and returned to control levels within 5 min.

Infusion rates as low as 8 μg/kg/min result in a 30—100% increase of pulmonary arterial pressure, and in a 55% increase in the difference of pressure between the pulmonary artery and the left atrium, with only a 16% increase in pulmonary blood flow (RUDOLPH and PAUL 1957a, 1957b; SHEPHERD et al. 1959; CRUMPTON et al. 1959). Infusion rates of 150 μg/kg/min 5-HT base produce a 300% increase in the mean pulmonary pressure, a 28% drop in systemic arterial mean pressure and a 60% rise of cardiac output. Calculated pulmonary resistances markedly increase up to 500% of control levels but, in contrast, systemic resistances decrease by 55%. Arterial oxygen saturation is usually considerably reduced during 5-HT infusion. These effects persist as long as the drug is administered (RUDOLPH and PAUL 1957a, 1957b; MCGAFF and MILNOR 1962, ROWE et al. 1963).

As a consequence of pulmonary vasoconstriction, there is a considerable decrease in the pulmonary mean transit time, as measured by the dye dilution method (from 3.92 to 2.24 seconds following i.v. infusion of 0.06—0.4 mg/kg/min 5-HT base), and an appreciable reduction in the pulmonary blood volume (from 11 to 8.7 ml/kg). According to MCGAFF and MILNOR (1960, 1962) and MILNOR et al. (1962), the magnitude of the decrease in pulmonary blood volume indicates that a relatively large part of the pulmonary vascular bed is constricted by 5-HT, and provides an example of the shifting of blood from pulmonic to systemic circuits by reciprocal changes in the distensibility of these beds.

Injection of 5-HT into the left pulmonary artery of the unanaesthetized dog produces a decrease in the volume and rate of flow in this vessel and little or no change in main pulmonary artery flow; injection into the right ventricle causes a delayed response in which flow increases moderately in both vessels (RUDOLPH et al. 1962).

Although the principal site of the increased resistance to flow through the lungs appears to be in the pulmonary arterioles (GILBERT et al. 1957, 1958; KABINS et al. 1959) or pre-capillary vessels (SHEPHERD et al. 1959), pulmonary venules are also constricted by 5-HT, especially when given in large doses (KABINS et al. 1959, SHEPHERD et al. 1959, AVIADO 1960, BRAUN and STERN 1961).

Signs of increased arteriolar constriction are the increase in the pressure gradients between the pulmonary artery and pulmonary artery wedge pressures, as well as the reduction in the lung weight following injection of 14—100 μg 5-HT into the pulmonary artery; signs of increased venular constriction are the increase in the pressure gradients between the pulmonary artery wedge pressure and the left atrial pressure, the increase in venular pressure, as measured directly, and finally the increase in pulmonary capillary blood volume.

The rise in venular pressure following intravenous injection of 2—4 μg 5-HT base is 50—80% of the respective increase in arterial pressure (AVIADO 1960); the increase in pulmonary capillary blood volume following infusion of 100—200 μg/min of 5-HT base is 6—133% (YOUNG et al. 1962).

The increase in pulmonary vascular resistance caused by 5-HT can be reduced in the dog by augmenting the pulmonary blood flow as well as by raising the pulmonary venous pressure up to 25—30 mm Hg (RUDOLPH and AMAULD 1960).

According to BRAUN and STERN (1961) the rise in pulmonary artery and pulmonary venous pressures is due not only to a direct action of 5-HT on vascular smooth muscle but also to chemoreceptor stimulation.

This opinion is not shared by VITOLO et al. (1962) who affirm that the pulmonary vasoconstriction provoked by 5-HT is due neither to neurogenic mechanisms nor to humoral mechanisms, but only to a direct action on the pulmonary vessels.

Promethazine, BOL and LSD (0.4—0.6 mg/kg) effectively antagonize the constrictor action of 5-HT on pulmonary vessels (ROSE and LAZARO 1958). Vasoconstriction produced by continuous infusion of 5-HT is in part also antagonized by acetylcholine, histamine and adenosine-triphosphate (RUDOLPH et al. 1959).

The action of 5-HT on the pulmonary vascular area exceeds that of angiotensin (CARLIER et al. 1958), and of all other biogenic amines, including catecholamines (ROSE and LAZARO 1958, BORST et al. 1957).

Large doses of 5-HT (0.2—3 mg) injected into the dog pulmonary artery produce in 75% of the animals moderate to severe pulmonary oedema with occasional evidence of left heart failure. Without excluding the possibility of other indirect or reflex mechanisms, such as release of histamine or catecholamines, or the initiation of reflexes over the sympathetic nervous system, it seems probable that the change in capillary permeability provoked by 5-HT may be due to the direct action of 5-HT itself on the pulmonary capillary wall. On the basis of similarity of results, it is suggested by KABINS et al. (1959) that 5-HT may perhaps play a part in pulmonary oedema formation due to unilateral starch embolization.

Following intravenous injection of 10 μg 5-HT in cats and 50 μg 5-HT in dogs and rabbits, masses of whitish translucent material visibly embolize pulmonary arteries, observed by quartz-rod transillumination. From seconds to 15 min the material seems to become less rigid, breaks up, is pushed into smaller branches and passes through the capillaries (KNISELY et al. 1958).

The question whether 5-HT can initiate systemic vascular reflexes in the pulmonary vessels is answered negatively by ROSE and LAZARO (1958) on the basis of experiments carried out on an experimental preparation in which such reflexes are easily demonstrated.

The injection of 0.04—0.07 μg/kg 5-HT into the bronchial artery of the dog causes consistent bronchoconstriction accompanied by increase in bronchopulmonary flow. Blood flow in the bronchial artery is either increased or decreased (DE LETONA et al. 1961).

Cat. The intravenous injection of serum vasoconstrictor or of 5-HT (5—40 μg) into the cat causes a rise of pressure in the right ventricle and in the pulmonary artery, accompanied by a fall in the pulmonary vein. In the cat, too, this phenomenon is due to an increase in the pulmonary resistance and not to cardiac stimulation (COMROE 1952, COMROE et al. 1953, REID and RAND 1952, REID 1952b). It is not abolished by vagotomy nor by atropine, but can be in part antagonized by yohimbine (REID 1952b) and, more efficaciously, by ergotamine and LSD (GINZEL and KOTTEGODA 1953). The pressor response in the lesser circulation is lacking if 5-HT is injected into the pulmonary vein.

The action of tryptamine in the cat, dog, and rabbit is similar to that described for 5-HT (REID 1952a). According to GINZEL and KOTTEGODA (1953) 1 dose of 5-HT is equipotent, on the pulmonary vessels of the cat, to 2.4 doses of tryptamine and to 10—20 doses of adrenaline or noradrenaline.

Man. Using the technique of right heart catheterization, GROVER et al. (1958) infused 4 mg 5-HT base in 100 ml of isotonic saline directly into the main pulmonary artery of 7 patients with normal pulmonary arterial pressure. Infusion lasted 7 to 10 minutes. Mean pulmonary arterial pressure rose from 2 to 10 mm Hg, while the wedge pressure remained unchanged. The change in total pulmonary vascular resistance was variable, increasing in three cases and decreasing in three others.

HARRIS et al. (1960) infused i.v. 0.6—2.5 μg/kg/min 5-HT base into 7 patients with normal hearts and minimal healed tuberculous lesions of the lung, and injected 0.4—1.6 μg/kg 5-HT into the right atrium of 3 other patients. In only one instance was there pressure rise in the pulmonary artery after infusion and this was accompanied by a rise in brachial artery pressure. Injections into the right atrium caused sustained rise in pressure in pulmonary and brachial arteries.

Finally, STONE and NEMIR (1960) injected 5-HT (4—400 μg/kg) through the distal lumen of a catheter inserted into the pulmonary artery before and after unilateral balloon occlusion of the corresponding artery. Only minimal changes in mean pulmonary artery pressure, pulmonary capillary pressure and pulse rate were observed with no objective or subjective signs resembling those associated with pulmonary embolism.

The above results concordantly demonstrate that the pulmonary vascular bed presents in man poor sensitivity to 5-HT and that it is unlikely that 5-HT participates in the pathogenesis of the clinical picture of human pulmonary embolism.

Calf. Intravenous infusion of 5-HT into calves (0.2 mg/kg/min for 3 min) fails to alter significantly pulmonary artery pressure, pulmonary artery wedge pressure or pulmonary vascular resistance, as measured by cardiac catheterization techniques. The only statistically significant effect of the amine is to decrease cardiac output. KUIDA et al. (1961) conclude that in calves 5-HT is not an effective pulmonary vasoconstrictor agent and hence that it is unlikely that it plays a role in the pathogenesis of spontaneous pulmonary hypertension.

Sheep. Intravenous infusion of 5-HT into the sheep (25—50 μg/kg/min) produces a 20—30% rise in pulmonary pressure accompanied by a 7—30% fall in arterial oxygen saturation (HALMAGYI and COLEBATCH 1961).

3. Liver vessels

An injection of 15 μg 5-HT into the portally perfused canine liver produces a small increase in the resistance to blood flow through the liver. However, 1 mg 5-HT added to 500 ml of perfusing liquid causes no congestion. Increased resistance probably occurs in the portal vessels before the hepatic artery and the portal vein join. It is concluded that it is unlikely that the cause of hepatic congestion in perfused preparations is either 5-HT or histamine (ANDREWS and BUTTERWORTH 1958).

In substantial accordance with these findings, SHOEMAKER et al. (1961) observed that in unanaesthetized dogs whose hepatic vessels had previously been catheterized, hepatic plasma flow decreased to approximately half the control value 1 to 2 min after the injection of 0.1—0.2 mg/kg 5-HT base into the femoral vein. The lowest point was reached in 1 to 1.5 min. An increase in portal venous potassium, often over 2 meq/l, occurred 1 to 2 min after the injection, followed by an increase in hepatic venous potassium. Multiplication of concentration differences by flow values showed a marked output of potassium from the non-hepatic splancnic area, 1—2 min after injection, followed by hepatic potassium output. In addition, there was a fall in arterial, portal and hepatic venous glucose levels and uptake of glucose by the non-hepatic splancnic area.

The portal pressure in the dog is raised also by the systemic intravenous injection of tryptamine. According to REID (1952) this is not due to constriction of the hepatic sphincter but appears to be a passive result of increased arterial pressure.

The action of 5-HT on the veins of the rat liver was examined by JÄNKÄLÄ and VIRTAMA (1962) with the aid of direct observation and microangiographic technique. They found that doses of 5-HT base from 0.2 to 10 mg/kg injected into the portal vein caused a conspicuous reduction of the liver volume, as shown by the decrease of the liver weight as a percentage of the total body weight (after 10 mg/kg 5-HT from 4.9 to 3.1%), and a vigorous constriction of the portal and hepatic veins. Vasoconstriction was most marked in the small venules. Pretreatment with reserpine did not prevent the venoconstrictor effect of 5-HT.

Similar results were obtained by LEVINE et al. (1964) in the isolated rat liver. Injections of 5-HT into the portal vein cannula produced a prompt decrease of hepatic blood flow and decrease was approximately proportional to the dose (threshold 12 μg 5-HT base). However, tachyphylaxis was notable in this preparation.

In human subjects the intravenous infusion of 12 μg/kg/min 5-HT base does not affect portal venous pressure significantly. The estimated hepatic blood flow is reduced by 9.2% and the splancnic resistance is raised by 13% (CHIANDUSSI et al. 1962, 1963).

4. Spleen vessels

Intravenous injection of 10—30 μg/kg 5-HT base causes a 56% decrease in the venous outflow of the *in situ* dog spleen, which lasts 7—12 min. Flow reduction is preceded by a short-lived, 25% flow increase. Direct injection of 1—20 μg 5-HT into the artery of both *in situ* and isolated perfused spleen produces similar results (RIVA SANSEVERINO and URBANO 1962).

Spleen volume is generally reduced by 5-HT, but whereas reduction of spleen volume is the sole response of the isolated perfused spleen to intraarterial 5-HT (1—20 μg), the normally irrigated *in situ* spleen sometimes responds to intravenous 5-HT (5—10 μg/kg) with an occasional volume increase, following the contraction. Lower intravenous doses of 5-HT (1 μg/kg) cause small, unpredictable changes in the spleen volume. Splenocontraction is ascribed mainly to vasoconstriction and subordinately to contraction of the smooth muscles in the spleen capsule (RIVA SANSEVERINO and URBANO 1961, 1962).

0.5—2 mg of bufotenine injected intravenously provokes, like 5-HT, a contraction of the dog spleen, which lasts longer than the pressure rise (RAYMOND-HAMET and DUFAU 1942).

5. Vessels of the placenta

ELIASSON and ÅSTRÖM (1955) and ÅSTRÖM and SAMELIUS (1957) first observed that 5-HT injected into the umbilical artery of the perfused placenta displayed a potent constrictor action which was about 10 times stronger than that of L-adrenaline, and 20 times stronger than that of L-noradrenaline. Doses of 0.3—3 μg provided moderate vasoconstriction; doses of 5—10 μg often caused complete closure of the vessels. Tryptamine was 10 to 20 less times active than 5-HT.

The action of 5-HT was enhanced by cocaine and antagonized by dihydroergotamine, LSD, tryptamine, yohimbine and chlorpromazine. Ephedrine, propanidine, iproniazid, hexamethonium, phenbenzamine, reserpine and heparin (up to 30 mg) were ineffective. Owing to lack of nervous tissue in the umbilical cord and in the placenta the above effects of 5-HT must be considered as the expression of a direct action of 5-HT on the vascular smooth muscle.

The results of ÅSTRÖM and co-workers were confirmed by others.

GAUTIERI and CIUCHTA (1962) perfused human placenta at a pressure of 50—60 mm Hg and measured venous outflow directly. The injection into the umbilical artery of 20 μg 5-HT base in 0.5 ml liquid caused an immediate decrease in the flow rate, which ranged between 19 and 61%. Vasoconstriction was maximal during the first two minutes and almost complete recovery to the preinjection level was attained in 6—8 min. There was no tachyphylaxis.

The funicular portion of the umbilical vein behaved like the umbilical artery. Here again the most potent constrictor agent was 5-HT, active at concentrations as low as 0.1—0.25 μg/ml (PANIGEL and MAYER 1959).

RODEGRA et al. (1957) and SCHMERMUND et al. (1959) suggest that 5-HT liberated from blood platelets may participate in the spontaneous closure of the umbilical artery after birth.

6. Musculo-cutaneous vessels

Careful experiments have been carried out especially in the dog and in man.

Dog. 5-HT infused into the brachial artery of the foreleg of anaesthetized dogs at a rate of 4—5 μg/min does not significantly change the total resistance of the foreleg vessels, but increases large artery and sometimes vein resistance and decreases small vessels resistance. This means that 5-HT causes pronounced constriction of large arteries and large veins with concomitant dilatation of small vessels (probably arterioles) and fall of small vessel intraluminal pressures. HADDY and co-workers (HADDY et al. 1957a, HADDY et al. 1957b, HADDY 1959) are of the opinion that 5-HT-induced segmental resistance changes occur through active mechanisms. They further suggest that a function of 5-HT may be that of influencing volume distribution of blood within various segments of the circulatory system as well as influencing water and salt distribution between intravascular and extravascular compartments.

The directionally opposite changes in segmental resistance may explain how 5-HT produces peculiar skin colour changes without predictable blood pressure variations when injected into intact animals or man.

Besides small vessel dilatation, 5-HT also produces oedema of the dog forelimb when given by prolonged infusion into the brachial artery of denervated animals. During infusion small venous pressure rises from 10 to 16 mm Hg and weight gain of the forelimbs averages 0.4 g/min, instead of 0.1 g/min. According to HADDY (1960) these findings indicate that 5-HT produces oedema by raising capillary hydrostatic pressure.

Still owing to the opposite changes in segmental resistance it produces, 5-HT is capable of antagonizing extremes of vascular tone induced in the dog foreleg by neurogenic means. When small vessels are dilated following denervation of the foreleg, 5-HT (4 μg/min) cannot dilate them further, but continues to constrict large vessels, the net effect being constriction. When small vessels are highly constricted following bilateral vagotomy, 5-HT dilates small vessels more than it constricts large vessels, the net effect being dilatation. A similar antagonism is more difficult to demonstrate when tone is varied by humoral means (HADDY et al. 1959). The interaction of 5-HT with vasoconstrictor agents has been the object of a particularly thorough study by GORDON and co-workers (GORDON et al. 1958a, 1958b; HURWITZ et al. 1961). 5-HT (2.5—8 μg/min) in combination with noradrenaline, adrenaline, vasopressin and angiotensin was infused into the brachial artery of the denervated dog forelimb at rates which were effective locally but not effective generally. Pressures were measured at 4 sites along the length of the foreleg vascular bed while the rate of blood flow in the brachial artery was held constant. Each combination resulted in net constriction but in the case of catecholamines the constriction was less than the sum of the constrictions of the two agents administered separately owing to the antagonistic action of 5-HT and catecholamines upon small blood vessels. The venous constrictor action of 5-HT was potentiated by each of the examined pressor agents (HURWITZ et al. 1961).

Results of recent experiments by McCUBBIN et al. (1962) on the dog perfused hind leg and the dog perfused kidney again point to the importance of neurogenic vasoconstrictor tone in determining the vascular response to 5-HT and indicate that inhibition of neurogenic vasoconstriction by 5-HT, with ensuing vasodilatation, may be mediated through the adrenergic vasodilator receptors.

In fact, when 5-HT (1—12 μg of the base) is injected into the vessels of the hind leg perfused by the dog's own circulation during stimulation of the lumbar sympathetic trunk it causes relaxation of the constricted small arteries but further constriction of the large ones, the net effect being decrease in total vascular resistance; when 5-HT is injected in the absence of stimulation it causes constriction of both large and small arteries and increase in vascular resistance. Small veins respond to stimulation and 5-HT as do small arteries. Small arteries of the mesentery react to regional nerve stimulation as do those of the hind limb.

There is no evidence of interference of 5-HT with sympathetic vasoconstrictor pathways and 5-HT does not oppose vasoconstriction due to noradrenaline or tyramine but does, in part, oppose the vasoconstriction that is due to adrenaline which acts on both adrenergic constrictor and dilator receptors. Selective blockade of adrenergic dilator receptors with dichloroisoproterenol prevents the vasodilator activity of 5-HT and eliminates the ability of the amine to depress vasoconstrictor responses to neurogenic stimulation.

McCUBBIN and co-workers advance the working hypothesis that 5-HT affects adrenergic vasodilator receptors in a manner that causes them to have a more prominent effect when stimulated. The resultant decrease in total vascular resistance would be caused by dilatation of small arteries and veins.

RAYMOND-HAMET (1941) found that a first injection of 0.1 mg bufotenine into the dog femoral artery caused an 82% reduction in the venous outflow and that a subsequent injection of 5 mg/kg of the amine brought about a reduction of only 30%. The substance was 100 to 500 times less vasoconstrictor than adrenaline. These results were considered to be indicative of a nicotine-like action of bufotenine on the vessels.

Man. In human subjects 5-HT infused into the brachial artery in doses of 0.4—7.5 μg/min causes a reduction of blood flow through the forearm (30% with 0.4 μg/min, 50% with 1.6 μg/min and 70% with 7.5 μg/min) as well as through the hand (75 to 90%), with a concomitant volume increase (due to oedema formation) and a marked flushing of the skin. In the forearm the fall of flow is preceded by a transient increase and, as the infusion continues, cyanosis develops gradually in the skin of the fingers. Small petechiae are occasionally observed some hours after the infusion, indicating capillary damage. Soon after beginning the infusion of 5-HT a sensation of tingling is felt in the hand and lower forearm, which decreases somewhat throughout the infusion period and subsides within a few minutes of the end of the infusion. Large doses produce severe but fleeting pain.

The above phenomena have been ascribed to dilatation of capillaries or lower-pressure capacity vessels, mainly responsible for the colour of the skin, and to constriction of arterioles or higher-pressure capacity vessels, mainly responsible for resistance to flow.

These findings and interpretations by GLOVER, WHELAN and co-workers (RODDIE et al. 1955a, 1955b; GLOVER et al. 1957, 1958) are in substantial accordance with those of other research workers.

CALÌ and LOMEO (1955, 1957a, 1957b) and CALÌ, STRANO and LOMEO (1956) found that 20—40 μg 5-HT injected into the brachial artery produced the following changes in the capillaries of the nail bed, as observed capillariscopically: remarkable reddening of the field, conspicuous dilatation of the capillaries, increase of the number of visible capillaries. On pletismographic examination, the finger volume was seen gradually to increase, up to a maximum after 10 to 20 min, and amplitude of arterial pulse to decrease consistently. Venous pressure recorded at the elbow showed a conspicuous elevation, which was of the order of 50 cm of water and persisted as long as 30 min after 50—200 μg 5-HT.

MAGALINI et al. (1956) similarly observed that 0.4 mg 5-HT base given intraarterially caused disappearance of the radial pulse for 5 min with a short period of blanching, followed by flushing of the skin of the volar and dorsal surfaces of the hand for longer than 30 min. Pressure in the homolateral vein rose from 65 to 280 mm H_2O, whereas there was no rise of pressure in the controlateral vein.

The potent constrictor action of 5-HT on the veins upon continuous intraarterial infusion (10 μg/min) has been confirmed by SHARPEY-SCHAFER and GINSBURG (1962).

Both BOL and sodium salicylate appear to be specific antagonists of the constrictor response of the forearm and hand blood vessels to intraarterial infusion of 5-HT, but whereas BOL displays a direct antagonistic action, sodium salicylate acts only indirectly, possibly through release of, or synergism with, some other substance, probably a hormone (GLOVER et al. 1957).

Following intravenous administration of 5-HT, changes in human forearm vessels are in many respects different from those observed after intraarterial injection of the amine. In fact, intravenous infusion of 0.5—1.2 mg 5-HT base/min causes a dilator response of the forearm vessels consisting of a huge initial transient increase in flow (3 to 4-fold, commencing within 1 to 1.5 min), followed by a smaller but sustained increase (Fig. 5). The resting level is attained 5 to 10 min after the infusion ceases. A fall in forearm flow is never seen. It has been suggested by LEMESSURIER et al. (1959) that the sustained increase in flow probably represents a balance between the direct constrictor action of the drug and a secondary vasodilator effect.

Local venous pressure is transiently elevated by intravenous infusion of 5-HT: by 10 cm of water following 1.5 μg and by 16—18 cm of water following 15 μg given in 5 min. Pressure rise lasts 15 min. Elevation of systemic venous pressure is not obtained even with extremely large doses of 5-HT (10 mg in 15—30 min) (MAGALINI et al. 1956).

According to BOCK et al. (1957) both intravenous and intraarterial 5-HT constantly increase flow in the cutaneous vessels. Flow in muscular vessels is increased by intravenous 5-HT, in doses ranging from 0.1 to 3 mg, and by small doses of intraarterial 5-HT, but reduced by large doses of intraarterial 5-HT.

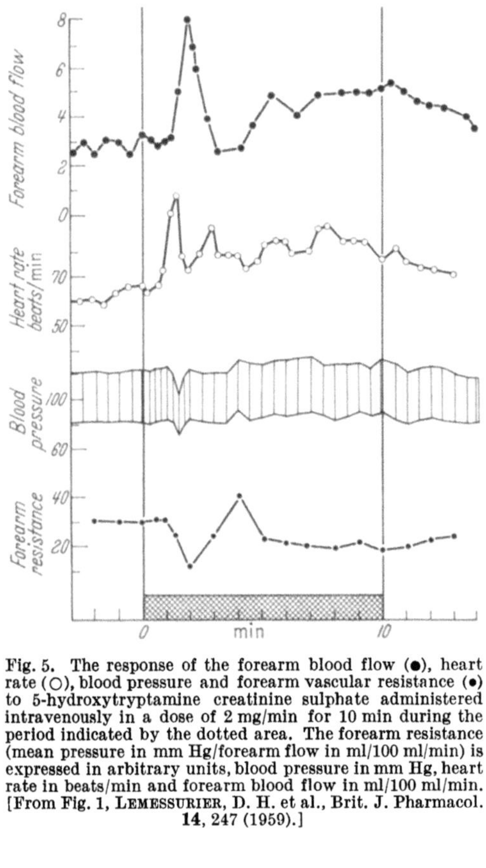

Fig. 5. The response of the forearm blood flow (●), heart rate (○), blood pressure and forearm vascular resistance (•) to 5-hydroxytryptamine creatinine sulphate administered intravenously in a dose of 2 mg/min for 10 min during the period indicated by the dotted area. The forearm resistance (mean pressure in mm Hg/forearm flow in ml/100 ml/min) is expressed in arbitrary units, blood pressure in mm Hg, heart rate in beats/min and forearm blood flow in ml/100 ml/min. [From Fig. 1, LEMESSURIER, D. H. et al., Brit. J. Pharmacol. 14, 247 (1959).]

Local subjective symptoms of the intravenous injection are pain along the course of the infused vein and heaviness in the infused limb. There is, in addition, an abnormally high incidence of thrombosis in the vein infused with 5-HT (LEMESSURIER et al. 1959).

Intradermal injection of 5-HT in concentrations up to 20 μg/ml produces no appreciable action on the skin over the front of the forearm. Concentrations greater than this (100—2500 μg/ml) generally cause the appearance of a red reaction, lasting 15—45 min; there is neither itching nor weal formation (REID 1952b, MOLLER and RORSMAN 1959, HERXHEIMER and SCHACHTER 1959, HEITE and KLEINHANS 1962). In subjects with clearly visible and raised subcutaneous veins, doses of 5-HT as small as 1 μg cause the total disappearance of the venous network and a sharp demarcation between the area with venoconstriction and the surrounding areas (REID 1952b, DEMIS et al. 1960). The intradermal injection of tryptamine in concentrations up to 0.5% causes no blanching, but a weak red reaction around the site of the injection (REID 1952a).

Following iontophoretic application, 5-HT (3.5 mg/cm^2) produces marked erythema, slight oedema and no cyanosis. There is also conspicuous constriction of both normal and varicose veins (STÜTTGEN and SCHIPPEL 1961).

Cat. The blood vessels of the hind leg of the cat constrict moderately after the injection of 1—10 μg 5-HT into the femoral artery. The vasoconstriction, lasting over a 5 min period is frequently preceded by vasodilatation, and usually declines after repeated injections (REID 1952a). Tryptamine is 0.3—1 times as active as 5-HT; adrenaline is 10 to 500 times more active than 5-HT but the constrictor response is of considerably shorter duration (GINZEL and KOTTEGODA 1953). Yohimbine and, more effectively, lysergic acid diethylamide antagonize 5-HT vasoconstriction (REID 1952a, GINZEL and KOTTEGODA 1953).

A more accurate and recent analysis of the effects of 5-HT on the musculo-cutaneous vascular area of the cat is lacking.

Guinea-pig. 5-HT produces, like adrenaline and histamine, a constriction of the vessels in the perfused hind leg of the guinea-pig. Lowering the concentration of calcium ions in the perfusion liquid causes only slight changes in the response to the three amines. This response, however, is completely inhibited by the addition to the calcium-free perfusion liquid of EDTA Na_2, which provokes a drainage of calcium from the irrigated territory (COHEN 1959, COHEN and BLANCHARD 1962).

Rat. Following intravenous or subcutaneous injection of adequate doses of 5-HT there appears, simultaneously with the changes in systemic blood pressure, a constriction of the tail artery, as evidenced by the absence of haemorrhage or shortening of bleeding time when the tail is severed. The local application of 5-HT onto the severed tail has no vasoconstrictor effect (CORRELL et al. 1952, CORREALE 1954).

5-HT is about twice as active on the intact hind leg vessels as on the abdominal aorta of the rat (STUDER and TRIPOD 1960). In rats made hypertensive through clipping of one renal artery, the vasoconstrictor action of 5-HT (0.5 μg/ml) on the perfused hind legs is the same as in control normotensive rats, but in hypertensive animals the amine counteracts oedema formation following perfusion more powerfully (TRIPOD and BEIN 1960).

When the nervous component of the vasomotor tone of the blood vessels of the innervated hind limb perfused with blood is reduced by ganglion blockade, by section of the nerves to the hind limb, or by the indirect effect of drugs, the vasoconstrictor response of the blood vessels to 5-HT (0.02 μg) is increased and perfusion pressure rises from 41.5 to 80.4 mm Hg. Similar results are obtained with adrenaline, noradrenaline, tyramine and ephedrine, but not with angiotensin or pitressin. Pretreatment with reserpine (3 mg/kg daily, for two days) reduces the mean response to 5-HT (15 mm Hg instead of 40). Results suggest that, in rats, activity in the sympathetic nervous system directly influences the reactivity of peripheral blood vessels to 5-HT and sympathomimetic drugs (LAVERTY 1962).

As in the case of the guinea-pig, the vasoconstrictor effect of 5-HT on the hind leg vessels of the rat is not affected by lowering the concentration of calcium in the perfusion liquid but is strongly reduced by drainage of calcium from the tissues produced by EDTA Na_2 (COHEN and BLANCHARD 1962).

Mouse. The effects of 5-HT on the vasculature of the mouse ear have been studied using a technique of freeze fixation which permits stereomicroscopic observation of the terminal vascular bed in a life-like state. It appears that single intravenous doses of 5-HT produce a) extravasation of parenerally administered Evans blue (after 50 or more μg 5-HT/kg), b) vasodilatation occurring directly after doses of 50—250 μg/kg or following an initial period of vasoconstriction after larger doses, and c) vasoconstriction, increasing in duration with dose (minimum 250 μg/kg). UML, 10 mg/kg, partially inhibits these effects. Local administration of 5-HT produces comparable results. Dye escape and vasoconstriction are most prominent in venules and are similar to the effects of 20 times the dose of histamine.

According to STROBEL et al. (1961) the above findings in mice provide additional evidence that concentrations of 5-HT within limits attainable from endogenous sources will produce the basic microcirculatory changes of early inflammation.

Rabbit ear preparation. The vessels of the rabbit's ear, prepared and perfused as described by PAGE (1942), are very sensitive to the constrictor action of 5-HT, the threshold dose being as low as 0.5—1 ng (BERTACCINI and ZAMBONI 1961). 0.15 μg of 5-HT were found by PAGE (1952) to be equivalent to about 0.025 μg of adrenaline. Similar results were obtained by GINZEL and KOTTEGODA (1953), who observed that the action of 5-HT on the ear vessels is usually even stronger than that of adrenaline, and that this action is not antagonized by hexamethonium or tolazoline.

GADDUM and HAMEED (1954) demonstrated that the action of 5-HT on the ear preparation is greatly increased when ephedrine (10 μg/ml) or choline-*p*-tolyl ether bromide (1 μg/ml) is present in the perfusion liquid. This potentiation has been ascribed to inhibition of monoamine oxidase.

Pig ear preparation. On the isolated pig ear 5-HT produces intense vasoconstriction, which is suitable for recording at 5-HT doses of 0.01 to 0.1 μg. Complete suppression of vasoconstriction is obtained with dihydroergotamine (GRETTE 1957).

7. Vessels of the kidney

See pages 285—297.

8. Brain vessels

Results obtained by different investigators are partly divergent, probably owing to different 5-HT dosage and route of administration, different experimental methods and different animal species.

SCARINCI (1955) found that intravenous or intracarotid injection of 5-HT (50—1000 μg/kg) produced in the dog blanching of the exposed cortical area, and BARUCCI (1956) obtained the same result in the rabbit, following 1 mg/kg of intravenous 5-HT. Ischemia lasted 15 to 25 min and was sometimes followed by hyperemia. However, results obtained in the cat were at complete variance. In fact, MALCOLM (1957) observed that intracarotid injection of 200—300 μg 5-HT produced marked dilatation of the vessels of the exposed area of the cortex, which began within 20—30 seconds of the injection and lasted 10—15 min. The surface veins appeared to be filled with bright red arterial blood. Vasodilatation was accompanied by permeability changes of the vessels with oedema.

CASELLA, FUMAGALLI and NOLI (1957) have tried to follow more exactly the changes in cerebral blood flow by means of thermofluximetric elements applied to the cortex of the temporal lobe. 5-HT was given intravenously in doses of 0.2—4 mg/kg.

In the rabbit 5-HT caused a moderate drop in cerebral blood flow which lasted 5 to 6 minutes and closely followed the fall of the systemic blood pressure. In the cat a first phase of decreased blood flow was followed by an increase in flow, which was independent of any change in systemic blood pressure and was possibly due to regional vasodilatation.

Finally CLINI et al. (1960) found that 1—80 μg 5-HT injected into the ipsilateral external carotid artery of the cat, the controlateral being closed, hardly modified the carotid blood flow. In the spinal cat, on the contrary, 1—5 μg 5-HT always produced a decrease of blood flow. The slow intravenous infusion of adrenaline, which increased blood pressure up to the values of the pretrigeminal cat, abolished or even inverted the effects of 5-HT.

Although it is evident that further studies are needed to solve the important problem of whether 5-HT is capable, especially when given by intraarterial injection, of provoking general or regional changes in the calibre and/or permeability of brain blood vessels, it seems that at present the conclusion by CLINI et al. that 5-HT plays little, if any part in the regulation of cerebral circulation is the most reasonable.

9. Vessels of the retina

Single intravenous injections of 4 mg/kg 5-HT produce a transient spasm of the retinal arteries in the rabbit; repeated doses also cause morphological changes consisting of a thickening of the muscular layer of the retinal vessels (MORLUNGHI and VOLPI 1959).

10. Vasa vasorum

5-HT causes a marked constriction of the vasa vasorum of both the swine carotid and coronary arteries (SMITH 1953).

11. Other vascular areas

Vessels of the rat mesoappendix. Intravenous injection of 0.1 mg of 5-HT or local application of 2—3 drops of a 0.1% solution at 37° provokes within a few seconds a constriction of the terminal arterioles and the arterial segment of the capillaries, accompanied by marked stasis in the remaining capillary bed (CORRELL et al. 1952).

It is well known that topically applied adrenaline constricts the arteriolar elements of the rat mesoappendix. Intravenous 5-HT tends to depress vascular reactivity to adrenaline in doses of 0.6 mg/kg, but renders the precapillaries hyperreactive to adrenaline in doses of 0.15—0.3 mg/kg (ZWEIFACH and METZ 1955).

Gastric vessels of the dog. Using the gated-sine electromagnetic flowmeter, gastric blood flow appears to be increased by administration of 5-HT (PETER et al. 1962).

Vessels of the hind leg of the frog and the toad. The outflow rate of the perfusion liquid from the frog hind leg shows rhythmical variations indicating an alternation of periods of vasoconstriction and periods of vasodilatation. This spontaneous rhythmical activity is stimulated, or evoked if lacking, by 5-HT at concentrations from 10^{-9} to 10^{-4}. Tryptamine is about 100 times less active than 5-HT (ZAMBONI and CARLEVARO 1954).

Apart from the above effect, 5-HT displays on the vessels of the hind leg of frogs and toads only a poor and variable constrictor action (ERSPAMER 1954, INOUE 1956). Bufotenine and gramine are even less active (HANDOVSKY 1920, POWELL and CHEN 1945).

12. Effect of local application of 5-HT

Mucous membranes. 5-HT applied topically onto the cheek pouch of the hamster produces intense vasoconstriction, the threshold concentration being 0.004—0.04 μg/ml. In half the experiments 5-HT is adrenaline-potentiating, in the other half it inhibits adrenaline (AKERS and ZWEIFACH 1955). However, a few drops of a 0.1% solution of 5-HT base cause hyperaemia of the conjunctiva, when introduced into the conjunctival sac of human subjects (CALÌ and LOMEO 1955).

Bleeding surfaces. 5-HT reduces haemorrhage of bleeding surfaces when put into direct contact with them in sufficient concentrations (0.02—0.1% solution). This has been demonstrated with musculo-cutaneous wounds in rats and guinea-pigs (FORNAROLI and KOLLER 1955, NIAUSSAT et al. 1958) and for wounds of parenchymatous organs, such as guinea-pig liver (CONTI and RICOTTI 1955) and rabbit kidney (BAZAN 1956).

The above experimental results represent the basis of the recommended therapeutic use of 5-HT in the control of bleeding from small vessels during surgical operations on eyes (PALIAGA 1956), tonsils (DEL BO 1956) and teeth (TORRIELLI and MINOLA 1956, RYSKY 1957) as well as during plastic surgery (BERGONZELLI and FONTANA 1957, VISETTI 1958).

So far there is not sufficient evidence that 5-HT has any advantage over, or is even at parity with, the classical haemostatic drugs.

13. Action of 5-HT on isolated artery strips or rings

Isolated rings or spiral strips of ox, dog and especially sheep carotid were used for several decades in qualitative demonstration and in quantitative titration of the serum vasoconstrictor. The preparation has been re-evaluated by RAND and REID (1951, 1952), REID (1952b and SHAW and WOOLEY (1953, 1954) for the study of 5-HT and 5-HT antagonists.

The arterial strips respond to 5-HT with a contraction which is, within certain limits, satisfactorily dependent upon the amount of substance introduced into the bath. The threshold dose varies for 5-HT from about 0.005 to 0.01 μg/ml of nutrient liquid; that for tryptamine is 17 times greater.

VACEK (1960) found that the susceptibility to 5-HT of rabbit aorta strips is considerably below that normal in animals made hypertensive by DOCA and NaCl. The cause of the phenomenon is supposed to be found in secondary changes in the aorta wall. In this regard it should be remembered that according to MILLAHN (1961) 5-HT increases the elasticity coefficient of pig and calf aorta, thus reducing the extensibility of the vasal segment.

The contractile response to 5-HT of strips of sheep aorta is inhibited by yohimbine, ergotoxine and antimetabolites of the 5-aminoindole type (SHAW and WOOLEY 1953, 1954); the contraction of spirally cut sections of horse carotid artery elicited by 5-HT (0.04—3 μg/ml) is non-specifically antagonized by reserpine (1—25 μg/ml) and hydralazine (25—500 μg/ml) (KIRPEKAR and LEWIS 1958).

Finally, contractions of strips of rabbit aorta can be blocked by pretreating with dibenamine. There is no "cross-protection" against dibenamine blockade between 5-HT on the one hand an histamine, acetylcholine and catecholamines on the other. It is concluded by FURCHGOTT (1955) that the aortic smooth muscle has specific sets of contraction receptors for 5-HT.

Spiral strips, 2.5—4 cm long, cut from the left circumflex artery of the sheep heart are contracted by 5-HT in concentrations of 0.3—1 μg/ml (KOVALČIK 1962).

The same concentrations of 5-HT are also active on coronary strips obtained from the pig heart. However, the response to 5-HT is less consistent than that to acetylcholine or to histamine (TAKENAKA 1959).

14. Conclusive remarks

Whereas at the beginning 5-HT was believed to be a pure, typical vasoconstrictor and hypertensive agent (hence the name "serotonin"), at present the decidedly dominant opinion is that the chief action of 5-HT on the vessels and, accordingly, one of the possible "physiological" functions of the circulating amine is to cause vasodilatation. The most authoritative sustainers of this theory are GORDON and co-workers (1958a, 1958b, 1959) and MCCUBBIN and co-workers (1962).

On the basis of synergistic and antagonistic actions manifested by 5-HT towards the adrenalines, GORDON et al. affirm that "a biological role of serotonin lies in its negative interaction with the adrenalines", and that 5-HT may decrease small vessel tone "through its capacity to antagonize the vasoconstrictor action of noradrenaline on small vessels". McCUBBIN et al., in their turn, suggest, as a working hypothesis, that the main action of 5-HT on the vascular smooth muscle is to affect the adrenergic vasodilator receptors in a manner that causes them to have a more prominent effect when stimulated, thus causing decrease in total vascular resistance. There would be no interference of the amine with sympathetic vasoconstrictor pathways.

It may be seen that the interpretation of the "vasodilator" action of 5-HT differs consistently from one group of research workers to the other. Moreover, results obtained in the musculo-cutaneous area under particular experimental conditions do not seem to be in accordance with other numerous results reported in detail in the preceding pages.

Actually, one cannot exclude the possibility that 5-HT may intervene, in particular vascular areas and in particular animal species, in the "physiological" regulation of tone and calibre of blood vessels, but this does not seem sufficient to allow us to draw conclusions of general value.

IV. Action on vascular permeability

ROWLEY and BENDITT (1956) first demonstrated that subcutaneous or intradermal injection of doses of 5-HT as small as 0.1—1 μg in 0.03—0.1 ml liquid produces oedema in rats, and that 10 times more tryptamine or 200 times more histamine is necessary to bring about oedema of equal severity.

These results were soon confirmed and extended by numerous research workers, especially using the Evans blue or Pontamine blue technique, and 5-HT oedema of the rat paw is now often employed in the study of 5-HT antagonists and in the evaluation of anti-inflammatory agents (GÖZSI and KÁTÓ 1957a, 1957b, SPARROW and WILHELM 1957, KELEMEN 1957, THEOBALD and DOMENJOZ 1958, PARRATT and WEST 1957b, 1958, DÖPFNER and CERLETTI 1958, CAUWENBERGE et al. 1959a, 1959b; MÖRSDORF and BODE 1959, STENGER 1959, GELFAND and WEST 1951, STONE et al. 1951, GIÃO and T. RICO 1962). Methods for a quantitation of 5-HT-induced oedema have been proposed by ECKHARDT et al. (1958), UNGAR et al. (1959), DOEPFNER and CERLETTI (1958), VOGIN and ROSSI (1963), and JAQUET (1963).

By far the most accurate study on the action of 5-HT on the permeability of rat vessels has been carried out, in the rat cremaster muscle, by MAJNO et al. (1961a, 1961b, 1961c).

0.3—2 μg 5-HT base or 18—180 μg histamine was injected subcutaneously into the scrotum, whence it spread into the underlying cremaster muscle. The cremaster vessels were "labelled" by intravenous injection of colloidal HgS or carbon. At electron microscopy examination numerous endotelial openings were present, in a diameter of 7 to 8 μ or more. These gaps were 0.1 to 0.8 μ in width. The underlying basement membrane was morphologically intact. The leaking vessels, as indicated by the HgS or carbon deposits, always belonged to the venous side of the circulation. The heaviest deposits were found in venules 20 to 30 μ in diameter. The deposits decreased towards larger venules up to a maximum diameter of 75 to 80 μ and towards the finer vessels until the calibre reached approximately 7 μ. Essentially spared by the deposits were the finest vessels, 4 to 7 μ in diameter. The changes induced by 5-HT and histamine were indistinguishable, except that the former was roughly 100 times more potent than the latter. With regard to the pathogenesis of the endothelial lacks, which disappear within 3 hr, the electron microscopic findings suggest that the endothelial cells become partially disconnected along the intercellular junctions.

General acral swelling (paws and snout) is also observed in rats and hamsters following subcutaneous or intraperitoneal injections of 5-HT (ASBOE-HANSEN and WEGELIUS 1956, BOIS and SELYE 1956).

In sharp contrast to some rodents, 5-HT has only negligible potency, if any, as a permeability factor in the skin vessels of other species.

In guinea-pigs the response to local injection of 5-HT is 500 times less than that to histamine, and in rabbits 20,000 times less (SPARROW and WILHELM 1957). Furthermore, no raised permeability is apparent in the guinea-pig either in the fore-paw vessels or in the vessels of the brain stem following intravenous injection of 0.2—0.8 mg/kg 5-HT base (BERKINSHAW-SMITH et al. 1962).

In man, intradermal 5-HT is actually capable of producing capillary dilatation, as shown by erythema and flare, but does not cause any whealing (HERXHEIMER and SCHACHTER 1959, TROMPIZ 1961). In atopic skin there is either no reaction or a reaction greatly diminished in intensity and evanescent (CLENDENNING et al. 1959). Given by intravenous injection, 5-HT (0.1 mg/kg) seems to inhibit in man wheal production by histamine (CENCIOTTI 1957) and tuberculin (MONCALVO and GIORDANO 1958).

The above findings once again emphasize the danger of generalizing results after experimentation in only one or a few species.

V. Action on capillary resistance

It has been repeatedly claimed that 5-HT increases capillary resistance both in man and in experimental animals and, on the basis of this claim as well as of the circumstance that 5-HT is contained in large amounts in blood platelets, the drug has been considered to be one of the physiological factors involved in the maintenance of normal capillary resistance and has been recommended in the treatment of morbid syndromes characterized by abnormal capillary fragility.

Actually, experimental and clinical results obtained in this field are often contradictory, and the bulk of evidence is against the hypothesis of any relationship between 5-HT and capillary resistance.

a) Action of endogenous 5-HT on capillary resistance

Animals and human beings whose platelets have been nearly completely depleted of their 5-HT through acute or chronic administration of reserpine do not show any significant change in capillary resistance (HAVERBACK et al. 1957, ZAMBONI 1957). The same is true of rats in which biosynthesis and metabolism of 5-HT is halved by removal of the large intestine (ZAMBONI et al. 1959).

BLAIR et al. (1955) observed that following iontophoresis of a 1% solution of LSD into the skin of the anterior aspect of the arm, a larger number of petechiae was produced at a given site by a given fall in pressure than would otherwise have been expected. It seems difficult to conclude from this finding that the lowered "capillary resistance" is due to the anti-5-HT action of LSD and hence that endogenous 5-HT may be concerned in preserving the integrity of small vessels.

b) Action of exogenous 5-HT on capillary resistance

According to BRACCO et al. (1954), 5-HT given intravenously in doses of 1 mg/kg produces in guinea-pigs and rats a marked increase in capillary resistance.

The effect appears after 10 min and lasts for about 3 hr. With daily injections of 5-HT the capillary resistance remains high throughout the treatment period. The capillary crisis following surgical stress is similarly prevented or removed by intraperitoneal injections of 2.5 mg/kg 5-HT. Under daily administration of the same dose of 5-HT no fall of the capillary resistance is observed during treatment. From the results of their experiments BRACCO and his colleagues conclude that 5-HT possesses not only a local vasoconstrictor effect but also a protective action on capillaries.

No attention whatever has been paid by the above investigators to the behaviour of the systemic blood pressure. Yet it is well known that the large doses of 5-HT they used provoke in guinea-pigs and especially in rats a conspicuous and prolonged fall in blood pressure, accompanied by important changes in the calibre of the cutaneous vessels. The possibility that the observed increase in capillary resistance is, at least in part, a direct or indirect consequence of these systemic circulatory changes cannot be excluded.

More recently, BRACCO et al. (1958a, 1958b, 1958c) lay stress on the possibility that 5-HT is active on capillary resistance and permeability mainly after its transformation, by plasma enzymes, into oxidation derivatives. In fact, two of these derivatives have been found to possess a positive action on capillary resistance in guinea-pigs, both normal and with C-avitaminosis, as well as in adrenalectomized rats (active dose 50 μg/rat), to display an antidiffusory action in the albino rabbit (300 μg i.v.), to antagonize experimental inflammation provoked by croton oil or formalin, and finally to accelerate the transformation of fibrinogen into fibrin.

Concerning man, results are at complete variance, apparently depending upon the basic conditions of the capillaries.

In subjects with normal capillary resistance there is no change following single or repeated intravenous or intramuscular doses of 2—5 mg 5-HT (ANNONI et al. 1955a, CALÌ and LOMEO 1956, FUGA 1959). On the other hand, in subjects showing an abnormal capillary fragility, petechial count appears to be consistently reduced following repeated doses of 5-HT. This has been observed in elderly people (ABBATI et al. 1956, FUGA 1959, BASSANI and FANTINI 1956), in children (LANCIANO and RESTANTE 1956) and in tuberculous patients (ROSSINI et al. 1956). Increase of capillary resistance sometimes persists for days or weeks (BASSANI and FANTINI 1956, ROSSINI et al. 1956), and this frankly casts some doubt not only upon the interpretation but also upon the credibility of experimental results.

c) Therapeutical trial of 5-HT in haemorrhagic syndromes ascribed to increased capillary fragility

5-HT has been used, especially in Italy, in the treatment of WERLHOF's disease and related haemorrhagic syndromes. The doses recommended were 2—4 mg 5-HT base, intravenously or intramuscularly, every 4—8 hours.

Unfortunately, the first enthusiastic reports (ALLEGRI and FERRARI 1954, BASERGA and BALLERINI 1955, BASERGA 1955, RAVETTA 1955, MARTINETTI and MARANGANI 1955, BARONI 1956) have not been confirmed by more accurate studies (MIESCHER 1955, SCHATZMANN 1955, SIEGENTHALER 1956, ZUCKER 1959, STEFANINI and MAGALINI 1956), and at the present time the use of 5-HT in the control of capillary fragility must be considered irrational.

Platelets and platelet derivatives have been used profitably in the management of thrombocytopoenic states. However, their beneficial effect is not due to their content of 5-HT (STEFANINI and KISTNER 1957).

VI. Participation in the mechanism of haemostasis

In vivo experiments. As early as 1912—1913 O'Connor and Zucker and Stewart advanced the hypothesis that the serum vasoconstrictor, released by the platelets at the moment of blood coagulation, might intervene in the process of haemostasis in consequence of its direct spasmogenic action on the vascular smooth muscle around the clot occluding the injured vessel. This hypothesis has been re-evaluated following the identification of the vasocontrictor with 5-HT and has been the object of extensive experimental work.

Correll et al. (1952) found that the injection of 0.01 to 1 mg 5-HT into the saphenous vein of the rat shortened significantly, though only transiently, the bleeding time following the severing of the tip of the tail. When applied topically, 5-HT had no effect. Similar haemostatic effects were observed in mice, guinea-pigs, hens and, to a lesser degree, in rabbits (0.25—1.5 mg/kg). The behaviour of the systemic blood pressure was not taken into consideration. Correll and co-workers conclude that the role of the substance in haemostasis is exclusively that of a humoral vasoconstrictor agent.

The above results have been generally confirmed in experimental animals. Correale (1954) stated that the haemostatic effect appearing in the rat after subcutaneous doses of 5-HT paralleled, in both intensity and duration, the hypotensive effect caused by the substance. There was no direct interdependence, however, between these two phenomena, as would be expected if the shortening of the bleeding time was caused by hypotension. Lecomte et al. (1954) found that the action of 5-HT (10 μg/kg or more, i.v.) on the bleeding time in the rabbit was at least 10 times less intense than that possessed by adrenaline or adrenochrome, and more fleeting.

Estève and Laporte (1957) were unable to detect any reduction of the prolongation of bleeding time induced in rabbits by sodium salicylate, even following intramuscular doses of 5-HT base up to 6 mg/kg. Prolongation of bleeding time caused by isoniazid, on the contrary, was diminished by 0.25 mg/kg 5-HT. Djerassi et al. (1958), in their turn, succeeded in increasing vascular resistance and shortening the duration of traumatic bleeding in irradiated thrombocytopoenic guinea-pigs and mice. The effect, however, was of short duration and was obtainable only with large doses of 5-HT (1.5 mg/kg, i.p., in guinea-pigs, and 12.5 mg/kg, i.p., in mice).

In five out of seven healthy persons, intravenous infusion of 0.2 mg/kg 5-HT base in 5% dextrose solution over a period of several hours caused significant reduction of bleeding time, from 4—6 min to 1—$2^1/_2$ min. The effect, however, was very fleeting and the bleeding time returned to pretreatment values within 15 min to 2 hr after suspension of the injection. These positive results of Stefanini and Magalini (1956) were confirmed by Bella and Rossi (1957) (2 mg 5-HT base, i.m.), but not by Siegenthaler (1956) (4 mg 5-HT by slow i.v. injection, or 8 mg 5-HT/hour by i.v. infusion) nor by Annoni et al. (1955) (2 mg 5-HT i.v. or i.m.).

In patients suffering from haemorrhagic disorders results were again at variance. A temporary reduction of bleeding time was observed by Stefanini and Magalini (1956) in patients with vascular pseudohaemophilia, but not in patients with thrombocytopoenic purpura, either idiopatic or secondary. Lewis (quoted by Zucker 1958) had short-lived positive results in thrombocytopoenic purpura. Finally, Siegenthaler (1956) obtained a reduction of the bleeding time only in the limited number of cases (5 out of 24) of essential or secondary thrombopoenia in which it was augmented.

The above data seem to be by themselves sufficient to prove the extremely erratic and inconstant character of the action of 5-HT on bleeding time, but the thesis that 5-HT in the platelets is important to the organism as a defence mechanism against bleeding has suffered the hardest and most definitive blow from experiments carried out in reserpinized human subjects and animals.

In fact, following nearly complete depletion of 5-HT provoked in animals and man by single or repeated doses of reserpine, no significant changes could be observed in constriction of cut vessels, as followed microscopically, in bleeding time, clotting time, prothrombin times, prothrombin consumption index, thromboplastin generation test with platelet dilutions, platelet adhesiveness or clot retraction (SHORE et al. 1956a, 1956b; WEINER and UDENFRIEND 1957, HUTCHISON et al. 1959, WITTE et al. 1961).

It is similarly highly improbable that death due to haemorrhage observed in rabbits subjected to a stress procedure plus reserpine administration is attributable, as suggested by JAQUES and FISHER (1960), to depletion of platelet 5-HT.

KWAAN et al. (1957) showed that intravenous or paravenous injection of 5-HT into human beings resulted in the development of fibrinolytic activity not only in the plasma of the blood within the vein but also within veins well removed proximally in the line of flow in the same arm and within veins of the opposite arm. Since this effect was abolished by atropine it was suggested that it was mediated through a cholinergic mechanism.

Similar results were obtained by the same research workers (KWAAN et al. 1958) in the marginal vein of the rabbit's ear in which experimental thrombi were produced by injection of 25 units thrombin in 0.05 cc ml liquid. Addition to the thrombin solution of 5-HT in amounts as low as 0.3—3 μg produced a significant acceleration of the lysis of the thrombi. Again a cholinergic mechanism was invoked, and it was suggested that 5-HT stimulated cholinergic effectors by producing constriction of the vasa vasorum and consequent ischaemia of the vein wall.

Unfortunately, these findings could not be duplicated by HOLEMANS and CHO (1962). In fact, no enhanced lysis of experimental thrombi in the marginal vein of the rabbit ear was observed by them following injection of 5-HT along the venous segment prior to, or after thrombus formation. Thus, the hypothesis of KWAAN et al. that a major function of the 5-HT liberated from disintegrating platelets *in vivo* is the stimulation of fibrinolytic activity must be accepted with much reservation.

In vitro experiments. According to FENICHEL and SEEGERS (1955) and to BALLERINI (1955), 5-HT enhances the retraction of bovine plasma clots in concentrations of 40 μg/ml and more, and must therefore be considered a clot retraction principle, possibly the only dialyzable one in platelets. On the other hand MAGALINI and STEFANINI (1955, 1956) failed to find any heightening by 5-HT of clot retraction or of prothrombin utilization during clotting of platelet-free human plasma.

The conversion of fibrinogen to fibrin in the presence of thrombin is accelerated by 5-HT (20—40 μg/ml of the base). However, in contrast to platelet factor 2, 5-HT inhibits the fibrinogen-fibrin reaction in a purified fibrinogen solution. It is postulated that 5-HT acts either through inhibition of an antithrombin which blocks the fibrinogen to fibrin reaction (MILNE and COHN 1957) or through a direct effect on fibrinogen (KÁTO and GÖZSY 1958).

In vitro 5-HT seems to inhibit fibrinolysis considerably. This was demonstrated by using two different procedures. In the first, solutions of a streptokinase activated human fibrinolysin in a PO_4-saline buffer were incubated with or without 5-HT for 30 min at 37° and then placed on opposite sides of a fibrin plate; in the second, a fibrinolytic system consisting of bovine fibrinogen, human thrombin, imidazole-saline buffer, thrombolysin and test solution was used.

5-HT caused clear inhibition of fibrinolysis in concentrations as low as 2 μg/ml. 5-HTP was less effective (threshold 100 μg/ml), and tryptamine practically inactive. Heated or unheated fibrin plates showed equal inhibition of fibrinolysis by 5-HT. There was no inhibition of proteolysis of casein. It was not possible to determine whether 5-HT achieved its inhibition of fibrinolysis by modifying the fibrin substrate, inhibiting the fibrinolytic enzyme or both (TSITOURIS et al. 1961, 1962).

The inhibition of fibrinolysis by 5-HT was confirmed by CHRYSSANTHOU and ANTOPOL (1964).

Of limited interest, because the enormous doses required (1 mg of either 5-HT or tryptamine against 1 μg of heparin), is the observation that indolealkylamines are capable of reducing the antithrombin time prolonged by the action of heparin (KELLER 1958).

Addition of small amounts of 5-HT to whole blood alters the tendency of the platelets, leucocytes, and red blood cells of dogs, cats and rabbits to aggregate. The magnitude of this response is dose-dependent and biphasic. Very small doses (0.1—0.2 μg/ml) seem to decrease the aggregation tendency; larger amounts (5—10 μg/ml) greatly increase this tendency. The effect is abolished by very slight reductions of pH, by addition of KCN to blood and by removing adhesive platelets from the blood. 5-Methoxytryptamine has effects comparable to those of 5-HT; 2,3-dihydro-5-HT, tryptamine, melatonin and 5-HIAA have no effect at doses 10 times higher than 5-HT. SWANK et al. (1963) suggest that 5-HT may be a factor in reducing peripheral resistance to the flow of blood through the smaller blood vessels including capillaries.

5-HT (0.15 μg/ml) does not prevent platelet aggregation induced by thrombin or adenosine diphosphate (O'BRIEN 1962).

Despite the very poor experimental evidence supporting the view that 5-HT interferes in haemostasis, the drug has been tried clinically in the control of surgical bleeding (ANNONI et al. 1955a; ANTONA 1955, 1959; SANZIO GRECO 1957; BERGONZELLI and FONTANA 1957; PEREZ-BUFILL PICHOT 1957; SALA 1956), as well as in spontaneous haemorrhages from nearly all organs and of the most varied etiology: uterus and genital tract (BELLA and ROSSI 1957, EL TORAEI 1956, CATALDI 1956c, FAWZI 1956), kidney and urinary tract (EL TORAEI 1956), gastrointestinal tube (EL TORAEI 1956), lung (DI PASQUALE 1956), meninges (BALDUINI et al. 1955) etc.

The results reported have often been satisfactory, but the writer's impression is that not infrequently clinical experimentation has been carried out with insufficient accuracy and critical evaluation. Consequently it is highly questionable whether 5-HT may be considered a useful drug in the prevention or treatment of haemorrhage.

VII. Action on the heart

1. Heart in situ

Effects of 5-HT on the heart of intact animals are variable depending on animal species and on route and rapidity of 5-HT administration.

Man. In man both rapid intravenous injection (ANNONI et al. 1955, BALDRIGHI and FERRARI 1955, HOLLANDER and MICHELSON 1956), intravenous infusion (LEMESSURIER et al. 1959, BOJS 1961) and infusion into the pulmonary artery (GROVER et al. 1958) generally produce an increase in heart rate (5 to 30 beats per minute) which precedes pressure changes by 10 to 20 seconds, suggesting a direct effect on the heart (LEMESSURIER et al. 1959). Although stroke volume is reduced (BALDRIGHI and FERRARI 1955), cardiac output rises (GROVER et al. 1958, BOJS 1961) or remains unchanged (HARRIS et al. 1960).

Dog. In the dog, rapid intravenous injection of 5-HT usually produces bradycardia (LOUBATIÈRES et al. 1955, JACOB and CUGURRA 1960) or initial bradycardia followed by marked tachycardia (BEN et al. 1962), or sinus tachycardia (McCAWLEY et al. 1952). Acute vagotomy and carotid sinus denervation produce the disappearance of bradycardia (JACOB and CUGURRA 1960). Heart contractile force is increased, at least initially (LOUBATIÈRES et al. 1955, BEN et al. 1962). Stroke volume and minute volume behave differently, depending upon anaesthesia: they are increased in the unanaesthetized dog and in the dog anaesthetized with chloralose, decreased in animals anaesthetized with barbiturates (HOTOVY and ROESCH 1958).

The main ECG changes produced by intravenous injection of 200 μg/kg 5-HT consist of a marked negative T wave during the phase of increased blood pressure, with disappearance of this wave during the phase of hypotension (WALAWSKI 1959).

5-HT (0.35—0.8 mg/kg, i.v.) does not affect the auricular fibrillation established by vagal stimulation in the thyrotoxic dog, and fails to produce ventricular tachycardia in the dog under chloroform anaesthesia or ventricular fibrillation under cyclopropane anaesthesia. In doses of 2.2 mg/kg, 5-HT causes respiratory arrest in the anaesthetized dog. When the animal is protected by artificial respiration the cardiac effects of this lethal dose consist merely of transitory ventricular extrasystoles originating from abnormal foci (McCAWLEY et al. 1952).

Working on a cord-transected dog, PAGE (1952) observed that after intravenous 5-HT stroke volume and minute output, measured from pressure-pulse tracing, are nearly doubled.

Upon rapid pulmonary arterial injection, 5-HT (200 μg of the base) causes bradycardia and electrocardiographic disturbances, quickly followed by a rise in cardiac output which helps to maintain the pressor response to 5-HT (MAC CANON and HORVATH 1954).

Given by infusion into the left or the right atrium of dogs anaesthetized with morphine and dial-urethane-nembutal, 5-HT (8 μg/kg/min) elicits a 21—61% increase in heart rate, an increase in right ventricular work and a 3% decrease in mechanical efficiency of the left ventricle. Cardiac output and stroke volume remain unchanged (MAXWELL et al. 1957, 1959; CRUMPTON et al. 1959) or show a significant increase (27.6%) (ROWE et al. 1963).

Finally, intravenously infused 5-HT gave completely different results at different dose levels and in the hands of different investigators. RUDOLPH and PAUL (1957) observed a 60% rise of cardiac output with an infusion rate of 60 μg/kg/min; McGAFF and MILNER (1962) found no significant changes in cardiac output, in stroke volume or in left atrium mean pressure with 0.06—0.4 mg/kg/min 5-HT; and NOBLE and NANSON (1959) noted a reduction of cardiac output, despite pronounced tachycardia, at an infusion rate as low as 2.5 μg/kg/min.

Psilocybin given intravenously into dogs anaesthetized with morphine and a dial-urethane-nembutal mixture at a dose of 0.5 mg/kg, depresses cardiac output. Tachycardia is constant, and cardiac work well maintained (MAXWELL et al. 1962). 5-acetyltryptamine causes bradycardia with slight and transient alterations in heart contractile force (BEN et al. 1962).

Cat. Using the technique of isolated heart perfusion, both REID (1952) and SCHNEIDER and YONKMAN (1953, 1954) showed that 2—200 μg of 5-HT in the cat heart causes an increase in heart rate, an increase in coronary flow and an increase in contractile force, which, in sensitive hearts, occasionally results in persistent systolic contraction. These data suggest that bradycardia observed in the intact cat after intravenous or intracoronary injection of 5-HT is caused by vagal reflexes masking the direct stimulant action of the substance on the heart. The fact that bradycardia is reduced or disappears following vagotomy, cooling of the vagi or intravenous injection of local anaesthetics has been considered direct evidence of the influence of 5-HT on vagal afferent fibres (SCHNEIDER and YONKMAN 1953, 1954; KOTTEGODA and MOTT 1955; WEIDMANN and CERLETTI 1955).

Pressure rise elicited by psilocybin (50—100 μg/kg, i.v.) is similarly accompanied by relative bradycardia (CERLETTI 1959).

Rabbit. Hypotension produced by 5-HT is regularly accompanied by transient slowing of the heart rate, associated with cardiac irregularities (SCHNEIDER and YONKMAN 1954). Psilocybin (50—100 μg/kg, i.v.), on the contrary, causes marked increase in the heart rate (CERLETTI 1959).

Calf. Cardiac output, as measured by the dye dilution method, is not changed in response to a 3-minute infusion of 0.2 mg/kg/min 5-HT (KUIDA et al. 1961).

Chicken. Both 5-HT (20—50 μg/kg) and tryptamine (100—500 μg/kg) produce a marked diminution in the height of ventricular contraction. This is followed by a brief period of myocardial stimulation in 56% of the animals (BUÑAG and WALASZEK 1961).

Rat. Fifteen to thirty minutes after intraperitoneal injection of 4 mg/kg 5-HT base cardiac output is unchanged, whereas blood flow in the myocardium is increased. Conversely, intravenous infusion of 2.3 μg/kg/min 5-HT produces an increase of cardiac output (TAKÁCS and VAJDA 1963).

2. Heart-lung preparation

Dog. FREYBURGER et al. (1952) found that 5-HT introduced into the circuit of a heart-lung preparation not only lacked any stimulant action but produced a certain decompensation, as shown by the rise of pressure in the left auricle. MAGGI and NOLI (1958) failed to detect any sign of cardiac decompensation, even at mg doses of 5-HT. 150—500 μg displayed a positive inotropic effect preceded by short-lived inhibition; 1—20 μg was completely inactive. Finally, DUTEIL (1962) and DUTEIL and AVIADO (1962) observed that the injection of 5-HT into the right atrium of the dog heart-lung preparation caused a rise in mean pulmonary arterial pressure, a rise in right ventricular systolic pressure, no change in left atrial pressure and transient fall in cardiac output. The lack of increase in cardiac output which is seen in the dog prior to conversion to a heart-lung preparation is interpreted as being due to the loss of cardioaccelerator mechanisms, particularly the sympathetic reflex induced by a rise in right intraventricular pressure.

Rabbit. In the rabbit heart-lung preparation 25 μg 5-HT produces the following changes: 10—15% reduction of the heart rate, decrease of the stroke volume, 30—50% reduction of the left ventricular work, 25—60% decrease of the coronary flow with increase in the coronary resistances, and finally a 25—30% increase in the O_2 consumption.

The above phenomena last 3 min, and there is evident tachyphylaxis. Doses of 0.5—5 μg 5-HT are completely inactive (MAGGI and NOLI 1958, MAGGI 1960).

Rat. On the heart-lung preparation of rats, 5-HT does not produce any change in heart rate or cardiac output in doses up to 40 μg/ml. Large doses cause the appearance of extrasystoles (MINELLI 1961).

3. Isolated heart

Rabbit. The effects of 5-HT on the isolated perfused rabbit heart have been thoroughly studied by JACOB and POITE-BEVIERRE (1960) over a wide dose range of 5-HT (2 μg to 5 mg of the base). In general three successive phases are observed:

a) irregular negative inotropic and chronotropic effect, antagonized by atropine;

b) positive inotropic and chronotropic effect, which disappears after pretreatment with reserpine and is considered to be mediated by catecholamines;

c) negative inotropic effect, resistant to atropine and often accompanied by a tonus increase. This effect is the predominant one for doses of 0.5 mg and more.

With 4 mg and more, atropine-resistant arrhythmias develop, consisting of cardiac arrest, atrioventricular block, flutter and fibrillation. BAS in this preparation appears to be an ambiguous 5-HT antagonist, sometimes mimicking rather than counteracting the 5-HT effects.

The positive inotropic and chronotropic effect of the medium doses of 5-HT (20—50 μg) has already been described by FREYBURGER et al. (1952) and by LOUBATIÈRES et al. (1955).

Bufotenidine is 50 times more potent than 5-HT. At 1—2 μg doses it causes an increase in amplitude of cardiac movements; at 5—10 μg doses the inotropic effect is accompanied by a positive chronotropic effect (UEDA et al. 1957).

Dog. 30—300 μg of 5-HT injected into the perfusion fluid of an isolated heart produce a marked increase in the heart rate and a clear increase in coronary flow, whereas the increase in amplitude of contractions is small (SCHNEIDER and YONKMAN 1954).

Cat. As already stated, both REID (1952) and SCHNEIDER and YONKMAN (1954) showed that 2—200 μg 5-HT infused into the isolated cat heart caused an increase in heart rate, an increase in coronary flow and an increase in contractile force which, in sensitive hearts, occasionally resulted in persistent systolic contraction.

Frog. On the frog heart 5-HT and tryptamine display a very moderate inotropic effect. This is potentiated by iproniazid and isoniazid, probably as a consequence not of MAO inhibition but of decreased penetration of the amines into the muscle cells (BURFORD et al. 1960). 56 μg of bufotenine has no effect on the preparation; 230 μg causes, after a latency period, a decrease in heart rate and a subsequent arrest of the organ (HANDOVSKY 1920). Gramine (500 μg) shows a similar negative inotropic and chronotropic action (POWELL and CHEN 1945).

4. Isolated atrium

Rabbit. Effects observed on the isolated rabbit atria are at variance. Whereas LOUBATIÈRES et al. (1955) could not see any influence of 5-HT (0.05—1 μg/ml) on the frequency and contractile strength of this preparation, others (McCAWLEY et al. 1952; SINHA and WEST 1953; LÉVY and MICHEL-BER 1956a, 1956b; TRENDELENBURG 1960) found that the amine (0.1—10 μg/ml) produced a pure stimulant effect (increase in amplitude of contraction and in rate of beat), or a stimulant effect which was preceded by short-lived inhibition and eventually followed by a more marked depression. Atropine (10^{-7}) and hexamethonium (10^{-5}) abolished the initial inhibiting effect, but not the subsequent one; procaine (0.5 γ/ml) caused a 50% reduction in 5-HT stimulation (SINHA and WEST 1953). It has been suggested that the initial inhibition is cholinergic in nature and that the predominant stimulant action of 5-HT is the result of the liberation of noradrenaline. In fact, atria of rabbits pretreated with reserpine show very little or no response to 5-HT (TRENDELENBURG 1960).

Guinea-pig. Guinea-pig atria respond to 5-HT (1—10 μg/ml) with a pronounced and regular increase in amplitude of contractions and in rate of beat. The effect of the amine is mainly direct (LSD-sensitive), but also indirect, morphine- and cocaine-sensitive effects may contribute to the stimulant response to 5-HT. The response of atria of animals pretreated with reserpine is not significantly different from the response of atria isolated from untreated animals (TRENDELENBURG 1960).

Cat. The response of cat atria to 5-HT (1 μg/ml) consists chiefly of an increase of rate. Changes in amplitude of contractions are seen, but are small and variable. The effect of 5-HT is blocked by LSD, but is not affected by pretreatment with reserpine (TRENDELENBURG 1960).

5. Papillary muscle

On papillary muscle preparations of cats, dogs and rabbits, LOUBATIÈRES et al. (1955) could not see any increase of the contractile strength at final concentrations of 5-HT ranging from 0.05 to 100 μg/ml. LEUSEN and LACROIX (1959), on the other hand, observed a positive inotropic effect on the cat papillary muscle at final concentrations of 1—100 μg/ml. This, however, was sometimes rather short-lived and was often preceded by a short depressive phase.

6. Strips of turtle and frog ventricle

Ventricular strips from turtle *(Pseudonymus elegans)* and frog *(Rana pipiens)* were isolated, suspended in air, superfused with buffered Ringer solution and driven at a constant frequency.

The force of mechanical contraction of turtle ventricular strips was not altered by 5-HT in concentrations from 0.1 to 100 μg/ml; at concentrations of 1000 μg/ml it was depressed. Moreover, no significant changes in refractory period, conduction time or stimulus threshold were seen.

Concerning the frog, concentrations of 5-HT from 1 to 10 μg/ml did not change the force of contraction of ventricular strips but, occasionally, periods of premature systoles and periods of autorhythmicity were seen.

5-HT did not alter the toxic effects of ouabain or procainamide (HANSON and MAGILL 1961, 1962).

7. Heart of molluscs

The stimulant action of 5-HT on the molluscan heart was first described by ERSPAMER and GHIRETTI (1951) who found that 5-HT provokes a marked increase in the amplitude and frequency of systolic contractions of *Octopus* and *Helix* hearts, whether isolated or *in situ*. The tonus, too, rises conspicuously, and with larger doses of the substance a persistent systolic arrest can be seen. The stimulant action extends over the pulsatile arteries, e.g. those of the kidney and gills, with reinforcement of their contractions or with renewal of their rhythmic activity if this has disappeared. The hearts of *Murex trunculus*, *Murex brandaris*, *Dolium galea* and *Aplysia limacina* are less sensitive than *Helix* or *Octopus* hearts. Tryptamine shows a similar action, which is, however, less prompt and 20 to 25 times less intense.

The above results were confirmed by all subsequent research workers and from extensive investigations it clearly appears that the sensitivity of the heart and regularity of its response varies a great deal in different molluscan species (BACQ et al. 1952, ZETLER and SCHLOSSER 1954, WELSH 1954, GADDUM and PAASONEN 1955, JAEGER 1962).

Since the studies of WELSH (1953, 1954, 1957) the heart of *Venus mercenaria* is considered one of the most suitable preparations and is largely used in the bioassay of 5-HT. The response of this heart to 5-HT shows, like that of the *Helix* and *Octopus* hearts, three components: an increase in amplitude, an increase in frequency and an increase in the resting tone of the muscle. The relative importance of these components varies with the concentration of 5-HT. At low to moderate concentrations (10^{-9} to 10^{-6} M) a positive inotropic effect is dominant; at high concentrations (10^{-5} M and more) a large increase in muscle tone.

Hearts exposed to high concentrations of 5-HT or other tryptamine analogues for long periods become tachyphylactic to low doses of these substances. However. large doses of 5-HT (about 2×10^{-5} M) still excite the tachyphylactic heart, but the response is then different (decrease in amplitude of beat) and like the response to catecholamines. When high bath temperatures render the heart insensitive to 5-HT, high concentrations of this compound again have the catecholamine effect (GREENBERG 1960a).

GREENBERG (1960b) and BERTACCINI and ZAMBONI (1961) have tested a number of tryptamine analogues on the isolated hearts of *Venus mercenaria* and *Helix luconum*, respectively. Results of these studies are in part summarized in Table 4 of chapter 3.

From the more numerous data obtained on the *Helix* heart, some prudent conclusions may be drawn concerning structure-activity relationship:

a) Shifting of the phenolic —OH group from position 5 to other positions regularly produces a decrease of biological activity, which is moderate when the transposition is to position 4, greater when it is to position 6, and tremendous when the transposition is to position 7.

b) Substitution on the indole nucleus of groups other than —OH groups does not always reduce biological activity. In fact 5-methoxytryptamine is more potent than 5-HT, 5-methoxy-α-methyltryptamine more potent than 5-hydroxy-α-methyltryptamine, and 5-aminotryptamine as potent as 5-HT.

c) The effect of alkyl substitution on the amino nitrogen is variable. In the case of 5-HT, substitution of two methyl groups (bufotenine) produces a 3-fold increase of activity, in the case of tryptamine a 5-fold decrease.

d) Substitution of an —OH group on the β-carbon of the side chain of bufotenine causes the disappearance of any activity.

e) Indazolealkylamines show a remarkable 5-HT-like activity, which is particularly evident for the first member of the series, more strictly related to 5-HT from a chemical point of view.

Table 4 further shows that results obtained with *Helix* heart are sometimes considerably different from those obtained with the *Venus* heart.

It should be added that, according to GREENBERG (1960b) congeners without a 5-hydroxy group and with methyl substitution tend to act not only less strongly than 5-HT, but also more slowly and irreversibly.

The effect of 5-HT is regularly antagonized by BOL, whereas LSD behaves in a strikingly different way: on the *Cyprina* and *Buccinum* hearts LSD acts as a good 5-HT antagonist, but on the *Venus* heart the drug displays a powerful irreversible 5-HT-like action (WELSH 1957, WELSH and MCCOY 1957, SHAW and WOOLEY 1956).

8. Heart of crustaceans

The response of the crustacean heart to 5-HT is strikingly different from one crustacean species to another not only from a quantitative but also from a qualitative point of view. In fact, whereas the heart of some crustacean species is potently stimulated by 5-HT, that of other species is potently inhibited.

Among the hearts which give a positive response to 5-HT the most sensitive are those of *Carcinus moenas* (threshold for 5-HT, 0.001 μg/ml; threshold for adrenaline, 0.1 μg/ml) and of *Cancer borealis* (threshold for 5-HT, 0.1 to 1 μg/ml) (Florey and Florey 1953, Welsh 1957).

Also in isolated lobster (*Homarus americanus*) hearts 5-HT causes an increase in rate and amplitude of beat. Experiments on isolated cardiac ganglia and on preparations in which simultaneous recordings of the heart beat and electrical activity of the ganglion are made show that all the effects of 5-HT can be explained as a primary action on the cardiac ganglion (Cooke 1962).

In evident contrast to the above findings, Sanborn and Pax (1962) observed that when the 8th and 9th pairs of nerves from the *Limulus* suboesophageal ganglion, which contain the inhibitory fibres to the heart, were stimulated with square-waves for 0.2 m sec duration, the action potentials in the cardiac ganglion decreased to less than half the frequency before stimulation and then gradually returned to their normal rate over a period of approximately 1 minute. Because this time course indicated chemical mediation a variety of compounds was tested. It was found that 5-HT produced the same cardiac effects as did nerve stimulation, the effective doses of 5-HT being 4 μg/kg when the drug was injected distant from the heart and 2 μg/kg when it was injected directly into the heart. Sanborn and Pax suggest that the rate of heart-beat of *Limulus* is controlled by neural secretion of indoleamine-like compounds.

These results confirm the previous ones of Burgen and Kuffler (1957) who noted that the rhythmic electrical bursts of activity of the isolated cardiac ganglion of *Limulus* were slowed or abolished by 5-HT, an effect which was blocked by BOL.

Recent reports have called attention to two other indolealkylamines occurring in the crustacean organism which are highly active on the crustacean heart.

On the one hand Kerkut and Price (1964) found that 6-HT, which seems to be a normal constituent of the *Carcinus* heart, is 10 times as active as 5-HT in exciting this heart, on the other hand Carlisle (1964) observed that 5,6-dihydroxytryptamine, which appears to be a normal constituent of the pericardial organ of *Cancer pagurus* and *Maia squinato*, is 100 times more active than 5-HT on the prawn (*Leander serratus*) heart.

Results described in this chapter do not support the eventual hypothesis that 5-HT plays a role in controlling normal cardiac activity in vertebrates. Hence, all the actions of 5-HT on the *in situ* and on the isolated vertebrate heart must be considered pharmacological actions.

Things are different in molluscan and crustacean hearts. The hearts of molluscs, at least those of some molluscs, contain detectable amounts of 5-HT and respond to the amine at extremely low, physiological dose levels with no sign of tachyphylaxis and with changes in their activity similar to those produced in the mammalian heart by catecholamines. Moreover, 5-HT is present, in considerable amounts, in the ganglia and nerves of molluscs.

All these findings support the view, originally advanced by Welsh (1954a, 1954b, 1956, 1957), and now shared by others (Meng 1958, 1960; Loveland 1963) that 5-HT in molluscs may be a humoral excitory agent released by cardioregulator nerves.

However, there are some other observations which are difficult to reconcile with the hypothesis that 5-HT is a cardiac neurohumor or a cardiovascular hormone in all molluscs (ERSPAMER and GHIRETTI 1951, BACQ et al. 1952). The most important of them is that the hearts of different species present conspicuous differences in their sensitivity to 5-HT. Whereas the hearts of *Venus mercenaria*, *Cyprina islandica*, *Octopus vulgaris*, *Helix pomatia* and *Spisula solida* are excited by concentrations of 5-HT as low as 0.1—1 ng/ml, those of numerous other molluscs show a considerably lower sensitivity and present irregular responses to the amine (ERSPAMER and GHIRETTI 1951, WELSH 1954, GADDUM and PAASONEN 1955).

As for the crustacean heart, the directionally opposite effects of 5-HT in different species, joined to the different sensitivity to the amine, represent serious obstacles against considering 5-HT a neurohumor or a transmitter substance of general significance. It is premature to say whether 6-HT or 5,6-dihydroxytryptamine is the sought-for neurohumor.

VIII. Action on the circulation and function of the kidney

Rat. The most extensive researches on the action of 5-HT on the function of the rat kidney have been carried out by the writer and his co-workers (ERSPAMER 1952a, 1954b, 1954c; ERSPAMER and OTTOLENGHI 1950, 1953; ERSPAMER and SALA 1954; ERSPAMER and CORREALE 1955; ERSPAMER et al. 1956).

Experiments performed on about 3500 groups of 4 rats each have made it possible to gather a number of data and to reach some definite conclusions.

5-HT displays in the rat a powerful antidiuretic action. This appears under most varied conditions of hydration, but is especially evident after a single oral dose of 5 ml tap water per 100 g of body weight (Fig. 6) (ERSPAMER 1952, ERSPAMER and OTTOLENGHI 1953). The substance inhibits not only water diuresis but diuresis produced by osmotic diuretics and xanthine derivatives. When 5-HT and posterior pituitary extracts are administered simultaneously the antidiuretic effect of the two hormones is simply additive (ERSPAMER 1953d).

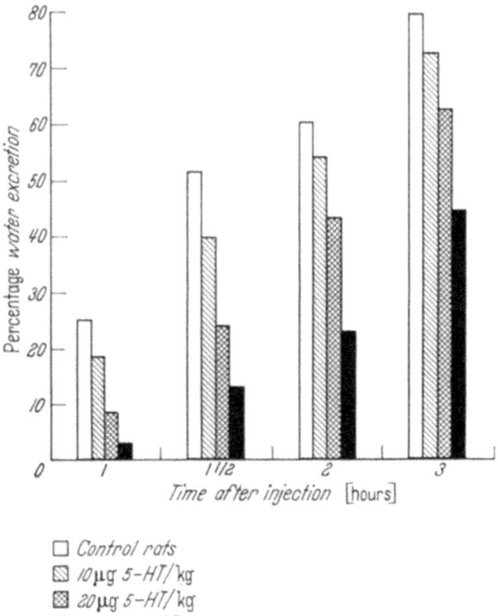

Fig. 6. Antidiuretic effect of subcutaneous 5-HT in hydrated rats. Each column represents the mean of results from 24—48 groups of 4 animals each. [From Fig. 8, ERSPAMER, V., Triangle (Basel) 2, 135 (1956).]

Among the species studied the rat is the most sensitive to 5-HT. It is sufficient to inject subcutaneously as little as 4 μg/kg 5-HT base to produce a significant reduction in the volume of urine during the first 60 min period following the water load. This dose is at least 50—100 times less than the minimum required to lower the systemic blood pressure (ERSPAMER 1952, CORREALE 1954) and at least 20,000 times less than the LD 50 by the subcutaneous route (FREYBURGER et al. 1952, Erspamer 1952). It corresponds to about 1/70 of the 5-HT content of the rat organism, per kg of body weight, and is certainly less than the quantity of endogenous 5-HT which is destroyed by amine oxidase every hour, as estimated by the urinary output of 5-HIAA (4—8 μg/kg/hr).

Higher doses cause a very conspicuous reduction in diuresis or even a virtual suppression of urine flow for several hours. The final result is that even 7 to 9 hr after the water load the animals treated with 5-HT excrete 10 to 20% less water than the control animals. The reduction in urine volume is accompanied by a simultaneous reduction in chloride excretion (Erspamer and Correale 1955).

The most appropriate and effective way of administering 5-HT is subcutaneously, as shown by the intensity, and still more by the duration of the antidiuretic effect. After intraperitoneal or intravenous injection the substance is several times less active; when given by mouth it is practivally inactive (Erspamer and Ottolenghi 1953, Erspamer and Sala 1954). These results explain why Ames and van Dyke (1952) did not succeed in producing antidiuresis by intravenous administration of 2—3 μg 5-HT base/rat.

Through the simultaneous evaluation of urine flow and renal excretion of test substances (thiosulphate, creatinine, PAH) in large groups of animals, it can be demonstrated that 5-HT antidiuresis in the rat is due primarily and essentially to a reduction in the glomerular filtration rate. This reduction, which is accompanied by a simultaneous reduction of the blood flow through the peritubular capillary network, must be ascribed, at least to a great extent, to a constriction of the afferent glomerular vessels, leading to a fall in intraglomerular hydrostatic pressure. The point of attack of 5-HT in the rat kidney is therefore the smooth muscle, or analogous contractile structures of the afferent glomerular system. Systemic hypotension and increase in the endocapsular pressure should really be listed among the factors causing a reduction in the filtration pressure, but neither of them can interfere when the dose of 5-HT is less than 0.4 mg/kg.

After 5-HT the percentage reduction in the urine volume is greater than that in the glomerular filtration rate and still more than that in the renal plasma flow, as measured by the PAH excretion. A higher percentage of the glomerular filtrate has therefore been reabsorbed by the tubules of the treated animals than by those of the controls. Even without excluding other possibilities, such as that of some direct or indirect stimulant effect of 5-HT on the tubular epithelium, a satisfactory explanation of the phenomenon may be based on the theory that, when the glomerular filtration rate is decreased, the reduced glomerular load is more completely reabsorbed during the slower passage down the nephron and less is excreted (Selkurt et al. 1952).

Other pieces of direct and indirect evidence in favour of a prevailingly vascular point of attack of 5-HT in the rat kidney, and hence of the possibility of a temporary, partial exclusion of the organ from the general circulation are as follows:

a) after the administration of high, unphysiological doses of 5-HT (2—10 mg/kg) the afferent vasoconstriction induced by the substance becomes visible even macroscopically through the mottled aspect of the kidney surface, due to the presence of ischemic cortical areas interposed between areas with an apparent normal blood supply. If the injury is particularly intense or repeated, ischemia results in degeneration and necrosis (Erspamer 1952, 1954d).

b) recovery in urine of subcutaneously injected thiosulphate is considerably higher (32.5%) in control rats than in rats given large doses of 5-HT (down to 9.3%). This means that the substance, owing to the more prolonged stay in the organism caused by renal ischemia, has been metabolized to a larger extent (Erspamer and Ottolenghi 1953).

c) sublimate intoxication is less severe in rats given repeated high doses of 5-HT than in control rats. This is so in spite of the nephrotoxicity of the high doses of 5-HT, on their own. The protection may be interpreted as being due to reduced flow of blood, and hence of the poison, through the kidney (ERSPAMER 1953b).

5-HT antidiuresis (0.1—0.5 mg/kg, s.c.) can be prevented but not suppressed once it has begun, by dibenamine, by the natural or hydrogenated ergot alkaloids of the ergotamine and ergotoxine groups, and by LSD (ERSPAMER 1953c, 1954b) and other lysergic acid derivatives. In the experiments of DE CARO (1963), confirmed by CHODERA (1963), none of the five investigated lysergic acid derivatives (100 μg/kg) were capable of completely blocking the antidiuretic action of 2 mg/kg 5-HT injected subcutaneously 30 min later. The relative potency of the compounds ranged in this order: MOB (1-methyl-BOL) = MLD (1-methyl-LSD) > UML (1-methyl-D-lysergic acid butanolamide) > BOL = LSD. Gramine and gramine derivatives (ERSPAMER, 1953c, 1955b), the N-methyltryptamines, the aminoindoles of WOOLEY and SHAW, including "medmain" and "1-methyl-medmain" (ERSPAMER, 1953c, 1954b), as well as some antihistaminic agents had a less consistent action (ERSPAMER, 1952c). The antidiuretic effect of 5-HT does not appear to be significantly affected by ganglion-blocking drugs, atropine, papaverine, nitrites, ethyl alcohol, 1-hydrazinophthalazine, histamine, adenosine or theophylline (ERSPAMER 1953d).

The fact that 5-HT is much more active when injected subcutaneously than when given intraperitoneally or intravenously and the fact that the majority of the drugs antagonistic to 5-HT are capable of preventing 5-HT antidiuresis but not of interrupting it is explained, without excluding alternative interpretations, by assuming that 5-HT occupies its receptors within the walls of the afferent renal vessels slowly and gradually, but very tenaciously. The gradual occupation would account for the necessity of a prolonged supply of small quantities of substance, as experimentally ensured by subcutaneous injection; the tenacity of occupation explains satisfactorily on the one hand the conspicuous duration of the antidiuretic effect and on the other the inability of some of the most powerful antagonists to remove 5-HT from its renal receptors (ERSPAMER 1954b, 1954c).

The writer's data on the powerful antidiuretic effect of 5-HT in the rat have been fully confirmed and the suggestion that this effect is mainly due to afferent glomerular vasoconstriction has been generally accepted (DEL GRECO and CORCORAN 1956, DEL GRECO et al. 1956).

VAN ARMAN and JENKINS (1956), for example, found that 5-HT had a highly significant ($P > 0.01$) antidiuretic effect in well-hydrated rats in subcutaneous doses as low as 10 μg/kg and that this effect could not be ascribed either to lowering of blood pressure or to painful sensations produced by the injection. Without excluding the possibility that 5-HT directly stimulated the kidney tubule to cause increased water reabsorption, the main cause of reduced diuresis was considered to be diminished glomerular filtration produced by changed blood flow. The frequently observed dissociation between diuresis and creatinine excretion, the latter being less reduced than the former, has been better explained by the assumption that a very slight drop in filtration can cause a large drop in water output (WHITE 1951). VAN ARMAN and JENKINS have criticized the conclusion of ERSPAMER (1954b) that dibenamine is incapable of removing 5-HT from its renal receptors once it has occupied them. Having found that dibenamine on it own has effects on the kidney which superficially resemble those of 5-HT, VAN ARMAN and JENKINS affirm that it would be difficult to say whether dibenamine can displace 5-HT from the renal receptors. We think that the most pertinent answer to the above criticism is the finding that lysergic acid derivatives also (LSD, BOL) given at dose levels which on their own completely lack any antidiuretic effect (e.g. 10 μg/kg, i.p.) consistently reduce 5-HT antidiuresis when administered prior to 5-HT injection, but have no effect at all when given after 5-HT (ERSPAMER 1954b, DEL GRECO and CORCORAN 1956, DEL GRECO et al. 1956).

Although subcutaneous administration of 5-HT is far more efficacious in producing antidiuresis than intraperitoneal or intravenous administration (AIRAKSINEN et al. 1960, ERSPAMER 1954b), a transient sharp drop in the rate of urine flow may be obtained in alcohol-anaesthetized hyperhydrated rats even by injection into the femoral vein of doses of 5-HT as low as 0.5 μg/100 g (SINCLAIR 1957), and in anaesthetized rats brought into osmotic diuresis with mannitol by intravenous infusion of 3—5 μg/kg/min 5-HT base. At this infusion rate a depression of glomerular filtration rate is observed, together with persistent decreases in urine volume, urinary osmolarity and urinary chlorides. Larger doses of 5-HT (6—8 μg/kg/min) cause severe and persistent depression of renal function, sometimes associated with macroscopic renal infarcts. These effects are largely independent of the changes in blood pressure (DEL GRECO and CORCORAN 1956, DEL GRECO et al. 1956).

Besides being decreased by sympatholytic drugs and lysergic acid derivatives, the antidiuretic effect of 5-HT (160 μg/kg, s.c.) is also significantly reduced by chlorpromazine (5—50 mg/kg) given 30 min before hydration. Antidiuresis produced by posterior pituitary extract (0.06 *u.*/kg) is not however counteracted by chlorpromazine (DASGUPTA 1957).

According to FRENKL et al. (1964) the antidiuretic effect of 5-HT is strongly reduced in rats trained for six weeks by forced swimming.

Isolated rat kidneys perfused with isotonic dextran solutions respond to 5-HT added to the perfusion liquid with reversible vasoconstriction, and within a certain range the degree of vasoconstriction depends on the concentration of 5-HT. For example, 0.034, 0.125 and 1 μg/ml 5-HT reduce the perfusion rate by 25—30, 60 and 70—75%, respectively. After a short initial period during which the vascular resistance rises, a constant vascular tone is reached and maintained for a long time. There is no significant tachyphylaxis up to 2 μg/ml 5-HT concentrations, but at a concentration of 10 μg/ml a slight effect of desensitization is noted. Even maximal effects of 5-HT can be fully reversed or suppressed with suitable doses of LSD (0.2 μg/ml) (PASSOW et al. 1960). The 5-HT constriction of the rat renal vessels is 5—10 times less than that produced by adrenaline (CERLETTI et al. 1955).

The opinion of BENDITT (1957) that trapping of fluid peripherally seems to offer an adequate explanation of the antidiuretic effect of 5-HT administered by the subcutaneous route cannot be seriously taken into consideration. Similarly, all the available experimental evidence is against the participation of post-pituitary ADH in the production of antidiuresis caused in rats and mice by single low doses of 5-HT (ERSPAMER and CORREALE 1955, DASGUPTA 1957, VAN ARMAN and JENKINS 1956). This statement is not in contrast with the histochemical findings of KIVALO et al. (1957, 1958b, 1959) that repeated subcutaneous doses of 5-HT (0.2 mg/kg of the base, daily for 7 days) cause depletion of the neurosecretory substance in the hypothalamus and in the posterior lobe of the hypophysis.

As already stated, the preliminary observations by ERSPAMER (1952a) on the nephrotoxic action of large doses of 5-HT have been fully confirmed by numerous other investigators (see p. 739) and this represents additional strong evidence supporting the view that the site of action of 5-HT in the rat kidney is mainly vascular.

Morphological studies on the effects of 5-HT upon the intrarenal circulation were carried out in the rat by DOLCINI et al. (1960) using a modified benzidine staining technique and intravascular injections of India ink. A marked vasodilatation with increased filling of glomeruli and peritubular capillaries was noted 15 min after the injection of 4 mg/kg 5-HT base, reaching a maximum at 30 min. At 90 and 180 min there was a striking change in the cortical zone, where the glomeruli appeared bloodless, while the circulation in the juxtamedullary area remained unaltered. According to DOLCINI and co-workers the glomerular filling effect is more likely to be on the basis of active vasodilatation rather than of stasis secondary to constriction and maintenance of juxtamedullary circulation throughout the experiment is due to a shunting of blood away from the cortex at the juxtamedullary area.

The above observations are, on the whole, in accordance with previous similar observations of FIORE-DONATI and ERSPAMER (1957) (Fig. 7). However, initial cortical blood filling is interpreted by these research workers as a frankly passive phenomenon, due to stasis secondary to afferent vasoconstriction. This is mainly based on the demonstration that at the time of maximal filling of the glomeruli there is complete block of glomerular filtration and diuresis, an event which evidently is incompatible with active vasodilatation.

It has been observed that several 5-HT antagonists (9-(N-methyl-piperidyliden-4′)thioxanthene, methysergide, cyproheptadine, imipramine) produce a more or less pronounced diuretic effect in non-hydrated and in hydrated rats. The question whether this diuresis could be related to a 5-HT mechanism was answered negatively, owing to lack of correlation between anti-5-HT and diuretic activity of these compounds (TRAPOLD and BRINER 1962).

Among the indolealkylamines, 5-HT is by far the most active on diuresis. The isomers of 5-HT are devoid, or nearly so, of any antidiuretic activity. In fact, 7-HT and 6-HT are ineffective in subcutaneous doses up to 20—40 mg/kg, and even 4-HT is more than 100 times less active than 5-HT (ERSPAMER and NOBILI 1962a, ERSPAMER unpublished observations).

The percentage activity of other indolealkylamines is a follows: N-methyl-5-HT 30—40, bufotenine 6—7, bufotenidine 0.3, 5-methoxytryptamine 25—40, tryptamine 0.3—0.5, 1-methyltryptamine 0.1—0.3, N-methyltryptamine and N,N-dimethyltryptamine 0.3.

No antidiuretic activity is shown by bufothionine, dehydrobufotenine, 6-methoxytryptamine, gramine, 2-methylgramine, 2-methyl-5-aminogramine, 2-methyl-5-nitrogramine, 2-methyl-5-chlorogramine, nor by indole derivatives lacking the amino group in the lateral chain (ERSPAMER 1952b, 1954b, and unpublished observations). Besides indolealkylamines some indoleaminoacids also produce antidiuretic effects, provided that they are transformed in the organism into active amines. So far, the aminoacids which have been found to comply with this condition are 5-HTP, 4-HTP (decarboxylation to 5-HT and 4-HT, respectively), 5-hydroxy-N-acetyltryptophan and 5-acetoxy-N-acetyltryptophan (hydrolysis to 5-HTP followed by decarboxylation), and tryptophan (direct decarboxylation to tryptamine or 5-hydroxylation to 5-HTP followed by decarboxylation to 5-HT) (ERSPAMER and BERTACCINI 1962, ERSPAMER and NOBILI 1962a, 1962b). None of the numerous other tryptophans investigated are decarboxylated in the organism to active amines (except, possibly, in traces) and hence, as expected, they are all completely inactive on diuresis (ERSPAMER et al. 1961, ERSPAMER unpublished observations).

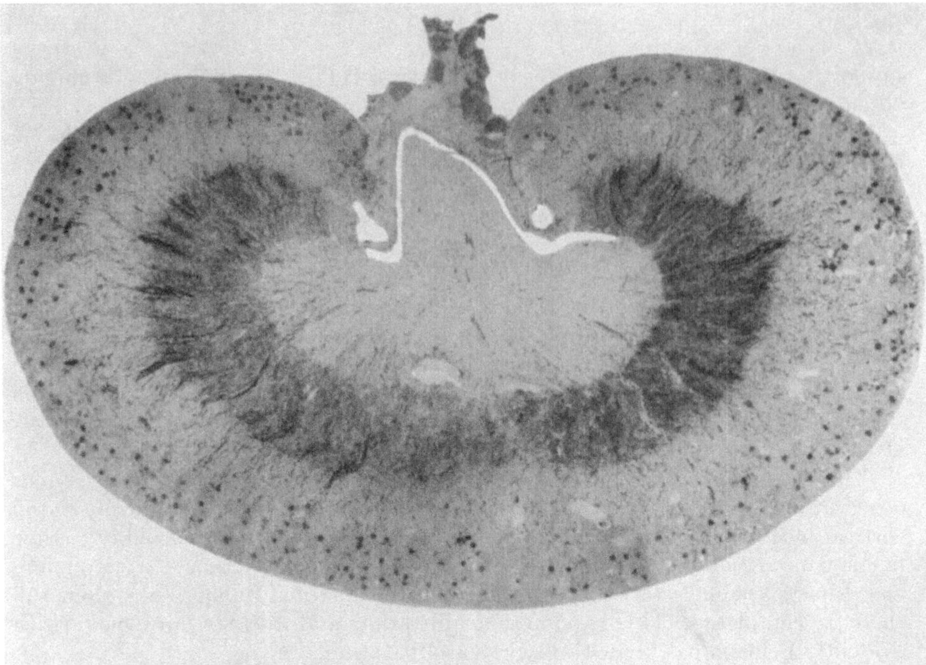

a

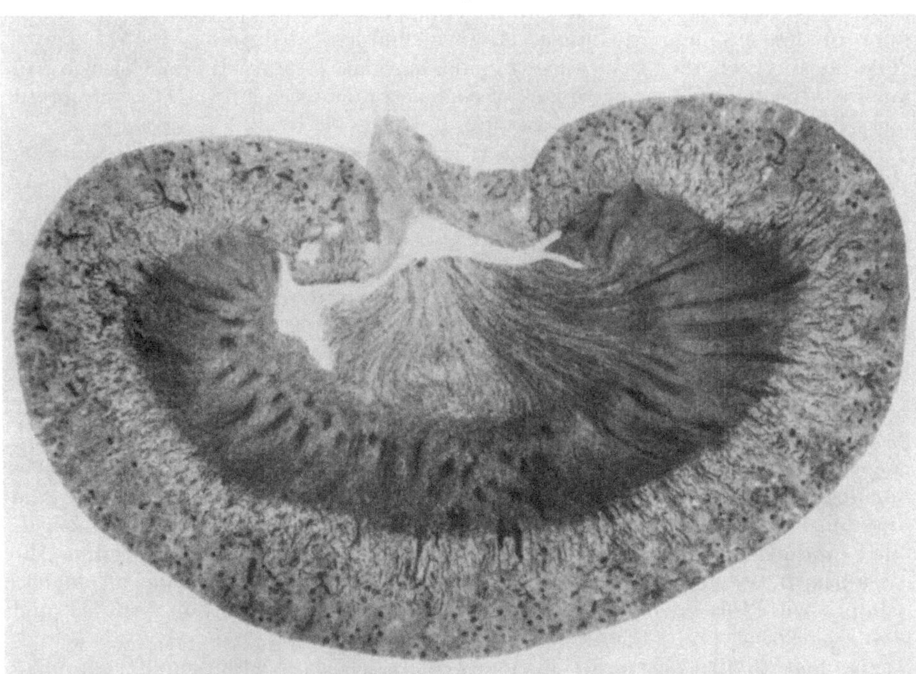

b

Fig. 7 a and b.. a Normal rat kidney stained with benzidine. The glomeruli are well filled with blood, whereas the filling of the inner band of the outer medullary zone is only a moderate one. b Kidney of a rat killed 60 min after a subcutaneous injection of 20 mg/kg 5-HT. Benzidine staining. Conspicuous congestion of the whole renal parenchyma: the peritubular capillary network, the outer and the inner bands of the outer medullary zone and the inner medullary zone are well filled with blood. ×6.5. [From Fig. 7, ERSPAMER, V., Triangle (Basel) **3**, 134 (1956).]

The minimum dose of DL-5-HTP and DL-4-HTP active on diuresis is approximately 10—20 mg/kg, by intraperitoneal or subcutaneous route. Oral amino-acids are at least 10 times less effective. Large doses of both 5-HTP and 4-HTP produce signs of cortical necrosis in a certain number of animals. The puzzling fact that exogenous 4-HT has, in sharp contrast to the 4-HT originating in the organism from 4-HTP, a very limited effect on diuresis, can be explained assuming that exogenous 4-HT, owing to its rapid inactivation, is not available for the renal receptors in sufficiently large amounts or, more probably, for a sufficiently long time to produce afferent vasoconstriction. The 4-HT originating from 4-HTP, on the other hand, may continue to circulate for long enough to allow firm occupation of the renal receptors (ERSPAMER et al. 1960, ERSPAMER and NOBILI 1962a).

5-Hydroxy-N-acetyltryptophan and 5-acetoxy-N-acetyltryptophan are considerably less effective than 5-HTP, even though they cause the appearance in the urine of large amounts of 5-HT (up to 50 μg/ml). This demonstrates that only 5-HT reaching the kidney via the blood is capable of reducing urine flow, whereas the amine generated within the kidney by decarboxylation of 5-HTP is inactive (ERSPAMER and NOBILI 1952b).

Although not directly pertinent to the topic dealt with in this chapter, some other experimental data are worth remembering. BERTACCINI and ERSPAMER (1962) have shown that single or repeated administration of tap water or of physiological NaCl solution produces in rats a conspicuous increase in urinary excretion of 5-HIAA which generally but not necessarily coincides with diuresis. One of the possible explanations of the phenomenon is that hydraemia and/or expansion of blood volume influence in some way renal excretion or reabsorption of 5-HIAA.

Mouse. Mice behave like rats in regard to the action of 5-HT on the kidney. The amount of urine collected in groups of mice after two hours, expressed as per cent of the water given, is 61% for the controls, but only 34% for the animals injected with 0.2 mg/kg 5-HT base. 2 mg/kg 5-HT has a more marked effect. Similar results are obtained with 0.5 μ/kg of posterior pituitary antidiuretic hormone, but whereas the chloride concentration in the urine of mice treated with 5-HT is significantly lower than that for the controls, the opposite may be seen for mice treated with antidiuretic hormone. It is suggested that the antidiuretic effect of 5-HT is the result of diminished blood flow through the kidney (WAAL and VEALE 1956).

Dog. The antidiuretic effect of 5-HT in the dog as well as in all other animal species examined is considerably less intense and constant than that observed in rats and mice. If we add that practically every research worker has used, in investigating the effect of 5-HT on the dog kidney, different doses of 5-HT, different routes of administration and different methods, it is small wonder that results have often been at apparent variance and that the mechanism of action of the drug in the dog kidney is controversial and largely obscure.

The minimum antidiuretic dose of 5-HT by single intravenous injection varies from 10 to 20 μg/kg (ABRAHAMS and PICKFORD 1956a) and by intravenous infusion from 3 to 10 μg/kg/min (SPINAZZOLA and SHERROD 1955, 1957, BLACKMORE 1958, LITTLE et al. 1961). The subcutaneous or intramuscular doses required to produce antidiuresis are considerably higher. SALA and CASTEGNARO (1953) obtained positive results with subcutaneous doses varying from 40 to 800 μg/kg; ABRAHAMS and PICKFORD (1956a) failed to produce antidiuresis with subcutaneous doses of 22—74 μg/kg and intramuscular doses of 14—36 μg/kg 5-HT.

5-HT is most effectively antidiuretic when injected into the cubital vein, less so when injected into the malleolar vein or carotid artery, and still less so when given into the aorta at a point above the origin of both renal arteries (ABRAHAMS and PICKFORD 1956a).

SALA and CASTEGNARO (1953) first injected 5-HT by subcutaneous route (0.04—0.8 mg/kg 5-HT base) into a series of 30 trained colpotomized bitches. They found that the amine constantly produced a more or less conspicuous reduction in urine volume, whereas the glomerular filtration rate remained unaltered for lower doses of 5-HT, while frequently showing a slight reduction for higher doses. The behaviour of the renal plasma flow was rather surprising: it remained unchanged or slightly diminished at first and increased, in the majority of cases, 20 to 30 minutes after the injection of the drug. These observations were largely confirmed by other research workers who gave 5-HT by single intravenous injections to anaesthetized dogs.

BARAC (1953a, 1955) noted that intravenous injections of 0.5—1 mg/kg 5-HT base elicited in dogs intravenously infused with saline a conspicuous reduction in the urine volume (80—100%), which was unaccompanied by any increase in chloride excretion and was largely independent of fluctuations of blood pressure. Antidiuresis was also evoked after adrenalectomy, after hypophysectomy as well as after section of the renal nerves. Ascorbic acid suppressed the antidiuretic effect of 5-HT (BARAC 1953b).

ABRAHAMS and PICKFORD (1956a) obtained similar results with lower doses of 5-HT (20—30 μg/kg). The amine not only reduced urine flow in both innervated and denervated kidneys, but also reduced the renal clearance of diodone and creatinine. One or both values, however, might increase towards and above preinjection level before urine flow recovered. The kidney surface became pale for several minutes, and injected bromophenol was found abundantly in the medullary zone, but only in a few radial streaks in the cortex. Juxtamedullary glomeruli were devoid of dye. 5-HT antidiuresis was always accompanied by obvious respiratory changes, by increase of systemic blood pressure and by changes in the colour of vaginal mucous membrane.

In a dog suffering from diabetes insipidus (daily elimination of 5—6 litres of urine), urine flow was reduced by 30 to 40% with 15 μg/kg 5-HT, and by 40—70% with 30 μg/kg 5-HT, given intravenously.

ABRAHAMS and PICKFORD (1956a) and PICKFORD (1957) repeatedly insist on the fact that the antidiuretic effect of 5-HT varies greatly from one animal to another and in the same animal from one observation period to another.

KHAZAN et al. (1962) injected 0.8 mg/kg 5-HT base into the veins of anaesthetized hydrated dogs (10 ml/kg water by stomach tube) and measured the volume of urine excreted through the ureters. A long-lasting, 30—40% reduction of urine volume was accompanied by a more conspicuous reduction in Na^+ and Cl^- excretion (from 80 ± 2.9 and 63 ± 2.4 to 38 ± 2.7 and 25 ± 0.26 meq/l, respectively) and by a consistent increase in K^+ excretion (from 223 ± 5.5 to 335 ± 3.4 meq/l). This pattern was the opposite of that caused by pitressin (2 u./kg) administration.

The renal venous pressure showed, after intravenous injection of 0.1 mg 5-HT base only a small transient reduction; then it increased at the same time with systemic pressure (MAZZELLA and MAQUIEIRA 1957).

Results obtained following intravenous infusion of 5-HT into unanaesthetized dogs were, on the whole, in good accordance.

SPINAZZOLA and SHERROD (1955, 1957) administered 5-HT to hydrated, trained female dogs in the postabsorptive state. A definite antidiuretic effect occurred at a threshold dose of 10 μg/kg/min 5-HT and became more pronounced until a dose of 20 μg/kg/min was administered. Increasing the dose to 25 μg/kg/min caused little or no further significant reduction in the rate of urine formation. Antidiuresis began within 15 min following start of the drug infusion, and lasted approximately 15 min following cessation of infusion. This was followed by a diuresis lasting 30 to 45 min. A reduction in GFR occurred beginning at a dose level of 15 μg/kg/min and it became more pronounced at the 20 μg/kg/min dose (maximum decrease = 30%). Increasing the dose up to 25 μg/kg/min resulted in little or no further decrease in GFR. An elevation of the effective renal plasma flow was noted beginning with the 10 μg/kg/min dose, which became quite significant (20—30%) and reached a plateau at about the 20—25 μg/kg/min dose. There was no important change in the mean arterial blood pressure at any of the above dose levels.

Working under similar experimental conditions, BLACKMORE (1957, 1958) found that 5 μg/kg/min 5-HT base produced as small but significant decrease in GFR, associated with increased RPF, and that 10 μg/kg/min caused the same changes plus a marked antidiuretic effect (from 3.5 to 0.6—0.9 ml urine/min). In all experiments there was a marked decrease in sodium excretion during 5-HT infusion, which returned to control values or above after cessation of the infusion. There were no changes in mean arterial blood pressure.

LITTLE and co-workers (1960, 1961) infused 5-HT into dogs infused with 0.9% NaCl solution at a rate of 0.5 ml/kg/min. At an infusion rate of 1.5 μg/kg/min 5-HT base only sodium ion excretion was significantly decreased; at a rate of 3 μg/kg/min there was a significant decrease in the renal excretion of sodium, chloride and potassium ions and a significant increase in sodium ion reabsorption. Rate of urine flow, GF and RPF were not changed during the infusion of 5-HT, but decreased significantly during the postinfusional period.

Finally, VILLAMIL et al. (1962) infused 5-HT creatinine sulphate at a rate of 30 to 60 μg/kg/min into dogs subjected to osmotic diuresis with 5% mannitol. Urine was collected from the bladder and blood samples were drawn from the femoral artery and the renal vein. 5-HT elicited a fall in the renal clearances and extractions of both creatinine and paraaminohippurate, as well as in total RPF and in the filtration fraction. Blood pressure fell slightly and renal resistance tended to increase.

A last set of experiments is concerned with the effects of 5-HT introduced directly into the artery of the *in situ* or the perfused kidney.

5-HT infused directly into the renal artery of laparotomized, anaesthetized dogs at a rate of 4—40 μg/min produced regularly an increase of the geometric component of renal vascular resistance through some mechanism unrelated to extrinsic nerves or to endogenous catecholamines. Dynamic changes in blood viscosity or interstitial pressure elevation were highly unlikely. The constriction of the renal vascular bed produced by 4 μg/min appeared to be nearly maximal. Urine flow rate did not appreciably change (EMANUEL et al. 1958, 1959).

Whereas single injections of 5-HT were found by PAGE (1957) to produce a strong and sustained constriction in perfused dog's renal vessels, the same injections (20 μg 5-HT base) appeared to possess, in the experiments of CERLETTI et al. (1955) only a slight and fleeting constrictor effect, which was less intense than that provoked by a 100 times smaller dose of adrenaline.

During stimulation of the peripheral end of a cut renal nerve, injection of 5-HT (0.3—7 μg) into the renal artery caused an initial rise of perfusion pressure approximately equal to that before stimulation, but this was followed by a sustained vasodilatation not present in the absence of stimulation (McCubbin et al. 1962).

5-HT perfused through a kidney transplanted to the neck in concentrations up to 7 μg/ml caused no significant change in the blood flow through the organ. This happened in sharp contrast to adrenaline which potently constricted renal vessels in concentrations as small as 0.02 μg/ml (Cuypers et al. 1957).

It is rather difficult to draw from the preceding data any definite conclusion about the mechanism of action of 5-HT on the dog kidney.

The only certain thing is that the renal effects of 5-HT are independent of the extrinsic innervation of the kidney and of the integrity of the posterior pituitary lobe (Barac 1955, Abrahams and Pickford 1956a, Blackmore 1958, Khazan et al. 1962), and that these effects, and hence the mechanism of action of 5-HT, may vary according to the dose and the way of administration of the drug. Whereas Abrahams and Pickford (1956a) and Pickford (1957) believe that it is necessary to look beyond the kidney for the effect of 5-HT on urine flow, suggesting that this is dependent on changes in the systemic blood pressure brought about by reflexes set up from the thorax, the great majority of investigators point to a direct action of 5-HT on the tubules and/or the intrarenal vascular bed. Concerning the possible vascular action of 5-HT, it should be stressed that a fall in intraglomerular pressure and, as a consequence, in GFR may be produced a) by an increase in renal vascular resistance due to constriction of afferent arterioles, b) by decrease in this resistance due to dilatation of both afferent and efferent arterioles, and finally c) by an intrarenal diversion of blood from the cortex towards the juxtamedullary zones and/or opening of vascular shunts simultaneously skipping glomeruli and proximal tubules. The last possibility has been proposed by Villamil et al. (1962).

It has been suggested that changes in renal haemodynamics and even moderate renal lesions found in dogs and rabbits subjected to extracorporeal circulation may be ascribed to 5-HT and ATP release following corpuscular blood thrauma (Frick 1960, Sarajas and Saure 1960). The amine, on the contrary, does not seem to play any role in the oliguria seen in dogs after burns (Renson et al. 1959).

Psilocybin provokes in the dog an active reduction of the kidney volume, when given intravenously in doses of 50—100 μg/kg (Weidmann et al. 1958).

Cat. In cats slightly anaesthetized with chloralose small intravenous doses of 5-HT (threshold 3 μg/kg) reduce the flow of urine into the bladder for $^1/_2$ to 2 minutes. Paling of the kidney and obvious spasms of the ureter are never observed. Antidiuresis is followed by a secondary diuresis.

The mechanism of this fleeting antidiuretic action is obscure. Reflex fall of blood pressure seems to play little part, and Fastier and Waal (1957) similarly hesitate to attribute the antidiuretic effect of 5-HT in the cat to either ureteral spasm or to constriction of renal blood vessels. In fact, if it is true that a moderate reduction of the blood flow through the kidney was observed by Cerletti et al. (1955) in direct perfusion experiments, it should be noted that the required dose of 5-HT was rather high (10—20 μg) and that adrenaline appeared, in this preparation too, to be 15—20 times as active as 5-HT.

Psilocybin produces, in doses of 50—100 μg/kg, an active increase in kidney volume, indicating vasodilatation (Weidmann et al. 1958, Cerletti 1959).

Rabbit. Intravenous doses of 5-HT of the order of 20—200 μg/kg constantly produce striking and persistent paling of the kidney. Ischemia is particularly evident in the cortex. Concomitantly there is a transient drop in the flow of urine from the ureters (Fastier and Waal 1957, Rovati et al. 1956).

In rabbits receiving chronic 5-HT treatment (3—5 mg/kg, over 13 to 23 days) a spotty ischemia of the renal cortex develops with both tubular and glomerular changes. Tubules present signs of hyaline degeneration; protein appears in the capsule of Bowmann and the basement membrane of the glomerular loops increases in thickness (ROVATI et al. 1956, BEREGI et al. 1962).

In contrast to the above results, VIRTAMA and JÄNKÄLÄ (1961) failed to demonstrate either in the rabbit or in the guinea-pig signs of constriction of the intrarenal arteries following injection of 5-HT (0.2—5 mg/kg) through a polyethylene catheter into the aorta just above the origin of the renal arteries. A radiographic contrast mass was injected immediately after or simultaneously with 5-HT.

In the writer's opinion these results only show that rapid intraaortic injection of 5-HT does not produce an immediate intrarenal vasoconstriction, as is necessary for arteriographic visualization.

Chicken. 60—80 μg 5-HT base injected into the leg vein of a chicken together with phenol red does not apparently affect the blood flow of the kidney, as shown by the normal phenol red excretion (SANNER 1963).

Man. Normal subjects. As in the case of the dog, the effect of 5-HT on diuresis and renal circulation varies conspicuously not only with the dose and the manner of administration of the drug, but also with the methods used in evaluating the effects of 5-HT on the kidney. Moreover, under exactly the same experimental conditions, striking differences in the reaction to 5-HT can be observed in different individuals.

HOLLANDER and MICHELSON (1956, 1957) found that following the intravenous injection of 0.5 mg 5-HT base (approximately 10 μg/kg) urine flow was reduced moderately but significantly for about 45 minutes. Concomitantly there was a slight but significant (30%) decrease in RPF often, but not necessarily, accompanied by a reduction in GFR and excretion of sodium and potassium. These changes were inconsistently related to changes in blood pressure. There is little possibility that reductions in renal functions might not have been due to actual reductions in renal haemodynamic function or electrolyte excretion but to inadequate washout of "dead space" consequent to the reduction in urine flow, because in some instances they occurred without any reduction of diuresis. HOLLANDER and MICHELSON conclude that 5-HT acts in man as a moderate antidiuretic but a weak renal vasoconstrictor agent.

DEL GRECO et al. (1956) and SCHNECKLOTH et al. (1957) observed that during osmotic diuresis 5-HT was marginally effective even when infused at a rate of 2 μg/kg/min and that doses of 4—9 μg/kg/min reduced not only urine flow, but also RPF and Na output. Maximum rate of water absorption was unchanged and K output increased.

SINCLAIR (1957) and AMBANELLI and SALVI (1960) showed that when doses of 4—8 mg 5-HT base were given by slow intravenous injection simultaneously with a rapid intravenous infusion of 850 ml of isotonic dextrose, the intensity of the diuretic response tended to be reduced, and the duration to be shortened. In two of the experiments of SINCLAIR reduction of urine volume after 90 min was from 1050 to 630 ml, and from 750 to 490 ml. In the experiments of AMBANELLI and SALVI on 18 normal subjects, average reduction in urine flow was 50, 30 and 20% after 30, 60 and 90 minutes, respectively.

ANNONI and LUCCHELLI (1955, 1957) observed that even intramuscular 5-HT (4 mg of the base) produced in 60% of hydrated subjects a significant reduction in urine volume, together with irregular changes in RPF and GFR. In some cases there was a conspicuous delay in the appearance in urine of injected phenolsulfonphthaleine. The effect of 5-HT was clearly appreciable also on diuresis produced by mercurial diuretics, while barely visible or lacking under conditions of normal hydration.

Bojs (1951), who has certainly carried out the most complete investigation on the action of 5-HT on the renal function in man, found that decreased renal sodium excretion was the most prominent finding during intravenous infusion of 5-HT (4.3—8.7 μg/kg/min). This effect was statistically highly significant ($P < 0.001$) even at the smallest 5-HT dose and often showed a close dose/response relationship. The average decrease at the largest 5-HT dose was 63%. The effect was rapid in onset (within 10 min) and reversal (within 20 min). Renal potassium excretion was not influenced by 5-HT. The fall in chloride excretion and osmolar clearance during 5-HT infusion was similar to the sodium decrease. The influence of 5-HT on water excretion was variable but antidiuresis was often observed when the initial urine flow was high. Parallel and small decreases in GFR and RPF were found during 5-HT infusion. However, these responses showed adaptation and were not statistically significant. Bojs suggests that augmented tubular sodium reabsorption is the main mechanism of 5-HT action, although decreased tubular sodium load may sometimes be a contributing factor.

To the above positive results, those of other investigators should be added, confirming that antidiuresis produced by 2—4 mg 5-HT given by the intravenous or intramuscular route is particularly evident after a water load (Correale 1957), and showing that GFR varies rather slightly, in general in the direction of a diminution (Cenacchi and Cariani 1958, Cenacchi et al. 1959), that RPF changes insignificantly in some cases, but presents a clear decrease in others (Cenacchi et al. 1959), and finally that there is generally a reduction in NaCl excretion (Hulet and Perera 1956, Correale 1957).

At complete variance with the preceding data are those of other investigators who found that 5-HT does not produce any change in the renal function or circulation of normal subjects (Curti and Fornaroli 1955, Carretti and Ronchetti 1955, Calì et al. 1956, Notter 1956, Corà et al. 1957, Vercillo and Mazzetti 1957). However, in this regard it immediately must be stressed that some of the negative results cannot be taken into consideration because of unsuitable experimental procedure, e.g. determination of urine volume and composition only at the end of a 24 hr observation period (Carretti and Ronchetti 1955, Vercillo and Mazzetti 1957), and that in other cases negative conclusions are not in accordance with partly positive experimental results. Calì, Lomeo and Bompiani (1956), for example, while affirming that 5-HT does not display any effect on the kidney function of normal subjects, present a table showing that 90 min after the administration of 6 mg 5-HT base, 6 subjects out of 10 showed a reduction in urine volume, 2 no change, and 2 an increase in urine volume.

Frick et al. (1961) suggest that the 5-HT released into plasma after major operations may participate in postoperative antidiuresis.

Diabetes insipidus. Serravalli (1955) and Curti and Fornaroli (1955) could not demonstrate any appreciable action of 5-HT on the diuresis. Erspamer (unpublished observation) and Annoni and Lucchelli (1955, 1957), on the contrary, found a consistent reduction of polyuria and polydipsia following single or repeated intramuscular injections of 2—5 mg 5-HT. In a case of juvenile diabetes mellitus with polyuria, 5-HT (2 mg every 8 hours) reduced not only diuresis (from 5—6 to 1.5—2 litres *pro die*), but also glycosuria (from 60—80 to 15—30 g) and albuminuria, with unchanged glycaemia.

Carcinoidosis. In some cases of carcinoidosis occasional periodic oliguria was observed clinically, often preceding flushing attacks (Sinclair 1957). During study of kidney function, severe renal vasoconstriction has been found in some instances unassociated either with hypertension or with abnormalities of renal function (Del Greco et al. 1956, Schneckloth et al. 1957).

It is difficult from the above data to draw definite conclusions on the site and mechanism of action of 5-HT in the human kidney. Evidence in favour of a direct vascular action of the amine is balanced by evidence in favour of a direct action on the tubules.

5-HT has been considered for some years by the writer (Erspamer 1954b, 1954c) to be a hormonal substance participating in the regulation of the intrarenal circulation and the function of the kidney. In spite of the fact that the existence of an antidiuretic effect of 5-HT has been generally confirmed in all the mammals studied, it must be admitted that so far only for rats do the renal actions of 5-HT fulfil the main conditions necessary for them to be considered "physiological". For all the other mammalian species, the renal effects, besides being more irregular, short-lasting and inconstant, are obtained with high, unphysiological doses of 5-HT.

Thus the theory of a specific renal effect of 5-HT should be dropped or drastically limited as lacking sufficient experimental evidence.

IX. Action on cellular permeability

This has been investigated in several representative cell models.

1. Slices of red beetroot. 5-HT, indoleacetic acid and, to a lesser degree, tryptamine (1—100 μg/ml) increase the effusion of pigment from beetroot slices, and strongly inhibit sodium uptake by this material, although they display little effect on the potassium efflux. These effects are not necessarily associated with any appreciable change in the rate of oxygen consumption by the tissue. They are generally irreversible in experiments lasting only a few hours, but may be completely reversible over long periods of time (Pickles 1955, Pickles and Sutkliff 1955).

2. Erythrocytes. Pretreating human erythrocytes with 5-HT (0.1—1 mM) accelerates their subsequent hypotonic haemolysis as shown by the haemoglobin release, but diminishes the amount of potassium lost in proportion to haemoglobin. Similarly, 5-HT pretreated erythrocytes lose potassium more slowly in cold-storage than controls do. Tryptamine in similar concentrations does not have either of these effects. LSD (0.1—1 mM) inhibits the effects of 5-HT (Pickles 1955, 1956).

Addition of 0.4—20 μg 5-HT to 100 ml normal human blood causes increase of serum bilirubin, as a consequence of increased escape of the pigment from the red blood cells (Nilsson et al. 1960).

3. Blood platelets. The movement of potassium (^{42}K) from plasma into blood platelets is increased when 5-HT is added to the plasma at a concentration of 1 to 10 μg/ml. 5-HT which is bound to the platelets does not display this effect (Born 1958).

4. Amphibian skin. Addition of 5-HT (15—400 μg/ml of the base) to distilled water used to bathe the outer surface of isolated abdominal frog or toad skin produces no significant effect on the net water flux from the outer surface inward, while increasing the net fluxes of sodium and potassium from the inner surface bathed in Ringer's solution outward. In skin showing very high initial Na and K fluxes, the addition of 5-HT decreases rather than increases the net movements. Addition of 5-HT does not alter the short-circuit current but does decrease the skin electrical potential difference, confirming that the increase in net Na efflux results from increased passive efflux and not from decreased active influx. Tryptamine has effects similar to those of 5-HT, whereas bufotenine is practically inactive (PICKLES 1957a, 1957b).

It has been suggested by PICKLES (1956) that the above effects may be explained by a selective alteration in cell-membrane permeability and that this may be relevant to the problem of the physiological function of 5-HT.

In the intact frog even large doses of 5-HT (0.1—8 mg/kg, into the dorsal lymphatic sac) fail to affect significantly the passage of water through the skin. It is, therefore, doubtful whether the substance plays any part in the cutaneous regulation of water metabolism (ERSPAMER 1954a). This conclusion is of interest because only in amphibians among the vertebrates does the skin play a highly important role in regulating water metabolism, and only in amphibians does the skin contain 5-HT or related indolealkylamines, which are often present in enormous amounts.

5. Amphibian urinary bladder. Concentrations of 5-HT up to 0.2 g/ml do not affect the permeability of the isolated frog urinary bladder (RASMUSSEN et al. 1963).

X. Action on extravascular smooth muscles

1. Gastro-intestinal tract

Man. Single intravenous injections of 5-HT produce in normal volunteers, studied by the balloon-kymographic method, a sharp rise in intestinal tone and the disappearance of mixing waves. In 25% of the subjects doses as low as 0.4 mg 5-HT base have a pronounced effect: however in another 15% doses up to 1.5 mg are ineffective and in yet another 10—15% 5-HT produces a decrease in tone. The stimulant effect appears 30 sec after the injection and disappears within 3—4 min, followed by a period of hypomotility and refractoriness to 5-HT. The increase in tone is accentuated by prior administration of monoamine oxidase inhibitors, inhibited by anticholinergic drugs and BAS (benzyl analogue of serotonin) and left unchanged by hexamethonium. 5-HT in doses up to 13 mg of the base fails to elicit any intestinal response when given intrajejunally to normal volunteers. However, 12 cirrhotic patients and two patients with non-tropical sprue showed a typical response when 5-HT was instilled into the jejunum (CLIFTON et al. 1956, HENDRIX et al. 1957).

It has been suggested that 5-HT stimulates intestinal motor activity through cholinergic nerves at a site distal to the ganglionic synapse (HENDRIX et al. 1957), and that hypersensitivity to oral 5-HT seen in certain pathological conditions may be due to a deficit in monoamine oxidase (CLIFTON et al. 1956).

In patients with ileostomies the intravenous injection of 1 mg 5-HT base produces an initial spasm of the intestine, followed by rhythmic contractions which last several minutes and then by a period of mechanical inactivity. The electrical activity of the ileal bud just distal to the intestinal segment containing the balloon is characterized by an initial continuous burst of action potentials followed by inhibition of electrical activity and then by intermittent bursts of action potentials. The effect of 5-HT is not inhibited by atropine, morphine or promethazine, but is blocked by large doses of LSD (3 mg, i.v.) (DANIEL et al. 1960).

The above observations have been substantially confirmed by experiments in which 5-HT was given by intravenous infusion, at rates of 2—10 μg/kg/min for 7—18 min. It was seen, however, that 5-HT, while stimulating the musculature of the jejunum and the ileum (in half of the cases the amine elicited contraction waves lasting 2—3 min, in the other half spasms), frequently reduced

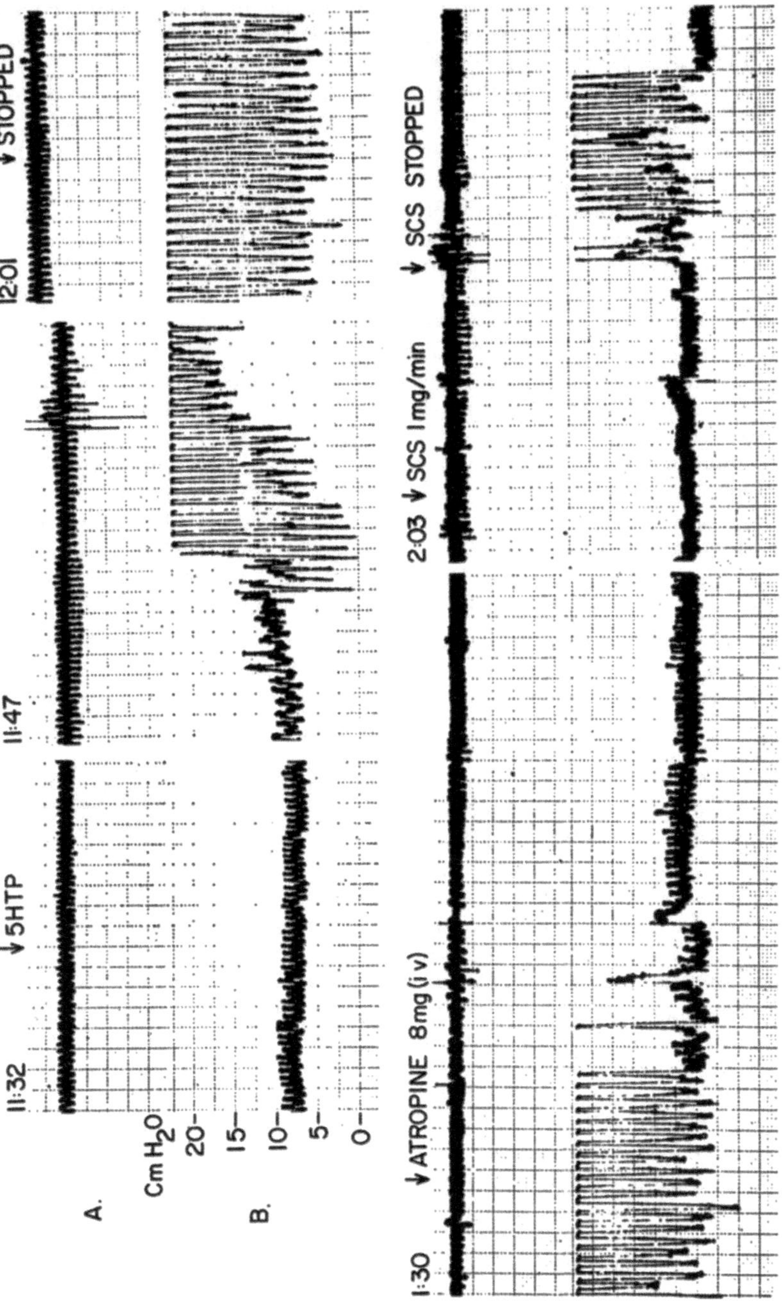

Fig. 8. Respiration (tracing A) and jejunal motility (tracing B) in a human subject. Following administration of 5-HTP in a dose of 40 mg over a period of 30 min (1.33 mg/min) a marked and sustained stimulus to motility occurred. Atropine sulphate inhibited motility stimulated by 5-HTP but not that stimulated by 5-HT creatinine sulphate (SCS: 1 mg/min for 2 min). A large division represents 10 seconds. [From Fig. 4, HAVERBACK, B. J., and S. K. WIRTSCHAFTER, Advanc. Pharmacol. 1, 318 (1962).]

tonus and spontaneous movements of the stomach, and constantly inhibited the movements of the large intestine. Inhibition lasted 10—20 min. BOL (2 mg/

orally) effectively counteracted the effects of 5-HT; atropine (1 mg, i.v.), reserpine, chlorpromazine, diphenhydramine and tripelennamine were inactive. Tachyphylaxis developed during the continuous intravenous infusion of 5-HT irrespective of dose, but within 10 min after cessation of the infusion the bowel regained its former sensitivity (HAVERBACK and DAVIDSON 1958, HAVERBACK and WIRTSCHAFTLER 1962, SCHMID and KINZLMEIER 1959).

Inhibition of movements of the large intestine and the appearance of tachyphylaxis could explain the failure by O'HARA and COLE (1959) to observe any change in intestinal transit time following infusion of 5-HT into human subjects at a rate of 15 to 260 μg/min for 1 hr.

The effects of intravenous infusion of 5-HTP differ from those of 5-HT in that the aminoacid provides a more sustained stimulation of the small intestine with no tachyphylaxis. Within 6 to 40 min after the start of the 5-HTP infusion (25—50 mg over a 30 min period) a marked increase in intestinal motility is observed in normal subjects (Fig. 8). Usually there is no marked increase in the intraluminal pressure, but in a few instances a pressure rise of up to 15 cm of water is noted and abdominal cramping is experienced. The pressure of the motility waves increases up to approximately 25—30 cm of H_2O. The increased motility persists for at least 90 min following the start of the 5-HTP infusion. At the employed 5-HTP dose no effect on pulse, blood pressure, respiration or mental status is noted. The stimulant action of 5-HTP is partially inhibited by BOL in an oral dose of 2—6 mg, and almost completely blocked by 1 mg of atropine sulphate, given subcutaneously. In one patient with non-tropical sprue, the response of the intestine to 5-HT and 5-HTP was identical with that in the normal subject. However, in another patient the intestinal response to 5-HTP was markedly diminished (HAVERBACK and DAVIDSON 1958, HAVERBACK and WIRTSCHAFTLER 1962).

In contrast to the small intestine, stomach and colon are again inhibited by the drug (SCHMID et al. 1960).

HAVERBACK and WIRTSCHAFTLER (1962) tend to explain the differences noted between 5-HT and 5-HTP in their effects on intestinal motility (unlike that of the latter, the action of the former shows tachyphylaxis and is resistant to atropine) by possible differences in dosage and in the site of action, intracellular or extracellular, of the two compounds.

In accordance with the results of CLIFTON et al. (1956), HAVERBACK and WIRTSCHAFTLER (1962) failed to elicit any intestinal stimulation following intraluminal introduction of 10 mg 5-HT or 30 mg 5-HTP. Similarly, the writer could not see any obvious effect on gastro-intestinal motility following oral introduction of 200—1000 mg of DL-4-HTP (ERSPAMER and NOBILI 1961).

The incapacity of 5-HT to stimulate all segments of the alimentary canal was confirmed by several other research workers both *in vivo* and *in vitro*.

FINK and FRIEDMAN (1960) made simultaneous intraluminal pressure measurements, in 16 human subjects, in two colonic segments 40 cm apart, using a perforated polyvinyl tube connected to an external electrical transducer system. They found that intravenous injection of 1.5 mg 5-HT increased the phasic activity of the proximal colon and depressed, for 4—6 min, that of the distal colon. 5-HT stopped not only spontaneous distal colon motility but also motility induced by prior administration of neostigmine.

SHEPHERD (1963) observed that 5 μg 5-HT either injected, during laparatomy, into an artery adjacent to the colon or applied directly to the surface failed to elicit any local increase of activity, whereas the same procedure applied to an ileal loop in another patient produced profound and prolonged contractions.

Finally, BESANÇON (1961) and DEBRAY and BESANÇON (1961) found that in intubated patients, whose intestinal motility was recorded by an electromanometric method, rapid intravenous injection of 0.2—0.45 mg 5-HT base was followed by an evident stimulation of the motility of the duodenum, the jejunum and the middle small intestine in 83, 63 and 47% of the experiments, respectively. The effect lasted 3 to 6 min. The ileum responded only in 15% of the experiments, and the large intestine never. There were striking differences from one patient to another even in the response of the more sensitive intestinal loops. A second injection of 5-HT administered 1 to 5 min after the disappearance of the response to a first injection was nearly always ineffective.

In spite of the above rather ambiguous results, DEBRAY and BESANÇON suggest that 5-HT may play a physiological role in controlling the motility of the duodenum and the jejunum, more precisely in provoking movements which cause an evacuation of these segments. This is based on the analogy existing on the one hand between motor responses to 5-HT and certain prolonged sequences of spontaneous waves, and on the other hand between the physiological refractory state seen after spontaneous contractions and the tachyphylaxis seen after 5-HT injections.

ADAMS (1960) found that in subjects given either 0.2 mg carbachol subcutaneously or 30 g magnesium sulphate orally serum 5-HT increased from 0.14 to 0.18 μg/ml, and from 0.184 to 0.2 μg/ml, respectively. He concludes that during increased small bowel activity a larger quantity of 5-HT is released into the circulation. Similar results were reported by BOJS (1961).

However, neither PAASONEN et al. (1960) nor BOJS could observe any increase in the urinary excretion of 5-HIAA after administration of cholinergic drugs or cathartics.

Concerning experiments *in vitro* it was found that the circular muscle of human ileum contracted in the presence of 5-HT in concentrations of 5 ng/ml upward, whereas the circular muscle of all regions of the colon relaxed in the presence of 5-HT (100 ng/ml upwards). The ascending colon appeared to be the least sensitive, and the change in response occurred sharply in the ileocaecal region (FISHLOCK and PARKS 1963, FISHLOCK 1964).

Dog. 5-HT, in intravenous doses as low as 4 μg/kg/min of the base, is a potent stimulus to jejunal motility in dogs in which an open end tube has been passed through a gastrostomy into the upper jejunum. The response is not modified by bilateral vagotomy. In all instances, increasing doses of 5-HT (4—32 μg/kg/min) evoke increasingly greater responses in jejunal motility. Tachyphylaxis develops during the continuous infusion of 5-HT irrespective of dose, and the increased motility elicited by a given dose usually ceases within 5 min. Within 10 min after cessation of the infusion, the bowel regains its former sensitivity. The action of 5-HT is not blocked by atropine (0.75 mg/kg, i.v.), hexamethonium (4 mg/kg, i.v.), mepyramine (5 mg/kg, i.v.) or reserpine (0.5 mg/kg). Compound 48/80 (0.5 mg/kg, i.v.) produces an inconstant inhibition of the 5-HT response; LSD (50 μg/kg, i.v.) potentiates it markedly and hinders the appearance of tachyphylaxis (HAVERBACK et al. 1957, HAVERBACK and WIRTSCHAFTLER 1962).

Given by injection into a terminal artery of the colon, 5-HT is as potent as acetylcholine in its contractile effect upon the intestinal musculature, the threshold dose varying from 0.001 to 1 μg. However, even with 1—10 μg doses the effect is short-lasting, not exceeding 30—90 sec. Atropine is 100 times more active towards acetylcholine than against 5-HT. The spasmogenic effect of 5-HT is enhanced by monoamine oxidase inhibitors and blocked by BAS and prochlorperazine. Hexamethonium is ineffective. SLEISENGER et al. (1958, 1959) suggest that 5-HT, although not directly acting via a cholinergic pathway, may be a modulator of the cholinergic system.

When 5-HT is applied (filter paper soaked with 0.1% solution of the amine) to the mucosal or serosal surface of a denervated dog's jejunal loop the intestinal motility is stimulated above and inhibited below the stimulated spot. This response is left unchanged by removal of the villi, but is abolished by cauterization of the basal part of the mucosa surrounding the crypts as well as by application of ganglion blocking agents. Evident tachyphylaxis occurs after repeated application of 5-HT. HUKUHARA et al. (1960) suggest, on the basis of the above results, that 5-HT acts upon the peripheral nerve endings distributed in the tunica propria surrounding the crypts.

The intestinal villi are stimulated in their rhythmic automatic activity both by intraarterial and intravenous injections of 5-HT (4—40 μg base), as well as by direct application of the drug to the exposed mucosa (4 μg/ml). Simultaneously there is an enhancement of the peristalsis of the intestinal muscle layer and a constriction of the capillaries. The effect lasts for about 10 min and is reversible. It is blocked by LSD (10 μg/kg, i.v.) and chlorpromazine (5 mg/kg, i.v.), but not by atropine. Tryptamine is 100 times less active (LUDÁNY et al. 1959).

Hypermotility of the intestinal tract occurring in dogs above an intestinal obstruction, and present also after hepatectomy or Eck fistula, was found by TYCE et al. (1961, 1964) to be accompanied by a marked increase (up to 500% !) of the 5-HT content in the pyloric mucosa, and by a slight increase in the duodenal mucosa. No changes were appreciable in the 5-HT content of jejunal or ileal mucosas, nor in the blood or brain 5-HT levels. Similarly, the urinary excretion of 5-HIAA was normal.

SIGEL et al. (1960) noted that urinary excretion of 5-HIAA in large dogs did not change in the first 4 hours after severe bowel ischemia, as produced by ligation of the arterial supply to the mesenteric small bowel followed by strangulation of the mid two feet of small intestine by a cord. However, analytical data are not in full accordance with the above statement.

Cat. The isolated small intestine responds to 5-HT with a prompt but transient tonus increase, the threshold dose being 10 μg/ml (ERSPAMER 1952a). Tryptamine and gramine, too, increase the tonus of this preparation (CHEN and CHEN 1933, SUPNIEWSKI and SERAFINOWNA 1938).

The cat bowel *in situ* seems to be more sensitive to 5-HT. In fact, an increase in intestinal motility may be produced by intraarterial administration of amounts of 5-HT as low as 1—2 μg/kg. The onset of the action begins 2—3 min after the injection and lasts 2—4 min (LEMBECK 1957).

Sheep. 5-HT stimulates in concentrations of 0.2—2 μg/ml isolated strips of sheep reticulum, abomasum and rumen, but is ineffective on omasum (SANFORD 1958).

Rabbit. The small intestine reacts to 5-HT (threshold concentration 0.01 to 0.1 μg/ml), as well as to bufotenine (0.01—0.1 μg/ml), bufotenidine (0.01 μg/ml) and tryptamine (2—10 μg/ml) with a short-lived tonus increase and with an increase in the amplitude of the pendulum movements. The reproducibility of the response is, however, unsatisfactory and so the preparation may be used only as a subsidiary test-object in the quantitative titration of the 5-hydroxyindolealkylamines (ERSPAMER 1946a, 1952a; SINHA and WEST 1953; POWELL 1955; UEDA et al. 1957).

The 5-HT stimulation of the rabbit intestine is not inhibited by sympatholytic drugs, nor by hexamethonium 10^{-4} or atropine 10^{-6}; higher concentrations of this alkaloid may, however, exert a partial antagonism (FINGL and GADDUM 1953, ROBERTSON 1953).

In contrast to the above indolealkylamines, gramine may produce moderate depressive effects (POWELL and CHEN 1945, POWELL 1955).

The rabbit rectum is less sensitive than the small intestine (ERSPAMER 1952a).

The rabbit intestine *in situ* shows a poor sensitivity to 5-HT. In fact, to obtain a clear stimulant action on the intestinal tone, intravenous doses as high as 0.2 mg/kg 5-HT base are required, the threshold dose being 10 μg/kg. Even at enormous dose levels (5 mg/kg, i.v.) tonus increase lasts less than one minute and tachyphylaxis appears with subsequent doses. The spasmogenic activity of 5-HT is abolished by banthine (5 mg/kg) and atropine (0.12 mg), but not by LSD (100 μg). GEORGES and HEROLD (1957, 1958) suggest that 5-HT acts on the rabbit intestinal smooth muscle both directly and indirectly, through central tvagal stimulation.

As in guinea-pigs, 5-HT in rabbits is also released from the intestinal wall into the lumen during peristalsis. However, the amount released by the caudal portion of the distal colon is barely 10% of that released by the small intestine (9.1 ng/min).

At partial variance with the guinea-pig, in the rabbit 5-HT, applied either outside or inside the intestine (1—10 μg/ml), stimulates propulsive activity after an initial contraction, although the stimulant effect is less rapidly obtainable if 5-HT is applied inside. Serosal application of 5-HT also facilitates the response to pelvic nerve stimulation (LEE 1960).

According to KÄRKI et al. (1960), when the intraluminal pressure and/or motility in a section of the ileum of anaesthetized splenectomized rabbits is elevated by intravenous injection of neostigmine or by direct introduction of air or paraffin into the intestinal lumen, the plasma 5-HT level of venous blood coming from this section shows a 2- to 4-fold increase for 10 min or longer. The interest of these results is obvious, but it seems that they should be accepted with caution, owing to the ambiguous significance of small changes in plasma 5-HT levels.

Guinea-pig. Very important work has been devoted to the study of the influence of 5-HT on intestinal motility in this species and results obtained in the guinea-pig constitute the basis for the theory which considers 5-HT to be a hormone participating in the physiological regulation of peristalsis.

The isolated small intestine of the guinea-pig responds to 5-HT, in dilutions down to 1 in 10^8—10^9, with a contraction resembling that produced by histamine. Even the most intense spasmogenic effects, however, e.g. those provoked by 2—4 μg/ml of 5-HT, are transitory and the smooth muscle becomes refractory to further doses of the substance (FREYBURGER et al. 1952, GADDUM 1953, GADDUM and PICARELLI 1957, GADDUM and HAMEED 1954). Guinea-pig ileum exposed to large doses of 5-HT not only becomes desensitized to subsequent doses of 5-HT, but its response to histamine, nicotine and to a lesser extent to acetylcholine is depressed (SZERB 1958). Gradual cooling of the bath temperature from 35° to 20—17° first abolishes the emptying phase of the peristaltic reflex, then progressively inhibits the longitudinal contraction due to intestinal distension and also the action of 5-HT (0.025—0.1 μg/ml) (INNES et al. 1957). While it is generally accepted that the spasmogenic action of 5-HT is diminished by atropine (0.01 to 1 μg/ml), there is no agreement about the degree of the antagonism (GADDUM 1953, RAPPORT and KOELLE 1953, ROCHA E SILVA et al. 1953). A partial explanation of the discrepancies existing in the literature is suggested by ROBERTSON (1953), who found that 0.01—0.1 μg/ml of atropine blocked the action of 2 ng of 5-HT, but not that of 20 ng of 5-HT.

HARRY (1963) has recently described a preparation of circular muscle from the guinea-pig isolated ileum which differs from the longitudinal muscle in that it is insensitive to drugs which act on autonomic effector tissues but, after inhibition of cholinesterase, it responds readily to choline esters, 5-HT, histamine and nicotine.

Before application of N,N-diisopropylphosphodiamidic fluoride (100 μg/ml) the strip does not respond even to 100 μg/ml 5-HT, but after 90 min exposure to the anticholinesterase drug it reacts readily to 0.5—4 μg/ml 5-HT.

The contraction of the strip is depressed, although less readily than the contraction by histamine or nicotine, by procaine, botulinum toxin, morphine and hemicholinium, as well as by atropine and hyoscine.

The point of attack of 5-HT in the guinea-pig ileum is controversial in spite of accurate studies on the interference, in 5-HT action, of procaine, cocaine. β-tubocurarine, hexamethonium, atropine, morphine, LSD, dibenzyline and other compounds as well. According to ROCHA E SILVA et al. (1953), 5-HT acts upon the post-ganglionic cholinergic fibres of the intramural nervous system; according to LÉVY and MICHEL-BER (1956), 5-HT stimulates both post-ganglionic cholinergic and post-ganglionic adrenergic fibres, without excluding the existence of particular receptors in the intramural ganglia; finally, according to GADDUM and HAMEED (1954) and GADDUM and PICARELLI (1957), there are two kinds of tryptamine receptors in the guinea-pig ileum, namely the M receptors which can be blocked with morphine and the D receptors which can be blocked with dibenzyline. Atropine, cocaine and methadone inhibit effects due to the M receptors even after dibenzyline, but have no additional effects after morphine; LSD, dihydroergotamine and 5-benzyloxygramine inhibit effects due to the D receptors, even after morphine, but have no additional effect after dibenzyline. The M receptors are probably in the nervous tissue and the D receptors are probably in the muscle.

In the case of the longitudinal muscle of the ileum, stimulation of receptors in nervous tissue, more precisely of specific receptors sited at the intramural parasympathetic ganglion cell, seems to be decidedly predominant (DAY and VANE 1963, BROWNLEE and JOHNSON 1963). Smooth muscle receptors are considered to be of negligible importance unless the neuronal mechanisms have been inactivated.

For the relative potency of other indolealkylamines on the isolated guinea-pig ileum see Table 4 of chapter 3.

In recent years the action of exogenous 5-HT and 5-HTP on intestinal motility has been thoroughly reinvestigated using accurate methods for recording the different phases of the peristaltic activity. Moreover, particular attention has also been paid to the influence of peristalsis on liberation of endogenous intestinal 5-HT.

The main results obtained by BÜLBRING and co-workers, LEMBECK, GINZEL and other research workers are as follows:

a) 5-HT (0.5—10 μg/ml) introduced into the bath in which an intestinal loop is suspended causes a transient muscle contraction followed by abolition of the peristaltic reflex (KOSTERLITZ and ROBINSON 1957, BÜLBRING and CREMA 1958, BÜLBRING and LIN 1958, LEMBECK 1958, GINZEL 1957a, 1957b). This predominant inhibitory effect is constant for the small intestine, whereas as a rule the colon ascendens shows increased propulsive work (LEMBECK 1958). Initial stimulation of peristalsis is rapid in onset but of shorter duration than that caused by mucosal application of 5-HT.

When the peristaltic reflex is blocked by introducing procaine into the lumen or by serosal application of 5-HT, morphine, dibenzyline or dihydroergotamine, serosal application of 5-HT has no effect; when the reflex is blocked by the presence in the bath of atropine or hexamethonium, serosal application of 5-HT restores peristalsis more effectively than mucosal application (BÜLBRING and CREMA 1958).

5-HT added in low concentration (0.005—0.02 μg/ml) to the fluid outside the intestine restores slight peristaltic activity after this activity has been abolished by cooling. If the peristalsis has been depressed but not abolished by cooling, 5-HT in the bath sometimes abolishes it (BELESLIN and VARAGIĆ 1958).

The transient or persistent facilitation of peristalsis produced by 5-HT applied to the serosal surface has been interpreted as being due to sensitization of the muscle to the transmitter substance acetylcholine (BÜLBRING and CREMA 1958) or to facilitation of transmission at synapses involved in the peristaltic reflex arc (BELESLIN and VARAGIĆ 1958); the inhibition of peristaltic reflex has been attributed to ganglionic block (BÜLBRING and CREMA 1958, LEMBECK 1958).

b) Introduction of 5-HT into the lumen of the isolated guinea-pig intestine stimulates peristalsis in concentrations from 10^{-9} to 10^{-5}. The threshold of the intraluminal pressure required to elicit peristaltic waves is lowered, the contractions are more frequent, and a larger volume of fluid is propelled (BÜLBRING and LIN 1957, 1958). LEMBECK (1958), for example, found that the frequency of peristaltic waves is increased by 90 and 200% after intraluminal infusion of 5-HT at a rate of 1.7 and 4.8 μg/min, respectively.

Stimulation of peristalsis can be observed in isolated strips of both ileum and colon. During irregular muscular activity of this last intestinal section, 5-HT applied intraluminally abolishes non-propulsive contractions and produces coordinate waves; however, higher concentrations of 5-HT cause an initial contraction and stimulation of peristalsis which is followed by depression (LEE 1960).

Mucosal application of 5-HT is highly effective in restoring the block of the peristaltic reflex produced by morphine, dibenzyline, procaine and 5-HT applied to the serosa, less effective in removing the block produced by atropine and hexamethonium and completely ineffective towards that caused by BOL and LSD (BÜLBRING and CREMA 1958).

c) When peristalsis is recorded from loops of *in situ* intestines with their normal blood supply, it can be seen that in the absence of spontaneous activity at low intraluminal pressure, intraarterial (0.1—0.2 μg), intravenous (4—10 μg) and intraluminal (100—200 μg) injections of 5-HT cause the appearance of short bursts of peristalsis (Fig. 9). Similarly, slow intraarterial infusion of 5-HT (0.2 to 1 μg/min) and 5-HTP (0.1 to 2.4 μg/min) causes vigorous peristalsis at pressure 10 mm below the normal threshold. However, tachyphylaxis occurs readily with all three routes of administration and large doses of 5-HTP always cause a diminution of fluid transport. Desensitization is more evident *in vivo* than *in vitro* (BÜLBRING and CREMA 1958b).

d) Small amounts of 5-HT (0.1—0.2 μg in 30 min) were found to be released into the fluid flowing through the lumen of an isolated or *in situ* loop of small intestine at an intraluminal pressure subthreshold for the initiation of peristaltic waves. When the intraluminal pressure is raised and the fluid is actively pushed out by peristalsis, the amount of 5-HT increases 2—8 times (BÜLBRING and LIN 1957, 1958). A further increase occurs in the presence of iproniazid, but the most striking increase (up to 2000 times the normal) is observed following intraluminal or intraarterial administration of 5-HTP. It should be emphasized that 5-HTP produces only a small increase in the mucosal 5-HT content (BÜLBRING and CREMA 1958b).

At a constant filling pressure the 5-HT release is very much greater during bursts of peristaltic activity than during the intervening periods of rest. When the augmentation of intraluminal pressure caused by muscle contraction is excluded by blocking the reflex with hexamethonium or by inverting the intestine, a residual 3-fold increase of 5-HT release is observed when the pressure is raised (BÜLBRING and CREMA 1958a). However, if the peristaltic contractions are abolished either by adrenaline or by asphyxiation of the muscular layer no 5-HT release occurs (LEE 1960).

The amount of 5-HT released into the lumen during peristalsis of the oral portion of the guinea-pig distal colon (6.3 ng/min) is of the same order of magnitude as in the small intestine (5.7—9.6 ng/min), whereas the amount released from the caudal portion is considerably smaller (1.6 ng/min). Sympathetic nerve stimulation reduces the amount of 5-HT on the average by only 30% whereas pelvic nerve stimulation causes no significant change (LEE 1960).

e) Peristalsis is abnormally active in reserpine-treated animals and occurs at low threshold. It declines gradually but does not stop in spite of extremely low mucosal 5-HT content (1 to 10% of the normal) and very small amounts of 5-HT being released. Peristalsis does not stop even when in these animals BOL is introduced into the lumen (BÜLBRING and CREMA 1959b).

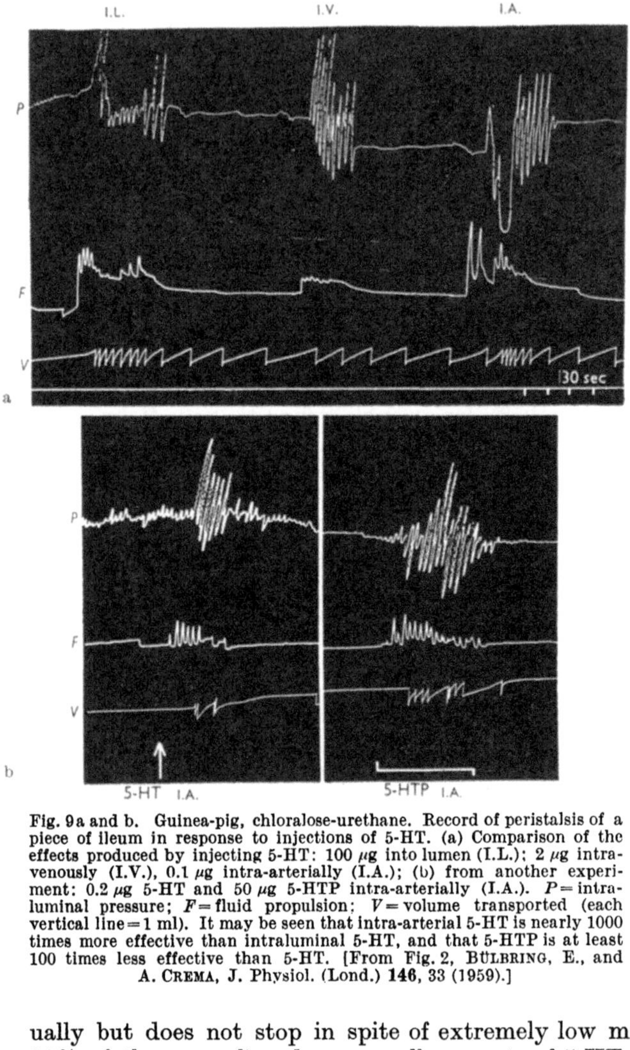

Fig. 9a and b. Guinea-pig, chloralose-urethane. Record of peristalsis of a piece of ileum in response to injections of 5-HT. (a) Comparison of the effects produced by injecting 5-HT: 100 μg into lumen (I.L.); 2 μg intravenously (I.V.), 0.1 μg intra-arterially (I.A.); (b) from another experiment: 0.2 μg 5-HT and 50 μg 5-HTP intra-arterially (I.A.). P = intraluminal pressure; F = fluid propulsion; V = volume transported (each vertical line = 1 ml). It may be seen that intra-arterial 5-HT is nearly 1000 times more effective than intraluminal 5-HT, and that 5-HTP is at least 100 times less effective than 5-HT. [From Fig. 2, BÜLBRING, E., and A. CREMA, J. Physiol. (Lond.) **146**, 33 (1959).]

According to BÜLBRING and LIN (1957, 1958) and to LEMBECK (1958), 5-HT stimulates intestinal motility mainly by sensitizing the sensory receptors in intestinal mucosa which are sensitive to pressure and trigger the peristaltic reflex. In addition, 5-HT might also stimulate chemoreceptors whose fibres converge on the same motor ganglion cells on which the fibres from pressure receptors impinge. The stimulation of both types of receptors would be additive and the reflex would thus be triggered off more readily.

However, on the basis of results listed under e), BÜLBRING and CREMA (1958b) themselves have recently advanced the opinion that 5-HT might not be of primary importance in initiating and maintaining peristalsis.

At this point it seems pertinent to recall that DOUGLAS and RITCHIE (1957) found that intravenous injection of 10—100 μg 5-HT causes in the cat firing of non-medullated afferent fibres in the cervical vagus which come from the gastro-intestinal tract. The effect is exerted at the endings of the fibres but it is not possible to establish whether these endings are excited directly by 5-HT, or indirectly as a consequence of some change in the gastrointestinal tract, such as muscular contraction.

Careful experiments have been carried out by BÜLBRING and BURNSTOCK (1960) on the membrane potential changes associated with tachyphylaxis produced in smooth muscle by application of 5-HT and other stimulant drugs for short periods in rapid succession. In the ganglion-free intestinal smooth muscle taken from the taenia coli of the guinea-pig, 5-HT (2×10^{-9}—1×10^{-6}), like acetylcholine and histamine, causes depolarization and, after removal of the drug, hyperpolarization, which is followed by a sequence of damped oscillation of the membrane potential. The average rate of depolarization is slowest with 5-HT and fastest with acetylcholine; the readiness with which tachyphylaxis occurs is, on the contrary, maximal with 5-HT. Increasing concentrations of 5-HT cause a progressively slower rate of depolarization and it is possible that 5-HT produces some more permanent alteration of the membrane properties than acetylcholine or histamine.

The taenia coli preparation is capable of taking up radioactive 5-HT from the bathing solution for about 120 min at both 0^0 and 37^0. But whereas the radioactivity is not concentrated at 0^0, at 37^0 its concentration is up to 5 times higher in the taenia than in the bathing fluid. Radioactivity taken up by the taenia is lost from it into the bathing fluid at two successive exponential rates, the half time of the first rate being ca. 4 min (5-HT in the extracellular space), and that of the second rate about 32 min (5-HT diffused into the smooth-muscle cell). According to BORN (1962), who made these observations, tachyphylaxis to 5-HT may be explained by the assumption that the continued presence of the amine in the tissue, on or near the receptors, brings about a reduction in its responsiveness.

Rat. The rat duodenum is a very sensitive test-object for 5-HT (0.001—0.01 μg/ml), bufotenine and bufotenidine, to which it responds, even when atropine is present, with a short-lived increase of tonus frequently accompanied by a reinforcement of spontaneous movements (ERSPAMER 1940b, 1946a, 1952a). The duodenal smooth muscle, however, seldom shows that reproducibility of response which is indispensable for an acceptable quantitative titration. Tachyphylaxis is particularly evident with bufotenine and bufotenidine (ERSPAMER 1946a). The stimulant action of 5-HT is strongly and irreversibly reduced by dibenamine. A clear inhibition is also produced by bufotenine (ERSPAMER 1946a, 1953a).

The rat colon has been used successfully by FELDBERG and TOH (1953) not only in the qualitative demonstration but also in the quantitative estimation of 5-HT in crude tissue extracts. Though the sensitivity of the preparation is somewhat variable, good responses are usually to be obtained with 0.01—0.02 μg of the substance per ml of nutrient liquid, and sometimes with considerably smaller doses, too. On the isolated rat ileum the *O*-sulphate of 5-HT is 100 times less active than 5-HT (YOSHIKO 1961).

Both 5-HT (10 mg/kg, s.c.) and 5-HTP (100 mg/kg, s.c.) first increase (by 15—20 times during the first 30 min) and then reduce the number and weight of faeces produced. 1 mg 5-HT or 10 mg/kg 5-HTP is just effective and 0.1 mg or 1 mg/kg is ineffective (ERSPAMER 1946a, BRITTAIN and COLLIER 1958).

Concerning gastrointestinal propulsion, as followed by the distribution of a dye or of charcoal given by mouth, results are at partial variance.

BRITTAIN and COLLIER observed that whereas 5-HTP failed, in subcutaneous doses up to 100 mg/kg, to influence significantly the distance travelled by a 5% suspension of charcoal in 10% gum acacia, 10 mg/kg 5-HT reduced this distance by 30—50%. This retardation probably occurred at the pyloric sphincter, since the effect disappeared if charcoal was allowed to enter the duodenum before 5-HT was given.

LISH et al. (1959) noted that both 5-HT (threshold subcutaneous dose 0.1 mg/kg; threshold oral dose 10 mg/kg) and 5-HTP (threshold subcutaneous dose 0.4 mg/kg) produced a definite inhibition of intestinal transit. Stomach emptying, however, was stimulated by 5-HT and inhibited by 5-HTP.

Like 5-HT, 5-methoxytryptamine produces defaecation in rats. Subcutaneous doses of 10 mg/kg are highly effective, doses of 1 mg/kg are ineffective (ERSPAMER 1946a).

Mouse. The mouse jejunum is stimulated by 5-HT in dilutions down to 10^{-8} (ERSPAMER 1946a).

As in rats, 5-HTP produces in mice a conspicuous increase in the number and weight of faeces (WOOLEY 1959). The ED 50 by the intraperitoneal route is 25 μg/mouse, the ED 100 300 μg/mouse. 4-HTP gives very inconstant and variable effects, the ED 50 being not less than 400 μg/mouse (ERSPAMER et al. 1960).

Chicken. The 5-HT content of the small intestine was estimated comparatively in conventional, contaminated and in germ-free white Leghorn chicks at four weeks of age. It was found that germ-free animals showing poor tonus of the intestinal tract and distension of the caeca had a higher 5-HT content in their gut, especially in the ileum (11 μg as compared to 6.1 μg/g), than conventional animals possessing elevated tonus of the intestinal musculature (PHILLIPS et al. 1961).

Many preparations of fowl rectal caecum are rather insensitive to 5-HT, but a concentration in the bath of 0.1 to 2 μg/ml often produces a biphasic contraction. A concentration of 5 μg/ml tryptamine causes a prolonged contraction with little or no tachyphylaxis (CLEUGH et al. 1961).

Tortoise. The isolated small intestine of the land tortoise (*Cyclemis amboinensis*) does not contract to 0.01—0.1 μg/ml of 5-HT, but is slightly stimulated by 1 μg/ml. The same concentrations of 5-HT inhibit the contractions of the intestine to acetylcholine. Atropinization abolishes the stimulant effect of 5-HT (TOH and MOHIUDDIN 1958).

Frog. The frog rectum (*Rana esculenta*) has been extensively used by VOGT (1954) in his researches on "Substanz DS", a principle which has been identified as 5-HT. The preparation seems to be highly sensitive to 5-HT (threshold concentration 0.01 μg/ml), to which it responds with the appearance of rhythmic movements and increase in tone. Atropine (1 μg/ml) and dibenamine do not influence the spasmogenic effect of 5-HT; dihydroergotamine 5×10^{-6} produces a reversible blockade.

Of the same sensitivity is the intestine of *Rana pipiens* (FÄNGE 1962).

The stomach of *Rana esculenta* is insensitive to bufotenine and bufotenidine in concentrations up to 10 μg/ml (ERSPAMER 1946a).

Fish. Fish afford another very impressive example of species difference in the sensitivity of the gut to 5-HT. In fact, whereas concentrations of 5-HT as low as

0.001—0.005 μg/ml are sufficient to stimulate the isolated intestine of *Pleuronectes platessa, Labrus bergylta* and *Salmo trutta*, concentrations 100—200 times higher are barely effective on the intestine of *Squalus acanthias, Raja batis, Myxine glutinosa* and *Tinca vulgaris* (EULER and ÖSTLUND 1957, BURNSTOCK 1958, VALETTE and AUGEREAU 1958).

Cyclostomata. The rectal part of the intestine of *Lampetra fluviatilis* shows strong rhythmic contractions in response to 100 μg/ml of 5-HT (JOHNELS and ÖSTLUND 1958).

Invertebrates. Peristalsis of the foregut of larvae of *Galleria melonella* is stimulated both by 5-HT and adrenaline (BEARD 1960).

The isolated stomach of *Helix pomatia* is potently contracted by 5-HT at exceptionally low concentrations (threshold 5×10^{-8} to 1×10^{-7} μg/ml). The response is not affected by atropine. LSD imitates the action of 5-HT (GRYGLEWSKI and SUPNIEWSKI 1963a). The *Helix* oesophagus is 10^5 times less sensitive than the stomach and the ileum 10^7 less sensitive (GRYGLEWSKI and SUPNIEWSKI 1963b).

The rectum of *Mercenaria mercenaria* is similarly stimulated by 5-HT, threshold being about 0.05 μg/ml. Small doses, usually below 1—2 μg/ml, often induce rhythmical activity; higher concentrations inhibit the beat while greatly increasing the tone. Tachyphylaxis occurs readily at high doses. Tryptamine is 10 to 100 times less effective than 5-HT. 5-HT appears to stimulate cholinergic nerves as well as directly exciting the rectal musculature. Its effects are mimicked by LSD and antagonized by UML (GREENBERG and JEGLA 1963).

The role of 5-HT in the physiological control of intestinal peristalsis. Since the main site of production and storage of 5-HT in the mammalian organism is the enterochromaffin cell of the gastrointestinal mucosa, and since 5-HT in several species has a powerful stimulating action on intestinal motility, it has been suggested that the chief physiological function of 5-HT, or at least one of its functions, is to control the motor activity of the gut. SMITH et al. (1957) and LEMBECK (1958) go even further, since they believe that the effects of 5-HT outside the gastrointestinal tract are always unphysiological, because they become apparent only after administration of exogenous 5-HT or following hyperproduction of 5-HT by malignant argentaffinomas.

The hypothesis of a local function of 5-HT within the gastrointestinal mucosa soon after its release from the enterochromaffin cells is at first sight very attractive, and it has been substantiated recently by the important results reported in detail in the preceding pages. On the basis of these results, BÜLBRING and LIN (1958), LEMBECK (1958) and HAVERBACK and WIRTSCHAFTLER (1962) maintain that the formation of 5-HT by the enterochromaffin cells could be part of the physiological mechanism required for peristalsis; more precisely, that 5-HT has a physiological modulating function in peristalsis.

The results and conclusions of BÜLBRING and co-workers are undoubtedly of great importance. However, once again extreme caution seems to be necessary in generalizing results obtained in one or two animal species or in transferring experimental data obtained on isolated intestines, or even on intestinal loops *in situ*, to the gastrointestinal tract of the intact animal. In fact, if we assume that the 5-HT which enhances the peristaltic reflex has a local origin, then it is rather difficult to give an acceptable explanation of the conspicuous differences in the distribution of the enterochromaffin cell system and of 5-HT along and outside the gastrointestinal tract of the various vertebrate species. What is the meaning of the enormous accumulation of enterochromaffin cells and 5-HT in the intramural portion of the pancreatic duct of the rabbit? What is the reason for the predominant accumulation of 5-HT in the stomachs of mice, hedgehogs and dogs, in the small intestines of guinea-pigs and chickens, and in the large intestines of rats, horses and cows? What, finally, is the significance of the enterochromaffin cells in the pancreatic islets of some mammals, and in the thymus of some birds? Moreover, if the 5-HT introduced into the lumen of an isolated guinea-pig intestine produces a stimulation of peristalsis in very low concentrations, the same 5-HT requires a decidedly larger dosage to produce short bursts of peristalsis when introduced into a loop of the guinea-pig intestine *in situ*, and requires a dosage far beyond any physiological limit to influence the motility of the intestine in the intact animal. In fact, the threshold oral dose capable of accelerating intestinal transit in rats is 4 mg/kg of the base, and doses of 5-HT or 5-HTP up to 10—15 mg given intrajejunally to normal volunteers fail to elicit any intestinal or systemic response.

Similarly, the stomach of the guinea-pig is, in sharp contrast to the ileum, very insensitive to 5-HT, as shown by the observation that 5-HT applied to the mucosal side of the stomach produces no effects with concentrations up to 100 μg/ml, and applied to the serosal side only sometimes does a concentration of 10 μg/ml elicit a slight contraction followed by a slight relaxation (PATON and VANE 1963).

This is not all. In fact, in man only the upper part of the small intestine seems to be stimulated by 5-HT, whereas stomach, ileum and large intestine are not affected by the amine, or are even inhibited. Yet all the sections of the gastrointestinal tract contain enterochromaffin cells and 5-HT and it is difficult to imagine how the same substance could carry out different functions in the different segments of a single apparatus.

Finally, nobody has so far brought any decisive evidence to demonstrate that distension or hypermotility of the intestines, kept within physiological limits, actually produces in the intact animal a local discharge of 5-HT from the enterochromaffin cells into the interstitial liquid of the mucosa, which evidently represents an essential condition for the stimulation of neuronal elements.

PATON and VANE (1963) did not succeed in controlling the factors governing the output of histamine and 5-HT in the stomach. They suggest that any procedure which changes the tone of the stomach, whether this is produced by transmural or vagal stimulation, by drugs or by mechanical distension may affect the amine output, possibly through the simple mechanical action of the smooth muscle in the stomach wall on the histamine- and 5-HT-containing cells in it.

It is evident that the above findings and considerations are not in favour of the hypothesis that 5-HT has a *general* significance as a *local* hormone modulating peristalsis.

Of course, 5-HT could also act on the gastrointestinal tract via the blood. But, frankly, it would be rather surprising if the 5-HT released from the intestines had to return to the same intestines, after having been exposed to severe enzymatic attacks and to large losses, to carry out there its main physiological action.

At any rate, if there are experimental results which demonstrate that stimulation of intestinal motility may be produced in some mammalian species by physiological amounts of 5-HT injected intravenously or intraarterially, there are other results which show that in other species parenteral 5-HT acts on peristalsis only at very high dosage levels, considerably exceeding those required to produce other biological effects, e.g. antidiuresis in rats.

Furthermore, there is as yet no proof that diurnal variations in the urinary excretion of 5-HIAA, indicative of variations in 5-HT release, may be correlated with gastrointestinal secretory or motor activity, nor that mechanical distension of the intestines or hyperperistalsis produced by drugs or toxic agents produces a discharge of 5-HT into the blood.

Whereas Peltola and Leppänen (1960) and Bettendorf et al. (1962) concordantly observed that as much as 50% of the daily amount of 5-HIAA is excreted during the night between 10 p.m. and 7 a.m., there are striking discrepancies concerning the period of maximum excretion of 5-HIAA during the day. The peak occurs in the 3-hour period on either side of noon according to Johnsen et al. (1958), between 1 and 4 p.m. according to Bettendorf et al. (1962), and finally between 5 and 9 p.m. according to Peltola and Leppänen (1960).

Bertaccini and Erspamer (1962) were unable to detect any increase in urinary 5-HIAA excretion in rats given by mouth 4 ml/100 g of paraffin oil, in spite of evident distension and hyperperistalsis of the intestine; Paasonen et al. (1960) found that cholinergic drugs and cathartics did not increase the urinary excretion of 5-HIAA in man; finally, several research workers (Haverback 1961, Kowlessar et al. 1958, Schmid et al. 1961) concordantly demonstrated that by chronic diarrhoea and cholitis ulcerosa urinary 5-HIAA was within normal limits.

The obvious conclusion is that before the hypothesis of a *general* significance of 5-HT in controlling intestinal motility can be accepted, additional positive experimental evidence is required, obtained, if possible, in representatives of all vertebrate classes, because all vertebrates contain enterochromaffin cells and 5-HT in their gastrointestinal mucosa.

2. Extrahepatic biliary tract

5-HT does not display, in concentrations up to 1 mg/ml, any effect on the isolated guinea-pig biliary bladder nor, *in vivo*, on the human biliary tract, as explored radiographically (2 mg 5-HT base, i.v.). The volume of the rabbit gall-bladder, on the contrary, is reduced by the i.v. administration of 0.4 mg/kg 5-HT base (Giro et al. 1960).

Given intravenously, in doses of 20—40 μg/kg, 5-HT causes a short-lasting but complete interruption of the flow through the cat sphincter of Oddi perfused from the choledocus, leaving unaffected the gall bladder (Granser et al. 1956).

On the calf isolated Oddi's sphincter 5-HT displays a strong contractile action in doses as low as 0.01—1 μg/ml. There is an increased tone of the longitudinal fibres and a block of the flow through the sphincter (Crema et al. 1962).

3. Bronchial smooth muscle

Guinea-pig. To Herxheimer (1953a, 1953b, 1955, 1957) belongs the credit for having carried out the first and most complete study on the bronchial actions of 5-HT administered by inhalation in guinea-pigs.

Guinea-pigs exposed to a 1% aerosol of 5-HT develop severe dispnoea, followed by convulsions. The shock syndrome resembles that produced by histamine, acetylcholine and anaphylaxis, but the animal does not usually die. If the guinea-pigs are exposed to 5-HT at intervals ranging from several hours to two days, they become tolerant to it after three to four exposures.

When guinea-pigs actively sensitized to egg albumin are desensitized by repeated exposure to the antigen, their tolerance to 5-HT increases. When they are resensitized, their tolerance to 5-HT falls to the previous value. Conversely, if guinea-pigs are made tolerant to 5-HT, they become less sensitive to egg albumin. When they lose their tolerance to 5-HT, their previous sensitivity to egg albumin returns.

Nicotine sulphate aerosol elicits a shock syndrome similar to that caused by 5-HT. Again, tolerance develops after repeated exposure and, at the same time, desensitization to anaphylaxis develops, as with 5-HT. Conversely, desensitization to anaphylaxis also causes tolerance to nicotine.

The mechanism responsible for the development of mutual tolerance must therefore be regarded as non-specific and it may be concluded that if there exists some relationship between the mechanism of 5-HT shock and anaphylactic shock, the same relationship exists between nicotine shock and anaphylactic shock.

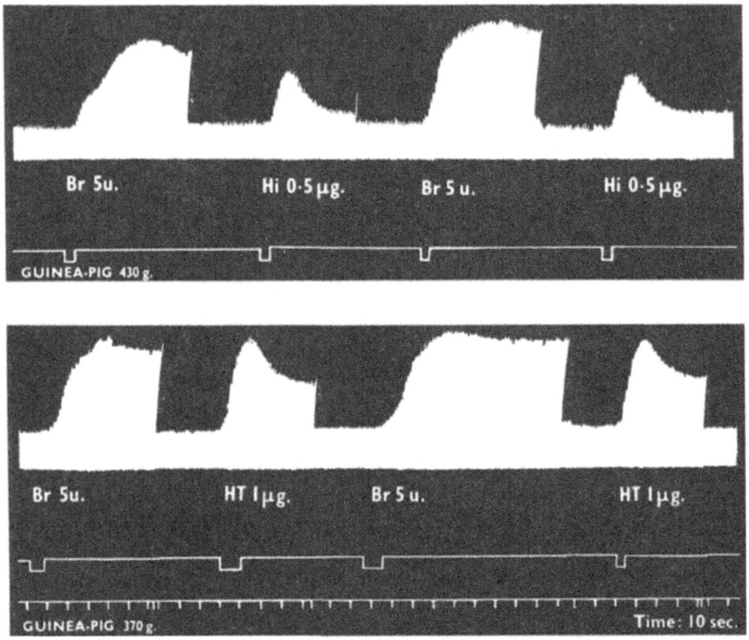

Fig. 10. Resistance to inflation of guinea-pig lungs *in vivo*. Increased resistance caused by bradykinin (Br), histamine (Hi), and 5-hydroxytryptamine (HT). Doses were administered intravenously at 10 min intervals. It may be noted that 5-HT is approximately as active as histamine, and that the response to bradykinin is more sustained than that to either 5-HT or histamine. [From Fig. 1, Collier, H. O. J. et al., Brit. J. Pharmacol. 15, 291 (1960).]

0.16 mg/kg atropine or 5 µg/kg LSD affords weak and inconstant protection against 5-HT; 0.65—1.3 mg atropine and 50—200 µg LSD a 60—75% protection; 400 µg LSD complete or nearly complete protection. Mepyramine, 1 mg/kg, has no effect.

The above results were generally confirmed. Frahm (1957) found that with aerosols containing 0.5—0.7% 5-HT initial hyperpnoea turned into definite asthmatic attacks only in 30—40% of the animals and that, despite continuous administration of the aerosol, these attacks resolved spontaneously. Atropine (300 µg/kg) and isopropylnoradrenaline (0.2—1% aerosol) displayed a more or less intense protective effect against 5-HT attacks, nembutal and local anaesthetics (pantocaine aerosol) aggravated them.

Tuberculous guinea-pigs tolerate 5-HT inhalations better than healthy animals and bronchial spasm is delayed from 2 to 15 min and more (Földes et al. 1959). Similarly, the average preconvulsion time is prolonged from 1 to 3 min in splenectomized animals (Sanyal and West 1959).

It is of interest that parenterally administered 5-HT is capable of affording complete protection against 5-HT bronchospasm, but not against bronchospasm produced by histamine or acetylcholine. This paradoxical auto-antagonistic action seems to be unique (COURVOISIER and LEAU 1959).

Bronchoconstriction can easily be elicited also upon intravenous injection of 5-HT (KONZETT 1956, MEIER et al. 1956, BALZER et al. 1956, JÄNKÄLÄ and VIRTAMA 1961).

In producing resistance to inflation of guinea-pig lungs *in vivo*, 5-HT is as potent as histamine. The response to bradykinin differs slightly in its slower onset and longer persistence at or near peak level (COLLIER et al. 1960) (Fig. 10).

Reduction of spontaneous respiration, increase of endotracheal pressure and decrease of tidal air are produced by doses of 5-HT as low as 2—10 μg/kg 5-HT base. Bronchial spasm is inhibited by lysergic acid derivatives (LSD, BOL, l-acetyl-LSD) adrenaline, regitine and dihydroergotamine, whereas section of the vagi, atropine and antihistaminic drugs yield inconstant or no effect (BALZER et al. 1956, KONZETT 1956).

A moderate protective action is also shown by heparin and related anti-coagulant drugs administered by 5% aerosols (SCHMID et al. 1959).

The isolated guinea-pig lung behaves like the *in situ* lung. Here again the bronchoconstrictor action of 5-HT (10—40 μg) is strongly antagonized by UML, LSD (0.25—4 μg), adrenaline and isopropylnoradrenaline (5 μg) and moderately so by dihydroergotamine (25 μg), dibenamine and regitine. Atropine, even at 0.5 mg doses, BAB and BAS are feeble antagonists and antihistamines show no action whatsoever (BHATTACHARYA 1955, SICUTERI et al. 1960, STORMORKEN 1959). Chlorpromazine is effective when given prior to the administration of 5-HT, but only weakly active in reversing 5-HT bronchoconstriction (KING 1957).

When perfused through a cannula in the pulmonary artery, the broncho-constrictor action of 5-HT (0.2—0.4 μg) is 2 times as intense as that of histamine (GREEFF and MOGG 1964).

Whereas the isolated intact trachea of the guinea-pig gives a contractile response to very low concentrations of 5-HT, the threshold being 0.05 μg/ml (JAMIESON 1962), the isolated tracheal chain is contracted only by large doses of the amine (SINHA and WEST 1953, BALZER et al. 1956). Surprisingly enough, the medium-sized bronchioles respond to the amine (threshold 0.4 μg/ml) with relaxation (BROCKLEHURST 1957).

Man. In normal human subjects inhalation of a 0.7% aerosol of 5-HT does not modify the vital capacity of the lung nor the respiratory rate. However, in asthmatic patients the same inhalation produces a prompt fall in vital capacity and decrease in respiratory flow rate sometimes resulting in a severe attack of bronchospasm, which regresses spontaneously or is abolished by isopropyl-noradrenaline (HERXHEIMER 1953b, MICHELSON et al. 1958).

Other mammalian species. REID and RAND (1952b) and COMROE et al. (1953) showed that intravenous 5-HT provokes a moderate bronchoconstrictor action in the cat. This has been confirmed by KONZETT (1956) in intact and spinal cats. In intact anaesthetized cats the reduction of tidal air due to 5-HT (threshold dose 3—35 μg/kg, i.v.) is usually identical before and after vagotomy, as well as before and after section of the spinal cord at C_1, suggesting mainly a direct action on the bronchi, and not a reflex effect. LSD, BOL and acetyl-LSD specifically antagonize the effect of 5-HT on tidal air; atropine and anti-histamines are incomplete and non-specific antagonists.

The spasmogenic action of 5-HT on the bronchial musculature of the dog has not been studied in detail, but it does not seem to be conspicuous (BALZER et al. 1956, NOBLE and NANSON 1959).

In the isolated rat lung perfused through the pulmonary artery 5-HT displays a very moderate bronchoconstrictor effect. In fact, with 100 μg 5-HT respiratory amplitude is reduced only by 23% (GREEFF and MOOG 1964).

As in the guinea-pig, so in all other examined species, 5-HT causes a relaxation of the medium-sized bronchioles. The most sensitive bronchioles are those of rats and cats (0.01 μg/ml), followed by those of dogs (0.05 μg/ml). The bronchioles of rabbits, monkeys and man are practically insensitive (5—20 μg/ml) (BROCKLEHURST 1957).

In sharp contrast to the above relaxing effect, 5-HT appears to be a potent contractile agent on the isolated intact trachea of the rat. The amine is almost as active as acetylcholine and some 100,000 times more potent than histamine (JAMIESON 1962).

Frog. 5-HT was found to cause a relaxation of the smooth muscle of the frog lung at extremely low concentrations (10^{-5} μg/ml), and within the region of low concentrations the amplitude of relaxation was nearly proportional to the logarithm of the concentration. Catecholamines were approximately 1000 times less potent. Atropine, morphine, cocaine, LSD, dibenzyline and iproniazid did not show any anti-5-HT action and the only certain antagonist of 5-HT appeared to be acetylcholine which caused contraction of the lung smooth muscle. BRECHT and JESCHKE (1960, 1962) suggest that 5-HT may display on the frog lung the function of "adjusting substance" or inhibitory neurohormone.

4. Uterus

Rat. The isolated diestrous uterus is barely sensitive to 5-HT and related indolealkylamines and shows marked tachyphylaxis. The estrous uterus and, less regularly, the uterus removed in advanced pregnancy or immediately after delivery is, on the contrary, highly sensitive. The introduction into the bath of as little as 2 to 10 ng of 5-HT per ml of nutrient liquid is enough to produce a noticeable response, i.e. appearance or reinforcement of movements. Higher doses not only cause increased motility, but also provoke a tonus increase, which is, within ample limits, proportional to the dose (Figs. 11, and 1 of chapter 1). On washing out with fresh nutrient solution, relaxation is immediate and the original reactivity of the preparation is promptly restored (ERSPAMER 1940b, 1940c, 1954c, 1956; GADDUM and HAMEED 1954).

Table 3 of chapter 1 shows the activity of a number of indolealkylamines, as compared to that of 5-HT. It is interesting to note that even 5-HTP possesses a very small stimulant action on the uterus, which, however, is at least 10,000 times smaller than that displayed by 5-HT. Since incubation of the isolated uterus with α-methyldopa (a potent dopadecarboxylase inhibitor) completely inhibits the oxytocic action of 5-HTP, this activity must be ascribed to the minute amounts of 5-HT formed by decarboxylation in uterine tissue (LOVAŠEN et al. 1961).

Owing to its high sensitivity to 5-HT, the conspicuous specificity of its response to the substance, and the easy reproducibility of this response, the estrous uterus of the rat has become one of the most often used preparations in the quantitative and qualitative assay of 5-HT, and in the study of substances antagonistic to 5-HT. For further details turn to pages 115—117.

When non-pregnant rats, either normal or pretreated with estrogens, gonadotropic hormones or estrogens + progesterone, are given intramuscularly 6—9 mg/kg of 5-HT base, no gross morphological alterations are visible in the uteri (CATALDI 1956b).

1.6 to 6.4 mg/kg 5-HT injected i.m., in 4 divided doses at 2-hr intervals, in pregnant rats at various stages of pregnancy fail to interrupt pregnancy and do not produce appreciable alterations of the uterus or the placenta. Interruption of pregnancy, on the other hand, is observed following larger doses of the amine (14—17 mg/kg given i.m. in divided doses over a period of 2 hours, or 3—5 mg/kg given by single intravenous injection). Generally foetal death, which is caused by vasoconstriction and severe placental haemorrhage, is not followed by premature delivery (CORRELL et al. 1952, CATALDI 1956a, MAROIS 1960, CRAIG 1962).

Subcutaneous administration of 1.2—4 mg/kg 5-HT base daily for 4 days to 25-day-old rats, together with 0.1 μg estradiol in 0.1 ml of sesame oil enhances the effect of estradiol, as demonstrated by increase in uterine wet weight and percent uterine water (ZILBERSTEIN 1962).

0.1—0.25 mg 5-HT given to rats by intrauterine administration produces acute vasodilatation, hyperaemia and increase in capillary permeability, with consequent rise of uterine water concentration from 78.6 to 83—84%. In producing

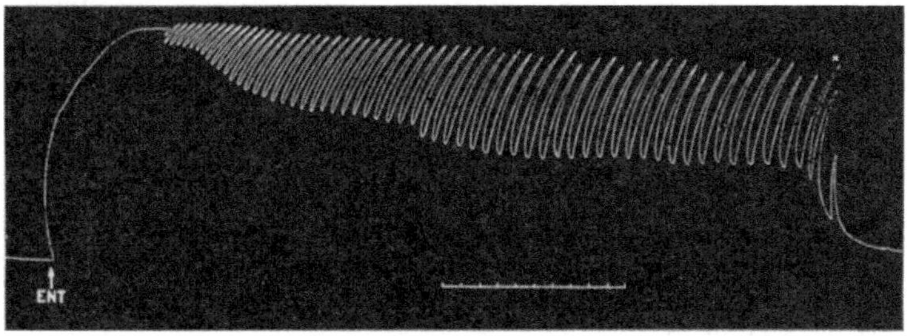

Fig. 11. Isolated oestrus-uterus of a rat. suspended in a 10 ml bath of Tyrode solution at 30°. Time in min. 40 μg of 5-HT base produced a tremendous tonus increase accompanied, after a few minutes, by lively rhythmic movements. The sustained response was immediately interrupted by washing with fresh nutrient liquid (x). [From Fig. 19, ERSPAMER, V., R. C. sci. Farmitalia **1**, 65 (1954).]

the above effects 5-HT is approximately 17 times as effective as histamine. However, 5-HT has less intense an influence on epithelial mitoses. According to SZEGO and SLOAN (1961) it is possible that 5-HT acts through histamine release, thus augmenting the action of estrogen.

Mouse. The isolated mouse uterus behaves in a manner exactly similar to that of the rat (ERSPAMER 1952a).

When administered subcutaneously at high dose levels (1 mg/mouse/day divided into two injections) 5-HT interrupts pregnancy both in its early and its later stages. Only a limited number of mice become pregnant (prevention of implantation?), and pregnancy is discontinued in all mice given 5-HT during the 11th to 16th day of pregnancy. At this time a single subcutaneous dose of 1 mg 5-HT is sufficient to produce death of the foetuses within half an hour. At autopsy death of foetuses is found to be caused by contraction of the blood vessels supplying the placenta with ensuing haemorrhage and disorganization of the placenta (POULSON et al. 1960a, 1960b; ROBSON and SULLIVAN 1963).

The effect of 5-HT in early pregnancy can be antagonized by progesterone and prolactin, as can the toxic effects of the drug on experimental decidual reaction. In late pregnancy progesterone produces little, and prolactin no reversal of the toxic action of 5-HT. It is suggested that in early pregnancy 5-HT interferes with the hormonal mechanisms responsible for the maintenance of gestation, while later on its main toxic action is exerted directly onto the uterine contents (LINDSAY et al. 1963).

Pretreatment (30 min) of the females with D-lysergic acid derivatives preserves the life of the young, the ED 50 for LSD being of 30 μg/kg and that for UML of only 3.7 μg/kg (FLÜCKIGER and SALZMANN 1961, POULSON and ROBSON 1963).

Smaller doses of 5-HT (0.05—0.25 mg/mouse, s.c. or i.v.) have no effect whatever on pregnancy (SAVI 1956, POULSON et al. 1960b).

Rabbit and guinea-pig. The non-pregnant isolated uteri of these animals respond only to large doses of 5-HT, with contractions which are irregular both in appearance and amplitude. On washing out, relaxation is slow (FREYBURGER et al. 1952, REID and RAND 1952). The stimulant action possessed by bufotenine, bufotenidine, tryptamine and gramine is still weaker. Threshold concentrations on the rabbit uterus are 2×10^{-5} to 5×10^{-6} for 5-HT, 1×10^{-5} to 2×10^{-6} for bufotenine, 1×10^{-5} for bufotenidine, and 1×10^{-4} to 1×10^{-5} for tryptamine and gramine (POWELL and CHEN 1945, ERSPAMER 1946, POWELL 1955); on the guinea-pig uterus 1×10^{-6} for 5-HT, 1×10^{-5} to 3×10^{-6} for bufotenine, 1×10^{-5} to 1×10^{-7} for bufotenidine, and 5×10^{-5} to 1×10^{-5} for gramine and tryptamine (POWELL and CHEN 1945, ERSPAMER 1946, POWELL 1955, UEDA et al. 1957).

Tryptamine shows on the rabbit uterus preparation a specific adrenolytic effect which is some 50 times weaker than that possessed by ergotamine. 5-HT and N,N-diethyltryptamine are even more potent, but their adrenolytic action does not seem to be specific (GLAZ et al. 1956).

A daily subcutaneous dose of 2—2.5 mg/kg 5-HT causes foetal death in rabbits, as in mice and rats, when given in late pregnancy (25th to 30th day), but has no effect on implantation and early foetal development. In late pregnancy, foetal death also occurs when 5-HT is administered by intravenous infusion (10 mg over 45 min), and large haemorrhagic areas become visible in the placenta (POULSON et al. 1960a).

It seems probable that the interruption of pregnancy seen in rats, mice and rabbits following large doses of 5-HT is due to a direct action of the amine on the placental vessels which are known to be particularly sensitive to the drug.

Cat. According to REID and RAND (1952) the *in situ* uterus of the non-gravid, adrenalectomized cat relaxes on intravenous injection of 24 μg of 5-HT or on the introduction of 9 μg of the substance into the low thoracic aorta. Tryptamine, too, relaxes the cat uterus *in situ* (LAIDLAW 1912).

The isolated cat uterus is contracted by 5-HT, tryptamine and gramine, but relaxed by bufotenine (POWELL 1955).

Dog. The *in situ* uterus of both conscious animals and of animals anaesthetized with chloralose responds to an intravenous injection of as little as 1 μg/kg 5-HT with a contraction, followed by a period of inhibition lasting up to 7 min. The action appears to be wholly peripheral (ABRAHAMS and PICKFORD 1956c).

Hamster. The isolated uterus is stimulated by large doses of gramine (POWELL and CHEN 1945).

Man. 5-HT seems to be poorly active both on the isolated and the *in situ* human uterus. Concentrations of 10 μg/ml 5-HT cause an increase in amplitude with a reduction in frequency of contractions; 100 μg/ml produces a frank stimulation of excised human myometrium.

By intravenous infusion 5-HT has no definite effect on uterine activity in pregnancy or labour when given at a rate of 100—300 μg/min for 1 to 14 min, but often produces transitory stimulation when infused at higher dose levels.

It is concluded that 5-HT holds little place in the physiology of human myometrial contraction (GARRETT 1958) and that the use of the substance as an oxytocic agent is highly questionable (VALSECCHI 1959).

Dogfish. Isolated uterine horns of the spiny dogfish which do not show spontaneous contractions respond upon addition of 0.2—1.6 μg/ml 5-HT base with powerful contractions often followed by smaller periodically occurring movements. A similar response is elicited by the clasper-siphon secretion of the fish, which is an extremely rich source of 5-HT. It is suggested that by eliciting uterine contractions, the clasper-siphon secretion may well play a physiological role during copulation, perhaps by facilitating sperm ascent to the site of fertilization (MANN and PROSSER 1963).

5. Urinary bladder

Dog. The isolated dog urinary bladder responds to 5-HT and related indolealkylamines with a tonus increase which is roughly proportional to the dose. At the beginning the sensitivity is 1 to 3 in 10^5, then it declines (ERSPAMER 1952a) (Fig. 1).

The *in situ* bladder of the anaesthetized dog reacts to intravenous 5-HT with an increase of tonus and with the appearance or reinforcement of rhythmic motility. The minimum active dose of 5-HT is 1 to 4 μg/kg. The stimulant action of 4-HT is approximately half as intense as that of 5-HT, but is more sustained. The percentage activity of other indolealkylamines, in comparison with 5-HT, is as follows: 5-methoxytryptamine 30—35; bufotenine 5—10; tryptamine 1.5; 1-methyltryptamine 1—1.5; N-methyltryptamine and N,N-dimethyltryptamine <0.5. Bufothionine, dehydrobufotenine and, possibly, bufotenidine are inactive (ERSPAMER 1952a, 1952d; ERSPAMER et al. 1960). Another indolealkylamine mimicking 5-HT already at low microgram levels is 5-acetyltryptamine (OSBORNE et al. 1962). Even 5-HTP and 4-HTP produce a remarkable contraction of the bladder, which is evidently caused by the amines originating from the decarboxylation of the precursor aminoacids. The contraction produced by 2—4 mg/kg of intravenous 4-HTP is 3 to 4 times more intense and considerably more sustained than that caused by the same dose of 5-HTP (ERSPAMER et al. 1960).

When 5-HT is injected into the abdominal aorta it produces a biphasic response: at first a transient, twitch-like reaction, then a second contraction of longer duration. Moreover, it enhances the action of various stimuli, such as pelvic nerve stimulation, methacoline, acetylcholine and KCl. 5-HT is 20 times more potent than acetylcholine, but 5 times less potent than muscarine.

The bladder contraction caused by 5-HT is highly resistant to atropine and hexamethonium, but is more or less completely blocked by dibenamine, 2-methyl-5-chlorogramine, chlorpromazine, BOL, LSD, imipramine and papaverine (ERSPAMER 1952a, 1952e, 1953a, 1954; GYERMEK 1962a, 1962b).

GYERMEK (1962b) suggests, on the basis of the above findings, that normal, physiological fluctuations of the 5-HT level in the organism may markedly influence the sensitivity of the bladder.

It does not seem conceivable that released 5-HT plays an important role in the urinary bladder tension produced by the intravenous injection of 0.5—1 mg/kg of reserpine (MAXWELL et al. 1956).

Given by subcutaneous route to the anaesthetized dog, 5-HT is practically devoid of any stimulant action, up to doses of 1 mg/kg. Intravenous doses of 5-HT greater than 50 μg/kg and subcutaneous doses greater than 200—400 μg/kg regularly provoke micturition and resistance to vesical catheterization in the intact conscious dog (ERSPAMER 1952a, 1954c).

Other animals. The rat urinary bladder and, still more, that of the guinea-pig are insensitive to 5-HT (ERSPAMER 1952a). The same may be said of the rabbit urinary bladder, in contact with bufotenine or bufotenidine (ERSPAMER 1946a). The cat bladder is weakly stimulated by tryptamine (LAIDLAW 1912).

6. Ureter

The perfused *in situ* dog ureter, with blood supply intact, responds to intravenous 5-HT (threshold dose 3—4 µg/kg) with a contraction which completely prevents the passage of fluid through its lumen for 1 to 2 min and slows the flow for a further period of 1 to 2 min (ABRAHAMS and PICKFORD 1956b).

The isolated dog ureter, on the other hand, does not react to 5-HT, even at concentrations up to 4—30 µg/ml (BORGSTEDT 1959, SPIRITO and TEODORO 1959).

7. Seminal vesicles

When added to the nutritive bath, 5-HT contracts the seminal vesicles of castrated rats but is practically inactive on the same organs excised from normal animals. However, 5-HT (1—10 µg/ml) added to the nutrient bath 30—60 seconds prior to adrenaline or noradrenaline (0.05—4 µg/ml) increases by 2—2.5 times the stimulant action of the catecholamines even on the seminal vesicles taken from normal rats. Synergism is not due to antioxidant action of 5-HT nor to inhibition of monoamineoxidase. It is possible that it depends on inhibition of catechol-O-methyl transferase. Low concentrations of tryptamine (20 µg/ml) do not affect the response to adrenaline, higher concentrations (200 µg/ml) diminish it (PICARELLI et al. 1962).

8. Spleen

5-HT (100 µg/ml) produces a contraction of isolated strips of cat spleen. Since the sensitivity to 5-HT of spleen strips from cats treated 24 hr earlier with reserpine is only one-fiftieth of that of normal strips, and the effects of tyramine on spleen strips almost exactly parallel the effects of 5-HT, it is suggested by INNES (1962b) that 5-HT has a dual action, viz. a major action due to release of stored noradrenaline and a minor direct action on adrenaline receptors.

9. Nictitating membrane

5-HT and related indolealkylamines contract both the *in situ* and the isolated nictitating membrane of the cat. This was first observed by REID and RAND (1952) and by ERSPAMER (1952a).

The retraction produced by 5-HT is 3 to 25 times smaller but more prolonged than that caused by adrenaline or noradrenaline (ERSPAMER 1954, LECOMTE 1955, TRENDELENBURG 1956, SCHAEPPI 1962, 1963). The denervated membrane is more sensitive than the innervated membrane (REID and RAND 1952). According to COSTA and ZETLER (1958, 1959) the threshold intravenous doses causing the normal and denervated membrane to contract are 14.4 and 1.69 µg/kg for 5-HT, and 30.8 and 4.27 µg/kg for bufotenine. However, large amounts of 5-HT (100 to 300 µg) cause a greater contraction of the normal membrane. This does not apply to the perfused cat head preparation, in which 5-HT in all doses causes a larger response on the denervated than on the normal side (TRENDELENBURG 1956). The chronically denervated membrane is 50 times more sensitive to 5-HT than the acutely denervated membrane (SCHAEPPI 1962, 1963).

Cocaine and other local anaesthetics moderately enhance the response to 5-HT, but, in every instance, less than that to catecholamines (ERSPAMER 1954, GYERMEK and POSSEMATO 1961); imipramine, on the contrary, potentiates the effect of 5-HT more markedly than that of catecholamines. Following administration of 0.15—2.4 mg/kg imipramine the membrane becomes 3 to 7 times more sensitive than before (SOFFER and GYERMEK 1961, GYERMEK and POSSEMATO 1961, SIGG et al. 1963).

Previous administration of 5-HT or bufotenine potentiates the retraction produced by subsequent injection of adrenaline and noradrenaline (LECOMTE 1953, 1955). The minimum intravenous dose potentiating the response of normal nictitating membrane to intravenous adrenaline is 88 μg/kg for 5-HT and 4.8 μg for bufotenine. For the denervated membrane the values are 23.9 and 6.6 μg/kg, respectively (COSTA and ZETLER 1958, 1959). The effect is generally ascribed to an inhibition of the enzymic inactivation of catecholamines. However, small doses of 5-HT (10—25 μg/kg) are found to decrease rather than to potentiate the action of catecholamines (SCHMITT and SCHMITT 1959). Besides that of adrenaline, intravenous 5-HT (10—200 μg/kg) increases the effect on the nictitating membrane of pre- or postganglionic stimulation of adrenergic nerves (BACQ and RENSON 1961).

On the innervated membrane 5-HT is consistently more potent than N-methyltryptamine or N,N-dimethyltryptamine, some 5 times more potent than tryptamine, and 2—5 times more potent than 4-HT. Bufotenidine, on the contrary, is more active than 5-HT (RAND and REID 1952, REID and RAND 1952, ERSPAMER 1954c, LECOMTE 1955, ERSPAMER et al. 1960, SCHAEPPI 1963). The tryptamine contraction is potentiated by cocaine and diphenhydramine, but depressed by yohimbine (REID and RAND 1952). Small doses of tryptamine (10—30 μg) appear to be slightly more effective on the chronically than on the acutely denervated membrane, whereas large doses (100—300 μg) retract both membranes equally (SCHAEPPI 1962). Single intravenous doses of 2—5 mg/kg 5-HTP do not contract the membrane; the same doses of 4-HTP produce a contraction lasting 30 to 50 min (ERSPAMER et al. 1960).

The isolated membrane brought into contraction by 5-HT (threshold dose (0.05—0.1 μg/ml) relaxes only slowly after washing out the drug and tachyphylaxis appears following successive administration of the same amount of 5-HT. It is not possible to obtain maximum contraction of the muscle even with large doses of 5-HT. Contractions are potentiated by cocaine and antagonized by atropine, dibenamine, dibenzyline, hyoscine, dihydroergotamine and LSD (THOMPSON 1958).

10. Iris smooth muscle

Isolated iris. D'ERMO and BONOMI (1961) first demonstrated that the isolated constrictor pupillae of the horse eye possessed very high sensitivity to 5-HT, the threshold concentration varying between 0.001 and 0.1 μg/ml. The response, which showed a good relationship with the dose, was not affected by atropine or mepyramine, up to 10^{-4}, but was partially inhibited by promethazine.

These results have been confirmed and extended by KOELLA and SCHAEPPI (1962) who thoroughly investigated the reaction to 5-HT of the isolated cat iris. The reaction of the pupillary opening on the intact iris was recorded by means of a photoelectric technique. The reaction of the isolated muscles was measured by means of isometric mechanoelectric transducers. 5-HT acted on the isolated iris as a powerful constrictor. The threshold dose appeared to be 0.15 μg 5-HT base. Doses as small as 2.5 and 5 μg often induced complete or almost complete closure of the pupil. Two-peaked pattern occurred often with larger doses. The pupillary constriction and ensuing dilation lasted up to 15 or more min. 5-HT treatment desensitized the preparation to later injections of 5-HT.

The isolated constrictor pupillae reacted to 5-HT with contraction. Threshold was less than 1 ng/ml, and maximal degree of contraction was obtained with 0.03—0.5 μg/ml. Repeated application of the same dose did not reveal desensitization. The isolated dilator pupillae reacted to 5-HT usually with dilatation (threshold 0.3 ng/ml), followed with larger doses by a prolonged slight contraction. It is suggested, from the above data, that pupillary constriction in response to 5-HT is the result of a dual mechanism, namely contraction of the constrictor muscle and relaxation of the radial dilator muscle, and that the basis for the constrictive effects of 5-HT is a direct action of the drug on the smooth muscle.

In contrast to the isolated cat iris, where 5-HT imitates the action of acetylcholine, the isolated pig iris responds to 5-HT doses as small as 0.025 μg with a decrease of the tone and a reduction of the amplitude of contractions produced by electrical stimulation (SCHAEPPI 1963).

In situ iris. Intravenous (100—500 μg/kg) or intracarotid (0.5—5 μg/kg) injection of 5-HT provokes in the anaesthetized cat a conspicuous constriction of the pupil, sometimes preceded by a transient dilatation. The action appears also in the decerebrated animal with sectioned oculomotor nerves and cervical sympathetic fibres (RAND and REID 1952, REID and RAND 1952a, REID 1952). Intracarotid administration of 5-HT to a waking cat induces a slight dilatation of the pupil immediately followed by a marked myosis (PAGE 1952). This effect is restricted to the eye ipsilateral to the site of injection. The contralateral iris usually reacts with a slight dilatation. Furthermore, constriction is obtained only if fairly large doses of 5-HT are used, whereas with smaller doses bilateral dilatation ensues in the waking animal. According to KOELLA and SCHAEPPI (1962) this rather complex pattern defies a simple explanation on the basis of one locus of action of the drug. The pupillary response could be interpreted as a resultant of at least two competing influences: a direct constrictive effect of 5-HT upon the iris restricted to the side of injection and a shift towards sympathetic preponderance and thus bilateral pupilla-dilating outflows paralleling a generalized central arousal, this latter effect being the result of drug action in the carotid sinus area as well as at intracranial sites. Furthermore it is possible that 5-HT acts upon the ciliary and the superior cervical ganglion and thus, by alteration of synaptic transmission, introduces two complicating factors.

20 μg 5-HT injected into the anterior chamber of the rabbit eye does not affect the musculature of the iris (SCHUMACHER and CLASSEN 1962a).

In the anaesthetized cat tryptamine has essentially the same effect as 5-HT, but in 10 times larger doses (LAIDLAW 1912, REID 1952). Gramine causes a transient pupillary constriction only at very high dose levels (v. EULER et al. 1936).

Bufotenine (up to 20 mg, i.v.) produces mydriasis in man (TURNER and MERLIS 1959) and the same effect is observed, both in man and in the waking experimental animal, following administration of psilocybin. Doses were 5—30 mg in man, by mouth or by parenteral route (DELAY et al. 1959), at least 10 mg/kg in mice, subcutaneously, and at least 20 μg/kg in rabbits, intravenously (CERLETTI 1959).

Large doses of 5-HTP (30—100 mg/kg), given intravenously or intraperitoneally, generally produce mydriasis in dogs, cats and rabbits (BOGDANSKI et al. 1958). However, in the rabbit also a slowly-appearing but long-lasting myosis has been described (SCHUMACHER and CLASSEN 1962a). In man the intravenous injection of 10—120 mg 5-HTP has no effect on pupillary size, evidently owing to insufficient dosage (DAVIDSON et al. 1957a, 1957b). Administered by intracarotid injection, 5-HTP (10—100 mg) elicits mydriasis in man, but striking myosis in the cat. The effect is ipsilateral to the site of injection (MANTEGAZZINI, personal communication).

11. Chick amnion

Preparations of the amnion of the developing chick are of interest because it is devoid of nervous elements of any description. Generally 5-HT increases motility in a rhythmic preparation already at concentrations as low as 0.01 μg/ml; quiescent strips require higher concentrations. Low or moderate doses of 5-HT cause responses which are reproducible without any sign of tachyphylaxis, at high doses the responses are variable and difficult to evaluate. However, at no concentration does the drug depress activity. Atropine decreases the responsiveness of the preparation; hexamethonium shows no effect (EVANS and SCHILD 1953. FERGUSON 1957).

12. Molluscan smooth muscle

Mytilus edulis. 5-HT concentrations as low as 0.01 μg/ml display a powerful relaxing action on the anterior bissus retractor muscle of *Mytilus edulis* when

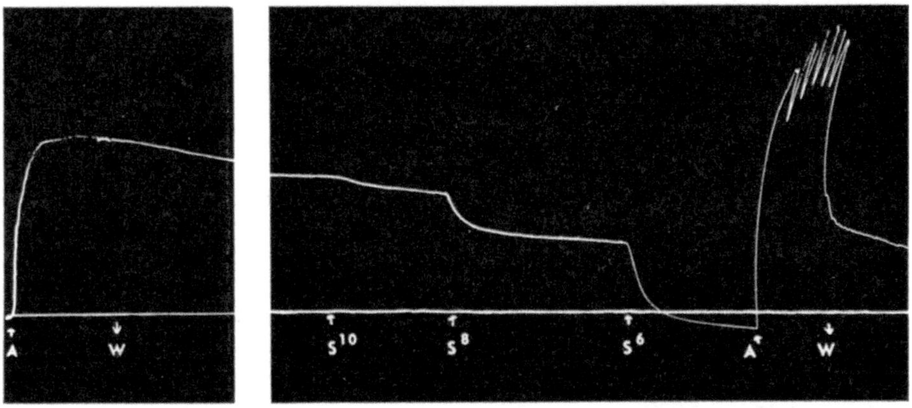

Fig. 12. Anterior bissus retractor muscle of *Mytilus edulis.* The interaction of 5-HT and acetylcholine. A, acetylcholine 4×10^{-6} M; W, wash; S^{10}, S^{8}, S^{6}, 5-HT 10^{-10}, 10^{-8}, and 10^{-6} M. It may be noted that 5-HT produces marked relaxation in a muscle tonically contracted by acetylcholine and that after full relaxation responses to acetylcholine are potentiated. [From Fig. 5, TWAROG, B. M., J. cell. comp. Physiol. **44**, 151 (1954).]

this muscle is contracted by acetylcholine (Fig. 12), electric stimulation, or electric stimulation plus adrenaline (TWAROG 1954, 1958, 1960a, 1960b; HOLGATE and CAMBRIDGE 1958; CAMBRIDGE and HOLGATE 1958; LOWY and MILLMAN 1959). In the presence of 5-HT, tension development by electrical stimulation or acetylcholine is not blocked, but potentiated, while the prolonged phase of contraction which usually may be seen after washing of the stimulating agent is abolished. Moreover, in the presence of 5-HT acetylcholine evokes a succession of spike-like electrical discharges. 5-HT itself, up to 10 μg/ml, does not interfere with neural excitation (TWAROG 1960a, 1960b). LSD (1 μg/ml) is ineffective as an antagonist of 5-HT on this muscle (CAMBRIDGE 1959).

It has been suggested that the relaxing effect of 5-HT involves an alteration of membrane properties which is expressed variously as increased synchronization and recruiting of previously non-spiking elements in response to stimulation (TWAROG 1960a). TWAROG maintains that acetylcholine and 5-HT should be considered as mediators released by the nerve supplying the bissal retractor muscle, with 5-HT being the transmitter involved in neurally-induced relaxation. This opinion, which is shared by others (HOLGATE and CAMBRIDGE 1958, LOWY and MILLMAN 1959), is strongly supported by the presence in the muscle of 5-HT and acetylcholine, as well as of cholinesterase and monoamine oxidase. LOWY and MILLMAN think that the kind of response, tonic or phasic, given by the retractor muscle on nervous stimulation is determined by the amount of 5-HT-like substance present.

Anodonta cygnea. The application of 5-HT (threshold 1 μg/ml) to the cerebral ganglia of this mollusc is followed, within 1 min, by relaxation of the tonically contracted adductor muscle. At the same time there is a considerable increase in the rhythmic activity of the muscle, the duration of which varies according to the concentration of 5-HT (up to $2^1/_2$ hr after 10 μg). The same effect is exerted by adrenaline, noradrenaline, LSD, tryptamine, 5-HTP and tryptophan. Surprisingly enough, there is no difference between the time elapsing between administration of 5-HT and the administration of the other indoles and the time of relaxation and similarly there is no difference in the efficacy of these substances. SÁLANKI and KOSCHTOJANZ (1962) and SÁLANKI (1963) suggest that indolealkylamines and phenylalkylamines may play an important part in the regulation of the periodic activity of *Anodonta*.

5-HT, 5-HTP, tryptophan and tryptamine all increase the rhythmic activity in the glochidia of fresh-water mussel. Tryptamine is the most effective agent (threshold 0.01 μg/ml water), and the increase of activity produced by it is long lasting, keeping on for over 30 min. It is suggested that in the early ontogenetic stage of *Anodonta cignea* tryptamine plays the role of a local hormone in the regulation of the "spontaneous" rhythmic activity (LABOS et al. 1964).

Busycon canaliculatum. The radula protractor muscle of this mollusc can be contracted by acetylcholine and can then be relaxed rhythmically by 5-HT and, even more effectively, by tryptamine. It is probable that indolealkylamines act, like acetylcholine, on the muscle rather than on the nerve (HILL 1958).

Strophocheilos oblongus. 5-HT 10^{-7} induces rhythmic contractions or "beating" of the penis retractor muscle. Graded responses may be obtained with increasing concentrations of 5-HT. Bufotenine and LSD cause irreversible rhythmic contraction (JAEGER 1963).

13. Muscles of worms

Leech dorsal muscle. According to POLONI (1955) the dorsal muscle of the leech responds to 5-HT with a relaxation which is proportional to the dose within astonishingly wide limits (from 0.001 ng to 1 mg/ml!). Relaxation is even more pronounced and proportional if the muscle has been previously contracted by acetylcholine (0.1—10 ng/ml). The effect of 5-HT is inhibited by LSD.

The above results have been generally confirmed by SCHAIN (1961), who similarly observed that 5-HT diminishes the size of acetylcholine contraction and accelerates relaxation of the muscle after washing out acetylcholine. The threshold concentration of 5-HT necessary to reduce the size of contraction produced by 3—5 ng/ml acetylcholine is 25—50 ng/ml. The relaxing effect is also seen in a muscle not contracted by acetylcholine but the effect is less pronounced and it has not been found suitable for the assay of 5-HT because of the difficulty of establishing a stable base line for comparison of relaxations. The nicotine contractions of the leech muscle are inhibited by 5-HT in the same way as acetylcholine contractions are, but potassium contractions are affected to a much lesser degree.

Liver fluke musculature

5-HT and related indolealkylamines, as well as LSD have a stimulatory effect on the rate and amplitude of contractions and on the tone of the musculature of the liver fluke *(Fasciola hepatica)*. The effect is peripheral and not mediated through the central ganglion; it persists, in fact, after removal of the ganglion. LSD is more than 100 times as active as 5-HT (threshold concentration of the amine 10 μg/ml), and this in its turn is 5—10 times more active than tryptamine or bufotenine and 100 times more active than 5-HTP.

BOL, yohimbine, harmine and dopamine depress rhythmical movements and antagonize the stimulant action of 5-HT and LSD.

On the basis of the above effects and on the occurrence of 5-HT in the organism of *Fasciola hepatica*, Mansour (1956, 1957) suggests that 5-HT or a related compound may be the humoral transmitter for the peripheral receptors of this worm.

14. Muscles of sea anemones

Column preparations. 5-HT has no significant effects on the tone, activity or responses of column preparations from *Calliactis parasitica* or *Metridium senile*. Tryptamine, on the contrary, causes, at concentrations of 100 μg/ml, direct contractions, high tonus and enhanced responses to stimulation. 5-Methoxytryptamine has similar effects. Treatment must be applied directly to the contractile part of the preparation; applying the active drugs to attached strips of column has no effect (Ross 1957, 1960a).

Sphincter preparations. 5-HT has no effect on either quick or slow contractions. Tryptamine (10—100 μg/ml) causes direct quick contraction of the sphincter and somewhat enhances both quick and slow responses to stimuli (Ross 1960b).

XI. Action on respiration

It is commonly observed that the intravenous injection of adequate doses of 5-HT and other indolealkylamines provokes transient respiratory effects in the experimental animal and in man. These effects may be different in different animal species. In spite of careful and extensive studies there is as yet no complete accordance of opinion in regard to the site and mechanism of action of 5-HT.

Cat. Reid and Rand (1952a, 1952b) and Reid (1952b) first found that intravenous injections, as well as direct introduction into the right heart of crude serotonin preparations and of pure 5-HT (10—200 μg) caused in the cat under chloralose anaesthesia and with intact vagi, a brief period of apnoea, lasting up to 30 seconds. This was frequently followed by tachypnoea and simultaneous bronchoconstriction, as shown by remarkable fluctuation in intrapleural pressure, reduced amplitude of the respiratory movements, and increase in the chest volume. The observations of the Australian investigators have been regularly confirmed (Fig. 13).

Schneider and Yonkman (1953, 1954) have analyzed the frequency of the vagal afferent impulses during the respiratory responses provoked by 5-HT in the normal cat and in the cat treated with ganglion-blocking agents and local anaesthetics. Following intravenous administration of 20—40 μg/kg 5-HT base there was at first respiratory arrest in expiratory position, then tachypnoea. In both conditions an increase in the frequency of afferent vagal impulses was recorded. Ganglion blockade (3 mg/kg hexamethonium) prolonged the period of respiratory arrest; local anaesthetics (procaine 10 mg/kg, nupercaine 0.5—0.7 mg/kg) shortened it. Schneider and Yonkman concluded that 5-HT has a peripheral point of attack on autonomic sensory nerve endings in the cardio-pulmonary region, including the pulmonary stretch receptors.

These conclusions have been accepted in part by other research workers.

COMROE and collaborators (COMROE 1952, COMROE et al. 1953) found that in the cat under slight chloralose anaesthesia, introduction of 20—40 μg 5-HT base directly into the right heart produced vehement circulatory and respiratory changes, including apnoea and both direct and reflex bronchospasm. With larger doses apnoea was persistent. They suggest that apnoea is due to stimulation of receptors situated in the ascending aorta, which are probably different from veratridine-sensitive receptors.

MOTT and co-workers (MOTT and PAINTAL 1953, KOTTEGODA and MOTT 1955) observed that reflex apnoea produced by intravenous injection of 20—40 μg 5-HT base was usually abolished by cooling the vagi to 1.5—2^0 or by vagotomy.

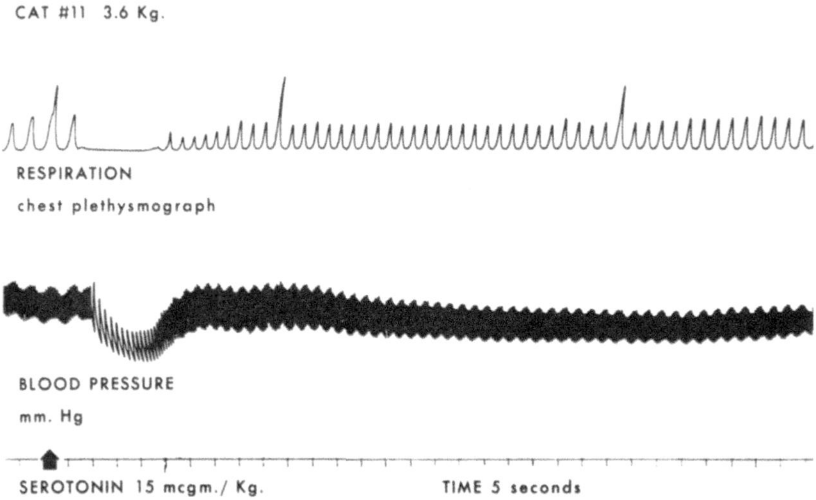

Fig. 13. Effect of a single intravenous injection of 15 μg/kg 5-HT on respiration and blood pressure of a cat anaesthetized with chloralose. The initial brief period of respiratory arrest is followed by a period of moderate tachypnoea (Courtesy Dr. D. C. KROEGER)

However, in some cases a brief apnoea was still produced after vagotomy. Respiratory arrest is interpreted by MOTT and co-workers as being caused by stimulation of receptors situated in the circulation between the large veins and the left atrium (pulmonary pain receptors ?). These receptors are thought to give origin to afferent vagal fibres having a conduction velocity of 5—6 m/sec. There is no evidence that doses of 5-HT less than 40 μg/kg stimulate or sensitize pulmonary stretch endings, nor right or left atrial or depressor nerve endings. However, intravenous injection of 40—85 μg/kg 5-HT base into vagotomized cats given artificial positive-pressure ventilation at constant stroke-volume caused a small increase in peak intra-tracheal pressure accompanied by changes in the rate of discharge of pulmonary stretch fibres. It is suggested by KOTTEGODA and MOTT (1955) that these changes are secondary to direct broncho-constriction caused by 5-HT.

The above results give an explanation of the finding of WEIDMANN and CERLETTI (1955) that vagotomy and cooling of the vagi reduced but did not abolish apnoea produced by 5-HT, and justifies the statement of WESTERMANN (1958) that apneic reactions produced by large doses of 5-HT are due to stimulation of both intrapulmonary receptors with vagal afferencies and the bulbo-inhibitory system of the reticular formation.

Ginzel and Kottegoda (1954) have investigated more closely the action of 5-HT on aortic and carotid sinus receptors. They observed that small amounts of 5-HT (2—10 μg) injected into the carotid sinus region caused fall of blood pressure and stimulation of respiration usually preceded by a short period of apnoea. After section of the sinus nerves only the apneic response remained. The same stimulant action, but no apnoea, was noted following introduction of 5-HT into the aortic body region. The effect was abolished after section of the vagus nerves, but remained unaffected after hexamethonium and atropine. Both 5-HT and tryptamine produced temporary desensitization to their own actions. Ginzel and Kottegoda believe that the excitation of respiration is due to

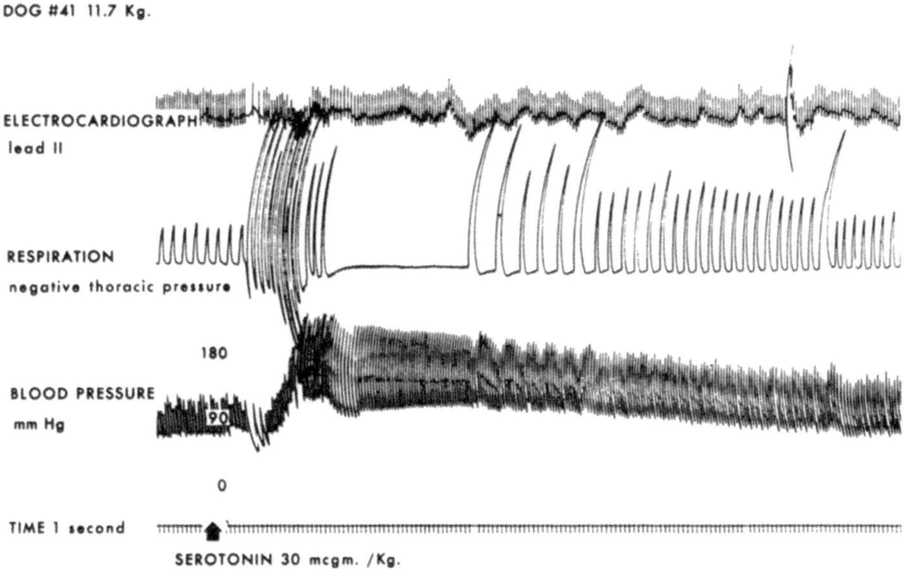

Fig. 14. Effect of a single intravenous injection of 30 μg/kg 5-HT on electrocardiogram, respiration and blood pressure of a dog anaesthetized with pentobarbital-morphine. Note the initial brief period of extreme respiratory effort (hyperpnoea and tachypnoea) followed by a period of respiratory arrest in the expiratory stage, followed in its turn by another period of inspiratory stimulation. [From Fig. 1, Kroeger, D. C., and L. J. Lucco, J. Amer. pharm. Ass., sci. ed. **49**, 171 (1960).]

chemoreceptor stimulation, and that the apnoea, a phenomenon quite independent of the preceding one, is probably of central origin.

Tryptamine (Ginzel and Kottegoda 1954, Reid 1952a), bufotenine and bufotenidine (Raymond-Hamet 1953a, 1954) act on respiration like 5-HT. Tryptamine is however about 20 times less active than 5-HT (Reid 1952a).

Dog. Numerous concordant observations demonstrate that the predominant respiratory response of the anaesthetized dog to single intravenous injections of 5-HT (5—100 μg/kg) is transient hyperpnoea followed in the majority of the animals by a period of apnoea (Douglas and Toh 1952, 1953, Page 1952b, Heymans and van den Heuvel-Heymans 1953, Schneider and Yonkman 1954, MacCanon and Horvath 1954, McCubbin et al. 1956, Westermann 1958). There are, however, also more or less divergent results. Kroeger and Lucco (1960), for example, found that most frequently three respiratory events were obtained with intravenous 5-HT: transient gasping and a slower developing hyperpnoea which was generally interrupted by apnoea (Fig. 14). Schmid, Waltz and Freund (1956) noted that whereas small doses of 5-HT displayed in the waking dog a prevalent depressive effect on respiration, quickly injected large doses produced respiratory stimulation. An initial decrease in respiratory movements resulting in marked tachypnoea was also observed by BEN, BOXILL and WINBURY (1962).

HARASAWA and RODBARD (1961) injected 4 μg/kg 5-HT base, or more, into the pulmonary artery of the anaesthetized dog. The respiratory cycle began to shorten about 10 seconds after the injection and became shortest in 15 to 45 seconds. The respiratory cycle then lengthened gradually to control values over the course of about 5 min. The effects on the respiratory cycle were reduced but not entirely abolished by vagotomy even though changes in heart rate were eliminated.

When 5-HT is infused into the right atrium at a rate of 4 μg/kg/min there is an increase in respiratory volume associated with a significant reduction in CO_2 content of arterial, mixed venous and coronary sinus blood (MAXWELL et al. 1957, CRUMPTON et al. 1959). Similarly, 5-HT produces in the intact dog a rise in the arterial oxygen saturation, as measured by the cuvette oximeter (NIDEN and BARKLAY 1959). Concerning the interpretation of the mechanism and sites of action of 5-HT in producing the above respiratory changes, there are still some obscure and controversial points.

On the basis of the observations a) that respiratory stimulation elicited by the introduction of 5-HT into the common carotid artery remains unchanged after ligation of the internal carotid, the external carotid and the occipital arteries but is abolished by section of the carotid sinus nerves and of the IX cranic nerve, and b) that respiratory effects produced by intravenous 5-HT are reduced or abolished by vagotomy and by bilateral ablation of carotid sinus and glomus, DOUGLAS and TOH (1952, 1953) believe that 5-HT exerts its respiratory effects mainly through stimulation of afferent fibres in the vagus and sinus nerves. A direct stimulation of the respiratory centre is not completely excluded, but it is considered of secondary importance. This view has not been accepted by HEYMANS and VAN DEN HEUVEL-HEYMANS (1953), who failed to confirm that denervation of the carotid sinus and section of the sinus-carotid and vago-aortic nerves caused a reduction in the respiratory response to 5-HT. Accordingly, they consider 5-HT hyperpnoea predominantly due to central stimulation. Another opinion is held by SCHNEIDER and YONKMAN (1953) who maintain that the initial respiratory stimulation in the dog is primarily due to a cardio-pulmonary reflex, since it is greatly diminished or abolished after bilateral vagotomy and only a short period of respiratory depression is observed when the spinal cord is sectioned at C_6. Again stimulation of vago-aortic and carotid sinus afferents appears to be of minor importance.

MCCUBBIN et al. (1956) seem to have resolved the problem by showing that small doses of 5-HT fail to stimulate respiration unless the drug reaches chemoreceptors. In fact, whereas 5 μg 5-HT given into the common carotid artery causes pronounced increase in chemoreceptor impulse traffic in the carotid sinus nerve, the same dose of the amine is ineffective when injected into a perfusion system permitting chemoreceptors to be excluded from the natural circulation. Much larger doses (100—220 μg 5-HT base) cause the reappearance of some respiratory stimulation, which persists after cervical section of the spinal cord with section of the vagus-aortic and sinus nerves. The mechanism of this residual effect is assumed to be central. On a weight basis, 5-HT appears to be a much more powerful chemoreceptor stimulant than lobeline, tryptamine or 1,1-dimethyl-4-phenylpiperazinium iodide.

The theory of a double or treble point of attack of 5-HT (carotid body chemoreceptors, respiratory centre and, eventually, cardiopulmonary receptors) is shared by WESTERMANN (1958) and by KROEGER and LUCCO (1960).

The above explanations, however, apply only to the stimulant action of 5-HT on respiration. Origin of secondary apnoea is largely obscure. KROEGER and LUCCO have called attention to the direct bronchoconstrictor effect possessed by 5-HT and have presented evidence that preventing bronchoconstriction reduced the occurrence of apnoea in the dog.

What has been said for 5-HT applies also to 7-HT and to tryptamine, administered in large doses. Initial hyperpnoea is always the most prominent response, sometimes followed or interrupted by periods of apnoea or reduced respiration (PAGE 1952b, REID 1952a). Psilocybin (0.5 mg/kg, i.v.) given to dogs premedicated with morphine and anaesthetized with a dial-urethane-nembutal mixture decreases respiratory volume from 2.7 to 2.1 l/min and respiratory rate from 19 to 17 movements per minute. There is a definite decrease in arterial oxygen content and arterial saturation also falls (MAXWELL et al. 1962). Little is known about gramine, which seems however to increase depth and rate of respiratory movements and to cause bronchoconstriction (SUPNIEWSKI and SERAFINOWNA 1938).

In marked contrast to the normal dog, but like the cat, the dog with neurogenic hypertension responds to 5-HT and tryptamine with a period of apnoea, followed by deep, forced breathing (PAGE 1962b).

Man. 0.5—1.5 mg 5-HT given by rapid intravenous administration produces in normal subjects a short-lasting (20—40 seconds) increase in depth and rate of respiration with elevation of the mid position of the chest. There are no signs of bronchial obstruction. The respiratory response is potentiated by pyrilamine maleate (25 mg), inhibited by BAS (50—100 mg, i.v.) and left unchanged by anticholinergic drugs, and by ganglionic or adrenergic blockade (HOLLANDER et al. 1957, MICHELSON et al. 1958).

The effect of 5-HT given by intravenous infusion in doses of 1—3 mg/minute is essentially the same. Stimulation of respiration is most marked in the first 5 min but persists to a lesser degree throughout the remainder of the 10- or 20-min infusion. Tidal air always increases but respiratory rate shows a variable change. Apnoea is not seen. On repeated infusion tachyphylaxis of the hyperpnoea is observed. Neither release of adrenaline nor increased metabolic rate seems to be responsible for the stimulatory effect of 5-HT (PARKS et al. 1960).

In asthmatic patients aerosolized 5-HT produces a prompt fall in vital capacity and a decrease in respiratory flow rate (MICHELSON et al. 1958).

Whereas MICHELSON and co-workers think that it is probable that the respiratory effect of 5-HT is due to direct stimulation of the central nervous system, PARKS et al. believe that 5-HT stimulates receptors situated in the systemic arterial circulation. This is based on the observation that the onset of hyperpnoea corresponds in time with the initial effect on the forearm blood flow.

Bufotenine produces, when blown into the nostrils (10 mg) or given intravenously by quick injection (10 mg in 50 seconds), hyperventilation eventually followed by apnoea (TURNER and MERLIS 1959). Given by slow intravenous injection (0.06—0.25 mg/kg over 3 to 20 min) it causes only slight variation in respiration with a tendency to increase (FABING et al. 1956).

Rabbit. The injection of 5-HT (50—100 μg/kg, i.v.) into the anaesthetized animal causes a marked immediate stimulation of breathing, followed in 50% of the animals by respiratory arrest in inspiratory position. A diminution of the respiratory response is evident after spinal cord section (SCHNEIDER and YONKMAN 1954). Respiratory arrest is not due to bronchospasm, since 5-HT has little or no effect on the bronchi of rabbits in doses up to 2.5 mg/kg given intravenously or endobronchially (JÄNKÄLÄ and VIRTAMA 1961). Like 5-HT, psilocybin (threshold dose 20 μg/kg, i.v.) and bufotenidine (threshold 5 μg/kg, i.v.) produce predominant respiratory stimulation (CERLETTI 1959, UEDA et al. 1957).

Guinea-pig. An analysis of the respiratory effects of 5-HT in the guinea-pig is made very difficult by the potent direct bronchoconstrictor action of the amine (HERXHEIMER 1955, 1957; BHATTACHARYA 1955; BALZER et al. 1956; JÄNKÄLÄ and VIRTAMA 1961). Intravenous 5-HT generally provokes hyperpnoea over a wide dosage range (WESTERMANN 1958). Tidal air, however, is decreased at constant stroke volume, both in anaesthetized and in spinal guinea-pigs. Threshold dose is 3 to 22 μg/kg (KONZETT 1956). 0.5—0.7% 5-HT aerosols administered to unanaesthetized animals provoke tachypnoea followed in 30—40% of the animals by an asthmatic attack, succeeded, in its turn, by deep and frequent respiration and then, in spite of continuous inhalation of aerosol, by normal breathing (FRAHM 1957). 1% 5-HT aerosols given to urethane-anaesthetized

Table 1. *Action on respiration of indolealkylamines administered intravenously to different animal species*

	5-HT	Bufotenine	Psilocybine	Bufotenidine	Tryptamine	Gramine
Man	+	+ (—)				
Dog normal	+ —		—		+ (—)	—
hypertensive	— (+)				— (+)	
Cat	— (+)	— (+)		— (+)	— (+)	
Rabbit	+ (—)		+	+		
Guinea-pig	+					
Rat	+ — +					
Chicken	—				—	

+ indicates respiratory stimulation,
— indicates reduced respiratory rate or apnoea.
Occasional or minor effects are given in brackets.

guinea-pigs induce characteristic changes in the expiratory reflexes and inspiratory dispnoea. Vagotomy largely reduces this response suggesting that 5-HT affects respiration not only through a direct peripheral action on the bronchi but also through vagal reflexes (MEIER et al. 1956).

Rat. The respiratory response of the rat to intravenous 5-HT shows remarkable individual variations (WESTERMANN 1958). Generally a brief initial stimulation is followed by apnoea in the expiratory position and then, sometimes, by moderate tachypnoea. The respiratory stimulant effect of 5-HT (4—10 μg/kg, i.v.) is abolished by inactivation of the carotid sinuses but not by vagus section or ganglionic blockade. It seems to depend on stimulation of carotid and probably aortic chemoreceptors, as well as, with larger doses, on a central mechanism (SALMOIRAGHI et al. 1956).

Chicken. 5-HT (5—50 μg/kg, i.v.) and tryptamine (25—500 μg/kg, i.v.) decrease both rate and amplitude of breathing. Antihistaminic drugs or atropine do not alter these respiratory effects (BUÑAG and WALASZEK 1961c).

It clearly appears from the preceding data that respiratory changes elicited by 5-HT and other indolealkylamines are consistently different in different animal species, and even, to some degree, in the same species according to experimental conditions. Table 1 summarizes the most common features of the respiratory effects of indolealkylamines.

According to WESTERMANN (1958) animal species whose respiratory centre possesses an elevated activity of its own, largely independent of vagal afferent impulses (e.g. cat) respond to 5-HT with predominant apnoea; animal species, on the contrary, with a respiratory centre largely dependent on vagal afferent impulses (e.g. guinea-pig) respond to the amine with hyperpnoea and/or tachypnoea.

There is no evidence that 5-HT participates in the physiological control of respiration. Hence, all actions described in this chapter should be considered pharmacological actions.

XII. Action on external secretions

1. Salivary secretion

Dog submaxillary gland. According to PETRUCELLI et al. (1961) single injections of 50—100 μg 5-HT into the common carotid artery via the cranial thyroid artery produce potentiation of salivation caused by continuous electrical stimulation of the chorda tympani. 5-HT in this dose range causes no salivation by itself. The intravenous administration of iproniazid further increases the potentiation observed with identical doses of 5-HT. The intravenous administration of reserpine in single doses which by itself produce salivation also further potentiates 5-HT after cessation of reserpine-induced salivation. Moreover, it appears that 5-HT by subminimal infusion potentiates the sialagogue effect of acetylcholine. PETRUCELLI and co-workers suggest that 5-HT, while not strictly necessary for neural transmission, may facilitate transmission at parasympathetic ganglia and/or neuroeffectors.

At complete variance with the above results are those of CALDARERA et al. (1961a, 1961b), who found that both the intravenous injection of 20—120 μg/kg 5-HT base and the intravenous infusion of 5—20 μg/kg/min 5-HT caused a complete or partial inhibition of the secretory response of the dog submaxillary gland to electrical stimulation of the chorda tympani as well as to intravenous infusion of pilocarpine. The inhibitory effect lasted 3—15 min and was sometimes preceded by transient potentiation of salivation. Enervation of the gland did not alter the effect of 5-HT. There was no definite correlation between reduction of salivation and the observed decrease in blood flow through the gland.

Posterior salivary glands of octopoda. Perfusion of the isolated posterior salivary glands of *Octopus vulgaris* and *Octopus macropus* with sea water containing 1—10 μg/ml 5-HT produces, together with a decrease in the perfusion rate and a conspicuous increase in the rhythmic movements of the gland and the ducts, the secretion of a liquid which greatly differs from that obtained by electrical stimulation of the gland. In fact, the secretion is clear, limpid, not viscous, rich in chlorides, poor in proteolytic enzymes and lacking any toxicity towards the crab. GHIRETTI (1953a, 1953b) suggests that 5-HT may act through changes in the permeability of the cellular elements of the gland.

2. Gastric secretion

Man. At variance with CALÌ and CORDOVA (1956a, 1956b) who found that intravenous 5-HT (2 mg) displayed in man a stimulant action on gastric secretion, which was inhibited by antihistaminic drugs and therefore did not appear to be mediated through liberation of histamine, all other research workers (ROSA et al. 1957—1958; SCHMID et al. 1959, 1960; PICHEL WARNER et al. 1959; HAVERBACK and DAVIDSON 1958) observed that 5-HT and 5-HTP inhibited the volume and acidity of both spontaneous and histamine-induced gastric secretion while at the same time increasing production of mucus. Following the intravenous infusion of 1.5—15 μg/kg/min 5-HT maximum effects (rise of pH values by 0.5 to

1.5) appear after 5—25 min and the secretory response wears off within 15—20 min after the infusion has been discontinued (SCHMID et al. 1959); 5-HTP infused intravenously for 5 min at a rate of 10—80 μg/kg/min produces a more intense and sustained reduction of gastric secretion. The pH of the gastric juice rises by 3.5 and the inhibitory effect lasts up to 60 min (SCHMID et al. 1960).

Dog. BLACK et al. (1956, 1958) and SMITH (1957) examined the effect of 5-HT on gastric secretion in dogs anaesthetized with chloralose and urethane, starved for al least 12—24 hours and prepared with a stomach fistula and a ligature at the pylorus-duodenal junction. They found that intravenous infusions of 5-HT, at a rate of 2.5—20 μg/kg/min for 45—90 min did not stimulate any gastric secretion whatever, but caused the production of an alkaline juice rich in mucus. During this infusion the arterial plasma pH fell, unlike the plasma pH during histamine infusion. When an acid gastric secretion was stimulated by a continuous intravenous infusion of histamine (e.g. 5 μg/kg/min) concurrent infusion of 5-HT (15 μg/kg/min) for 30 minutes was found to inhibit the secretion. Recovery from the inhibition usually began within 60 min after stopping the 5-HT infusion. Infusion of 5-HT at the start of histamine-stimulated gastric secretion failed to prevent the onset of secretion due to infusion of histamine.

However, the effect of 5-HT on histamine-induced gastric secretion was greatly influenced by the previous dietary history of the animals. In dogs which were not starved completely but were given a fatty meal in the 12 hours preceding the experiment, 5-HT elicited a much more striking inhibitory response and all acid secretion was abolished, whereas in dogs in which the period of starvation was prolonged to 36 hours, 5-HT did not inhibit and in several cases stimulated the acid secretion.

When 5-HT was given after bilateral cervical vagotomy it was found to be ineffective in inhibiting histamine-stimulated secretion. This has been considered evidence in favour of the suggestion that 5-HT might exert its effects on gastric secretion reflexly, through stimulation of vagal receptors in the stomach wall.

The above observations were, on the whole, confirmed by several research workers.

HAMMOND (1956) observed that in dogs receiving 5-HT intravenously in doses which stimulated intestinal motility, no gastric secretion ensued and that stimulation of gastric secretion by reserpine was not affected by the simultaneous injection of 5-HT.

WHITE and MAGEE (1958) found that intravenous infusion of 10—30 μg/kg/min 5-HT increased by 200% the secretion of mucin from the pyloric mucosa of the dog and that this effect was regularly reduced by the administration of 1 mg atropine intravenously. The action of 5-HT was not dependent on increased motility since it was present in the everted pouch and was not abolished by hexamethonium, which decreased motility.

Finally, HAVERBACK et al. (1957, 1958) noted that whereas 5-HT base in a dose up to 4 μg/kg/min had no marked transient or sustained effect on the volume and pH of gastric secretion from the denervated Heidenhain pouch, a dose of 16 μg/kg/min produced a rise of the pH of the reduced volume of gastric juice.

In acute observations on dogs anaesthetized with pentobarbital, bearing a tube in the stomach introduced through a duodenostomy, 3 subcutaneous doses of 10 μg/kg 5-HT base given every 15 min, single intravenous doses of 25 μg/kg and intravenous infusions of 13 μg/kg/min for 45 min failed to cause any appreciable change in the gastric secretion (HAVERBACK and WIRTSCHAFTLER 1962).

The variable effect of 5-HT on histamine-stimulated gastric secretion is again emphasized in recent experiments by SOSIN et al. (1962). They observed that whereas significant elevation of free HCl (177% of controls) occurred in Heidenhain pouches of dogs receiving an intravenous infusion of 4 μg/kg/min histamine plus 8 μg/kg/min 5-HT base, no significant changes in free HCl were noted in dogs receiving the same dose of histamine plus 16, 25 and 32 μg/kg/min 5-HT. Dogs receiving 5-HT alone produced virtually no free HCl. The volume of gastric juice paralleled free HCl, and pepsin activity was not altered in any test group.

Results obtained with the precursor aminoacid 5-HTP were on the whole in accordance with those obtained with 5-HT, with an important partial discrepancy, however, concerning the effect of 5-HTP on the histamine-induced gastric secretion.

Smith et al. (1957) and Black et al. (1958, 1959) found that the intravenous infusion of doses of 5-HTP as low as 5—20 μg/kg/min produced, after a latent

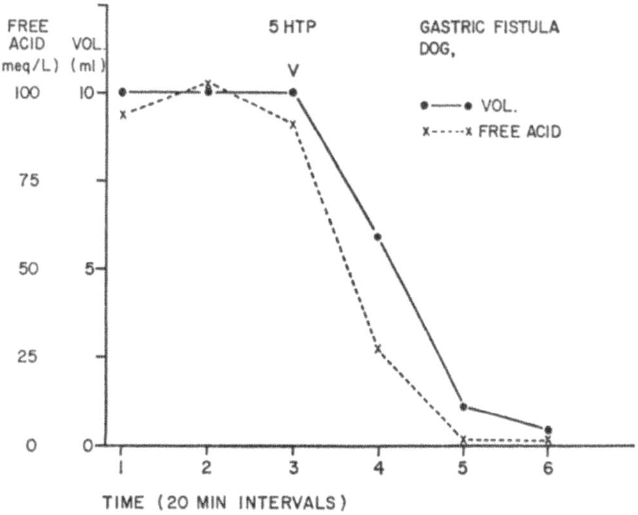

Fig. 15. The inhibitory effect of 5-HTP (25 mg/kg, i.v.) on spontaneous gastric secretion in a dog with gastric fistula and intact vagal nerves. Each value represents the mean of three studies on different days. [From Fig. 6, Haverback, B. J., and S. K. Wirtschaftler, Advanc. Pharmacol. 1, 323 (1962).]

period of 15—30 min, a marked fall in secretory acid output elicited by histamine. Occasionally 5-HTP stimulated gastric acid secretion for a short time as the first action. The effect was maximal when 5-HTP was given 2 hours after histamine stimulation. Bilateral cervical vagotomy markedly reduced the inhibitory effect of 5-HTP.

Haverback and co-workers (Haverback 1958, Haverback et al. 1958, Haverback and Wirtschaftler 1962) observed that 5-HTP in a single intravenous dose of 25 mg/kg inhibited spontaneous gastric secretion in dogs with Heidenhain pouches and with simple gastric fistulae and intact vagal nerves (Fig. 15). Volume of gastric juice fell from 10 to 1.5 ml/20 min, and free acid from 93 to 0 meq/litre within 40 min after 5-HTP administration. The aminoacid was equally effective in inhibiting gastric acid secretion stimulated by insulin-induced hypoglycaemia and by urecholine infusion (3.5 μg/kg/min) (Fig. 16). However, it did not inhibit gastric secretion stimulated by reserpine or histamine (2 μg/kg/min). In each instance, following inhibition of gastric acid secretion, there was a marked increase in the quantity of mucus secreted by the stomach.

It is suggested that 5-HTP does not directly affect the mechanism of acid formation, but probably interrupts the pathway for the transmission of stimuli to gastric secretion.

Of considerable interest is the observation of BLACK et al. (1959) that in previously starved anaesthetized dogs, feeding of tryptophan (300—1000 mg)

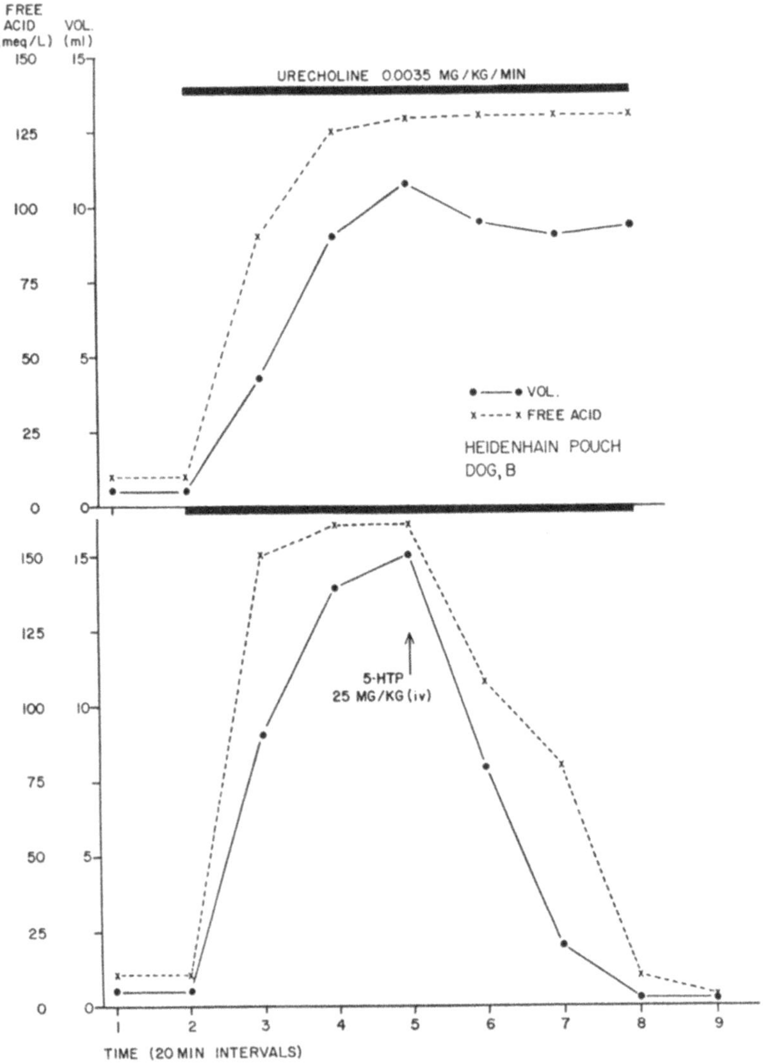

Fig. 16. (Above) Stimulus of urecholine to gastric secretion in a dog with a Heidenhain pouch. (Below) Inhibition of this secretion in the same dog by 5-HTP (25 mg/kg, i.v.) [From Fig. 7, HAVERBACK, B.J., and S. K. WIRTSCHAFTLER, Advanc. Pharmacol. 1, 324 (1962).]

before the start of an experiment led to a fall in acid output between 1 and 3 hours after the onset of histamine-stimulated secretion.

Guinea-pig. Given to unanaesthetized guinea-pigs in intraperitoneal doses of 1 to 20 mg/kg, 5-HT reduces the concentration of free acid and raises the concentration of Na in the gastric secretion induced by histamine. Like other inhibitors of gastric secretion, 5-HT causes the replacement of Cl ions with Na ions, leaving unaffected the concentration of potassium. Small doses of 5-HT increase and larger doses decrease the peptic activity of the juice (WILSON 1957).

Rat. Both 5-HT (4—8 mg/kg of the base, subcutaneously) and 5-HTP (10 to 20 mg/kg) produce a significant depression in volume, acid and pepsin output of the interdigestive gastric secretion in the Shay-rat, as well as a depression of gastric secretion stimulated by urecholine. Doses of 5-HT lower than 10 mg/kg are ineffective. Following 5-HTP, inhibition of gastric secretion occurs after a considerable latency (SHAY et al. 1957, 1958; HAVERBACK and DAVIDSON 1958; HAVERBACK et al. 1958).

These results were confirmed in chronic gastric fistula rats prepared by implanting stainless steel cannulae in the rumen portion of the stomachs. 5-HT (8 mg/kg, s.c.) significantly reduced, 2 hr after the injection, the volume of gastric juice and the output of free and total acid (MARSHALL et al. 1962).

To explore whether inhibition of gastric secretion observed following HCl perfusion of the small intestine was due to release of 5-HT by the upper intestine, gastric secretion in the pyloric-ligated rat was studied by RESNICK and GRAY (1961) after the administration of varying quantities of 5-HT through the rat portal vein. It was found that infusion of 5-HT (2—20 μg 5-HT base in 1-hr experiments, and 4—180 μg in 3-hr studies) did not alter either gastric pH or secretory volume. Similarly, neither partial depletion of intestinal 5-HT by reserpine nor use of 5-HT antagonists prevented the suppression of gastric secretory function caused by HCl perfusion of the small intestine.

The above experiments are more than ever pertinent since RESNICK and GRAY (1962) demonstrated that perfusion of 0.1 N HCl (3 ml for a period of 15 min) through the upper intestine of the rat or introduction of HCl into an obstructed intestinal loop, produced a decrease in the 5-HT concentration from 2.4 to 1.8 μg/g and from 3.4 to 1 μg/g, respectively.

At intraperitoneal doses of 15 mg/kg, 5-HT does not produce any significant increase in plasma pepsinogen, i.e. it does not stimulate gastric endocrine function (KOWALEWSKI 1960).

Cat. The effect of intravenous 5-HT (1—6 mg base/cat) on the secretion of gastric pouches is variable, in part depending upon the integrity of the vagus nerves. With intact vagi, spontaneous secretion is but little affected by 5-HT (production of a small amount of non-acid juice), and histamine-induced secretion (40 μg histamine/min) is generally reduced in both volume and acidity. With cut vagus nerves non-acid spontaneous secretion is more abundant, for 10 minutes, and reduction of histamine-induced secretion is preceded by an increase of secretion. When vagus nerves are cut at the cardias instead of at the neck, there is always an immediate reduction in both volume and acidity of the histamine-induced secretion (DE CORRAL SALETA 1956, 1960).

3. Pancreatic and biliary secretions

Rats given daily injections of 2 mg/kg 5-HT base for 3 days present a slight decrease in the lipase and protease activity of the pancreatic juice, whereas the amylase activity remains unchanged (MIGLIETTA and SALVADÈ 1959).

No significant changes in bile flow occur during and after 4 to 6 hr of perfusion of 5-HT (2 to 100 μg/min) through the portal vein cannula of an isolated rat liver (LEVINE et al. 1964).

In dogs with total pancreatic fistulae, 5-HT (0.2 mg base/kg, i.v.) reduces both food-stimulated and non-stimulated flow of pancreatic juice. Whereas pH or amylase activity of the juice is not affected, bicarbonate level is decreased. 5-HTP (25 mg/kg, i.v.) produces similar but slower and less pronounced effects

(DRAPANAS and POLLACK 1960). Pancreatic secretion provoked by intravenous infusion of pilocarpine (5—25 μg/kg/min) is reduced both by single intravenous injections (40—60 μg/kg of the base) and by intravenous infusion of 5-HT (10 μg/kg/min). Inhibition of pancreatic flow is sometimes preceded by short-lived stimulation (RIVA SANSEVERINO and URBANO 1961c, 1961d, 1963), Concerning the influence of 5-HT and 5-HTP on flow rate of secretin-stimulated pancreatic juice results are at variance. DRAPANAS and POLLACK observed no action, RIVA SANSEVERINO and URBANO a clear inhibitory effect.

5-HT (0.7—1 mg/kg of the base, i.v.) elicits in the majority of the experiments a temporary diminution of the bile flow in the dog. The effect on bile concentration is variable (SEFERIAN 1962).

In man, intravenous infusion of 4 μg/kg/min 5-HT for 60 min does not affect significantly external pancreatic secretion (volume, bicarbonate and amylase concentration of the duodenal aspirate), but partially inhibits the bile pigment flow (PICHEL WARNER et al. 1959).

Intramuscular injection of 10 mg 5-HT base, repeated after 1 hr, provokes in man a more rapid disappearance of sulfobromophthalein from plasma, i.e a more prompt extraction of the dye by the hepatocytes (TURA et al. 1960)

It appears from the preceding data that 5-HT and 5-HTP display on the secretions of the alimentary canal a prevalently depressive effect. Now, the problem arises as to whether or not this pharmacological action elicited by hexogenous 5-HT or 5-HTP is indicative of a possible physiological function displayed on gastrointestinal secretions by strictly endogenous 5-HT. In other words, considering for the sake of simplicity the stomach only, does the 5-HT produced and stored within the stomach mucosa contribute to a local regulation of the gastric secretion, or does the 5-HT circulating in the blood display the same function ?

In the writer's opinion evidence so far available is insufficient for an answer to the above questions. However, a few considerations can be made:

a) There is no direct proof whatever demonstrating that a *local* release of 5-HT by the enterochromaffin cells of the gastric mucosa occurs at the time of gastric secretion and may exert any influence upon this secretion. In fact, no changes in the 5-HT content of the stomach have been described which could be referred to the phases of the secretory activity of the organ.

The suggestion that reserpine may stimulate gastric secretion through local release of 5-HT is hardly tenable because 5-HT, in contrast to reserpine, inhibits gastric acid secretion, and because reserpine is active even after pretreatment with 5-HTP which is a potent inhibitor of gastric secretion (HAVERBACK et al. 1958, HAVERBACK and WIRTSCHAFTLER 1962, NEČINA and KREJČI 1961).

b) BLACK et al. (1959) affirm that 5-HT levels in portal blood are higher in fed (0.24—0.39 μg/ml) than in starved dogs (0.13 μg/ml). These observations, which would indicate a release of 5-HT by the gastrointestinal mucosa in connection with presence of food in the alimentary canal, await confirmation before they can be accepted. In fact, keeping in mind the rate of blood flow through the portal vein, excess 5-HT liberated by the intestines of fed animals would be enormous, far beyond any reasonable expectation. Caution is more than ever justified since no relationship between meals and the peak in the diurnal variation in 5-HT metabolism, as inferred from the urinary excretion of 5-HIAA, could be demonstrated in man.

It should be added that increased liberation into the blood of 5-HT produced by food would neither prove nor disprove that released 5-HT acts on secretory processes.

c) Although the 5-HT content of the gastric mucosa is generally maximum in the red, glandular portion of the stomach, even the white, non-glandular portion may contain large amounts of the amine. In *Ameiurus catus*, a fish belonging to the Teleostei, enterochromaffin cells are localized only near the pylorus, while completely lacking in the glandular portion of the stomach.

These species differences in the gastric distribution of enterochromaffin cells and 5-HT are not in favour of a direct local action of 5-HT on gastric secretion.

d) Accepting the view that 5-HT may exert its physiological action on the gastric secretion via the blood, then it should be stressed that the intravenous doses of exogenous 5-HT required to produce changes in the gastric secretion are always considerably high [in the rat doses of 5-HT base infused into the portal vein for 1—3 hours at a rate of up to 20—50 μg/rat/hour failed to alter either gastric pH or secretory volume (RESNICK and GRAY 1961)] and that changes in the stomach secretion are accompanied by changes in gastrointestinal motility and by a more or less conspicuous involvement of the vascular system.

So far, information is lacking about the behaviour of gastric secretion following close intraarterial injection or infusion of physiological doses of 5-HT.

e) As already stated, BLACK et al. (1959) observed that feeding of tryptophan to dogs produced, after a latency period, a reduction in histamine-stimulated gastric secretion. The confirmation of these results appears to be of the greatest interest and it would be important to try separately L-tryptophan and D-tryptophan and to follow up the urinary excretion of 5-HIAA during the experiment. It is evident that the demonstration that endogenous 5-HT originating from dietary L-tryptophan is capable of influencing gastric secretion would offer strong support to the hypothesis that 5-HT is involved in the physiological control of this secretion.

4. Sweat secretion

In man intramuscular doses of 2 mg 5-HT are sufficient to depress sweat secretion. The effect, which reaches its maximum during the second hour, wears off within 4 to 5 hours. In 50% of the cases inhibition is preceded by stimulation (MORSIANI and MARTELLI 1955). In mice complete inhibition of plantar transpiration is observed only with doses of 5-HT base as high as 5—6 mg/kg (BLOZOVSKI and SIVADJIAN 1959), which are known to produce conspicuous vascular effects.

XIII. Metabolic effects. Action on enzymes

1. Action on carbohydrate metabolism

Mammals. CORRELL et al. (1952) first found that the intravenous injection of 10 mg/kg 5-HT into non-anaesthetized rats produced an increase of plasma glucose level from 157 to 269 mg per cent, and that the injection of 2.5 mg/kg 5-HT into rabbits brought the level from 120 to 193 mg per cent. The presence of the adrenal medulla was not essential for the hyperglycaemic response. These data have been generally confirmed.

In rats, hyperglycaemia produced by 5-HT (0.4 mg/rat, i.v.) may by preceded by a hypoglycaemic phase which is potentiated by pentobarbital anaesthesia. Insulin-induced hypoglycaemia is enhanced by 5-HT, whereas adrenaline-induced hyperglycaemia is reduced by the amine. Chronic administration of 5-HT for 50 days increases insulin sensitivity and glucose tolerance (KOBAYASHI et al. 1960a).

Furthermore, 0.1—0.4 mg 5-HT base/rat given by intraperitoneal or intravenous route depletes liver glycogen, decreases glycogen levels (by 35—50%)

and phosphorylase activity of uterine smooth muscle, decreases glycogen concentration in the diaphragm (25—30%) and rapidly elevates glycogen in heart muscle (30%), while leaving phosphorylase activity unaltered in both instances (KOBAYASHI et al. 1960b, LEONARD and DAY 1960).

However, when given subcutaneously to adrenodemedullated rats, 5-HT increases the glycogen content of the diaphragm, the effects of 5-HT and insulin being additive when given together (KOBAYASHI 1960).

The intravenous injection of 20—200 μg 5-HT base/rat causes a rapid rise of blood lactate both in intact and adrenodemedullated animals. This is due both to enhancement of extrahepatic production and to retardation of hepatic utilization of lactate (UI et al. 1960a, 1960b).

LEVINE et al. (1964) administered 5-HT into the portal vein cannula of an isolated rat liver, either by rapid injection over a 2-min period (7—700 μg 5-HT base) or by constant infusion (1.6—100 μg/min). They observed that the amine produced glycogenolysis, hyperglycaemia and stimulation of hepatic phosphorylase activity. The increase in blood glucose was not dose-related and was variable. These actions were independent of observed vasomotor effects of 5-HT on hepatic blood flow. Similar effects were produced by 5-HTP (8—26 mg/hr).

A more precise analysis of the effects of 5-HT in stimulating phosphorylase activity in the rat uterus was carried out by LEONARD (1963). He found that 5-HT administered either intraperitoneally (5 mg/kg every 30 min for 6 hr) or by intraluminal uterine injection (0.5 mg/uterine horn) did not increase uterine weight or activity of *a*(active)-phosphorylase. Intraperitoneally-injected 5-HT produced, however, a decrease in total-phosphorylase activity which was similar though smaller than that caused by histamine.

After intraperitoneal injection of 2 mg 5-HT base/rat there is a significant increase in the P^{32} uptake by adrenal cortex and medulla, pancreas, liver and diaphragm, and a significant decrease in the spleen and testis. This signifies that 5-HT, according to different tissues, increase or decreases the rate of metabolic phosphorylation (LINGJAERDE and SKAUG 1957).

5-HT at 10 mM concentrations abolishes the oxidative phosphorylation of guinea-pig liver mitochondria. This can be observed when either L-glutamate or β-hydroxybutyrate is used as substrate. Tryptamine is approximately half as active as 5-HT, IAA possesses the same activity as tryptamine, 5-HTP is inactive (ALIVISATOS et al. 1964).

In rabbits both 5-HT and 5-HTP elicit a predominant hyperglycaemic response. Rise in blood sugar level is by 10, 40 and 60% after 2, 4 and 12 mg/kg 5-HT base, respectively (MAZZONE et al. 1959a, 1959b), and by 40% after 5 to 20 mg/kg 5-HTP (KONZETT 1958). Hyperglycaemia may be preceded by a fleeting hypoglycaemic phase (—10%). Diabetic rabbits behave like normal rabbits (NIAUSSAT et al. 1961). 5-HT-induced hyperglycaemia is antagonized by dihydroergotamine and probital anaesthesia, whereas pretreatment with 5-HT (1 mg/kg) has little influence on hyperglycaemia produced by LSD (MAZZONE et al. 1959b, KONZETT 1956, 1958).

2.5—25 mg/kg 5-HT given intravenously in the rabbit produces an important decrease in the brain consumption of oxygen and glucose, a mobilization of brain glycogen and a reduction in brain production of pyruvate as well as an increase in the consumption of lactate and inorganic phosphate (CAHN et al. 1957, 1958).

Glucose content of the cortex of the perfused cat brain is higher when 25 to 44 mg 5-HTP or 40—300 μg 5-HT are added to the perfusion liquid. However, neither glucose uptake nor oxygen consumption are affected whereas there are some indications that 5-HTP tends to depress aerobic glycolysis (MAGNES and HESTRIN-LERNER 1960).

In normal dogs intravenous doses of 5-HT base as low as 5 μg/kg fail, as expected, to produce hyperglycaemia. However, when the same or even half the amount of 5-HT is injected into depancreatized dogs, there is a significant rise in blood sugar level during the first 40—60 min. This preliminary observation of SIREK (1957) still awaits confirmation.

Large doses of 5-HT (2 mg/kg of the base, i.v.) produce even in normal dogs a 30% rise in blood glucose, a decrease in liver glycogen and an increase in liver phosphorylase activity. Since 5-HT fails to prevent the progressive decrease in blood sugar and liver glycogen seen in adrenalectomized dogs treated with saline, it is suggested that the changes in carbohydrate metabolism observed in normal dogs are secondary to a release of adrenaline from the adrenal glands and not due to a direct stimulation of liver phosphorylase by 5-HT (COLOMBO et al. 1960).

Intravenous injection of STH, ACTH or deserpidine does not cause any significant rise of catecholamines or 5-HT in the blood of the pancreato-duodenal vein of the dog. Thus, the hyperglycemia which sometimes follows intravenous injection of STH cannot be explained by a release of 5-HT (GALANSINO et al. 1963).

In human subjects, 4 mg 5-HT given intramuscularly or intravenously does not appreciably affect blood sugar level (SCALTRINI 1956).

At least 3 mg/kg of intravenous psilocybin is required to give in rabbits a moderate hyperglycaemic response (CERLETTI 1959, STEINER and SULMAN 1963). Intravenous doses of 50—500 μg/kg tryptamine are inactive on the blood sugar level of the rabbit (WEITZEL et al. 1956). Gramine doses as large as 5—20 mg/kg have no effect on the plasma glucose level of fasting rabbits (POWELL and CHEN 1945).

In thyroid slices or homogenates of beef, pig, sheep and dog, 5-HT (0.2—1 mg/ml) stimulates the oxidation of glucose-1 and 6-^{14}C to $^{14}CO_2$. Tryptamine and 5-methoxytryptamine are approximately half as active as 5-HT. N-acetyl-5-HT, melatonin, 5-HTP and 5-HIAA are inactive. The effects of 5-HT and adrenaline are additive. In a cell-free system fortified with TPNH, 5-HT augments the oxidation of TPNH to TPN (PASTAN and FIELD 1962, HUPKA and DUMONT 1963).

Molluscs. When an excised gill of *Mytilus edulis* or *Modiolus demissus* is incubated in sea water, both the rate of endogenous respiration and the rate of anaerobic glycolysis are stimulated promptly by the addition of 5-HT. Concomitantly there is an increase in lactic acid production. Glucose uptake, on the contrary, is not enhanced by 5-HT. A similar stimulation has been observed to develop slowly in the presence of 5-HTP. In contrast, neither acetylcholine nor adrenaline influence the respiration of excised gill. 5-HT 10^{-5} causes a 75% increase in oxygen consumption, a 30—70% increase in glycolysis and a 50—150% increase in lactic acid production; 5-HT 10^{-7} is completely inactive. 5-HTP is approximately 30—100 times less active than 5-HT and maximal response is not reached until the second hour after addition of the compound. The actions of 5-HT on the carbohydrate metabolism of excised lamellibranch gill cannot be ascribed to an activation of the gill phosphorylase. Similarly, the glycogen that is degraded during incubation of the gill cannot account for all the oxygen that is consumed, indicating that some other substrate within the gill is also oxidized. BOL 10^{-4} M inhibits the effects of 5-HT, while LSD 10^{-4} M mimicks them. It is suggested that the action of 5-HT on carbohydrate metabolism may be responsible for the accelerated ciliary activity that is observed after the addition of the amine (MILTON and GOSSELIN 1960a, 1960b; MOORE et al. 1961; MOORE and GOSSELIN 1962).

The addition of 10^{-6} M 5-HT to the anterior byssus retractor muscle of *Mytilus edulis* produces a gradual increase in the oxygen consumption, which reaches a maximum (40%) after 45 min. It is suggested that the effect is due to an interference of 5-HT in oxydative phosphorylation (BAGUET and GILLIS 1964).

Liver fluke. It has been reported elsewhere that 5-HT stimulates the rhythmical movement of this parasite. This stimulation is accompanied by the following biochemical events when 5-HT is put into contact with *Fasciola hepatica* at concentrations of 10^{-5} M to 10^{-3} M:

a) An increase in the rate of anaerobic glucose uptake.

b) An increase in glycogen breakdown when the organisms are cultured in media containing no glucose. Stimulation of glycolysis also occurs in homogenates of flukes which have previously been incubated with 5-HT when glucose, glucose-6-phosphate or fructose-6-phosphate are used as substrate.

c) A 2- to 10-fold increase in lactic acid production with little or no change in the production of propionic and acetic acids.

d) An increase in phosphorylase activity, with a rapid and specific increase in the formation of adenosine-3′,5′-phosphate or cyclic 3′,5′-AMP.

e) An increase in the activity of phosphofructokinase, the activating effect of 5-HT being dependent upon the presence of a heavy particulate fraction, ATP and Mg^{++} (MANSOUR and LAGO 1958, MANSOUR 1959, MANSOUR and MENARD 1960, MANSOUR et al. 1960, 1961a, 1961b, MANSOUR and MANSOUR 1962).

Stimulation of phosphofructokinase activity can account, at least in part, for the increase in glycolysis by 5-HT in intact flukes (MANSOUR 1962).

It has been suggested that 5-HT may have a direct effect on mechanisms concerned with the uptake and utilization of glucose by flukes (MANSOUR and LAGO 1958, MANSOUR 1959), and that some actions of 5-HT in the liver fluke appear analogous to some actions of catecholamines and glucagon in mammalian liver and to some actions of catecholamines in mammalian skeletal and cardiac muscle (MANSOUR et al. 1960).

2. Action on oxygen consumption

RAPPORT and VIRNO (1952) first observed that 5-HT reduced the rate of oxygen consumption of the rat when injected intraperitoneally in doses of at least 1 mg/kg. The reduction varied in intensity between 24 and 61%, and in duration between 12 and 120 min. A similar effect was obtained with tryptamine and histamine at much higher dose levels. The effect was not observed in other experimental animals, even with enormous amounts of 5-HT. The phenomenon was attributed, at least to a great extent, to the action of the drug on the central nervous system or on the arterial vessels of the brain.

BIANCHI (1957) showed that mice behaved like rats in their response to 5-HT. In fact, 0.85 mg/kg 5-HT given by subcutaneous route lowered the oxygen consumption of the animals by 20—25%.

Similarly, FÖLDES and KOMLÓS (1959) found that 0.4—4 mg/kg 5-HT base, given by the subcutaneous route, produced in rats a significant and prolonged decrease in O_2 consumption and a fall in body temperature when the environmental temperature was 20°, but had no effect when the animals were kept at 30°. Neither adrenalectomy nor previous administration of chlorpyramine, chlorpromazine or reserpine appreciably influenced the action of 5-HT on oxygen consumption while iproniazid pretreatment enhanced it both in normal and adrenalectomized rats. It is suggested that reduction of oxygen consumption is secondary to the vascular effects of 5-HT (FÖLDES and PALINKAS 1960, FÖLDES 1961).

Decrease of oxygen consumption and fall of body temperature produced by 0.8 mg/kg 5-HT at 20° is much more marked in 6-month-old than in 2-year-old rats (FÖLDES et al. 1961, 1962).

DL-5-Iodotryptophan has no significant effect on the oxygen consumption or weight of guinea-pigs (HARVEY 1959).

Results obtained *in vitro* are partly at variance, possibly depending on the different 5-HT dosage. SALGARELLO (1955) and STARBUCK and HEIM (1959) noted an evident depressive action of 5-HT (0.2 mg/ml) on the respiration of liver (—55%) and brain homogenates (—16 to —32%). However, chronic intraperitoneal administration of 5-HT (2 mg/kg daily for 32 days) produced an increase in the oxidative metabolism of liver and brain (SALGARELLO and TURRI 1958). MIETKIEWSKI and JANKOWSKA (1960) found that oxygen consumption of slices of rat brain, kidney, liver and diaphragm was augmented when the animals were killed 15 min after intravenous injection of 4 mg/kg 5-HT base. Similarly, there was an increase in respiration when slices of kidneys or brains taken from untreated rats were incubated with 20—200 μg/ml 5-HT.

3. Action on fat content in peripheral blood

5-HT given subcutaneously to dogs in doses of 0.1 mg/kg increases in peripheral blood neutral fats by 20% after 15 min and decreases phospholipids by 25% over a period of 3 hr. Free cholesterol is slightly above initial levels (MARKIEWICZ 1959).

Oral administration of 0.05—0.2 mg/kg psilocybin produces in human subjects a 100—200% increase in circulating non-esterified fatty acids (KEELER 1963).

4. Action on intestinal absorption of calcium and water

5-HT seems to facilitate the intestinal absorption of calcium. In fact the increase in calcium blood level produced in man by administration of calcium aspartate is further augmented when 40 mg 5-HT base is given by mouth at the same time (TESSARI and PARRINI 1961).

5-HT given to rats intraluminally (2.5 mg) or by i.v. infusion (5 μg/min for 65 min) reduces the speed of tritium-water absorption to about 50%. This effect may be caused by a change in intestinal capillary blood flow or an inhibition of active water transport.

When 5-HT is infused intravenously, but not when it is given into the intestinal lumen, the concentration of tritium-water in blood is found to be higher than in controls. This reduction of the tritium-water space can be explained by concomitant vasoconstriction (LEMBECK et al. 1964).

5. Miscellaneous metabolic effects

5-HT (1 mg/kg), LSD and BOL (0.25 mg/kg), all decrease the incorporation of ^{35}S-methionine into brain proteins. The ATP content of the rat brain is greatly reduced following administration of 5-HT alone, much less reduced in groups of animals receiving 5-HT plus LSD, and is increased in groups given 5-HT plus BOL (KRAWCZYNSKI et al. 1958, KRAWCZYNSKI 1961).

6. Inhibition of lipide peroxide formation in tissues

5-HT is a very powerful inhibitor, as an anti-oxidant, of lipide peroxide formation in tissues. 6—10 μg/ml 5-HT completely blocks the lipide peroxide formation by rat liver mitochondria, and 1 μg/ml still shows appreciable activity.

5-Hydroxyindoleacetaldehyde has approximately the same activity as 5-HT; tryptamine, bufotenine and adrenaline are less active; tyramine, dopa, mescaline and indoleacetic acid are essentially without effect.

According to BERNHEIM et al. (1957) it is not possible to state that the antioxidant activity of 5-HT explains any of its physiological actions. This activity, however, may be of some importance in the radiation protection given by 5-HT injected immediately before exposure.

7. Action on cholinesterases

The hydrolysis of acetylcholine, butyrylcholine, procaine and murexine by plasma cholinesterase is inhibited by high concentrations of 5-HT (50% inhibition of the enzyme is attained at 7.1×10^{-4} M to 3.2×10^{-3} M concentrations of the amine, depending on the substrate), tryptamine (5.6×10^{-4} M to 5×10^{-3} M) and gramine (1.3—6.3×10^{-4} M) (LANGEMANN 1954, ERDÖS et al. 1956, 1957), but markedly potentiated by lower concentrations of 5-HT (31% augmentation at 5×10^{-6} M) (FRIED and ANTOPOL 1957). Bufotenine has been recognized as a strong inhibitor of serum cholinesterase since 1937 by SOBOTKA and ANTOPOL, who called attention to the structural analogy between this indolealkylamine and eserine. ZSIGMOND et al. (1961a) have now shown that bufotenine and psilocybin inhibit plasma cholinesterase more than 5-HT. An inhibitory effect of 5-HT is also seen on hydrolysis of acetylcholine by red cell cholinesterase (LANGEMANN 1954). On this enzyme tryptamine and psilocybin are approximately as active as 5-HT, bufotenine and gramine 20 times more active (ERDÖS et al. 1956, ZSIGMOND et al. 1961a, 1961b).

Surprisingly enough the hydrolysis of benzoylcholine by plasma cholinesterase is conspicuously activated by tryptamine, whereas 5-HT, 5-HTP and N,N-dimethyltryptamine possess no marked activating effect (ERDÖS et al. 1957a, 1957b).

On the cholinesterase from rabbit caudate nucleus homogenates, 5-HT produces at final concentrations of 10^{-3} M, 5×10^{-3} M, and 10^{-2} M an inhibition of 29, 63 and 100%, respectively. Since marked inhibition occurs only at fairly high concentrations of 5-HT, APRISON (1960) suggests that the action of the amine at normal physiological levels might be to compete with acetylcholine for acetylcholine-receptor proteins, whereas at elevated levels, such as after administration of large doses of 5-HTP, the amine would inhibit cholinesterase. Thus the sedative effect seen after moderate doses of 5-HTP might be the result of the block of normal acetylcholine action, whereas the stimulatory effect seen after large doses of 5-HTP might be due to the increased accumulation of acetylcholine after cholinesterase inhibition.

The rat brain cholinesterase is inhibited by large concentrations of 5-HT (0.5 mg/ml and more) when the amine is added to the incubation mixture prior to the substrate, but is activated, with a maximum in the first 5 min (20—150%), when the amine is added at the same time as the substrate (TONINI 1955).

Human grey matter cholinesterase requires a 10^{-2} M concentration of 5-HT for a 50% inhibition (ZSIGMOND 1961b).

5-HT has no inhibitory effect, up to 10^{-3} M concentration, on brain cholinesterases, as evidenced by the KOELLE's histochemical method (FÖLDES et al. 1959).

The inhibitory effect of psilocybin and 5-HT on grey matter cholinesterase is identical. This indicates that there is no correlation between the *in vitro* anticholinesterase activity of indolealkylamines and their hallucinogenic effekt (ZSIGMOND et al. 1961a).

8. Action on ceruloplasmin

5-HT, 5-HTP, 5-HIAA and bufotenine (0.38 μM/ml), but not tryptamine, indole acetic acid and indole propionic acid are capable of inhibiting the oxidation of N,N-dimethylparaphenylendiamine by purified plasmin and serum oxidase (APRISON et al. 1959).

Like catecholamines, 5-HT (1.5×10^{-4} M) is capable of mediating the oxidation of reduced phosphoridine nucleotides, DPNH and TPNH, in the presence of ceruloplasmin. It is suggested that the free radical semiquinones of the amines formed by the action of ceruloplasmin are the possible electron acceptors during the oxidation of DPNH and TPNH (WALAAS and WALAAS 1961a, 1961b).

9. Action on phenol oxidases

5-HT and, to a lesser degree, other indolealkylamines, inhibit the phenol oxidases of *Fasciola hepatica* and *Tenebrio molitor* (competitive inhibition) as well as the melanoma phenol oxidase (non-competitive inhibition), but display no effect on mushroom and potato phenol oxidases. For total inhibition of liver fluke phenol oxidase 2 mg/ml 5-HT is required, but partial inhibition is already appreciable with 0.02 mg/ml. 5-HT, 5-HTP and bufotenine are not oxidized by the liver fluke oxidase (MANSOUR 1957, 1958).

The tyrosinase prepared from mouse melanoma is significantly inhibited by 5-HT, 5-HTP, 5-HIAA and also by 5-hydroxyindole at relatively low concentrations ($< 10^{-4}$ M). Melatonin, indoleacetic acid and other tryptophan metabolites exert some inhibitory effect only at higher concentrations (10^{-2} M) (SEIJI 1961).

10. Miscellaneous effects on enzymes

Tryptophan pyrrolase. Many tryptophan analogs effectively block the conversion of tryptophan to kynurenine in the tryptophan pyrrolase reaction. Among the most effective are 5-HT, 5-HTP and tryptamine, which produce 81, 79 and 48% inhibition, respectively, at a 5×10^{-4} M concentration (FRIEDEN et al. 1961).

Tyrosine transaminase. 5-HT and 5-HTP are much more potent inhibitors *in vitro* of tyrosine transaminase of rat liver than catecholamines. Tryptophan, tryptamine and 5-HIAA also have some inhibitory activity but indole is inactive (JACOBY and LA DU 1962).

Brain enzymes other than cholinesterase. 5-HT (10 mM) shows no action either on the alkaline phosphatase or on the lactic or malic dehydrogenase of rat brain homogenates (CLARK et al. 1956), nor does it inhibit *in vivo* oxidative phosphorylation in the rat brain, as determined by the uptake of ^{32}P (LINGJAERDE and SKAUG 1957).

However, subcutaneous administration for 7 days of 0.2 mg/kg 5-HT, seems to increase moderately both phosphatase and acetylcholinesterase activity in the hypothalamic magnocellular nuclei of the rat brain, leaving unaffected succinic dehydrogenase activity, as shown by histochemical methods (KIVALO et al. 1958a). Bufotenine slightly inhibits brain lactic dehydrogenase (CLARK et al. 1956), while activating alkaline phosphatase. Oxidative phosphorylation in preparations of brain mitochondria is, on the contrary, unaffected by concentrations of bufotenine as high as 10^{-3} M (BAIN 1957).

Psilocybin does not display any effect on choline acetylase at a concentration of 10^{-7} M; however, at a 10^{-8} M concentration it potentiates the action of the enzyme. 5-HT is without effect in concentrations of 10^{-7}—10^{-6} M. At the same concentrations 5-HT inhibits coenzyme A while psilocybin has no effect (Bošković and Pržić 1961).

Thyroxine-degrading enzymes. 5-HT, 5-HTP, 5-HIAA, 3-hydroxyanthranilic acid, xanturenic acid and reserpine (2×10^{-3} M) all depress the degradation of thyroxine to inorganic iodide by homogenates of mammalian and amphibian tissues. In the presence of 5-HT increased amounts of tetraiodothyroacetic acid are formed in certain tissues. Both 5-HT and reserpine also inhibit the formation of iodide from triiodothyronine, whereas the deiodination of mono- and diiodotyrosine by mouse liver homogenate is not altered by the presence of 5-HT. Deiodination *in vitro* is not influenced significantly by the administration of tryptophan derivatives *in vivo* (Galton and Ingbar 1961).

Hyaluronidase. Hyaluronidase effects are inhibited by 5-HT (Ezer and Szporny 1961).

XIV. Action on chromatophores

1. 5-Hydroxytryptamine

Frog skin chromatophores. Both in *Rana esculenta* and in *Rana pipiens* high doses of 5-HT injected into the dorsal lymph espace produce a dispersion of the pigment in the melanocytes, i.e. a darkening of the skin. In *Rana esculenta* doses of 5-HT base above 0.5 mg/frog are required to produce this effect, which reaches its maximum within $1^1/_2$ hr and disappears after 5—6 hr (Kahr and Fischer 1957). In *Rana pipiens* the effect is apparent within 15 min after injection of 0.1—1 mg 5-HT or tryptamine and lasts an additional 15—30 min, then the pigment returns to its normal contracted condition (Davey 1959). According to Kahr (1957) the phenomenon is mediated through release of the melanocyte-stimulating hormone, but Davey has observed darkening of the skin even in hypophysectomized specimens of *Rana pipiens.* Davey (1960) suggests that not 5-HT but rather intermedin may act on the frog skin indirectly, through release of an indolealkylamine.

Van de Veerdonk (1960) and Burgers et al. (1962) have confirmed the pigment-dispersing activity of 5-HT also on the melanophores of *Xenopus laevis.*

Fish cromatophores. The effect of 5-HT on fish chromatophores seems extremely variable depending upon the species. Whereas the drug is completely inactive, both *in vivo* and *in vitro*, on the melanophores of *Lebistes reticulatus* (Cerletti and Berde 1955, Berde and Cerletti 1957) it appears highly active on the chromatophores of other species. Turner (1958), for example, observed that 2—3 μg 5-HT base injected just beneath the scales produced a local constriction lasting half an hour, and that on the dilated chromatophores of the tail fin, which had been cut off, a 5-HT solution of 0.5 μg/ml led to contraction beginning within 10 min.

Although per se inactive, 5-HT and 2,3-dihydro-5-HT are capable, given in high doses, of antagonizing the chromatophore-expanding action of LSD and BOL, as seen in *Lebistes reticulatus* (Cerletti and Berde 1955, Berde and Cerletti 1957, Fellman et al. 1962).

Chromatophores of cephalopoda. Both the chromatophores of *Loligo pealii* (Rosenblum and Zweifach 1959) and those of *Octopus vulgaris* (Kahr 1958) are closed by 5-HT and tryptamine, the threshold concentration for 5-HT and *Octopus* chromatophores being 0.01 μg/ml. The same effect is produced by LSD and by MAO inhibitors. It has therefore been suggested that chromatophore control is achieved in cephalopoda by an amine-amineoxidase system (closure) opposed by an acetylcholine-cholinesterase system (expansion) (Rosenblum and Zweifach 1959).

2. Melatonin

Melatonin, 5-methoxy-N-acetyltryptamine, while apparently devoid of any other important pharmacological activity, possesses a tremendously intense effect of lightening or paling on frog, toad and fish melanocytes.

The most sensitive preparation seems to be the skin of *Rana pipiens*, previously darkened with caffeine or MSH. For measurable lightening of this skin the following concentrations of melatonin and related amines are required, in μg per ml: melatonin 1×10^{-7}, tryptamine 2×10^{-1}, N-acetyltryptamine 5×10^{-2}, 5-HT 1, 5-hydroxy-N-acetyltryptamine 6×10^{-3}, 5-methoxytryptamine 2×10^{-6}, 5-ethoxytryptamine 5×10^{-2}, 5-ethoxy-N-acetyltryptamine 10^{-5}, 5-methoxy-N-methyltryptamine 2×10^{-1}, 5-methoxy-N-formyltryptamine 2×10^{-4}, 5-methoxy-N-propionyltryptamine 1×10^{-7}, 5-methoxy-N-butyryltryptamine 1×10^{-7}, 5-acetoxy-N-acetyltryptamine 5×10^{-3} (Lerner et al. 1958, Case and Wright 1960, Lerner and Case 1960). By microscopic bioassay 0.01 ng melatonin can be detected (Mori and Lerner 1960). In lightening the chromatophores of *Rana pipiens* melatonin is far more potent than adrenaline or triiodothyronine.

On the melanophores of *Scardinius erythrophtalmus* pretreated with caffeine the closing effect of melatonin reaches its maximum at concentrations ranging from 1 ng to 1 μg/ml. Melatonin, however, seems to be less potent than adrenaline (Mira 1962).

Intracutaneous injections of 50 μg melatonin into an adult man produced erythema, which faded within an hour. However, when 100 μg was given a punched-out ulcer appeared at the injection site 2—4 days later. No depigmentation was observed and there was no increase in local sweating. One patient, given 200 mg melatonin intravenously experienced mild sedation. Numerous metabolic tests made before and after the patient received 200 mg melatonin daily for 5 days revealed no change (Lerner and Case 1960).

The enormous interest in the discovery of melatonin is obvious, and future studies will solve the fascinating problem of whether this hormone is involved in the function of chromatophores in human skin and in the pathogenesis of vitiligo and malignant melanomas (Lerner and Case 1959, 1960; Lerner et al. 1959).

XV. Action on endocrine glands. Inter-endocrine correlations

1. Anterior hypophysis

ACTH. Bertelli et al. (1954) first observed that 5-HT given intravenously or injected into the cisterna magna of the dog in doses of 20—40 μg/kg significantly reduced the number of circulating eosinophils, and injected intraperitoneally into the rat in doses of 0.2—0.8 mg/kg moderately reduced the ascorbic acid content of the adrenal glands. The effects were ascribed to a stimulation of the anterior pituitary with ensuing release of ACTH.

The results of Bertelli and co-workers were generally confirmed. Concerning the ascorbic acid depletion of the adrenal glands, Moussatchè and Alvares Pereira (1956) claim to have obtained in the rat a 20% depletion (from 338 to 267 mg/100 g) with intravenous 5-HT doses as low as 10 μg/kg, and a 30—35% depletion with doses of 250 μg/kg, whereas Smelik and de Wied (1958a, 1958b) obtained only a 15% reduction with 100 μg/kg 5-HT base. Reduction of the ascorbic acid in the adrenals was missing in hypophysectomized rats, in rats with hypothalamo-hypophysial connections interrupted by electrolytic lesions in the caudal eminence one week previously, and in rats whose hypothalamus was blocked by intraperitoneal injection of 50 mg/kg prednisone 24 hr previously.

Fiore-Donati, Pollice and Chieco-Bianchi (1959) similarly observed a remarkable decrease in the ascorbic acid content of the adrenal and the preputial glands of rats sacrificed 2 hr after the subcutaneous injection of 4 mg/kg 5-HT base. Decrease in adrenal glands was similar both in intact and ovariectomized rats (23.4 and 23%, respectively), decrease in preputial glands was greater in ovariectomized rats. The weight of the adrenals remained unchanged.

In regard to the eosinopenic action of 5-HT, Halberg (1954) found that in the mouse 5-HT and cortisone acted reciprocally to potentiate their eosinopenic effects. Indeed, the combined administration of non-eosinopenic doses of cortisone reinforced the eosinopenic effect manifested by 5-HT doses of 0.125, 1.25 and 12.5 mg/kg, and conversely the effect upon the number of eosinophils induced by cortisone in 0.3 and 3 mg/kg doses was strengthened by a non-eosinopenic dose of 5-HT (21.5 μg/kg). Halberg considers the eosinopenic effect of large doses of 5-HT as a pure pharmacological effect, but believes that the synergism between 5-HT and cortisone may have physiological significance and may be listed among the factors interfering with the production of "eosinophil responses".

Milković and Supek (1956) confirmed in the rat the eosinopenic effect of large doses of 5-HT (3 mg/kg) and further stated that LSD (20—120 μg/kg) failed to prevent the eosinopenic action of the amine. 5-HT doses of 150 to 300 μg/kg were completely ineffective.

Finally, reduction in the number of circulating eosinophils following 5-HT administration was observed in the rat also by Steiner and Hedinger (1956) [from 1000 to 600 per mm^3 after 50 mg/kg 5-HT] and by Serra and Bruni (1957) [from 150 to 90—100 eight hours after subcutaneous injection of 2—20 mg 5-HT].

At variance with the above results which, on the whole, are suggestive of a possible "pharmacological" activation of the hypophysary-adrenocortical axis, are the experimental data of Georges (1957) and Georges and Herold (1958). These investigators found that following repeated administration of large doses of 5-HT (2—8 mg/kg daily for 5 successive days, intraperitoneally) there was an inhibition of the reduction of ascorbic acid in the adrenal glands produced by adrenaline, vasopressin, histamine and formalin. They suggest that 5-HT provokes an elective inhibition of the ACTH secretion by the anterior pituitary.

The reason for these strikingly divergent results is not clear. It is possible that it resides in the different dosage schedule of 5-HT. It is perhaps a matter of dosage also that led to the negative finding of Scheiffarth et al. (1961) and of Schwemmle et al. (1961) who could not detect in man any significant change either in the number of eosinophils or in the excretion of 17-ketosteroids following intravenous administration of 10 to 40 mg 5-HTP.

Growth or somatotropic hormone. Laborit and co-workers (1959a, 1959b, 1959b, 1959d, 1959e) found that growth hormone given subcutaneously to rabbits increased urinary excretion of 5-HIAA, the smaller doses being more effective than the larger ones. With a single injection of 2 Evans u. urinary 5-HIAA rose from the normal 32 ± 16 μg per day and per rabbit to 305 μg (!), with 4 u. to 111 μg, with 20 u. to 161 μg. Isoniazid, administered as a MAO inhibitor (6—12 mg/kg), antagonized the effect of STH. Repeated administration of 2 u. STH on successive days produced effects of decreasing intensity (305 μg 5-HIAA during the first day, 60 μg during the third day).

The above rather surprising observations, together with the observation that 5-HT stimulates the growth of young plants and possesses anti-oxidant properties, are at the root of Laborit's theory that 5-HT is an essential growth factor favouring anaerobic processes. However, it seems that more evidence must be gathered before LABORIT'S data and conclusions can be accepted.

In dogs the injection of STH into the femoral vein causes no significant rise of 5-HT in the pancreatic blood. This makes it unlikely that the type of hyperglycaemic substance which is released by growth hormone from the area drained by the pancreato-duodenal vein is 5-HT (FOÀ et al. 1962).

Gonadotropins. ROBSON and BOTROS (1960, 1961) found that the administration of 5-HT to immature, 3-weeks-old female mice (1—25 mg/kg 5-HT base, s.c., daily for 18—35 days) produced a marked depression of the growth of the ovaries, uterus and vagina as well as a delay in the opening of the vagina and in the onset of vaginal oestrus. There was little or no effect on body growth. Given to mature female mice, at daily doses of 20—25 mg/kg for 2 weeks, 5-HT produced some inhibition of the oestrus cycle and marked depression of the weight of the sex organs.

ROBSON and BOTROS conclude that the above results strongly suggest that the effect of 5-HT is exerted either on the pituitary itself or on some part of the brain which controls pituitary gonadotropic secretion.

On the other hand, the same group of research workers (BOTROS et al. 1961, LINDSAY et al. 1961, 1962) observed that 5-HT and iproniazid were capable of producing not only interruption of pregnancy, possibly through an action on the placenta, but also marked disorganization of experimental deciduomata in mice. In order to elicit experimental decidual reaction, the females were mated with castrated males implanted with testosterone propionate pellets and on the fourth day after mating the uteri were traumatized by passing a double cotton thread along both horns. 5-HT was given subcutaneously or intraperitoneally at doses of 0.2—0.4 mg base per mouse.

The toxic effects of 5 HT could be prevented by the simultaneous administration of progesterone and, to a lesser extent, of luteotrophin.

ROBSON and co-workers were unable to decide whether 5-HT acted directly on the placenta or the corpus luteum, or indirectly through the pituitary or the centres in the brain responsible for controlling pituitary activity.

However, not all the above experimental results could be duplicated by other investigators. DE MELLO (1957) failed to detect any change in the macroscopic or microscopic aspect of the ovaries or any sign of follicular haemorrhage or follicular increase in the ovaries of rabbits treated, 48 hr previously, with intravenous or intracarotid injections of 0.2—5 mg/kg 5-HT base. He concluded that 5-HT does not play any role in the mechanism of liberation of gonadotropic hormones.

DISCHLER (1960) could not find any influence on the oestrus cycle of the mouse of either 5-HT (20—40 mg/kg, subcutaneously or intramuscularly, daily for 4 weeks) or iproniazid (120 mg/kg per os daily for 8 weeks) alone, or of the combination of the two drugs.

CZYBA and CHIRIS (1962), on the other hand, observed that whereas 5-HT hindered experimental traumatic decidual reaction in rats, it had no effect on rabbits and enhanced decidual reaction in hamsters. The doses of 5-HT base administered daily for 11 days were 10 mg/kg i.p. in rats, 2—5 mg/kg i.v. in rabbits and 4—10 mg/kg i.p. in hamsters.

Prolactin. POLLICE and MAIORANO (1958) first observed that daily subcutaneous administration, for 20 days, of 4 mg/kg 5-HT base displayed in the rat an evident stimulant effect on the growth of mammary glands, with hyperplasia of the duct system and lobulo-alveolar development. Effects were particularly evident in ovariectomized animals.

MEITES and co-workers (MEITES et al. 1959, MEITES and HOPKINS 1960) noted that in mature virgin rats, daily subcutaneous injections of 20 μg reserpine or 0.2 mg 5-HT base/kg for 5 days, preceded by daily injections of 10 μg estradiol for 10 days, initiated milk secretion and induced growth of mammary lobulo-alveolar tissue. When either drug was injected with estradiol for 10 days, mammary growth was greater than with estradiol alone, but there was little evidence of milk secretion. Injections of 5-HT and reserpine alone for 21 days failed to elicit mammary growth or secretion. Injections of 5-HT or reserpine for 10 days following litter removal on 4th day after parturition retarded mammary involution and maintained secretory function. In rats hypophysectomized after estrogen-priming the drugs were inactive in provoking mammary responses.

Induction of mammary growth and lactation is provoked by 5-HT (2 mg 5-HT base once daily, for 5 days, s.c.) also in estrogen-primed rabbits. 5-HT is more active than adrenaline or acetylcholine (MEITES et al. 1960).

Finally, lactation may be induced in normal rabbits by daily intracranial injection, into the hypothalamic region, of 4 mg 5-HT base in 1 ml physiological saline (KEHL et al. 1962).

It is concluded from the above results that 5-HT and reserpine stimulate in rats and rabbits secretion of prolactin and perhaps other factors by the pituitary favourable to mammary growth and lactation.

Effects of hypophysectomy. The influence of lack of all the hormones of the hypophysis, as produced by hypophysectomy, on the level of 5-HT in rat tissues is controversial.

DE MAIO (1959) found a reduction of the 5-HT concentration in serum (from 0.5 to 0.2 μg/ml) and an increase of the 5-HT level in the medulla oblongata (from 0.37 to 0.84 μg/g) and brain stem (from 0.97 to 1.54 μg/g), but these results could not be duplicated by YEH et al. (1959). GHIRINGHELLI et al. (1961b) observed that both the number of enterochromaffin cells and 5-HT concentration were decreased in the small intestine 28 days after hypophysectomy, and that intraperitoneal administration of STH (15 Evans units in the last 7 days) prevented to some extent the effects of hypophysectomy, but RESNICK et al. (1961) were unable to detect any change in brain or tissue 5-HT, including gastro-intestinal 5-HT, either following removal of hypophysis or administration of corticotropin (10 units for 10 days).

2. Supraoptico-hypophyseal tract

Daily subcutaneous doses of 0.2 mg/kg 5-HT base administered for 7 days produce in rats:

a) A decrease of the neurosecretory material in the posterior lobe of the hypophysis as well as in the cells of the supraoptic and paraventricular nuclei, with no change or even increase of the quantity of neurosecretory material going into the portal vessels in the region of the median eminence.

b) An increase in the nucleus and nucleolus volume in the cells of the nucleus supraopticus (KIVALO et al. 1958a, 1958b, HECKMANN et al. 1964).

c) A moderate increase of acetylcholinesterase and phosphatase activity of the hypothalamic magnocellular nuclei (KIVALO and RINNE 1959).

KIVALO and co-workers conclude from the above findings that 5-HT stimulates the activity of the supraoptico-hypophyseal tract, and that 5-HT antidiuresis seen in rats after 5-HT administration is due, at least in part, to an increased release of antidiuretic hormone.

3. Adrenals

ROSENKRANTZ and LAFERTE (1959, 1960) observed that the *in vitro* addition of 5-HT (40—400 μg base per pair of adrenals) produced the release of a blue tetrazolium-reactive reducing material, possibly steroid in nature, from the adrenals of rabbits, guinea-pigs, rats and cows, as well as from a human adrenal tumour which appeared cortical in nature. The releasing-activity of 5-HT, which was protected by iproniazid but completely inhibited by amphenone, appeared to be highly specific, as demonstrated by the failure of several other indolealkylamines, among which were 4-HT and 6-HT, to imitate the effect of 5-HT.

28 to 54% of added exogenous 5-HT was taken up by the adrenal tissue. Rabbit adrenal showed the least uptake in comparison with that of the dog, the cow and the rat, but released the greatest amount of blue-tetrazolium reducing materials. 5-HT was found to elevate oxygen consumption of the adrenals from all species. None of the observations on the uptake of 5-HT, release of reducing material or stimulation of oxygen consumption could be correlated with the dietary habits of the animals. The 5-HT action on the adrenals appeared to be dependent upon a functional oxidative phosphorylating system since the absence of oxygen and the presence of cyanide or dinitrophenol abolished the 5-HT response, whereas adenosine diphosphate augmented it. The optimal concentration for stimulation of adrenals was 80 μg 5-HT base/100 g tissue, and the optimal incubation period for the 5-HT stimulated release of reducing material was 90 min (CONNORS and ROSENKRANTZ 1962).

The above observations have been substantially confirmed and extended by others. CORMIER and JOUAN (1962) found that addition of 5-HT to the incubation liquid of slices of rat adrenals (65 μg 5-HT base per 100 mg adrenal tissue) produced a 30% increase in the secretion of aldosterone and steroid X2, leaving unaffected that of corticosterone, 11-deidrocorticosterone and steroid X3. It is concluded that 5-HT possesses a direct and selective action on corticogenesis. VERDESCA et al. (1961), in their turn, noted that 5-HT given by direct arterial perfusion of the adrenal glands of the hypophysectomized dog (20 μg/min) stimulated the secretion of hydrocortisone to a degree comparable to that seen during ACTH stimulation (1 u/min). Measurable quantities of corticosterone were also secreted. It is suggested that these findings offer a possible explanation of the sodium and chloride retention seen in man and animals following 5-HT administration.

It has been claimed that adrenalectomy produces in rats a decrease of 5-HT in serum (from 0.5 to 0.12 μg/ml) and an increase of 5-HT levels in the hemispheres (from 0.85 to 1.95 μg/g), brain base (from 0.97 to 1.15 μg/g) and medulla oblongata (from 0.37 to 1.4 μg/g) (DE MAIO 1959, SOFER and GUBLER 1962) as well as a progressive increase in the urinary excretion of 5-HIAA, the average 24 hr output being about 70% higher on the 4th and 5th day after adrenalectomy than during the four days before the operation (ENERBACK 1960).

Similarly, HICKS and WEST (1958) found that adrenalectomized rats given water presented a two-fold increase of the 5-HT levels in skin, ears, feet, liver and lung, whereas amine levels in adrenalectomized rats given saline remained normal. Not all the above results could be confirmed. TOWNE and SHERMAN (1960), for example, were unable to detect in rats any influence of acute bilateral adrenalectomy on brain 5-HT level, RESNICK et al. (1961) failed to reveal any change in the 5-HT content of brain and gastrointestinal tract, PFEIFER et al. (1963) found 3—7 days after adrenalectomy a decrease in the rat brain 5-HT from 0.69 to 0.31 μg/g.

PUT and MEDUSKI (1962b) observed in rats subjected to acute bilateral adrenalectomy a biphasic change in the metabolism of 5-HT. In the first post-operative phase (up to 24 hr after surgery) there was an immediate increase in urinary 5-HIAA excretion (up to 200%) with unchanged brain 5-HT level; in the second post-operative phase 5-HIAA returned, more or less promptly, towards normal whilst brain 5-HT level appeared reduced to 12—15% of that of control rats. On the basis of these results PUT and MEDUSKI put forward a questionable theory on probable mechanism of binding and release of 5-HT by tissues.

Daily intramuscular injections of cortisone, prednisolone, triamcinolone, dexamethasone, fludrocortisone and 2-methylfludrocortisone are found to lower the 5-HT level in the skin and small intestine of normal rats (in spleen no 5-HT depletion is noted and the stomach presents, instead of a decrease, an increase in the amine content), to retard the recovery of 5-HT in the skin depleted of the amine by prolonged treatment with polymyxin or with compound 48/80, and to restore to normal the increased 5-HT concentration seen in the skin of adrenalectomized rats. Sex hormones are weaker in these effects, while mineralocorticoids and corticotrophin are inactive. Corticosteroids have no effect on the dopa-decarboxylase activity either of kidney or of liver (HICKS and WEST 1958; WEST 1959; TELFORD and WEST 1960, 1961; CASS and MARSHALL 1962). On the basis of all these results, TELFORD and WEST (1961) suggest that the tissue reserves of 5-HT, like those of histamine, may be in part regulated in rats by the secretion of the adrenal cortex.

Adrenalectomized rats given saline and DOCA show after 10 days a 45% increase of the 5-HT content of the small intestine, accompanied by a similar increase in the number and granular charge of the enterochromaffin cells of the duodenum (GHIRINGHELLI et al. 1961a).

In man glucocorticoids produce an increase in the urinary excretion of 5-HIAA, both following single and repeated doses (SCHWEMMLE et al. 1961).

It is well known that large doses of subcutaneous 5-HT are capable of eliciting in rats acral swelling. BOIS and SELYE (1956) observed that oedema produced by 5-HT (10 mg/kg, s.c.) in adrenalectomized animals was most pronounced after administration of DOCA, 100 μg/day, slightly less so after maintenance on 1% NaCl only or administration of DOCA plus cortisol, and almost completely absent after administration of cortisol acetate, 400 μg/day.

The report of DAVIS and KENNEDY (1962) concerning a case of carcinoid syndrome associated with adrenal hyperplasia is of interest.

4. Thyroid

ZIZINE (1959) and D'ADDARIO et al. (1963) found that single or repeated injections of 5-HT (e.g. 1—2 mg/kg 5-HT base s.c. every second day for 20 days) produced in rats a decrease of thyroid activity, as studied by means of radioactive iodine, and histological signs of atrophy of the parenchymal cells. SALABE' et al. (1963), on the contrary, were unable to detect any significant difference in the ^{131}I uptake by the thyroid gland of rats given 5-HT (3 mg/kg i.m. for 7 days) and of control rats.

In the rabbit, daily intramuscular administration for 4 months of 2 mg/kg 5-HT produces, according to CARLIER et al. (1960) increase in weight and vascularity of the thyroid gland with histological signs of hyperactivity. Similar, but less pronounced results, may be obtained with 5-HTP.

40 μg 5-HT base put onto the surface of a chicken embryo on the 3rd or 9th day of incubation causes a significant increase in the uptake of radioactive iodine

by the thyroid tissue, eventually preceded by a decrease. MARAUD et al. (1962) suggest that this effect may be secondary to the vascular changes produced by the amine.

All research workers agree that thyroidectomy does not change the 5-HT content of brain and other tissues of the rat (TOWNE et al. 1959, RESNICK et al. 1961, PUT and HOGENHUIS 1962). On the other hand, administration of thyroid hormone or antithyroid compounds seems to produce different results in different tissues.

The 5-HT level in the rat brain, for example, is significantly increased (from 0.56 to 1.01 and 0.92 μg/g, respectively) both after subcutaneous injection of L-thyroxine (500 μg/kg daily for 14 days) and after administration ad libitum, for 14 days, of a 0.075% solution of propylthiouracil (TOWNE et al. 1959, PUT and HOGENHUIS 1962). However, feeding for 21 days a meal containing 0.15% strong desiccated thyroid produces a decrease of heart 5-HT only in female rats (from 0.8 to 0.54 μg/g) with no significant effect in males, and feeding a meal containing 0.15% propylthiouracil causes no significant change of heart 5-HT either in male or female rats (SKILLEN et al. 1962).

Similar ambiguous results have been reported in man. In fact, the increased urinary excretion of 5-HIAA seen in thyrotoxic patients by SKANSE and HANSON (1962) has not been observed by KUSCHKE et al. (1962).

The subcutaneous administration of 1 mg/kg melatonin, every day for 10 days, produces in the rat a 20% reduction in thyroid weight, a decrease of nearly 50% in cell height, a prevention of thyroid hyperplasia by methylthiouracil and finally a drastic reduction (from 42.2 to 2%) in the uptake of radioactive iodine by the thyroid gland. This inhibitory effect of melatonin on thyroid function is ascribed by BASCHIERI et al. (1963) to an inhibition of either the secretion of the thyrotropic hormone or the action of this hormone on the thyroid gland.

5. Pineal gland

It has been suggested by JOUAN (1963), without any persuasive evidence, that the factor secreted by the pineal gland which induces secretion of aldosterone is closely related to 5-HT.

6. Testes

5-HT (3—6 mg/kg, s.c.) and histamine (100—200 mg/kg) when administered either separately or in combination, cause weight increase of the mouse prostate gland (from 33.4 to 68.3 mg/100 g) and histological changes indicative of edema or vascular defect. Pathological changes in testes of treated mice include degenerating seminiferous tubules that contain spermatogonial cells with pyknotic nuclei and giant multinucleate cells. O'STEEN (1963) suggests that the above histological changes are not necessarily dependent upon vascular effects of the two amines.

Rats subjected to orchidectomy or injected with testosterone cyclopentylpropionate (three 7 mg doses, one dose every three weeks) show no change in tissue 5-HT (RESNICK et al. 1961).

Male specimens of *Rana esculenta* present in 73% of cases an ejaculation when 5 mg 5-HT is injected into the dorsal lymphatic sac. Maximum response is observed after 5 hr. This gametokinetic activity is ascribed to pituitary stimulation (SALVADORI et al. 1962).

7. Ovary

Daily injections, for 28 days, of microgram amounts of melatonin (20 to 200 μg/kg, i.p.) in rats decrease the incidence of oestrus and reduce ovarian weight. This effect is reduced by exposure of the rats to constant light. Circulating exogenous melatonin is selectively taken up and retained by the ovary and pineal gland. On the basis of these and other experimental results (cf. pag. 152—153) WURTMAN et al. (1963, 1964) and AXELROD et al. (1964) suggest that it is possible that some of the effects of the pineal gland on gonad function of rats are mediated by melatonin, and similarly that some of the effects of lighting on bird gonads are mediated by alterations in the rate of synthesis of melatonin in the pineal gland.

This may certainly be true, but it should be pointed out, however, that in spite of all appearance, the doses of melatonin injected into the rat by WURTMAN and his colleagues are very high, if compared with the content of endogenous melatonin in the rat pineal gland [1—3 ng/pineal, according to QUAY (1964)], and with the melatonin-synthesizing capacity of the rat pineal gland [2.5—5 ng/hr/pineal, according to WURTMAN et al. (1964)].

8. Pancreas

On the basis of experiments carried out *in vitro* on the rat diaphragm, UI (1962b) suggests that 5-HT is a physiological "accelerator" of insulin secretion in the organism.

The concentration of 5-HT in the dog blood is not affected by total pancreasectomy (LOUBATIÈRES et al. 1963).

It is highly probable that endocrine glands, neurohormones and tissue hormones interfere in the biosynthesis, release and metabolism of 5-HT, as well as in the physiological actions of the amine. However, up to the present time, meagre information is available on the most intimate biochemical and functional correlations existing between 5-HT and other hormones or active tissue products. In fact, very often doses of 5-HT which have been found to elicit responses by endocrine glands are far beyond physiological limits and, on the other hand, removal of endocrine glands or administration of hormones have frequently given conflicting or ambiguous results.

XVI. Protective action of indolealkylamines in experimental tissue injury

1. Radiation injury

Since the first communication by GRAY et al. (1962) a considerable number of research papers has been devoted to the description of the protective effects of 5-HT and related indolealkylamines against ionizing radiations. In addition to the authors quoted in the text see also, for complete information on the topic, BRAUN et al. (1960), HIETBRINK et al. (1961), PANASEWICZ et al. (1961), TRICOU and DOULL (1960b, 1961), WANG et al. (1961), VENINGA and BRINKMAN (1962). FRANZEN (1962), VITTORIO et al. (1963), DOULL et al. (1963), ZHEREBCHENKO et al, (1963).

a) Reduction of radiation lethality

Mouse. The most extensive investigation on the protective effect of indolealkylamines has been carried out in the mouse.

Protection afforded by different intraperitoneal doses of 5-HT against whole-body irradiation with 810 r is as follows, according to LANGENDORFF et al. (1958):

5-HT dose	Survival rate (%) after 30 days
Nil (controls)	2
0.2 mg/mouse	31
0.4 mg/mouse	80
0.6 mg/mouse	53
0.8 mg/mouse	72
1.0 mg/mouse	82
1.5 mg/mouse	58

Essentially similar results have been obtained by BACQ (1954), TRICOU and DOULL (1960a, 1960c), PANASEWICZ and LOPACIUK (1960), LEITSCH (1961), WANG and KEREIAKES (1962) and COHEN and COHEN (1962).

Protection is maximal when 5-HT is administered 0—5 min before irradiation, negligible when the amine is given more than 30 min before irradiation or after irradiation (MELCHING et al. 1958, LANGENDORFF et al. 1958, DUKOR 1962).

Table 2. *Radioprotective action of indolealkylamines* (DUKOR and SCHÜPPLI 1961)

Compound (50 mg/kg, i. p.)	Survival rate (%) after 30 days	
	900 r	1050 r
5-HT and creatinine sulphate	100	65
N-methyl-5-HT dioxalate	100	
N,N-dimethyl-5-HT dioxalate	5	
1-methyl-5-HT and creatinine sulphate	0	
5-methoxytryptamine base	80	60
5-methoxy-N-acetyltryptamine base	0	
4-HT oxalate	12.5	5
N-methyl-4-HT oxalate	0	
N,N-dimethyl-4-HT base	0	
α-methyl-4-HT dimaleinate	0	
Controls	2.5	0

5-HT is active not only against a single exposure to X-irradiation, but also against repeated whole-body irradiation with lethal doses (LANGENDORFF et al. 1959a).

The protective effect of 5-HT is reinforced by simultaneous administration of adenosine triphosphate or adenosine monophosphate (LANGENDORFF et al. 1960). Similarly, survival rate from radiation is increased by combination of 5-HT with either AET (aminoethylisothiouronium) or MEA (mercaptoethylamine) (MAISIN and DOHERTY 1960, LEITCH 1961, WANG and KEREIAKES 1962, LANDAHL and HASEGAWA 1962, 1963). For example, whereas at 1100 r no protection is afforded by 88 mg/kg of 5-HT alone, the same dose of 5-HT administered together with AET or MEA gives 70—80% protections (WANG and KEREIAKES 1962).

However, combined treatment with AET (8.8 mg/mouse, i.p.) and 5-HT (0.4 mg/mouse, i.p.) while providing better protection to the bone marrow than either alone, does not increase intestinal protection beyond that of AET alone (MAISIN and DOHERTY 1963, MAISIN et al. 1963).

Combination of 5-HT with MAO inhibitors causes a significant increase in the survival time of irradiated mice (DUKOR 1962), combination with LSD, BOL, BOL + LSD or UML (Deseril) strongly reduces or even completely abolishes the protective effect of 5-HT (LANGENDORFF et al. 1959, VAN DEN BRENK and HAAS 1961, DUKOR 1962).

The radioprotective activity of a number of indolealkylamines related to 5-HT is summarized in Table 2. The drugs were given intraperitoneally, in doses of 50 mg/kg, 5 min before exposure to whole-body irradiation with 900 and 1050 r.

In other experiments N-ethyl-5-HT proved to be as effective as 5-HT and 5-benzyloxytryptamine as effective as 4-HT. N-acetyl-5-HT, β-methyl-5-HT, β-dimethyl-5-HT, 6-HT and 7-HT showed no radioprotective activity (DUKOR 1962). Protection afforded by 100 mg/kg tryptophan and 20 mg/kg 5-HTP given 60—90 min prior to irradiation was moderate (LANGENDORFF 1959). The combination of 5-HTP with either pyridoxal-5-phosphate or adenosinetriphosphate, or of 5-HTP and tranylcypromine, a MAO inhibitor, was more active than 5-HTP alone (LANGENDORFF and MELCHING 1959, COEN and WHITEHEAD 1962).

On examination of the blood and tissues of protected animals, eventually in comparison with the tissues of non-protected animals, it emerged that: a) none of the 5-HT-protected mice developed leucaemia, b) lymphocytosis and leucocytosis seen soon after irradiation showed complete regression later on, c) whereas the red blood count was only slightly decreased 7—9 months after irradiation, haemoglobin was significantly reduced (MIYATA et al. 1960), d) whereas the decrease of reticulocytes in the peripheral blood produced by whole-body irradiation with 75 r was to a great extent prevented by 5-HT, the disturbance in the incorporation of ^{59}Fe into young erythrocytes was not corrected by the amine (ELTGEN et al. 1961), e) whereas radiation injury seen in spleen and thymus was the same during the first few days both in protected and non-protected mice, later on the organs of the protected animals showed faster recovery, and finally f) there was an immediate partial protection of the bone marrow, as shown by a smaller reduction of the cell count in the marrow of protected animals (LANGENDORFF and HAGEN 1962, HAGEN and FLEMMING 1963).

Besides increasing survival time, large doses of 5-HT and tryptamine (6 to 200 mg) are capable of protecting mice effectively against epilation caused by X-irradiation (RADIVOJEVIĆ et al. 1960).

It has been demonstrated that splenectomy increases the survival rate of irradiated mice. Surprisingly, this protective effect is reduced by administration of 5-HT (MELCHING et al. 1961).

Rat. GRAY et al. (1952) first observed that the survival rate of rats exposed to lethal X-ray dosage is significantly increased after intraperitoneal pretreatment with 9 mg/kg 5-HT. This observation was soon confirmed by others.

Following intraperitoneal injection of 8 mg/kg 5-HT base 5 min prior to whole-body irradiation with 690 and 800 r, survival rate after 30 days increases from 4—16 to 57—58%, and from 0 to 13—33%, respectively (KRIEGEL and MELCHING 1959). At the same time a reduction of incidence of diarrhoea may be observed in the survivors (VAN DEN BRENK and ELLIOTT 1958).

Intraperitoneal administration of 8 mg/kg 5-HT base 30 min prior to whole body irradiation with 1000 r displays an evident protective effect against depletion of Gomori-positive neurosecretory material in the posterior lobe of the hypophysis produced by irradiation (HECKMANN et al. 1964).

The radioprotective action of 5-methoxytryptamine (10 mg/kg, i.p., 5 min before exposure to 900 r) seems to be greater than that of 5-HT. 5-Benzyloxytryptamine, 4-hydroxy-N,N-dimethytryptamine and tryptamine, on the contrary, do not show any protective effect (SUPEK et al. 1961).

Guinea-pig. 6 mg/kg of 5-HT base given by intraperitoneal route 5 min before irradiation of a guinea-pig flank completely prevents the temporary epilation produced by 800 r and changes into temporary the persistent epilation produced by 1600 r. On histological examination carried out 23—35 days after irradiation the skin of protected animals shows well-preserved hair bulbs together with numerous mitoses. Acanthosis is less pronounced (MAGGIORA 1960, 1962a).

The protective effect of 5-HT is manifested only if the amine is administered not more than 3 hr before irradiation (MAGGIORA 1962b).

Following administration of 5-HT by ionophoresis (2 mg 5-HT, 20 min) it may be observed, surprisingly enough, that the treated flank is less protected against the epilatory effect of X-rays than the opposite flank, where 5-HT arrives via the blood (MAGGIORA 1963).

Bufotenine, like 5-HT, shows a strong protective action. Feeble protection is afforded by 5-HTP and tryptophan and no protection by 5-HIAA, IAA, psilocine, psilocybine, tryptamine and 5-indoleacetamide (15 mg/animal, i.p.). Surprisingly enough, UML (10 mg, s.c.) does not counteract the protective effect of 5-HT (MAGGIORA and BRUN 1963).

Dog. Chemical mixtures including 5-HT reduce radiation lethality in dogs also (WANG and DAVIDSON 1961).

b) Effects of 5-HT on response of tumours to in vivo irradiation

5-HT (0.4 mg/mouse, i.p., 8—10 min before irradiation) has been found by COHEN and COHEN (1962) to inhibit the response of the isogenic mammary carcinoma to doses of radiation which are normally curative in non-medicated controls, reducing the cure-rate to about half of its control level. On the other hand, whereas direct transthoracic irradiation of both tumour and host tissues with the standard test dose of 7500 r was uniformly lethal to unprotected controls, 5-HT appeared to protect mice from the early mortality associated with the visceral phase of the postirradiation syndrome.

A similar reduction of the radiosensitivity of tumours was produced by 5-HT in the case of Ehrlich ascites and of Ehrlich solid carcinoma. The irradiated Crocker sarcoma, on the contrary, was not protected by 5-HT (KOCH 1962).

It seems pertinent to remember here that 5-HT produces a much greater fall of oxygen tension in tumoral tissue, as followed by a polarographic method, than in bone marrow and muscle (CATER 1962).

c) Radioprotective action of 5-HT in vegetables

When seeds of *Vicia faba* are exposed to an X-ray dose of 400 r the growth of accessory roots is completely inhibited. However, seeds plunged into a 5-HT solution (concentration ?) for 30 min and then irradiated develop accessory roots, at least to a certain extent, after an inhibitory phase of 6 to 8 days (LOZERON et al. 1964).

d) Effect of 5-HT on irradiation-induced mutation rate of bacteria

Following addition of 5-HT, up to 0.01 M concentrations, to a suspension of *E. coli* (strain B/r and its leucine-dependent mutant) irradiated with 40000 r (800 r/min) survival rate increases from 6.5 to 17.7% and irradiation-induced back-mutation to prototrophy is halved (KÜNKEL and TRAMS 1963).

e) Mechanism of the radioprotective action of 5-HT

According to GRAY et al. (1952), VAN DEN BRENK and MOORE (1958), VAN DEN MEER et al. (1961) and BOOZ and BETZ (1961), protection afforded by 5-HT against ionizing radiation is mainly due to vasoconstriction with ensuing temporary tissue anoxia. This view is strongly supported by the experimental results of VAN DEN BRENK and MOORE (1958) showing that increase in respired oxygen pressure to 4 or 5 atmospheres absolute pressure almost completely reverses the protective action of 5-HT, and by the observation of Booz and Betz (1961) that 5-HT and tryptamine do not protect thymocytes *in vitro* against radiation injury.

However, other investigators maintain that the anoxic mechanism is insufficient to explain the protective effect of 5-HT and suggest that the amine may also act via the central nervous system (Langendorff and Koch 1957), through neutralization of free radicals of water (Alexander et al. 1955) or through a more specific protection of the radio-sensitive substrate against reactive radicals (Dukor 1962). Langendorff and Melching (1959) further suggest that exogenous 5-HT may compensate for lack of endogenous 5-HT due to hindered decarboxylation of 5-HTP (Langendorff and Hagen 1963).

Dukor (1962) affirms that there is no parallelism between the pharmacological effects of indolealkylamines and radioprotection. In the writer's opinion rather the opposite is true, unless a strictly quantitative parallelism is demanded. Furthermore, no comparative data are available on the pharmacological effects (vasoconstriction!) of the different indolealkylamines on the most radiosensitive tissues, such as, for example, intestines and bone marrow.

For description of the effects of X-irradiation on 5-HT levels in tissues and 5-HIAA excretion see pages 373—375.

2. Liver cirrhosis

5-HT administered subcutaneously every other day in doses of 4 mg/kg during the early phase of cirrhogenic treatment, inhibits liver cirrhosis induced by carbon tetrachloride. No comparable effect is observed in rats treated with 5-HT at a more advanced stage of CCl_4 administration. Combined administration of 5-HT and CCl_4 results in 50% reduction of hepatic cellular damage (Fiore-Donati et al. 1958, 1959b; Fiore-Donati and Chieco-Bianchi 1960).

Similarly, 5-HT (13 mg/kg of the base, i.p.) affords considerable protection against liver damage provoked in rats by allyl alcohol, provided that it is administered 15—30 min prior to the poison. No protection is seen when 5-HT is given 2 hr before allyl alcohol (Eger 1958).

5-HT does not influence fatty liver, leading to cirrhosis, when produced with a choline-deficient, high-fat, high-caloric diet (MacDonald et al. 1958).

Fiore-Donati et al. (1959b) suggest that the hepatoprotective effect of 5-HT may be due to liberation of ACTH or adrenocortical steroids rather than to any vascular effect of 5-HT.

3. Cardiac and renal necroses

5-HT injected subcutaneously at a dose of 0.4 to 0.6 mg/animal twice daily, prevents renal and cardiac calcifications induced in rats by dihydrotachysterol administered per os at a dose of 0.25 mg for 5 consecutive days. This preventive action is also demonstrable with regard to cardiac calcifications produced by plasmocid and coronary vein ligature, as well as to skeletal muscle calcifications produced by paraphenylendiamine. 5-HT diminishes but does not prevent degenerative and necrotic lesions associated with these calcifications. On the other hand, the development of massive cardiac infarcts that follows the occlusion of the left main coronary artery cannot be influenced by 5-HT.

Similar protection is afforded by 5-HTP and nialamide, in daily doses of 200 and 30 mg/kg, respectively.

The mode of action of these agents is obscure because 5-HT prevents the deposition of calcium salts without changing calcium blood level. It may be that 5-HT acts through vasoconstriction or through decrease of the oxygen requirements of the myocardium (BAJUSZ and JASMIN 1962, JASMIN and BAJUSZ 1962).

XVII. Miscellaneous effects

1. Action on striated muscle

a) Crustaceans. The injection of 1 μg 5-HT into the musculature of the pincers of *Potamoebius*, through the tip of the propodite, causes, after a short latency, an abrupt powerful closing of the pincers which lasts for several minutes. An exactly similar result is produced by extracts of nervous tissue of cephalopods and decapod crustaceans, extracts which like 5-HT are also active on the heart (FLOREY and FLOREY 1954).

b) Insects. The effect of tryptamine analogues on the neuromuscular transmission of impulses in the jumping leg of the locust *Schnistocerca gregaria* has been studied by recording action potentials and active membrane responses with intracellular micro-electrodes, and by recording tension with a mechano-electronic transducer.

High concentrations of 5-HT and tryptamine (10^{-2} to 10^{-3} M) block the development of an action potential and of tension in fibres of the metathoracic extensor tibialis and flexor tibialis muscles, but do not block the action potential in the fibres of the crural nerve which supplies "fast" motor axons to the extensor and flexor tibialis. Tryptamine analogues do not inhibit the active membrane response in the fibres of the extensor or flexor tibialis, or alter their membrane resistance. It is concluded by HILL and USHERWOOD (1961) that 5-HT and tryptamine block neuromuscular transmission in the locust.

LSD and BOL do not antagonize 5-HT but, on the contrary, have effects similar to those of the amine and in similar concentrations.

c) Mammals. The statement of PHILIPPOT and DALLEMAGNE (1956) and of SALA and PERRIS (1958) that 5-HT (25—400 μg/kg, i.v.) is caprable of moderately antagonizing, in the cat and in the rabbit, the neuro-muscula block produced by tubocurarine, but not that produced by decamethonium was not confirmed in man by FROSALI et al. (1961).

Artificial actomyosin threads are poorly sensitive to 5-HT. In fact, the threshold dose for actomyosin prepared from ox heart is 50 μg/ml, that for actomyosin obtained from bovine striated muscle 250 μg/ml (KURIAKI and INOUE 1955, INOUE 1956).

2. Action on the gill cilia of molluscs

Both 5-HT (threshold concentration 0.1 μg/ml, optimum concentration 10 μg/ml) and 5-HTP (5—100 μg/ml) stimulate the activity of lateral gill cilia of *Mytilus edulis* and of other lamellibranchiates.

Beat frequency of the cilia and velocity of the metachronal wave increase, while the average wave length remains unchanged (AIELLO 1957, 1960a, 1960b; GOSSELIN and ERNST 1958; GOSSELIN 1961). The acceleration, as measured in stroboscopic light, is prompt, sustained, and graded over a wide range of drug concentrations. Maximal frequencies, however, are not greater than those sometimes encountered in untreated gills. Different gill preparations may vary widely in sensitivity and summer *Mytilus* is more sensitive to 5-HT than winter *Mytilus*. In summer *Mytilus* high concentrations of 5-HT inhibit the ciliary activity, instead of increasing it (GOSSELIN 1961).

The action of 5-HTP is less prompt than that of 5-HT but lasts longer, up to several hours (Milton and Gosselin 1960b). LSD and BOL block the action of 5-HT, but at the same time are effective accelerators of gill cilia (Gosselin and Ernst 1958). According to Aiello (1963), 5-HT affects ciliary activity by some action at or near the cell surface.

Since the gills of lamellibranchiates contain detectable amounts of 5-HT, it has been suggested that this endogenous 5-HT is concerned in the physiological regulation of ciliary activity (Aiello 1960b, 1962; Milton and Gosselin 1960b; Gosselin et al. 1962).

Similarly, it is possible that 5-HT plays a role in the motor activity of embryos of some marine gastropods, through stimulation of their cilia (Koshtoyants et al. 1961).

3. Action on lymph flow

5-HT infused intravenously into unanaesthetized dogs at a rate of 20 μg/kg/min produces a 115% increase in lymph flow from the thoracic duct cannulated with a polyethylene catheter, with a 20% decrease in total protein concentration. According to Shim et al. (1961) these effects are brought about by a probable selective alteration of capillary permeability rather than by increasing intestinal motility.

4. Action on intra-ocular pressure

The intravenous injection of 7 μg/kg 5-HT base produces in the dog an evident reduction of intra-ocular pressure which does not parallel systemic hypotension.

Intra-ocular pressure of the rabbit is not affected by the introduction of 5-HT into the conjunctival sac but is consistently reduced following subconjunctival or retrobulbar injection of 90—450 μg 5-HT. This effect is not changed by antihistamine compounds and is only slightly increased following pretreatment with iproniazid (Schumacher and Classen 1962b).

5. Histamine-releasing activity

Tryptamine and 5-HT, according to Feldberg and Smith (1953), are to be listed among the drugs able to release histamine. This property of the indolealkylamines has been shown experimentally on perfused isolated skin flaps and gastrocnemius muscles of the cat and the dog after arterial injections of 1 to 5 mg of the substance (estimation of histamine in the venous effluent), as well as on rat tissues after subcutaneous or intraperitoneal injections of 2 mg 5-HT or 13 mg tryptamine (estimation of tissue histamine). The activity of the indolealkylamines is somewhat greater than that of propamidine, but about 100 times less than that of compound 48/80. Feldberg and Smith suggest that histamine release may be at the root of certain phenomena resembling effects of histamine which are seen in the intact animal after injection of tryptamine compounds. This opinion is shared by several research workers. Scarinci (1955b, 1955c) and Buñag and Walaszak (1962b), for example, believe that hypotension seen in dogs and chickens following intravenous injection of 5-HT is largely due to liberation of histamine.

6. Action on phagocytosis

Ludány et al. (1958) observed that 5-HT enhanced phagocytosis by rat leucocytes obtained from the peritoneal cavity by injection of bouillon, and by circulating rabbit leucocytes. Increase in phagocytosis was 25% at 100 μg/ml concentration of 5-HT, and 13% at 10 μg/ml concentration. Lower concentrations were ineffective and so was tryptamine at concentrations up to 1 mg/ml. LSD (1 μg/ml) did not inhibit the stimulant action of 5-HT.

These observations were confirmed and extended by NORTHOVER (1961), who found that, at concentrations as low as 1—10 μg/ml, 5-HT stimulated phagocytosis both by rabbit neutrophil polymorphonuclear leucocytes (obtained from the peritoneal cavity by injection of sterile isotonic saline solution) and by rabbit macrophages (obtained by intraperitoneal injection of a mixture of liquid paraffin, peptone water and acacia solution). 5-HTP acted similarly in somewhat higher concentrations and 1 μg/ml appeared to stimulate significantly only phagocytosis by macrophages. BOL was not found capable of preventing the phagocytosis-stimulating action of 5-HT and 5-HTP.

7. Action on tumour growth

When 1.3 mg of 5-HT or 1.1 mg histamine is administered to rats daily, starting 2 days prior to sarcoma implantation, the animals have larger tumours than their controls (0.4 g as compared to 0.3 g). 5-HT depletion with reserpine decreases tumour growth and/or the percentage of takes. Lysergic acid derivatives (LSD, BOL and MLD) antagonize the action of 5-HT. These results suggest that 5-HT and histamine are beneficial to tumour growth (SCOTT et al. 1958, SCOTT and STONE 1959).

In sharp contrast to the above observations, PURKHALSKAIA et al. (1961), SOKOLOFF et al. (1961) and PURKHALSKAIA (1962) found that large doses of 5-HT (3—200 mg/kg, i.p. or s.c.) inhibited by 42 to 97% the growth of 7 out of 9 varieties of tumour in mice and rats. The tumours, however, did not resolve completely in any instance, and oral administration of 5-HT produced no effect.

Similarly, 1 mg 5-HT injected directly into S-91 melanoma or S-180 sarcoma implanted on the feet of mice immediately before exposure of the feet to heat (44° for from 30 to 40 min) increased the "curative" effect of heating. Moreover, 1 mg 5-HT injected daily into tumours for from 2 to 3 weeks and accompanied by no heating "cured" 7 out of 55 mice with S-91 melanoma, as compared with one "cure" in 46 mice given injections of saline. If the tumour did not disappear, the rate of growth was greatly reduced (CRILE 1963).

Indoleacetic acid inhibits mitotic activity in LIEBERKÜHN's crypts, as studied by the DUSTIN's colchicine method, when injected intraperitoneally to mice in doses of 2—10 mg/kg (LEAHU 1961).

8. Action on pigment formation

Coats of yellow Ay/a mice given subcutaneous injections of 1 mg/g of DL-5-methyltryptophan daily for a period of 7—10 days, starting at 3—4 days of age, appear darker in colour than those of controls. These results support the idea that tryptophan or a derivative may be utilized for pigment formation by these mice (NACHMIAS 1961).

Utilization of 5-HT in the synthesis of plant pigments is indirectly suggested by the distribution of 5-HT in the vegetable kingdom, and more directly proved by the observation of BROWN and NICHOLS (1958) that addition of 5-HT to an aqueous medium (10—250 μg/ml) results in increased pigmentation of surviving slices of potato tuber.

9. Action on bioluminescence

5-HT introduced into sea water to give a concentration of 20 μg free base/ml initiates prolonged luminescence of the euphausiid crustacean *Meganyctiphanes norvegica* without apparently damaging the creature. Lower concentrations stimulate no luminescence. However, 5-HT concentrations insufficient to initiate luminescence facilitate the luminescent glow following exposure to room light or to electronic flash. There is reduction in the delay of response and increase in duration and/or intensity of the luminescent response. According to KAY (1963) it is possible that the third step in the chain retina → nervous system → transmitter → photophore luminescence is represented by 5-HT.

10. Action on growth of plant tissues

5-HT (1—100 μg/ml) seems slightly to enhance the growth of plant tissues (NIAUSSAT and DUBOIS 1962, PILET 1962). It may be that the amine acts upon water uptake, by regulating cellular permeability (PILET 1962).

On the elongation of the coleoptiles of *Triticum sativum*, 5-HT is the least active of the four examined indole derivatives, the most active being IAA, followed in order by tryptamine and 5-HIAA. PILET (1963) suggests that indoles other than IAA may act after partial transformation in vivo into IAA.

11. Action on food intake

5-HT injected subcutaneously in daily doses of 1.2 mg/kg for 10 days, decreases food and caloric intake, but not glucose intake in the rat (SOULAIRAC and SOULAIRAC 1960).

12. Action on metamorphosis in amphibians

Tadpoles of *Rana temporaria* injected every other day with 40 μg 5-HT base grow and overcome the metamorphosis crisis exactly as the controls do. Larger doses of the amine (200 μg) are, on the contrary, fatal to the larvae (KEHL et al. 1961).

13. Inhibition of mitochondria swelling

The observation of CASU (1960) that 5-HT has a protective action on liver mitochondria swelling in 0.25 M sucrose is apparently of only slight interest, owing to the enormous concentrations of 5-HT required to elicit the effect (200 μg/ml).

14. Action on brain microsomes

AGHAJANIAN (1963) observed that ascorbic acid produces in specially prepared rat brain microsomes (membrane fragments) a gradual decrease of light scattering and protein fluorescence, and that 5-HT is a powerful inhibitor of these structural changes. There is complete inhibition at about 4×10^{-4}, with graded lesser effects down to 5×10^{-6} or lower.

15. Action on cerebro-spinal fluid pressure

Small doses of 5-HT (2—10 μg/kg, i.v.) initially cause a drop, later on an increase in cerebro-spinal fluid pressure (animal species not indicated!). This biphasic reaction is still more obvious in the case of greater doses (100—1000 μg/kg). The initial phase is very short (10—20 seconds), the second one lasts longer (20—35 min) and occurs when the blood pressure is about to return to its original level (KELENTEY 1963).

16. Action on collagen

5-HT consistently reduces the shrinkage temperature of normal human collagen obtained from the tendo Achillis of people who had died in accidents. With 0.02 M 5-HT reduction is by 1.5—4^{0} from the normal shrinkage temperature of 60^0, with 0.08 M by 7 to 12^0, with 0.32 M by up to 30^0. 5-Methoxytryptamine and tryptamine produce only a slight reduction; 5-HTP and 5-HIAA, on the contrary, raise the shrinkage temperature. The electron-microscopic appearances of specimens of collagen affected by 5-HT show progressive disorganization. These results suggest that 5-HT may have a direct and important effect on collagen in some disorders, such as rheumatoid arthritis and carcinoid syndrome (Highton and Garrett 1963).

17. Teratogenic effect

The subcutaneous injection of single doses of 5-HT (0.2—0.8 mg 5-HT base/animal) into pregnant mice produces a large number of foetal abnormalities, mostly of the eyes (absence of one or both eyes, absence of eyelids, one cyclops), limbs (polydactily and syndactily, phocomelia) and tail (absence of tail). The skull and the central nervous system are also sometimes affected (exencephaly, exomphalos). The incidence of abnormalities reaches a maximum of about 30% of surviving foetuses when the injection is given on the 9th to 10th day of pregnancy. The teratogenic effect of 5-HT is inhibited by the administration of 5-HT antagonists, but not by the simultaneous administration of progesterone (Poulson et al. 1963a, 1963b; Robson and Sullivan 1964).

Similar results have been obtained, again in the mouse, by Seller (1964), and in the rat by Reddy et al. (1963) following subcutaneous administration of 5-HT during pregnancy, in daily doses of 1.5—15 mg/kg. Reddy and co-workers briefly describe also two cases of carcinoid syndrome in human beings, in which pregnancy resulted in abortion, in infants who died within a few hours after birth, and in an infant presenting multiple congenital malformations.

According to Robson and Sullivan (1964) there is quite clear evidence that 5-HT interferes with the blood supply to the placenta and with the nutrition of the foetus and it seems likely that this effect is responsible for the development of abnormalities. Thus, as the majority of teratogens, also 5-HT acts on some point in the uterus or the placenta or the umbilical vessels.

(For References see at the end of Chapter 8)

Chapter 8

Participation of 5-hydroxytryptamine in physiopathological processes

By

Vittorio Erspamer

With 1 Figure

I. Anaphylaxis

1. Mouse

Starting from the observations that both egg-white sensitized and normal mouse uteri are 1000 times more sensitive to 5-HT than they are to histamine and that LSD and reserpine always completely prevent anaphylactic contraction on strips of sensitized uteri, Fink (1956) first suggested that the Schultz-Dale reaction and, more generally, the systemic anaphylactic reaction in the mouse was dependent on the release of 5-HT.

This view has been accepted by other investigators. Sanyal and West (1959) confirmed that the anaphylactic reaction of the isolated actively sensitized uterus was blocked by BOL but not by mepyramine; Gershon and Ross (1961) found that depletion of body depots of 5-HT produced by reserpine (5 mg/kg, i.p.) or α-methyl DOPA (nine injections of 400 mg/kg each, at 6 hr intervals) afforded protection against anaphylactic shock and that the effect of shock on behaviour and body temperature was similar to the effect on behaviour and temperature produced by reserpine.

Tokuda and Weiser (1960, 1961) studied the anaphylactic response of the mouse to challenge with a soluble antigen-antibody complex composed of bovine serum albumin — antibovine serum albumin. They observed that protection against anaphylaxis was afforded by prechallenge treatment with either reserpine, LSD, BOL, chlorpromazine, epinephrine, norepinephrine, dopamine, histamine or sodium salicylate, and that the protective effect of reserpine could be abolished with 5-hydroxytryptophan but not with DOPA. Prechallenge treatment with 5-HT or 5-HTP increased the susceptibility of the animals to anaphylaxis. Reduction of the mortality rate on challenge with horse serum by lysergic acid derivatives (UML and PML, viz. butanolamide and propanolamide of 1-methyllysergic acid; 1 and 5 mg/kg, i.v., respectively) was confirmed by Gelfand and West (1961).

However, other evidence is less compatible with the hypothesis that 5-HT serves as an important mediator in anaphylaxis of the mouse.

Higginbotham (1960) noted that adrenalectomy decreased resistance to anaphylaxis more markedly than to 5-HT (100 times as compared to 6—7 times), and that anaphylaxis was more resistant to cortisol therapy than 5-HT intoxication was. Waalkes and Coburn (1960) found that whereas histamine rose in the lung of sensitized mice during anaphylaxis, no significant changes occurred in the 5-HT content of mouse blood and tissues. Moreover, 5-HT was not released, as it was in the rabbit, into the plasma when whole blood of sensitized mice was incubated with horse serum. They conclude that whilst histamine appears to be of distinct importance in mouse anaphylaxis, the role of 5-HT is questionable.

DONALDSON et al. (1960) studied anaphylaxis in mice bearing a transplantable mastocytoma potentially capable of secreting large quantities of 5-HT. They noted that in spite of the fact that anaphylactic shock produced a significant decrease in the 5-HT level of kidneys (from 39.8 to 9.9 μg/g), lungs (from 27.1 to 3.5 μg/g), intestine (from 12.9 to 1.1 μg/g) and liver (from 81.6 to 20.9 μg/g), and consequently the liberation into the blood stream of unusually large amounts of 5-HT, neither the tumour nor its secretory products had any influence on the course of anaphylaxis.

Another position has recently been taken up by HALPERN et al. (1963). Having observed that passive cutaneous anaphylaxis in the mouse is strongly inhibited by chlorpromazine and promethazine as well as by the simultaneous injection of mepyramine and LSD, whereas the two latter antagonists, each injected alone, affect the anaphylactic reaction only weakly, they suggest that this reaction in mice is the result of simultaneous release of both histamine and 5-HT, each of them strengthening the effect of the other.

2. Rat

Results obtained by BROCKLEHURST (1957) on the rat uterus removed from animals sensitized passively to ovoalbumin are completely at variance with what FINK (1956) described in the mouse.

In fact, the contraction of the rat uterus caused by anaphylactic shock persists in the presence of 2 μg/ml LSD, although this concentration of antagonist reduces the response to 5-HT by a factor of 400. A difference of this magnitude makes it unlikely that 5-HT is responsible for the anaphylactic contraction.

This conclusion is supported by the observation that when no antagonist is present, the sensitivity of the tissue to 5-HT is greater shortly after anaphylactic shock than it was previously; this is in contrast with the tachyphylaxis which persists after a large dose of applied 5-HT.

Moreover, BROCKLEHURST et al. (1960) could not demonstrate — following depleting the skin of histamine and 5-HT by compound 48/80 and/or reserpine, or following pretreatment with mepyramine and/or BOL — any significant change either in the reversed passive cutaneous anaphylactic reactions produced in passively or actively sensitized rats or in the direct cutaneous anaphylactic reactions produced in passively and actively sensitized rats. BROCKLEHURST and co-workers conclude that histamine and 5-HT are not primary mediators of anaphylactic reaction in the rat skin but play only a secondary part and, more generally, that there is no evidence that 5-HT plays any part in the smooth muscle spasm seen in rat anaphylaxis.

Exactly the same results have been obtained by SANYAL and WEST (1958) who found that severity of the anaphylactic shock in the rat, characterized by progressive circulatory collapse, was not modified in animals whose skin and intestinal histamine and 5-HT had been depleted, nor in animals pretreated with 5-HT and histamine antagonists. *Haemophilus pertussis* vaccine aggravated anaphylactic shock in the rat, the target organ being the small intestine. However, once again, neither histamine nor 5-HT seemed to play major roles in this aggravation. In fact, treatment with vaccine did not alter the content of histamine and 5-HT in the tissues, nor did it alter the release of histamine and 5-HT either from perfused tissues on addition of antigen, or from the tissues from an animal undergoing anaphylactic shock (SANYAL and WEST 1958).

Finally, MOTA (1957) is against the participation of 5-HT in rat anaphylaxis because of the absence in the plasma of shocked rats of any activity that could not be inhibited by antihistamines and of the protection afforded by these drugs against the shock.

However, other investigators are of partly divergent opinions.

WEISSBACH et al. (1957) believe that in rats and rabbits and in other species in which both 5-HT and histamine are present in the lung, both agents should be considered in explaining the pulmonary effects seen in anaphylaxis.

Similarly, GARCÍA-AROCHA (1957, 1959, 1961) maintains that both 5-HT and histamine play an important role in rat anaphylaxis, and that, whereas the anaphylactic response of the rat uterus depends mainly on the release of 5-HT, both histamine and 5-HT participate in the anaphylactic response of other rat tissues. The following evidence is brought by GARCÍA-AROCHA in support of his view: a) both 5-HT and histamine are released when antigen is added to peritoneal cell suspensions or to fluid perfusing the small intestine of sensitized rats. Isolated peritoneal fluid cells release 50—60% of their histamine and all their 5-HT when incubated at 38° and pH 7.8 for 30 min in the presence of 5% horse serum. The 5-HT and histamine release from the small intestine reaches a peak within 2 min after the injection of the antigen and is usually complete within 10 min (0.34—0.89 μg histamine and 0.11—0.16 μg 5-HT); b) similar results are obtained from the perfused hindquarters of the rat; c) in parallel experiments with minced uterine tissue the antigen fails to release significant amounts of histamine, but does release 5-HT (0.01—0.25 μg); d) pretreatment with either the combination of mepyramine and BOL or with chlorpromazine results in substantially complete protection of 25% of the rats against haemorrhagic infiltrations of the small intestine, and partial protection of the other 75%.

GARCÍA-AROCHA (1962) found that the concentration of the antigen was of decisive importance for the release of 5-HT and histamine from suspensions of peritoneal cells of sensitized rats. In the case of horse serum, the effective concentration was found at a dilution of 1:20; with bovine plasma albumin the critical concentration was found in the range of 2—5 mg per ml of cell suspensions. Adjusting the concentration of these antigens to higher or lower values repeatedly failed to produce any recognizable effect on these preparations. Thus, in the case of isolated cells, the exact ratio of antigen to antibody appeared to be an essential condition for the anaphylactic response.

This statement by GARCÍA-AROCHA may at least in part explain the contrasting results obtained by different investigators. To quote some other most recent data on the role of 5-HT in the Schultz-Dale reaction, BORÉUS and WESTERHOLM (1962) observed that whereas a decrease of the very low 5-HT content of rat uterus was noted when uteri from many sensitized animals were pooled and incubated with the antigen (from 0.15—0.17 to 0.09 μg/g or less), this decrease was not noted in other rat tissues (ileum, spleen and skin), and no release of a substance stimulating the highly 5-HT-sensitive rat uterus was noted when the Schultz-Dale reaction was produced in the uterus or ileum of the rat. The difficulty of drawing definite conclusions from the above results is evident.

3. Guinea-pig

The great majority of investigators share the opinion that 5-HT plays only an unimportant part, if any, in the systemic or local anaphylactic reaction of the guinea-pig.

FINK and GARDNER (1958) and SANYAL and WEST (1958) observed that the Schultz-Dale reaction in egg-white or bovine serum albumin sensitized guinea-pig uterus or ileum persisted in the presence of LSD and BOL and that it was impossible to demonstrate any release of 5-HT from sensitized guinea-pig lung, uterus or ileum into the nutrient liquid. DWORETSKY (1959) concluded from his experiments that no more than 10% of the total anaphylactic contraction in the isolated sensitized guinea-pig ileum could be accounted for by liberation of histamine or any other substance into the bath fluid. GIERTZ et al. (1961) failed to detect any 5-HT in the lung perfusate of guinea-pigs subjected to anaphylactic shock or injected with anaphylotoxin and, similarly, FEIGEN, PETERSON and NIELSEN (1959) could not detect any 5-HT in the perfusate of the isolated guinea-pig heart during anaphylaxis. The pharmacological assay of the perfusate showed that the substance or substances liberated were histamine or histamine-like.

INOUE and KURIAKI (1958), in their turn, could not find, during anaphylactic shock, any statistically significant increase in the 5-HT content of venous blood coming from different organs, except for portal blood.

At variance with some positive findings by PALLOTTA and WARD (1957) who claimed that LSD given intravenously (1—100 μg/kg) 1 hour prior to the antigen showed significant protection against fatal anaphylaxis, HERXHEIMER (1955, 1957) failed to observe any protective effect of LSD (up to 100—400 μg/kg) in the anaphylactic shock of the guinea-pig, and GIERTZ et al. (1961) found that pretreatment with LSD produced some delay but did not abolish the anaphylactic bronchoconstriction nor did it influence the reduced perfusion rate through the lung observed in anaphylaxis.

A lesser number of investigators hold the view that the part played by 5-HT in the pathogenesis of anaphylactic shock in the guinea-pig is not so negligible as would appear from the preceding data. GEIGER and ALPERS (1959), for example, conclude from their experiments that at least three humoral agents are involved in the contraction of ileum from sensitized guinea-pigs, upon re-exposure to antigen *in vitro*: 5-HT, histamine and acetylcholine, the liberation of acetylcholine being apparently a result, rather than a cause of the contraction. This conclusion is mainly based on the fact that the Schultz-Dale reaction is suppressed completely only in the presence of a combination of drugs capable of blocking not only the histamine receptors (antihistaminic agents), but also the two kinds of 5-HT receptors in the guinea-pig ileum (LSD and atropine).

On the other hand, ENGELHARDT (1960) found that in the acute anaphylactic shock of the guinea-pig there was release of 5-HT both from the enterochromaffin cells and the spleen, as shown by the significant reduction of the 5-HT content of the jejunum (— 24%), the ileum (— 28%) and the spleen (— 45%). No change was observed in the 5-HT content of the stomach. In the chronic anaphylactic shock only spleen 5-HT presented a significant reduction.

Of doubtful significance is the observation of GIERTZ and HAHN (1959) that 100 mg/kg azulene SN applied in the form of aerosol affords a significant protection against 5-HT and anaphylactic shock, but no protection against histamine shock, and the observation of FEIGEN et al. (1957) that whereas pretreatment of the isolated guinea-pig ileum with ammonium chloride abolishes the Schultz-Dale effect and strongly reduces the response to 5-HT, it scarcely affects the spasmogenic action of histamine.

Similarly, it is not clear why before and after sensitization only 30 to 40% of the guinea-pig uteri respond to 5-HT (7 μg base/ml!), whereas after shocking by exposure of the animal to the antigen the percentage of the uteri which respond maximally to 5-HT increases to 61% (MACHAFFIE et al. 1958).

4. Rabbit

Important changes in 5-HT and histamine distribution are observed in the rabbit during anaphylactic shock: whole blood 5-HT and histamine decrease, plasma 5-HT and histamine increase and the lung content for these amines is transiently elevated; the 5-HT content of other tissues remains practically unchanged (Table 1) (WAALKES and COBURN 1959, JOHANSSON 1960). The drop in whole blood 5-HT and histamine is due to the disappearance of the platelets which are caught in the lung, the increase in plasma 5-HT to the release of the amine from the platelets. The maximum 5-HT level in plasma is attained in one minute, and in those animals which survive, the value returns to normal in two minutes. In comparison, the histamine levels rise to higher maximum values and return to normal more slowly. Whole blood 5-HT and histamine levels fall to minimum values within four minutes, with a gradual rise thereafter (WAALKES et al. 1957). Injection of the antigen-antibody precipitate into a normal rabbit causes changes in the 5-HT content of blood and organs similar to those provoked by intravenous injection of the antigen (2 ml horse serum) into sensitized rabbits, thus demonstrating that effects seen in sensitized rabbits are mediated through the formation of the antigen-antibody complex (WAALKES and COBURN 1959).

Table 1. *The 5-HT content of rabbit tissues and blood during anaphylaxis* (WAALKES and COBURN 1959)

	5-HT content (in μg/ml or μg/g)	
	Control	Experimental (4 min after horse serum)
Intestine	9.3—22	19
Liver	1.3—3.2	3.9
Heart	0.2—0.7	0.4
Brain	0.3—0.6	0.5
Lung	2.2—4.7	18
Whole blood	4.2—5.7	0.5
Plasma	0.05—0.1	0.5[1]

[1] 1 min after horse serum.

As a consequence of the release of conspicuous amounts of 5-HT from platelets there is an increase in the urinary excretion of 5-HIAA soon after anaphylactic shock (FISCHER and LECOMTE 1956, JOHANSSON 1960). Pretreatment of the animals with heparin (3000—4000 I.U./kg, i.v.) prevents increase of 5-HT in plasma and lung tissue, increase in urinary 5-HIAA excretion and also release of 5-HT from platelets in sensitized blood after addition of the specific antigen. Similarly, heparin inhibits the ability of platelets to absorb 5-HT *in vitro* (JOHANSSON 1960).

HUMPHREY and JAQUES (1955) found that free calcium ions and normal plasma were necessary for the release of 5-HT and histamine from platelets incubated with purified antibody and antigen, and that the rate of release increased with increasing amounts of plasma in the system (with 2 ml plasma, 5-HT released after 30 min from 3×10^9 platelets was 95%; with 0.5 ml and 0.1 ml plasma, 57 and 5%, respectively). Plasma heated at 55° for 30 min was only a quarter as effective.

In spite of the observed changes in 5-HT distribution and the fact that some cardiovascular phenomena seen in anaphylaxis are similar to those seen after intravenous injections of 5-HT (fall of the systemic blood pressure and rise of the pulmonary arterial pressure) (LECOMTE and FISCHER 1958), the amine is generally believed to be, in the rabbit too, of minor importance in the pathogenesis of the anaphylactic reaction.

In fact, depletion of tissue 5-HT and, still more, of platelet 5-HT (over 95%) produced by pretreatment with reserpine (2.5—3.5 mg/kg) does not affect either course or severity of the anaphylactic manifestations provoked by subsequent administration of the antigen (FISCHER and LECOMTE 1956). The intervention of 5-HT in shock is even more questionable as sensitized rabbits pretreated with reserpine have an elevated plasma level of histamine, but not of 5-HT during anaphylaxis (WAALKES et al. 1957).

Moreover, cutaneous vascular reactions seen in anaphylaxis (vasoconstriction followed by vasodilatation) strikingly differ from those provoked by 5-HT (vasodilatation followed by vasoconstriction) (LECOMTE and VAN DE BERG 1957) and neither lysergic acid derivatives nor phenotiazines display an antianaphylactic activity proportional to their anti-5-HT activity (LECOMTE and FISCHER 1957, 1958).

Similarly, 5-HT does not seem to play any essential role in local anaphylactic reactions. In fact, pretreatment of sensitized rabbits with 5-HT, or with dihydroergotamine and promethazine, which are peripheral antagonists of 5-HT, does not modify allergic vascular reactions produced by exposure to test antigen (LECOMTE and HUGUES 1958).

This does not, however, rule out the possibility that 5-HT may participate in some of the toxic phenomena seen in rabbit anaphylaxis. MARCELLE and LECOMTE (1959), for example, suggest that the intestinal hyperperistalsis seen in rabbits during anaphylactic shock may be due to liberation of 5-HT, but the low sensitivity of the rabbit intestine towards 5-HT is against this suggestion; WAALKES and COBURN (1959) believe that in those animal species in which both 5-HT and histamine are present and accumulate in the lung it is difficult to attribute the pulmonary anaphylactic manifestations to histamine alone, and that both amines may contribute to the reaction. Changes similar to those provoked when antigen is injected intravenously into a sensitized rabbit or when an antigen-antibody complex precipitate is injected into a normal rabbit can be obtained by intravenous injection of glycogen (100 mg/kg) into normal rabbits. There is the usual marked fall in whole blood concentration of 5-HT, a release of 5-HT into the plasma and a rise in the lung content of the amine (from 2.6 to 13 μg/g). When glycogen is incubated with normal rabbit blood both histamine and 5-HT are released from the platelets (WAALKES and COBURN 1959).

5. Dog

In dogs a release of histamine but not of 5-HT seems to occur as a result of anaphylactic reaction (SANYAL and WEST 1958). However, according to NITZESCO et al. (1959) bronchoconstriction seen in the dog during anaphylactic shock cannot be ascribed entirely to histamine. Other factors, for instance 5-HT and bradykinin, may play a part in the phenomenon.

6. Man

HERXHEIMER and SCHACHTER (1959) believe that it is unlikely that the release of 5-HT is of significance in reactions involving wealing or angio-oedema in man. In fact, 5-HT which, in high concentrations (100—2500 μg/ml), is an effective flaring agent when given intradermally in man, fails to cause whealing or other evidence of increased capillary permeability.

7. Chicken

Owing to dissimilarity of effects produced by 5-HT to symptoms of anaphylactic shock in chickens, LECOMTE and BEAUMARIAGE (1957) doubt whether 5-HT plays any important part in the pathogenesis of anaphylactic reaction in this animal species.

To conclude, it may well be that 5-HT plays some role in the anaphylactic reaction, at least in some animal species or in some particular tissues. But the actual importance of this role is unknown. Anaphylaxis, even local anaphylaxis, is a complex phenomenon which involves contemporaneous or successive liberation not only of histamine and 5-HT but also of polypeptides (e.g. bradykinins) and of lipid-soluble organic acids (e.g. slow-reacting substance A), and probably of other substances too. It is extremely difficult to discern the essential links in this chain of biochemical events (ERSPAMER 1961).

II. Anaphylactoid reaction

1. Egg-white, ovomucoid, dextran, polyvinylpyrrolidone, compound 48/80

Local or systemic administration of egg-white, ovomucoid, dextran, polyvinylpyrrolidone or compound 48/80 produces hyperaemia and oedema of paws and snout in rats. This is the so-called anaphylactoid reaction.

It has been suggested by an important group of research workers that this reaction is mediated mainly by 5-HT, or by both 5-HT and histamine, and the following data have been brought in support of this opinion:

a) Subcutaneous 5-HT is about 30—200 times more potent than histamine in producing oedema, doses as low as 0.2—0.4 μg being effective (ROWLEY and BENDITT 1956, LIACOPOULOS et al. 1957).

b) Pretreatment of the rats with repeated injections of reserpine (5—10 mg/kg $\times$ 2, i.p.; 3 mg/kg $\times$ 3, s.c.) prevents dextran oedema and greatly reduces the oedema following local injections of compound 48/80 and egg-white (PARRATT and WEST 1956, 1957a, 1957b, 1957d; ARRIGONI-MARTELLI and KRAMER 1958; MÖRSDORF 1959, 1960). Similarly, local injections of reserpine (0.1 mg $\times$ 5) inhibit oedema produced by local injections of egg-white (MEDAKOVIĆ 1959). The same protection towards egg-white oedema is observed following prolonged treatment with compound 48/80 (PARRATT and WEST 1957b, 1957d).

c) Pretreatment with polymyxin B, which can release a maximum of histamine from the skin with little or no action on tissue 5-HT, fails to modify the response to any of the above oedema-producing substances (PARRATT and WEST 1957b, 1957c, 1957d).

d) The known 5-HT antagonists LSD (4 mg/kg, i.p., or 10 μg locally), BOL (4 mg/kg, i.v.), UML (1 mg/kg, i.p.) and PML (5 mg/kg i.p.) completely prevent the oedema produced by 5-HT, compound 48/80, egg-white or dextran without altering the response to histamine (PARRATT and WEST 1957b, 1957d, 1958; STENGER 1958, 1959; MEDAKOVIĆ 1959; GELFAND and WEST 1961). Antihistamine drugs (mepyramine 4 mg/kg, s.c.) are inactive or afford only slight protection (PARRATT and WEST 1957b, ROWLEY and BENDITT 1956). However, combinations of anti-5-HT drugs and antihistamines or, even more so, antagonists possessing both anti-5-HT and antihistamine properties (dibenamine 5 mg/kg + mepyramine 4 mg/kg, i.v.; chlorpromazine 0.5—2 mg/kg, i.v., or 25 mg/kg, s.c.; methotrimepazine 0.25 mg/kg) are the most potent inhibitors of the alterations in capillary permeability caused by oedema-producing substances (PARRATT and WEST 1957b, 1958; STENGER 1959; STUCKI and THOMPSON 1958).

e) The areas most prone to the production of increased capillary permeability by 48/80 are rich in both histamine and 5-HT. Other areas containing histamine but less 5-HT exhibit this response weakly (PARRATT and WEST 1958).

f) The oedema fluid contains detectable amounts of 5-HT, but no histamine (PARRATT and WEST 1957).

g) Local injection into the rat paw of dextran produces a significant reduction (from 0.75 to 0.22 μg/g) of the 5-HT content not only in the injected paw, but also in the opposite untreated paw, thus demonstrating a generalized liberation of 5-HT (SUPEK et al. 1961). Local depletion of 5-HT (30%) has been confirmed by MÖRSDORF (1959).

h) Perfusion of rat tissues with dextran or 48/80 produces a simultaneous release of both 5-HT and histamine, the ratio of the two amines being 1:17 for dextran (HALPERN et al. 1957, SPARROW and WILHELM 1957). Identical results are obtained following incubation of isolated rat mast cells with dextran or 48/80 (ARCHER 1961). Similarly, incubated rat skin releases a substance which appears to be 5-HT. This spontaneous release is increased in the presence of egg-white (MEDAKOVIĆ 1959).

However, in spite of the above copious evidence, not all the research workers seem to be disposed to accept the view that "oedema-producing substances bring about in the rat a sequence of events which is primarily due to the release of 5-HT from the stores in the skin" (WEST 1957). In fact the following important data are in favour of the theory that agents other than 5-HT must be involved, and probably play a decisive role, in the pathogenesis of the anaphylactoid reaction:

1. Oedema produced by 5-HT, even after the highest doses that can be tolerated, is never as marked as that obtained with egg-white, dextran, 48/80 or other substances capable of producing an anaphylactoid inflammation (BOIS and SELYE 1956).

2. The capacity of oedema-producing substances to cause an oedematous swelling of the rat paw bears no relation to their ability to liberate 5-HT as observed *in vitro*. In fact, only egg-albumin has been shown to cause a liberation of 5-HT from homogenates of the rat paws. Compound 48/80, dextran and histamine are inactive. *In vivo* a fall in the tissue concentration of 5-HT has been demonstrated solely after marked tissue reactions to egg-albumin and dextran (MÖRSDORF 1961).

3. The preventive effect of 5-HT antagonists and 5-HT releasers could be confirmed only in part and with limitations. MÖRSDORF and FEHRES (1959) found that local injection of 10 μg LSD failed to inhibit increase in capillary permeability produced by dextran, while completely blocking oedema produced by 5-HT; PARRATT and WEST (1958) and VOGEL and MAREK (1961) observed that doses of BOL or LSD necessary to afford complete protection against oedema provoked by dextran, egg-white or compound 48/80 were considerably higher than doses necessary for inhibiting 5-HT oedema. Finally, results obtained by FRANCHIMONT et al. (1961, 1962) were even more surprising. They noted that both reserpine (1 mg/kg$\times$5, i.p.) and BOL (1 mg/kg$\times$4, i.p.) or UML treatment failed to modify dextran oedema, while producing an evident reduction of the oedema provoked by local injection of histamine.

4. Iproniazid, the potent monoamineoxidase inhibitor, does not enhance, as one would have expected according to the 5-HT theory, dextran or ovomucoid oedema, but rather reduces its intensity (ARRIGONI-MARTELLI and KRAMER 1958, KRAMER 1959, SETNIKAR et al. 1958). On the basis of these data, SETNIKAR and co-workers suggest that iproniazid may display its antiphlogistic activity by inhibiting the inactivation of tissue 5-HT. This suggestion is perhaps less conjectural that it may appear at first sight. In fact, GEORGES and HEROLD (1957) observed that 5-HT (1.5—8 mg/kg) given by intraperitoneal route 30 min before dextran significantly reduced oedema produced by the polysaccaride, the afforded protection being greater following bilateral nephrectomy. This is similar to the observation by FRANCHIMONT et al. (1961) concerning the inhibition of histamine and formol oedema by the intraperitoneal injection of 5-HT (4 mg/kg).

5. Oedema produced by histamine, dextran or formaldehyde is inhibited to a great extent by pretreatment with glucagon (1 mg/kg), whereas 5-HT oedema is not significantly changed (LEFEBVRE 1961).

6. Protection afforded by phenotiazine derivatives against anaphylactoid reaction does not parallel their anti-5-HT activity (KRAMER and ARRIGONI-MARTELLI 1958).

7. Intraperitoneal injection into rats of anti-mast-cell serum is followed by reddening and swelling of the muzzle, ears, feet and scrotum and by simultaneous destruction of all the mast cells of the mesentery and of the majority of mast cells in the ear, scrotum and abdominal skin. Attending the disruption of mast cells the levels of tissue histamine drop sharply, whereas in the scrotum and abdominal skin 5-HT not only does not fall below normal, but is markedly above normal at the time when histamine and mast cell content are lowest (SMITH and LEWIS 1961).

8. Anaphylactoid reaction produced by dextran and egg-white in the perfused hindquarters of the rat (reduction of the perfusion rate) is not changed by pretreatment with reserpine (5 mg/kg) or with morphine (30 mg/kg); similarly, anaphylactoid reaction elicited by the above agents in the isolated rat uterus and gut (contraction or inhibition) is not affected by contact of the tissues with 48/80 (3.10^{-5}) (LENDLE and WEISSER 1962).

9. 48/80, even when given repeatedly, does not produce any change in the urinary excretion of 5-HIAA, and rats given compound 48/80 in increasing doses for 8 days excrete as much 5-HIAA after injection of reserpine as untreated controls do (JASMIN 1961). This is certainly not in favour of the hypothesis that anaphylactoid reaction produced by 48/80 is mediated by 5-HT.

Besides provoking the typical anaphylactoid reaction, dextran (20—160 mg/kg, i.p.) causes in the rat also a dose-dependent inhibition of diuresis. Since dextran antidiuresis, unlike that of 5-HT, is prevented by pretreatment with 48/80 and by antihistamine agents devoid of anti-5-HT properties, it is suggested that it is mediated mainly by histamine (GREEFF and CONTZEN 1960).

Before concluding this survey of different data and opinions, it should be stressed that there are many important dissimilarities between dextran oedema and egg-white oedema, and between oedema produced by 48/80 on the one hand and dextran or egg-white oedema on the other. KRAMER (1956a, 1956b) found that whereas procainamide inhibited egg-white oedema it was ineffective against dextran oedema, and that, on repeated administration, egg-white became inactive whereas no resistance appeared against dextran. On the other hand, in rats treated with repeated intraperitoneal injections of egg-white until the injections no longer produced skin oedema, an intraperitoneal injection of 48/80 still caused oedema and accumulation of circulating dye as in normal rats (GÖZSY and KÁTO 1957).

Similarly, LENDLE and WEISSER (1962) found that whereas egg-white contracted the rat uterus, dextran relaxed it, as histamine does, and that even in the perfused hindquarters of the rat, the action of the two substances might be different.

Summing up, the same conclusive remarks which were made when the role of 5-HT in anaphylaxis was discussed seem to be equally applicable to the anaphylactoid reaction.

2. Formalin

Local reaction produced by formalin injection into the rat foot is sharply different, in many respects, from the reaction provoked by local or systemic administration of compound 48/80 and of the highmolecular weight substances considered in the preceding pages, and the term "anaphylactoid reaction" is probably being improperly used for formalin.

The possible mediation of 5-HT in producing oedema and other aspects of vascular injury seen after local injection of formalin into the rat or mouse foot is again controversial, and experimental results are often at complete variance. Pretreatment of the animals with reserpine has little or no effect on formalin oedema according to PARRATT and WEST (1957) and MÖRSDORF (1959), but significantly diminishes oedema according to FRANCHIMONT et al. (1962) and NORTHOVER and SUBRAMANIAN (1962). 5-HT antagonists are ineffective according to STENGER (1958) (10 μg LSD injected locally together with formalin), but inhibit oedema according to VOGEL and MAREK (1961) (local injection of LSD), FRANCHIMONT et al. (1961, 1962) and NORTHOVER and SUBRAMANIAN (1962) (systemic administration of BOL or UML).

Other relevant observations are that administration of 5-HTP (100 mg/kg, s.c.) does not influence formalin oedema (MÖRSDORF 1958); that chlorpromazine (25 mg/kg), a powerful 5-HT and histamine antagonist, displays only a weak protective effect towards the lesions produced by formalin (STENGER 1959); finally, that iproniazid reduces, instead of increasing, formalin oedema. With 200 mg/kg complete inhibition is observed, with 50—100 mg/kg partial inhibition (MÖRSDORF 1959, SETNIKAR et al. 1959). Moreover, following formalin injection the 5-HT content of the inflamed skin is not significantly reduced (MÖRSDORF 1959, SUPEK et al. 1961).

NORTHOVER and SUBRAMANIAN (1962) suggest that formaldehyde-induced inflammation in the mouse foot may be conveniently divided into two parts, the first involving 5-HT as mediator and the second some mediator (plasma globulin permeability-enhancing enzymes) which is unrelated to 5-HT.

The bulk of the experimental data is rather against than in favour of any important 5-HT mediation.

Even the histamine theory seems to be hardly tenable, since formalin oedema is unaffected by depletion of tissue histamine (PARRATT and WEST 1957).

III. Other immunological reactions

1. Rabbit

Lesions of hypersensitivity vasculitis (pulmonary periarteritis and panarteritis) provoked by passive reversed subanaphylactic sensitization techniques with bovine serum antigens are scarcely attenuated by pretreatment with LSD, chlorpromazine, reserpine and antihistaminic drugs. This points to minor importance of release of 5-HT and histamine in the pathogenesis of the lesions (COHEN and SAPP 1960).

Similarly, the possibility that 5-HT might be an ethiological factor in the development of the Arthus phenomenon is excluded by WAALKES and COBURN (1960) on the basis of the fact that the reaction develops readily in rabbits depleted of 5-HT by reserpine.

5-HT injected intravenously or locally into the abdominal skin of rabbits treated 24 hr previously with an intradermal injection of an active polypeptide prepared from *Serratia marcescens* does not provoke any local reaction. Typical haemorrhagic-necrotic lesions result, on the contrary, from locally injected adrenaline, noradrenaline and pitressin (RALL and GASKIN 1956).

According to POPENENKOVA (1961) intravenous injection of typhoid vaccine into the rabbit produces a long-lasting decrease of the 5-HT concentration in blood and tissues. Unfortunately the credibility of this observation is impaired by the apparent inaccuracy of the bioassay method used by the investigator (the 5-HT content of the normal rabbit skin is given the unacceptable value of 8 μg/g!).

2. Guinea-pig

Tri-weekly injections of LSD (20 and 50 μg/kg, starting on the day of inoculation of brain homogenate) reduce the incidence of paralysis, mortality and histopathologic lesions of experimental allergic encephalomyelitis in guinea-pigs. Reserpine given tri-weekly in doses of 0.1 mg/kg, s.c., increases mortality and histopathologic lesions. This is most evident when injections of the drug are commenced several weeks after injection of the brain homogenate. The effectiveness of an anti-5-HT compound to inhibit the development of the disease coupled with the increased severity of the disease by release of 5-HT is taken by HUGHES et al. (1962) as evidence that 5-HT is implicated in the pathogenesis of experimental allergic encephalomyelitis in the guinea-pig.

3. Rat

The severe cutaneous inflammation which develops on challenging with *H. pertussis* vaccine the skin of rats treated, 6 to 28 days previously, with the same vaccine, is not inhibited by anti-5-HT and/or antihistamine drugs, nor by disruption of mast cells. Similarly, sensitization does not enhance the oedema-producing activity of histamine, 5-HT, or 48/80 given by subcutaneous route. These findings suggest that this cutaneous hypersensitive inflammation is not mediated by tissue 5-HT and/or histamine (ROWLEY 1959).

4. Mouse

Mice injected with a rabbit antiserum to EHRLICH'S ascites tumour develop haemorrhagic oedematous lungs with markedly increased 5-HT content (from 2.59 ± 0.37 to 11.78 ± 1.65 μg/g). Cyproheptadine effectively blocks the pathologic manifestations. In spite of the above, a supposed role of 5-HT in the ethiology of pulmonary oedema is a doubtful matter (KIND et al. 1961).

Injections of pertussis vaccine produce in mice, independently of their strain, increased sensitivity to 5-HT. In the experiments of FISHEL et al. (1962) the LD 50 of 5-HT base dropped from 350 to 13 mg/kg.

Hypersensitivity appears 24 hr after the injection of the vaccine, reaches its peak after 3—4 days, and disappears within 25 days. Ability to induce 5-HT sensitivity seems to be characteristic of *H. pertussis*. Desensitization of pertussis-treated animals may be obtained by acute exposure to progressively increasing amounts of 5-HT or by pretreatment with dibenzyline or LSD (MUNOZ and GREENWALD 1957, MUNOZ 1957, KALLOS and KALLOS-DEFFNER 1957, FISHEL et al. 1962).

Starting from the observation that there are no gross differences between normal mice and pertussis-treated mice in the urinary excretion of the metabolites of exogenous radioactive 5-HT, FISHEL et al. conclude that hypersensitivity to 5-HT is the result of a localized hyperreaction of the effector cells to normally non-toxic concentrations of 5-HT.

IV. Response to bacterial toxins

Intravenous injections of a heat-killed suspension of *E. coli* into a rabbit provokes a febrile reaction which is accompanied by two phases of constriction in the vessels of the denervated ear, one early and the other delayed. Both phases, which are independent of the rise of body temperature, are due to the appearance of filtrable substances in the circulating blood. The substance in the early phase resembles 5-HT (0.1 μg/litre); those in the delayed phase resemble adrenaline and 5-HT (0.5—1 μg/litre). The phases are modified when the pyrogen is injected again after an interval. The early phase is exaggerated and is due to the release of substances resembling 5-HT (10—20 μg/litre) and possibly histamine; the delayed phase is diminished (ARMIN and GRANT 1957a, 1957b).

The release of 5-HT from rabbit platelets upon injection of *E. coli* endotoxin was confirmed by DAVIS et al. (1961a, 1961b, 1961c) and by MEEKER and DAVIS (1961). Fifteen seconds after the injection, platelet 5-HT drops to 10% of the control, whereas plasma 5-HT increases from 0.03—0.08 to 2.25 μg/ml. The magnitude of the release is correlated with the amount of endotoxin administered.

Similar results are obtained in the dog. Following rapid intravenous injection of crude *E. coli* endotoxin (1 mg/kg) there is a precipitous fall in circulating platelets followed by a decline of 5-HT concentration in serum (from 0.55 to 0.11 μg/ml after 5 min), which remains low throughout the shock state (DAVIS et al. 1959, ROSENBERG et al. 1960).

Rapid amine release occurring in vivo following administration of *E. coli* endotoxin is probably secondary to the action of thrombin on platelets, and is inhibited in animals pretreated with warfarin or heparin. Tolerance and immaturity of the animals decrease, but do not prevent amine release (DAVIS et al. 1963).

In the cat, pretreatment with dibenamine and pyrilamine, dibenamine alone or LSD with or without pyrilamine diminishes or prevents the acute hypotensive response to small doses of *E. coli* endotoxin (GILBERT 1959).

It is evident that the above observations are compatible with the view that histamine and 5-HT are released and play a role in the early stages of the vascular reactions provoked by *E. coli* endotoxin in the rabbit, dog and cat (see also KOBOLD et al. 1963, and TSAGARIS et al. 1963).

For the mouse things may be different and 5-HT involvement in toxicity of endotoxin is not clear. In fact, increased resistance to lethal doses of endotoxin is observed both after administration of 5-HTP (250 mg/kg × 2, i.p.), which produces a 5-HT excess, and BAS (benzylanalogue of serotonin: 20 mg/kg × 2, i.p.) which antagonizes 5-HT, and increased susceptibility to endotoxin is manifest after phenylisopropylhydrazine (25 mg/kg × 2, i.p.) which, like 5-HTP, is expected to raise 5-HT levels (DES PREZ et al. 1961).

The beneficial effect of 5-HT (1—2 mg, s.c.) on *E. coli* endotoxin mortality has been confirmed by GORDON and LIPTON (1957), who further observed that protection afforded by 5-HT was enhanced by the simultaneous injection of 1 mg/kg compound F.

Finally, it is worth remembering that WIEGERSHAUSEN (1961) suggests that some of the pharmacological actions displayed by the staphylococcical toxin (e.g. stimulant action on the rat uterus) are mediated by the liberation of 5-HT from the smooth muscle.

V. Inflammatory processes

1. Bacterial inflammation

Lethal infections were induced in the rat by *Ps. pyocyanea* and *C. ovis*, and lethal intoxication by *Staphylococcus aureus* α-toxin. Only negligible amounts of 5-HT (total less than 1 μg) and no more than 10% of the liberable histamine were found in the peritoneal fluid and their release appeared to be epiphenomenal.

The mast cells were morphologically unchanged. It was concluded that the role of the two amines in the early reaction to the acute infection was unessential (SMITH and MILES 1960).

On the other hand, depletion of histamine by repeated injections of polymyxin B, or of 5-HT by injections of reserpine causes in the rat a breakdown of the resistance against infection by *Staphylococcus aureus* (MISHRA and SANYAL 1959).

It remains to be demonstrated that resistance of rats to infection and the presence of amines in the tissues may be related.

2. Turpentine inflammation

Pleural exsudates were produced by injections of turpentine into the pleural cavity of rats. Thirty minutes after turpentine administration they contained 1—3 μg/ml 5-HT, and 0.2 μg/ml or less after 1 hr. Moreover, 5-HT activity (1 μg/ml) was found to develop in platelet- and 5-HT-free exudate from resolving pleurisy incubated with washed mitochondria isolated from rat lungs. On the basis of these data, SPECTOR and WILLOUGHBY (1957a, 1957b) suggested at first that 5-HT might be a mediator of increased capillary permeability in the earliest phases of acute inflammation, and that the release of the amine might depend partly or wholly on interaction of plasma either with platelets or with tissue cells and their constituents. However, later on, they changed this idea, because both BOL (3—4 mg/kg, i.v.) and reserpine (7 mg/kg × 4, i.p.) failed to influence accumulation of exsudate (SPECTOR and WILLOUGHBY 1958) and iproniazid and other MAO inhibitors reduced the increased capillary permeability in inflammation due to thermal injury or turpentine-induced pleurisy, while leaving unaffected the increased capillary permeability due to 5-HT and histamine. In their last paper, SPECTOR and WILLOUGHBY (1960) conclude that after injury there is a local destruction of vasoconstrictor substances, probably by MAO. MAO inhibitors would then act by preserving these vasoconstrictor agents from inactivation.

According to BASSOLI and BENATI (1956) 5-HT (1 mg/kg × 3) displays an evident inhibitory effect on the inflammatory reaction produced in guinea-pigs by injections of tuberculine or intrapleural administration of irritant substances.

Injection of turpentine oil into the rat skin causes a significant reduction of the 5-HT content of the inflamed area (SUPEK et al. 1961). Chlorpromazine (25 mg/kg, s.c.) potently antagonizes turpentine oedema (STENGER 1959).

3. Thermal injury

Results of studies concerning the possible intervention of 5-HT in the response to thermal injury have been partly at variance but the bulk of available evidence supports the view of WILHELM and MASON (1960) and of GANLEY (1962) that 5-HT does not seem to play any part either in the immediate or in the delayed response to burning. This does not rule out the possibility that thermal injury may produce an alteration in the metabolism of 5-HT.

Two points have been mainly investigated: the 5-HT content of tissues and blood, and the urinary excretion of 5-HIAA following burns.

BALLANI and co-workers (1959a, 1959b) found no changes in the 5-HT content of the skin, spleen or lungs of anaesthetized rats and mice immersed in hot water at 60° for 10 seconds. 5-HT content was determined 10 min, 2 hr, 7 hr and 7, 12, 21 days after scalding. SPECTOR and WILLOUGHBY (1958) observed that BOL caused only a slight and inconstant delay in the onset of increased capillarity following thermal injury, as shown by dye-leakage. The results obtained by BALLANI and co-workers are not in accordance with those of JOHANSSON (1960), who found an increased 5-HT content of the rat skin (from 0.8—1.1 to 1.4—1.8 μg/g) 1 and 6 hr after scalding. JOHANSSON further noted that in the scalded rabbit there was a decrease of 5-HT in whole blood, accompanied by a decrease in circulating platelets.

Concerning the influence of burns on the urinary excretion of 5-HIAA, GOLDSMITH et al. (1961) observed that the output of 5-HIAA in rat urine presented a conspicuous drop immediately after thermal injury (from 24 to less than 5 μg/rat/day) and then rose by the fourth post-burn day to 73 μg. Cyproheptadine, a potent 5-HT antagonist, altered neither the mortality, nor the 5-HIAA excretion of the burned animals. Results were similar in ten burned patients followed for periods of 4 to 117 days. It was noted that 5-HIAA excretion remained persistently low (often less than 1 mg/day) from shortly after the burning until convalescence ensued.

Again completely at variance were the results of JOHANSSON (1960) who found in five burned patients an increase in urinary 5-HIAA, up to 35 mg/day, and small amounts of 5-HT (about 0.1 μg/ml) in the blister fluid.

4. Ultraviolet irradiation

A significant increase in blood levels of 5-HT (from 2.52 to 5.18 μg/ml after 16 hr) and histamine (from 8 to 13 μg/ml after 24 hr) is found in skin inflammation elicited in rabbits by ultraviolet irradiation. On a second irradiation, repeated 14 days later, 5-HT increase is higher (6.14 μg/ml). The skin 5-HT content does not show any appreciable change. If 0.5 ml/kg of a 10% solution of calcium gluconate is administered intravenously to rabbits prior to irradiation blood levels of 5-HT and histamine increase much less markedly (CERHOVÁ et al. 1962).

5. X-ray irradiation

RENSON and FISCHER (1959) found a 50 to 80% decrease in the 5-HT content of the rat hypothalamus 2 hr after whole-body irradiation with 1000 r, and a reduction of brain 5-HT levels was observed also by ROYAL et al. in the mouse (1959) one week after exposure to 900 r and by SPECK (1962) in the rat immediately after exposure to 9000 r (from 0.53 to 0.42 μg/g) and 18 hr after exposure to 4500 r (from 0.53 to 0.44 μg/g), coinciding with EEG slowing and lethargy.

Similarly, EGAÑA (1963) noted that the content of 5-HT in the central nervous system of rats exposed to internal irradiation with ^{32}P was decreased, the hypothalamus, mesencephalon and rhinencephalon being the most affected areas.

On the other hand, ERSHOFF and GAL (1961) failed to detect any significant difference in brain 5-HT concentration between X-irradiated (900 r total-body irradiation) or gamma-irradiated rats and untreated pair-fed controls, with values for all three groups, however, reduced below that of untreated, ad-libitum-fed controls. Similar negative results were obtained by MELCHING et al. (1960) in mice exposed to 810 r whole-body irradiation and by RANDIĆ et al. (1962) in rats exposed to the same dose (900 r) of X-irradiation. However, adrenalectomized rats presented immediately after irradiation a significant decrease in their brain content of 5-HT.

In contrast to the above findings, TCHERNOW (1960) reported an immediate increase in the 5-HT content of brain homogenates of rats and guinea-pigs exposed to 500—1000 r, and RANDIĆ and SUPEK (1962) a 24—63% increase in the 5-HT content of the brain of rats administered high doses (8000—12000 r) of whole-body irradiation and killed immediately after irradiation.

Neither shielding of the head or body nor pretreatment with iproniazid or reserpine interfered with the 5-HT increase. The dose of 3000 r did not elicit any regular increase in the concentration of brain 5-HT (PALAIĆ et al. 1963).

In recent experiments, PALAIĆ et al. (1964), while confirming that whole-body irradiation with 900 r did not produce any immediate change in the 5-HT and 5-HIAA content of the rat brain stem, found an increase of total 5-OR indoles (from 1.22 to 1.74 μg/g) which was probably due to neutral 5-OR indoles of unknown nature and origin. No other brain area presented this increase.

Concerning other tissues, a significant reduction of the 5-HT content of lung, kidney, spleen and liver of mice and of blood, spleen and small intestine of rats was observed 3 and 6 days after exposure to 450—900 r total-body irradiation by a number of research workers (ROYAL et al. 1959, RAUSHENBAKH and TCHERNOW 1960, ERSHOFF and GAL 1961, ERSHOFF et al. 1962, MATSUOKA et al. 1962). However, in the early phase after irradiation (24—48 hr after exposure to 900 r) the 5-HT content of the rat gut did not appear appreciably changed in the experiments of VARAGIĆ et al. (1963), while the 5-HT content of the spleen was nearly doubled.

MATSUOKA et al. (1962) affirm that there are considerable species differences in the behaviour of the intestinal 5-HT towards X-irradiation (maximal reduction in rats, minimal in rabbits), and that the radiation sensitivity of the intestine seems to be closely related with its 5-HT content.

It is noteworthy that whole-body irradiation with 600 and 1200 r causes a loss of granules in the enterochromaffin cells and their disappearance in the guinea-pig duodenum and upper ileum. Maximum reduction, 50—70%, may be observed after 3—4 hr. After 12 hr number and aspect of the enterochromaffin cells are again normal (ANSARI et al. 1962).

Urinary excretion of 5-HIAA appears to be significantly increased both in normal and in adrenalectomized rats during the first 24-hr period following whole-body X-irradiation with 800—1000 r (RENSON and FISCHER 1959, MELCHING et al. 1960, RANDIĆ and SUPEK 1961), as well as in rabbits after 700 r (RENSON 1960) and in hypophysectomized frogs after 400 r (BRINKMAN and VENINGA 1962).

DEANOVIĆ et al. (1963) have carried out an excellent study on the relationship between the dose of whole-body X-irradiation and the urinary excretion of 5-HIAA in rats. It was shown (Fig. 1) that 5-HIAA excretion in the first postoperative day increased with the dose of X-irradiation, the threshold dose being 100—150 r, and that the increase in 5-HIAA output was considerably greater in female rats than in male rats at all doses of X-irradiation.

Cystamine (100 mg/kg, i.p.) partially inhibited this effect.

According to DEANOVIĆ and SUPEK (1964) the groups of rats which, following exposure to 800 r whole-body irradiation, showed a greater increase in the excretion-rate of 5-HIAA, presented a longer survival time. This observation, which is not in contrast with that of FRANZEN (1962) and FRANZEN et al. (1963) that irradiated rats which excreted more 5-HT in urine showed a more severe radiation syndrome, raises the important problem of whether 5-HT release produced by irradiation should be considered beneficial or harmful.

Like ionizing radiation, nitrogen mustard and urethane produce in rats a moderate but significant increase of 5-HIAA urinary excretion on the second day after injection. Chloral hydrate is ineffective (SUPEK et al. 1963).

In human patients results are divergent. BETTENDORF et al. (1962) found that in 9 out of 17 female patients suffering from carcinoma of the genitals,

X-ray irradiation produced a decrease in the daily urinary excretion of 5-HIAA while in the other 8 patients effects were equivocal. NAFTALIN (1962), on the contrary, observed an increase in 5-HIAA excretion in patients therapeutically irradiated with X-rays.

From the above results it is difficult to decide whether and to what extent 5-HT participates in the production of gastrointestinal, haematologic or cerebral manifestations of radiation injury.

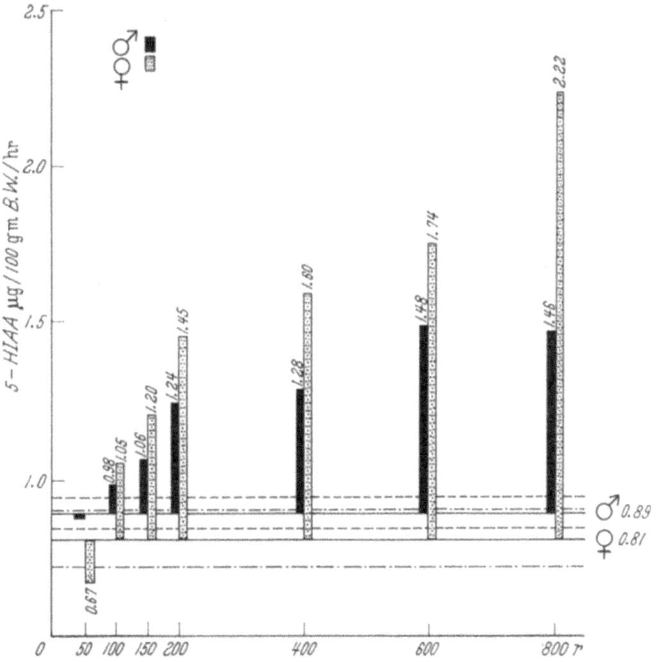

Fig. 1. Relationship between dose of X-irradiation and urinary 5-HIAA excretion in the first postirradiation day. Increase in 5-HIAA excretion was remarkably higher in female rats than in male rats at any dose of X-irradiation. [From Fig. 3, DEANOVIĆ, Z. et al., Internat. J. Radiat. Biol. 7, 4 (1963).]

6. Response to snake venoms

On the basis of the observations that RUSSELL's viper venom and saw-scaled viper venom have equal capillary permeability effects in mice, rats, guinea-pigs and rabbits and that these effects are completely prevented by drugs possessing both antihistamine and anti-5-HT properties, FEARN et al. (1964) conclude that the increased capillary permeability induced by the venoms is largely mediated through the release of histamine and 5-HT.

However, owing to the enormous species differences in the capillary responses to 5-HT and histamine, the above conclusion does not seem persuasive.

In an excellent review article on substances which affect capillary permeability, SPECTOR (1958) concludes that "it seems at the moment that the importance of 5-HT as a mediator substance of altered vascular permeability in inflammation is likely to be confined to certain tissues, perhaps only the skin of the rat and possibly of the mouse".

This conclusion represents the maximum concession which may reasonably be made to the 5-HT theory in inflammation.

VI. Formation of granulation tissue and healing of wounds

Two sponge-pellets were implanted symmetrically under the skin of the rat; one was kept as control, the other was injected with single or repeated doses of 10 μg 5-HT.

Single injections produced an increase of the amount of total and neutro-soluble hexosamines as well as of haemoglobin in the interstitial liquids. Collagen tissue was not appreciably affected. Histological examination of the newly-formed connective tissue revealed capillary dilatation without oedema, numerous haemorrhagic dots and a moderate infiltration of leucocytes. Metachromasy was not changed (LAPIÈRE 1961a).

Repeated injections of 5-HT caused an increase of the soluble fractions of the collagen and of the insoluble hexosamine fraction. Weight of wet and dry tissue was not significantly changed. Infiltration by leucocytes was conspicuous, and the newly-formed tissue appeared more basophilic upon staining with toluidine blue. Some fibroblasts showed the characteristics of young cells with large nucleus and basophilic cytoplasma (LAPIÈRE 1961b, 1961c).

Instead of injecting 5-HT locally, FRANCHIMONT et al. (1961) administered 5-HT by intraperitoneal route, at daily doses of 10 mg/kg for 9—10 successive days. Under these conditions they noted a reduction of the liquid contained in the SELYE's granulomatous pocket and an inhibition of the growth of the connective shell which usually surrounded, after some days, the cotton-pellets implanted under the skin.

The effect of 5-HT on early inflammatory reaction and on connective tissue regeneration was also studied by SAXENA (1960) and by FIORE-DONATI and MOLTKE (1960). SAXENA found that intraperitoneal 5-HT (0.4 mg/kg), like histamine and hyaluronidase, increased exudate formation. FIORE-DONATI and MOLTKE observed that 5-HT, administered by i.p. route at daily doses of 4 mg/kg for 8 consecutive days, caused a significant decrease in the tensile strength of the wounds resulting from standard incisions of the skin, with no significant changes in the mast cell morphology. They suggest that this negative influence upon connective tissue regeneration might be due to release of adrenocortical steroids.

The recent statement by BHATT and SANYAL (1963, 1964) that depletion of tissue 5-HT produced in the rat by reserpine provokes both a reduction in exudate formation (granuloma pouch method) and in development of fibrous tissue (cotton wool pellet method) and, consequently, that 5-HT depletion adversely affects the exudative or reparative phases of inflammation in the rat is based on the assumption that the only effect of reserpine is to cause a depletion of 5-HT.

VII. Reaction to stress

According to WEST (1957), 5-HT plays a major role in the rat in the reaction of the organism to the stress and strain of life, particularly with respect to its location in the skin, in areas which are in contact with the outside world. In fact, 5-HT increases in concentration under physiological conditions involving a fresh environment — two days after weaning the 5-HT values of the skin are about double those found in unweaned rats of the same age (PARRATT and WEST 1956) — or an increased use of the tissue — the tongue of females has more than twice the amount of 5-HT found in the tongue of males (PARRATT and WEST 1957a). From the above data it would appear that endogenous 5-HT interferes favourably in the reaction of animals to stress. Other data, however, suggest rather an unfavourable influence of both exogenous and endogenous 5-HT on the resistance of animals to cold and trauma.

Rats treated with intramuscular injections of 5-HT (0.1—1 mg/kg) prior to exposure to a standard amount of Noble-Collip trauma present mortality which significantly exceeds that of controls. When rats receive 5-HT intravenously (10—200 μg/kg) no differences from controls are seen following trauma (McNeil and Hampton 1959).

Jones and Ripstein (1958) not only confirmed that 5-HT (0.5—10 mg/kg, s.c.) failed to increase the resistance of rats against drum shock, but found that it apparently antagonized the protective action of promethazine at certain combinations of doses of the two drugs.

In adrenalectomized rats subjected to shock by limb ischaemia produced by rubber tourniquets applied for 2 hr on both hind legs, 5-HT level of blood samples taken 45 min later increases from 0.096 to 0.37 μg/ml (Medaković and Spužik 1959).

Zilberstein (1960) studied the effects of reserpine, 5-HT and vasopressin on the survival of cold-stressed rats. He found that all drugs lowered the ability of intact rats to withstand cold stress applied immediately or 18 hr after injections (4—8 mg 5-HT/kg). On the basis of similarity of the survival times of adrenalectomized rats, Zilberstein suggests that treatment with these drugs results in temporary functional adrenalectomy through action on the pituitary-adrenal system.

Concerning the influence of temperature on the 5-HT content of tissues, Toh (1960) observed that the 5-HT content of the brain of rats exposed to extreme heat or cold was lower than that of control rats (0.2—0.24 μg/g as compared with 0.38 μg/g), whereas no significant alteration could be observed in the 5-HT content of spleen, stomach or small intestine. On the other hand, Gordon (1961) found a consistent increase in whole blood 5-HT of female rats exposed to cold: in one experiment, for example, from 0.43 to 1.08 μg/ml after a 5—11 min exposure. Gordon thinks that these perturbations in 5-HT concentration may indicate a participation of the amine in cardiovascular and/or metabolic adjustment to cold.

According to Miline et al. (1958) stress due to the presence of a dog caused in a hare at first a transient increase (from 0.075 to 0.1 μg/g), and then a decrease (down to 0.04 μg/g) in the concentration of brain 5-HT. Concluding from these meagre results that 5-HT is highly engaged in the adaptation syndrome seems frankly to be excessive.

VIII. Miscellaneous experimental pathological processes

1. Haemorrhagic shock

5-HT concentration in peripheral blood of dogs subjected to haemorrhagic shock does not differ significantly from 5-HT concentration in blood of control animals (Rosenberg et al. 1960, Rosenberg 1961). However, rabbits and rats subjected to a 10 ml/kg bleeding at room temperature present a 50% increase of whole blood 5-HT. This elevation persists, according to Gordon (1961) at least for a week and does not simply depend on elevation of blood platelets. Rabbits bled from the xylene-dilated ear at 3^0 show, within the first minute, a 50% fall in whole blood 5-HT which is followed by a rising and falling of 5-HT of sinoid character with 2-min periods.

2. Transfusional reaction

In man the 5-HT concentration in whole blood decreases from 0.1—0.6 to 0—0.02 μg/ml during the acute phase of the transfusional reaction. However, since this decrease parallels the decrease in blood platelets and is accompanied by a reduction in the 5-HIAA concentration in the post-transfusional urine samples, it appears that the fall of blood 5-HT level is not due to a release of 5-HT from the platelets, but rather to a sequestration of the platelets in the lung or liver (SILVER et al. 1961).

3. Complications in extracorporeal circulation

SARAJAS et al. (1959) found in model experiments in rabbits and dogs with a simple extracorporeal circuit suggestive evidence that 5-HT and ATP were released from the platelets into the plasma as a result of corpuscular blood trauma. In fact, whole blood 5-HT decreased, while plasma 5-HT increased and, concurrently, the urinary excretion of 5-HT was markedly increased, while that of 5-HIAA showed the opposite trend. SARAJAS and co-workers and HOLLENBERG et al. (1963) suggest that release of 5-HT and ATP may explain some features associated with perfusion experiments in general and some complications including fatalities following the use of heart-lung machines for open cardiac surgery.

SCHIEVELBEIN et al. (1962), however, obtained divergent results. In fact, whereas no significant changes in blood 5-HT level were observed in dogs subjected to cardiac surgery with extracorporeal circulation, in human patients blood 5-HT level increased by 100% during "by-pass" and 2 hr later a significant increase in urinary 5-HIAA was also noted.

4. Pulmonary thromboembolism

According to SMITH and SMITH (1955) the signs and symptoms of experimental pulmonary embolism in the cat may depend on the release to some considerable extent of 5-HT from both the blood clot and the infarcted area of the lung. In fact, both 5-HT and blood clot cause, on systemic injection, a rise in the pulmonary arterial pressure and a fall in the systemic pressure which is not abolished by vagotomy or antihistamine drugs, is potentiated by cocaine and is minimized by dibenamine, yohimbine and 5-HT antagonists.

The above results have been essentially confirmed in the dog by COBB and NANSON (1960), who further found that the effects of intravenous infusion of 5-HT (25—50 μg/kg/min) were antagonized by heparin (200 u./kg). In reality, it appears from the figures illustrating the paper by COBB and NANSON that heparin antagonizes only the effect of 5-HT on systemic blood pressure, not that on pulmonary pressure.

On the basis of the ambiguous circumstance that gaseous embolism causes in the rabbit a decrease in the 5-HT content of the lung, it is suggested by MONTANARI and GIAROLI (1962) that in the rabbit, too, bronchoconstriction and pulmonary hypertension seen after pulmonary embolism may be ascribed to release of 5-HT.

SANDERS et al. (1959) are of a completely divergent opinion. Following a well-documented study they affirm that the pressure changes due to thromboembolism in the anaesthetized dog can be explained on the basis of mechanical occlusion and do not resemble the changes elicited by 5-HT injections. Consequently, the role of 5-HT in the picture of pulmonary thromboembolism, in the dog and in man, is probably negligible.

A particular type of embolism has been studied by DUSEK et al. (1963), namely that produced in rabbits by intravenous injection of human amniotic liquid (1—3 ml/kg). A conspicuous increase in free plasma 5-HT is observed, but it is questionable whether 5-HT release plays any role in the pathogenesis of the cardiovascular phenomena elicited by amniotic liquid.

Considering experimental thromboses in other vascular areas, BAUMGARTNER et al. (1963) found that i.p. administration of 10 mg/kg 5-HT 17 and 1 hour before traumatization of the intima of the marginal vein of the rabbit ear significantly reduced development of platelet deposits, and hence formation of thrombi, on the intimal surface of the traumatized vein. The effect of 5-HT was reinforced by the contemporaneous administration of MAO inhibitors, and abolished by 5-HT antagonists. It is suggested that the inhibition of the formation of thrombotic deposits is caused by accumulation of 5-HT in the platelets and possibly in the vessel wall.

5. Ozone-induced pulmonary oedema

Rats exposed to 6 parts per million of ozone by volume for 4 hours develop severe pulmonary oedema and haemorrhage with significant increase in lung weight, lung protein content and lung 5-HT (13.3 μg/kg body weight, instead of 5.6 μg/kg). Ozone exposure does not alter blood 5-HT content. The origin of excess 5-HT in the lung is obscure, and participation of the amine in the pathogenesis of the oedema is questionable (SKILLEN et al. 1961a).

6. Decompression sickness

The mean levels of 5-HT in tissues of albino rats subjected to rapid decompression from high ambient pressure (5 atm.) shows no significant change even when decompression time is short enough to cause immediate death. It is concluded that it is improbable that the release of 5-HT plays a role in decompression sickness (KINDWALL et al. 1962).

7. Reaction to air ions and microparticle inhalation

Exposure of rabbits and guinea-pigs to positive air ions, in special ionizing cages, produces depression of ciliary activity in the trachea, contraction of the posterior tracheal wall, exaggerated response of the tracheal mucosa to trauma, marked vasoconstriction in the tracheal wall and finally increased respiratory rate.

Since these changes are very similar to those obtained with intravenous administration of 5-HT, it is suggested by KRUEGER and SMITH (1960a) that (+) air ion effects are mediated by the release of 5-HT.

Negative air ions are capable not only of reversing all the effects produced by (+) ions but also of decreasing 5-HT concentrations in extirpated strips of rabbit trachea and in the respiratory tract of the mouse. KRÜGER and SMITH (1960b) conclude that (—) air ion effects may depend on their ability to accelerate enzymatic breakdown of 5-HT.

Inhalation of aluminium or iron oxide submicronic particles possesses strong constricting properties upon guinea-pig lungs, which are prevented by cyproheptadine. The content of 5-HT of the lungs increases from 0.21 to 1.55 μg/g following inhalation of aluminium oxide, but shows no change following inhalation of iron oxide. Yet both aluminium and iron oxide conspicuously increase the histamine content of the lung. The obvious conclusions is that histamine and not 5-HT is responsible for the constriction of the lungs (ROBILLARD and ALARIE 1963).

8. Dumping-syndrome

After the rapid instillation of hypertonic glucose into the proximal intestine of the dog there is an acute elevation in portal blood 5-HT which parallels the appearance of the dumping syndrome (DRAPANAS et al. 1962).

Intraduodenal introduction of 200 ml of a 40% glucose solution produces in man a 50% reduction in the urinary excretion of 5-HIAA, lasting 4—8 hours, accompanied by reduction in urine flow; intraduodenal introduction of 200 ml of 0.1 N HCl or 500 ml of distilled water is without any effect on 5-HIAA excretion or reduces it slightly. From these results SCHMID et al. (1962) conclude that there is no obvious relationship between dumping-syndrome and 5-HT metabolism.

9. Calciphylactic muscular distrophy

In rats sensitized by a single oral dose of 10 mg/kg dihydrotachysterol, a single subcutaneous injection of 10 mg/kg 5-HT base given during the critical period (2 to 4 days after dihydrotachysterol administration) produces a widespread and often fatal muscular distrophy. However, a similar 5-HT injection is capable of causing some muscular lesions even as late as 11 days after a single dose of dihydrotachysterol. The muscular changes provoked by 5-HT do not exhibit a significant amount of calcification (SELYE et al. 1962a, 1962b).

10. Osteolathyrism

5-HT administered for 3 weeks in daily doses of 10 mg/kg (2×5 mg/kg, i.p.) increases the severity of the bone lesions provoked in the rat by administration of aminoacetonitrile. UML, given at repeated doses of 0.1 mg reduces severity of lesions (FRANCHIMONT et al. 1961).

11. Reactive hyperaemia

Butanol extracts of dogs' whole blood contain an oxitocic substance closely resembling 5-HT. The butanol-extractable 5-HT represents about 2.5% of total blood 5-HT. Now, it has been found that whereas blood collected from the hind limbs during reactive hyperaemia contained no detectable plasma kinins and showed no increase in total 5-HT, it presented a conspicuous increase, up to 7-fold, of the butanol-extractable 5-HT. In spite of this observation, it seems improbable that 5-HT is the mediator of the vascular changes observed in reactive hyperaemia (HORTON 1964).

12. Poisoning produced by putrefied fish

The hypothesis advanced by JANTSCHEW and NATSCHEW (1963) that 5-HT plays a role in the production of symptoms observed following ingestion of bad gone fish lacks any evidence.

References

ABBATI, A., A. T. FAGGIONI e G. LENZI: Modificazioni della resistenza dei più piccoli vasi cutanei in seguito a somministrazione di 5-idrossitriptamina. Arch. Pat. Clin. med. **32**, 265—268 (1955).

ABRAHAMS, V. C., and M. PICKFORD: The effect of 5-hydroxytryptamine on the excretion of water in conscious dogs. Brit. J. Pharmacol. **11**, 35—43 (1956a).

— — The effect of 5-hydroxytryptamine on the ureter and on the blood pressure of dogs; and of adrenaline, noradrenaline and posterior pituitary extracts on the ureter. Brit. J. Pharmacol. **11**, 44—49 (1956b).

— — The effect of 5-hydroxytryptamine on the uterus of conscious and anaesthetized dogs. Brit. J. Pharmacol. **11**, 50—51 (1956c).

ADAMS, B. G.: Serum 5-hydroxytryptamine levels following experimental increase in gastrointestinal activity in man. Lancet **1960 I**, 207—208.

— The measurement of intestinal sounds in man and their relationship to serum 5-hydroxytryptamine. Gut **2**, 246—251 (1961).

AGHAJANIAN, G. K.: The effect of serotonin and norepinephrine on structural changes induced in brain microsomes. Fed. Proc. **22**, 450 (1963).

AIELLO, E. L.: Influence of the branchial nerve and of 5-hydroxytryptamine on the ciliary activity of *Mytilus* gill. Biol. Bull. **113**, 325 (1957).
— Factors affecting ciliary activity on the gill of the mussel. Fed. Proc. **19**, 282 (1960a).
— Factors affecting ciliary activity on the gill of the mussel *Mytilus edulis*. Physiol. Zool. **33**, 120—135 (1960b).
— Relationship of 5-hydroxytryptamine to ciliary activity in the mussel. Fed. Proc. **22**, 625 (1963).
AINSWORTH, C.: Substituted β-aminoethylindazoles. J. Amer. chem. Soc. **80**, 965—967 (1958).
AIRAKSINEN, M. M.: Studies of the metabolism and antidiuretic action of 5-hydroxytryptamine and the effect of the mode of administration. Ann. Med. exp. Fenn. **41**, Suppl. 4, 1—91 (1963).
— M. K. PAASONEN and P. PELTOLA: New aspects in the 5-hydroxyindoleacetic acid excretion after administration of 5-hydroxytryptamine. Ann. Med. exp. Fenn. **38**, 237—241 (1960).
AKERS, R. P., and B. W. ZWEIFACH: Effect of vasoactive materials on the peripheral blood vessels in the hamster. Amer. J. Physiol. **183**, 529—534 (1955).
AKKERMAN, A. M., D. K. DE JONGH and H. VELDSTRA: Synthetic oxytocics. I. 3-(Piperidyl-(N)-methyl-)indoles and related compounds. Rec. Trav. chim. Pays-Bas **70**, 899—908 (1951).
ALEXANDER, P., Z. M. BACQ, S. F. COUSENS, M. FOX, A. HERVE and J. LAZAR: Mode of action of some substances which protect against the lethal effects of X-rays. Radiat. Res. **2**, 392—415 (1955).
ALIVISATOS, S. G. A., F. UNGAR and C. BIAVA: Effect of indoles and imidazoles, including serotonin and histamine, on the morphology and oxidative phosphorylation of guinea pig liver mitochondria. Nature (Lond.) **201**, 47—49 (1964).
ALLEGRI, A., e V. FERRARI: Esperienze cliniche con la 5-ossitriptamina (serotonina) in alcune forme di diatesi emorragica. Minerva med. **45**, 1660—1663 (1954).
AMBANELLI, U., e G. SALVI: L'antidiuresi da enteramina. G. Clin. med. **40**, 1499—1513 (1960).
AMES, R. C., and H. B. VAN DYKE: Antidiuretic hormone in the serum or plasma of rats. Endocrinology **50**, 350—360 (1952).
ANDREWS, W. H. H., and K. R. BUTTERWORTH: The vascular action of 5-hydroxytryptamine on the canine liver. J. Physiol. (Lond.) **141**, 38—38P (1958).
ANNONI, G., M. LEONE, A. LONGARETTI, G. LONGO e P. D. LUCCHELLI: Prime ricerche cliniche con la serotonina. Clin. ter. **8**, 125—133 (1955a).
—, and P. D. LUCCHELLI: Ulteriori osservazioni sull'azione della 5-idrossitriptamina (enteraminaserotonina) sulla diuresi nell'uomo. Nota II. Farmaco, Ed. sci. **12**, 362—369 (1957).
— — e G. BARBIERA: L'azione della 5-idrossitriptamina (enteramina-serotonina) sulla diuresi nell'uomo. Farmaco, Ed. sci. **10**, 306—311 (1955b).
ANSARI, M., H. EDER u. W. NAEGELE: Die Strahlenwirkung auf die enterochromaffinen (Kultschitsky-)Zellen des Darmes. Strahlentherapie **117**, 191—200 (1962).
ANTONA, G.: Rilievi preliminari sulle possibilità d'impiego della 5-ossitriptamina per la prevenzione del sanguinamento nel corso di interventi chirurgici. Farmaco, Ed. sci. **10**, 86—89 (1955).
— Utilità della 5-ossitriptamina in ostetricia e ginecologia. Minerva ginec. **11**, 350—356 (1959).
ANTOPOL, W., and C. CHRYSSANTHOU: Effect of bradykinin and serotonin inhibitors on the Schwartzman phenomenon. Fed. Proc. **23**, 563 (1964).
APRISON, M. H.: Effect of 5-hydroxytryptamine on cholinesterase activity. Fed. Proc. **19**, 275 (1960).
— K. M. HANSON and D. C. AUSTIN: Studies on serum oxidase (ceruloplasmin) inhibition by tryptophan metabolites. J. nerv. ment. Dis. **128**, 249—255 (1959).
ARCHER, G. T.: Release of 5-hydroxytryptamine from rat mast cells *in vitro*. Nature (Lond.) **190**, 350 (1961).
ARMAN, C. G., VAN, and B. A. JENKINS: The antidiuretic effect of 5-hydroxytryptamine in the rat as influenced by dibenamine. Arch. int. Pharmacodyn. **108**, 356—365 (1956).
ARMIN, J., and R. T. GRANT: Further observations on vasoconstrictor substances in blood of rabbit and man. J. Physiol. (Lond.) **138**, 401—416 (1957).
— — The vasoconstriction caused by a pyrogen. J. Physiol. (Lond.) **138**, 417—433 (1957).
ARRIGONI-MARTELLI, E., e M. KRAMER: Significato della liberazione di serotonina da dextran, ovomucoide, ovalbumina nella cute del ratto per la patogenesi dell'edema provocato. Boll. Soc. ital. Biol. sper. **34**, 1130—1132 (1958).
ASBOE-HANSEN, G., and O. WEGELIUS: Serotonin and connective tissue. Nature (Lond.) **178**, 262 (1956).

Åström, A., and U. Samelius: The action of 5-hydroxytryptamine and some of its antagonists on the umbilical vessels of the human placenta. Brit. J. Pharmacol. **12**, 410—414 (1957).
Aviado, D. M.: Pulmonary venular responses to anoxia, 5-hydroxytryptamine and histamine. Amer. J. Physiol. **198**, 1032—1036 (1960).
Axelrod, J., R. J. Wurtman and Ch. M. Winget: Melatonin synthesis in the hen pineal gland and its control by light. Nature (Lond.) **201**, 1134 (1964).
Bachur, N. R., H. Weissbach and S. Udenfriend: Enzymatic formation of fatty acid amides of physiologically active amines. Fed. Proc. **22**, 415 (1963).
Bacq, Z. M.: The amines and particularly cysteamine as protectors against roentgen rays. Acta radiol. (Stockh.) **41**, 47—55 (1954).
— P. Fischer et F. Ghiretti: Action de la 5-hydroxytryptamine chez les céphalopodes. Arch. int. Physiol. **60**, 165—171 (1952).
—, et J. Renson: Tyramine, 5-hydroxytryptamine et excitation des nerfs adrénergiques. Arch. int. Pharmacodyn. **130**, 464—466 (1961).
Baguet, F., et J. M. Gillis: Stimulation de la respiration des muscles de Lamellibranches par la 5-hydroxytryptamine. Arch. int. Physiol. Biochim. **72**, 351—352 (1964).
Bain, J. A.: A review of the biochemical effects *in vitro* of certain psychotomimetic agents. Ann. N.Y. Acad. Sci. **66** (3), 459—467 (1957).
Bajusz, E., and G. Jasmin: Protective action of serotonin against certain chemically and surgically induced cardiac necroses. Rev. canad. Biol. **21**, 51—62 (1962).
Baldrighi, V., e V. Ferrari: Risposte emopressorie sistemiche e polmonari alla serotonina (5-idrossitriptamina) nell'uomo. Folia cardial. (Milano) **14**, 7—23 (1955).
Balduini, M., L. Boari e F. Tiepolo: L'uso terapeutico di un nuovo emostatico, la 5-idrossitriptamina. Esperienze cliniche. Boll. Soc. med.-chir. Cremona **9**, 25—35 (1955).
Ballani, G. K., C. D. Jha and R. K. Sanyal: Histamine and 5-hydroxytryptamine after cutaneous burns in mice and rats. J. Pharm. Pharmacol. **11**, 512 (1959).
Ballerini, G.: 5-OH-triptamina e retrazione del coagulo. Progr. med. (Napoli) **11**, 455—456 (1955).
Balzer, H., K. Greeff u. E. Westermann: Die bronchoconstrictorische Wirkung des Serotonins. Klin. Wschr. **34**, 1204 (1956).
Banerjee, A. K., and J. J. Lewis: Influence of drugs upon $^{47}Ca^{2+}$ uptake in depolarised intestinal smooth muscle. J. Pharm. Pharmacol. **16**, 439—440 (1964).
Barac, G.: Recherches sur la brûlure. Sur l'effet antidiurétique de la 5-hydroxytryptamine chez le Chien. Arch. int. Physiol. **61**, 403—406 (1953a).
— Recherches sur la brûlure. Suppression de l'action antidiurétique de la 5-hydroxytryptamine par l'acide ascorbique. Arch. int. Physiol. **61**, 400—402 (1953b).
— Recherches sur la brûlure. 5-hydroxytryptamine et élimination rénale du chlore chez le Chien. C. R. Soc. Biol. (Paris) **149**, 1523—1525 (1955).
Bargiel, Z., et W. Kadziela: Réactions vasomotrices du réseau vasculaire de l'oreille du Lapin au cours de la fatigue aiguë sous l'influence de certaines substances neurovasotropes. J. Physiol. (Paris) **55**, 192—193 (1963).
Barlow, R. B., and I. Khan: Actions of some analogues of tryptamine on the isolated rat uterus and on the isolated rat fundus strip preparations. Brit. J. Pharmacol. **14**, 99—107 (1959a).
— — Actions of some analogues of 5-hydroxytryptamine on the isolated rat uterus and the rat fundus strip preparations. Brit. J. Pharmacol. **14**, 265—272 (1959b).
Baroni, G.: Diatesi emorragiche sintomatiche: loro trattamento con 5-idrossitriptamina. Gazz. med. ital. **115**, 51—56 (1956).
Barucci, M.: Ricerche sperimentali su alcuni effetti della 5-idrossitriptamina sul sistema nervoso centrale di conigli. Rass. Studi psichiat. **45**, 893—898 (1956).
Baschieri, L., F. de Luca, C. de Martino, A. Oliverio and M. Negri: Modifications of thyroid activity by melatonin. Experientia (Basel) **19**, 15—17 (1963).
Baserga, A.: Les facteurs plaquettaires. Sang **25**, 742—751 (1955).
—, et G. Ballerini: La 5-hydroxytryptamine dans la thérapie des hémorragies thrombocytopéniques. Schweiz. med. Wschr. **85**, 914—915 (1955).
Bassani, A., e S. Fantini: Effetti della somministrazione di 5-idrossitriptamina nei vecchi con positività delle prove del laccio. G. Geront. **4**, 130—138 (1956).
Bassoli, G., e E. Benati: Serotonina e reazioni allergiche alla tubercolina nella cavia sensibilizzata. G. ital. Chemioter. **2**, 88—91 (1956).
Baumgartner, H. R., A. Studer u. K. Reber: Über Methoden zur Erzeugung experimenteller Thrombosen am Kaninchenohr und die Bedeutung von 5-Hydroxytryptamin bei deren Entstehung. Thrombos. Diathes. haemorrh. (Stuttg.) **9**, 485—511 (1963).
Bazan, P.: Influenza del fattore vasocostrittore serico (5-idrossitriptamina) sull'emostasi renale. Arch. E. Maragliano Pat. Clin. **12**, 643—653 (1956).

BEARD, R. L.: Electrographic recording of foregut activity in larvae of *Galleria melonella*. Ann. Amer. Soc. Entomol. **53**, 346—351 (1960).

BELESLIN, D., and V. VARAGIĆ: The effect of cooling and of 5-hydroxytryptamine on the peristaltic reflex of the isolated guinea-pig ileum. Brit. J. Pharmacol. **13**, 266—270 (1958).

BELLA, U., e R. ROSSI: Possibilità di impiego del fattore vasocostrittore piastrinico nelle emorragie ginecologiche. Riv. Pat. Clin. **12**, 1—22 (1957).

BEN, M., G. C. BOXILL and M. M. WINBURY: The comparative cardiovascular activity of 5-acetyltryptamine (5-AT) with 5-hydroxytryptamine (5-HT). Fed. Proc. **21**, 113 (1962).

BENDITT, E. P., J. HOLCENBERG and D. LAGUNOFF: The role of serotonin (5-hydroxytryptamine) in mast cells. Ann. N.Y. Acad. Sci. **103**, 179—184 (1963).

BERDE, B., u. A. CERLETTI: Über den Angriffspunkt von D-Lysergsäurediäthylamid und 5-Hydroxytryptamin im Melanophorentest. Z. ges. exp. Med. **129**, 149—153 (1957).

BEREGI, E., I. FÖLDES, R. JANKOVICS and L. CSÖTÖRTÖK: Serotonin-induced renal changes in the rabbit and in the rat. Arch. int. Pharmacodyn. **138**, 268—275 (1962).

BERGAMASCO, G. I., G. BINDA e A. AGOSTINI: Inversione dell'effetto pressorio della 5-idrossitriptamina (serotonina) ad opera del fegato nel cane anestetizzato. Atti Soc. lombarda Sci. med. biol. **11**, 215—221 (1956).

BERGONZELLI, V., e A. M. FONTANA: L'azione emostatica della 5-ossitriptamina in chirurgia plastica. Minerva chir. **12**, 958—962 (1957).

BERKINSHAW-SMITH, E. M. I., R. S. MORGAN and G. PAYLING WRIGHT: Permeability response of cerebral and cutaneous blood vessels to vasoactive agents. Nature (Lond.) **196**, 173 (1962).

BERNHEIM, M. L. C., A. OTTOLENGHI and F. BERNHEIM: The anti-oxidant effect of serotonin. Biochim. biophys. Acta (Amst.) **23**, 431—432 (1957).

BERTACCINI, G., and V. ERSPAMER: The effect of the administration of water or isotonic NaCl solution on the urinary excretion of 5-hydroxyindoleacetic acid in the rat. J. Pharm. Pharmacol. **14**, 687—697 (1962).

—, and M. B. NOBILI: Effect of L-tryptophan on diuresis and 5-hydroxyindoleacetic acid excretion in the rat. Brit. J. Pharmacol. **17**, 519—525 (1961).

BERTELLI, A., G. CANTONE e L. MARTINI: Azione della serotonina sull'asse ipofisi-surrene. Atti Soc. lombarda Sci. med.-biol. **9**, 10—12 (1954).

BESANÇON, F.: Le rôle physiologique de la sérotonine (5-hydroxytryptamine) dans la motricité de l'intestin grêle humain. C. R. Soc. Biol. (Paris) **154**, 1771—1776 (1961).

BETTENDORF, G., A. P. MOJE u. H.-J. SCHMERMUND: Der Einfluß der Strahlenbehandlung auf die 5-Hydroxy-Indol-Essigsäure-Ausscheidung. Strahlentherapie **117**, 370—376 (1962).

BHATT, K. G. S., H. R. K. ARORA, H. L. DHAR and R. K. SANYAL: Changes in serotonin content in the heart following acute myocardial infarction in the dog. Med. exp. **9**, 46—48 (1963).

—, and R. K. SANYAL: Association of histamine and 5-hydroxytryptamine with the inflammatory processes. J. Pharm. Pharmacol. **15**, 78—79 (1963).

— — The role of histamine and 5-hydroxytryptamine in inflammatory processes. J. Pharm. Pharmacol. **16**, 385—393 (1964).

BHATTACHARYA, B. K.: A pharmacological study on the effect of 5-hydroxytryptamine and its antagonists on the bronchial musculature. Arch. int. Pharmacodyn. **103**, 357—369 (1955).

BIANCHI, C.: Valutazione dell'attività calmante di alcuni depressivi del SNC. Arch. int. Pharmacodyn. **111**, 227—238 (1957).

BINET, L., et M. BURSTEIN: Sur les effets vasculaires périphériques du 5-hydroxytryptamine créatinine sulfate (sérotonine). C. R. Soc. Biol. (Paris) **149**, 1860—1866 (1955).

BLACK, J. W., E. W. FISHER and A. N. SMITH: The effect of 5-hydroxytryptamine on gastric secretion. XXth Internat. Physiol. Congr. Bruxelles 1956. Abstr. Comm. p. 102—103.

— — — The effects of 5-hydroxytryptamine on gastric secretion in anaesthetized dogs. J. Physiol. (Lond.) **141**, 27—34 (1958).

— — — The effects of 5-hydroxytryptophan (5-HTP) on acid gastric secretion in anaesthetized dogs. J. Physiol. (Lond.) **143**, 21—22P (1958).

— — — The effect of precursors of 5-hydroxytryptamine on gastric secretion in anaesthezized dogs. J. Physiol. (Lond.) **146**, 10—17 (1959).

BLACKMORE, W. P.: Effect of serotonin on water and electrolyte excretion. Fed. Proc. **16**, 282 (1957).

— Effect of serotonin on renal hemodynamics and sodium excretion in the dog. Amer. J. Physiol. **193**, 639—643 (1958).

BLAIR, E. L., M. WAKEFIELD, G. I. C. INGRAM and P. ARMITAGE: Lowered "capillary resiststance" after iontophoresis of lysergic acid diethylamide. Nature (Lond.) **176**, 563 (1955).

BLOZOVSKI, M., et J. SIVADJIAN: Action de la sérotonine, de la réserpine et d'autres agents pharmacologiques sur la sécrétion sudorale. Etudes hygrophotographiques. Arch. int. Pharmacodyn. **123**, 58—66 (1959).
BOCCABELLA, A. V., E. D. SALGADO and E. A. ALGER: Testicular function and histology following serotonin administration. Endocrinology **71**, 827—837 (1962).
BOCK, K. D., H. DENGLER, H. M. KUHN u. K. MATTHES: Die Wirkung von 5-Hydroxytryptamin auf Blutdruck, Haut- und Muskeldurchblutung des Menschen. Naunyn-Schmiedeberg's Arch. exp. Path. Pharmak. **230**, 257—273 (1957).
—, and M. MEIER: The effect of atropine on cardiovascular reactions elicited by catecholamines, angiotensin, histamine, serotonin, and acetylcholine in the conscious dog. Arch. int. Pharmacodyn. **142**, 444—456 (1963).
BOGDANSKI, D. F., H. WEISSBACH and S. UDENFRIEND: Pharmacological studies with the serotonin precursor, 5-hydroxytryptophan. J. Pharmacol. exp. Ther. **122**, 182–194 (1958).
BOIS, P., and H. SELYE: Production of anaphylactoid inflammation and gastric ulcers with 5-hydroxytryptamine. Rev. canad. Biol. **15**, 238—239 (1956).
BOJS, G.: An experimental study on serotonin (5-HT) on man, with special reference to renal function. Scand. J. clin. Invest. **13**, Suppl. 55, 1—88 (1961).
BOLLARD, B., e A. GIUDITTA: Effetto della serotonina (5-OH-triptamina) su alcuni sistemi enzimatici. Boll. Soc. ital. Biol. sper. **39**, 1714—1716 (1963).
BONACCORSI, A., and G. B. WEST: Absence of capillary permeability response in rats to dextran and egg-white. J. Pharm. Pharmacol. **15**, 372—378 (1963).
BOOZ, G., et E. H. BETZ: Action de la tryptamine et de la 5-hydroxytryptamine sur les thymocytes irradiés in vitro. C. R. Soc. Biol. (Paris) **155**, 197—199 (1961).
BORÉUS, L. O., and B. WESTERHOLM: 5-Hydroxytryptamine in the Schultz-Dale reaction. Acta physiol. scand. **56**, 17—25 (1962).
BORGSTEDT, H. H.: The effect of serotonin and LSD on the isolated dog ureter. Fed. Proc. **18**, 370 (1959).
BORN, G. V. R.: The effect of 5-hydroxytryptamine on the movement of potassium into the blood platelets. IV. Internat. Congr. Biochemistry Vienna 1958. Abstr. Comm. p. 81.
— The fate of 5-hydroxytryptamine in a smooth muscle and in connective tissue. J. Physiol. (Lond.) **161**, 160—174 (1962).
BORST, H. G., E. BERGLUND and M. MCGREGOR: The effect of pharmacologic agents on the pulmonary circulation in the dog. Studies on epinephrine, norepinephrine, 5-hydroxytryptamine, acetylcholine, histamine and aminophylline. J. clin. Invest. **36**, 669—675 (1957).
BÔSKOVIĆ, B., and R. PRŽIĆ: The influence of some indole derivatives on the activity of choline acetylase and CoA. Biochem. Pharmacol. 8, 33 (1961).
BOTROS, M., D. LINDSAY, E. POULSON and J. M. ROBSON: Mode of action of 5-HT and iproniazid on pregnancy. Biochem. Pharmacol. 8, 102 (1961).
—, and J. M. ROBSON: The effects of 5-hydroxytryptamine and iproniazid on sexual development. J. Endocr. **20**, XP (1960).
BRACCO, M., and P. C. CURTI: The vasoconstrictor factor of platelets. Experientia (Basel) **10**, 71—72 (1954).
— — Nuovi derivati dell'ossidazione biologica della 5-ossitriptamina. III. Prime esperienze sull'attività biologica. Boll. Soc. ital. Ematol. **6**, 31—33 (1958b).
— — e G. BALLERINI: Azione del fattore vasocostrittore piastrinico (5-idrossitriptamina) sulla resistenza capillare. Farmaco, Ed. sci. **9**, 318—327 (1954).
— — V. GIULIANO e G. PESSINA: Nuovi derivati dell'ossidazione biologica della 5-ossitriptamina. I. Isolamento dal materiale biologico. Boll. Soc. ital. Ematol. **6**, 26—27 (1958a).
BRAUN, K., and S. STERN: Pulmonary and systemic blood pressure response to serotonin: role of chemoreceptors. Amer. J. Physiol. **201**, 369—374 (1961).
BRAUN, W., E.-J. KIRNBERGER, G. STILLE u. V. WOLF: Vergleich einiger Sulfhydrylverbindungen im Strahlenschutz und Wirkungsgrad und Zeitabhängigkeit. Strahlentherapie **108**, 262—268 (1960).
BRECHT, K., u. D. JESCHKE: Über die Wirkung des Serotonins auf die Froschlunge. Naturwissenschaften **47**, 20—21 (1960).
— — Wirkungen von 5-Hydroxytryptamin auf die glatte Muskulatur der Froschlunge. Pflügers Arch. ges. Physiol. **274**, 385—400 (1962).
BRENK, H. A. S., VAN DEN, and K. ELLIOT: Radioprotective action of 5-hydroxytryptamine. Nature (Lond.) **182**, 1506—1507 (1958).
— and M. HAAS: Studies of mechanism of chemical radiation protection in vivo. I. 5-Hydroxytryptamine in relation to effect of antimetabolites, antagonists and releasing agents. Int. J. Radiat. Bioll **3**, 73—94 (1961).
—, and R. MOORE: Effect of high oxygen pressure on the protective action of 5-hydroxytryptamine and cystamine in irradiated rats. Nature (Lond.) **183**, 1530—1531 (1958).

BRINKMAN, R., and T. S. VENINGA: Contribution to the study of immediate and early x-ray reactions with regard to chemoprotection. V. Liberation of serotonin (and other amines) in the frog after x-irradiation. Int. J. Radiat. Biol. **4**, 249—254 (1962a).
— — Contribution to the study of immediate and early x-ray reactions with regard to chemoprotection. VI. Random liberation of biogenic amines as a cause of early irradiation effects. Int. J. Radiat. Biol. **5**, 283—289 (1962b).
BRITTAIN, R. T., and H. O. J. COLLIER: Effects of 5-hydroxytryptamine and 5-hydroxytryptophan on defecation and propulsion of a charcoal meal in intact mice. J. Physiol. (Lond.) **141**, 14—15P (1958).
BROCKLEHURST, W. E.: The action of 5-HT on smooth muscle. In: G. P. LEWIS, 5-Hydroxytryptamine, p. 172—176. London: Pergamon Press 1957.
— J. H. HUMPHREY and W. L. M. PERRY: Cutaneous antigen-antibody reactions in the rat. J. Physiol. (Lond.) **150**, 489—500 (1960).
BROWN, R. G., and B. J. NICHOLS: The effect of 5-hydroxytryptamine creatinine sulfate on pigmentation of surviving tuber slices of *Solanum tuberosum*. Fall Meeting Amer. Soc. Pharmacol., Ann Arbor 1958. Abstr. Pap. p. 7.
BROWNLEE, G., and E. S. JOHNSON: The site of the 5-hydroxytryptamine receptor on the intramural nervous plexus of the guinea-pig isolated ileum. Brit. J. Pharmacol. **21**, 306—322 (1963).
BÜLBRING, E., and G. BURNSTOCK: Membrane potential changes associated with tachyphylaxis and potentiation of the response to stimulating drugs in smooth muscle. Brit. J. Pharmacol. **15**, 611—624 (1960).
—, and A. CREMA: Observations concerning the action of 5-hydroxytryptamine on the peristaltic reflex. Brit. J. Pharmacol. **13**, 444—457 (1958).
— — The release of 5-hydroxytryptamine in relation to pressure exerted on the intestinal mucosa. J. Physiol. (Lond.) **146**, 18—28 (1959).
— — The action of 5-hydroxytryptamine, 5-hydroxytryptophan and reserpine on peristalsis in anaesthetized guinea-pigs. J. Physiol. (Lond.) **146**, 29—53 (1959).
—, and R. C. Y. LIN: The action of 5-hydroxytryptamine (5-HT) on peristalsis. J. Physiol. (Lond.) **138**, 12P (1957).
— — The effect of intraluminal application of 5-hydroxytryptamine and 5-hydroxytryptophan on peristalsis; the local production of 5-HT and its release in relation to intraluminal pressure and propulsive activity. J. Physiol. (Lond.) **140**, 381—407 (1958).
BUÑAG, R. D., and E. J. WALASZEK: Mechanism of the serotonin depressor response following BAS-phenol administration in the dog. Experientia (Basel) **17**, 503—504 (1961a).
— — The mechanism of the depressor response to tryptamine and serotonin in the chicken. Fed. Proc. **20**, 111 (1961b).
— — The depressor effect of serotonin and tryptamine on chicken blood pressure. J. Pharmacol. exp. Ther. **133**, 52—56 (1961c).
— — Blockade of depressor responses to serotonin and tryptamine by lysergic acid derivatives in the chicken. Arch. int. Pharmacodyn. **135**, 142—151 (1962a).
— — The mechanism of serotonin and tryptamine induced vasodepression in the chicken. J. Pharmacol. exp. Ther. **135**, 150—155 (1962b).
— — Differential antagonism by BAS-phenol of responses to indolealkylamines. J. Pharmacol. exp. Ther. **136**, 59—67 (1962c).
— — The latent vasopressor effect of serotonin in the chicken. Arch. int. Pharmacodyn. **143**, 108—118 (1963).
BURFORD, H., J. LEICK and E. J. WALASZEK: Modification of the effects of biogenic amines on the heart by iproniazid. Arch. int. Pharmacodyn. **128**, 39—50 (1960).
—, and E. J. WALASZEK: Modification of the pressor effects of tyramine and tryptamine by iproniazid and reserpine. Fed. Proc. **19**, 124 (1960).
BURGEN, A. S. V., and S. W. KUFFLER: The inhibition of the cardiac ganglion of *Limulus polyphemus* by 5-hydroxytryptamine. Biol. Bull. **113**, 336 (1957).
BURGERS, A. C. J., D. I. ZANDEE, J. M. M. VAN BAKEL, G. M. L. HILLEMANS and G. J. VAN OORDT: The effect of LSD-derivatives and serotonin on the melanophores of the toad, *Xenopus laevis*. Acta physiol. pharmacol. neerl. **11**, 431—442 (1962).
BURNSTOCK, G.: The effect of drugs on spontaneous activity and on response to stimulation of the extrinsic nerves of the gut of a teleostean fish. Brit. J. Pharmacol. **13**, 216—226 (1958).
CAHN, J., G. GEORGES, M. HÉROLD et R. PIERRE: Influence de la sérotonine sur le métabolism cérébral et la narcose barbiturique, au cours de 24 heures suivant l'injection intraveineuse de 12.5 mg/kg chez le lapin in vivo. Thérapie **13**, 62—65 (1958).
— H. HÉROLD, M. DUBRASQUET et J. P. BURET: Effets de la 5-hydroxytryptamine (5-HT), de la diethylamide de l'acide D-lysergique (LSD 25), du phénobarbital, du nembutal et de 2 dérivés de la phénothiazine sur le métabolisme cérébral in vivo. C. R. Soc. Biol. (Paris) **151**, 82—85 (1957).

Caldarera, G., E. Riva Sanseverino e A. Urbano: Azione della 5-idrossitriptamina sulla secrezione salivare del cane. Boll. Soc. ital. Biol. sper. **37**, 1080—1083 (1961a).
— — — Modificazioni della secrezione salivare provocate dalla 5-idrossitriptamina sulla ghiandola sottomascellare di cane priva dell'innervazione simpatica ovvero totalmente enervata. Boll. Soc. ital. Biol. sper. **37**, 1083—1085 (1961b).
— — — Azione della 5-idrossitriptamina sul flusso venoso e sulla secrezione della ghiandola sottomascellare di cane. Boll. soc. ital. Biol. sper. **37**, 1085—1088 (1961c).
— — — Effetti della 5-idrossitriptamina sull'attività secretoria della ghiandola sottomascellare di cane. Arch. Sci. biol. (Napoli) **47**, 115—132 (1963).
Calì, G., e C. Cordova: 5-Ossitriptamina e secrezione gastrica. Progr. med. (Napoli) **12**, 752—757 (1956a).
— — Influenza degli antiistaminici di sintesi sulla curva di secrezione gastrica da 5-ossitriptamina. Rass. Fisiopat. clin. ter. **28**, 1072—1085 (1956b).
—, e G. Lomeo: Azione della 5-ossitriptamina sui capillari. Progr. med. (Napoli) **11**, 743—747 (1955).
— — 5-Ossitriptamina e fattori vascolari dell'emostasi. Rass. Fisiopat. clin. ter. **27**, 1092—1105 (1956).
— — Azione distrettuale della 5-ossitriptamina sulle arterie periferiche nell'uomo. Boll. Soc. ital. Biol. sper. **33**, 271—272 (1957a).
— — Comportamento della pressione venosa in un territorio vascolare periferico sotto l'azione distrettuale della 5-ossitriptamina. Boll. Soc. ital. Biol. sper. **33**, 272—273 (1957b).
— — e G. D. Bompiani: 5-Ossitriptamina e secrezione renale. Rass. Fisiop. clin. ter. **27**, 1079—1092 (1956).
— A. Strano e G. Lomeo: Influenza della 5-ossitriptamina sul pletismogramma digitale. XVIII Congr. Soc. ital. Cardiologia, Riass. Comun. pp. 136—137 (1956).
Cambridge, G. W.: Further investigations of the mechanisms of contraction and relaxation of *Mytilus* muscle. XXI Internat. Congr. Physiol. Sci. Buenos Aires 1959. Abstr. Commun. p. 49—50.
—, and J. A. Holgate: Responses of muscle from *Mytilus edulis* to drugs. J. Physiol. (Lond.) **142**, 41P (1958).
Carbonin, P. U., S. Sensi, A. Piffanelli, A. V. Greco and G. Gambassi: Aspects of the 5-hydroxytryptamine (HT) action on the perfused heart. Biochim. Biol. sper. **2**, 90—93 (1962—1963).
Carlier, J., G. Lejeune-Ledant et G. Barac: Angiotensine, 5-hydroxytryptamine et circulation pulmonaire chez le Chien. C. R. Soc. Biol. (Paris) **152**, 1034—1038 (1958).
— — et Ch. Keil: Action de la 5-hydroxytryptamine et du 5-hydroxytryptophane sur la thyroide du Lapin. J. Physiol. (Paris) **52**, 42—44 (1960).
Carlisle, D. B.: The neurohumoral control of heart rate in crustaceans. In: D. Richter Ed., Comparative Neurochemistry, pp. 323—328. Oxford: Pergamon Press 1964.
Carretti, D., e G. Ronchetti: L'influenza dell'enteramina sulla diuresi nell'uomo. Boll. Soc. med.-chir. Modena **55**, 581—583 (1955).
Case, J. D., and M. R. Wright: Effect of O-methylation and other substitutions of indoles on lightening of frog melanocytes. Fed. Proc. **19**, 282 (1960).
Casella, C., B. Fumagalli e S. Noli: Effetti della 5-idrossitriptamina sul circolo cerebrale nel coniglio e nel gatto. Boll. Soc. ital. Biol. sper. **33**, 1550—1552 (1957).
Cass, R., and P. B. Marshall: Effect of adrenocortical hormones on tissue histamine and 5-hydroxytryptamine in the rat. Arch. int. Pharmacodyn. **136**, 311—332 (1962).
Casu, A.: Serotonin inhibition of liver mitochondria swelling *in vitro*. Experientia (Basel) **16**, 489—490 (1960).
Cataldi, G.: Azione della 5-idrossitriptamina sull'utero gravido. Riv. ital. Ginec. **39**, 3—22 (1956a).
— Azione sull'utero, in particolari condizioni sperimentali, della 5-idrossitriptamina. Riv. ital. Ginec. **39**, 204—212 (1956b).
— Possibilità terapeutiche della 5-idrossitriptamina nel campo ostetrico e ginecologico. Riv. ital. Ginec. **34**, 298—314 (1956c).
Cater, D. B.: The effect of breathing oxygen, injection of serotonin and changes of systemic blood pressure upon the oxygen tension in tumours. G. ital. Chemioter. **6—9**, 240 (1962).
Cato, J., and E. J. Cafruny: Effects of tetrazotized diorthoanisidine on depressor response to 5-hydroxytryptamine in the rabbit. Proc. Soc. exp. Biol. (N.Y.) **104**, 103—105 (1960).
Cauwenberge, H., van, C. Lapière, J. Lecomte et F. Halkin: Modifications pharmacodynamiques et hormonales de l'oedème provoqué chez le rat par la 5-hydroxytryptamine. C. R. Soc. Biol. (Paris) **153**, 189—192 (1959b).
— — — et J. Renson: Modifications pharmacodynamiques et hormonales de l'augmentation de la perméabilité vasculaire provoquée par la 5-hydroxytryptamine. C. R. Soc. Biol. (Paris) **152**, 1848—1851 (1959a).

Cenacchi, G. C., e A. Cariani: Influenza della 5-idrossitriptamina sulla funzionalità renale nell'uomo. Boll. Soc. ital. Biol. sper. **34**, 569—570 (1958).
— — e L. Rosa: Contributo allo studio degli effetti della serotonina sulla funzione renale dell'uomo. Arch. Fisiopat. Clin. Ricambio **23**, 14—23 (1959).
Cenciotti, L.: Influenza della 5-idrossitriptamina sul pomfo da istamina. Boll. Sci. med. **128**, 281—285 (1957).
Cerhová, M., A. Šídlova and A. Zelený: The effect of skin inflammation on skin content of serotonin and histamine. Physiol. bohemoslov. **11**, 136—141 (1962).
Cerletti, A.: Pharmacology of psilocybin. In: B. B. Bradley, P. Deniker and C. Radouco-Thomas: Neuro-Psychopharmacology, pp. 291—294. Amsterdam: Elsevier Publ. Co. 1959.
—, u. B. Berde: Die Wirkung von D-Lysergsäure-diäthylamid (LSD 25) und 5-Oxytryptamin auf die Chromatophoren von *Poecilia reticulatus*. Experientia (Basel) **11**, 312—313 (1955).
— A. Carpi u. E. Rothlin: Über die Wirkung von 5-Oxytryptamin (Serotonin) auf die Diurese und Nierendurchblutung. Helv. physiol. Acta **13**, C 8—9 (1955).
—, u. H. Weidmann: Untersuchungen zur Differenzierung des vasokonstriktorischen Effektes von Serotonin. Arch. int. Pharmacodyn. **139**, 177—186 (1962).
Chen, K. K., and A. L. Chen: The pharmacological actions of ten amines related to ephedrine and tryptamine. J. Amer. pharm. Ass., sci. Ed. **22**, 813—819 (1933).
Chiandussi, L., F. Greco, D. Indovina, L. Cesano, A. Vaccarino and F. Muratori: Effect of drug infusion on splancnic circulation. II. Serotonin infusion in normal and cirrhotic subjects. Proc. Soc. exp. Biol. (N.Y.) **112**, 326—328 (1963).
Chodera, A.: Blockade of 5-hydroxytryptamine antidiuresis in rats by 2-bromlysergic acid diethylamide tartrate and 1-methyllysergic acid butanolamide. J. Pharm. Pharmacol. **15**, 386—389 (1963).
Chryssanthou, C., and W. Antopol: Inhibition of fibrinolysis by endotoxin, bradykinin and serotonin. Fed. Proc. **23**, 240 (1964).
Clark, L. C., R. P. Fox, R. Morin and F. Benington: Effect of psychotomimetic compounds on certain oxidative and hydrolytic enzymes in mammalian brain. J. nerv. ment. Dis. **124**, 466—472 (1956).
Clendenning, W. E., G. A. Deoreo and R. B. Stoughton: Serotonin. Its effect in normal and atopic skin. Arch. Derm. **79**, 503—511 (1959).
Cleugh, J., J. H. Gaddum, P. Holton and E. Leach: Assay of substance P on the fowl rectal caecum. Brit. J. Pharmacol. **17**, 144—158 (1961).
Clifton, J. A., M. Atkinson, T. R. Hendrix and F. J. Ingelfinger: The effect of 5-hydroxytryptamine upon small intestine motility in man. J. Lab. clin. Med. **48**, 796 (1956).
Clini, V., G. B. Ferrara, A. Glässer e P. Mantegazzini: Effetti della 5-idrossitriptamina (enteramina) sul circolo cerebrale del gatto. Arch. ital. Sci. farmacol. **10**, 110—114 (1960).
Cobb, B., and E. M. Nanson: Further studies with serotonin and experimental pulmonary embolism. Ann. Surg. **151**, 501—506 (1960).
Coen, E. D., and R. W. Whitehead: Certain MAO inhibitors as protectors vs total body X-irradiation of mice. Fed. Proc. **21**, 423 (1962).
Cohen, A., and L. Cohen: Effects of aminoethylisothiouronium bromide and 5-hydroxytryptamine on the response of C^{31} mammary tumour isografts to irradiation in vivo. Brit. J. Radiol. **35**, 200—204 (1962).
Cohen, S. G., and T. M. Sapp: Serotonin- and histamine-affecting agents and experimental vascular sensitization. J. Allergy **31**, 248—256 (1960).
Cohen, Y.: Étude comparative des effets de la chélation sur les proprietés de quelques amines vasoactives. XXI Internat. Congr. Physiol. Sci. Buenos Aires 1959. Abstr. Com. pp. 66—67.
—, et P. Blanchard: Effets comparès de la chélation du calcium sur les propriétés de l'histamine et de l'hydroxy-5-tryptamine sur la vaso-motricité *in vitro* du cobaye et du rat. J. Physiol. (Paris) **54**, 316—318 (1962).
Collier, H. O. J., J. A. Holgate, M. Schachter and P. G. Shorley: The bronchoconstrictor action of bradykinin in the guinea-pig. Brit. J. Pharmacol. **15**, 290—297 (1960).
Colombo, J.-P., J. W. Weber, G. Guidotti, D. Kanameishi and P. P. Foa': Liver phosphorylase in normal and adrenalectomized dogs treated with serotonin. Endocrinology **67**, 693—697 (1960).
Comroe, jr. J. H.: Direct and reflex cardiopulmonary effects of serotonin (5-OH-tryptamine); their relation to pulmonary embolism. Amer. J. Physiol. **171**, 715 (1952).
— B. van Lingen, R. C. Stroud and A. Roncoroni: Reflex and direct cardiopulmonary effects of 5-HO-tryptamine (serotonin). Amer. J. Physiol. **173**, 379—389 (1953).

CONNORS, M., and H. ROSENKRANTZ: Serotonin uptake and action on the adrenal cortex. Endocrinology 71, 407—413 (1962).
CONTI, U., e G. F. RICOTTI: L'azione della 5-ossitriptamina sulle emorragie parenchimali (a nappo). Farmaco, Ed. sci. 10, 637—640 (1955).
COOKE, I.: Effects of the pericardial organ neurosecretory substance on the crustacean heart. Gen. comp. Endocrin. 2, 29 (1962).
CORA', D., F. ALBRIGNANI e S. DEBIASI: Influenza della 5-idrossitriptamina sulla diuresi. Minerva nefrol. 4, 21—23 (1957).
CORMIER, M., et P. JOUAN: Action de la 5-hydroxytryptamine sur la sécrétion in vitro des corticostéroides par les capsules surrénales du rat. C. R. Acad. Sci. (Paris) 254, 3444—3445 (1962).
CORREALE, P.: Azione dell'enteramina (5-idrossitriptamina) sulla pressione sistemica e sull'emostasi del ratto. Arch. int. Pharmacodyn. 97, 106—114 (1954).
— Azione della 5-idrossitriptamina (enteramina) sulla diuresi nell'uomo. Arch. ital. Sci. farmacol. 7, 153—165 (1957).
CORRELL, J. T., L. F. LYTH, S. LONG and J. C. VANDERPOEL: Some physiologic responses to 5-hydroxytryptamine creatinine sulfate. Amer. J. Physiol. 169, 537—544 (1952).
COSTA, E., and G. ZETLER: Interactions between epinephrine and psychotomimetic drugs on cat nictitating membrane. Fed. Proc. 17, 360 (1958).
— — Interactions between epinephrine and some psychotomimetic drugs. J. Pharmacol. exp. Ther. 125, 230—236 (1959).
COURVOISIER, S., et O. LEAU: Action protectrice de la 5-hydroxytryptamine (5-HT) administrée par voie parénterale vis-à-vis du bronchospasme provoqué chez le cobaye par la 5-hydroxytryptamine en aérosols. Specificité de cette action. In: B. B. BRADLEY, P. DENIKER and C. RADOUCO-THOMAS: Neuro-Psychopharmacology, pp. 303—307. Amsterdam: Elsevier Publ. Co. 1959.
CRAIG, J. M.: The mechanism of serotonin induced abortion in the rat. Fed. Proc. 21, 276 (1962).
CREMA, A., G. BENZI and F. BERTE': The action of some natural substances on the terminal portion of the common bile duct isolated "in toto". Arch. int. Pharmacodyn. 137, 307—317 (1962).
CRILE jr., G.: The effects of heat and radiation on cancers implanted on the feet of mice. Cancer Res. 23, 372—380 (1963).
CRONHEIM, G. E., and J. T. GOURZIS: Cardiovascular effects of serotonin in dogs premedicated with reserpine. Fed. Proc. 15, 414 (1956).
— — Cardiovascular and behavioral effects of serotonin and related substances in dogs without and with reserpine premedication. J. Pharmacol. exp. Ther. 130, 444—449 (1960).
CRUMPTON, C. W., C. A. CASTILLO, G. G. ROWE and G. M. MAXWELL: Serotonin and the dynamics of the heart. Ann. N.Y. Acad. Sci. 80 (3), 960—963 (1959).
CURTI, P. C., e P. FORNAROLI: Sulla tollerabilità della 5-ossitriptamina nel corso di trattamenti prolungati. Farmaco, Ed. sci. 10, 965—969 (1955).
CUYPERS, Y., A. NIZET et G. BARAC: Action directe de la 5-hydroxytryptamine, de l'adrénaline, de l'artérénol et de l'histamine sur le débit sanguin rénal chez le chien. C. R. Soc. Biol. (Paris) 151, 1768—1770 (1957).
CZYBA, J. C., et M. CHIRIS: Action de la sérotonine sur l'endomètre de quelques Rongeurs. C. R. Soc. Biol. (Paris) 156, 856—858 (1962).
— — et P. DUBOIS: Décidualisation chez la lapine castrée soumise à un conditionnement par la progestérone et la sérotonine. C. R. Soc. Biol. (Paris) 157, 295—297 (1963).
D'ADDABBO, A., R. GIORGINO e G. FANFANI: Studio di una nuova azione della 5-idrossitriptamina: inibizione della captazione di ^{131}I nel ratto. Folia endocr. (Roma) 16, 577—590 (1963).
DANIEL, E. E., A. J. HONOUR and A. BOGOCH: Antagonism of serotonin-induced contraction and electrical activity in the ileum. Gastroenterology 39, 62—73 (1960).
DASGUPTA, S. R.: The effect of chlorpromazine on antidiuresis produced by 5-hydroxytryptamine (serotonin) in rats. Fed. Proc. 16, 290 (1957); — Arch. int. Pharmacodyn. 112, 264—271 (1957).
DAVEY, K. G.: Serotonin and change of colour in frogs. Nature (Lond.) 183, 1271—1272 (1959).
— Intermedin and change of color in frogs: a new hypothesis. Canad. J. Zool. 38, 715—721 (1960).
DAVIDSON, J. D., A. SJOERDSMA, L. N. LOOMIS and S. UDENFRIEND: The effects of 5-hydroxytryptophan, the precursor of serotonin, in experimental animals and man. Clin. Res. Proc. 4, 304 (1957a).
— — — — Studies with the serotonin precursor, 5-hydroxytryptophan, in experimental animals and man. J. clin. Invest. 36, 1594—1599 (1957b).

DAVIS, R. B., W. L. BAILEY and N. P. HANSON: Comparative effects of lethal amounts of endotoxin on platelets, serotonin, and histamine concentrations in tolerant and nontolerant rabbits. J. Labor. clin. Med. **58**, 811 (1961c).

— — — Modification of serotonin and histamine release after *E. coli* endotoxin administration. Amer. J. Physiol. **205**, 560—566 (1963).

—, and B. J. KENNEDY: Carcinoid syndrome associated with adrenal hyperplasia. Arch. intern. Med. **109**, 192—200 (1962).

— D. G. MCQUARRIE and W. R. MEEKER: Immediate effects of *Escherichia coli* endotoxin administration on platelets and serotonin concentration. Fed. Proc. **18**, 211 (1959).

— W. R. MEEKER jr and W. L. BAILEY: Serotonin release after injection of *E. coli* endotoxin in the rabbit. Fed. Proc. **20**, 261 (1961a).

— — — Serotonin release by bacterial endotoxin. Proc. Soc. exp. Biol. (N.Y.) **108**, 774—776 (1961b).

DAY, M., and J. R. VANE: An analysis of the direct and indirect actions of drugs on the isolated guinea-pig ileum. Brit. J. Pharmacol. **20**, 150—170 (1963).

DEANOVIĆ, Ž., and Z. SUPEK: Relationship between urinary excretion-rate of 5-hydroxyindoleacetic acid and survival time of X-irradiated rats. Int. J. Radiat. Biol. **7**, 569—574 (1963).

— — and M. BULAT: Effect of chemoprotection by cystamine on urinary excretion of 5-hydroxyindoleacetic acid in X-irradiated rats. Int. J. Radiat. Biol. **7**, 109—111 (1963).

— — and M. RANDIĆ: Relationship between the dose of whole-body X-irradiation and the urinary excretion of 5-hydroxyindoleacetic acid in rats. Int. J. Radiat. Biol. **7**, 1—9 (1963).

DEBRAY, CH., et F. BESANÇON: L'intervention de la sérotonine (5-hydroxytryptamine) dans la motricité physiologique de l'intestin grêle de l'homme. Recherches électromanométriques. J. Physiol. (Paris) **53**, 525—541 (1961).

DE CARO, G.: Azione antagonista di alcuni derivati dell'acido lisergico sull'antidiuresi da 5-idrossitriptamina. Arch. int. Pharmacodyn. **141**, 54—61 (1963).

DE CORRAL SALETA, J.: Action de la sérotonine sur la sécrétion gastrique du chat. XX. Internat. Physiol. Congr. Bruxelles 1956. Abstr. Comm., pp. 225—226.

DE CORRAL SALETA, J. M.: Action of serotonin on gastric secretion. Rev. exp. Physiol. **16**, 217—230 (1960).

DELAY, J., P. PICHON, T. LEMPERIÈRE, P. NICHOLAS-CHARLES et A.-M. QUETIN: Les effets somatiques de la psilocybine. Ann. méd. psychol. **117**, 891—899 (1959).

DEL BO, M.: L'uso della 5-ossitriptamina associata ad anestetici locali nella tonsillectomia. Farmaco, Ed. sci. **11**, 506—509 (1956).

DE LETONA, J. M. L., R. C. DE LA MATA and D. M. AVIADO: Local and reflex effects of bronchial arterial injection of drugs. J. Pharmacol. **133**, 295—304 (1961).

DEL GRECO, F., and A. C. CORCORAN: Arterial pressure and renal functions during intravenous infusions of serotonin in rats. Fed. Proc. **15**, 415—416 (1956).

— G. M. C. MASSON and A. C. CORCORAN: Renal and arterial effects of serotonin in the anaesthetized rat. Amer. J. Physiol. **187**, 509—514 (1956).

DE MAIO, D.: Influence of adrenalectomy and hypophysectomy on cerebral serotonin. Science **129**, 1678—1679 (1959).

DE MELLO, W. C.: Serotonin and ovulation. Naturwissenschaften **44**, 587—588 (1957).

DEMIS, D. J., M. J. DAVIS and J. C. LAWLER: A study of the cutaneous effects of serotonin. J. invest. Derm. **34**, 43—56 (1960).

D'ERMO, F., e L. BONOMI: Ricerche farmacologiche sull'azione della serotonina (enteramina) sulla muscolatura iridea isolata. Boll. Oculist. **40**, 483—491 (1961).

DES PREZ, R. M., N. FALLON and E. W. HOOK: Modification of lethal effect of bacterial endotoxin by substances altering the metabolism of 5-hydroxytryptamine. Proc. Soc. exp. Biol. (N.Y.) **107**, 529—532 (1961).

DI PASQUALE, S.: Trattamento delle emottisi tubercolari con 5-OH-triptamina (Antemovis). Ann. med. Sondalo **4**, 40—45 (1956).

DISCHLER, W.: Der Einfluß langdauernder Behandlung mit Reserpin, Iproniazid und 5-Oxytryptamin auf den Oestrus-Zyklus von Mäusen erbreiner Stämme. Naturwissenschaften **47**, 401—402 (1960).

DJERASSI, I., E. KLEIN, S. FARBER and D. PALMER: Effects of 5-hydroxytryptamine on some aspects of hemorrhagic state in radiation-induced thrombocytopenia. Proc. Soc. exp. Biol. (N.Y.) **97**, 552—554 (1958).

DOEPFNER, W., and A. CERLETTI: Comparison of lysergic acid derivatives and antihistamines as inhibitors of the edema provoked in the rat's paw by serotonin. Int. Arch. Allergy **12**, 89—97 (1958).

DOLCINI, H. A., I. ZAIDMAN, F. LICHTENBERG and S. J. GRAY: Effects of serotonin on circulation in the rat kidney. Amer. J. Physiol. **199**, 1153—1156 (1960).

DOMBRO, R. S., L. S. BRADHAM, N. K. CAMPBELL and D. W. WOOLLEY: Serotonin receptors. III. The role of salt formation. Biochim. biophys. Acta (Amst.) **54**, 516—524 (1961).

DONALDSON jr., R. M., S. MALKIEL and S. J. GRAY: Serotonin studies on mouse tissues. Proc. Soc. exp. Biol. (N.Y.) **103**, 261—263 (1960).

DONTAS, A. S.: Effects of protoveratrine, serotonin and ATP on afferent and splanchnic nerve activity. Circulat. Res. **3**, 363—373 (1955).

DOUGLAS, W. W., and J. M. RITCHIE: On excitation of non-medullated afferent fibres in the vagus and aortic nerves by pharmacological agents. J. Physiol. (Lond.) **138**, 31—43 (1957).

— , and C. C. TOH: The effect of 5-hydroxytryptamine (serotonin) on respiration in the dog. J. Physiol. (Lond.) **117**, 71—72P (1952).

— — The respiratory stimulant action of 5-hydroxytryptamine (serotonin) in the dog. J. Physiol. (Lond.) **120**, 311—318 (1953).

DOULL, J., V. PLZAK and J. COWAN: Pharmacological and toxicological compounds as protective or therapeutic agents against radiation injury in experimental animals. III. The effect of chemical protection on life-span shortening in x-irradiated mice. USAF Radiat. Lab. Univ. Chic. Quart. Rep. **47**, 77—91 (1963).

DRAPANAS, TH., and J. C. McDONALD: The direct removal of portal blood serotonin by the liver. Surg. Gynec. Obstet. **116**, 481—485 (1963).

— — and J. D. STEWART: Serotonin release following instillation of hypertonic glucose into the proximal intestine. Ann. Surg. **156**, 528 (1962).

—, and E. L. POLLACK: The effect of serotonin and serotonin precursor on pancreatic secretion in the dog. Surgery **48**, 854—861 (1960).

DUKOR, P.: Versuche zum Mechanismus der Strahlenschutzwirkung von Oxytryptaminderivaten. Strahlentherapie **117**, 330—355 (1962a).

— Weitere Untersuchungen über die Wirksamkeit von Oxytryptaminderivaten im Strahlenschutzversuch. Experientia (Basel) 18, 513—515 (1962b).

—, and R. SCHUPPLI: Konstitutionschemische Bedingungen für die Wirksamkeit von Oxytryptaminderivaten im Strahlenschutzversuch. Experientia (Basel) **17**, 257—258 (1961).

DUSEK, J., J. JEZDINSKY, J. RESSL u. T. PRASILOVA: Der Spiegel des freien Serotonins im Plasma der Kaninchen bei der Experimentalembolie durch Fruchtwasser. Gynaecologia (Basel) **155**, 242—254 (1963).

DUTEIL, J. J.: Pulmonary vasoconstriction by 5-hydroxytryptamine in heart-lung preparation. Fed. Proc. **21**, 128 (1962).

—, and D. M. AVIADO: Factors influencing pulmonary hypertensive response to 5-hydroxytryptamine. Circulat. Res. **11**, 466—473 (1962).

DWORETSKY, M.: Role of histamine or other released substances in anaphylaxis in isolated guinea-pig ileum. Amer. J. Physiol. **197**, 31—33 (1959).

EBLE, J. N.: The depressor effect of tryptamine in the chicken: absence of tachyphylaxis and reversal following monoamine oxidase inhibitors. Fed. Proc. **21**, 330 (1962).

— An analysis of the depressor and pressor effects of tryptamine in the chicken. J. Pharmacol. exp. Ther. **139**, 31—37 (1963).

ECKARDT, E. T., G. B. THOMAS and W. M. GOVIER: Comparison of circumferimetry with observation in quantitation of serotonin-induced edema in rat paw. Proc. Soc. exp. Biol. (N.Y.) **98**, 211—212 (1958).

EDERY, H., and G. SCHATZBERG-PORATH: Some biological properties of two fluoro-derivatives of tryptamine. Experientia (Basel) **16**, 200 (1960).

EGAÑA, E.: Variations in CNS 5-HT during internal (β-particle) irradiation. Biochem. Pharmacol. **12**, Supplement, 155 (1963).

EGER, W.: Serotonin und Histamin als Leberschutzstoffe im Tierexperiment. Naturwissenschaften **45**, 442—443 (1958).

ELIASSON, R., and A. ÅSTRÖM: Pharmacological studies on the perfused human placenta. Acta pharmacol. (Kbh.) **11**, 254—264 (1955).

ELTGEN, D., R. KOCH u. H. LANGENDORFF: Untersuchungen über einen biologischen Strahlenschutz. XXXVIII. Mitt. Der Einfluß von Cysteamin und Serotonin auf die Retikulozyten und den Eisenstoffwechsel bestrahlter Tiere. Strahlentherapie **114**, 118—127 (1961).

EL TORAEI, I.: The antihemorrhagic factor of the blood platelets, 5-hydroxytryptamine, and its therapeutic use in surgery. Gazette Kasr-El-Aini Fac. Med. **22**, 51 (1956).

EMANUEL, D. A., J. SCOTT, R. COLLINS and F. J. HADDY: Effect of serotonin on renal vascular resistance and urine flow rate. Fed. Proc. **17**, 42 (1958).

— — — — Local effect of serotonin on renal vascular resistance and urine flow rate. Amer. J. Physiol. **196**, 1122—1126 (1959).

ENERBACK, L.: Influence of adrenalectomy on urinary excretion of 5-hydroxyindole acetic acid in the rat. Endocrinology **67**, 717—719 (1960).

Engelhardt, G.: Über eine Serotoninfreisetzung unter der anaphylaktischen Reaktion des Meerschweinchens. Naunyn-Schmiedeberg's Arch. exp. Path. Pharmak. **238**, 99—100 (1960).
Erdös, E. G., N. Baart, F. F. Földes and E. K. Zsigmond: Activation of enzymatic hydrolysis of benzoylcholine by tryptamine. Science **126**, 1177—1178 (1957b).
— — S. P. Shanon and F. F. Földes: The inhibitory effect of chlorpromazine and indolealkylamines on human cholinesterases. XX. Internat. Physiol. Congr. Bruxelles 1956. Abstr. Comm. pp. 274—275.
— F. F. Földes, N. Baart and S. P. Shanor: Activating effect of tryptamine, benzylamine and histamine on plasma cholinesterase. Fed. Proc. **16**, 294 (1957a).
Ershoff, B. H., and E. M. Gal: Effects of radiation on tissue serotonin levels in the rat. Proc. Soc. exp. Biol. (N.Y.) **108**, 160—162 (1961).
— R. Hellmers and A. F. Wells: Effects of a radioprotective agent on tissue serotonin levels in the X-irradiated rat. Proc. Soc. exp. Biol. (N.Y.) **110**, 536—538 (1962).
Erspamer, V.: Pharmakologische Studien über Enteramin. I. Über die Wirkung von Acetonextrakten der Kaninchenmagenschleimhaut auf den Blutdruck und auf isolierte überlebende Organe. Naunyn-Schmiedeberg's Arch. exp. Path. Pharmak. **196**, 343—365 (1940a).
— Pharmakologische Studien über Enteramin. II. Über einige Eigenschaften des Enteramins sowie über die Abgrenzung des Enteramins von den anderen kreislaufwirksamen Gewebsprodukten. Naunyn-Schmiedeberg's Arch. exp. Path. Pharmak. **196**, 366—390 (1940b).
— Ricerche farmacologiche sulle indolalchilamine del veleno di rospo. Bufotenina e bufotenidina. Arch. Sci. biol. (Napoli) **31**, 63—85 (1946a).
— Ricerche farmacologiche sull'enteramina. VII. Enteramina e indolalchilamine del veleno di rospo. Arch. Sci. biol. (Napoli) **31**, 86—95 (1946b).
— Enteramina e 5-metossitriptamina. Tossicità. Azione sulla diuresi, sulla pressione del sangue e su alcuni organi a muscolatura liscia. Ric. Sci. **22**, 694—702 (1952a).
— Biological activity of some enteramine-related substances. Nature (Lond.) **170**, 281—282 (1952b).
— Modificazioni delle azioni dell'enteramina ad opera degli agenti antiistaminici. Ric. Sci. **22**, 2148—2153 (1952c).
— Pharmacological studies on enteramine. IX. Influence of sympathomimetic and sympatholytic drugs on physiological and pharmacological actions of enteramine. Arch. int. Pharmacodyn. **93**, 293—316 (1953a).
— Influence of 5-hydroxytryptamine (enteramine) on the course of the acute lethal sublimate intoxication in the rat. Experientia (Basel) **9**, 186—187 (1953b).
— Azione antienteraminica di alcune indolalchilamine, del 2-metil-3-etil-5-aminoindolo e degli alcaloidi del gruppo dell'armina. Ric. Sci. **23**, 1203—1207 (1953c).
— Influenza di droghe ganglioplegiche, di agenti parasimpaticolitici e miolitici, di sostanze diuretiche e antidiuretiche sull'antidiuresi e su alcuni effetti farmacologici dell'enteramina (5-idrossitriptamina). Ric. Sci. **23**, 2250—2257 (1953d).
— Influence of 5-hydroxytryptamine (enteramine) on the regulation of water exchange through the skin of the frog. Acta pharmacol. (Kbh.) **10**, 1—6 (1954a).
— Il sistema cellulare enterocromaffine e l'enteramina (5-idrossitriptamina). Rend. sci. Farmitalia **1**, 1—193 (1954b).
— Pharmacology of indolealkylamines. Pharmacol. Rev. **6**, 425—487 (1954c).
— Observations on the fate of indolalkylamines in the organism. J. Physiol. (Lond.) **127**, 118—133 (1955a).
— Gramine derivatives antagonistic to 5-hydroxytryptamine (enteramine). Science **121**, 369—370 (1955b).
— Some observations on the fate of exogenous 5-hydroxytryptamine (enteramine) in the rat. J. Physiol. (Lond.) **133**, 1—9 (1956).
— Pharmacologically active substances of mammalian origin. Ann. Rev. Pharmacol. **1**, 175—218 (1961).
—, and G. Bertaccini: Observations on the antidiuretic action and the fate of 5-hydroxy-DL-tryptophan in the rat organism. Arch. int. Pharmacodyn. **137**, 6—23 (1962).
—, and P. Correale: Further observations on the action of 5-hydroxytryptamine (5-HT) on the urine flow and chloride excretion in the rat. Arch. int. Pharmacodyn. **101**, 99—112 (1955).
— — and L. Fiore-Donati: Pharmacodynamic and biochemical responses to 5-hydroxytryptamine (enteramine) of rats treated chronically with the substance. Arch. int. Pharmacodyn. **106**, 122—140 (1956).
—, and F. Ghiretti: The action of enteramine on the heart of molluscs. J. Physiol. (Lond.) **115**, 470—481 (1951).

ERSPAMER, V., A. GLÄSSER and P. MANTEGAZZINI: Pharmacological actions of 4-hydroxytryptamine and 4-hydroxytryptophan. Experientia (Basel) **16**, 505—506 (1960).
— — C. PASINI and G. STOPPANI: *In vitro* decarboxylation of tryptophans by mammalian decarboxylase. Nature (Lond.) **189**, 483 (1961).
—, and M. B. NOBILI: Observations on the fate of 4-hydroxy-DL-tryptophan in the organism of rat and man. Arch. int. Pharmacodyn. **137**, 24—38 (1962a).
— — Observations on the fate of DL-5-hydroxy-N-acetyltryptophan and DL-5-acetoxy-N-acetyltryptophan in the rat organism. Arch. int. Pharmacodyn. **139**, 304—317 (1962b).
—, and A. OTTOLENGHI: Antidiuretic action of enteramine. Experientia (Basel) **6**, 428 (1950).
— — Pharmacological studies on enteramine. VIII. Action of enteramine on the diuresis and the renal circulation of the rat. Arch. int. Pharmacodyn. **93**, 177—201 (1953).
—, and G. SALA: Identification of the stable antidiuretic substance ("stable ADS") of serum with 5-hydroxytryptamine. Brit. J. Pharmacol. **9**, 31—36 (1954).
—, and A. TESTINI: Observations on the release and turnover rate of 5-hydroxytryptamine in the gastrointestinal tract. J. Pharm. Pharmacol. **11**, 618—623 (1959).
ESTÈVE, A., et J. LAPORTE: L'action de certains antihemorragiques sur le prolongement du temps de saignement provoqué par quelques médicaments. Thérapie **12**, 510—520 (1957).
EULER, H. V., H. ERDTMAN u. H. HELLSTRÖM: Über das Alkaloid Gramin. Ber. dtsch. chem. Ges. **69**, 743—747 (1936).
EULER, U. S. VON, and E. ÖSTLUND: Effects of certain biologically occurring substances on the isolated intestine of fish. Acta physiol. scand. **38**, 364—372 (1957).
EVANS, D. H. L., and H. O. SCHILD: Reactions of nerve-free and chronically denervated plain muscle to drugs. J. Physiol. (Lond.) **122**, 63P (1953).
EZER, E., and L. SZPORNY: Inhibition of hyaluronidase effects by serotonin. Acta physiol. Acad. Sci. hung. **20**, 171—176 (1961).
FABING, H. D., E. L. KROPA, J. R. HAWKINS and C. D. LEAKE: Bufotenine effects in humans. Fed. Proc. **15**, 421 (1956).
FÄNGE, R.: Pharmacology of poikilothermic vertebrates and invertebrates. Pharmacol. Rev. **14**, 281—316 (1962).
—, and A. MATTISSON: Studies on the physiology of the radula-muscle of *Buccinum undatum*. Acta zool. **39**, 53—54 (1954).
FASTIER, F. N., M. A. MCDOWALL and H. WAAL: Pharmacological properties of phenyldiguanide and other amidine derivatives in relation to those of 5-hydroxytryptamine. Brit. J. Pharmacol. **14**, 527—535 (1959).
—, and H. WAAL: The antidiuretic action of 5-hydroxytryptamine in cats in relation to the production of certain chemoreflexes. Brit. J. Pharmacol. **12**, 484—488 (1957).
FAWZI, S.: Effect of 5-hydroxytryptamine (Antemovis) as an antihemorrhagic in various cases of bleeding in gynaecology. J. Egypt. med. Ass. **33**, 74—77 (1956).
FEARN, H. J., C. SMITH and G. B. WEST: Capillary permeability responses to snake venoms. J. Pharm. Pharmacol. **16**, 79—84 (1964).
FEIGEN, G. A., C. B. NIELSEN and G. B. SUTHERLAND: Differential action of ammonium chloride on the response of the sensitized gut to ovalbumin, serotonin, and histamine. J. Immunol. **78**, 240—245 (1957).
— J. K. PETERSON and C. B. NIELSEN: Anaphylaxis in isolated guinea-pig heart. XXI. Internat. Congr. Physiol. Sci. Buenos Aires 1959. Abstr. Com. p. 88.
FELDBERG, W., and A. N. SMITH: Release of histamine by tryptamine and 5-hydroxytryptamine. J. Physiol. (Lond.) **122**, 62P (1953); — Brit. J. Pharmacol. **8**, 406—411 (1953).
FELLMAN, J. H., T. S. FUJITA and C. J. BELBER: 2,3-Dihydro-5-hydroxytryptamine. Biochem. Pharmacol. **11**, 557—561 (1962).
FENICHEL, R. L., and W. H. SEEGERS: Bovine platelets, serotonin and the retraction of bovine plasma clots. Amer. J. Physiol. **181**, 19—20 (1955).
FERGUSSON, J.: Action of serotonin on motility of aneural smooth muscle. Fed. Proc. **16**, 37 (1957).
FINGL, E., and J. H. GADDUM: 5-Hydroxytryptamine blockade by dihydroergotamine in vitro. Fed. Proc. **12**, 320 (1953).
FINK, M. A.: Anaphylaxis in the mouse: possible relation of the Schultz-Dale reaction to serotonin release. Proc. Soc. exp. Biol. (N.Y.) **92**, 673—675 (1956).
—, and CH. E. GARDNER: Anaphylaxis in guinea-pig: improbability of release of serotonin in the Schultz-Dale reaction. Proc. Soc. exp. Biol. (N.Y.) **97**, 554—557 (1958).
FINK, S., and G. FRIEDMAN: The differential effect of drugs on the proximal and distal colon. Amer. J. Med. **28**, 534—540 (1960).
FIORE-DONATI, L., and L. CHIECO-BIANCHI: Effect of 5-hydroxytryptamine on the development of the carbon-tetrachloride-induced cirrhosis in rats. Lab. Invest. **9**, 625—638 (1960).

FIORE-DONATI, L., L. CHIECO-BIANCHI e G. BERTACCINI: Effetto protettivo della 5-idrossitriptamina sul danno epatocellulare da tetracloruro di carbonio nel ratto. Arch. int. Pharmacodyn. **123**, 115—131 (1959b).

— G. MAIORANO e L. CHIECO-BIANCHI: Interferenza della 5-idrossitriptamina sullo sviluppo della cirrhosi epatica da CCl_4. Boll. Soc. ital. Biol. sper. **34**, 1493—1494 (1958).

— and E. MOLTKE: Effect of reserpine, 5-hydroxytryptamine, and polymyxin B on mast cells and tensile strength of healing wounds. Acta endocr. (Kbh.) **34**, 430—436 (1960).

— L. POLLICE and L. CHIECO-BIANCHI: Response of adrenal and preputial glands of rats to administration of 5-hydroxytryptamine. Experientia (Basel) **15**, 193—195 (1959a).

FISCHER, P., et J. LECOMTE: Choc anaphylactique chez le lapin traité par la réserpine. C. R. Soc. Biol. (Paris) **150**, 1026—1028 (1956a).

— — Hyperexcrétion urinaire d'acide 5-hydroxyindolacétique au cours du choc anaphylactique. C. R. Soc. Biol. (Paris) **150**, 1649—1650 (1956b).

FISHEL, CH. W., A. SZENTIVANYI and D. W. TALMAGE: Sensitization and desensitization of mice to histamine and serotonin by neurohumors. J. Immunol. **89**, 8—18 (1962).

FISHLOCK, D. J.: The action of 5-hydroxytryptamine on the circular muscle of the human ileum and colon in vitro. J. Physiol. (Lond.) **170**, 11—12P (1964).

—, and A. G. PARKS: Study of human colonic muscle *in vitro*. Brit. med. J. 1936 **II**, 666—667.

FLOREY, E., u. E. FLOREY: Über die mögliche Bedeutung von Enteramin (5-Oxy-Tryptamin) als nervöse Aktionssubstanz bei Cephalopoden und decapoden Crustaceen. Naturwissenschaften **40**, 413—414 (1953); — Z. Naturforsch. **9**b, 58—68 (1954).

FLÜCKIGER, E., u. R. SALZMANN: Serotoninantagonismus an der Placenta. Experientia (Basel) **17**, 131 (1961).

FOÁ, P. P., G. GALANSINO and R. LITTA-MODIGNANI: Release of serotonin and catecholamines by growth hormone and by deserpidine. Proc. int. Union Physiol. Sci. **2**, Abstr. 429 (1962).

FÖLDES, I.: Die Wirkung von Serotonin auf den O_2-Verbrauch von Ratten. Acta physiol. Acad. Sci. hung. **18**, 105 (1961).

— L. HARANGHY, L. CSÖTÖRTÖK and E. BEREGI: Comparative studies of different effects of exogenous serotonin (5-hydroxytryptamine) on young and old rats. Acta biol. Acad. Sci. hung. **12**, Suppl. 4, 32 (1962); — Gerontologia (Basel) **5**, 19—24 (1961).

—, u. E. KOMLÓS: Die Wirkung von Serotonin (5-Hydroxytryptamin) auf den Gasstoffwechsel und die Körpertemperatur weißer Ratten. Arch. int. Pharmacodyn. **120**, 121—129 (1959).

— — and J. PÁLINKÁS: Effect of tuberculosis on serotonin-induced bronchial spasm in guinea-pigs. Lancet **1959**a **I**, 154.

—, u. J. PALINKAS: Weitere Untersuchungen über die Wirkung von Serotonin (5-Hydroxytryptamin) auf den Gasstoffwechsel weißer Ratten. Arch. int. Pharmacodyn. **127**, 331—336 (1960).

— E. K. ZSIGMOND, E. G. ERDÖS and F. F. FÖLDES: Histochemical demonstration of the inhibitory effect of d-lysergic acid diethylamide (LSD) and its congeners on brain cholinesterases. Fed. Proc. 18, 389 (1959b).

FORNAROLI, P., e M. KOLLER: Prove sperimentali sull'azione emostatica della 5-ossitriptamina nell'animale normale. Farmaco, Ed. sci. **10**, 91—96 (1955).

FRAHM, M.: Beeinflussung der Meerschweinchenatmung durch 5-Hydroxytryptamin (5-HT). Naunyn-Schmiedeberg's Arch. exp. Path. Pharmak. **232**, 286—287 (1957).

— F. H. VAN CAUWENBERGE et J. LECOMTE: Action de la sérotonine (5-HT) et d'un de ses inhibiteurs, l'UML 491, sur le développement des réactions granulomateuses chez le rat. C. R. Soc. Biol. (Paris) **155**, 432—435 (1961c).

— — — Action de la réserpine sur les réactions oedémateuses locales chez le rat. C. R. Soc. Biol. (Paris) **156**, 186—190 (1962a).

— U. CH. LASSEN u. K. SOEHRING: 5-Hydroxytryptamin und Bezold-Jarisch-Effekt. Naturwissenschaften **44**, 264 (1957).

FRANCHIMONT, P., J. LECOMTE et H. VAN CAUWENBERGE: Influence de la sérotonine et d'un de ses antagonistes sur le développement des réactions oedémateuses locales provoquées chez le rat par divers agents. C. R. Soc. Biol. (Paris) **155**, 180—184 (1961a).

— J. LECOMTE et H. VAN CAUWENBERGE: Action de la 5-HT sur l'évolution de l'oédème de la patte chez les rats normaux et surrénalectomizés. C. R. Soc. Biol. (Paris) **156**, 400—402 (1962b).

— P. LEFEBVRE et H. VAN CAUWENBERGE: Effects de la sérotonine, d'un de ses inhibiteurs, l'UML 491, et du glucagon sur l'ostéolathyrisme expérimental du rat. C. R. Soc. Biol. (Paris) **155**, 427—431 (1961b).

FRANZEN, F.: Biologic amines in urine and blood following subletha :total-body irradiation. 10th Internat. Congr. Radiology Montreal-Quebec 1962. Abstr. pp. 187—188.

— H. GROSS u. G. THIELICKE: Biogene Amine im Urin und Blut von Ratten nach subletaler Ganzkörperbestrahlung. Strahlentherapie **120**, 598—610 (1963).

Frenkl, R., L. Cslaay, G. Makara, Z. Somfai et L. Selmeci: L'effet de l'activité musculaire régulière sur la sensibilité à la sérotonine des rats. Med. exp. **10**, 190—194 (1964).

Freyburger, W. A., B. E. Graham, M. M. Rapport, P. H. Seay, W. M. Govier, O. F. Swoap and M. J. van der Brook: The pharmacology of 5-hydroxytryptamine (serotonin). J. Pharmacol. exp. Ther. **105**, 80—86 (1952).

Frick, M. H.: Influence of 5-hydroxytryptamine on renal function in extracorporeal circulation. Nature (Lond.) **187**, 609—610 (1960).

— L. Virkkula and M. K. Paasonen: 5-Hydroxytryptamine and antidiuresis after operation. Surgery **50**, 447—451 (1961).

Fried, G. H., and W. Antopol: Potentiation of pseudocholinesterase by serotonin and LSD. Fed. Proc. **16**, 357 (1957).

Frieden, E., G. W. Westermark and J. M. Schor: Inhibition of tryptophan pyrrolase by serotonin, epinephrine and tryptophan analogs. Arch. Biochem. **92**, 176—182 (1961).

Frosali, L., L. Salvini et A. M. Pacetti: Ricerche cliniche sulla attività anticurarica della 5-idrossitriptamina. Acta anaesth. (Padova) **12**, 441—448 (1961).

Fuga, G. C.: Azione della 5-ossitriptamina sulla funzione dei capillari cutanei dei senescenti. Dermatologia (Napoli) **10**, 80—88 (1959).

Furchgott, R. F.: Dibenamine blockade in strips of rabbit aorta and its use in differentiating receptors. J. Pharmacol. exp. Ther. **111**, 265—284 (1955).

Gaddum, J. H.: Tryptamine receptors. J. Physiol. (Lond.) **119**, 363—368 (1953).

—, and K. A. Hameed: Drugs which antagonize 5-hydroxytryptamine. Brit. J. Pharmacol. **9**, 240—248 (1954).

—, and Z. P. Picarelli: Two kinds of tryptamine receptor. Brit. J. Pharmacol. **12**, 323—328 (1957).

Galansino, G., R. Litta-Modignani, F. Berlinger, D. Billinger and P. P. Foá: Studies on release of serotonin and catecholamines in the pancreatic-duodenal area. Proc. Soc. exp. Biol. (N.Y.) **112**, 542—544 (1963).

Galton, V. A., and S. H. Ingbar: The influence of reserpine, serotonin and metabolites of tryptophane on the degradation of thyroxine and its derivatives. Endocrinology **68**, 435—449 (1961).

Ganley, O. H.: Protective effect of cyproheptadine, a new antihistamine-antiserotonin compound on lethal burns in the mouse. Arch. int. Pharmacodyn. **138**, 125—132 (1962).

Garcia-Arocha, H.: Histamine and 5-HT release from rat peritoneal cells. Rev. canad. Biol. **16**, 483—484 (1957).

— Chemical mediators of the anaphylactic reaction in the rat. Fed. Proc. **18**, 50 (1959).

— Release of histamine and 5-hydroxytryptamine from cells of the peritoneal fluid of rats. Canad. J. Biochem. **39**, 395—402 (1961a).

— Liberation of 5-hydroxytryptamine and histamine in the anaphylactic reaction of the rat. Canad. J. Biochem. **39**, 403—416 (1961b).

— Role of the antigen concentration in the anaphylactic response of isolated cells. Proc. int. Union Physiol. Sci. **2**, Abstr. 596 (1962).

Garrett, W. J.: The action of 5-hydroxytryptamine on the human uterus. Arch. int. Pharmacodyn. **117**, 435—443 (1958).

Gautieri, R. F., and H. P. Ciuchta: Effect of certain drugs on perfused human placenta. I. Narcotic analgesics, serotonin and relaxin. J. pharm. Sci. **51**, 55—58 (1962).

Geiger, W. B., and H. S. Alpers: The mechanism of the Schultz-Dale reaction. J. Allergy **30**, 316—328 (1959).

Gelfand, M. D., and G. B. West: Experimental studies with the butanolamide and propanolamide of 1-methyl-lysergic acid. Int. Arch. Allergy **18**, 286—291 (1961).

Georges, G.: Influence de la 5-hydroxytryptamine sur la réactivité du couple hypophysosurrénalien chez le rat. R. C. Soc. Biol. (Paris) **151**, 692—695 (1957b).

—, et M. Hérold: Influence de la sérotonine sur l'oedème plantaire au dextran chez le rat. C. R. Soc. Biol. (Paris) **151**, 695—698 (1957c).

— — Effets de la 5-hydroxytryptamine sur la motilité intestinale chez le lapin in vivo. C. R. Soc. Biol. (Paris) **151**, 77—79 (1957a).

— — Effets de la 5-hydroxytryptamine sur la motilité intestinale chez le lapin "in vivo". Thérapie **13**, 56—61 (1958a).

— — Influence de la sérotonine et du marsilid sur la réactivité de l'axe hypothalamo-hypophyso-surrénalien chez le rat. II. C. R. Soc. Biol. (Paris) **152**, 436—440 (1958b).

Gershon, M. D., and L. L. Ross: Studies on the relationship of 5-hydroxytryptamine and the enterochromaffin cells to anaphylactic shock in mice. J. exp. Med. **115**, 367—382 (1961).

Gessner, P. K., W. M. McIsaac and I. H. Page: Pharmacological actions of some methoxyindolealkylamines. Nature (Lond.) **190**, 179—180 (1961).

GHIRETTI, F.: Les excitants chimiques de la sécrétion salivaire chez les Céphalopodes octopodes. Arch. int. Physiol. **61**, 10—21 (1953a).
— Enteramina, octopamina e tiramina nelle secrezioni esterna ed interna delle ghiandole salivari posteriori dei cefalopodi. Arch. Sci. biol. (Napoli) **37**, 435—441 (1953b).
GHIRINGHELLI, F., E. MIRA e G. BERTACCINI: Le cellule enterocromaffini e la 5-idrossitriptamina nell'intestino del ratto surrenectomizzato. Folia endocr. (Roma) **14**, 571—580 (1961a).
— — — Le cellule enterocromaffini e la 5-idrossitriptamina nell'intestino di ratti ipofisectomizzati e trattati con ormone somatotropo. Arch. Biol. (Liège) **72**, 485—499 (1961b).
GIÃO, J. M., et T. RICO: Action de quelques dérivés de la phénotiazine sur l'oedème provoqué par la sérotonine chez le rat, étudiée avec des isotopes radioactifs. C. R. Soc. Biol. (Paris) **156**, 207—209 (1962).
GIERTZ, H., u. F. HAHN: Die Wirkung von Azulen auf den Histamin-, den Serotonin- und den anaphylaktischen Schock des Meerschweinchens. Arzneimittel-Forsch. **9**, 553—555 (1959).
— — W. OPFERKUCH u. W. SCHMUTZLER: Vergleichende Untersuchungen über den anaphylaktischen Schock und den Anaphylotoxinschock an der isolierten Meerschweinchenlunge. Naunyn-Schmiedeberg's Arch. exp. Path. Pharmak. **242**, 42—64 (1961).
GILBERT, R. P.: Effect of antihistaminic and antiserotonin drugs on vascular responses to *E. coli* endotoxin in the cat. Proc. Soc.exp. Biol. (N.Y.) **100**, 346—349 (1959).
— L. B. HINSLAW, H. KUIDA and M. VISSCHER: Effects of histamine, 5-hydroxytryptamine and epinephrine on pulmonary hemodynamics with particular reference to arterial and venous segment resistances. Amer. J. Physiol. **194**, 165—170 (1958).
— H. KUIDA, L. B. HINSLAW and M. VISSCHER: The effects of histamine and serotonin on pulmonary arterial and venous resistances. Clin. Res. Proc. **5**, 225 (1957).
GINZEL, K. H.: The action of lysergic acid diethylamide (LSD 25), its 2-brom derivative (BOL 148) and of 5-hydroxytryptamine (5-HT) on the peristaltic reflex of the guinea-pig ileum. J. Physiol. (Lond.) **137**, 62—63P (1957a).
— Die Wirkung von 5-Oxytryptaminen und Antagonisten auf den peristaltischen Reflex. Naunyn-Schmiedeberg's Arch. exp. Path. Pharmak. **232**, 287—288 (1957b).
— The effects of 5-hydroxytryptamine on peripheral receptors of cardiovascular and respiratory reflexes. In: G. P. LEWIS, 5-Hydroxytryptamine, p. 131—135. London: Pergamon Press 1957 (c).
—, and S. R. KOTTEGODA: A study on the vascular actions of 5-hydroxytryptamine, tryptamine, adrenaline and noradrenaline. Quart. J. exp. Physiol. **38**, 225—231 (1953).
— — The action of 5-hydroxytryptamine and tryptamine on aortic and carotid sinus receptors in the cat. J. Physiol. (Lond.) **123**, 277—287 (1954).
GIRO, C., A. BARONCHELLI, G. D'ANTUONO e E. PIERAGNOLI: Effetti della serotonina sul tono e sulla motilità delle vie biliari extraepatiche. Boll. Soc. ital. Biol. sper. **36**, 1345—1347 (1960).
GLAZ, T., L. GYERMEK and T. NOGRADI: The adrenolytic activity of tryptamine and related compounds on isolated organs. Arch. int. Pharmacodyn. **108**, 420—430 (1956).
GLOVER, W. E., A. D. M. GREENFIELD, B. S. L. KIDD and R. F. WHELAN: The reactions of the capacity blood vessels of the human hand and forearm to vasoactive substances infused intraarterially. J. Physiol. (Lond.) **140**, 113—121 (1958).
— R. J. MARSHALL and R. F. WHELAN: The antagonism of the vascular effects of 5-hydroxytryptamine by BOL 148 and sodium salycilate in the human subjects. Brit. J. Pharmacol. **12**, 498—503 (1957).
GOLDBERG, L. I., and A. SJOERDSMA: Effects of several monoamine oxidase inhibitors on the cardiovascular actions of naturally occurring amines in the dog. J. Pharmacol. exp. Ther. **127**, 212—218 (1959).
GOLDSMITH, R. S., B. W. EVANS and J. P. ROBERTS: Excretion of 5-hydroxyindoleacetic acid (5-HIAA) following burns. Clin. Res. **9**, 179 (1961).
GORDON, P.: Non-drug induced changes in blood serotonin. Fed. Proc. **20**, 315 (1961a).
— Changes in blood serotonin during exposure to cold. Nature (Lond.) **191**, 183—184 (1961b).
—, F. J. HADDY and M. A. LIPTON: Serotonin antagonism of noradrenaline in vivo. Science **128**, 531—532 (1958b).
— — — Serotonin-adrenaline interaction in vivo. Fed. Proc. **18**, 397 (1959).
—, and M. A. LIPTON: Beneficial effect of serotonin and compound F on *E. coli* endotoxin mortality in mice. Fed. Proc. **16**, 301 (1957).
— — and F. J. HADDY: Interaction of serotonin and the adrenalines upon limb resistance, cardiac rate and systemic arterial blood pressure. Fed. Proc. **17**, 58 (1958a).
GOSSELIN, R. E.: The cilioexcitatory activity of serotonin. J. cell. comp. Physiol. **58**, 17—25 (1961).
—, and M. M. ERNST: Action of serotonin on the gill cilia of lamellibranchiates. Fall Meet. Amer. Soc. Pharmacol., Ann Arbor 1958. Abstr. Pap. p. 15.

GOSSELIN, R. E., K. E. MOORE and A. S. MILTON: Physiological control of molluscan gill cilia by 5-hydroxytryptamine. J. gen. Physiol. **46**, 277—296 (1962).
GÖZSY, B., and L. KÁTO: Role of 5-hydroxytryptamine in the inflammatory process. Science **125**, 934—936 (1957a).
— — Changes in the permeability of the skin capillaries of rats after histamine depletion with 48/80, dextran or egg white. J. Physiol. (Lond.) **139**, 1—9 (1957b).
— — Investigations into the mechanism of dextran-induced edema in the rat. Canad. J. Biochem. **41**, 1855—1863 (1963).
— — The role of histamine and serotonin in alterations of capillary permeability following injury. Dermatologica (Basel) **127**, 403—409 (1963).
— — Effect of histamine, serotonin and catecholamines depletors on the capillaries in the rat skin. Arch. int. Pharmacodyn. **148**, 243—254 (1964).
GRANSER, G., G. HERTTING, E. RISSEL u. F. WEWALKA: Untersuchungen über die Beeinflußbarkeit des Sphinkter Oddi. Arch. int. Pharmacodyn. **105**, 389—402 (1956).
GRAY, J. L., J. T. TEW and H. JENSEN: Protective effect of serotonin and of paraaminopropiophenone against lethal doses of x-radiation. Proc. Soc. exp. Biol. (N.Y.) **80**, 604—607 (1952).
GREEFF, K., u. C. CONTZEN: Über den Mechanismus der diuresehemmenden Wirkung des Dextrans bei Ratten. Naunyn-Schmiedeberg's Arch. exp. Path. Pharmak. **239**, 35—53 (1960).
—, u. E. MOOG: Vergleichende Untersuchungen über die bronchoconstrictorische und gefäßconstrictorische Wirkung des Bradykinins, Histamins und Serotonins an isolierten Lungenpräparaten. Naunyn-Schmiedebergs Arch. exp. Path. Pharmak. **248**, 204—215 (1964).
GREENBERG, M. J., and T. C. JEGLA: The action of 5-hydroxytryptamine and acetylcholine on the rectum of the Venus clam, *Mercenaria mercenaria*. Comp. Biochem. Physiol. **9**, 275—290 (1963).
GRIGGS jr., D. M., and R. B. CASE: Effect of serotonin on coronary vascular resistance and myocardial oxygen consumption. Circulation **22**, 758—759 (1960).
GROVER, R. F., S. K. OLSON and S. G. BLOUNT jr.: Pulmonary vascular response to serotonin in man. Clin. Res. **6**, 62 (1958).
GRYGLEWSKI, R., and J. SUPNIEWSKI: Influence of 5-hydroxytryptamine and other biologically active substances on the movements of the isolated stomach of *Helix pomatia*. Bull. Acad. pol. Sci., Ser. Sci. biol. **11**, 53—56 (1963).
— — Action of chemical transmitters on the isolated internal organs of snail *Helix pomatia*. Biochem. Pharmacol. **12**, Supplement, 39 (1963).
GYERMEK, L.: Beiträge zur Pharmakologie von Tryptamin, Tyramin und Phenylaethylamin. Acta physiol. Acad. Sci. hung. **4**, 323—332 (1953).
— Cholinergic stimulation and blockade on urinary bladder. Amer. J. Physiol. **201**, 325—328 (1962a).
— Action of hydroxytryptamine on the urinary bladder of the dog. Arch. int. Pharmacodyn. **137**, 137—144 (1962b).
—, and C. POSSEMATO: Potentiation of 5-hydroxytryptamine by imipramine. Med. exp. **3**, 225—229 (1961).
HADDY, F. J.: Further evidence that arteries, arterioles and veins are independent resistances. XXI. Internat. Congr. Physiol. Sciences, Buenos Aires 1959. Abstr. Comm. p. 116.
— The mechanism of edema production by acetylcholine, serotonin, histamine and norepinephrine. Fed. Proc. **19**, 93 (1960).
— M. FLEISHMAN, D. A. EMANUEL and J. B. SCOTT: The effect of serotonin upon systemic small and large vessel resistances. Clin. Res. Proc. **5**, 174—175 (1957a).
— — — Effect of epinephrine, norepinephrine and serotonin upon systemic small and large vessel resistance. Circulat. Res. **5**, 247—251 (1957b).
— P. GORDON and D. A. EMANUEL: The influence of tone upon responses of small and large vessels to serotonin. Circulat. Res. **7**, 123—130 (1959).
HAGEN, U., u. K. FLEMMING: Zum Wirkungsmechanismus des Serotonins als Strahlenschutzstoff. Naturwissenschaften **50**, 303 (1963).
HALBERG, F.: Eosinopenic effects of tryptamines in mice. Synergism of effects of serotonin and cortisone. Amer. J. Physiol. **179**, 309—313 (1954).
HALMAGYI, D. F. J., and H. J. H. COLEBATCH: Serotonin-like cardiorespiratory effects of a serotonin antagonist. J. Pharmacol. exp. Ther. **134**, 47—52 (1961).
HALPERN, B. N., P. LIACOPOULOS et M. LIACOPOULOS-BRIOT: Libération de 5-hydroxytryptamine chez le rat sous l'influence de substances histamino-libératrices. C. R. Soc. Biol. (Paris) **151**, 1692—1696 (1957).
— T. NEVEU and S. SPECTOR: On the nature of the chemical mediators involved in anaphylactic reactions in mice. Brit. J. Pharmacol. **20**, 389—398 (1963).

HALPERN, B. N., M. LIACOPOULOS-BRIOT, V. SPICAK, T. NEVEU, M. F. PERRAMANT et A. BRANELLEC: Mécanisme de libération de l'histamine et de la 5-hydroxytryptamine au cours de la réaction anaphylactique et sous l'action de substances histamino-libératrices (S.H.L.) chez le rat. Arch. int. Pharmacodyn. **147**, 431—449 (1964).
HAMMOND, J. B.: The effect of serotonin and lysergic acid diethylamide on the secretory response to reserpine. Clin. Res. Proc. **4**, 247 (1956).
HANDOVSKI, H.: Ein Alkaloid im Gifte von *Bufo vulgaris*. Naunyn-Schmiedeberg's Arch. exp. Path. Pharmak. **86**, 138—158 (1920).
HANSON, A. S., and TH. A. MAGILL: Electrical and mechanical actions of 5-hydroxytryptamine, epinephrine, ouabain, and procainamide on strips of turtle ventricle. Fed. Proc. **20**, 122 (1961).
— — Effects of epinephrine and 5-hydroxytryptamine on strips of frog and turtle ventricle. Proc. Soc. exp. Biol. (N.Y.) **109**, 329—333 (1962).
HARASAWA, M., and S. RODBARD: Estimation of airway responses to physiological stimuli and drugs. J. Pharmacol. exp. Ther. **133**, 246—252 (1961).
HARDING-GAUDIN, F.: Excrétion urinaire d'acide 5-hydroxyindolylacétique chez le rat albinos carencé ou non en riboflavine. Acta vitamin. (Milano) **15**, 193—196 (1961).
HARRIS, P., H. W. FRITTS jr. and A. COURNAND: Some circulatory effects of 5-hydroxytryptamine in man. Circulation **21**, 1134—1139 (1960).
HARRY, J.: The action of drugs on the circular muscle strip from the guinea-pig isolated ileum. Brit. J. Pharmacol. **20**, 399—417 (1963).
HARVEY, D. G.: The quantitative response of the oxygen consumption and weight of guinea pigs to some metabolic stimulants, with a note on DL-5-iodotryptophan. J. Pharm. Pharmacol. **40**, 681—688 (1959).
HAVERBACK, B. J.: Serotonin and gastrointestinal tract. Clin. Res. **6**, 57 (1958a).
— Effect of the serotonin precursor, 5-hydroxytryptophan, on gastric secretion and gastric mucosa in animals. Clin. Res. **6**, 100 (1958b).
— Discussion of the paper presented by E. P. BENDITT "Mechanism of inflammation". Gastroenterology **40**, 338—343 (1961).
— D. F. BOGDANSKI and C. A. M. HOGBEN: Inhibition of gastric acid secretion in the dog by the precursor of serotonin, 5-hydroxytryptophan. Gastroenterology **34**, 188—195 (1958).
—, and J. D. DAVIDSON: Serotonin and the gastrointestinal tract. Gastroenterology **35**, 570—578 (1958).
— F. T. DUTSCHER, P. A. SHORE, E. G. TOMICH, L. L. TERRY and B. B. BRODIE: Serotonin changes in platelets and brain induced by small daily doses of reserpine. Lack of effect of depletion of platelet serotonin in hemostatic mechanisms. New Engl. J. Med. **256**, 343—345 (1957b).
— C. A. M. HOGBEN, N. C. MORAN and L. L. TERRY: Effect of serotonin (5-hydroxytryptamine) and related compounds on gastric secretion and intestinal motility in the dog. Gastroenterology **32**, 1058—1065 (1957a).
—, and S. K. WIRTSCHAFTLER: The gastrointestinal tract and naturally occurring pharmacologically active amines. Advanc. Pharmacol. **1**, 309—348 (1962).
HECKMANN, U., H. A. KUNKEL u. E. LAPPE: Über den Einfluß von 5-Hydroxytryptamin und die strahleninduzierten Veränderungen im neurosekretorischen Zwischenhirnsystem der Ratte. Naturwissenschaften **51**, 219 (1964).
HEITE, H.-J., u. D. KLEINHANS: Zur diagnostischen Bedeutung des quantitativ erfaßten Serotonin-Erythems bei verschiedenen Ekzemformen. Arch. klin. exp. Derm. **214**, 573—581 (1962).
HENDRIX, T. R., M. ATKINSON, J. A. CLIFTON and F. J. INGELFINGER: The effect of serotonin on intestinal motor function in man. Clin. Res. Proc. **5**, 19 (1957a).
— — — — The effect of 5-hydroxytryptamine on intestinal motor function in man. Amer. J. Med. **23**, 886—893 (1957b).
HERXHEIMER, H.: The bronchial reaction of guinea-pigs to 5-hydroxytryptamine. J. Physiol. (Lond.) **120**, 65P (1953a).
— Influence of 5-hydroxytryptamine on bronchial function. J. Physiol. (Lond.) **122**, 49—50P (1953b).
— The 5-hydroxytryptamine shock in the guinea-pig. J. Physiol. (Lond.) **128**, 435—445 (1955).
— The 5-HT shock in the guinea-pig. In: G. P. LEWIS, 5-Hydroxytryptamine, p. 163—167. London: Pergamon Press 1957.
—, and M. SCHACHTER: Weal and flare in human skin produced by hystamine and other substances. Nature (Lond.) **183**, 1510—1511 (1959); — J. Physiol. (Lond.) **145**, 34—35P (1959).
HEYMANS, C., et G. VAN DEN HEUVEL-HEYMANS: Sur la pharmacologie de l'hydroxytryptamine (sérotonine) et d'une substance analogue. Arch. int. Pharmacodyn. **93**, 95—104 (1953).

HICKS, R., and G. B. WEST: Adrenal cortical hormones and the formation of histamine and 5-hydroxytryptamine. Nature (Lond.) **181**, 1342—1343 (1958a).
— — Adrenalectomy and tissue amines. Nature (Lond.) **182**, 401—402 (1958b).
HIETBRINK, B. E., A. B. RAYMUND and K. B. DUBOIS: The effects of ionizing radiations on the biochemistry of mammalian tissues. I. The influence of cysteine, 2-mercaptoethylamine and 5-hydroxytryptamine in the radiation-induced changes in enzyme activities of hematopoietic tissues and small intestine of rats. USAT Radiat. Lab. Univ. Chicago Quart. Rep. **38**, 1—14 (1961).
HIGGINBOTHAM, R. D.: Effect of compound 48/80 on toxicity of histamine and of serotonin in mice. Proc. Soc. exp. Biol. (N.Y.) **102**, 4—8 (1959).
— Histamine, 5-hydroxytryptamine and cortisol in mouse anaphylaxis. Fed. Proc. **19**, 215 (1960).
HIGHTON, T. C., and M. H. GARRETT: Some effects of serotonin and related compounds on human collagen. Lancet **1963 I**, 1234—1236.
HILL, R. B.: The effects of certain neurohormones and of other drugs on the ventricle and radula protractor of *Busicon canaliculatum* and on the ventricle of *Strombus gigas*. Biol. Bull. **115**, 471—482 (1958).
—, and P. N. R. USHERWOOD: The action of 5-hydroxytryptamine and related compounds on neuromuscular transmission in the locust *Schnistocerca gregaria*. J. Physiol. (Lond.) **157**, 293—401 (1961).
HOLEMANS, R., and M. H. CHO: Local influence of certain drugs on thrombolysis. Fed. Proc. **21**, 63 (1962).
HOLGATE, J. A., and G. W. CAMBRIDGE: Responses of the anterior retractor muscle of the byssus of *Mytilus edulis*. Nature (Lond.) **182**, 34—35 (1958).
HOLLANDER, W., and A. L. MICHELSON: The effects of serotonin and antiserotonins in hypertensive man. J. clin. Invest. **35**, 712—713 (1956).
— — and R. W. WILKINS: Serotonin and antiserotonins. I. Their circulatory, respiratory, and renal effects in man. Circulation **16**, 246—255 (1957).
HOLLENBERG, G. M., R. PRUETT and A. THAL: Vasoactive substances liberated by prolonged bubble oxygenation. J. thorac. cardiovasc. Surg. **45**, 402—411 (1963).
HONUS, E.: Das Verhalten des 5-Hydroxytryptamins des Magen-Darm-Traktes nach experimentellem Ileus. Wien. klin. Wschr. **75**, 765—768 (1963).
HORITA, A., and J. H. GOGERTY: The pyretogenic effect of 5-hydroxytryptophan and its comparison with that of LSD. J. Pharmacol. exp. Ther. **122**, 195—200 (1958).
HORTON, E. W.: An increase in butanol-extractable 5-hydroxytryptamine in venous blood during reactive hyperaemia. J. Physiol. (Lond.) **170**, 101—109 (1964).
HOTOVY, R.: Diskussionsbemerkung zum Vortrag von A. CERLETTI u. H. KONZETT. Naunyn-Schmiedeberg's Arch. exp. Path. Pharmak. **228**, 148 (1956).
—, u. E. ROESCH: Zur Pharmakologie der Kreislaufwirkung von 5-Hydroxytryptamin. Naunyn-Schmiedeberg's Arch. exp. Path. Pharmak. **232**, 369—386 (1958).
HUDOCK, I. I., A. KHENTIGAN, R. CRAMTON, P. VANAMEE and W. LAWRENCE jr.: Serotonin and pancreatic secretion. Surg. Forum **12**, 362—364 (1961).
HUGHES, W. F., D. J. O'BRIEN and J. W. NEWBERNE: Influence of lysergic acid diethylamide (LSD) and other centrally active agents on experimental allergic encephalomyelitis. Fed. Proc. **21**, 16 (1962).
HUGUES, J.: Contribution à l'étude des facteurs vasculaires et sanguins dans l'hémostase spontanée. Arch. int. Physiol. **61**, 565—711 (1953).
HUKUHARA, T., S. NAKAYAMA and R. NAUBA: The effects of 5-hydroxytryptamine upon the intestinal motility, especially with respect to the intestinal mucosal intrinsic reflex. Jap. J. Physiol. **10**, 420—426 (1960).
HULET, W. H., and G. A. PERERA: Effect of serotonin on renal excretion of sodium; possible relation to Rauwolfia action. Proc. Soc. exp. Biol. (N.Y.) **91**, 512—514 (1956).
HUMPHREY, J. H., and R. JAQUES: Liberation of histamine and serotonin from platelets by antigen-antibody reaction. J. Physiol. (Lond.) **119**, 43P (1953).
— — The release of histamine and 5-hydroxytryptamine (serotonin) from platelets by antigen-antibody reactions (in vitro). J. Physiol. (Lond.) **128**, 9—27 (1955).
HUPKA, S., and J. E. DUMONT: *In vitro* effect of adrenaline and other amines on glucose metabolism in sheep thyroid, heart, liver, kidney and testicular slices. Biochem. Pharmacol. **12**, 1023—1036 (1963).
HURWITZ, R., R. W. CAMPBELL, P. GORDON and F. J. HADDY: Interaction of serotonin with vasoconstrictor agents in the vascular bed of the denervated dog forelimb. J. Pharmacol. **133**, 57—62 (1961).
HUTCHISON, H. E., J. M. STARK and J. A. CHAPMAN: Platelet serotonin and normal haemostasis. J. clin. Path. **12**, 265—267 (1959).

INNES, I. R.: Smooth muscle receptors for amphetamine and 5-hydroxytryptamine. Proc. Int. Union Physiol. Sci. **2**, Abstr. 591 (1962).
— An action of 5-hydroxytryptamine on adrenaline receptors. Brit. J. Pharmacol. **19**, 427—441 (1962b).
— H. W. KOSTERLITZ and J. A. ROBINSON: The effects of lowering the bath temperature on the responses of the isolated guinea-pig ileum. J. Physiol. (Lond.) **137**, 397—409 (1957).
INOUE, T.: Pharmacology of 5-hydroxytryptamine. The mechanism of contracting action of 5-hydroxytryptamine on muscle. Nippon Yakurigaku Zasshi **52**, 41—45 (1956).
—, et K. KURIAKI: Teneur en 5-hydroxytryptamine du plasma sanguin lors du choc anaphylactique. C. R. Soc. Biol. (Paris) **151**, 1470—1471 (1958).
JASMIN, G., et E. BAJUSZ: Action de la sérotonine, du 48/80 et de la réserpine sur les lésions de calcinose provoquées par divers agents chez le rat. Rev. canad. Biol. **21**, 135—143 (1962).
JACOB, J., et F. CUGURRA: Actions de la benzyl-1-dimethyl-2,5 sérotonine (B.A.S.) sur l'activité cardiaque chez le chien et chez le lapin. Arch. int. Pharmacodyn. **123**, 362—376 (1960).
—, et G. MICHAUD: Effets de la 5-hydroxytryptamine et de la nicotine sur les hypertensions provoquées par la 5-hydroxytryptamine, la nicotine, la tryptamine et l'acétaldéhyde. Arch. int. Pharmacodyn. **140**, 92—104 (1962).
—, et M. POITE-BEVIERRE: Actions de la sérotonine et de la benzyl-1-diméthyl-2,5 sérotonine sur le coeur isolé de lapin. Arch. int. Pharmacodyn. **127**, 11—26 (1960).
JACOBY, G. A., and B. N. LA DU: Inhibition of tyrosine transaminase by serotonin and related compounds. Fed. Proc. **21**, 238 (1962).
JAEGER, C. P.: Physiology of mollusca. II. Action of serotonin and other amines on the heart of *Strophocheilos oblongus*. Comp. Biochem. Physiol. **6**, 243—246 (1962).
— Physiology of mollusca. IV. Action of serotonin on the penis retractor muscle of *Strophocheilos oblongus*. Comp. Biochem. Physiol. **9**, 131—136 (1963).
JAMIESON, D.: A method for the quantitative estimation of drugs on the isolated intact trachea. Brit. J. Pharmacol. **19**, 286—294 (1962).
JÄNKÄLÄ, E. O., and P. VIRTAMA: On the bronchoconstrictor effect of serotonin. Bronchographic studies on rabbits and guinea-pigs. J. Physiol. (Lond.) **159**, 381—383 (1961).
— — Action of serotonin and reserpine on the veins of the rat liver. Ann. Med. exp. Fen. **40**, 110—117 (1962).
JANTSCHEW, W., u. T. NATSCHEW: Ein Beitrag zum klinischen Bild, zur Behandlung und zum vermutlichen toxikologischen Mechanismus der Fischvergiftung (speziell Vergiftung an Pelamys sarda-Bloch). Z. ges. inn. Med. **18**, 219—224 (1963).
JAQUES, L. B., and L. M. FISHER: Platelet serotonin as a factor in hemostasis. Arch. int. Pharmacodyn. **123**, 325—333 (1960).
JAQUET, H.: Versuch einer Interpretation des Reaktionsmechanismus der durch Liberationsvorgänge ausgelösten entzündlichen Hautreaktion. Arch. int. Pharmacodyn. **144**, 161—184 (1963).
JOHANSSON, S.-A.: 5-Hydroxytryptamine in burns. Acta physiol. scand. **48**, 126—132 (1960a).
— Inhibition of thrombocytopenia and 5-hydroxytryptamine release in anaphylactic shock by heparin. Acta physiol. scand. **50**, 95—104 (1960b).
JOHNELS, A. G., and E. OSTLUND: Anatomical and physiological studies on the enteron of *Lampetra fluviatilis*. Acta zool. **39**, 9—12 (1958).
JOHNSEN jr., H. A., R. E. SMITH and W. SIMON: Diurnal variations in the excretion of urinary 5-hydroxyindoles. Clin. Res. **6**, 268—269 (1958).
JOHNSON, L. P., R. D. SLOOP and J. E. JESSEPH: Serotonin, duodenal hyperosmolarity and the enterogastrone concept of gastric motor inhibition. Rev. Surg. (Philad.) **20**, 91—94 (1963).
JONES, C. J., and CH. B. RIPSTEIN: The action of meprobamate and other compounds on nonhemorrhagic shock in the rat. Sect. Meeting, New York City, Amer. Col. Surgeons March 1958.
JOUAN, P.: Épiphyse, 5-hydroxytryptamine et corticoidogenèse *in vitro*. Ann. Endocr. (Paris) **24**, 365—370 (1963).
KABINS, S. A., C. MOLINA and L. N. KATZ: Pulmonary vascular effects of serotonin (5-OH-tryptamine) in dogs: its role in causing pulmonary edema. Amer. J. Physiol. **197**, 955—958 (1959).
KÄRKI, N. T., M. K. PAASONEN and P. PELTOLA: Factors influencing the release of 5-hydroxytryptamine from the rabbit intestine into the venous blood. Ann. Med. exp. Fenn. **38**, 231—236 (1960).
KAHR, H.: Zur Diagnose, zur allgemeinen und experimentellen Pathologie des Carcinoidsyndroms. Acta neuroveg. (Wien) **16**, 324—335 (1957).

KAHR, H.: Die Bedeutung des Serotonins für die Melanophorenreaktion des Octopus vulgaris. Naturwissenschaften **45**, 243 (1958).
—, u. W. FISCHER: Die Wirkung des 5-Oxytryptamins auf das Pigmentsystem der Haut. Klin. Wschr. **35**, 41—44 (1957).
KALLOS, P., and L. KALLOS-DEFFNER: Effect of inoculation with *H. pertusis* vaccine on susceptibility of albino mice to 5-hydroxytryptamine (serotonin). Int. Arch. Allergy (N.Y.) **11**, 327—345 (1957).
KANAI, T., G. MISRAHY and L. C. CLARK: Neuropharmacological effects of O-methyl-bufotenine. Fed. Proc. **21**, 322 (1962).
KAPILA, K., and R. B. ARORA: Effectiveness of 5-hydroxytryptamine in ectopic ventricular tachycardia resulting from acute myocardial infarction in the dog. J. Pharm. Pharmacol. **14**, 831—832 (1962).
KÁTO, L., and B. GÖZSY: Action of serotonin on conversion of fibrinogen to fibrin. Amer. J. Physiol. **195**, 66—68 (1958).
KAY, R. H.: Bioluminescence of the euphausiid crustacean *Meganyctiphanes norvegica*: the influence of 5-hydroxytryptamine. J. Physiol. (Lond.) **165**, 63P (1963).
KEASLING, H. H., R. R. RUSSELL and H. J. TREIZENBERG: The overt effects of tryptamine and their antagonism in the mouse. Fed. Proc. **22**, 624 (1963).
KEELER, M. H.: Inter-relations of the effects of psilocybin on subjective sensation, photopic critical frequency of fusion, and circulating non-esterified fatty acids. Experientia (Basel) **19**, 37—38 (1963).
KEHL, R., J. C. CZYBA, G. ARNAUD et H. GUEYFFIER: Déclenchement de la sécrétion lactée, chez la lapine, par injection de 5-hydroxytryptamine dans la région de l'hypothalamus. C. R. Soc. Biol. (Paris) **156**, 1414—1415 (1962).
— L. DUMONT et J. C. CZYBA: Action comparée de la réserpine, de la chloropromazine et de la sérotonine sur la métamorphose du têtard de *Rana temporaria*. C. R. Soc. biol. (Paris) **155**, 1667—1669 (1961).
KELEMEN, E.: The inhibition by sodium salicylate of oedema of the hind-paw of the rat induced by 5-hydroxytryptamine. Brit. J. Pharmacol. **12**, 28—29 (1957).
KELENTEY, B.: Effect of serotonin on CSF pressure. Biochem. Pharmacol. **12**, Suppl., 209 (1963).
KELLER, R.: Beeinflussung der Gerinnungswirkung von Heparin durch Serotonin und Tryptamin. Experientia (Basel) **14**, 181—182 (1958).
KERBY, G. P., and S. M. TAYLOR: Solubilization of serotonin and related compounds in benzene-*n*-butanol in presence of human plasma. Proc. exp. Soc. Biol. (N.Y.) **107**, 936—941 (1961).
KERKUT, G. A., and M. A. PRICE: Chromatographic separation of cardiaccelerators (6 HT and a mucopeptide) from *Carcinus* heart. Comp. Biochem. Physiol. **11**, 45—52 (1964).
KHAZAN, N., J. ADIR, Y. PFEIFER and F. G. SULMAN: Mechanism of the antidiuretic action of reserpine. Proc. Soc. exp. Biol. (N.Y.) **109**, 32—35 (1962).
KIND, L. S., A. BURKHALTER and R. SHERINS: Increased lung serotonin and pulmonary edema in mice injected with antiserum to EHRLICH's ascites tumor. Proc. Soc. exp. Biol. (N.Y.) **108**, 735—737 (1961).
KINDWALL, E. P., L. O. BORÉUS and B. WESTERHOLM: Failure to show change in rat tissue histamine and serotonin after rapid decompression. Amer. J. Physiol. **203**, 389—390 (1962).
KIRPEKAR, S. M., and J. J. LEWIS: Effects of reserpine and hydralazine on isolated strips of carotid arteries. J. Pharm. Pharmacol. **10**, 255—259 (1958).
KIVALO, E., P. MARJANEN and U. K. RINNE: Response of the hypothalamic neurosecretory substance to serotonin. Acta endocr. (Kbh.) **28**, 553—565 (1958b).
—, and U. K. RINNE: Effect of 5-hydroxytryptamine on the nucleus supraopticus. Ann. Med. exp. Fenn. **37**, 262—267 (1959).
— — and S. MAKELA: Acetylcholinesterase, acid phosphatase, and succinic dehydrogenase in the hypothalamic magnocellular nuclei after serotonin administration. Experientia (Basel) **14**, 408—409 (1958a).
— — and P. MARJANEN: Response of the neurohypophysis to serotonin, reserpine and chlorpromazine. Ann. Med. intern. Fenn. **46**, 191—197 (1957).
KNISELY, W. H., J. M. WALLACE and W. A. ADDISON: "Temporary" pulmonary embolization caused by intravenous injection of 5-hydroxytryptamine. Fed. Proc. **17**, 89 (1958).
KOBAYASHI, B.: The role of serotonin in carbohydrate metabolism. V. Enhanced glycogenesis by serotonin in rat diaphragm. Endocr. jap. **7**, 279—283 (1960).
— M. UI and Y. WARASHINA: The role of serotonin in carbohydrate metabolism. I. Glycemic effect of serotonin in rats. Endocr. jap. **7**, 225—238 (1960a).
— — — The role of serotonin in carbohydrate metabolism. II. The effect of serotonin on glycogen content of liver, heart and diaphragm in rats. Endocr. jap. **7**, 239—248 (1960b).

KOBOLD, E., W. KATZ and A. P. THAL: Vasoactive mechanisms in endotoxin shock. Fed. Proc. **22**, 430 (1963).
KOCH, R.: Der Einfluß verschiedener Strahlenschutzstoffe auf die Strahlenempfindlichkeit von Tumoren. Nucl. Med. (Stuttg.) **2**, 265—271 (1962).
KOELLA, W. P., and U. SCHAEPPI: The reaction of the isolated cat iris to serotonin. J. Pharmacol. exp. Ther. **138**, 154—158 (1962).
KONZETT, H.: The effects of 5-hydroxytryptamine and its antagonists on tidal air. Brit. J. Pharmacol. **11**, 289—294 (1956a).
— Zur Wirkung von LSD (und LSD-Derivaten) auf den Blutzucker. XXth Internat. Physiol. Congr. Bruxelles 1956b. Abstr. Comm. p. 518—519.
— Hyperglycaemia induced in rabbits by 5-hydroxytryptophan. Nature (Lond.) **182**, 1168—1169 (1958).
KOSHTOYANTS, K. S., G. A. BUZNIKOV and B. N. MANUKHIN: The possible role of 5-hydroxytryptamine in the motor activity of embryos of some marine gastropods. Comp. Biochem. Physiol. **3**, 20—26 (1961).
—, and K. S. RÓZSA: Comparative pharmacological data on the effect of serotonin, noradrenaline and chlorpromazine on mollusc *Helix pomatia* ganglia. Acta physiol. Acad. Sci. hung. **19**, 189—197 (1961).
KOSTERLITZ, H. W., and J. A. ROBINSON: Inhibition of the peristaltic reflex of the isolated guinea-pig ileum. J. Physiol. (Lond.) **136**, 249—262 (1957).
KOTTEGODA, S. R., and J. C. MOTT: Cardiovascular and respiratory actions of 5-hydroxytryptamine in the cat. Brit. J. Pharmacol. **10**, 66—72 (1955).
KOVALČIK, V.: Effect of bradykinin on isolated coronary arteries. Nature (Lond.) **196**, 174 (1962).
KOWALEWSKI, K.: Effect of a histamine liberator and of serotonin on plasma pepsinogen in rats. Arch. int. Pharmacodyn. **129**, 71—76 (1960).
KOWLESSAR, O. D., R. C. WILLIAMS, D. H. LAW and M. H. SLEISENGER: Urinary excretion of 5-hydroxyindoleacetic acid in diarrheal states, with special reference to nontropical sprue. New Engl. J. Med. **259**, 340—341 (1958).
KOZNIEWSKI, S., and W. BAREY: Effect of acetylcholine, adrenaline and serotonin on movements of the rumen in sheep. Acta physiol. pol. **11**, 291—303 (1950).
KRAMER, M.: Pharmakologische Differenzierung des Eiklar- und Dextranödems der Ratte. Naunyn-Schmiedeberg's Arch. exp. Path. Pharmak. **228**, 302—306 (1956a).
— Die Bedeutung der Histaminfreisetzung durch Compound 48/80, Dextran und Eiereiweiß für die Ödementstehung bei der Ratte. Naunyn-Schmiedeberg's Arch. exp. Path. Pharmak. **228**, 340—346 (1956b).
— Discussion of the paper presented by K. MÖRSDORF. Naunyn-Schmiedeberg's Arch. exp. Path. Pharmak. **236**, 46—49 (1959).
—, e E. ARRIGONI-MARTELLI: Significato dell'attività antiserotoninica e sedativa centrale di derivati fenotiazinici, per la loro azione inibitrice sull'edema da dextran nel ratto. Boll. Soc. ital. Biol. sper. **34**, 1128—1130 (1958).
KRAWCZYNSKI, J.: The influence of serotonin, D-lysergic acid diethylamide and 2-brom-LSD on the incorporation of 35 S methionine into brain proteins and on the level of ATP in the brain. J. Neurochem. **7**, 1—4 (1961).
— S. WISZNIOWSKA, I. DREWNOWSKA and R. KUJAWA: The influence of lysergic acid diethylamide (LSD-25) on the incorporation of (35 S) methionine in the protein of the central nervous system of rabbits. IV. Internat. Congr. Biochem. Vienna 1958, Abstr. p. 155.
KRIEGEL, H., u. H.-J. MELCHING: Zur Strahlenschutzwirksamkeit des 5-Hydroxytryptamins bei Ratten. Naturwissenschaften **46**, 652—653 (1959).
KROEGER, D. C., and L. J. LUCCO: Serotonin-induced apnea. J. Amer. pharm. Ass., sci. Ed. **49**, 170—175 (1960).
KRUEGER, A. P., and R. F. SMITH: The biological mechanisms of air ion action. I. 5-Hydroxytryptamine as the endogenous mediator of positive air ion effects on the mammalian trachea. J. gen. Physiol. **43**, 533—540 (1960a).
— — The biological mechanisms of air ion action. II. Negative air ion effects on the concentration and metabolism of 5-hydroxytryptamine in the mammalian respiratory tract. J. gen. Physiol. **44**, 269—276 (1960b).
KÜNKEL, H. A., u. A. TRAMS: Über den Einfluß von 5-Hydroxy-Tryptamin (Serotonin) auf die strahleninduzierte Mutationsrate bei E. coli. Naturwissenschaften **50**, 666 (1963).
KUIDA, H., A. M. BROWN, J. L. THORNE, R. L. LANGE and H. H. HECHT: Pulmonary vasomotor response to 5-OH-tryptamine (5-HT) and acetylcholine (Ach) in calves. Fed. Proc. **20**, 106 (1961).
KURIAKI, K., et T. INOUE: Mécanisme de l'action excitante de la 5-hydroxytryptamine sur le muscle. C. R. Soc. Biol. (Paris) **149**, 2053—2055 (1955).

KUSCH, T.: Glutamic acid-pyruvic acid transaminase and glutamic acid-oxalacetic acid transaminase under the influence of chlorpromazine, reserpine, serotonin and physical strain. Acta biol. med. germ. **11**, 485—493 (1963).
KUSCHKE, H. J., H. WERNZE and A. IGATA: Increased thyroid function and urinary excretion of 5-hydroxyindoleacetic acid. Lancet **1962 II**, 360.
KWAAN, H. C., R. LO and A. J. S. MCFADZEAN: The production of plasma fibrinolytic activity in vivo by serotonin (5-hydroxytryptamine) creatinine sulphate. Clin. Sci. **16**, 255 (1957).
— — — On the lysis of thrombi experimentally produced within veins. Brit. J. Haemat. **4**, 51—62 (1958).
LABORIT, H., J. M. JOUANY et P. NIAUSSAT: Excrétion d'acide 5-hydroxy-indolylacétique dans l'urine du lapin après injection de somatotrophine hypophysaire. C. R. Soc. Biol. (Paris) **153**, 549—551 (1959a).
— P. NIAUSSAT, B. BROUSSOLLE et J. M. JOUANY: Sur la signification biologique de la sérotonine. Presse méd. **67**, 927—928 (1959b).
— — — — On the biological significance of serotonin. Int. Rec. Med. **172**, 361—366 (1959c).
— — — — Exposé de résultats expérimentaux concernant certaines proprietés originales de la sérotonine. Med. exp. (Basel) **1**, 27—33 (1959d).
— — — — Discussion de faits expérimentaux amenant a proposer une signification biologique nouvelle de la sérotonine. Med. exp. (Basel) **1**, 78—84 (1959e).
LÁBOS, E., J. SALÁNKI and K. S. RÓZSA: Effect of serotonin and other bioactive agents on the rhythmic activity in the glochidia of fresh-water mussel (*Anodonta cygnea* L.) Comp. Biochem. Physiol. **11**, 161—172 (1964).
LAIDLAW, P. P.: The physiological action of indoleethylamine. Biochem. J. **6**, 141—150 (1912).
LANCIANO, O., e A. RESTANTE: Azione del solfato doppio di 5-ossitriptamina sui capillari della superficie corporea. Arch. ital. Pediat. **18**, 119—133 (1956).
LANDAHL, H. D., and A. T. HASEGAWA: Pharmacological and toxicological compounds as protective or therapeutic agents against radiation injury in experimental animals. III. Protection by mercaptoethylamine (MEA) and serotonin against radiation to gastrointestinal tract of mice. USAF Radiat. Lab. Univ. Chicago Quart. Rep. **42**, 81—85 (1962).
— — Pharmacological and toxicological compounds as protective or therapeutic agents against radiation injury in experimental animals. IV. Effect of various radioprotective treatments in mice. USAF Radiat. Lab. Univ. Chic. Quart. Rep. **47**, 92—102 (1963).
LANGEMANN, H.: 5-Oxy-Tryptamin als Anticholinesterase. Helv. physiol. Acta **12**, C 28 (1954).
LANGENDORFF, H., u. U. HAGEN: Untersuchungen über einen biologischen Strahlenschutz. XLV. Mitteilung. Wirkung von Schutzsubstanzen auf die Strahlenschädigung von Knochenmark, Milz und Thymus. Strahlentherapie **117**, 321—329 (1962).
—, u. R. KOCH: Untersuchungen über einen biologischen Strahlenschutz. XVIII. Die Wirkung zentralerregender Pharmaka auf das bestrahlte Tier. Strahlentherapie **102**, 58—64 (1957).
—, u. H.-J. MELCHING: Untersuchungen über einen biologischen Strahlenschutz. XXXIII. Weitere Untersuchungen über den Wirkungsmechanismus des 5-Hydroxytryptamins im Strahlenschutzversuch. Strahlentherapie **110**, 505—509 (1959).
— — u. H.-A. LADNER: Untersuchungen über einen biologischen Strahlenschutz. XXX. Mitteilung. Über die Strahlenschutzwirkung des 5-Hydroxytryptamins im Tierversuch. Strahlentherapie **108**, 251—256 (1958).
— — — Untersuchungen über einen biologischen Strahlenschutz. XXXI. Mitteilung. Zum Wirkungsmechanismus des 5-Hydroxytryptamins im Strahlenschutzversuch. Strahlentherapie **109**, 554—560 (1959a).
— — — Untersuchungen über einen biologischen Strahlenschutz. XXXII Mitteilung. Zur Frage des biologischen Strahlenschutzes nach wiederholter Ganzkörperbestrahlung mit letal wirkenden Strahlendosen. Strahlentherapie **110**, 34—40 (1959b).
— — u. H. RÖSSLER: Untersuchungen über einen biologischen Strahlenschutz. XXXVII. Über den Anteil des Adenylsäuresystems und des Pyridoxal-5-phosphats am Strahlenschutzeffekt des Serotonins. Strahlentherapie **113**, 603—609 (1960).
LAPIÈRE, C. M.: Action de la 5-hydroxytryptamine sur le tissu conjonctif du rat. C. R. Soc. Biol. (Paris) **155**, 1145—1148 (1961a).
— Action de l'histamine et de la 5-hydroxytryptamine, en injections locales répétées, sur la composition du tissu conjonctif néoformé du rat. C. R. Soc. Biol. (Paris) **155**, 1610—1612 (1961b).
— Etude histologique des modifications provoquées localement par l'histamine et la 5-hydroxytryptamine au niveau du tissu conjonctif néoformé de l'éponge d'Ivalon. C. R. Soc. Biol. (Paris) **155**, 1723—1726 (1961c).

LAVERTY, R.: Relation in rat hind-limb blood vessels between nervous vasomotor tone and the response to vasoconstrictor drugs. Brit. J. Pharmacol. **18**, 451—464 (1962).
LEAHU, L.: The action of β-indoleacetic acid (IAA) on animal cell mitotic activity. Naturwissenschaften **48**, 575—576 (1961).
LECOMTE, J.: Sensibilisation à l'adrénaline par la 5-hydroxytryptamine. Arch. int. Physiol. **61**, 84—85 (1953).
— 5-Hydroxytryptamine et membrane nictitante du chat. Arch. int. Pharmacodyn. **100**, 457—464 (1955).
—, et M.-L. BEAUMARIAGE: Propriété pharmacodynamiques de la 5-hydroxytryptamine chez le Coq. C. R. Soc. Biol. (Paris) **151**, 1641—1643 (1957).
—, et L. VAN DE BERG: Sur les propriétés vasomotrices de la 5-hydroxytryptamine chez le lapin. C. R. Soc. Biol. (Paris) **151**, 1639—1641 (1957).
— Y. BOUNAMEAUX, P. FISCHER et P. OSTERRIETH: Action de la 5-hydroxytryptamine sur le temps de saignement moyen chez le lapin. Arch. int. Pharmacodyn. **97**, 389—394 (1954).
— H. VAN CAUWENBERGE et M. VILIERS: Oedème au dextran et médications anti-inflammatoires. Arch. int. Pharmacodyn. **121**, 65—70 (1959).
—, et P. FISCHER: Dérivés de l'ergot et choc anaphylactique du lapin. C. R. Soc. Biol. (Paris) **151**, 1279—1281 (1957).
— — 5-Hydroxytryptamine et choc anaphylactique du lapin. Arch. int. Physiol. **66**, 50—61 (1958).
—, and J. HUGUES: Influence of 5-hydroxytryptamine and of reserpine on allergic vascular reactions in the rabbit. Int. Arch. Allergy **13**, 364—369 (1958).
LEE, C. Y.: The effect of stimulation of extrinsic nerves on peristalsis and on the release of 5-hydroxytryptamine in the large intestine of the guinea-pig and the rabbit. J. Physiol. (Lond.) **152**, 405—418 (1960).
LEFEBVRE, P.: Influence du glucagon sur l'oedème local provoqué chez le rat par certaines substances phlogistiques. C. R. Soc. Biol. (Paris) **104**, 2154—2156 (1965).
LEITSCH, J. L.: X-irradiation protection studies. III. Modification of the radiation syndrome in female DAL-Swiss mice by AET and 5-HT. Radiat. Res. **15**, 641—647 (1961).
LEMBECK, F.: Carcinoids and the significance of 5-hydroxytryptamine. In: G. P. LEWIS, 5-Hydroxytryptamine, p. 147—152. London: Pergamon Press 1957.
— Die Beeinflussung der Darmmotilität durch Hydroxytryptamin. Pflügers Arch. ges. Physiol. **265**, 567—574 (1958).
— K.-FR. SEWING u. D. WINNE: Der Einfluß von 5-Hydroxytryptamin auf die Resorption von Tritium-Wasser (HTO) aus den Dünndarm der Ratte. Naunyn-Schmiedebergs Arch. exp. Path. Pharmak. **247**, 100—109 (1964).
LEMESSURIER, D. H., C. J. SCHWARTZ and R. F. WHELAN: Cardiovascular effects of intravenous infusions of 5-hydroxytryptamine in man. Brit. J. Pharmacol. **14**, 246—250 (1959).
LENDLE, L., u. U. WEISSER: Anaphylaktoide Reaktionen von Hühnereiweiß und Dextran an isolierten Organen von Ratten. Int. Arch. Allergy **20**, 143—173 (1962).
LEONARD, L. S., and H. T. DAY: Effect of 5-hydroxytryptamine on phosphorylase and glycogen levels in muscle tissue. Proc. Soc. exp. Biol. (N.Y.) **104**, 338—341 (1960).
LEONARD, S. L.: Effect of histamine and serotonin in stimulating phosphorylase activity in the rat uterus. Endocrinology **72**, 865—870 (1963).
LERNER, A. B., and J. D. CASE: Pigment cell regulatory factors. J. invest. Derm. **32**, 211—221 (1959).
— — Melatonin. Fed. Proc. **19**, 590—592 (1960).
— — W. MORI and M. R. WRIGHT: Melatonin in peripheral nerves. Nature (Lond.) **183**, 1821 (1959).
— — Y. TAKAHASHI, T. H. LEE and W. MORI: Isolation of melatonin, the pineal gland factor that lightens melanocytes. J. Amer. chem. Soc. **80**, 2587 (1958).
LEUSEN, I., and E. LACROIX: Influence of 5-hydroxytryptamine (serotonin) on the cat papillary muscle. Arch. int. Physiol. **67**, 93—96 (1959).
LEVINE, R. A., L. A. PESCH, G. KLATSKIN and N. J. GIARMAN: Effect of serotonin on glycogen metabolism in isolated rat liver. J. clin. Invest. **43**, 797—809 (1964).
LÉVY, J., et E. MICHEL-BER: Analyse des effets exercés par la sérotonine sur l'oreillette isolée de lapin. C. R. Acad. Sci. (Paris) **243**, 326—329 (1956a).
— — Contribution a l'action pharmacologique exercée par la sérotonine sur quelques organes isolès (intestin et oreillette). J. Physiol. (Paris) **48**, 1051—1084 (1956b).
LIACOPOULOS, P., B. N. HALPERN et M. LIACOPOULOS-BRIOT: Modalités de l'inhibition des effets de l'histamine, des substances histamino-libératrices et de la 5-hydroxytryptamine sur la perméabilité capillaire par leurs antagonistes. C. R. Soc. Biol. (Paris) **151**, 1661—1666 (1957).

LINDSAY, D., E. POULSON and J. M. ROBSON: The effect of 5-hydroxytryptamine and of an amine oxidase inhibitor on experimental deciduomata in mice. J. Endocr. **23**, 209—215 (1961).
— — — Interrelation between progesterone, 5-hydroxytryptamine and HP 1325 in the decidual response in ovariectomized mice. J. Endocr. **25**, 53—56 (1962).
— — — The effect of 5-hydroxytryptamine on pregnancy. J. Endocr. **26**, 85—96 (1963).
LINGJAERDE, P., and O. E. SKAUG: Effect of 5-hydroxytryptamine on the uptake of P^{32} in the rat. J. biol. Chem. **226**, 33—36 (1957).
LISH, P. M., B. B. CLARK and S. I. ROBBINS: Effects of some physiologic substances on gastrointestinal propulsion in the rat. Amer. J. Physiol. **197**, 22—26 (1959).
LITTLE, J. M., E. A. ANGELL, W. HUFFMAN and W. BROOKS: The effect of 5-hydroxytryptamine (5-HT) on renal hemodynamics, water and electrolyte excretion. Fed. Proc. **19**, 367 (1960).
— — — — The effect of 5-hydroxytryptamine (serotonin) on renal hemodynamics, water and electrolyte excretion. J. Pharmacol. exp. Ther. **131**, 44—48 (1961).
LOUBATIÈRES, A., M. M. MARIANI, P. BOUYARD, A. M. RONDOT, J. CHAPAL et R. ALRIC: Effets de la pancréasectomie totale sur le taux de la sérotonine sanguine chez le Chien. C. R. Soc. Biol. (Paris) **157**, 1655—1657 (1963).
— A. SASSINE et J. MAUCHE: Contribution a l'étude sur le coeur de la 5-hydroxytryptamine (sérotonine). C. R. Soc. Biol. (Paris) **149**, 1634—1636 (1955).
LOVAŠEN, Ž., Z. SUPEK and M. RANDIĆ: The oxitocic activity of DL-5-hydroxytryptophan. J. Pharm. Pharmacol. **13**, 565—566 (1961).
LOVELAND, R. E.: 5-Hydroxytryptamine, the probable mediator of excitation in the heart of *Mercenaria (Venus) mercenaria*. Comp. Biochem. Physiol. **9**, 95—104 (1963).
LOWY, J., and B. M. MILLMAN: Tonic and phasic responses in the anterior byssus retractor muscle (ABRM) of Mytilus. J. Physiol. (Lond.) **149**, 68—69P (1959).
LOZERON, H., A. MAGGIORA and W. JODASSOHN: Protection of *Vicia faba equina* against X-rays by serotonin. Experientia (Basel) **20**, 390—391 (1964).
LUDÁNY, G., T. GÁTI, ST. SZABÓ u. J. HIDEG: 5-Hydroxytryptamin (Enteramin, Serotonin) und die Darmzottenbewegung. Arch. int. Pharmacodyn. **118**, 62—69 (1959).
— J. VAJDA, J. RIGO u. HAN TU VU: 5-Hydroxytryptamin und die Phagozytose der Leukozyten. Acta physiol. Acad. Sci. hung. **14**, 371—373 (1958).
MACCANON, D. M., and S. M. HORVATH: Hemodynamic effects of serotonin (5-hydroxytryptamine) injected into the pulmonary artery of anesthetized dogs. Fed. Proc. **13**, 92—93 (1954a).
— — Some effects of serotonin in pentobarbital anesthetized dogs. Amer. J. Physiol. **179**, 131—134 (1954b).
MACDONALD, R. A., S. L. ROBBINS and G. K. MALLORY: Morphologic effects of serotonin (5-hydroxytryptamine). Arch. Path. **65**, 369—377 (1958).
MACHAFFIE, R. A., A. J. BARAC and R. L. O'BRIEN: Studies in allergy. I. Serotonin, histamine and antigen-antibody complex activity in isolated sensitized guinea-pig uteri. J. Allergy **29**, 545—552 (1958).
MAGALINI, S. I., and M. STEFANINI: Failure of synthetic 5-hydroxytryptamine creatinine sulfate to enhance clot retraction of platelet-poor human plasma. Proc. Soc. exp. Biol. (N.Y.) **90**, 615—617 (1955).
— — A platelat factor responsible for clot retraction. Lancet **1956a I**, 246—247.
— — Clot retraction promoting factor in platelets and tissues. Fed. Proc. **15**, 123—124 (1956b).
— — and F. E. SMITH: Vasopressor effect of synthetic 5-hydroxytryptamine creatinine sulfate in man. Proc. Soc. exp. Biol. (N.Y.) **92**, 433—436 (1956).
MAGGI, G. C.: L'azione della 5-HT sulla portata coronarica e sul consumo di O_2 nel preparato cuore-polmoni. Boll. Soc. ital. Biol. sper. **36**, 1850—1852 (1960).
—, e S. NOLI: L'azione della 5-idrossitriptamina sul preparato cuore-polmoni. Boll. Soc. ital. Biol. sper. **34**, 1290—1294 (1958).
MAGGIORA, A.: Sérotonine et effet local des rayons X. Expériences sur la peau du cobaye. Bull. schweiz. Akad. med. Wiss. **16**, 315—319 (1960).
— Sérotonine et effet local des rayons X. II. Sérotonine et effet des rayons X sur les mitoses du bulbe pileux et l'acanthose radiologique. Dermatologica (Basel) **124**, 183—188 (1962a).
— Sérotonine et effet local des rayons X. III. De la durée de la protection due à la sérotonine vis-à-vis de l'effet épilateur chez le cobaye. Dermatologica (Basel) **124**, 385—388 (1962b).
— Sérotonine et effet local des rayons X. V. Application de la sérotonine par ionophorèse chez le cobaye. Dermatologica (Basel) **127**, 398—402 (1963).
—, et R. BRUN: Sérotonine et effet local des rayons X. IV. Effet protecteur de substances apparentées à la sérotonine envers les rayons X. Dermatologica (Basel) **126**, 30—39 (1963).

MAGNES, J., and S. HESTRIN-LERNER: Effect of 5-hydroxytryptophan and serotonin on glucose content and functional activity of the perfused cat brain. J. Neurochem. **5**, 128—134 (1960).

MAISIN, J. R., and D. G. DOHERTY: Chemical protection against radiation damage. Fed. Proc. **19**, 356 (1960).

— — Comparative chemical protection to the intestinal and hematopoietic systems of whole-body irradiated mice. Radiat. Res. **19**, 474—484 (1963).

— A. LEONARD, M. LAMBIET et G. MATTELIN: Action de la 2-β-aminoéthylisothiourée (AET) et de la 5-hydroxytryptamine (sérotonine) sur l'intestin grêle et le système hématopoietique des Souris irradiées. C. R. Soc. Biol. (Paris) **157**, 1525—1529 (1963).

MAJNO, G., and G. E. PALADE: Studies on inflammation. The effect of histamine and serotonin on vascular permeability: an electron microscopy study. J. biophys. biochem. Cytol. **11**, 571—605 (1961).

— — and G. I. SCHOEFL: Studies on inflammation. II. The site of action of histamine and serotonin along the vascular tree: a topographic study. J. biophys. biochem. Cytology **11**, 607—626 (1961b).

— G. I. SCHOEFL and G. E. PALADE: Effect of histamine and serotonin on vascular permeability. Fed. Proc. **20**, 119 (1961a).

MALCOLM, J. L.: Effects of 5-hydroxytryptamine on evoked responses in the brain of anaesthetized cats. In: G. P. LEWIS, 5-Hydroxytryptamine, p. 221—228. London: Pergamon Press 1957.

MANN, T., and L. C. PROSSER: Uterine response to 5-hydroxytryptamine in the clasper-siphon secretion of the spiny dogfish, *Squalus acanthias*. Biol. Bull. **125**, 384—385 (1963).

MANSOUR, T. E.: The effect of lysergic acid diethylamide, serotonin and related compounds on a parasitic trematode, *Fasciola hepatica*. Fed. Proc. **15**, 454—455 (1956).

— The effect of serotonin and related amines on the activity of phenol oxidases. J. Pharmacol. exp. Ther. **119**, 164 (1957a).

— The effect of lysergic acid diethylamide, 5-hydroxytryptamine, and related compounds on the liver fluke, *Fasciola hepatica*. Brit. J. Pharmacol. **12**, 406—409 (1957b).

— Effect of serotonin and phenol oxidase from the liver fluke *Fasciola hepatica* and from other sources. Biochim. biophys. Acta (Amst.) **30**, 492—500 (1958).

— The effect of serotonin and related compounds on the carbohydrate metabolism of the liver fluke, *Fasciola hepatica*. J. Pharmacol. exp. Ther. **126**, 212—216 (1959).

— Effect of serotonin on glycolysis in homogenates from the liver fluke *Fasciola hepatica*. J. Pharmacol. exp. Ther. **135**, 94—101 (1962).

—, and A. D. LAGO: Biochemical effects of serotonin on *Fasciola hepatica*. J. Pharmacol. exp. Ther. **122**, 48A (1958).

— N. A. LEROUGE and J. M. MANSOUR: Effect of serotonin and of cyclic 3—5 AMP on phosphofructokinase from the liver fluke *Fasciola hepatica*. Fed. Proc. **20**, 226 (1961a).

— — — Activation of phosphofructokinase from the liver fluke *Fasciola hepatica* by serotonin and cyclic 3:5-AMP. Biochem. Pharmacol. **8**, 5 (1961b).

—, and J. M. MANSOUR: Effects of serotonin (5-hydroxytryptamine) and adenosine 3',5'-phosphate on phosphofructokinase from the liver fluke *Fasciola hepatica*. J. biol. Chem. **237**, 629—634 (1962).

—, and J. S. MENARD: Effect of serotonin on glycolysis in homogenates from the liver fluke *Fasciola hepatica*. Fed. Proc. **19**, 50 (1960).

— E. W. SUTHERLAND, T. W. RALL and E. BUEDING: The effect of serotonin (5-hydroxytryptamine) on the formation of adenosine 3',5'-phosphate by tissue particles from the liver fluke, *Fasciola hepatica*. J. biol. Chem. **235**, 466—470 (1960).

MARAUD, R., R. STOLL et A. SPARFEL: Action de la sérotonine sur la thyroide de l'embryon de poulet. C. R. Soc. Biol. (Paris) **156**, 1375—1377 (1962).

MARCELLE, R., et J. LECOMTE: Sur l'origine de l'hyperpéristaltisme intestinal du choc anaphylactique du lapin. C. R. Soc. Biol. (Paris) **153**, 1889—1891 (1959).

MARKIEWICZ, L.: On the effect of adrenaline and serotonin on fat content in peripheral blood. Bull. Acad. pol. Sci., Ser. Sci. biol. **7**, 79—82 (1959).

MAROIS, M.: Sérotonine et accouchement. C. R. Soc. Biol. (Paris) **154**, 1200—1203 (1960).

MARSHALL, R. W., O. M. MORENO and D. A. BRODIE: The effect of ulcerogenic drugs on gastric acidity in the chronic fistula rat. Fed. Proc. **21**, 256 (1962).

MARTINETTI, L., e U. MARANGANI: Rilievi preliminari sull'impiego della 5-idrossitriptamina in terapia antiemorragica. Farmaco, Ed. prat. **10**, 122—130 (1955).

MASHKOVSKII, M. D., and G. S. ARUTYUNYAN: Pharmacology of 5-methoxytryptamine hydrochloride (mexamine). Fed. Proc. **23**, No 1, Part 2, T 125 (1964).

MATSUOKA, O., T. TSUCHIYA and Y. FURUKAWA: The effect of X-irradiation on 5-hydroxytryptamine (serotonin) contents in the small intestines of experimental animals. J. Rad. Res. **3**, 104—108 (1962).

MAXWELL, D. R., W. R. GRAY and E. M. TAYLOR: Relative activity of some inhibitors of mono-amine oxidase in potentiating the action of tryptamine in vitro and in vivo. Brit. J. Pharmacol. **17**, 310—320 (1961).

MAXWELL, G. M., C. A. CASTILLO, J. E. CLIFFORD, C. W. CRUMPTON and G. G. ROWE: Effect of serotonin (5-hydroxytryptamine) on the systemic and coronary vascular bed of the dog. Amer. J. Physiol. **197**, 736—738 (1959).

— — D. H. WHITE jr. and C. W. CRUMPTON: The effects of serotonin (5-hydroxytryptamine) upon systemic, pulmonary, and coronary hemodynamics and metabolism. Clin. Res. Proc. **4**, 294—295 (1957).

— G. M. KNEEBONE and R. B. ELLIOTT: The effect of psilocybin upon the systemic, pulmonary, and coronary circulation of the intact dog. Arch. int. Pharmacodyn. **137**, 108—115 (1962).

MAXWELL, R. A., A. J. PLUMMER, S. D. ROSS and M. W. OSBORNE: Effects of reserpine on urinary bladder tension. Proc. Soc. exp. Biol. (N.Y.) **92**, 227—230 (1956).

MAZZELLA, H., and C. MAQUIEIRA: Continuous record of renal vein pressure. Arch. int. Physiol. **65**, 27—35 (1957).

MAZZONE, R., N. SOZIO e N. PADOLECCHIA: Processi neuroumorali di reazione agli stimoli. Ricerche su una possibile mediazione 5-idrossitriptaminica. Boll. Soc. ital. Biol. sper. **35**, 1050—1052 (1959a).

— — — Ulteriori indagini sulle modificazioni glicemiche indotte dalla 5 HTA. Boll. Soc. ital. Biol. sper. **35**, 1273—1274 (1959b).

MCCAWLEY, E. L., P. E. LEVEQUE and H. L. H. DICK: Certain actions of serotonin (5-hydroxytryptamine creatinine sulfate) on cardiac rhythm. J. Pharmacol. exp. Ther. **106**, 406 (1952).

MCCUBBIN, J. W., J. H. GREEN, G. C. SALMOIRAGHI and I. H. PAGE: The chemoreceptor stimulant action of serotonin in dogs. J. Pharmacol. exp. Ther. **116**, 191—197 (1956).

— Y. KANEKO and I. H. PAGE: Inhibition of neurogenic vasoconstriction by serotonin: vasodilator action of serotonin. Circulat. Res. **11**, 74—83 (1962).

—, and I. H. PAGE: Renal inhibition of pressor responses to drugs. Circulat. Res. **2**, 35—40 (1954).

MCGAFF, CH. J., and W. R. MILNOR: Effects of serotonin on pulmonary blood volume and flow in the dog. Fed. Proc. **19**, 96 (1960).

— — Effects of serotonin on pulmonary blood volume in the dog. Amer. J. Physiol. **202**, 957—960 (1962).

MCNEIL, J. P., and J. K. HAMPTON: Effects on homeostasis of 5-hydroxytryptamine, lysergic acid diethylamide and 2-brom-d-lysergic acid. Amer. J. Physiol. **197**, 1191—1194 (1959).

MEDAKOVIĆ, M.: Egg white reaction in rats and 5-hydroxytryptamine. Arch. int. Physiol. **67**, 294—305 (1959).

—, and L. SPUŽIĆ: 5-Hydroxytryptamine in blood during experimental traumatic shock in rats. Nature (Lond.) **183**, 1685 (1959).

MEEKER jr., W. R., and R. B. DAVIS: The role of serotonin in anaphylaxis and endotoxin shock. Minn. Med. **44**, 417—421 (1961).

MEER, C. VAN DER, and D. W. VAN BEKKUM: A study on mechanism of radiation protection by 5-hydroxytryptamine and tryptamine. Int. J. Radiat. Biol. **4**, 105—110 (1961).

MEIER, R., H. J. BEIN u. H. G. KRAFT: Zur Charakterisierung der durch 5-Hydroxytryptamin bedingten Atemreaktion. Helv. physiol. Acta **14**, C 74—75 (1956).

MEITES, J., and T. F. HOPKINS: Release of prolactin from the anterior pituitary by neurohormones, drugs, hypothalamic tissue and other agents. Fed. Proc. **19**, 156 (1960).

— C. S. NICOLL and P. K. TALWALKER: Effects of reserpine and serotonin on milk secretion and mammary growth in the rat. Proc. Soc. exp. Biol. (N.Y.) **101**, 563—565 (1959).

— P. K. TALWALKER and C. S. NICOLL: Induction of mammary growth and lactation in rabbits with epinephrine, acetylcholine and serotonin. Proc. Soc. exp. Biol. (N.Y.) **104**, 192—194 (1960).

MELCHING, H.-J., H. ERNST u. H. RÖSSLER: Untersuchungen über einen biologischen Strahlenschutz. XXXVI. Zum Stoffwechsel des 5-Hydroxytryptamins bei der Ganzkörperbestrahlung weißer Mäuse und Ratten. Strahlentherapie **113**, 394—401 (1960).

— M. LANGENDORFF u. H. A. LADNER: Über die Abhängigkeit der Strahlenschutzwirksamkeit des 5-Hydroxytryptamins von Konzentration und Zeitfaktor. Naturwissenschaften **45**, 545 (1958).

— O. MESSERSCHMIDT u. CH. STREFFER: Untersuchungen über einen biologischen Strahlenschutz. XXXIX. Mitteilung. Über die Bedeutung der Milz bei Strahlenschaden. Strahlentherapie **114**, 179—186 (1961).

MENG, K.: 5-Hydroxytryptamin und Acetylcholin als Wirkungsantagonisten beim Helix-Herzen. Naturwissenschaften **45**, 470 (1958).

— Untersuchungen zur Steuerung der Herztätigkeit bei *Helix pomatia* L. Zool. Jb. **68**, 539—566 (1960).

MICHELSON, A. L., W. HOLLANDER and F. C. LOWELL: The effect of 5-hydroxytryptamine (serotonin) on the respiration of nonasthmatic subjects. I. J. Lab. clin. Med. **51**, 57—62 (1958).

MIDDLETON jr., E., and G. B. PHILLIPS: Effect of lysolecithin on the smooth muscle stimulating activity of histamine, acetylcholine, 5-hydroxytryptamine, anaphylactic slow-reacting substance and bradykinin. Nature (Lond.) **198**, 758—760 (1963).

MIESCHER, P.: Diskussionsbemerkung zum Vortrag von A. BASERGA and G. BALLERINI, La 5-hydroxytryptamine dans la thérapie des hémorragies thrombocytopéniques. Schweiz. med. Wschr. **85**, 915 (1955).

MIETKIEWSKI, E., u. I. JANKOWSKA: Über den Einfluß von Serotonin und Reserpin auf den Sauerstoffverbrauch der Gewebe von Ratten. Wien. klin. Wschr. **72**, 642—643 (1960).

MIGLIETTA, M., e P. SALVADÈ: Effetto della serotonina sulla secrezione pancreatica. Rass. ital. Chir. Med. **8**, 615—622 (1959).

MILINE, R., P. STERN et S. HUKOVIĆ: Sur les variations stressogènes quantitatives de la sérotonine dans le cerveau. Experientia (Basel) **14**, 415—416 (1958).

MILKOVIĆ, S., u. Z. SUPEK: Über die Wirkung von 5-Oxytryptamin (Serotonin) und Lysergsäurediäthylamid (LSD) auf das Hypophysen-Nebennierenrinde-System. Naunyn-Schmiedeberg's Arch. exp. Path. Pharmak. **228**, 146 (1956).

— — u. J. TABORSKY: Über den Einfluß des Ferro-Ions auf 5-Oxytryptaminwirkungen. Naunyn-Schmiedeberg's Arch. exp. Path. Pharmak. **227**, 221—223 (1955).

MILLAHN, H. P.: Der Einfluß von Histamin und Serotonin auf das Druckvolumdiagramm und die Elastizität isolierter Rinder- und Schweineaorten. Pflügers Arch. ges. Physiol. **274**, 39 (1961).

MILNE, W. L., and S. H. COHN: Role of serotonin in blood coagulation. Amer. J. Physiol. **189**, 470—474 (1957).

MILNOR, W. R., J. W. FEELY and T. D. LEE: Physical and pharmacological factors that influence pulmonary blood volume. XXII. Congr. Physiol. Sci. Leiden 1962. Abstr. Comm. p. 137.

MILTON, A. S., and R. E. GOSSELIN: Effect of 5-hydroxytryptamine (5-HT) on the carbohydrate metabolism of the gill plates of *Mytilus edulis*. Pharmacologist **2**, 68 (1960a).

— — Metabolism and cilio-accelerator action of 5-hydroxytryptophan (5-HTP) in gill plates of *Mytilus* and *Modiolus*. Fed. Proc. **19**, 126 (1960b).

MINELLI, R.: L'azione della 5-idrossitriptamina sul preparato cuore-polmoni di ratto. Boll. Soc. ital. Biol. sper. **37**, 345—347 (1961).

MIRA, E.: Prime osservazioni sull'attività della melatonina sui cromatofori di *Scardinius erythrophtalmus* L. Arch. int. Pharmacodyn. **138**, 41—49 (1962).

MISHRA, B. P., and R. K. SANYAL: Staphylococcal infection in histamine and 5-hydroxytryptamine depleted rats. J. Pharm. Pharmacol. **11**, 127—128 (1959).

MIYATA, H., H.-J. MELCHING u. H. RÖSSLER: Untersuchungen über einen biologischen Strahlenschutz. XXXV. Mitteilung. Zur Frage hämatologischer Spätveränderungen nach wiederholter Ganzkörperbestrahlung weißer Mäuse unter Serotoninschutz. Strahlentherapie **113**, 193—200 (1960).

MÖRSDORF, K.: Zur Frage einer möglichen Bedeutung des 5-Hydroxytryptamins (5-HT) bei der experimentellen Entzündung. Naunyn Schmiedeberg's Arch. Path. Pharmak. **236**, 46—49 (1959a).

— Spectrofluorometrische Bestimmung des 5-Hydroxytryptamingehaltes der Rattenpfote bei experimentellen „Entzündungen". Med. exp. (Basel) **1**, 87—90 (1959b).

— Die Oedembereitschaft der Rattenpfote in Abhängigkeit ihres Gehaltes an 5-Hydroxytryptamin (5-HT). Naunyn-Schmiedeberg's Arch. exp. Path. Pharmak. **240**, 29—30 (1960).

— Die serotoninfreisetzende Wirkung einiger zur Auslösung experimenteller „Entzündungen" verwendeter Stoffe in vitro. Med. exp. (Basel) **4**, 293—297 (1961).

—, u. H. H. BODE: Zur Beeinflussung der permeabilitätssteigernden Wirkung des Serotonins durch verschiedenartige Pharmaka. Arch. int. Pharmacodyn. **118**, 292—297 (1959).

—, u. L. FEHRES: 5-Hydroxytryptamin (5-HT) und hyperergische Reaktion. Med. exp. (Basel) **1**, 58—63 (1959).

MOLLER, H., and H. RORSMAN: Studies on vascular permeability factors with sodium fluorescein. III. The effect in man of intracutaneously injected 5-hydroxytryptamine. Acta derm.-venereol. (Stockh.) **39**, 12—16 (1959).

MONCALVO, F., e M. GIORDANO: Modificazioni indotte dalla 5-idrossitriptamina e dalla vitamina P sulla reattività, cutanea tubercolinica in ammalati di tubercolosi polmonare. Riv. Pat. Clin. Tuberc. **31**, 19—26 (1958).

MONNIER, M.: Action de la psilocybine sur le cerveau du lapin. Experientia (Basel) **15**, 321—323 (1959).

MONTANARI, C., e M. GIAROLI: Intorno alla identificazione del fattore umorale dell'embolia gassosa sperimentale con la enteramina. Arch. ital. Sci. biol. **46**, 11—23 (1962).

MOORE, K. E., and R. E. GOSSELIN: Effects of 5-hydroxytryptamine on the anaerobic metabolism and phosphorylase activity of lamellibranch gill. J. Pharmacol. exp. Ther. **138**, 145—153 (1962).
— A. S. MILTON and R. E. GOSSELIN: Effect of 5-hydroxytryptamine on the respiration of excised lamellibranch gill. Brit. J. Pharmacol. **17**, 278—285 (1961).
MORI, W., and A. B. LERNER: A microscopic bioassay for melatonin. Endocrinology **67**, 443—450 (1960).
MORLUNGHI, C., e U. VOLPI: Azione della serotonina (5-idrossitriptamina) sui vasi oculari in coniglie normali, castrate e gravide. Ann. Oftal. **85**, 453—460 (1959).
MORSIANI, M., e G. MARTELLI: 5-Idrossitriptamina e sudorazione. G. Psichiat. Neuropat. **83**, 951—962 (1955).
MOTA, I.: Action of anaphylactic shock and anaphylatoxin on mast cells and histamine in rats. Brit. J. Pharmacol. **12**, 453—456 (1957).
MOTT, J. C., and A. S. PAINTAL: The action of 5-hydroxytryptamine on pulmonary and cardiovascular vagal afferent fibres and its reflex respiratory effects. Brit. J. Pharmacol. 8, 238—241 (1953).
MOULIN, G., M. CROISILLE et G. LAPICOREY: Effets de l'administration prolongée de sérotonine chez le jeune rat wistar. C. R. Soc. Biol. (Paris) **156**, 676—678 (1962).
MOUSSATCHÉ, H., and N. ALVARES PEREIRA: Adrenocorticotropin liberation by 5-hydroxytryptamine. Naturwissenschaften **43**, 517 (1956).
— — Release of adrenocorticotrophin by 5-hydroxytryptamine. Acta physiol. lat.-amer. **7**, 71—75 (1957).
MUNOZ, J.: Effect of *H. pertussis* on sensitivity of mice to serotonin. Proc. Soc. exp. Biol. (N.Y.) **95**, 328—331 (1957).
—, and M. A. GREENWALD: Effect of *H. pertussis* on sensitivity of mice to serotonin. Fed. Proc. **16**, 427 (1957).
NACHMIAS, V. T.: 5-Methyltryptophan and darkening of the hair in yellow Ay/a mice. Nature (Lond.) **191**, 934—935 (1961).
NAFTALIN, L.: Urinary excretion patterns during therapeutic irradiation. 2nd Internat. Congr. Radiat. Research, Harrogate 1962. Abstracts p. 88.
NAHAS, G. G.: Effects of norepinephrine and 5-HT on pulmonary circulation of the spinal dog. Fed. Proc. **17**, 115 (1958).
—, and I. MACDONALD: Effects of norepinephrine and 5-hydroxytryptamine on the pulmonary circulation of the spinal dog. Amer. J. Physiol. **196**, 1045—1048 (1959).
NATOFF, I. L., and M. F. LOCKETT: The assay of histamine, 5-hydroxytryptamine, adrenaline, and noradrenaline, on the blood pressure of the fowl. J. Pharm. Pharmacol. **9**, 464—468 (1957).
NEČINA, J., and I. KREJČI: On the role of serotonin and catecholamines in relation to some effects of reserpine. Biochem. Pharmacol. **8**, 35 (1961).
NIAUSSAT, P., J. DROUET et J. BERTHOU: Influence de la 5-hydroxytryptamine utilisée à doses pharmacologiques sur la glycémie du lapin normal ou expérimentalment diabétique. Med. exp. (Basel) **4**, 197—206 (1961).
—, et C. DUBOIS: Influence comparée de la sérotonine (5-hydroxytryptamine) et de l'acide naphthalène-acétique utilisés aux mêmes concentrations, sur la croissance pondérale d'explantats de tubercules d'hiver de topinambur cultivés en présence ou en l'absence de glucose. C. R. Acad. Sci. (Paris) **254**, 4068—4070 (1962).
—, et H. LABORIT: Nouveaux résultats expérimentaux concernant certaines propriétés de la sérotonine. Med. exp. (Basel) **1**, 207—214 (1959).
— — et C. BARON: Contribution à l'étude du rôle de la sérotonine (5-hydroxytryptamine) sur le temps de saignement moyen du cobaye non anesthésié. C. R. Soc. Biol. (Paris) **152**, 1100—1103 (1958).
NICOLOFF, D. M., H. SOSIN, E. T. PETER, E. F. BERNSTEIN and O. H. WANGENSTEEN: The effect o f serotonin on gastric secretion. Amer. J. dig. Dis. **8**, 267—272 (1963).
NIDEN, A. H., and W. R. BARKLAY: The effect of drugs on pulmonary ventilation and circulation as reflected by changes in arterial oxygen saturation. Fed. Proc. 18, 114 (1959).
NILSSON, I. M., B. SKANSE, S. E. BJORKMAN and F. SERIN: Platelet function in thrombocythemia. The effect of platelets and serotonin on serum potassium and bilirubin. Acta med. scand. **167**, 353—368 (1960).
NITZESCO, I. I., M. D. CIRSTEA et M. GRUENSPAN: Sur le mécanisme de la bronchoconstriction anaphylactique chez le chien. XXI. Congr. Internat. Physiol. Sciences Buenos Aires 1959. Abstr. Comm. p. 200.
NIZET, E., L. WILSENS et G. BARAC: Recherches sur la brûlure. XXX. La 5-hydroxytryptamine provoquet-elle une constriction des artères glomérulaires afférentes chez le chien ? Arch. int. Pharmacodyn. **96**, 76—78 (1953).

NOBLE, J. G., and E. M. NANSON: An investigation of the effects of 5-hydroxytryptamine (serotonin) on the cardiovascular system of the dog. Ann. Surg. **150**, 846—853 (1959).
NORTHOVER, B. J.: The effect of histamine and 5-hydroxytryptamine on phagocytosis of staphylococci *in vitro* by polymorphs and macrophages. J. Path. Bact. **82**, 354—361 (1961).
—, and G. SUBRAMANIAN: A study of possible mediators of inflammatory reactions in the mouse foot. Brit. J. Pharmacol. **18**, 346—355 (1962).
NOTTER, B.: Der Einfluß von 5-Hydroxytryptamin (Serotonin) auf die Nierenfunktion beim Menschen. Schweiz. med. Wschr. **85**, 481—483 (1956).
O'BRIEN, J. R.: Platelet aggregation. J. clin. Path. **15**, 446—455 (1962).
O'CONNOR, J. M.: Über den Adrenalingehalt des Blutes. Naunyn-Schmiedeberg's Arch. exp. Path. Pharmak. **67**, 195—232 (1912).
O'HARA, R. S., and J. W. COLE: The effect of serosal application of serotonin on intestinal motility. Surgery **46**, 688—691 (1959).
— R. O. FOX and J. W. COLE: Serotonin release mediated by intraluminal sucrose solutions. Surg. Forum **10**, 214—218 (1960).
OSBORNE, M., R. DETAR and L. GABEL: Comparison between the autonomic pharmacology of 5-hydroxytryptamine and 5-acetyltryptamine (5-AT). Fed. Proc. **21**, 324 (1962).
O'STEEN, W. K.: Serotonin and histamine: effects of a single injection on the mouse testis and prostata gland. Proc. Soc. exp. Biol. (N.Y.) **113**, 161—163 (1963).
OUTSCHOORN, A. S., and J. JACOB: A study of antagonists of 5-hydroxytryptamine and catecholamines on the rat's blood pressure. Brit. J. Pharmacol. **15**, 131—139 (1960).
PAASONEN, M. K., P. PELTOLA and P. A. VANHAKARTANO: The effect of reserpine and neostigmine on the excretion of 5-hydroxytryptamine and 5-hydroxyindoleacetic acid in rabbits. Ann. Med. esp. Fenn. **38**, 220—226 (1960).
PAGE, I. H.: A method for perfusion of rabbits' ears, and its application to the study of the renin-angiotonin vasopressor system, with a note on angiotonin tachyphylaxis. Amer. Heart J. **23**, 336—348 (1942).
— Cardiovascular effects of serotonin, 5- and 7-hydroxytryptamine and tryptamine. Fed. Proc. **11**, 116 (1952a).
— The vascular action of natural serotonin, 5- and 7-hydroxytryptamine and tryptamine. J. Pharmacol. exp. Ther. **105**, 58—73 (1952b).
— Certain aspects of neurogenic and humoral control of blood vessels. Ciba Foundation. Symposium on Hypertension, p. 3—30. London: J. and A. Churchill 1954.
— Cardiovascular actions of serotonin (5-hydroxytryptamine). In: G. P. LEWIS, 5-Hydroxytryptamine, p. 93—108. London: Pergamon Press 1957.
— and J. W. MCCUBBIN: The variable arterial pressure response to serotonin in laboratory animals and man. Circulat. Res. **1**, 354—362 (1953a).
— — Modification of vascular response to serotonin. Amer. J. Physiol. **174**, 436—444 (1953b).
— — Arterial pressure response to infused serotonin in normotensive dogs, cats, hypertensive dogs and man. Amer. J. Physiol. **184**, 256—270 (1956).
— — The advancement of the concept of clinical pharmacology. Arch. int. Pharmacodyn. **140**, 251—257 (1962).
PAINTAL, A. S.: Impulses in vagal afferent fibres from specific pulmonary deflation receptors. The response of these receptors to phenyl diguanide, potato starch, 5-hydroxytryptamine and nicotine, and their role in respiratory and cardiovascular reflexes. Quart. J. exp. Physiol. **40**, 89—111 (1955).
PALAIĆ, D., Ž. DEANOVIĆ and Z. SUPEK: 5-Hydroxyindolyl compounds in the rat brain after X-irradiation. J. Neurochem. **11**, 761—763 (1964).
—, M. RANDIĆ and Z. SUPEK: X-radiation and 5-hydroxytryptamine content in the brain of rats and mice. J. Rad. Biol. **6**, 241—246 (1963).
PALIAGA, G. P.: Sulle possibilità di impiego in oculistica della 5-idrossitriptamina. G. ital. Oculist. **9**, 617—627 (1956).
PALLOTTA, A. J., and J. W. WARD: Protection against anaphylaxis by LSD. J. Pharmacol. exp. Ther. **119**, 174 (1957).
PANASEWICZ, J., and S. LOPACIUK: On protective effects of 5-hydroxytryptamine (serotonin) in lethal-dose roentgen irradiation of mice. Acta physiol. pol. **11**, 856—858 (1960).
— — and F. LUBIARZ: Studies on the role of 5-hydroxytryptamine (serotonin) in the pathogenesis of haematological disorders during the acute irreversible radiation sickness. Pol. Tyg. lek. **16**, 1270—1274 (1961).
PANIGEL, M., et M. MAYER: Reactions vasomotrices de la veine du cordon ombilical humain. C. R. Acad. Sci. (Paris) **248**, 1031—1033 (1959).
PARKS, V. J., A. G. SANDISON, S. L. SKINNER and R. F. WHELAN: The stimulation of respiration by 5-hydroxytryptamine in man. J. Physiol. (Lond.) **151**, 342—351 (1960).

PARRATT, J. R., and G. B. WEST: Influence of age on tissue histamine and 5-hydroxytryptamine. J. Physiol. (Lond.) **133**, 71—72 P (1956).
— — Oedema-producing substances in the rat. J. Physiol. (Lond.) **135**, 10—11 P (1957a).
— — Inhibition of oedema production in the rat. J. Physiol. (Lond.) **135**, 24—25 P (1957b).
— — 5-Hydroxytryptamine in tissue mast cells. J. Physiol. (Lond.) **137**, 169—178 (1957c).
— — 5-Hydroxytryptamine and the anaphylactoid reaction in the rat. J. Physiol. (Lond.) **139**, 27—41 (1957d).
— — Inhibition by various substances of oedema formation in the hind-paw of the rat induced by 5-hydroxytryptamine, histamine, dextran, eggwhite and compound 48/80. Brit. J. Pharmacol. **13**, 65—70 (1958).
PASSOW, H., H. SCHNIEWIND u. C. WEISS: Die Wirkung von 5-Hydroxytryptamin auf das Gefäßsystem der isolierten Rattenniere. Naunyn-Schmiedeberg's Arch. exp. Path. Pharmak. **240**, 179—186 (1960).
PASTAN, I., and J. B. FIELD: *In vitro* stimulation of glucose oxidation in thyroid by serotonin. Endocrinology **70**, 656—659 (1962).
PATON, W. D. M., and J. R. VANE: An analysis of the responses of the isolated stomach to electrical stimulation and to drugs. J. Physiol. (Lond.) **165**, 10—46 (1963).
PELTOLA, P., and V. LEPPÄNEN: Studies in the excretion of 5-hydroxyindoleacetic acid. Ann. Med. intern. Fenn. **49**, 283—291 (1960).
PEREZ-BUFILL PICHOT, G.: La serotonina en oftalmologia. Práct. méd. (Barcelona) **5**, 5 (1957).
PETER, E. T., D. M. NICOLOFF, H. SOSIN, A. I. WALDER and O. H. WAGENSTEEN: Relationship between gastric blood flow and secretion. Fed. Proc. **21**, 264 (1962).
PHILIPPOT, E., et M. J. DALLEMAGNE: L'action anti-curare de la 5-hydroxytryptamine. Arch. int. Pharmacodyn. **105**, 426—428 (1956).
PHILLIPS, A. W., H. R. NEWCOMB, J. E. SMITH and R. LACHAPELLE: Serotonin in the small intestine of conventional and germ-free chicks. Nature (Lond.) **192**, 380 (1961).
PETRUCELLI, L. M., P. H. BULLE and M. OSKOUI: Effects of 5-HT, iproniazid and reserpine on submaxillary salivation. Fed. Proc. **20**, 318 (1961).
PFEIFER, K. A., E. SZ. VIZI, E. SATORY and E. GALAMBOS: The effect of adrenalectomy on the norepinephrine and serotonin content of the brain and on reserpine action in rats. Experientia (Basel) **19**, 482—483 (1963).
PICARELLI, Z. P., N. HYPPOLITO and J. R. VALLE: Synergistic effect of 5-hydroxytryptamine on the response of rats' seminal vesicles to adrenaline and noradrenaline. Arch. int. Pharmacodyn. **138**, 354—363 (1962).
PICHEL WARNER, R. R., H. D. JANOWITZ and D. A. DREILING: The effect of serotonin on human gastric and pancreatic secretion and bile flow. Clin. Res. **7**, 32 (1959).
PICKFORD, M.: The effect of 5-hydroxytryptamine on renal circulation and function. In: G. P. LEWIS, 5-Hydroxytryptamine, p. 109—115. London: Pergamon Press 1957.
PICKLES, V. R.: Effect of 5-hydroxytryptamine, tryptamine and indolylacetic acid on the release of pigment from beetroot disks. J. Physiol. (Lond.) **127**, 34—35 P (1955a).
— Acceleration by 5-hydroxytryptamine of haemolysis in hypotonic solutions. J. Physiol. (Lond.) **128**, 22—23 P (1955b).
— The effects of 5-hydroxytryptamine on hypotonic haemolysis, and on the potassium loss from erythrocytes during cold storage. J. Physiol. (Lond.) **134**, 484—496 (1956).
— The effects of 5-hydroxytryptamine on the passage of water, sodium and potassium through the isolated amphibian skin. J. Physiol. (Lond.) **135**, 59—60 P (1957a).
— The effects of 5-hydroxytryptamine on the movement of sodium and potassium through the isolated amphibian skin. J. Physiol. (Lond.) **138**, 495—505 (1957b).
—, and J. F. SUTKLIFF: The effects of 5-hydroxytryptamine, indole-3-acetic acid, and some other substances, on pigment effusion, sodium uptake, and potassium efflux, by slices of red beetroot in vitro. Biochim. biophys. Acta (Amst.) **17**, 244—251 (1955).
PIERRE, R., et J. CAHN: Etude du mécanisme d'action de la 5-hydroxytryptamine (sérotonine) sur la tension artérielle et la respiration. XXth Internat. Physiol. Congr. Bruxelles 1956, Comm. p. 726—727.
PILET, P. E.: Propriétés phytobiologiques de la sérotonine. Experientia (Basel) 18, 169—170 (1962).
— Action auxinique comparée de la tryptamine et de la sérotonine. Pharmaceut. Acta helv. **39**, 312—326 (1964).
POLLICE, L., e G. MAIORANO: Modificazioni della ghiandola mammaria del ratto dopo somministrazione prolungata di 5-idrossitriptamina. Boll. Soc. ital. Biol. sper. **34**, 1491—1492 (1958).
POLONI, A.: Il muscolo dorsale di sanguisuga quale test biologico per l'evidenziamento dell'attività serotoninica nei liquidi organici. Cervello **31**, 472—476 (1955).
POPENENKOVA, Z. A.: Change in the serotonin content of the blood of rabbits following thyphoid intoxication. Bull. exp. Biol. Med. **51**, 157—161 (1961).

Poulson, E., M. Botros and J. M. Robson: The effects of 5-hydroxytryptamine and iproniazid on pregnancy. J. Endocr. **20**, XI P (1960a).
— — — Effect of 5-hydroxytryptamine and iproniazid on pregnancy. Science **131**, 1101—1102 (1960b).
—, and J. M. Robson: Prevention by antagonists of the toxic action of 5-hydroxytryptamine on pregnancy. Brit. J. Pharmacol. **21**, 150—154 (1963).
— — and F. M. Sullivan: Effects of 5-hydroxytryptamine on pregnancy and foetal development in mice. J. Endocr. **26**, XXV (1963a).
— — — Teratogenic effect of 5-hydroxytryptamine in mice. Science **141**, 717—718 (1963b).
Powell, C. E.: The pharmacologic action of indole compounds. J. Amer. pharm. Ass., sci. Ed. **44**, 399—404 (1955).
—, and K. K. Chen: Action of gramine. Proc. Soc. exp. Biol. (N.Y.) **58**, 1—4 (1945).
Purkhalskaia, E.: The mechanism of action of serotonin on tumors. Protection from the oxidation of the organism by active groups of 5-hydroxytryptamine. Vop. med. Khim. 8, 42—47 (1952).
— M. F. Petrova and G. P. Menshikov: A 5-hydroxytryptamine from Hippophae rhamnoides as an antitumor preparation in experiments on animals. Bull. exp. Biol. Med. **50**, 1076—1080 (1961).
Put, T. R., and L. A. H. Hogenhuis: Brain serotonin and thyroid function. Acta physiol. neerl. **10**, 343—352 (1962).
—, and J. W. Meduski: The effect of adrenalectomy on the 5-hydroxytryptamine metabolism in the rat. Acta physiol. neerl. **11**, 240—256 (1962).
Quay, W. B.: Circadian and estrous rhythms in pineal melatonin and 5-hydroxy-indole-3-acetic acid. Proc. Soc. exp. Biol. (N.Y.) **115**, 710—713 (1964).
Quivy, D.: La sérotonine intervient-elle dans l'hémostase? Hémostase **1**, 193—200 (1961).
Radivojević, D. V., M. L. Beaumariage et Z. M. Bacq: Histamine, 5-hydroxytryptamine et protection du système pileux des souriceaux irradiés in toto. C. R. Soc. Biol. (Paris) **144**, 1489—1493 (1960).
Rall, D. P., and J. R. Gaskin: Local vasoconstrictors as provoking agents in local Schwartzman reaction. J. Pharmacol. exp. Ther. **116**, 47—48 (1956).
Rand, M., and G. Reid: On the presence in rabbit serum of thrombotonin (thrombocytin or serotonin). Aust. J. exp. Biol. med. Sci. **30**, 153—161 (1952).
Randić, M., and Z. Supek: Urinary excretion of 5-hydroxyindoleacetic acid after a single whole-body X-irradiation in normal and adrenalectomized rats. Int. J. Radiat. Biol. **4**, 151—153 (1961).
— — Influence of high doses of X-radiation on 5-hydroxytryptamine in the brain of rats. Int. J. Radiat. Biol. **4**, 637—638 (1962).
— — and Z. Lovasen: The influence of total-body X-irradiation on the 5-hydroxytryptamine content of the brain in normal rats. In: Effects of ionizing radiation on the nervous system, p. 263—265. Vienna: Int. Atomic Energy Agency 1962.
Rapport, M. M., and G. B. Koelle: The action of antihistaminics and atropine in blocking the spasmogenic activity of serotonin on the guinea pig ileum. Arch. int. Pharmacodyn. **92**, 464—490 (1953).
—, and M. Virno: Metabolic effect of serotonin in the rat. Proc. Soc. exp. Biol. (N.Y.) **81**, 203—205 (1952).
Rasmussen, H., I. H. Schwartz, R. Young and J. Marc-Aurele: Structural requirements for the action of neurohypophyseal hormones upon the isolated amphibian urinary bladder. J. gen. Physiol. **46**, 1171—1189 (1963).
Raushenbakh, M. O., and G. A. Tchernov: Probl. Gemat. **4**, 3 (1959).
Ravenna, F.: Sintesi e attività biologica del 5-ammino-triptofano. Experientia (Basel) **14**, 273—274 (1958).
Ravetta, A.: Rilievi sul trattamento sintomatico antiemorragico del morbo di Werlhof con 5-idrossitriptamina (Antemovis). Minerva med. **46**, 1193—1195 (1955).
Raymond-Hamet: Dans quel group pharmacologique faut-il ranger la donaxine? C. R. Soc. Biol. (Paris) **126**, 859—862 (1937).
— Sur les propriétés adrénalinolytiques de la donaxine. C. R. Soc. Biol. (Paris) **130**, 1218—1220 (1939).
— Indoléthylamine et phényléthylamine. C. R. Soc. Biol. (Paris) **135**, 1322 (1941a).
— Sur l'action vasculaire locale de la bufoténine. C. R. Soc. Biol. (Paris) **135**, 1414—1461 (1941b).
— Sur une propriété non encore connue de la bufoténine. C. R. Soc. Biol. (Paris) **136**, 318 (1942a).
— Sur les effets vasculaires de la bufoténine introduite dans la circulation générale. C. R. Acad. Sci. (Paris) **214**, 506—508 (1942b).

Raymond-Hamet: Sur le méchanisme de l'action vasoconstrictrice de la bufoténine. C. R. Acad. Sci. (Paris) **214**, 687—688 (1942c).
— Sur la bufoténidine, principe extrêmement actif du venin du crapaud commun. C. R. Soc. Biol. (Paris) **137**, 74—75 (1943a).
— Effets tenseurs de la bufoténidine avant et après yohimbinisation. C. R. Soc. Biol. (Paris) **137**, 744—746 (1943b).
— Sur les effets tenseurs et respiratoires de la bufoténidine basique dissoute dans le diméthyl-acétonyl-carbinol. C. R. Acad. Sci. (Paris) **218**, 54—56 (1944).
— Spartéine et bufoténine. C. R. Acad. Sci. (Paris) **222**, 691—693 (1946).
—, et R. Dufau: Le venin du crapaud commun et la bufoténine. Bull. Soc. Chim. biol. (Paris) **24**, 190—194 (1942).
Reddy, D. V., F. H. Adams and C. Baird: Teratogenic effects of serotonin. J. Pediat. **63**, 394—397 (1963).
Redisch, W., F. F. Tangco, A. J. Lewis and J. M. Steele: Vasomotor responses to reserpine in man. XXth Internat. Physiol. Congr. Bruxelles 1956, p. 755—756.
Reid, G.: The pharmacology of tryptamine. Aust. J. exp. Biol. med. Sci. **29**, 101—116 (1952a).
— Circulatory effects of 5-hydroxytryptamine. J. Physiol. (Lond.) **118**, 435—453 (1952b).
—, and M. Rand: Pharmacological actions of 5-hydroxytryptamine (serotonin, thrombocytin). Nature (Lond.) **169**, 801—802 (1952).
Renson, J.: Radioprotection de la souris par la 5-hydroxytryptamine et quelques substances voisines. Arch. int. Physiol. **68**, 531—533 (1960).
— Excrétion urinaire d'acide 5-hydroxyindolacétique chez le mammifère irradié. J. Physiol. (Paris) **52**, 208—209 (1960).
— Y. Bounameaux et G. Barac: 5-hydroxytryptamine et oligurie aigue du chien brûlé. Arch. int. Pharmacodyn. **119**, 492—494 (1959).
—, et P. Fischer: Libération de 5-hydroxytryptamine par le rayonnement X. Arch. int. Physiol. **67**, 142—144 (1959).
— H. Weissbach and S. Udenfriend: Studies on the biological activities of the aldehydes derived from norepinephrine, serotonin, tryptamine and histamine. J. Pharmacol. exp. Ther. **143**, 326—331 (1964).
Resnick, R. H., and S. J. Gray: Serotonin release by hydrochloric acid: possibility of a feed-back mechanism. Amer. J. Physiol. **201**, 1017—1019 (1961).
— — Serotonin release by hydrochloric acid. I. In vivo and in vitro demonstration. J. Lab. clin. Med. **59**, 462—468 (1962a).
— — Chemical and histologic demonstration of hydrochloric acid induced release of serotonin from intestinal mucosa. Gastroenterology **42**, 48—55 (1962b).
— G. T. Smith and S. J. Gray: Endocrine influences on tissue serotonin content of the rat. Amer. J. Physiol. **201**, 571—573 (1961).
Riva Sanseverino, E., e A. Urbano: Modificazioni del volume della milza di cane per effetto della 5-idrossitriptamina. Boll. Soc. ital. Biol. sper. **37**, 1552—1554 (1961a).
— — Effetti della 5-idrossitriptamina sul volume della milza di cane artificialmente perfusa. Boll. Soc. ital. Biol. sper. **37**, 1554—1556 (1961b).
— — Effetti della 5-idrossitriptamina sul flusso provocato di succo pancreatico di cane. Boll. Soc. ital. Biol. sper. **37**, 1556—1557 (1961c).
— — Modificazioni della secrezione esterna del pancreas di cane per effetto della infusione intravenosa di 5-idrossitriptamina. Boll. Soc. ital. Biol. sper. **37**, 1557—1559 (1961d).
— — Variazioni circolatorie della milza di cane per effetto della 5-idrossitriptamina. Boll. Soc. ital. Biol. sper. **38**, 518—521 (1962a).
— — Azione della 5-idrossitriptamina sulla milza di cane. Arch. Sci. biol. (Napoli) **46**, 419—431 (1962b).
— — Azione della 5-idrossitriptamina sulla secrezione esterna del pancreas di cane. Arch. Sci. biol. (Napoli) **47**, 181—192 (1963).
Robertson, P. A.: An antagonism of 5-hydroxytryptamine by atropine. J. Physiol. (Lond.) **121**, 54—55P (1953).
Robillard, E., and Y. Alarie: Mechanical properties and histamine and serotonin content of guinea pig lungs as influenced by microparticles inhalation. Canad. J. Biochem. **41**, 2177—2182 (1963).
Robson, J. M., and M. Botros: The effect of 5-hydroxytryptamine and of monoamine oxidase inhibitors on sexual maturity. J. Endocr. **22**, 165—175 (1961).
—, and F. M. Sullivan: Mechanism of lethal action of 5-hydroxytryptamine on the foetus. J. Endocr. **25**, 553—554 (1963).
— — Serotonin as a teratogen. Brit. med. J. **1964 I**, 370.
Rocha e Silva, M., J. R. Valle and Z. P. Picarelli: A pharmacological analysis of the mode of action of serotonin (5-hydroxytryptamine) upon the guinea-pig ileum. Brit. J. Pharmacol. 8, 378—388 (1953).

RODDIE, I. C., J. T. SHEPHERD and R. F. WHELAN: The effects of 5-hydroxytryptamine on the peripheral blood vessels of the human subject. J. Physiol. (Lond.) **130**, 8—9P (1955a).
— — — The action of 5-hydroxytryptamine on the blood vessels of the human hand and forearm. Brit. J. Pharmacol. **10**, 445—450 (1955b).
RODEGRA, H., G. ROEDER, H. J. SCHMERMUND u. K. SOEHRING: Wirkung von 5-Hydroxytryptamin auf die isolierte Nabelschnurarterie. Naunyn-Schmiedeberg's Arch. exp. Path. Pharmak. **232**, 285—286 (1957).
ROOS, B.-E.: On the occurrence and distribution of 5-hydroxyindoleacetic acid in brain. Life Sci. **1**, 25—27 (1962).
ROSA, L., G. C. CENACCHI e G. P. TOSCHI: L'influenza della 5-idrossitriptamina sul gastroacidogramma istaminico. Bologna med. **4**, 73—76 (1957—1958).
ROSE, J. C., and E. J. LAZARO: Pulmonary vascular responses to serotonin and effects of certain serotonin antagonists. Circulat. Res. **6**, 283—288 (1958).
ROSENBERG, J. C.: Sympathoadrenal response and serotonin release during hemorrhagic shock in epinephrine- and endotoxin-tolerant dogs. Circulation **24**, 1023—1024 (1961).
— R. C. LILLEHEI, W. H. MORAN and B. ZIMMERMANN: A comparison of the effects of irreversible hemorrhagic and endotoxin shock on serotonin concentration in blood. Surg. Forum **10**, 397—400 (1960a).
— — — — Effect of endotoxin on plasma catechol amines and serum serotonin. Proc. Soc. exp. Biol. (N.Y.) **102**, 335—337 (1960b).
ROSENBLUM, W., and B. W. ZWEIFACH: Action of biogenic amines, amine oxidase inhibitors, and other agents on chromatophores of Squid, *Loligo pealii*. Proc. Soc. exp. Biol. (N.Y.) **100**, 448—454 (1959).
ROSENKRANTZ, H.: A direct influence of 5-hydroxytryptamine on the adrenal cortex. Endocrinology **64**, 355—362 (1959).
—, and R. O. LAFERTE: Further observations on the relationship between serotonin and the adrenals. Endocrinology **66**, 832—841 (1960).
ROSS, D. M.: The action of tryptamine and 5-hydroxytryptamine on muscles of sea anemones. Experientia (Basel) **13**, 192—194 (1957).
— The effects of ions and drugs on neuro-muscular preparations of sea anemones. I. On preparations of the column of *Calliactis* and *Metridium*. J. exp. Biol. **37**, 732—752 (1960a).
— The effects of ions and drugs on neuro-muscular preparations of sea anemones. II. On sphincter preparations of *Calliactis* and *Metridium*. J. exp. Biol. **37**, 753—774 (1960b).
ROSSINI, G., P. CATTANEO, G. NESSI e G. PIAZZA: Attività della 5-ossitriptamina sulla fragilità capillare dei tubercolotici. Minerva med. **47**, 1793—1794 (1956).
ROVATI, V., C. MORLUNGHI e T. PICOTTI: Contributo allo studio dell'attività della serotonina sulla diuresi e sulla circolazione intrarenale. Boll. Soc. med.-chir. Pisa **24**, 295—307 (1956).
ROWE, G. G., S. ALFONSO, C. A. CASTILLO, J. C. KYLE, TH. R. LEICHT and CH. W. CRUMPTON: Systemic and coronary hemodynamic effects of an amine oxidase inhibitor and of serotonin. Clin. Pharmacol. Therap. **4**, 467—475 (1963).
ROWLEY, D. A.: Severe active cutaneous hypersensitivity in the rat. Fed. Proc. **18**, 503 (1959).
— Venous constriction as the cause of increased vascular permeability produced by 5-hydroxytryptamine, histamine, bradykinin and 48/80 in the rat. Brit. J. exp. Path. **45**, 56—67 (1964).
—, and E. P. BENDITT: 5-Hydroxytryptamine and histamine as mediators of vascular injury produced by agents which damage mast cells in rats. J. exp. Med. **103**, 399—411 (1956).
ROYAL, G. W., C. CONGDON and C. G. ROYAL: A comparison of 5-hydroxytryptamine (serotonin) levels in tissues from lethally irradiated mice after isologous or heterologous bone marrow treatment. Radiat. Res. **11**, 464 (1959).
RUDOLPH, A. M., and P. A. AMAULD: Physical factors affecting normal and serotonin-constricted pulmonary vessels. Amer. J. Physiol. **198**, 864—872 (1960).
— M. D. KURLAND, P. A. AMAULD and M. H. PAUL: Effects of vasodilator drugs on normal and serotonin-constricted pulmonary vessels of the dog. Amer. J. Physiol. **197**, 617—623 (1959).
—, and M. H. PAUL: Pulmonary and systemic vascular responses to 5-hydroxytryptamine (serotonin). Fed. Proc. **16**, 110 (1957a).
— — Pulmonary and systemic vascular response to continuous infusion of 5-hydroxytryptamine (serotonin) in the dog. Amer. J. Physiol. **189**, 263—268 (1957b).
— E. M. SCARPELLI and E. MESEL: Differential pulmonary blood flows in the unanesthetized animal. Fed. Proc. **21**, 108 (1962).
RUTLEDGE, R. A., W. E. BARRETT and A. J. PLUMMER: Alterations in the blood pressure response to serotonin caused by methylphenidate and reserpine. Fed. Proc. **18**, 441 (1959).

RYSKY, S. D.: L'Antemovis (5-idrossitriptamina) in odontoiatria. Rass. trim. Odontoiat. 38, 16—19 (1957).
SADRE, N. I., and B. B. GAITONDE: Some aspects of tracheal chain responses to various spasmogenic drugs. J. postgrad. Med. 7, 130—134 (1961).
SALA, E., e C. PERRIS: Ricerche sull'attività della 5-idrossitriptamina a livello della giunzione neuromuscolare. Neurone (Mantova) 6, 127—136 (1958).
SALA, G., and E. CASTEGNARO: Influence of enteramine (5-hydroxytryptamine) on renal function of the dog. Proc. Soc. exp. Biol. (N.Y.) 82, 621—623 (1953).
SALABE', G. B., A. OLIVERIO, P. ROSSI e F. DE LUCA: Effetti della serotonina sulla captazione tiroidea del 131 I nel ratto. Boll. Soc. ital. Biol. sper. 39, 969—971 (1963).
SALÁNKI, J.: The effect of serotonin and catecholamines on the nervous control of periodic activity in fresh-water mussel (*Anadonta cygnea*). Comp. Biochem. Physiol. 8, 163—171 (1963).
—, u. CH. S. KOSCHTOJANZ: Untersuchung der Wirkungen von Serotonin, Tryptamin, Adrenalin, Noradrenalin und LSD auf die Neuroregulation der periodischen Aktivität von Süßwassermuscheln (Anodonta cygnea). Acta physiol. Acad. Sci. hung. 20, Suppl., 45 (1962).
SALGARELLO, G.: Azione della 5-idrossitriptamina sulla respirazione dei tessuti. Esperimenti in vitro. Boll. Soc. ital. Biol. sper. 31, 786—787 (1955).
—, e E. TURRI: Comportamento della respirazione tessutale nel trattamento cronico con atropina, enteramina e misolina. Boll. Soc. ital. Biol. sper. 34, 628—629 (1958).
SALMOIRAGHI, G. C., J. W. MCCUBBIN and I. H. PAGE: Effects of d-lysergic acid diethylamide and its brom derivative on cardiovascular responses to serotonin and on arterial pressure. J. Pharmacol. exp. Ther. 119, 240—247 (1957).
— I. H. PAGE and J. W. MCCUBBIN: Cardiovascular and respiratory response to intravenous serotonin in rats. J. Pharmacol. exp. Ther. 118, 477—481 (1956).
SALVADORI, B., G. CAGNAZZO and G. BERNARDINI: The gametokinetic activity of serotonin in the male of *Rana esculenta*. Acta endocr. (Kbh.), Suppl. 7, 146 (1962).
SANBORN, R. C., and R. A. PAX: Regulation of the rate of heart-beat of Limulus. Proc. int. Union Physiol. Sci. 2, Abstr. 71 (1962).
SANDERS, R., T. P. WAALKES, J. W. GILBERT jr. and L. L. TERRY: Serotonin (5-hydroxytryptamine) and pulmonary thromboembolism. Surg. Gynaec. Obstet. 109, 455—459 (1959).
SANFORD, J.: The response of isolated strips of sheep's stomach to histamine and other substances. J. Physiol. (Lond.) 143, 82—83 (1958).
SANNER, E.: Studies on the excretion mechanism of serotonin (5-hydroxytryptamine) in the chicken kidney. Acta physiol. scand. 58, 330—341 (1963).
SANYAL, R. K.: Histamine and 5-hydroxytryptamine metabolism after superficial skin burn. Int. Arch. Allergy 21, 326—334 (1962).
—, and G. B. WEST: 5-Hydroxytryptamine and anaphylactic shock. Nature (Lond.) 180, 1417 (1957).
— — Anaphylactic shock in the albino rat. J. Physiol. (Lond.) 140, 47—48P (1958); 142, 571—584 (1958a).
— — The relationship of histamine and 5-hydroxytryptamine to anaphylactic shock in different species. J. Physiol. (Lond.) 144, 525—531 (1958b).
— — The effect of splenectomy on the production of anaphylactic shock in the guinea pig and the rat. J. Pharm. Pharmacol. 11, 17—25 (1959).
SANZIO GRECO, A.: Impiego del solfato doppio di 5-ossitriptamina e creatinina (Antemovis) in soggetti con emostasi normale operati di tonsillectomia. Minerva otorinolaring. 7, 26—27 (1957).
SARAJAS, H. S. S., R. KRISTOFFERSON and M. H. FRICK: Release of 5-hydroxytryptamine and adenosinetriphosphate in extracorporeal circulatory system as a result of corpuscular blood trauma. Amer. J. Physiol. 197, 1195—1198 (1959); — Nature (Lond.) 184, 1127—1128 (1959).
—, and L. SAURE: Renal affection resulting from blood trauma in extracorporeal circuits. Nature (Lond.) 185, 768—770 (1960).
SÁTORY, E., A. K. PFEIFER and E. SZ. VIZI: Pharmacological and biochemical effects of diethyltryptamine. Arch. int. Pharmacodyn. 147, 400—407 (1964).
SAVI, C.: Influenza della 5-ossitriptamina sulla evoluzione della gravidanza nel mus musculus albinus. Attual. Ostet. Ginec. 2, 625—630 (1956).
SAXENA, P. N.: Effect of drugs on early inflammatory reaction. Arch. int. Pharmacodyn. 126, 228—237 (1960).
SCALTRINI, G. C.: Il quadro emocitario periferico e la glicemia dopo 5-idrossitriptamina. Haematologica 41, 681—687 (1956).
SCARINCI, V.: Ricerche farmacologiche sulla 5-idrossitriptamina. I. Azione sulla epilessia riflessa. Arch. ital. Sci. farmacol. 5, 265—270 (1955a).

Scarinci, V.: Ricerche farmacologiche sulla ossitriptamina. II. Azione sulla pressione arteriosa. Farmaco, Ed. sci. **10**, 783—792 (1955b).
— Osservazioni preliminari sul meccanismo di azione della 5-idrossitriptamina sulla pressione arteriosa. Boll. Soc. ital. Biol. sper. **31**, 777—778 (1955b).
Schaeppi, U.: Effect of neurohumors on the nictitating membrane of the cat. Fed. Proc. **21**, 330 (1962).
— Comparison of serotonin with directly and indirectly acting compounds in their effect on the nictitating membrane of spinal cats. J. Pharmacol. exp. Ther. **139**, 330—336 (1963a).
— Effects of electrical stimulation and serotonin on the contractility of the isolated pig iris. Fed. Proc. **22**, 461 (1963b).
Schain, R. J.: Effects of 5-hydroxytryptamine on the dorsal muscle of the leech *(Hirudo medicinalis)*. Brit. J. Pharmacol. **16**, 257—261 (1961).
Schatzmann, H. J.: Tödliche thrombocytopenische Purpura bei Benzolvergiftung. Schweiz. med. Wschr. **85**, 1123—1126 (1955).
Scheiffarth, F., L. Zicha u. W. Forster: Vergleichende Untersuchungen über die eosinopenische Wirkung verschiedener Glucocorticoidester sowie des 5-Hydroxytryptophans beim Menschen. Arzneimittel-Forsch. **11**, 602—606 (1961).
Schievelbein, H., F. Sebening, U. Surberg u. I. Trautschold: Freisetzung von Serotonin bei Operationen unter Verwendung des extrakorporalen Kreislaufs. Klin. Wschr. **40**, 919—920 (1962).
Schmermund, H. J., H. Rodegra u. K. Soehring: Über die Beteiligung von 5-Hydroxytryptamin beim physiologischen Verschluß der Nabelschnurgefäße post partum. Arch. Gynäk. **191**, 457—462 (1959).
Schmid, E., u. H. Kinzlmeier: Das Verhalten der Magenacidität und der Motilität im Verdauungstrakt des Menschen bei Infusion von Serotonin. Naunyn-Schmiedeberg's Arch. exp. Path. Pharmak. **236**, 51—54 (1959).
— K. Meythaler jr., H. Schön u. H. Henning: Untersuchungen über die Ausscheidung von 5-Hydroxyindolessigsäure im Harn beim experimentell ausgelösten Dumping-Syndrom. Klin. Wschr. **40**, 908—911 (1962).
— U. Rosenbusch, K. Heinkel, K. Schwemmle u. H. Schön: 5-Hydroxytryptamin und Erkrankungen der Verdauungsorgane. 2. Mitteilung. Ausscheidung von 5-Hydroxyindolessigsäure im Harn, klinische und bioptisch-morphologische Untersuchungsergebnisse. Gastroenterologia (Basel) **96**, 275—290 (1961).
— F. Scheiffarth, W. Roschinsky u. L. Zicha: Über Histamin- und Serotonin-antagonistische Effekte von Antikoagulantien. Wirkungsmechanismus und pathophysiologische Bedeutung. Int. Arch. Allergy **14**, 292—301 (1959).
— H. Waltz u. G. Freund: Zur Kreislauf- und Atmungswirkung von Serotonin (5-Hydroxytryptamin) am wachen Hund. Naunyn-Schmiedeberg's Arch. exp. Path. Pharmak. **228**, 307—313 (1956).
— L. Zicha u. F. Scheiffarth: Über die Wirkung von 5-Hydroxytryptophan auf den Magendarmtrakt des Menschen. Med. exp. (Basel) **2**, 266—269 (1960).
Schmitt, H., et H. Schmitt: Modifications de l'action des catécholamines sur la membrane nictitante du chat par la 5-hydroxytryptamine. C. R. Soc. Biol. (Paris) **153**, 917—919 (1959).
Schneckloth, R. E., I. H. Page and A. C. Corcoran: Depressed renal function in the carcinoid syndrome: effects of serotonin in normal subjectes and of an antiserotonin (Bromo-LSD). Clin. Res. Proc. **4**, 308 (1957).
Schneider, J. A., R. Gaunt and A. E. Earl: Effect of adrenal cortical and medullary factors on the cardiovascular response to serotonin (5-hydroxytryptamine) in the dog. J. Pharmacol. exp. Ther. **110**, 45—46 (1954).
—, and R. K. Rinehart: Circulatory interactions of serotonin and reserpine (serpasil) in dogs. Arch. int. Pharmacodyn. **105**, 253—268 (1956); — J. Pharmacol. exp. Ther. **116**, 51 (1956).
—, and F. F. Yonkman: Action of serotonin (5-hydroxytryptamine) on vagal afferent impulses in the cat. Fed. Proc. **12**, 128 (1953); — Amer. J. Physiol. **174**, 125—134 (1953).
— — Species differences in the respiratory and cardiovascular response to serotonin. J. Pharmacol. exp. Ther. **111**, 84—98 (1954).
Schötensack, W., P. Bischler u. G. Richarz: Vergleich pharmakologischer Wirkungen von Indol- und Benzofuranalkylamines. Naunyn-Schmiedeberg's Arch. exp. Path. Pharmak. **245**, 120—121 (1963).
Schofield, B. M., and J. M. Walker: Perfusion of the coronary arteries of the dog. J. Physiol. (Lond.) **122**, 489—497 (1953).
Schumacher, H., u. H.-G. Classen: Neuropharmakologische Untersuchungen zur Analyse der Pupillomotorik. Albrecht v. Graefes Arch. Ophthal. **164**, 533—537 (1962a).
— — Der Einfluß von 5-Hydroxytryptamin auf den Augeninnendruck. Albrecht v. Graefes Arch. Ophthal. **164**, 538—542 (1962b).

SCHWEMMLE, K., E. SCHMID, F. SCHEIFFARTH, L. ZICHA u. E. SCHICHOR: Zur Frage der gegenseitigen Beziehungen zwischen adrenocorticotropem Hormon bzw. Glucocorticoiden und dem Serotonin-Stoffwechsel. Arzneimittel-Forsch. **11**, 616—619 (1961).

SCOTT, K. G., R. R. SCHELINE and R. S. STONE: Mast cells and sarcoma growth in the rat. Cancer Res. **18**, 927—931 (1958).

—, and R. S. STONE: The anti-tumor action of lysergic acid derivatives and their serotonin-blocking effect as reflected by the I^{131} distribution in rats. Cancer Res. **19**, 783—787 (1959).

SEFERIAN, V.: Sérotonine et cholérèse. Thérapie **17**, 185—187 (1962).

SEIJI, M.: The effect of tryptophan metabolites on melanin formation. Fed. Proc. **20**, 6 (1961).

SELLER, M. J.: Serotonin as a teratogen. Brit. med. J. **1964 I**, 308—309.

SELYE, H., J.-M. DIEUDONNÉ and G. GABBIANI: The critical period in calciphylaxis. Fed. Proc. **21**, 168 (1962a).

— — and R. VEILLEUX: Calciphylactic muscolar dystrophy induced by DHT plus 5-HT. Proc. Soc. exp. Biol. (N.Y.) **109**, 232—233 (1962b).

SERRAVALLI, S.: 5-Idrossitriptamina e diabete insipido. Atti Accad. Sci. Ferrara **32**, 67—71 (1954—1955).

SETNIKAR, I., M. SALVATERRA and O. TEMELCOU: Antiphlogistic activity of iproniazid. Brit. J. Pharmacol. **14**, 484—487 (1959).

SHARPEY-SCHAFER, E. P., and J. GINSBURG: Humoral agents and venous tone. Effects of catecholamines, 5-hydroxytryptamine, histamine and nitrites. Lancet **1962 II**, 1337—1340.

SHAW, E., and D. W. WOOLLEY: Yohimbine and ergot alkaloids as naturally occurring antimetabolites of serotonin. J. biol. Chem. **203**, 979—989 (1953).

— — Pharmacological properties of some antimetabolites of serotonin having unusually high activity on isolated tissues. J. Pharmacol. exp. Ther. **111**, 43—53 (1954).

— — Some serotoninlike activities of lysergic acid diethylamide. Science **124**, 121—122 (1956).

SHAY, H., D. C. H. SUN and M. GRUENSTEIN: Effect of serotonin and reserpine on interdigestive gastric secretion in the rat. Fed. Proc. **16**, 118 (1957).

— — — Effect of serotonin and its precursor on interdigestive gastric secretion in the rat. Fed. Proc. **17**, 146 (1958).

SHEPHERD, J. J.: Serotonin and gut motility. Brit. med. J. **1963 II**, 1589.

—, D. E. DONALD, E. LINDER and H. J. C. SWAN: Effect of small doses of 5-hydroxytryptamine (serotonin) on pulmonary circulation in the closed-chest dog. Amer. J. Physiol. **197**, 963—967 (1959).

SHIM, W. K. T., E. L. POLLACK and TH. DRAPANAS: Effect of serotonin, epinephrine, histamine and hexamethonium on thoracic duct lymph. Amer. J. Physiol. **201**, 81—84 (1961).

SHOEMAKER, W. C., H. KLECKNER, M. PERLOW and G. GALANSINO: Effect of serotonin on regional metabolism. Fed. Proc. **20**, 314 (1961).

SHORE, P. A., A. PLETSCHER and B. B. BRODIE: Release of platelet serotonin by reserpine-effect on hemostasis. J. Pharmacol. exp. Ther. **116**, 51—52 (1956).

SIEGENTHALER, W.: Zur Behandlung der thrombocytopenischen hämorrhagischen Diathese mit 5-Oxytryptamin (Serotonin). Schweiz. med. Wschr. **86**, 1443—1446 (1956).

SIGEL, B., I. M. POTASH and M. W. WOLCOTT: Excretion of 5-hydroxyindoleacetic acid following bowel ischemia in dogs. Proc. Soc. exp. Biol. (N.Y.) **105**, 237—238 (1960).

SIGG, E. B., L. SOFFER and L. GYERMEK: Influence of imipramine and related psychoactive agents on the effect of 5-hydroxytryptamine and catecholamines on the cat nictitating membrane. J. Pharmacol. exp. Ther. **142**, 13—20 (1963).

SILVER, D., W. DEMARIA and W. G. ANLYAN: Hemodynamic and humoral changes during the acute phase of transfusion reaction. Surg. Gynec. Obstet. **113**, 705—710 (1961).

SINCLAIR, I. S. R.: Some aspects of intestinal and renal function in metastasizing argentaffinoma. Proc. roy. Soc. Med. **50**, 447—451 (1957).

SINHA, Y. K., and G. B. WEST: The antagonism between local anesthetic drugs and 5-hydroxytryptamine. J. Pharm. Pharmacol. **5**, 370—374 (1953).

SIREK, A.: Nature and site of origin of the hyperglycaemic substance released following an injection of growth hormone. Nature (Lond.) **179**, 376 (1957).

SKANSE, B., and A. HANSON: Increased thyroid function and the urinary excretion of 5-hydroxyindole acetic acid. Lancet **1962 I**, 1072.

SKILLEN, R. G., C. H. THIENES, J. CANGELOSI and L. STRAIN: Lung 5-hydroxytryptamine and ozone induced pulmonary edema in rats. Proc. Soc. exp. Biol. (N.Y.) **107**, 178—180 (1961a).

— — — — Brain 5-hydroxytryptamine in ozone-exposed rats. Proc. Soc. exp. Biol. (N.Y.) **108**, 121—122 (1961b).

— — and L. STRAIN: 5-Hydroxytryptamine, 5-hydroxytryptophan decarboxylase and monoamine oxidase in hearts of normal, thyroid-fed and propylthiouracil-fed male and female rats. Endocrinology **70**, 743—747 (1962).

Sleisenger, M. H., D. H. Law, Ch. M. Lewis and J. H. Pert: Comparative effect of parasympathomimetic agents and 5-hydroxytryptamine upon colon contractility in dogs. Clin. Res. **6**, 276—277 (1958).
— — F. W. Smith, J. H. Pert and Ch. M. Lewis: Studies of colon contractility in dogs. I. Description of method and effect of parasympathomimetic agents and serotonin. J. clin. Invest. **38**, 2119—2130 (1959).
Smelik, P. G., and D. de Wied: Corticotropin-releasing action of adrenaline, serotonin and pitressin. Experientia (Basel) **14**, 17—18 (1958a).
— — The corticotropin-releasing action of adrenaline and pitressin. Acta physiol. neerl. **7**, 154—155 (1958b).
Smith, A. N.: The effect of 5-hydroxytryptamine on acid gastric secretion. In: G. P. Lewis, 5-Hydroxytryptamine, p. 183—190. London: Pergamon Press 1957.
— J. W. Black and E. W. Fisher: Inhibitory effect of 5-hydroxytryptophan on acid gastric secretion. Nature (Lond.) **180**, 1127 (1957).
Smith, D. D., and A. A. Miles: The role of histamine in early bacterial inflammation of the rat peritoneal cavity. Brit. J. exp. Path. **41**, 305—312 (1960).
Smith, D. E., and Y. S. Lewis: Preparation and effects of an anti-mast cell serum. J. exp. Med. **113**, 683—692 (1961).
Smith, D. J.: Physiology of the vasa vasorum. Fed. Proc. **12**, 133—134 (1953).
Smith, G., and A. N. Smith: The role of serotonin in experimental pulmonary embolism. Surg. Gynec. Obstet. **101**, 691—700 (1955).
Smyth, Ch. J., O. B. Gum and P. K. Hamilton: Effects of intra-articular serotonin and competitive amines on connective tissue proliferation in rabbit joints. J. Lab. clin. Med. **60**, 492—503 (1962).
Sobotka, H., and W. Antopol: Inhibitors of choline esterase. Enzymologia **4**, 189—191 (1937).
Sofer, S., and C. J. Gubler: Studies on effect of various procedures in the 5-OH tryptamine (5-HT) levels in the brain of rats. Fed. Proc. **21**, 340 (1962).
Soffer, L., and L. Gyermek: The interaction of imipramine, its derivatives, and phenotiazines with 5-HT, epinephrine and norepinephrine. Fed. Proc. **20**, 396 (1961).
Sokoloff, B., K. Funaoka, M. Fujisawa, C. C. Saelhof, E. Taniguchi, L. Bird and C. Miller: An oncostatic factor present in the bark of Hippophae rhamnoides. Growth **25**, 401—409 (1961).
Sosin, H., D. M. Nicoloff, E. T. Peter, A. I. Walder and O. H. Wangensteen: Effect of serotonin on histamine stimulated secretion in canine Heidenhain pouches. Fed. Proc. **21**, 264 (1962).
Soulairac, A., et M. L. Soulairac: Action de la réserpine, de la sérotonine et de l'iproniazide sur le comportement alimentaire du rat. C. R. Soc. Biol. (Paris) **154**, 510—513 (1960).
Sparrow, E. M., and D. L. Wilhelm: Species differences in susceptibility to capillary permeability factors: histamine, 5-hydroxytryptamine and compound 48/80. J. Physiol. (Lond.) **137**, 51—65 (1957).
Speck, L. B.: Effects of massive X-irradiation on rat electroencephalograms and brain serotonin. J. Neurochem. **9**, 573—574 (1962).
Spector, W. G.: Substances which affect capillary permeability. Pharmacol. Rev. **10**, 475—505 (1958).
—, and D. A. Willoughby: 5-Hydroxytryptamine in acute inflammation. Nature (Lond.) **179**, 318 (1957a).
— — Histamine and 5-hydroxytryptamine in acute experimental pleurisy. J. Path. Bact. **74**, 57—65 (1957b).
— — Experimental suppression of the early inflammatory phenomena of turpentine pleurisy in rats. Nature (Lond.) **181**, 708—709 (1958a).
— — Experimental suppression of increased capillary permeability in thermal burns in rats. Nature (Lond.) **182**, 949—950 (1958b).
— — Suppression of increased capillary permeability in injury by monoamine oxidase inhibitors. Nature (Lond.) **186**, 162—163 (1960).
Spencer, P. S. J., and G. B. West: Sensitivity of the hyperthyroid and hypothyroid mouse to histamine and 5-hydroxytryptamine. Brit. J. Pharmacol. **17**, 137—413 (1961).
Spies, T. D., and R. E. Stone: Effect of serotonin on blood pressure and lack of effect of antimetabolite. J. Amer. med. Ass. **150**, 1599—1600 (1952).
Spinazzola, A. J., and T. R. Sherrod: Serotonin on renal hemodynamics. J. Pharmacol. exp. Ther. **113**, 49 (1955).
— — The effects of serotonin (5-hydroxytryptamine) on renal hemodynamics. J. Pharmacol. exp. Ther. **119**, 114—121 (1957).
Spirito, A., e U. Teodoro: Interferenza dell'attività serotoninica sulla motilità ureterale (ricerche sperimentali). Inform. med. (Genova) **14**, 141—150 (1959).

SPIRITO, A., U. TEODORO e G. VANNI: Interferenza dell'eparina e della 5-ossitriptamina sul tasso plasmatico e tissurale della glucosamina nelle ustioni sperimentali. Inform. med. (Genova) **14**, 163—168 (1959).

STARBUCK, W. C., and H. C. HEIM: Some *in vitro* effects of chlorpromazine, lysergic acid diethylamide, and 5-hydroxytryptamine on the respiration of rat brain. J. Amer. pharm. Ass., sci. ed. **48**, 251—253 (1959).

STEFANINI, M., and S. KISTNER: Use of platelet derivatives and platelet substitutes in the management of thrombocytopenic states. Clin. Res. Proc. **5**, 151—152 (1957).

—, and S. I. MAGALINI: Evaluation of hemostatic properties of synthetic serotonin. Arch. intern. Med. **98**, 23—27 (1956).

STEINBERG, M. S., A. WALLACE and P. WILSON: Pulmonary vascular responses to serotonin and effects of hypertonic sodium chloride solution in the rabbit. J. Amer. osteopath. Ass. **61**, 127—129 (1961).

STEINER, J. E., and F. G. SULMAN: Simultaneous studies of blood sugar, behavioural changes and EEG on the wake rabbit after administration of psilocybin. Arch. int. Pharmacodyn. **145**, 301—308 (1963).

STENGER, E. G.: Zur Frage des Entstehungsmechanismus der experimentellen Dextran-Schwellung der Rattenpfote. Arzneimittel-Forsch. 8, 693—694 (1958).

— Zum Wirkungsmechanismus des Chlorpromazins. Arzneimittel-Forsch. **9**, 190—191 (1959).

STORMORKEN, H.: The antiserotonin effects of the benzyl analog of bufotenin (BAB) and the benzyl analog of serotonin (BAS) in the isolated guinea pig lung. Arch. int. Pharmacodyn. **119**, 232—237 (1959).

STONE, C. A., H. C. WENGER, C. T. LUDDEN, J. M. STAVORSKI and CH. A. ROSS: Anti-serotonin-antihistaminic properties of cyproheptadine. J. Pharmacol. exp. Ther. **131**, 73—84 (1961).

STONE, H. H., and P. NEMIR jr.: Study of the role of 5-hydroxytryptamine (serotonin) and histamine in the pathogenesis of pulmonary embolism in man. Ann. Surg. **152**, 890—900 (1960).

STROBEL, G. E., J. MCINTOSH and J. P. KULKA: Effects of serotonin and their inhibition: morphologic observations on the vasculature of the mouse ear. Fed. Proc. **20**, 118 (1961).

STUCKI, J. C., and CH. R. THOMPSON: A screeining procedure for substances which inhibit dextran edema in the rat. Amer. J. Physiol. **193**, 275—282 (1958).

STUDER, A., u. J. TRIPOD: Verschiedene Reaktivität isolierter Gefäße auf verengernde und erweiternde Pharmaka. Helv. physiol. pharmacol. Acta **18**, 384—393 (1960).

STÜTTGEN, G., u. M. SCHIPPEL: Die pharmakologische Serotoninwirkung an der menschlichen Haut unter verschiedenen Applikationsformen. Arch. klin. exp. Derm. **212**, 180—193 (1961).

SUPEK, Z., M. JOVIĆ u. S. KECKES: Der 5-Hydroxytryptamin-Gehalt der Haut der Ratte bei experimenteller Entzündung. Arzneimittel-Forsch. **11**, 132—133 (1961).

— M. RANDIĆ and Z. LOVASEN: Radioprotective action of some indolealkylamines. Int. J. Radiat. Biol. **4**, 111—112 (1962).

— B. UROIĆ and M. RABADJIJA: The effect of some nucleotoxic agents on urinary excretion of 5-hydroxyindoleacetic acid in rats. Biochem. Pharmacol. **12**, 759—761 (1963).

SUPNIEWSKI, J. V., and M. SERAFIN-GAJEWSKA: 2-Methylgramine. Acta Pol. pharm. **2**, 125—129 (1938).

—, and M. SERAFINOWNA: Pharmacological properties of gramine. Bull. int. Acad. Cracovie, Cl. Méd., Nr 7/8, 479—486 (1938).

SWANK, R. L., J. H. FELLMAN and W. W. HISSEN: Aggregation of blood cells by 5-hydroxytryptamine (serotonin). Circulat. Res. **13**, 392—400 (1963).

SZARVAS, F., u. K. KOVACZ: Die Untersuchungen der Serotoninwirkung bei der mit Hormonen hervorgerufenen Nierenrindennekrose bei Ratten. Med. exp. **9**, 241—248 (1963).

SZEGO, C. M., and S. H. SLOAN: The influence of histamine and serotonin in promoting early uterine growth in the rat. Gen. comp. Endocr. **1**, 295—305 (1961).

SZERB, J. C.: Non-specific depressant effect of 5-hydroxytryptamine on guinea-pig ileum. Fed. Proc. **17**, 160 (1958).

TAKÁCS, L., and V. VAJDA: Effect of serotonin on cardiac output and organ blood flow of rats. Amer. J. Physiol. **204**, 301—303 (1963).

TAKENAKA, F.: Response of coronary strips to acetylcholine, histamine, 5-hydroxytryptamine and adrenaline. Jap. J. Pharmacol. **9**, 55—60 (1959).

TAPANI, T.: The acute toxicity of 5-HT in anaesthetized rats. Biochem. Pharmacol. **12** (Suppl.), 38 (1963).

TCHERNOW, G. A.: Med. Radiol. (Moskva) **5**, 75 (1960).

—, and L. M. MOROZOVSKAIA: On the mechanism of serotonin metabolism disorders in acute radiation sickness. Med. Radiol. (Moskva) **6**, 59—62 (1961).

TCHERNOW, G. A., and M. O. RAUSHENBAKH: Study of the role of serotonin in the pathogenesis of acute radiation sickness. 2. Change in the content of serotonin in the intestine and brain of guinea-pigs and rats in acute radiation sickness. Probl. Gemat. **5**, 3—7 (1960).

TELFORD, J. M., and G. B. WEST: The effects of corticosteroids and related compounds on the histamine and 5-hydroxytryptamine content of rat tissues. Brit. J. Pharmacol. **15**, 532—539 (1960).

— — Some effects of corticosteroids on the metabolism of histamine and 5-hydroxytryptamine in the rat. Brit. J. Pharmacol. **16**, 360—368 (1961).

TESSARI, L., e L. PARRINI: Effetto della 5-HT sull'assorbimento intestinale del calcio. Arch. Ortop. (Milano) **74**, 228—232 (1961).

THEOBALD, W., u. R. DOMENJOZ: Das Serotonin-Oedem der Ratte und seine Beeinflussung durch Antiphlogistica. Arzneimittel-Forsch. **8**, 18—19 (1958).

THOMPSON, J. W.: Studies on the responses of the isolated nictitating membrane of the cat. J. Physiol. (Lond.) **141**, 46—72 (1958).

TODA, N.: Effects of 5-hydroxytryptamine on the isolated atrium of rabbit. Jap. J. Pharmacol. **13**, 82—103 (1963).

TOH, C. C.: Effect of temperature on the 5-hydroxytryptamine (serotonin) content of tissue. J. Physiol. (Lond.) **151**, 410—415 (1960).

—, and A. MOHIUDDIN: Vasoactive substances in the nasal mucosa. Brit. J. Pharmacol. **13**, 113—117 (1958).

TOKUDA, S., and R. S. WEISER: Studies on the mechanism of anaphylaxis in the mouse. Fed. Proc. **19**, 214 (1960).

— — Studies on the role of serotonin and mast cells in anaphylaxis of the mouse produced with soluble antigen-antibody complexes. J. Immunol. **86**, 292—301 (1961).

TONINI, G.: Effetti della 5-idrossitriptamina sulla attività colinesterasica del cervello di ratto *in vitro*. Boll. Soc. ital. Biol. sper. **31**, 766—768 (1955).

TORRIELLI, F. C., e G. MINOLA: La 5-ossitriptamina in anestesia locale. Minerva stomat. **5**, 234—237 (1956).

TOWNE, J., T. PUT and N. SCHWARTZ: Brain serotonin and thyroid function. Fed. Proc. **18**, 452 (1959).

TOWNE, J. C., and J. O. SHERMAN: Failure of acute bilateral adrenalectomy to influence brain serotonin levels in the rat. Proc. Soc. exp. Biol. (N.Y.) **104**, 721—722 (1960).

TRAPOLD, J. H., and U. BRINER: Diuretic activity of 9-(N-methyl-piperidyliden-4′) thioxanthene (BP-400) a serotonin-histamine antagonist. Fed. Proc. **21**, 430 (1962).

TRENDELENBURG, U.: The action of histamine and 5-hydroxytryptamine on isolated mammalian atria. J. Pharmacol. exp. Ther. **130**, 450—460 (1960).

TRICOU, B. J., and J. DOULL: Pharmacological and toxicological compounds as protective or therapeutic agents against radiation injury in experimental animals. I. Pharmacological studies on the radioprotective activity of serotonin. USAF Radiat. Lab. Univ. Chicago Rep. **34**, 46—61 (1960a).

— — Pharmacological and toxicological compounds as protective or therapeutic agents against radiation injury in experimental animals. II. Mechanism of the radioprotective effect of serotonin. USAF Radiat. Lab. Univ. Chicago Rep. **35**, 70—88 (1960b).

— — Pharmacological and toxicological compounds as protective or therapeutic agents against radiation injury in experimental animals. III. Further studies on the radioprotective effects of serotonin in mice. USAF Radiat. Lab. Univ. Chicago Rep. **36**, 85—106 (1960c).

— — Pharmacological and toxicological compounds as protective or therapeutic agents against radiation injury in experimental animals. IV. Further studies on the mechanism of the radioprotective action of serotonin. USAF Radiat. Lab. Univ. Chicago Rep. **38**, 42—59 (1961).

TRIPOD, J., et H. J. BEIN: Modification de la réactivité vasculaire périphérique dans l'hypertension rénale du rat. Helv. physiol. pharmacol. Acta **18**, 394—403 (1960).

TROMPIZ, G.: Ensayo de una intradermoreaccion con serotonina. Estudio en 332 casos. Folia clín. int. (Barcelona) **11**, 63—69 (1961).

TSAGARIS, T. J., J. A. KOEHLER, F. L. ANDERSON, H. KUIDA and H. H. HECHT: Drug inhibition of circulatory responses to endotoxin. Fed. Proc. **22**, 630 (1963).

TSITOURIS, G., S. BELLET, J. SCHRAEDER and L. FEINBERG: The anti-fibrinolytic properties of serotonin. Fed. Proc. **20**, 59 (1961).

— H. SANDBERG, S. BELLET, L. FEINBERG and J. SCHRAEDER: The effects of serotonin on inhibition of the plasmin-plasminogen fibrinolytic system in vitro. J. Lab. clin. Med. **59**, 25—39 (1962).

TSUCHIYA, M., and C. J. KENSLER: The effect of autonomic drugs and 2-amino-2-methylpropanol, a choline antagonist, on ciliary movement. Fed. Proc. **18**, 453 (1959).

TURA, S., E. PIERAGNOLI, P. R. DAL MONTE e C. GIRO: Effetti della serotonina sulla captazione epatica della bromosulftaleina. Boll. Soc. ital. Biol. sper. **36**, 1352—1353 (1960).
TURNER, W. J.: Effect of Rauwolfia alkaloids and related substances on chromatophores. Dis. nerv. Syst. **19**, 1—8 (1958).
—, and S. MERLIS: Effect of some indolealkylamines on man. Arch. Neurol. Psychiat. (Chic.) **81**, 121—129 (1959).
TWAROG, B. M.: Response of a molluscan smooth muscle to acetylcholine and 5-hydroxytryptamine. J. cell. comp. Physiol. **44**, 141—164 (1954).
— Nervous control of a molluscan smooth muscle. Fed. Proc. **17**, 165 (1958).
— 5-Hydroxytryptamine as a relaxing agent. In: Inhibition in the Nervous System and γ-Aminobutyric Acid, p. 97—101. London: Pergamon Press 1960a.
— Effects of acetylcholine and 5-hydroxytryptamine on the contraction of molluscan smooth muscle. J. Physiol. (Lond.) **152**, 236—242 (1960b).
TYCE, G. M., G. H. C. STOBIE and J. L. BOLLMAN: 5-Hydroxytryptamine content of gastrointestinal mucosa. Fed. Proc. **20**, 252 (1961).
UEDA, M., S. TAKAHASHI and T. MINESHITA: Pharmacological studies on bufotenidine. Ann. Rep. Shionogi Res. Lab. **7**, 109—122 (1957).
UI, M.: The role of serotonin in carbohydrate metabolism. VI. Serotonin-stimulated glycogen formation and its relation to insulin effect in isolated rat diaphragm. Endocr. jap. **9**, 12—21 (1962a).
— The role of serotonin in carbohydrate metabolism. VII. *In vitro* observations suggesting enhanced release of insulin in response to serotonin treatment. Endocr. jap. **9**, 22—32 (1962b).
—, and B. KOBAYASHI: The role of serotonin in carbohydrate metabolism. VIII. *In vitro* effect of serotonin on lactate production of rat diaphragm. Endocr. jap. **9**, 33—40 (1962).
— U. WASASHINA and B. KOBAYASHI: The role of serotonin in carbohydrate metabolism. III. The effect of serotonin on blood lactate level of rats. Endocr. jap. **7**, 261—270 (1960a).
— — — The role of serotonin in carbohydrate metabolism. IV. Mechanism of serotonin hyperlactacidemia. Endocr. jap. **7**, 271—278 (1960b).
UNGAR, G., S. KOBRIN and B. R. SEZESNY: Measurement of inflammation and evaluation of anti-inflammatory agents. Arch. int. Pharmacodyn. **123**, 71—77 (1959).
UROIĆ, B., M. RABADJIJA and Z. SUPEK: Toxicity of a nucleotoxic agent, mustine hydrochloride, and its enhancement by 5-hydroxytryptamine pretreatment. J. Pharm. Pharmacol. **16**, 61—62 (1964).
VACEK, L.: Susceptibility of rabbit aorta strips to serotonin in endocrine hypertension. Arch. int. Pharmacodyn. **124**, 461—465 (1960).
VALETTE, G., et P. AUGEREAU: Réactivité des muscles lisses des poissons a l'histamine et a d'autres agents contracturants (5-hydroxytryptamine, acétylcholine et chlorure de barium). J. Physiol. (Paris) **50**, 1067—1074 (1958).
VALSECCHI, A.: Influenza dell'apporto di serotonina sul travaglio di parto nella donna. Minerva ginec. **10**, 898—901 (1959).
VANE, J. R.: The relative activities of some tryptamine analogues on the isolated rat stomach strip preparation. Brit. J. Pharmacol. **14**, 87—98 (1959).
VARAGIĆ, V., M. KRSTIĆ, S. STEPANOVIĆ and HAJDUKOVIĆ: The effect of γ-irradiation on the amount of 5-hydroxytryptamine in the gut and spleen in the early phase after irradiation. Experientia (Basel) **19**, 647—648 (1963).
VEERDONK, F. C. G. VAN DE: Serotonin, a melanocyte-stimulating component in the dorsal skin secretion of *Xenopus laevis*. Nature (Lond.) **187**, 948—949 (1960).
VENINGA, T. S., and R. BRINKMAN: Contributions to the study of immediate and early x-ray reactions with regard to chemoprotection. VI. Random liberation of biogenic amines as a cause of early irradiation effects. Int. J. Radiat. Biol. **5**, 283—289 (1962).
VERCILLO, L., e G. M. MAZZETTI: Comportamento della diuresi e di alcuni indici di funzionalità renale in soggetti normali sottoposti a trattamento con 5-ossitriptamina. Minerva med. **48**, 1217—1220 (1957).
VERDESCA, A. S., C. D. WESTERMANN, R. S. CRAMPTON, W. C. BLACK, B. J. NEDELJKOVIC and J. G. HILTON: Direct adrenocortical stimulatory effect of serotonin. Amer. J. Physiol. **201**, 1065—1067 (1961).
VIALLI, M.: Azione della bufotalina sull'occhio enucleato di rana. Biochim. Terap. sper. **30**, 186—189 (1943).
VILLAMIL, M. F., N. YEYATI, P. GARRAHAM and A. C. TAQUINI: Renal circulatory effect of serotonin. Proc. Int. Union Physiol. Sci. **2**, Abstr. 234 (1962).
VIRTAMA, P., and E. JÄNKÄLÄ: Effect of serotonin on the renal arteries of the guinea-pig and the rabbit. Arteriographic studies. Angiology **12**, 372—375 (1961).
VISETTI, M.: Su un particolare modo di impiego della 5-ossitriptamina in chirurgia plastica. Minerva derm. **33**, 505—507 (1958).

VITOLO, E., M. OBBIASSI, G. P. ZOCCHI and G. C. SCOTTI: Mechanism of pulmonary vasoconstriction after injection of 5-hydroxytryptamine in the dog. Brit. Heart J. **24**, 422, 430 (1962).
VITTORIO, P. V., and E. W. WIGHT: The effect of X-irradiation and serotonin on Cr^{51} uptake in mouse bone, muscle, and brain. Canad. J. Biochem. **41**, 1525—1530 (1963).
— — and B. E. SINNOTT: A study of the protective action of serotonin (5-hydroxytryptamine) against whole-body X-irradiation in mice with the aid of chromium 51. Canad. J. Biochem. **41**, 347—360 (1963).
VOGEL, G., u. M. L. MAREK: Über die Hemmung verschiedener Rattenpfoten-Oedeme durch Serotonin-Antagonisten. Arzneimittel-Forsch. **11**, 1051—1054 (1961).
VOGIN, E. E., and G. V. ROSSI: Radiometric quantitation of the inhibition of 5-hydroxytryptamine-induced edema in mice. Arch. int. Pharmacodyn. **144**, 151—160 (1963).
VOGT, W.: Identifizierung von Substanz DS mit 5-Oxytryptamin. Naunyn-Schmiedeberg's Arch. exp. Path. Pharmak. **222**, 427—430 (1954).
WAAL, H. J., and A. M. O. VEALE: Antidiuretic effect of serotonin. Proc. Univ. Otago med. School **34**, 12 (1956).
WAALKES, T. PH., and H. COBURN: Comparative effects of glycogen and antigen-antibody reactions on serotonin and histamine in the rabbit. Proc. Soc. exp. Biol. (N.Y.) **101**, 123—125 (1959a).
— — The role of platelets and the release of serotonin and histamine during anaphylaxis in the rabbit. J. Allergy **30**, 394—407 (1959b).
— — The role of histamine and serotonin during anaphylaxis in the mouse. J. Allergy **31**, 151—161 (1960a).
— — Serotonin, histamine, and the Arthus phenomenon. J. Allergy **31**, 181—184 (1960b).
— H. WEISSBACH, J. BOZICEVICH and S. UDENFRIEND: Release of serotonin and histamine from rabbit platelets during anaphylaxis. J. Pharmacol. exp. Ther. **119**, 191 (1957a).
— — — — Further studies on the release of serotonin and histamine during anaphylaxis in the rabbit. Proc. Soc. exp. Biol. (N.Y.) **95**, 479—482 (1957b).
WALAAS, E., and O. WALAAS: Oxidation of reduced diphosphopyridine nucleotide (DPNH) by adrenaline, noradrenaline and serotonin in the presence of ceruloplasmin. V. Int. Congr. Biochem., Moscow 1961a, Abstr. Comm., p. 102.
— — Oxidation of reduced phosphopyridine nucleotides by p-phenylenediamines, catecholamines and serotonin in the presence of ceruloplasmin. Arch. Biochem. **95**, 151—162 (1961b).
WALASZEK, E. J., and H. BURFORD: Modification of the vasopressor effect of tryptamine and tyramine by reserpine. Arch. int. Pharmacodyn. **143**, 543—549 (1963).
WALAWSKI, J.: The role of serotonin in the tonus regulation of the vegetative nervous system. XXI. Int. Congr. Physiol. Sciences, Buenos Aires 1959, Abstr. Comm., p. 292.
WANG, R. I. H., and J. BALLANTYNE: Chemical protection against repetitive supralethal doses of X-irradiation in mice. Fed. Proc. **21**, 421 (1962).
—, and D. E. DAVIDSON jr.: Reduction of radiation lethality in dogs by chemical mixture. US Army Med. Res. Lab. Rep. **484**, 1—17 (1961).
—, and J. G. KEREIAKES: Increased survival from radiation by mixtures of radioprotective compounds. Acta radiol. (Stockh.) **58**, 99—104 (1962).
— — R. R. ANDERSON and R. A. POTTS: Organ weight changes in chemically protected and non-protected x-irradiated rats. US Army Med. Res. Lab. Rep. **449**, 1—9 (1961).
WARNER, R. R. P.: Serotonin and gastrointestinal tract function. J. Mt. Sinai Hosp. **26**, 45—63 (1959).
WEIDMANN, H., u. A. CERLETTI: Differenzierung der reflektorischen Atmungs- und Kreislaufwirkungen von Serotonin und Veratridin. Helv. physiol. pharmacol. Acta **13**, C 38—C 40 (1955).
— — Untersuchungen über die pressorische Wirkung des 5-Hydroxytryptamins (Serotonin). Arch. int. Pharmacodyn. **111**, 98—107 (1957).
— — Zur pharmakodynamischen Differenzierung der 4-Oxyindolderivate Psilocybin und Psilocin im Vergleich mit 5-Oxyindolkörpern (Serotonin, Bufotenin). Helv. physiol. pharmacol. Acta **17**, C 46—48 (1959).
— — Studies on psilocybin and related compounds. I. Structure/activity relationship of oxyindole-derivatives with regard to their effect on the knee jerk of spinal cats. Helv. physiol. pharmacol. Acta **18**, 174—182 (1960).
— — Vasoconstrictor effects of 5-hydroxytryptamine and related substances. Biochem. Pharmacol. **8**, 165 (1961).
— M. TAESCHLER u. H. KONZETT: Zur Pharmakologie von Psilocybin, einem Wirkstoff aus *Psilocybe mexicana* Heim. Experientia (Basel) **14**, 378—379 (1958).
WEINER, M., and S. UDENFRIEND: Relationship of platelet serotonin to disturbances of clotting and hemostasis. Circulation **15**, 353—357 (1957).

WEISSBACH, H., T. PH. WAALKES and S. UDENFRIEND: Presence of serotonin in lung and its implication in the anaphylactic reaction. Science **125**, 235—236 (1957).
WEITZEL, G., U. ROESTER, E. BUDDECKE u. F.-J. STRECKER: Zinkgehalt und blutzuckersteigernde Wirkung von Organextrakten. Hoppe-Seylers Z. physiol. Chem. **303**, 161—175 (1956).
WELSH, J. H.: Excitation of the heart of *Venus mercenaria*. Naunyn-Schmiedeberg's Arch. exp. Path. Pharmak. **219**, 23—29 (1953).
— Hydroxytryptamine: a neurohormone in the invertebrates. Fed. Proc. **13**, 162—163 (1954a).
— Marine invertebrate preparation useful in the bioassay of acetylcholine and 5-hydroxytryptamine. Nature (Lond.) **173**, 955—956 (1954b).
— Neurohormones of invertebrates. I. Cardio-regulators of *Cyprina* and *Buccinum*. J. mar. biol. Ass. U.K. **35**, 193—201 (1956).
— Serotonin as a possible neurohumoral agent: evidence obtained in lower animals. Ann. N.Y. Acad. Sci. **66** (3), 618—630 (1957).
WEST, G. B.: Oedema and 5-hydroxytryptamine in the rat. In: G. P. LEWIS: 5-Hydroxytryptamine, p. 168—171. London: Pergamon Press 1957.
— Glucocorticoids and tissue amines. XXI. Congr. Physiol. Sciences, Buenos Aires 1959, Abstr. Comm., p. 295.
WESTERMANN, E.: Über die Wirkung vom 5-Hydroxytryptamin (Serotonin) auf die Atmung. Naunyn-Schmiedeberg's Arch. exp. Path. Pharmak. **233**, 518—530 (1958).
WHITE, H. L.: Renal function. Trans. 2nd Conference, p. 127. New York: Josiah Macy & Co. 1951.
WHITE, T. T., R. A. MCALEXANDER and D. F. MAGEE: Effects of serotonin precursors on gastric secretion in the dog. Surg. Gynec. Obstet. **109**, 168—172 (1959).
—, and D. F. MAGEE: The influence of serotonin on gastric mucin production. Gastroenterology **35**, 289—291 (1958).
WIEGERSHAUSEN, B.: Zur Pharmakologie von Staphylokokkentoxin. Wiss. Z. Humbold-Univ. Berlin, math.-nat. R. **10**, 589—640 (1961).
WILHELM, D. L., and B. MASON: Vascular permeability changes in inflammation: the role of endogenous permeability factors in mild thermal injury. Brit. J. exp. Path. **41**, 487—506 (1960).
WILLIAMS, B. B., and S. T. COKER: Role of serotonin in the thyroid action of reserpine. J. pharm. Sci. **52**, 568—571 (1963).
WILSON, C. W. M.: Discussion. In G. P. LEWIS: 5-Hydroxytryptamine, p. 191—192. London: Pergamon Press 1957.
WITTE, S., K. T. SCHRICKER u. E. SCHMID: Mikroskopische Befunde über die Blutstillung bei Serotoninausschaltung. Thrombos. Diathes. haemorrh. (Stuttg.) **5**, 505—518 (1961).
WOOLLEY, D. W.: Probable evolutionary relationship of serotonin and indoleacetic acid, and some practical consequences therefrom. Nature (Lond.) **180**, 630—633 (1957).
— Highly potent antimetabolites of serotonin with little serotoninlike action. Biochem. Pharmacol. **1**, 51—59 (1959).
—, and N. K. CAMBPELL: Serotonin receptors. II. Calcium transport by crude and purified receptor. Biochim. biophys. Acta (Amst.) **40**, 543—544 (1960).
— — Serotonin-like and antiserotonin properties of psilocybin and psilocin. Science **136**, 777—779 (1962).
—, and E. SHAW: Differentiation between receptors for serotonin and tryptamine by means of the exquisite specificity of antimetabolites. J. Pharmacol. exp. Ther. **121**, 13—17 (1957).
— — J. R. VANE, H. O. J. COLLIER, S. J. CORNE, E. MARLEY and P. B. BRADLEY: Tryptamine and serotonin receptors. Nature (Lond.) **194**, 486—487 (1962).
—, and B. W. GOMMI: Transport of calcium into muscles in response to serotonin and other hormones. Biochim. biophys. Acta (Amst.) **74**, 781—782 (1963).
WURTMAN, R. J., J. AXELROD and E. W. CHU: Melatonin, a pineal substance: effect on the ovary. Science **141**, 277—278 (1963).
— — and L. T. POTTER: The uptake of H^3-melatonin in endocrine and nervous tissue and the effects of constant light exposure. J. Pharmacol. exp. Ther. **143**, 314—318 (1964).
YEH, S. D. J., J. D. SOLOMON and B. F. CHOW: Influence of vitamin B_6 on tissue serotonin levels in rats. Fed. Proc. **18**, 357 (1959).
YOSHIKO, K.: Synthesis and properties of serotonin-O-sulfate. J. Biochem. **49**, 436—440 (1961).
YOUNG jr., R. C., H. NAGANO, T. R. VAUGHAN and N. C. STAUB: Effect of serotonin (5-HT) on pulmonary capillary blood volume (Vc) in dogs. Fed. Proc. **21**, 442 (1962).
— — — — Pulmonary capillary blood volume in dogs: effects of 5-hydroxytryptamine. J. appl. Physiol. **18**, 264—268 (1963).

ZAMBONI, P.: The capillary resistance in rats treated with reserpine. Arch. int. Pharmacodyn. **113**, 203—208 (1957).
— G. BERTACCINI e M. B. NOBILI: Ulteriori ricerche sulla interferenza dell'enteramina (5-HT) del sangue nel controllo della resistenza capillare del ratto. Arch. ital. Sci. farmacol. **9**, 389—393 (1959).
—, e G. C. CARLEVARO: Sostanze regolatrici degli autoritmi vasali. Boll. Soc. ital. Biol. sper. **30**, 1011—1013 (1954).
ZETLER, G., u. L. SCHLOSSER: Über das Vorkommen von 5-Hydroxytryptamin (Enteramin oder Serotonin) im Gehirn von Säugetieren. Naunyn-Schmiedeberg's Arch. exp. Path. Pharmak. **222**, 345—351 (1954).
ZHEREBCHENKO, O. G., I. G. KRASNYKH, E. I. KUZNETS, N. N. SUVOROV, V. S. SHASHKOV and S. P. YARMOTENKO: Protective effect of combinations of amines against radiation. Fed. Proc. **22**, T 836—839 (1963).
ZIEMLANSKI, S.: Effect of serotonin on post-histamine gastric juice secretion. Acta physiol. pol. **10**, 59—65 (1959).
ZILBERSTEIN, R. M.: Effects of reserpine, serotonin and vasopressin on the survival of cold-stressed rats. Nature (Lond.) **185**, 249 (1960).
— Reserpine- and serotonin-estrogen interactions on the uterus of the rat. Life Sci. No 7, 281—283 (1962).
ZIZINE, L.: Action de la sérotonine sur l'activité thyroidienne du rat. C. R. Soc. Biol. (Paris) **153**, 1156—1158 (1959).
ZSIGMOND, E. K., F. F. FÖLDES and W. M. FÖLDES: The inhibitory effect of psilocybin and related compounds on human cholinesterase. Fed. Proc. **20**, 393 (1961 a).
— — — The *in vitro* inhibitory effect of LSD, its congeners and 5-hydroxytryptamine on human cholinesterases. J. Neurochem. **8**, 72—80 (1961 b).
ZUCKER, F. T., u. G. N. STEWART: Beobachtungen über vasokonstriktorische Wirkungen des Blutes. Zbl. Physiol. **27**, 85—87 (1912).
ZUCKER, M. B.: Serotonin (5-hydroxytryptamine): hematologic aspects. Progr. Hemat. **2**, 206—224 (1959).
ZWEIFACH, B. W., and D. B. METZ: Relation of blood-borne agents acting on mesenteric vascular bed to general circulatory reactions. J. clin. Invest. **34**, 653—672 (1955).

The survey of the literature was concluded in March-April 1964.

Chapter 9

Pharmacological actions of indolealkylamines and precursor aminoacids on the central nervous system*

By

PAOLO MANTEGAZZINI †

With 2 Figures

A. Effects on behaviour

I. 5-Hydroxytryptamine

1. Mouse

Simple behavioural observation showed that 5-HT had sedative or depressive effects on mice. The doses used were the following: 20 mg/kg i.p. (SHORE et al. 1955), 1—20 mg/kg i.v. (CHESSIN et al. 1956, 1957), 86—172 mg/kg i.p. (ASTON and CULLUMBINE 1960).

Behavioural examination with quantitative methods yielded results in agreement with those furnished by direct observation. BROWN (1957) and KOBINGER (1958a) investigated the effects of amine on the motility. BROWN observed reduction in the spontaneous motor activity of grouped mice with 5—320 mg/kg i.p. and KOBINGER obtained the same result in grouped or single mice with 4.55 mg/kg i.p. KOBINGER also reported that 5-HT (4.55 mg/kg) injected intraperitoneally together with D-methylamphetamine (3.3 mg/kg) or with cocaine (20 mg/kg) prevented the hyperactivity induced by these two drugs.

YEN et al. (1959) tried out the effect of the amine on the aggressivity. It is well known that prolonged isolation induces in the male mouse aggressive behaviour towards another mouse of the same sex temporarily placed in the same cage. Mice, after three weeks' isolation, were injected with 5-HT (50 mg/kg i.p.) and caged for five minutes with a mouse not previously isolated. Whereas before the injection all the mice attacked their cage-mates, after the injection only 10% of the animals maintained aggressive attitudes. The same results were obtained by prolonging the treatment with 5-HT for 14 days (50 mg/kg/day i.p.). MANTEGAZZINI and PEGRASSI (unpublished observations) observed extinction of the aggressive behaviour after intraperitoneal injection of 5 mg/kg of 5-HT. The body temperature of the injected animals was 3—4 °C lower than that of control animals.

---

* The coverage in this chapter extends, with a few later additions, to june 1963, when the manuscript was completed.

The doses of 5-HT are expressed in term of base, except when otherwise indicated.

The author wishes to thank dr. CAMILLO BIANCHI for offering many valuable suggestions during the preparation of this review and for translating it.

Haley (1957a, b) injected 5-HT into the cerebral ventricles, with the aim of by-passing the blood-brain barrier. After injection of 0.4 and 1.2 μg of 5-HT (volume of the injection = 0.05 ml), the author observed together with autonomic symptoms (micturition, defaecation and bristling) central depression, stupor and bouts of scratching. Normal activity resumed in 15—60 minutes.

According to the author, no motor disturbance appeared after 5-HT and control injection of saline had no effect. The size of the brain made it difficult to direct the tip of the needle without the aid of a stereotaxic instrument, and the mechanical trauma of the injection could have greatly interferred with the effects of the drug.

2. Rat

In rats, as in mice, 5-HT induces symptoms considered as expression of sedation (reduction of motor activity and aggressivity) and moreover blocks the conditioned-reflexes and self-stimulation behaviour.

Depression of spontaneous motor activity and sedation (or prostration) have been observed by Erspamer since 1952 and subsequently by Cook and Weidley (1957) (0.5—40 mg/kg s.c.), by Hoffman (1958b) (5 mg/kg s.c.) and by Kärki and Paasonen (1959) (4.3 mg/kg i.v.).

Brunaud and Siou (1959) reported that 5-HT reduced aggressivity in rats. In these experiments two male rats caged together were electrically stimulated at regular intervals through the floor. The painful stimulation evoked the fighting behaviour. 5-HT at a dose of 20 mg/kg blocked it. Lower doses were inactive. 5 mg/kg of chlorpromazine had the same effect as 20 mg/kg of 5-HT.

Winter and Flataker (1956) administered 5-HT to rats trained to climb a vertical rope under the double incentive of food at the top and noxious stimuli at the bottom. 5-HT (0.9 mg/kg i.p.) did not reduce the animal performance; LSD-25 (0.5 mg/kg i.p.) markedly prolonged climbing time; 5-HT (0.9 mg/kg i.p.) injected 30 minutes before LSD-25 strongly antagonised the effect of the latter.

The action of 5-HT on the conditioned avoidance responses was examined by Cook and Weidley (1957), by Grandjean and Bättig (1957), by Pletscher et al. (1959) and by Gessner et al. (1961). Cook and Weidley reported that 5-HT (0.5—40 mg/kg s.c.) blocked the pole-climbing responses to a conditioned stimulus (a buzzer). 0.5 and 2 mg/kg knocked out the conditioning in 10% of the animals. The maximum effect observed (after 10 mg/kg or more) was a block of responses in 50% of the animals only and occurred 1 and 2 hours after treatement. The deconditioning was accompained by falling off in spontaneous motor activity; the unconditioned responses were unaffected. The effects of the 5-HT were antagonized by 0.5 mg/kg of LSD-25. The well-known blocking actions of chlorpromazine and reserpine were also antagonized by the LSD-25; a fact supporting the idea that the LSD-25—5-HT antagonism is not specific. Grandjean and Bätting (1957) reported that 5-HT (0.5—5 mg/kg i.p.) prolonged the reaction time and partly abolished the conditioned avoidance responses. The deconditioning effect increased linearly with the logarithm of the dose; 0.25 mg/kg were ineffective. According to the authors, neither hypothermia nor gross behavioural changes occurred after deconditioning doses. Pletscher et al. (1959) obtained a 25% block of conditioned pole climbing responses with 4 mg/kg i.p. of 5-HT (unconditioned responses were unaffected). Adrenaline, noradrenaline and dopamine had qualitatively the same effect as 5-HT. Gessner et al. (1961) observed a partial block of the conditioned responses together with paresis of the hind legs in rats injected with 17.6 mg/kg of 5-HT. The research workers did not report if the unconditioned responses were blocked or not when the neurological disturbances appeared.

The above results allow us to think that 5-HT blocks the conditioned avoidance responses and that the block is specific, i.e. it does not involve the unconditioned responses. This means that the deconditioning does not depend on an obstacle in the execution of the motor task.

The intracerebral injection route was used by OLDS and OLDS (1958). Electrodes and pipette were chronically implanted to stimulate the ventral posterior hypothalamus just in front of the mamillary body. The rats were at first trained to self stimulate by pressing a lever. When the animals had attained high rates of self stimulation, the electrical stimulus was replaced by a chemical one (self injection through the pipette of 0.6 μg of 5-HT base in 1/700 ml). The rate of self-injection quickly fell off and the animals lost muscular tone and apparently went to sleep. According to the authors, 5-HT had no rewarding effect. Acetylcholine behaved like the 5-HT; noradrenaline and saline did not show any effect.

Rats with electrodes implanted in the posterior hypothalamus and midbrain tegmentum were trained by STEIN (1960) to regulate the intensity of self-stimulation (reward threshold). 5-HT (4 mg/kg s.c.) increased the reward threshold or knocked out self stimulation behaviour. Chlorpromazine (1.5 mg/kg s.c.) had the same effect as 5-HT.

From the above data, it is clear that 5-HT, peripherally administered, produces marked behavioural changes in the mouse and in the rat: reduction of spontaneous motility and hostility and extinction of the conditioned reflexes and self-stimulation behaviour. The problem is now to find out if the behavioural effects depend on the direct action of 5-HT on the CNS or if they depend on the multiple effects of the amine on the extracerebral regions wich, in turn, act on the CNS.

Let us consider the facts:

I. In the unanaesthetised rat 5-HT (0.4 mg/kg or more s.c.) induces hypotension and marked cutaneous vasodilatation (ERSPAMER 1952; CORREALE 1954). After 2 mg/kg (the highest dose tried) the blood pressure falls to 60—70 mm Hg, recovery occurring only after 120—160 minutes. In the anaesthetised rat, the amine intravenously injected, induces, even at the dose of 0.8 μg/kg, marked hypotension lasting 3—4 minutes (SALMOIRAGHI et al. 1956a). The extent of hypotension induced by the amine in quantities as high as those generally used in behavioural studies is unknown, but it will probably be much higher than that induced by the relatively small doses quoted above, and therefore such as to interfere greatly with animal behaviour.

II. In rats and mice 5-HT induces marked hypothermia at doses within the range of those active on behaviour. It has been reported (LESSIN and PARKES 1957) that chlorpromazine and reserpine, two drugs which definitely act on the CNS, do not induce sedation in the mouse if the fall in body temperature is prevented by keeping the animals at a room temperature of 31° C. This means that the hypothermia largely contributes to produce sedation after chlorpromazine and reserpine. We may justly suspect that in the case of 5-HT hypothermia also plays an important part in inducing sedation, at least in the mouse.

To sum up: 5-HT peripherally administered markedly affects the behaviour; it is strongly to be suspected that the peripheral effects elicited by 5-HT are the determining factors in the behavioural responses to the drug. This suspicion is strengthened by the fact that up to now there is no evidence to show that 5-HT can cross the blood-brain barrier.

3. Rabbit

Reduction of spontaneous motility and of reactivity to acoustic and painful stimuli, together with a tendency to maintain forced positions were observed by BARUCCI (1956) in rabbits intravenously injected with 1 mg/kg of 5-HT. Recovery occurred within 20 to 40 minutes. Substantially the same symptoms, but preceded by transitory restlessness immediately after injection, were also observed by GANGLIOFF and MONNIER (1957) after i.v. injection of 0.1—1 mg/kg of amine.

The observations reported above would lead us to think that 5-HT has a sedative or depressive action on the rabbit, but it is wise to wait for quantitative results before accepting the conclusions drawn from visual observations.

4. Cat

The greater part of the observations reported in the literature refer to the injection of 5-HT into the lateral ventricle. This route has been proposed in order to bypass the blood-brain barrier and to avoid the peripheral effects of the amine. The injection was made through a permanently implanted canula and the animal was allowed freedom of movement during the observation period.

FELDBERG and SHERWOOD (1954) first described the pattern of behavioural effects of 5-HT intraventricularly injected. After 75—500 μg the cat lay down not asleep but with its eyes wide open and when compelled to walk, it did so unsteadily, as if it had muscular weakness. Tachypnea, bursts of profuse salivation, licking movements, tremors of the head and neck muscles and twitching of the eyelids appeared after large doses. These effects began to appear within ten minutes and lasted up to 1 hour and a half. A dose of 10 μg was ineffective.

FELDBERG and SHERWOOD's observations were confirmed by GADDUM and VOGT (1956), by SCHWARZ et al. (1956), by BRADLEY and HANCE (1956) and by SCHAIN (1961). GADDUM and VOGT moreover reported that LSD-25 (0.8 mg) and ergometrine (1.5 mg), injected into the lateral ventricle at the same time with of after 5-HT, delayed the appearance or interrupted the lethargy induced by the amine. LSD-25 and ergometrine, at the doses used, produced sham rage. Morphine (1 mg into the ventricle) methadone (10 mg s.c.) and amphetamine (15 mg s.c.) shared the antagonistic action of LSD-25 and ergometrine in spite of the fact that they have no anti-5-HT action on the peripheral organs. Bromo LSD (1 mg into the ventricle) and 5-benzyloxygramine (2.1 mg into the ventricle) did not prevent the appearance of the usual 5-HT effects although they had an anti-5-HT action on the peripheral organs. These results suggested that there was no relation between the antagonism observed on the behaviour and that observed on the peripheral organs.

No antagonism between 5-HT and LSD-25 intraventricularly injected was observed by SCHWARZ et al. (1956) with doses of LSD-25 (15 μg) much lower than those tried by GADDUM and VOGT. BRADLEY (1958) briefly reported that 5-HT had the same behavioural effects when it was injected in the ventricle as when it was injected peripherally.

DOMER and FELDBERG (1960a and b) examined the tremor produced by the intraventricular injection of 5-HT. The tremor started 1—2 minutes after injection of 110—215 μg of amine and lasted from 20 minutes to 2 hours. It appeared first in the ears, then in the hind legs and finally spread all over the body. Also in this set of experiments the animals were less alert after 5-HT injection than before. They sat or lay down in their cages.

In complete contrast with the results given till now are those reported by JOHN et al. (1958). These authors administered 5-HT intraventricularly to cats trained to avoid shock on the presentation of either an auditory or visual stimulus (conditioned avoidance response). Neither lethargy nor attenuation of the conditioned responses occurred after doses of amine as high as 270 μg even when iproniazid (135 μg) was simultaneously injected to block the amine metabolism. The authors reported that KILLAM and JOHN (unpublished data) had previously observed changes in drug action after avoidance conditioning. According to the authors this could account for the ineffectiveness of 5-HT in inducing lethargy and apathy in their experiments.

Administration into the ventricle has the double advantage of avoiding the blood-brain barrier and reducing the interference of the amine's peripheral effects on the central effects. It must however be remembered that as yet there is no direct evidence as to whether 5-HT can get into the brain tissue from the ventricles. Also admitting that 5-HT penetrates the brain, it remains to be seen to what extent the drug's action on the blood vessels in the region near the ventricle walls interferes with the direct action on the neurons. In our opinion the results obtained after intraventricular injection of 5-HT do not clarify the physiological meaning of the amine normally present in the CNS more than those obtained after peripheral administration.

5. Dog

Intravenous injection (0.6—2.5 mg/kg) (SACCHI et al. 1955b; BONAMINI and GARELLO 1956) or intravenous infusion of 5-HT (1.7 μg/kg/min, for three hours) (CRONHEIM and GOURZIS 1960) had no gross effects on the behaviour of the dog. On the other hand, in dogs treated with reserpine, intravenous administration of 5-HT changed the slight sedation into a very marked comatose state and at the same time caused a fall in blood pressure to about 40 mm Hg (CRONHEIM and GOURZIS 1960). Such a fall in blood pressure might well account for the deep sedation and the coma!

According to FLORU et al. (1959), salivary conditioned reflexes and conditioned behaviour were inhibited by 5-HT (0.5—2.5 mg/kg i.v.). The authors did not report data which clarify the part played on the genesis of the deconditioning by the peripheral effects of 5-HT.

SACCHI et al. (1955b) and BONAMINI and GARELLO (1956) reported that 5-HT directly injected into the Cisterna Magna produced marked behavioural and neurological changes; on the contrary it had no effect when intravenously injected. Catatonia occurred 10—15 minutes (rarely more) after the injection of 80—120 μg/kg. The symptomatology gradually increased until complete block of the motility; muscular tone was reduced and responsiveness to visual, acoustic and olfactory stimuli was abolished. Slight salivation and micturition were the only apparent vegetative symptoms. Adrenaline (0.1—2.5 mg) did not produce catatonia; a fact which led the authors to claim that vasoconstrinction was not responsible for catatonia. LSD-25 and methedrine prevented or abolished the 5-HT catatonia (SACCHI et al. 1955a).

With the aim of localising the regions responsible for catatonia, SACCHI et al. (1956) injected the amine through an outside loop of a canula permanently implanted along the Aqueduct of Sylvius in such a way that one tip was in III. ventricle and the other one in the Cisterna magna; 5-HT was administered into III. ventricle or into Cisterna magna, the passage of the drug from one place to the other being prevented by clamping the loop of the canula during the injection. The injection into the III. ventricle produced catatonia, whereas injection into the Cisterna magna had no effect whatsoever. This led to the claim that the structures responsible for the 5-HT catatonia were located near the walls of III. ventricle or lateral ventricles. No more can be said about the position of these structures nor about the mechanism of 5-HT action. What has been said about this technique when applied in the cat is valid also in the dog.

6. Pigeon

Aprison and Ferster (1961c) trained hungry pigeons to get food after pecking a disk for a fixed number of times or for a fixed period of time depending from the color of the disk. 5-HT (1.75 and 4.3 mg/kg i.m.) lowered the rate of pecking. It must be pointed out that the highest dose was sometimes lethal and that a dose of 0.86 mg/kg did not significantly interfere with the animal's performance.

7. Fish

5-HT (40—200 mg/kg i.m.) markedly reduced the motility of the *Carassius auratus*. The fish assumed abnormal positions: it stayed with its head up or down or it lay on one side, but resumed the normal behaviour after strong stimulation. The mortality was high (about 25%) (Sacchi and Gianniotti 1956a). LSD-25 prevented the effect of 5-HT (Sacchi and Gianniotti 1956b). In *Betta splendens* in a stress situation (hypoxia), 5-HT (13 mg/l) increased the motor activity (Trout 1957).

8. Frog

High doses of 5-HT injected into the linphatic sack (54—182 mg/kg) or the peritoneal cavity (54—108 mg/kg) or intramuscularly (43—108 mg/kg) did not impair the motor functions of *Rana esculenta*. The animal lost muscular tone when the amine (43 mg/kg) was put in direct contact with the brain through a breach in the frontal bones (Dolce and Garello 1956).

II. 5-Hydroxytryptophan

After the demonstration that the cerebral 5-HT increases following injection of its precursor, 5-hydroxytryptophan (5-HTP) (Udenfriend et al. 1956, 1957a), the latter has been used as a tool for investigating the physiological significance of cerebral 5-HT, in the hope that the effects of an excess of 5-HT might throw some light on the functions of the amine normally present in the brain.

1. Mouse and rat

Bogdanski et al. (1956, 1958) did not observe any marked behavioural change in animals intraperitoneally injected with doses of 5-HTP as high as 120 mg/kg (mice) and 300 mg/kg (rats). In rats, three hours after an intraperitoneal injection of 75 and 150 mg/kg of 5-HTP, the brain 5-HT level increased about 2 and 6 times respectively (Udenfriend et al. 1957a). Pretreatment with iproniazid increased the sensivity of the animals to the 5-HTP: 30—60 mg/kg i.p. in mice and 50—100 mg/kg in rats (i.e. doses inactive in normal animals) produced excitement, trembling, increase in motor activity, brief clonic convulsions, peripheral vaso-dilatation and mydriasis. The increased sensitivity was associated with an increased brain 5-HT level. According to the authors the 5-HTP grossly resembled LSD-25 in its effects. Chessin et al. (1957) confirmed 5-HTP (25 mg/kg i.v.) produced stimulation in mice pretreated with iproniazid; that in absence of iproniazid the amino acid produced slight sedation only, even at a very large dose (200 mg/kg i.v.). The neurological pattern after 5-HTP plus iproniazid was characterised by muscle tremors, preconvulsive twitches and loss of placing reactions; nor motor hyperactivity of a purposeful nature occurred. TEDESCHI et al. (1959a) observed hypotonia, decrease of motor activity and peripheral vaso-dilatation in rats after 100—400 mg/kg of 5-HTP i.v. Lower doses produced no overt effect.

HESS and DOEPFNER (1961) reported that 5-HTP (8 and 16 mg/kg i.p.) provoked headshake and aimless hypermotility in rats pretreated with JB 516 (5 mg/kg i.p.) (a MAO inhibitor). The amino acid alone (160 and 320 mg/kg i.p.) did not provoke any behavioural change in normal rats, in spite of the fact that in these animals it (320 mg/kg) increased the cerebral 5-HT more than it did at lower doses (8 and 16 mg/kg) in JB 516 pretreated rats. Furthermore the rats treated with JB 516 alone (5 mg/kg) showed a normal behaviour but had cerebral 5-HT level as high as that of rats treated with JB 516 + 5-HTP. From such a result it seems that the cerebral 5-HT increase is not the determining factor of the behavioural changes induced in rats by 5-HTP plus MAO inhibitors.

BROWN (1960) studied the effect of 5-HTP on the motility of grouped mice (photocell counter technique): doses between 0.1 and 100 mg/kg i.p. reduced spontaneous motility; 20 mg/kg i.p. prevented hyperactivity induced by cocaine and amphetamine.

PLETSCHER et al. (1959) and STEINER et al. (1959) briefly reported that 5-HTP (100 mg/kg i.p.) partially blocked the conditioned avoidance responses (pole climbing response) in rats.

ERSPAMER et al. (1960a) reported that 5-HTP reduced the aggressiveness induced in the male mouse by prolonged isolation: 100 mg/kg i.p. abolished the aggressive behaviour in 50% of the couples of males caged together following an isolation period.

WINTER and FLATAKER (1956) and MAHLER and HUMOLLER (1959) injected with 2 and 5 mg/kg and 100 mg/kg of 5-HTP respectively, rats trained to climb a vertical rope to reach food at the top. The animal performance was unaffected. Rats trained to cross a maze were given 100 mg/kg of 5-HTP intraperitoneally. After dosing, the animals made mistakes and took longer to reach the goal box (MANTEGAZZINI and PEGRASSI, unpublished data).

To sum up: 5-HTP, even at very high doses (200 mg/kg i.v. in mice and 400 mg/kg i.v. in rats) induces sedation, reduces motility and aggressiveness (in mice) and blocks the conditioned reflexes and worsens the performance of animals trained to cross a maze (in rats). After pretreatment with MAO inhibitors, 5-HTP, at much lower doses, produces excitement, motor hyperactivity, muscular trembling and preconvulsive twitches. It is doubtful if the differences in the 5-HTP behavioural effects in normal and in the MAO inhibitors pretreated rats may be ascribed to differences in the 5-HT cerebral level.

2. Rabbit

BOGDANSKI et al. (1956, 1958) observed motor excitement, muscular tremors, twitches and, occasionally, brief clonic convulsions together with symptoms of sympathetic stimulation after intravenous injection of doses of 5-HTP ranging from 40 to 100 mg/kg i.v. COSTA and RINALDI (1958) observed alertness, muscular tremors, chewing movements, uncoordinated movements of the legs, bristling, panting and unresponsiveness to auditory and tactile stimuli in rabbits intravenously injected with 75 mg/kg of 5-HTP. The effects appeared about 30 minutes after the injection and lasted about two hours. After such a dose of 5-HTP, the 5-HT concentration increased in the telencephalon, in the hippocampus, in the medulla-pons and in the midbrain and returned to normal within three hours in all structures but the mid-brain where the increase lasted longer than the behavioural effects. Chlorpromazine premedication prevented the behavioural effects of the 5-HTP but facilitated the increase of 5-HT concentration in brain tissue. MONNIER and TISSOT (1958) and MONNIER (1960) observed slight sedation in the rabbit after intravenous injection of 10—20 mg/kg of 5-HTP, and muscular tremors, motor excitement, mydriasis and transitory tachypnea after 30 mg/kg or more.

To sum up: in the rabbit 5-HTP produces different effects according to the dose. Low doses produce only slight sedation, high doses (generally more than 30 mg/kg i.v.) produce motor excitement, muscular trembling and twitches, uncoordinated movements of the limbs, chewing movements and some time brief clonic convulsions. Mydriasis, bristling and panting are the overt vegetative symptoms induced by high doses.

3. Cat

BOGDANSKI et al. (1956, 1958) first described the neurological and behavioural effects of 5-HTP in the cat. The neurological effects consisted in ataxia and other abnormalities in walking (for doses higher than 50 mg/kg i.v.) and in generalised tremors, extensory twitches, abolition of the patellar reflex and rigidity (for doses higher than 100 mg/kg i.v.). The behavioural effects consisted in sedation (for doses lower than 100 mg/kg i.v.) and in excitement, sham rage reaction, reduced responsiveness to painful stimuli and unresponsiveness to visual and auditory stimuli (for doses higher than 120 mg/kg i.v.). The vegetative symptoms were myosis that at the highest doses turned into mydriasis, nasal, lacrimal and salivary secretions, diarrhea and dispnea. Two hours after injection of 120 mg/kg i.v. the amine content increased two-threefold in the hypothalamus, in the midbrain, in the medulla, in the pons, in the thalamus and in the white matter (corpus callosum and internal capsule) and 4—6 times in the cerebellum, in the cortical grey matter and in the caudate nucleus. LEWIS (1958) reported that normal or iproniazidized cats injected with 30 mg/kg of 5-HTP showed no sign of excitement but lay slightly drowsy.

To produce an unilateral increase of the brain 5-HT level, ANTONELLI, BERTACCINI and MANTEGAZZINI (unpublished results) infused 5-HTP (20 mg in 20 min) into one of the carotid arteries of conscious cats through a canula tied in the lingual artery. No behavioural change nor neurological asymmetry occurred after the infusion, the only effects being a marked myosis on the infused side, salivation and some times vomiting. Two cats were killed ten minutes after dosing: the amine concentration of the caudate nucleus of the infused side was twofold that of the caudate nucleus of the opposite side and of the caudate nucleus of untreated animals.

From the above data it is clear that, in the cat, low doses of 5-HTP, which induce marked increases in the brain amine content and marked peripheral effects, do not affect the behaviour, or, at the most, produce a slight drowsiness; on the other hand, high doses produce excitement and sham rage.

4. Dog

BOGDANSKI et al. (1958) observed ataxia and other abnormalities in walking after 20 mg/kg or more of 5-HTP i.v. and trembling, extensory twitches, plastic rigidity, abolition of the patellar reflex and of the responsiveness to painful stimuli after 40 mg/kg or more. Doses between 40 and 60 mg/kg i.v. were often lethal. The animals seemed to be drowsy after 5—30 mg/kg and excited after 40—60 mg/kg i.v. During the excitement phase, the animals walked hesitatingly and although they had the eyes open, they did not avoid obstacles as blind. They did not show aggressive attitude, on the contrary they seemed to be terrified. Even after the lowest dose there was mydriasis that was not reduced by light. Other vegetative effects were dyspnea, increased nasal, salivary and lacrimal secretions and intestinal hyper-motility. Two hours after the injection of 60 mg/kg i.v. of 5-HTP the content of 5-HT increased about 4 times in the medulla, 7 to 10 times in the cortical grey matter, in the thalamus, in the hypothalamus, in the mid-brain, in the cerebellum and in the pons, and 15 times in the caudate nucleus. Cronheim and Gourzis (1960) injected dogs with 30 mg/kg i.v. of 5-HTP. During the first 15—30 minutes after injection, the animals appeared to be subdued; during the next two hours they still lay quietly without showing any interest in their surroundings, but reacted hostilely to the approach of persons or objects. There were no signs of blindness or of motor incoordination, but there was marked salivation and mydriasis and pupillary light reflex was depressed. Later on the animals frequently assumed a peculiar posture, hunching on their hindquarters, with their snouts touching the floor. Recovery took place within 4—6 hours. In dogs pretreated with reserpine (1 mg/kg i.v.) the 5-HTP (30 mg/kg i.v.) accentuated the reserpine induced sedation and transformed it into a comatose state.

Himwich and Costa (1960) injected 5-HTP into a vein or cranially into a common carotid or vertebral artery without interrupting the arterial blood flow, and compared the increase in the 5-HT content in certain brain structures with the severity of the symptomatology. The dogs were pretreated with tranylcypromine (a MAO inhibitor). 10—15 min after intravenous injection of 5-HTP (3—7 mg/kg) the animals appeared to be drowsy and showed no interest in their surroundings; after 20—30 min hypertonic extension of the legs occurred; after 40—50 min the animals showed motor hyperactivity and were more alert; there was motor incoordination accompanied by a hunched back and, then, by steppage gate. The syndrome developed gradually into a state so called as "obstinate progression": the animals walked constantly and aimlessly until they found an obstacle to push against obstinately. During this phase they were insensitive to light, sound and touch. Hostility and aggressiveness sometimes appeared before "obstinate progression". Salivation, hyperthermia and panting occurred inconstantly. Recovery started 3—4 hrs after the injection. Intrarterial injections gave the same symptomatology, but for the same dose of 5-HTP the severest symptoms occurred after intravertebral injection or after intracarotid injection in dogs with the basilar artery clipped at mid-medullary level. In the latter case the carotid blood reached all the regions placed cranially to the arterial block. These results suggested to the A.A. that the structures more involved in the 5-HTP syndrome are placed between the mid-medullary level and the area of the brain normally irrigated by carotid blood. Dogs injected with tranylcypromine and 5-HTP (5—7 mg/kg i.v.) were killed at definite stages of the syndrome. The contents of 5-HT in the pons, the extralaminar nuclei of the thalamus, the corpora quadrigemina and the hippocampus significantly increased when the dogs exhibited "ostinate progression"; the 5-HT content in the extralaminar nuclei of the thalamus, the piriform cortex and the amygdalae significantly increased when the dogs showed agressive behaviour; the 5-HT content in the caudate nucleus and the septum increased in all the stages of the syndrome so that no correlation could be made between the concentration of 5-HT in these structures and behaviour; no significant increase was observed in the frontal cortex, the mid-brain, the hypothalamus and in the medulla oblongata at any stage of the 5-HTP syndrome.

From the data given above it appears that 5-HTP gives different effects according to the dose; at low doses (between about 5 and 20 mg/kg i.v.) induces only sedation; at higher doses (above 40 mg/kg i.v.) it chiefly induces excitement and affects postural aptitude, motility and responsiveness to stimuli; at intermediate doses it induces sedation at first and excitement later. Tranylcypromine, a MAO inhibitor, increases sensitivity to 5-HTP.

5. Pigeon

APRISON and FERSTER (1960, 1961a) administered 5-HTP to pigeons trained to peck a key in order to gain access to food. Depending on the colour of the key the 50th peck (fixed ratio) or the first peck after 10 min (fixed interval) operated the food magazine. After 25, 50 and 75 mg/kg i.m. of 5-HTP the rate of pecking fell off proportionally to the dose. Lower doses had little or no effect. The treated pigeons showed tremors, head-shaking and continuous shifting from one leg to the other. Iproniazid potentiated the behavioural effects of 5-HTP (APRISON and FERSTER 1961b).

III. Bufotenine

1. Rat

MAHLER et al. (1958) and MAHLER and HUMOLLER (1959) injected bufotenine (8—27 mg/kg i.p.) into rats trained to climb a pole under the double incentive of food at the top and noxious stimuli at the bottom. After the injection, the animals seemed confused, often climbed only part way up and returned to the stimulating grid instead of making a systematic ascent to the food platform. The effect started 5—10 min after the injection and lasted 90—120 min. LSD-25 (0.3—0.7 mg/kg i.p.) produced the same effects. GESSNER et al. (1961) observed a partial block of the conditioned avoidance responses after 20.5 mg/kg of bufotenine.

2. Dog

FABING and HAWKINS (1956) reported that dogs intravenously injected with bufotenine (4 mg/kg) splayed out their hind legs, howled violently and exhibited indifference to noxious stimuli as well as to attacks from other dogs. The vegetative symptoms were salivation and piloerection.

HIMWICH and coll. (HIMWICH et al. 1959; COSTA et al. 1959; HIMWICH and COSTA 1960) injected bufotenine (1 mg/kg) into the vertebral artery, the internal carotid artery, the descending aorta or intravenously and compared the effects produced by the different routes. In some of the experiments the basilar artery was tied in order to separate the vertebral circulation from the carotid one. The carotid receptors were denerved. After the injection there was always marked muscular weakness, often unresponsiveness to visual or auditory stimulation and hypersensitivity to touch and, in the dogs most severely affected, inhability to stand up. The animals frequently responded to prodding by howling or crying and did not attempt to defend themselves. Later they howled even when they were not stimulated. A few animals responded by circling or by convulsing to the injection into the carotid artery. Salivation and mydriasis were the vegetative symptoms. The effects produced by the bufotenine appeared a few minutes after the injection and lasted up to 4 hrs. They were more pronounced after the injection into the vertebral artery than after the injection into a vein or into the descending aorta; the intracarotid route was the least effective. These results allow us to exclude the peripheral effects as the determining factor of the behavioural response to bufotenine and support the claim that the behavioural effects depend on the amine action on structures located in the regions irrigated by the vertebral artery.

3. Monkey

For about 20 min after intravenous administration of bufotenine (5 mg/kg) the monkeys *(Macaca mulatta)* maintained a prone position; afterwards they assumed a sitting posture and made attempts to move around. The movements were ataxic but within 1 hr ataxia faded out. Muscular power was unaffected by the bufotenine, while the reactions to visual and painful stimuli were abolished. The animals were unusually tame. Once ataxia had gone, the animals moved around, bumping headlong into any objects interposed in their path and showed no reactions to moving objects or lights. The bufotenine effects lasted from one and a half to two hours. Doses below 5 mg/kg produced weaker effects. LSD-25 behaved like bufotenine (EVARTS 1956).

To sum up: In the rat, bufotenine partially blocks the conditioned responses and impairs the performance of trained animals; in the dog and the monkey it reduces reactions to visual and auditory stimuli, defensive and aggressive reactions and affects motility and posture. It is proved that, in the dog, the behavioural effects are not dependent on the peripheral actions of the amine.

IV. Psilocybin

1. Mouse

10 and 50 mg/kg s.c. of psilocybin reduced spontaneous motor activity (light beam interruption method) and produced piloerection and mydriasis. Lower doses were ineffective. 50 mg/kg s.c. significantly reduced the reaction time to noxious stimulation in normal mice as well as in mice previously injected with morphine (WEIDMANN et al. 1958; CERLETTI 1959). Reduced motor activity after psilocybin was also observed by DELAY et al. (1959). The authors registered by actographic method the spontaneous motor activity and that induced by noxious stimuli both in normal mice and in mice pretreated with imino-$\beta\beta'$-dipropionitrile (IDPN) (souris tournante). In normal mice, 0.5 mg/kg of psilocybin i.p. had no effect, 5—50 mg/kg slightly reduced the spontaneous motility only, and 100 mg/kg markedly reduced spontaneous motility as well as that induced by noxious stimulation. The effect was more evident in the IDPN mice and lasted from 15 min to more than 1 hr according to the dose. LSD-25 had the same action as psilocybin on motility, but, at variance with the amine, produced bristling, salivation and tremors.

2. Rabbit

WEIDMANN et al. (1958) and CERLETTI (1959) briefly reported that psilocybin (1—3 mg/kg i.v.) produced slight sedation together with pupillary dilatation, increase in heart rate and hyperthermia. The hyperthermia appeared with doses as low as 0.02 mg/kg and increased rather slowly with the dose. Doses lower than 1 mg/kg i.v. did not modify the behaviour. Tameness or sedation, associated to slight hyper-excitability to stimuli, was also observed by MONNIER (1959) in rabbits intravenously injected with psilocybin (1.5—5 mg/kg). The vegetative effects were mydriasis, slight hypertension, long lasting hyperpnea and transitory bradycardia.

3. Monkey

In the monkey, psilocybin gives effects similar to those observed in the mouse and in the rabbit i.e. slight tranquillization after large doses (CERLETTI 1959).

4. Spider

Psilocybin (0.3—6 g/kg) given orally to *Araneus diadematus* stopped their web-building activity for 24 hrs in more than 90% of the animals (WITT 1960, CHRISTIANSEN et al. 1962). 150 mg/kg of amine given on 4 different days caused a delay in web-building. From the changes of the webstructure the AA. concluded that the treated spiders behaved as if they were heavier.

V. Tryptamine and tryptophan

In rats, intravenous tryptamine produced clonic convulsions localised in the forepaws or generalized, depending on the dose. 5 mg/kg gave convulsions in 4% and 40 mg/kg in 98% of the animals. The convulsive phase lasted, after the highest doses, 30—40 seconds. In rabbits (i.v. infusion for 5—10 min of 2—3 mg/kg/min) and in monkeys (10 mg/kg or more i.v.) tryptamine produced the same effects. Iproniazid enhanced the convulsant action of the amine (TEDESCHI et al. 1959a, 1959b). Tranylcypromine, another MAO inhibitor, behaved as iproniazid in the rat. Both inhibitors facilitated the accumulation in the brain of the amine injected i.v.; there was some relationship between brain tryptamine level and occurrence, duration and intensity of the convulsions (GREEN and SAWYER 1960).

In cats tryptamine caused convulsions, tonic extension of the limbs, hissing and snarling, piloerection, salivation and mydriasis. The animals behaved as angry or afraid. These effects lasted for about 5 min, but the animals remained subdued for some hours afterwards. Iproniazid premedication prolonged the phase of excitement (VANE et al. 1961).

HESS et al. (1959) reported that in rabbits pretreated with iproniazid, L-tryptophan (800 mg/kg i.p.) produced marked central effects, including convulsions, and marked increase in brain tryptamine level (more than 10 times the normal).

HESS and DOEPFNER (1961) described the behavioural effects of tryptophan in normal rats pretreated with iproniazid (150 mg/kg i.p.) or with nialamide (20 mg/kg) or with JB 516 (5 mg/kg i.p.), three MAO inhibitors. In normal rats and in rats pretreated with nialamide (1 or 16 hrs.) or with iproniazid (1 hr.) tryptophan (200 mg/kg i.p.) did not produce any behavioural change. In rats pretreated with JB 516 (1 or 16 hrs.) or with iproniazid (16 hrs.) the aminoacid at the same dose produced headshake and aimless, continuous motor hyperactivity. Larger doses of tryptophan (800 mg/kg i.p.) administered after iproniazid or JB 516 produced more striking behavioural effects: the rats exhibited a backward circling motion, generalized tremors and then convulsions, paralysis and death occurring within about 2 hours. In animals pretreated with MAO-inhibitors, the tryptophan (200 mg/kg i.p.) induced marked increase in brain concentrations of 5-HT and tryptamine, but there was no direct relationship between brain amine levels and behavioural changes.

According to CRONHEIM and GOURZIS (1960) i.v. infusion of L-tryptophan (0.1 mg/kg/min for 3 hrs.) in the dog did not induce any behavioural change. Tryptamine, when injected into lateral ventricles, produced in the dog (800 μg/kg) a catatonic-like state similar to that observed after injection of 5-HT into the third ventricle (EDERY and SCHATZBERG-PORATH 1960), and in the cat (200 μg) ataxia, tremor, loss of spontaneous motor activity and tachypnea, i.e. symptoms similar to those observed after 5-HT (SCHAIN 1961).

L-Tryptophan and tryptamine (as 5-HTP and 5-HT) markedly depressed motor activity of grouped mice (photocell counter technique) (BROWN 1960). The effect was already evident after 0.07 mg/kg i.p. of tryptophan, but it did not increase with the dose (up to 150 mg/kg i.p.). L-Tryptophan (0.018 mg/kg i.p.) also prevented the motor stimulation induced by cocaine, amphetamine and caffeine, but not that induced by pipradol. Depression of spontaneous locomotion in mice injected with tryptamine (50 mg/kg i.p.) was also observed by VANE et al. (1961) (photocell counter technique).

VI. Other indolealkylamines

GREIG et al. (1959) observed excitement and irritability in mice and rats treated with α-methyltryptamine and α-ethyltryptamine, two MAO inhibitors. They also observed that 5-hydroxy-α-methyltryptamine which is deprived of MAO blocking effect, did not change behaviour. Locomotor excitement was also observed by VAN METER et al. (1960) in rats after α-methyltryptamine (10 to 20 mg/kg i.p.), by GREIG et al. (1961) in mice after α-ethyltryptamine and by VANE et al. (1961) in mice injected with α-methyltryptamine (12.5 mg/kg i.p.), α-ethyltryptamine (12.5 mg/kg i.p.) or 5-methoxy-α-methyltryptamine (50 mg/kg i.p.). In cats, motor activity appeared to be reduced after α-ethyltryptamine (10 mg/kg i.p.; 5 mg/kg were ineffective); the animals walked without ataxia when prodded and exhibited a tipical defensive response when stimulated. The pupil was dilated and nictitating membrane contracted (MATTHEWS et al. 1961).

SAI-HALÁSZ and ENDRÖCZY (1959) administered N,N-dimethyltryptamine and N,N-diethyltryptamine (two tryptamine derivatives with psychotic effects on humans) to dogs trained to recognize the bell sound announcing a reward (access to food). The two amines (2 mg/kg and 1.5 mg/kg i.m. respectively) first impaired the discriminating ability and later knocked out the responsiveness to the stimuli. Furthermore animals injected with N,N-diethyltryptamine exhibited hallucinatory behaviour. Recovery occurred after 2 hrs or more.

N,N-diethyltryptamine affected the behavioural responses evoked in dogs by electrical stimulation of the reticular formation and of the amygdalae. Before the drug, stimulation of the reticular formation evoked a fear reaction; after the drug it evoked a reaction of rage and hostility. The stimulation of the amygdalae gave rise to a fear reaction which was enhanced by the N,N-diethyltryptamine (SAI-HALÂSZ and ENDRÖCZY 1959).

GESSNER et al. (1961) reported that 5-methoxygramine (17.5 mg/kg), 5 methoxytryptamine (19 mg/kg) and 5-methoxy-N,N-dimethyltryptamine (11 mg/kg) blocked the conditioned avoidance responses in the rat. The first two amines were just as active as the bufotenine (20.5 mg/kg), whereas the 5-methoxy-N,N-dimethyltryptamine was much more active. Melatonin (46 mg/kg) and gramine (14.5 mg/kg) were inactive.

EDERY and SCHATZBERG-PORATH (1960) injected 5-fluorotryptamine (1 mg/kg), 4-fluoro-7-methyltryptamine (2 mg/kg) and tryptamine (0.8 mg/kg) into the lateral ventricle of dogs. After the injection the animals fell into a catatonic-like state similar to that observed by SACCHI et al. (1956) after 5-HT injection.

CRONHEIM and GOURZIS (1960) infused intravenously 1-benzyl-2,5-dimethylserotonine (BAS), a 5-HT-antagonist, (100 μg/kg/min for 3 hrs.) into normal dogs and dogs treated with reserpine. In the normal dogs the BAS infusion produced mydriasis, skeletal muscle disturbance and apparent depression, without modifying the blood pressure or the heart rate; in the dogs treated with reserpine the BAS infusion (as with the 5-HT infusion) transformed the slight reserpine-induced sedation into a comatose state and made the blood pressure collapse to about 65 mm Hg (low enough to explain the deep sedation!).

Gaddum and Vogt (1956) injected 5-benzyloxygramine (2.1 mg), a 5-HT-antagonist, into the lateral ventricle of cats and did not observe any behavioural change or prevention of the lethargic action of 5-HT administered by the same route.

B. Passage of 5-HT through the blood-brain barrier

In the mouse Woolley and Shaw (1954) did not observe any detectable increase of the brain 5-HT level after intraperitoneal injection of 5 mg of 5-HT (chemical assay) and Shore et al. (1957) found a small increase (about 25%) 15 min after intraperitoneal injection of a large dose of amine (100 mg/kg).

In the rat Kärki and Paasonen (1959) found a conspicuous rise of the brain 5-HT concentration (from 0.5 μg/g to about 1.2 μg/g) 10 min after intravenous injection of 4.3 mg/kg of amine (biological assay). Similar percentage increase was also observed in animals preinjected with iproniazid. From these results it seems that in the rat the blood-brain barrier is largely permeable to 5-HT, but Bertaccini, Mantegazzini and Pegrassi (unpublished data) were not able to confirm the Kärki and Paasonen's data. They did not found any increase of the brain 5-HT level 10—15 min after intravenous injection of 10 mg/kg of amine in normal and iproniazidised rats (biological assay).

McIsaac and Page (1959) found significant amounts of radioactivity in the brains of rats i.p. injected with about 15 mg/kg of 5-hydroxytryptamine-C^{14}. They also observed the same fact in one rabbit 4 days after intraperitoneal administration of 8 mg/kg of amine. According to the AA. the significance of these data is doubtful because the radioactivity might depend on the extracerebral metabolites of the amine rather than on the intracerebral ones or on the amine itself. No detectable increase in 5-HT brain level was observed by Udenfriend et al. (1957b) in rabbits and dogs after 60 mg/kg and by Erspamer (1961) in rabbits after 10—20 mg/kg i.v. of 5-HT.

Costa and Aprison (1957, 1958), in the course of cross circulation experiments in rabbits, injected 2—4 mg of 5-HT into a common or internal carotid artery of the recipient animal. They observed that the amine level in some areas of the brain of the recipient animal was higher than that in the corresponding areas of the donor animal. The significance of this result cannot be generalized because some factors related to the experimental conditions (heparin or interruption of the blood circulation during the insertion of the canulas or reduction of arterial cerebral inflow and of the venous outflow caused by the ligature of some vessels) may have modified the capillary wall, facilitating the passage of the 5-HT into the brain.

To sum up: the proof that 5-HT can get through the blood-brain barrier is lacking. The data backing this suggestion have not been confirmed or are not convincing due to the possibility that the permeability of the capillary wall was modified by the experimental conditions.

C. Effects on body temperature

It has been frequently reported that 5-HT produces hypothermia and 5-HTP hyperthermia, but there is no evidence at all indicating the central origin of these effects.

In mice 5-HT (43 mg/kg i.p.) caused a fall in rectal temperature from 38° C to 33° C in 30 min (room temperature 22° C) (Lessin and Parkes 1957), and enhanced (20 mg/kg s.c.) (from 3° C to 10° C) the hypothermic response of animals exposed to a cold environment (Fastier et al. 1957).

In rats injected with 5-HT (5 mg/kg s.c.) the rectal temperature dropped about 2° C below normal in the 1st hr and gradually returned toward normal in the subsequent 3 hrs. A secondary hypothermia occurred 6 and 24 hrs after injection (HOFFMAN 1958b). Adrenalectomy markedly potentiated the effect of 5-HT in rats. Replacement therapy with adrenal cortical extracts prevented the potentiating effect of adrenalectomy and abolished the secondary hypothermia. Treatment with epinephrine prevented the primary hypothermia, not the secondary one, induced by 5-HT in adrenalectomized rats (HOFFMAN 1959). The meaning of these data is not clear. FÖLDES and KOMLÓS (1959) reported that 5-HT (2.1 to 4.3 mg/kg s.c.) induced hypothermia in rats kept at room temperature of 20° C, but not in animals kept at 30° C.

5-HT (5 mg/kg s.c.) lowered also the body temperature of pigeons. Maximal depression (1.6° C) occurred 0.5—1 hr after the injection and recovery was attained 24 hrs later (HOFFMAN 1958a).

5-HTP has an opposite effect to 5-HT, causing hyperthermia. HORITA and GOGERTY (1958) studied the pyretogenic effect of 5-HTP in rabbits kept at room temperature (24° C). 25 mg/kg i.v. had a slight effect; 50 mg/kg i.v. induced hyperthermia (1—1.5° C) lasting 3—4 hrs. 75—100 mg/kg i.v. caused an increase up to 43—44° C within 30—60 min, frequently followed by death. Iproniazid premedication potentiated the pyretogenic effect of 5-HTP. Doses of 5—10 mg/kg i.v. were large enough to give hyperthermia and 20 mg/kg i.v. caused death. Death occurred at the apex of the hyperthermia.

D. Interferences with central acting drugs

This section deals with the interferences at central level between indolealkylamines (and precursors) and central acting drugs. Drugs which antagonize or release the amines, or block the enzymes responsible for their metabolism are not considered here but in the chapters 10, 11 and 12 of this review.

I. Hypnotics and anesthetics

1. 5-Hydroxytryptamine

FORNAROLI and KOLLER (1954, 1955) first reported that 5-HT prolonged the hypnosis induced by barbiturates and ether, and that it induced hypnosis when injected after an ineffective dose of barbiturate. In these experiments, and in followings, the hypnosis was defined as absence of the righting reflexes. Many other AA. confirmed FORNAROLI and KOLLER'S observations. The results will be found in Table 1.

Summarizing we may say: I. 5-HT enhances the blocking action on the righting reflexes of many drugs with different chemical structure and different metabolism (barbiturates, ether, chloral hydrate, ethanol, mephenesin and meprobamate). II. 5-HT enhances the hypnotic action of barbiturates even when they are injected intravenously. III. Amine injected i.v. in animals just recovering from barbiturate hypnosis quickly re-induces the hypnosis; injected i.v. after a non-hypnotic dose of thiopental induces hypnosis. These data lead to the conclusion that the potentiating effect of 5-HT does not depend on interferences with the speed of adsorption and the rate of detoxication of the hypnotics. However its implication cannot be completely rouled out.

Hypothermia prolongs the duration of the hypnosis induced in mice by pentobarbital and allylbarbituric acid (FUHRMAN 1947); 5-HT produces hypothermia in mice and rats. FASTIER et al. (1957) and DANDIYA and SELLERS (1961)

Table 1

5-HT: Dose (mg/kg) and routes	5-HT: Time (in min) before or after drugs	Drugs tested: Dose (mg/kg) and route	Effects[1]	Animal	Authors
0.43—4.3 i.v.	after	kemithal 100 i.v. thiopental 40 i.v.	+	mouse	FORNAROLI and KOLLER (1954, 1955)
		thiopental 2.5; 5; 10; 15 i.v.	+	rat	
1.3—20	before	ether	+	rat	
0.86 i.p.	same time	urethan 700	0	rat	PIERRE and CAHN (1955)
0.86; 8.6 i.p. 0.86 i.v.	10 before or same time	pentobarbital 15; 30			
0.86 s.c.	10 before	kemithal 100			
8.6 i.p.	10 before	ether			
0.86; 8.6 s.c. 2.15 i.v.	5—10 before	thiopental 40	+		
5.4	2 after	thiopental 42 i.v.	0	rabbit	
0.54; 5.4	2 after or 10 before	pentobarbital 59; 65 i.v. kemithal 96; 106 i.v.	+		
20 i.p.	10 before	hexobarbital 100 i.p.	+	mouse	SHORE et al. (1955)
20 i.v.	after recovery				
20 i.p. 20 s.c.	before	cyclobarbital 100 i.p. chloral hydrate 250 i.p.	+	mouse	FASTIER (1956)
8.6 i.p.	10 before	hexobarbital 100 i.p.	+	mouse	SALMOIRAGHI et al. (1956b)
		hexobarbital 150 i.p.	+	rat	
10; 15 s.c.	30 before	pentobarbital i.v. infusion	+	rabbit	MANTEGAZZINI (1956)
8.6 i.p.	10 before	hexobarbital 70 i.p.	+	mouse	SALMOIRAGHI and PAGE (1957)
5—360 i.p.	60 before	hexobarbital 100 i.p.	+	mouse	BROWN (1957)
5 i.v.	after recovery				
4.5 i.v.	10 before	thiopental 20 i.v.	+	mouse	TAESCHLER and CERLETTI (1957)
8.6 i.p.	10 before	hexobarbital 100 i.p. butabarbital 56 i.p. mephenesin 320; 435 i.p. meprobamate 240; 280 i.p.	+	mouse	ZANOWIAK and RODMAN (1959)
10 i.p.	before	chloral hydrate 325 i.p.	+	mouse	LÉVY and MICHEL-BER (1960)
2.15—8.6 i.p.	10 before	hexobarbital 100 i.p.	+	mouse	ASTON and CULLUMBINE (1960)
8.6 i.p.	10 before	ethanol 5 i.p.			
9 i.p.	10 before	hexobarbital 105 i.p.	+	rat	GESSNER et al. (1960)
3.44 i.p.	10 before	pentobarbital 50 i.p.	+	mouse	DANDIYA and SELLERS (1961)
12.9	60 before	hexobarbital 90—100 i.p.	+	mouse	PENNEFATHER and THORP (1958)
4.3; 8.6 i.p.	3—5 before	hexobarbital 75 i.p.	+	mouse	HOLTZ et al. (1957)

[1] + = potentiating effect; 0 = no effect.

put in evidence the contribution of 5-HT hypothermia on the prolongation of the hypnosis. FASTIER et al. reported that amine (20 mg/kg s.c. in mice) prolonged the chloral hydrate sleeping time (200 mg/kg i.p. 10 min after 5-HT) and at the same time enhanced the fall in body temperature induced by the hypnotic. If the fall in body temperature was prevented by keeping the mice in a room at 38° C, the chloral hydrate sleeping time (about 15 min) did not change, while the chloral hydrate + 5-HT sleeping time was markedly reduced (from 82 to about 37 min). DANDIYA and SELLERS (1961) observed that 5-HT (3.44 mg/kg i.p.) prolonged the pentobarbital sleeping time (from about 25 to 64 min) and accentuated the fall in body temperature (11° C instead of 6.7° C) of mice kept at room temperature of 22° C. Keeping the mice at 38° C partly counteracted the potentiating effect of 5-HT on the pentobarbital sleeping time (from 64 to about 37.5 min), but did not modify the effect of pentobarbital alone. We may conclude that hypothermia largely, but not solely, contributes to the hypnosis-prolonging activity of 5-HT.

The speed of re-induction of hypnosis after 5-HT injection in animals recovering from barbiturates, or of induction in animals treated with an ineffective dose of barbiturates is another factor which leads us to think that the lowering of body temperature may not be the only factor responsible for the potentiating effect of 5-HT. In fact, hypothermia takes some time to set in, whereas hypnosis, in the conditions quoted above, almost immediately follows the 5-HT injection. In rabbits, 10 and 15 mg/kg s.c. of 5-HT, i.e. doses large enough to potentiate a non-hypnotic dose of pentobarbital caused a conspicuous fall in blood pressure (from about 110 mm Hg to 70—80 mm Hg) (MANTEGAZZINI 1956). In the rat 5-HT (2—3 mg/kg i.p.) injected immediately after recovery from a thiopental hypnosis, quickly re-induced the hypnosis and brought about a fall of 40—60 mm Hg in blood pressure. Hypotension was long lasting (MANTEGAZZINI and PEGRASSI, unpublished data). Not 5-HT only but many other vaso-active drugs (histamine, dopamine, epinephrine and norepinephrine) enhanced the barbiturates and chloral hydrate hypnotic activity in mice (FASTIER 1956; FASTIER et al. 1957; LÉVY and MICHEL-BER 1960; DANDIYA and SELLERS 1961). The suspect arises that vascular changes, apart from hypothermia, may play some role in prolonging the hypnosis.

To sum up: 5-HT potentiates blocking effects on the righting reflexes of hypnotic and anesthetic drugs. It is certain that hypothermia largely contributes to the production of the potentiating effect; it is also likely that the vascular effects of 5-HT (systemic hypotension or/and cerebral blood flow changes) may contribute to it. There is no proof that the potentiating activity depends on a direct action of 5-HT on the CNS.

2. 5-Hydroxytryptophan

HOLTZ et al. (1957) observed that 5-HTP prolonged, as 5-HT, the hexobarbital sleeping time in mice (15 mg/kg of 5-HTP i.v. 5—8 min before 75 mg/kg i.p. of barbiturate). In the same species, 5-HTP (50 and 40 mg/kg i.p.) also prolonged the hypnosis produced by pentobarbital (50 mg/kg i.p.) (KATO 1959) and chloral hydrate (325 mg/kg i.p.) (LÉVY and MICHEL-BER 1960). After iproniazid, 5-HTP showed an opposite effect, i.e. antagonized the hypnotic effect of hexobarbital (HOLTZ et al. 1957) and chloral hydrate (LÉVY and MICHEL-BER 1960).

3. Bufotenine and psilocybin

Prolongation of the chloral hydrate and hexobarbital sleeping time after bufotenine was observed by FASTIER (1956) (20 mg/kg of amine i.p. 10 min before 250 mg/kg of chloral hydrate i.p. in mice) and by GESSNER et al. (1960) (10.5 mg/kg of amine i.p. 10 min before 105 mg/kg of barbiturate i.p. in rats). According to SALMOIRAGHI and PAGE (1957) bufotenine in large doses (5 mg/kg i.p. in mice) blocked, and in small doses (2—100 μg/kg i.p.) enhanced the potentiating effect of 5-HT (8.3 mg/kg i.p.) on hexobarbital hypnosis. Psilocybin (11 mg/kg i.p.), like bufotenine, prolonged hexobarbital hypnosis in rats (GESSNER et al. 1960).

4. Tryptamine and tryptophan

Prolongation of the chloral hydrate sleeping time after tryptamine was observed by FASTIER (1956) (20 mg/kg of amine i.p. 10 min before 250 mg/kg of chloral hydrate i.p. in mice) and LÉVY and MICHEL-BER (1960) (50 mg/kg of amine i.p. before 325 mg/kg of chloral hydrate i.p. in mice). The latter AA. reported that tryptophan (600 mg/kg i.p.) behaved as tryptamine. Tryptamine (20 mg/kg i.p.) and tryptophan (20 mg/kg i.v.) also prolonged the hexobarbital sleeping time in mice (75 mg/kg i.p. 3—5 min after dosing); iproniazid potentiated the effect of the amine but inverted that of the aminoacid (HOLTZ et al. 1957).

II. Convulsants

5-HT (8.6 and 215 mg/kg s.c. 15 or 120 min before the convulsants) did not modify the clonic convulsive pattern of camphor (70 and 205 mg/kg i.p.) and leptazol (66 mg/kg i.p.) (BIANCHI 1957) nor (up to 300 mg/kg s.c.) did it afford any protection against the convulsant action of leptazol (40 mg/kg i.v.) in mice, whereas it protected rats from epileptic seizures induced by acoustic stimuli (DE 50 = 7 mg/kg s.c.) (TRIPOD et al. 1957).

5-HTP, even at doses (100 mg/kg i.p.) which induced marked increase in the 5-HT brain content, afforded little protection against the convulsant action of leptazol in rats (BONNYCASTLE et al. 1957) and mice (KOBINGER 1958) or against the lethal action of leptazol in mice (LESSIN and PARKES 1959) and did not modify the supramaximal electroshock seizure pattern in rats (PROCKOP et al. 1959). After iproniazid, 5-HTP (at doses between 25 and 50 mg/kg i.p.) raised the convulsant dose (KOBINGER 1958) and the lethal dose (LESSIN and PARKES 1959) of leptazol i.v. in mice, and prevented the tonic convulsions by electroshock in rats (PROCKOP et al. 1959).

III. Other central acting drugs

5-HT (5—10 mg/kg s.c.), 5-HTP (30—400 mg/kg s.c.) and tryptamine (100 mg/kg s.c.) but not tryptophan (100 mg/kg s.c.) enhaced and prolonged the analgesic effect of morphine in mice (reaction time to painful heat stimulation of the tail). 5-HT by itself (20 mg/kg s.c.) prolonged the reaction time to painful stimulation, whereas 5-HTP was ineffective even in very large doses (400 mg/kg s.c.) (SIGG et al. 1958). 5-HTP (15 mg/kg s.c.) potentiated the analgesic effect of morphine also in mice pretreated with iproniazid (reaction time to painful stimulation of the tail) (SCHAUMANN 1958).

5-HT, at a dose of 4.55 mg/kg i.p., partially blocked the motor hyperactivity induced by d-methylamphetamine (3.3 mg/kg i.p.) and by cocaine (20 mg/kg i.p.) (KOBINGER 1958a). At the dose of 10 mg/kg s.c. it completely prevented the hyperactivity produced by d-amphetamine (4 mg/kg s.c. in mice) (photocell counter technique), but even at high doses (up to 300 mg/kg s.c.) it did not protect grouped mice from the toxic effects of d-amphetamine (MAXWELL 1959). In mice, 5-HTP (20 mg/kg i.p.) and tryptophan (0.018 mg/kg i.p.) reduced spontaneous motor activity and antagonized the hypermotility induced by cocaine (2.5—10 mg/kg s.c.), by d-amphetamine (2—10 mg/kg s.c.) and by caffeine (20 mg/kg s.c.) (photocell counter technique) (Brown 1960).

E. Drugs and treatments affecting the brain 5-HT content

Some drugs or treatments affecting the brain functions also affects the 5-HT content. The study of the relationships between changes in brain 5-HT level and pharmacological effects induced by these treatments or drugs may throw some light on the physiological role played by 5-HT normally present in the brain. Drugs which antagonize or release 5-HT or block the enzymes responsible for its metabolism are excluded from this section as they are dealt with in chapters 10, 11 and 12 respectively of this review.

I. Electroshock and convulsants

Garattini and co-workers (Garattini et al. 1957, Garattini and Valzelli 1957, Jori et al. 1957) reported that after electroshock or leptazol shock (80 mg/kg i.p.) in rats there was a conspicuous increase in brain 5-HT level (spectrophotometric and biological methods). The increase reached the maximum (3.5 times the normal level in spectrophotometric assay and 27—40 times in biological assay) 10 min after electro- or chemo-shock; it gradually fell off and was no longer detectable after 24 hrs. A second increase was detectable between 36 and 72 hrs. after the electroshock. The first increase in brain 5-HT, but not the second one, was associated with a decrease in intestinal 5-HT.

Electroshock also induced an increase in brain 5-HT level (10 min and 40 hrs. after electroshock) in guinea-pigs, rabbits and dogs, but not in mice (Fresia et al. 1957). Significant increases in the amine level after electroshock in dogs were observed in the motor area of the cerebral cortex (51%), in the hypothalamus (38%) and in the mid-brain (60%) but not in the visual cortex, in the cerebellum and in the thalamus (spectrofluorimetric method) (Fresia et al. 1958) and in rats in the diencephalic (58%) and mesencephalic portions (93%) and in the cerebral hemispheres (43%) but not in the cerebellum (spectrofluorimetric method) (Garattini et al. 1960).

According to Garattini et al. (1960) there was no relationship between the increase in brain 5-HT and the intensity of the epileptic seizures after electroshock. In fact when the convulsions have been reduced or abolished pretreating the animals with barbiturates (phenobarbital 120 mg/kg i.p.; pentobarbital 35 mg/kg i.p.; hexobarbital 80 mg/kg i.p.) or with diphenylhydantoin (100 mg/kg i.p.) or using an intensity of current insufficient to induce typical convulsions, there was all the same an increase in brain 5-HT level as that observed after typical convulsions. Note, however, that the three barbiturates used and diphenylhydantoin induce by themselves an increase in the brain amine content (Bonnycastle et al. 1957).

Three reports have challenged the findings of Garattini and co-workers described above. Bonnycastle et al. (1957) briefly reported that convulsant procedures such as electroshock or the administration of leptazol, picrotoxin or CO_2 did not modify the brain 5-HT level in rats (biological method). Bertaccini (1959) repeated Garattini's experiments but did not find any significant increase in brain 5-HT level in rats 10, 30, 60 and 120 min after electroshock and 10 and 60 min after injection of a convulsant dose of leptazol (60 mg/kg i.p.) (biological method). Gal and Drewes (1961) dosed the brain 5-HT content of rats injected 1 hr. previously with a convulsant dose of leptazol (60 mg/kg i.p.) or of fluoroacetate (8 mg/kg i.p.). Even these AA. observed no deviations from normal values of the brain 5-HT level (spectrofluorimetric method).

The conclusion is that in rats leptazol and electroshock convulsions do not induce changes in brain 5-HT level.

II. Anticonvulsant drugs

Bonnycastle et al. (1957) (see also: Bonnycastle et al. 1956) observed that treatment of rats with various anticonvulsant drugs led to a significant increase in 5-HT level of the brain (from 0.34 to 0.5—0.6 μg/g) but not of the small intestine, spleen and venous blood. The drugs (injected i.p.) and the dosage regimens employed were as follows: diphenylhydantoin (100 mg/kg injected 16 times over 2 days), mesantoin (200 mg/kg injected once or 4 times over 2 days), trimethadione (150 mg/kg injected 4 times over 2 days), paramethadione (200 mg/kg injected once or 4 times over 2 days), epidon (400 mg/kg injected 4 times over 2 days), methylphenylsuccinimide (450 mg/kg injected once or 4 times over 2 days), phenacemide (500 mg/kg injected once or 4 times over 2 days), primidone (500 mg/kg injected once or 4 times over 2 days), phenobarbital (125 mg/kg), mephobarbital (125 mg/kg), and sodium bromide (1 g/kg injected 5 times over 2 days). Brain 5-HT levels were checked (biological method) 12 hrs. after the last dose, except in the case of sodium bromide (4 hrs. after the last dose) and of barbiturates (2.5 hrs after the injection). In a subsequent paper Anderson et al. (1962) reported that an increase in brain 5-HT level was evident even 30 min after 12.5 (biological method) and 50 mg/kg i.p. (spectrofluorimetric method) of diphenylhydantoin. Prockop et al. (1959) did not observe, in contrast with Bonnycastle and co-workers, any increase in cerebral 5-HT after doses of diphenylhydantoin (25 to 75 mg/kg) high enough to block the tonic extension component of electroshock in rats.

To sum up: it seems established that anticonvulsant drugs increase the brain 5-HT content in rats, but it has not yet been established whether there is correlation between the increase and the protection against convulsions. It is improbable that such increase may account for the protective action of the anticonvulsant, as 5-HTP which causes marked increase in brain 5-HT affords little protection against leptazol or electroshock convulsions (see D, II of this chapter).

III. Barbiturates and other central depressant drugs

Bonnycastle et al. (1957) reported that the treatment of rats with phenobarbital (125 mg/kg i.p.), mephobarbital (125 mg/kg i.p.), hexobarbital (100 mg/kg i.p.) or pentobarbital (50 mg/kg i.p.) resulted in increased 5-HT brain concentration (from 0.34 to about 0.52 μg/g) (biological method). Bonnycastle et al. (1962) reported also that many compounds whose common property is to depress the CNS shared in the ability to increase cerebral 5-HT (biological method): chloralose (100 mg/kg i.p.), ethyl urethan (1800 mg/kg i.p.), diethyl ether (administered by inhalation), chloral hydrate (300 mg/kg i.p.) and meperidine (25 mg/kg i.p.). The increase after pentobarbital or chloral hydrate was checked by both the biological and fluorimetric methods.

Anderson and Bonnycastle (1960) investigated the relationships between the increase in brain 5-HT (biological method) induced by pentobarbital, phenobarbital or ether in rats and the effects of these substances on the righting reflexes and spontaneous motility (photocell counter technique). 2.5 min after i.p. injection of 50 mg/kg of pentobarbital the brain 5-HT level slightly increased (from 0.33 to 0.36 μg/g), and the righting reflexes were blocked. The level reached the peak (0.754 μg/g) 5 min after the injection and then declined slowly. When the righting reflexes reappeared the level was lower than 0.5 μg/g. After i.p. injection of 25 mg/kg of pentobarbital the 5-HT level approached 0.5 μg/g when the righting reflexes disappeared and fell below 0.5 μg/g when they reappeared; there was a good co-relation between the elevation of brain 5-HT and depression of motor activity. After i.p. injection of 100 mg/kg of phenobarbital there was a slow increase in the brain amine content (up to a maximum of 0.572 μg/g 2 hrs. after the injection) accompanied by a slow falling-off in motor activity; the brain 5-HT level was about 0.5 μg/g when the righting reflexes disappeared, and fell below this value when they reappeared. Three min after the beginning of ethyl-ether inhalation the 5-HT content was still normal but the righting reflexes were blocked; the content started to increase only after 10 min inhalation and reached 0.611 μg/g after 20 min inhalation. From these results it seems that the rise in brain 5-HT is not related to the onset of central depression. The AA. suggest that "it is well to keep in mind that the rise in brain 5-HT that is associated with central-acting compounds may be a fortuitous event and no bearing on the mechanism by which these compounds act". SCHANBERG and GIARMAN (1962) observed that the increase in brain 5-HT concentration induced by phenobarbital (100 mg/kg) in rats was associated with an increase in the percentage of "free" 5-HT. Increase in the amount of "free" 5-HT was observed by the AA. after other CNS depressants (chlorpromazine, reserpine, α-methyl-DOPA) irrespective of the change of total 5-HT.

It was also reported that in rabbits i.v. injected with phenobarbital (100 mg/kg) or barbital (200 mg/kg) and killed 4 hrs after dosing (BRODIE et al. 1956) (spectrofluorimetric method) and in rats i.p. injected with phenobarbital (100 mg/kg) or pentobarbital (50 mg/kg) (EFRON and GESSA 1963) (spectrofluorimetric and biological methods) no significant change in brain 5-HT level was detected.

GURSEY and OLSON (1960) reported that ethanol (2 g/kg i.v. infused) reduced the 5-HT content in the brain stem of rabbits. The amine concentration declined to about 40% of control value 30 min after dosing, then increased slowly, reaching normal value in about 6 days. Brain stem noradrenaline concentration declined correspondingly. Alcohol disappeared from the blood in 6 hrs. HÄGGENDAL and LINDQVIST (1961) did not observe any modification of brain 5-HT level after ethanol in rabbits (1 and 12 hrs. after i.v. infusion of 2 g/kg) and in mice (2 hrs. after 2.5 g/kg i.p.). In mice only after 5 g/kg, i.e. after a dose very near the lethal one, there was a slight reduction in 5-HT concentration (spectrofluorimetric method). Cerebral noradrenaline behaved like 5-HT. EFRON and GESSA (1963) confirmed the results of HÄGGENDAL and LINDQVIST, but BONNYCASTLE et al. (1962) reported that in rats ethanol (4.5 g/kg i.p.) increased brain 5-HT level.

It is wise to wait further experimental results before concluding about the effects of barbiturates and ethanol on cerebral 5-HT.

IV. Cortisone

BRODIE et al. (1956) reported that in rabbits the brain 5-HT concentration was normal 4 hrs. after i.v. injection of 26 mg/kg of cortisone (spectrofluorimetric method). WEST (1958) reported that in rats cortisone (50 mg/kg i.m. per day over 14 days) lowered the 5-TH content of the skin and did not affect that of the brain (biological method). The animals were killed 24 hrs. after the last injection. KATO and VALZELLI (1958) obtained different results. They reported that in rats cortisone (50 mg/kg i.m. per day over 15 days) induced a slight but significant increase in brain 5-HT (from 0.48 to 0.57 μg/g). The increase was restricted to the cerebral hemispheres and to the mid-brain and pons. The content of the cerebellum and the diencephalic-hypothalamic region did not vary (spectrofluorimetric method). The animals were killed 6 hrs. after the last cortisone injection.

V. Central nervous system lesions

Toh (1960) checked the cerebral 5-HT content of rats 3 days after placing bilateral electrolytic lesions in the hypothalamus (biological method). The amine content did not significantly differ from that of control rats. Heller et al. (1962) checked the brain 5-HT content (spectrofluorimetric method) in rats 35 days after placing bilateral electrolytic lesions in the lateral hypothalamus, medial hypothalamus, septal region, hippocampus, ventral midbrain tegmentum, dorsomedial midbrain tegmentum, habenula, lateral pontine tegmentum, caudate nucleus or cortex of the dorsomedial aspect of the cerebral hemispheres. Reduction of the brain 5-HT level ranging from 12 to 15% was observed in rats with lesions in the septal region, the dorsomedial midbrain tegmentum and the ventral midbrain tegmentum. An higher reduction (36%) was observed in rats with lesions in the lateral hypothalamus. The lesions in the septal region, in the hypothalamus or in the hippocampus induced a short-lasting irritability to handling; the lesions in the dorsomedial midbrain tegmentum provoked a persistent aggressive behaviour towards an other rat caged together. There was no relationship between changes in the brain 5-HT content and behavioural changes. According to the AA. the fall in brain 5-HT level may be a result of a central denervation secondary to the section of fibres of the medial forebrain bundle within the lateral hypothalamus. In a subsequent paper the same AA. (Harvey et al. 1963) reported that a unilateral lesion in the lateral hypothalamus destroying the medial forebrain bundle, produced a 5-HT fall restricted to the lesioned hemi-brain. The effect of medial forebrain bundle lesion appeared 2—3 days after operation, reached its maximum 12 days after, remaining constant afterwards.

Antonelli et al. (1961) dosed the brain 5-HT content in cats with brainstem acutely transected at midpontine level just in front of the trigeminal rootlets, or at mesencephalic level 1—2 mm in front of the superior border of the pons. The pontine section induced an EEG and ocular pattern typical of the waking state, whereas the mesencephalic transection resulted in a sleeping pattern. 5-HT content (biological method) of the midbrain-hypothalamus did not differ in the two opposite states.

To sum up: there is no relationship between the concentration of brain 5-HT and behavioural changes induced by cerebral lesions in rats. In cats the concentration of 5-HT in the midbrain-hypothalamus does not differ in the two opposed states of sleeping and waking induced by brain-stem transections.

F. Effects on the electroencephalogram

I. 5-Hydroxytryptamine

1. Rabbit

Ferro Milone and Gomirato (1956) observed EEG activation and marked reduction of the frequency of the convulsive spikes induced by application of strychnine on motor area after 5-HT (43—215 μg/kg i.v.). The effect began immediately after the injection and lasted 1—3 min. Mantegazzini (1956) observed no change whatsoever in the synchronised EEG record, typical of the resting animal, after subcutaneous injection of 5-HT up to 10 mg/kg. Only after 15 mg/kg there were long periods of spontaneous activation. Such a dose of 5-HT resulted in severe hypotension which cast some doubt on the significance of EEG data. MONNIER and co-workers (GANGLOFF and MONNIER 1957; MONNIER and TISSOT 1958) observed after intravenous injection of 5-HT (0.1—1 mg/kg), a brief arousal reaction (lasting about 1 min) followed by a longer period of synchronisation (irregular highvoltage, slow waves in the cortex and subcortex with 12—14 c/sec spindle activity in sensory-motor cortex). 30—60 min after injection a "mixed arousal and relaxation pattern" appeared (low voltage fast activity in the sensory-motor cortex and a permanent, regular synchronised 3—5 c/sec rythm in the thalamus, rhinencephalon and parieto-occipital cortex). During this phase paroxysmal spike discharges spontaneously occurred in the hippocampus, and the arousal reaction to the stimulation of the midbrain reticular formation was reduced or abolished. DOMER and LONGO (1962) reported that 5-HT had no detectable effect on the electrical activity of the cerebral cortex, the hippocampus and the midbrain reticular formation up to 100 μg/kg i.v. Higher doses (up to 30 mg/kg i.v.) produced an overall diminution in the voltage of brain waves. According to the AA. the effect of the higher doses was doubtful as a severe and long-lasting hypotension was concomitant.

2. Cat

ROTHBALLER (1957) administered 5-HT (2.15—13 μg/kg i.v.) to curarized cats with intact nervous system and to cats with electrolytic lesions in the midbrain tegmentum. He observed a brief arousal reaction, followed by longer period of deactivation sometimes with abnormal slow waves. A second period of activation occurred only after high doses. There was a brief rise in blood pressure followed by long-lasting fall.

CREPAX and INFANTELLINA (1957) studied the effects of an intracarotid injection of 5-HT on the EEG of cats with intact nervous system. No change in the synchronised record occurred after doses up to 170 μg; after higher doses (up to 860 μg) it appeared a pattern attributed by the AA. to local vasomotor changes: periods of slow waves of simplified shape and low voltage, alternating with periods of electrical silence. The latency and duration of the effect depended on the dose: at 860 μg the effect appeared 10 sec after the injection and lasted up to 45 min. There was no relation between EEG changes and systemic blood pressure changes. MANTEGAZZINI (1957a, 1957b) injected 5-HT directly into the cerebral circulation (vertebral artery or bicarotid trunk) of the "encephale isolé" preparation. Vagi and in some of the experiments trigeminal nerves too, were bilaterally sectioned. 5-HT at 0.5—2 μg did not modify the desynchronized EEG pattern prevalent in the "encephale isolé" with trigeminal nerves intact, while at 0.25—1 μg it desynchronized the enduring sleeping pattern induced by trigeminal deafferentation. The arousal reaction began 3—12 sec after the end of the injection and lasted from tens of seconds to minutes; it was not accompaniep by changes in the systemic blood pressure. Carotid sinus denervation did not prevent the arousal effect, while brain stem transection at ponto-mesencephalic border did it. 5-HT ineffectiveness in arousing the sleeping pattern induced by a mesencephalic transection was confirmed by CREPAX and INFANTELLINA (1957). They observed a reduction in the amplitude of the cortical waves, but not arousal, after intracarotid injection of large doses of 5-HT (86—215 μg) in "cerveau isolé" preparations. Lower doses (8.3—43 μg) were totally ineffective.

Brain stem transection at midpontine level just in front of the trigeminal rootlets ("midpontine pretrigeminal preparation") brings about a persistent EEG activation (BATINI et al. 1959a); hemi-mesencephalic transection in "midpontine pretrigeminal preparation" results in a symmetrically or asymmetrically synchronized EEG record (CORDEAU and MANCIA 1958); combined olfactory and visual deafferentation changes the waking pattern of the "midpontine preparation" into that typical of sleep (BATINI et al. 1959b). GLÄSSER and MANTEGAZZINI (1960a, 1960b) described the effects of 5-HT on the EEG of the "midpontine pretrigeminal preparation". In some of their experiments mesencephalic hemisection or sensory deafferentation was performed. The amine was injected into a carotid artery (through the lingual artery), the other one being occluded. At doses of between 2 and 80 μg it did not change the activated pattern of the "midpontine pretrigeminal preparation". At lower doses (1—4 μg) it frequently activated the EEG synchronized by mesencephalic hemisection or by sensory deafferentation. The changes in blood flow in the common carotid artery of the injected side (REIN's Thermostromuhr method) and the changes in systemic blood pressure induced by 5-HT were often negligeable and in any case had nothing to do with the electroencephalographic changes.

Intraventricular injections of 5-HT (200—500 μg) in conscious cats (BRADLEY and HANCE 1956; SCHWARZ et al. 1956; BRADLEY 1958) or subcutaneous injection of a huge dose of amine (15 mg/kg) in "encephale isolé" preparation (MANTEGAZZINI 1956) had slight or no effects on the electrical activity of the cerebral cortex.

In the writer's opinion, the main effect of the 5-HT injected into the blood stream of the cat is an arousing one. Complete sensory deafferentation does not prevent it. This does not exclude that stimulation of the peripheral receptors may largely contribute to producing the EEG arousal in preparations not deafferented and with nervous system intact. Midbrain transection prevents the 5-HT arousal, a fact which indicates that the arousing action is mediated or conditioned by brain structures located below the midbrain. The arousal reaction occurs even in absence of detectable changes in carotid blood flow.

II. 5-Hydroxytryptophan

1. Rabbit

MONNIER and TISSOT (1958), COSTA and RINALDI (1958) and DOMER and LONGO (1962) studied the effects of intravenously injected 5-HTP on the electrocortical activity of rabbits. According to MONNIER and TISSOT low doses (10 to 20 mg/kg) produced EEG synchronization while higher doses (30 mg/kg or more) gave, within 10—20 min, EEG desynchronization, lasting about 2 hrs, together with spontaneous discharges in rhinencephalic leads. Mesencephalic transection did not prevent the 5-HTP arousal. According to COSTA and RINALDI 5-HTP (75 mg/kg i.v.) at first induced a pattern of slow waves of a very simplified shape; within the second half-hour after injection, an over-all diminution of the voltage of the cortical leads occurred with disappearance of hippocampal 5—7 c/sec waves (theta rhythm). Recovery occurred within the second hour after injection. According to DOMER and LONGO 20—30 mg/kg of 5-HTP produced a marked diminution in the voltage of the spindles and of the slow waves typical of the resting state. Reduction of electrical activity occurred even in the ventromedial nucleus of the thalamus and in the mesencephalic reticular formation, while in the dorsal hippocampus there was a disruption of the theta rhythm. Increasing the dose of 5-HTP (up to 50—100 mg/kg) cortical and subcortical records flattened until the isoelectric line, while bursts of spikes at 30—40 c/sec appeared in the hippocampus. Hyperpnea, tremors, struggling and hyperthermia accompanied the development of EEG changes. When a total dose of 150 mg/kg was reached the animals died. The same changes occurred when 5-HTP was intravenously infused (5 mg/min).

Costa et al. (1960) injected 5-HTP into a common carotid artery and tried to relate EEG changes to changes in 5-HT concentration in the mesencephalon-diencephalon, in the hippocampus and in the telencephalon. Both vagi were severed and carotid bodies inactivated. After 22 mg of 5-HTP the EEG synchronization typical of resting state was accentuated for about 30 min and then returned to normal level. After 44 mg some of the animals showed the same changes as those treated with lower doses but some developed, after an initial augmentation of synchronization, a persistent desynchronized pattern which lasted for 1 hr or more. There was no correlation between increases in 5-HT concentrations in the telencephalon and the hippocampus and EEG changes. The 5-HT content of the mesencephalon-diencephalon was higher in animals with an alerting pattern than in animals with a sleeping pattern, reaching values of more than 3 times above the control ones.

To sum up: some results indicate that 5-HTP in rabbits at low doses induces synchronization and at high doses desynchronization of the electrical activity of the cerebral cortex. Other results lead us to conclude that the main effect of 5-HTP is a flattening of EEG and the appearance of bursts of spikes in the hippocampus.

2. Cat

Glässer and Mantegazzini (1960a, 1960b) described the effects of 5-HTP on the EEG of the "midpontine pretrigeminal preparation". 5-HTP was infused through the lingual artery into the external carotid artery on one side, the common carotid artery on the opposite one being occluded during the infusion. The aminoacid (8—20 mg) changed the desynchronized pattern typical of this preparation to a pattern of marked synchronization similar to that produced by thiopental (Fig. 1). Higher doses (40—60 mg) also prevented the arousing effect of visual and olfactory stimulation. The synchronizing effect began within a few minutes after the infusion and lasted for more than 30—45 min. When the contralateral carotid artery was left open during the intracarotid infusion in order to obtain a difference in 5-HTP concentration in the areas irrorated by the two arteries, the hemisphere on the infusion side showed a greater synchronization than that of the other side. This means that the synchronization was not due to by-products of the extracerebral metabolism of the aminoacid nor to its peripheral effects, as these ought to have symmetrically affected the EEG. The electroencephalographic changes were wholly independent of the changes in the systemic blood pressure and in the carotid blood flow (Rein's Thermostromuhr method). Mesencephalic hemisection in the "midpontine pretrigeminal preparation" resulted in EEG synchronization which was sometimes confined to the hemisphere above the mesencephalic lesion. 5-HTP (5—20 mg) increased the synchronization induced by the lesion and blocked the arousal reaction to olfactory and visual stimulation, but never, even at lower doses (2—5 mg), it desynchronized the EEG. Antonelli et al. (1961) dosed the 5-HT content of the midbrain-hypothalamus in "midpontine pretrigeminal preparation" of cats after intracarotid infusion of the minimum synchronizing dose of 5-HTP (5 to 10 mg). The infusion brought about an EEG sleeping pattern in the hemisphere on the side of the infusion and left the activated pattern of the opposite hemisphere unchanged. When the EEG syndrome developped 5-HT concentration in the midbrain-hypothalamus on the side of the infusion was 50% higher than that on the opposite side and of non-injected preparations.

To sum up: 5-HTP induces in the "midpontine pretrigeminal preparation" of cat an EEG pattern resembling that of barbiturate sleep. The synchronizing

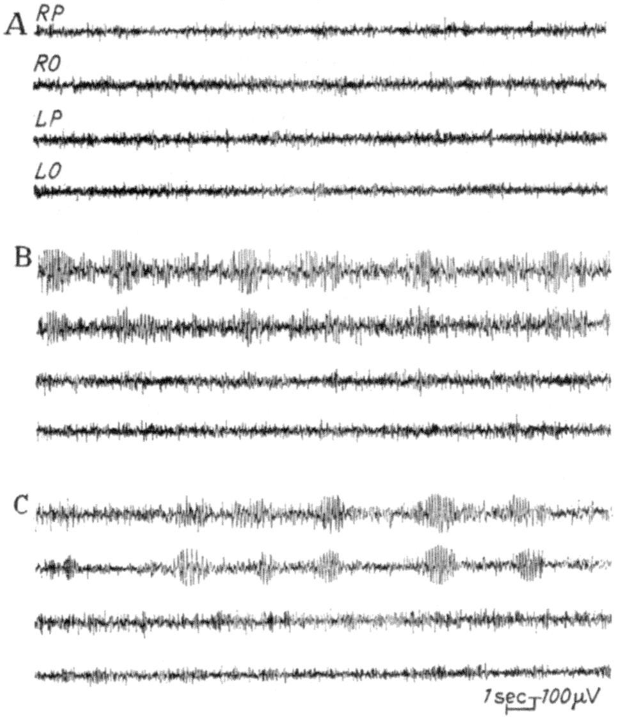

Fig. 1 A—C. Effects of 5-HTP on the EEG of the midpontine-pretrigeminal cat. A EEG pattern symmetrically activated, 2 hr after midpontine transection. B Clear EEG asymmetry produced by 1 mg of thiopental injected into the right carotid artery, the controlateral artery being open: only the hemisphere on the side of the injection shows synchronization. C The same EEG pattern produced by 20 mg of 5-HTP injected as in (B). (From GLÄSSER and MANTEGAZZINI 1960b)

effect is not due to the peripheral actions of 5-HTP nor to any gross alteration in cerebral circulation. The 5-HT content of the midbrain-hypothalamus increases by 50% after a minimum synchronizing dose of aminoacid.

III. Other indolealkylamines and precursor aminoacids

MONNIER (1959) reported that in rabbits psilocybin (1.5—5 mg/kg i.v.) induced, within a few minutes after injection, activation of the electrical activity in cortical leads, and deactivation in subcortical leads (hippocampus, caudate nucleus, thalamus and mesencephalic reticular formation). Mesencephalic transection partially blocked the amine arousing effect (2 mg/kg i.v.). CERLETTI (1959) also observed an arousal reaction after intravenous injection of 1—2 mg/kg of psilocybin in curarized rabbits. Bufotenine behaved as psilocybin (MONNIER and KRUPP 1960).

BRODEY et al. (1963) reported that in rabbits psilocybin (4—6 mg/kg), psilocin (0.5—2 mg/kg), 4-methyl-α-methyltryptamine (1—2 mg/kg), 4-hydroxy-α-methyltryptamine (5—7 mg/kg) and 1-methylpsilocybin (6.8—12.6 mg/kg) i.v. injected, produced EEG alert patterns lasting 45 min or more. Brain stem transection at precollicular level prevented the arousing effect of 4-methyl-α-methyltryptamine and psilocin. Pontine transection passing dorsally at retrocollicular level and ventrally at the posterior border of the pons raised the activating dose of the former drug (7 mg/kg) while prevented the arousing action of the latter one (3 mg/kg). In the AA. opinion these results demonstrate that 4-methyl-α-methyltryptamine act at midbrain level while psilocin does not.

Van Meter et al. (1960) reported that in rabbits α-methyltryptamine (2 mg/kg i.v.), an inhibitor of the MAO and 5-HTP decarboxylase, induced EEG desynchronization for more than 2 hrs. When the basilar artery was occluded, injection into a vertebral artery induced an arousal reaction, whereas injection of the same quantity of amine into a carotid artery was ineffective. I.v. injection did not affect the synchronized pattern of the "cerveau isolé". From this data the AA. inferred that the arousing effect was due to an action of the amine on the caudal portion of the brain stem reticular formation. Matthews et al. (1961) (see also Matthews 1963) studied the effects of DL-α-ethyltryptamine, a MAO inhibitor, on the cat EEG. In conscious animals and in "encéphale isolé" preparations, intravenous injection of 10 mg/kg of amine resulted in an EEG activation pattern. The behaviour revealed signs of alertness. The effects began within 60—90 min after the injection and lasted many hours. Rostropontine transection or mesencephalic transection at intercollicular level prevented the DL-α-ethyltryptamine arousal.

Domer and Longo (1962) reported that tryptamine (15—20 mg/kg i.v.) in rabbits produced a flattening of the cortical activity and a short-lasting spiking discharge in the hippocampus. The effect lasted only a few minutes. Subsequent injections were less active. Tryptamine was ineffective when slowly i.v. infused (1 mg/min for 90 min).

According to Vane et al. (1961) DL-α-methyltryptamine, DL-α-ethyltryptamine, DL-5-methoxy-α-methyltryptamine and N,N-dimethyltryptamine (2 mg/kg i.p.) did not produce EEG arousal in unrestrained conscious cats. Bursts of 6—10 c/sec high-voltage activity appeared within few min after injection and lasted for more than 6 hrs. In "encéphale isolé" preparation DL-α-methyltryptamine (0.5—2 mg/kg i.v.) produced a brief arousal reaction followed by a longer period of bursts of high-voltage cortical activity.

Erspamer et al. (1960a) described the effect of 4-HTP on the "midpontine pretrigeminal preparation" of the cat. 4-HTP penetrates into the brain and is there decarboxylated to 4-HT (Erspamer et al. 1960b). The aminoacid injected slowly into a carotid artery (25—40 mg) transformed the activated EEG pattern into a sleeping pattern. 5-HTP had the same effect, but at lower doses. Costa et al. (1960) injected rabbits intracarotidly with 44 mg of DL-5-methyltryptophan, an aminoacid not attacked "in vitro" by mammalian decarboxylase (Erspamer et al. 1961). No EEG change was detectable after the injection.

G. Effects on action potentials evoked in cerebral cortex and in subcortical structures

I. 5-Hydroxytryptamine

1. Responses of the cerebral cortex to direct electrical or chemical stimulation

Di Stefano et al. (1956) studied the effect of 5-HT on the action potentials evoked, by electrical stimulation, in neuronally isolated slab of cerebral cortex of cats. 5-HT (2.15—4.3 μg i.v.) gave transitory depression of the evoked potentials and caused a fall in cortical oxygen tension (polarographic technique), and in systemic blood pressure. Depression of cortical potentials occurred 1—3 min after the injection, when both the blood pressure and cortical oxygen tension had returned to normal, and persisted for 4—8 min. Cortical oxygen tension was not measured in the isolated slab but in the intact cortex; diminution in blood flow and hypoxia, probably more marked and long-lasting here than in the intact cortex, could account for the depression of the electrical response of the slab.

Crepax and Infantellina (1957) found that 5-HT applied on the isolated cerebral cortex of cats enhanced at low concentrations ($1:10^4$—$1:10^3$) and depressed at higher concentrations the spontaneous electrical activity of the slab. The amine differently affected the two components of the response set up by electrical stimulation (single shock). Surface-negative wave (superficial response) was unaffected by any concentration whatsoever of the amine between $1:10^4$ and $2:10^2$, whereas surface-positive wave (deep response) was enhanced by low concentrations ($1:10^4$—$5:10^4$) and was reduced both in amplitude and duration by higher concentrations ($1:10^3$—$1:10^2$) (5-HT concentrations expressed in terms of creatinine sulfate salt). 5-HT intracarotidly injected enhanced at doses of 2.15—4.3 μg, and depressed at higher doses (6.45—10.75 μg) the spontaneous electrical activity of the slab and the surface positive component of response to electrical stimulation (single shock). Even at the highest dose tested (10.75 μg) the amine did not affect the surface negative component of the response. Electrical responses to repetitive stimulation were blocked by amounts of 5-HT (locally applied or intracarotidly injected) lower than those depressing the response to single shock. In the AA. opinion 5-HT effects could be attributed to hypoxia affecting the postsynaptic potentials of deep-lying neurones (positive wave) more than that of apical dendrites of pyramidal cells (negative wave) and affecting repetitively stimulated neurones more than those submitted to a single shock. Ochs et al. (1960) reported that 5-HT ($5:10^3$—$1:10^2$) topically applied on the intact cerebral cortex of cats or rabbits diminished or eliminated the surface negative response to direct electrical stimulation. A fact which would indicate that the amine also affects the postsynaptic potential of the apical dendrites of pyramidal cells.

Rech and Domino (1960) explored the effects of 5-HT on the electrical activity induced by local application of strychnine or d-tubocurarine on the neuronally isolated cerebral cortex of dogs. 5-HT (20—60 μg/kg) intravenously or intracarotidly injected lowered the frequency of strychnine or d-tubocurarine spiking but the effect was variable and not significant. It did not depend on changes in blood pressure.

Crossland and Mitchell (1956) briefly reported that 5-HT (0.1—0.4 μg) injected into the internal carotid artery of decerebrated rabbits did not modify the electrical activity of the cerebellar cortex.

From the above data it appears that 5-HT mainly depresses the cortical response set up by direct electrical stimulation; there is no agreement between the authors as to the sensitivity of the single components of the response. It appears that the amine hardly affects the electrical activity induced in the isolated cortex by strychnine. The cortical origin of the effects observed is beyond dispute, as all the experiments were performed in neuronally isolated cortex or applying the amine directly on the cortex. The mechanism whereby 5-HT depresses cortical responses remains open to investigation. It may be thought that the amine acts directly on the nerve cells, but it can't be ruled out that it acts indirectly for instance through local blood flow changes in turn acting on the neurones. It must be stressed that the amine has the same effects either when it is locally applied or when it reaches the cortex through the blood. In the latter case the direct action on the neurones can be upheld only admitting that 5-HT passes the blood-brain barrier, that is to say accepting a fact not yet proved.

2. Cortical and subcortical responses evoked by afferent impulses

a) Transcallosal stimulation

Marazzi and Hart (1955) (see also: Hart et al. 1956 and Marazzi 1957) studied the effects of 5-HT on the response of the visual cortex to stimulation of the symmetrical point in the contralateral cortex, in cats lightly pentobarbitalized. 5-HT (1 μg) injected into the carotid artery of the recording side reduced the amplitude of the surface negative component of the response, and left the initial positive component unaffected. The effect began 30—40 sec after injection, reached the maximum after 1 min and disappeared after about 3 min. No pressure change occurred after such a dose of amine. The participation of the discharges of the carotid receptors to the inhibition of the transcallosal response which followed the intracarotid injection of 5-HT was ruled out in experiments in which glomus carotideus was by-passed (Rodriguez et al. 1961). Guth and Spirtes (1959) confirmed Marazzi's results. On the basis that the initial positive wave is the action potential of impulses propagating up to the afferent terminals in the cerebral cortex and that the secondary surface negative wave is the post-synaptic response of cortical neurones, Marazzi stated that 5-HT acts as an inhibitory synaptic neurohumor.

Koella et al. (1960) studied the effects of the amine on the transcallosal response of the cortex of the suprasylvian gyrus in cats anaesthetized with dial-urethan. 5-HT (4.3 μg) was injected into the common or into the external carotid artery (that is to say above or below the carotid sinus) of the recording or of the contralateral side (stimulating side). When the drug was injected into the external carotid artery it reached the brain, avoiding the carotid receptors. Peak-to-peak amplitude of the positive-negative transcallosal response was always reduced, but to various degrees, by 5-HT injected into each of the four points indicated. The injection into the external carotic artery of each side was more effective than the injection into the corresponding common carotids; data which allows us to suspect, in contradiction with that advanced by Rodriguez et al. (1961) that stimulation of the carotid receptors by 5-HT exercises a facilitatory action on the transcallosal response. The injection into the external or common carotid artery of the stimulating side, had the same effect, although of less importance, than the injection into the external or common carotid artery of recording side. Since the blood flowing through a carotid artery does not reach the hemicortex of the contralateral side, this data indicates that 5-HT may affect the transcallosal response acting on structures located elsewhere than at the recording point. It is possible that 5-HT may reduce the electrical excitability of the stimulated cortex reached by the drug injected on the same side and/or, as the AA. sustain, that it may activate inhibitory subcortical structures projecting on both sides of the cortex. Any way these results don't allow to affirm that 5-HT is a neurohumor with inhibitory effect on the cortical synapses.

b) Sensory nerves and sense organs stimulation

Malcolm (1958) studied the effect of 5-HT on the responses evoked in the sensory cortex, in the ventral thalamus and in the hypothalamus by stimulation of the sural nerve in chloralosated cats. The amine was locally applied on the exposed cortex or injected into a carotid artery or into a lateral ventricle. As arterial injection was made through a catheter tied into the artery, a part of the volume injected (about one third, according to the A.) was retained in the dead space of the canulation tubing and the artery. 5-HT locally applied (1:10^3) did not produce any detectable effect on the cortical evoked responses. 5-HT intracarotidly injected (200—300 μg) first depressed and then enhanced the surface negative component of the cortical response. The depression was over within 3 min, the enhancement was at the peak in 12—16 min but never completely disappeared. The effect on evoked responses in the subcortical structures was solely one of long-lasting depression. The amine (100—200 μg) also caused fall in the systemic blood pressure, marked dilatation of the cortical vessels and oedema of exposed cortex. The vasodilatation lasted 10—15 min; the oedema lasted longer and not easily reversed. 5-HT intraventricularly injected (50 and 200 μg) decreased the amplitude of the surface negative component of the cortical response, left unchanged the initial surface positive component as well as the responses evoked in deeper structures, and abolished (at 200 μg only) the marked facilitation of the thalamic response produced by repetitive stimulation of the sural nerve (10 shocks in 25 msec).

Koella and co-workers (Koella et al. 1959, 1960; Smythies et al. 1959) described the effects of 5-HT on the responses evoked in the visual areas I of both hemispheres by photic stimulation. The amine (0.53—4.3 μg) was injected into the right or left common carotid artery, one of the carotid sinuses being denervated. The injection into the innervated carotid artery reduced the peak-to-peak amplitude of the positive-negative response not only in the cortex of the injected side but also in the other one. The injection into the denervated carotid was much less effective than the injection into the innervated carotid. This suggests that stimulation of the presso- and/or chemo-receptors of the carotid sinus by 5-HT exercises a bilateral inhibitory effect on the visual areas. 5-HT, even when injected into the denervated artery, depressed the responses of both the visual areas, in spite of the fact that it did not reach the contralateral hemicortex. 5-HT effect on the contralateral cortex may be explained admitting that the amine acts on structures located elsewhere but projecting to the visual areas.

Evarts (1958) reported that 5-HT (0.1 mg or more) injected into the carotid artery of the recording side did not affect the synaptic transmission in the lateral geniculate nucleus of the cat.

II. 5-Hydroxytryptophan

Revzin and Costa (1960) studied, in the cat, the effects of 5-HTP on the potentials evoked in the hippocampus by stimulation of the amygdala. The aminoacid (100—200 mg/kg i.v.) caused a slight depression of the response. Premedication with tranylcypromine (a MAO inhibitor) markedly potentiated the depressant effect of 5-HTP. This potentiation was much more marked in chronic unanaesthetized animals than in "cerveau isolé" preparation. Monnier (1960) briefly reported that the injection of 5-HTP (50—85 mg/kg i.v.) into unanaesthetized rabbits caused depression of transcallosal responses of somaesthetic and visual cortex, but left unchanged the potentials evoked in the somaesthetic cortex by thalamic stimulation.

III. Other indolealkylamines

Evarts et al. (1955) studied the effects of bufotenine on the electrical activity in the visual system of anaesthetized cats. The amine was injected into the carotid artery on the recording side. 0.2 mg/kg caused marked depression of the postsynaptic response evoked in the lateral geniculate by optic nerve stimulation. The response of the visual cortex to stimulation of the optic radiations and the response of the optic tract to retinal photic stimulation were left unchanged by bufotenine even when injected in quantities many times higher than that sufficient to reduce the geniculate response. The effect was at the peak 20—60 sec after the injection and was over within 1 hr. It was independent of any blood pressure and respiratory changes.

Tryptamine and N,N-dimethyltryptamine behaved as bufotenine. N,N-dimethyltryptamine had approximately the same activity as bufotenine, both in terms of peak effect and in duration of action. Tryptamine had a short-lasting effect (about 3—6 min). 5-hydroxy-N,N-dibuthyltryptamine, 5,6-dimethoxy-N,N-dimethyltryptamine, bufotenidine and gramine were inactive (EVARTS 1958).

MONNIER (1959) reported that in rabbits psilocybin (1.5—5 mg/kg i.v.) caused a reduction of the amplitude of the potential evoked in the somato-sensory cortex by stimulation of the ventral-lateral nucleus of the thalamus, while it left unchanged the transcallosal response in the visual and somato-sensory cortex. MATTHEWS et al. (1961) (see also: MATTHEWS 1963) observed no change in the amplitude of the response evoked in the somato-sensory cortex by radial nerve stimulation after α-ethyltryptamine injection (20 mg/kg i.v.) in curarized cats.

H. Effects on the spinal reflexes

I. 5-Hydroxytryptamine

SLATER et al. (1955) briefly reported that intrarterial injection of 5-HT (43—430 μg) in spinal cats resulted in an increase, followed by a depression, of a flexor reflex. Hydrazinophtalazine blocked the pressor action of the amine but did not prevent that on the reflex. Increase in amplitude of the flexor reflex followed by depression was also observed by LITTLE et al. (1957) after 5-HT (50 μg/kg i.v.) in cats with spinal cord transected at T 13 and lightly anaesthetized with dial-urethan. The patellar reflex was momentarily inhibited. KISSEL and DOMINO (1957, 1959) studied the effects of 5-HT on the patellar reflex, the crossed extensor reflex and the reflex inhibition of the knee jerk and the neuro-muscular transmission in spinal cats. Patellar reflex was mechanically elicited, while the crossed extensor reflex and the inhibition of the patellar reflex were evoked by electrical stimulation of a sciatic nerve. 2.1—4.3 μg/kg of 5-HT i.v. produced a marked transitory inhibition followed by facilitation of the patellar and crossed extensor reflexes. 20 μg/kg blocked the patellar reflex as long as 40 sec. 5-HT did not affect the reflex inhibition and the neuro-muscular transmission. The stabilization of arterial pressure or the block of the vascular effects of 5-HT by dibenzyline (5 mg/kg i.v.) failed to prevent the 5-HT effect on the reflexes; chloralose reduced it. Inhibition of patellar reflex after 5-HT in spinal cat was also observed by WEIDMANN and CERLETTI (1959, 1960) (5—10 μg/kg i.v.) and enhancement of the flexor reflex by VANE et al. (1961) (1 mg/kg i.v.).

From the above results it appears that 5-HT injected into the blood stream of the spinal cat has, at first, an inhibitory action on the extensor reflexes (patellar and crossed extensor) and a facilitatory action on the flexor reflex, and later on an opposite action. Moreover these effects seem to be largely independent of the vascular effects of the amine.

In contrast with the above quoted authors, WEIDMANN and CERLETTI (1957) observed inconstant changes of the flexor and crossed extensor reflexes after

5 μg or more of 5-HT i.v. and VANE et al. (1961) obtained enhancement of the patellar reflex after a huge dose of 5-HT (1 mg/kg i.v.) in spinal cats.

As far as the mechanism of the action of 5-HT on the spinal reflexes is concerned, attempts to demonstrate any direct action of the amine on the neurones of the spinal cord were negative in outcome. CURTIS et al. (1955) studied the 5-HT effect on the ventral roots responses evoked in cats by electrical stimulation of the corresponding dorsal roots, the afferent inflow from other structures being prevented by crushing the remaining dorsal roots of the region. Close intrarterial injection of 50—200 μg of 5-HT occasionally depressed the mono- and polysynaptic responses, but, according to the AA., the effect was due to stimulation of the peripheral receptors.

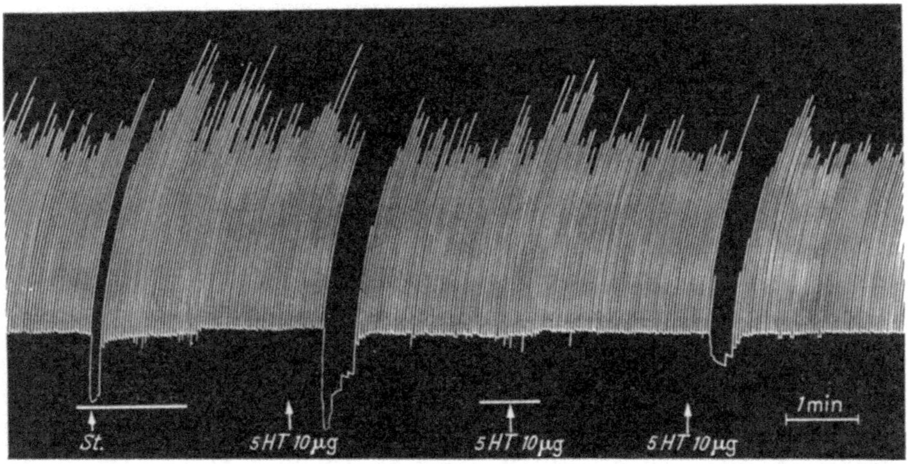

Fig. 2. Effect of the occlusion of the abdominal aorta on the block of the patellar reflex produced by 5-HT in the spinal cat. Aorta occlusion (during the signal line) does not affect the block of the reflex produced by noxious stimulation of the foot (St.), but prevents the blocking action of 5-HT (10 μg) injected into a brachial vein

To by-pass the blood-brain barrier, CURTIS et al. (1961) applied electrophoretically 5-HT on the environment of interneurones in spinal cord of cats, recording their activity with the aid of coaxial microelectrodes. The interneurones were identified by their responses to the stimulation of the dorsal and ventral roots. The inner barrel of the microelectrode, extruding 2—3 μ, was used to record the extracellular spike potentials; the outer barrel was filled with an aqueous solution of 5-HT. 5-HT was applied to 16 different interneurones with currents up to 200 nA for periods as long as 45 sec. In no case did the amine have any effect whatever on the spontaneous activity or on that evoked by the dorsal root stimulation. Diffusional barriers may prevent the 5-HT ejected from the microelectrode to bridge the gap (of a least 3—4 μ) between the tip of the barrel and the neuronal membrane. These results, therefore, do not permit to conclude that 5-HT has no effect at all on the spinal interneurones, but strongly strengthen the suspicion that the effects of 5-HT on the reflexes do not depend on the direct action of the amine on the neurones.

MANTEGAZZINI et al. (1963) observed that the injection of small doses of 5-HT (0.1—0.4 μg) into the femoral artery of the recording side (through a collateral) caused a clear transitory inhibition of the patellar reflex in spinal and eviscerated cats. The intravenous injection of the same doses was totally ineffective. I.v. injection of higher doses (5—10 μg) inhibited the reflex, but the inhibitory effect was completely prevented occluding for a few seconds after injection the abdominal aorta at the biforcation into the internal iliac arteries (Fig. 2). In such a way the amine reached the spinal cord but not the hind legs. The gentle touching of the foot had the same effect as 5-HT. These results led us to think that the inhibition of the patellar reflex in the cat may be accounted for by afferent impulses discharged by 5-HT in the territories irrorated by iliac arteries. It is quite likely that the effects on the flexor and extensor reflexes may be explained in the same way.

ANGELUCCI (1956) perfused the spinal cord of the frog through a cannula pushed into the vertebral canal; oxygen was supplied through the blood vessels. 5-HT added to the perfusion fluid (up to $1:10^4$) did not affect the flexor reflex nor alter the depressant action of reserpine. Biological assay of the effluent revealed that 5-HT-like substances were released from the spinal cord at rest. The release increased when the reflex was stimulated. CARELS (1962) applied 5-HT to the isolated spinal cord of the frog. 5-HT ($1:10^4$ to $1:10^2$ in the bath) inhibited the monosynaptic component of the response evoked in the ventral roots by stimulation of the dorsal roots or of the descending fibres in the lateral column, but did not affect the response of the motoneurones to antidromic stimulation. These results suggested to the author that the amine acted at presynaptic level.

II. Psilocybin and psilocin

Psilocybin intravenously injected into the spinal cat provoked a steady, long-lasting increase of the patellar reflex (5—10 μg/kg or more) and an increase (up to 0.1 mg/kg) or a decrease (higher doses) of the flexor reflex. The effects did not depend on the blood pressure or neuro-muscular transmission changes (WEIDMANN et al. 1958; WEIDMANN and CERLETTI 1959; CERLETTI 1959; WEIDMANN and CERLETTI 1960). Psilocin behaved like psilocybin, both theamines having an opposite effect on the patellar reflex of that of 5-HT (WEIDMANN and CERLETTI 1959, 1960). When electrophoretically applied on spinal interneurones in the cat, psilocybin and psilocin were inactive (CURTIS et al. 1961).

III. Bufotenine

WEIDMANN and CERLETTI (1959, 1960) reported that bufotenine (20—50 μg/kg i.v.) like 5-HT, temporarily inhibited the patellar reflex in the spinal cat. The esterification of bufotenine with phosphoric acid diminished the activity. CURTIS et al. (1955) failed to observe any change in the poly- and monosynaptic reflexes recorded from the ventral roots in spinal cats, following close intrarterial injection of bufotenine.

IV. Other indolealkylamines

WEIDMANN and CERLETTI (1960) reported that the i.v. injection of 4-HT (20—50 μg/kg), 4-hydroxy-N-methyltryptamine (20—50 μg/kg), 5-hydroxy-α-methyltryptamine (10—20 μg/kg), 5-hydroxy-α-methyl-N,N-dimethyltryptamine (20—50 μg/kg) and 5-hydroxy-β-methyltryptamine (> 50 μg/kg) depressed the patellar reflex in spinal cats, while the injection of 4-hydroxy-N-ethyltryptamine (20—50 μg/kg), 4-hydroxy-N,N-diethyltryptamine (20—50 μg/kg), 4-hydroxy-α-methyltryptamine (> 50 μg/kg), 4-hydroxy-α-methyl-N,N-dimethyltryptamine (> 50 μg/kg) and 4-hydroxy-β-hydroxy-N,N-dimethyltryptamine (> 50 μg/kg) enhanced it. The derivatives of N,N-dimethyltryptamine with the following groups — Br, CH_3, OCH_3, $OCH_2C_6H_5$, $OCOC_6H_5$ or $OCONHCH_3$ — in 4 position behaved like psilocybin, i.e. enhanced the patellar reflex.

Vane et al. (1961) reported that tryptamine, DL-α-methyltryptamine, DL-α-ethyltryptamine, N,N-dimethyltryptamine and DL-5-methoxy-α-methyltryptamine (0.5 mg/kg i.v.) facilitated both the patellar and the flexor reflex in spinal or chloralosed cats. They were more potent when injected into a spinal artery. Tryptamine at larger doses abolished the flexor reflex. Matthews et al. (1961), on the contrary, did not observe any change in mono- and poly-synaptic reflexes (dorsal root-ventral root preparation) after 5 and 10 mg/kg i.v. of DL-α-ethyltryptamine in spinal cats. 15 mg/kg gave a slight depression of the polysynaptic discharges.

Tryptamine and α-methyltryptamine were electrophoretically applied to interneurones located in the lumbar segments of cat spinal cord. They failed to affect the responses of the neurones to dorsal root stimulation, even when they were released by currents as large as 150—200 nA. (Curtis 1962).

To sum up: psilocybin, bufotenine and a number of other indolealkylamines affect the spinal reflexes. There is no proof that the synaptic transmission in the spinal cord is affected by the amines; furthermore any attempt to demonstrate any action on the interneurones was negative in outcome. It is conceivable that, as 5-HT, other indolealkylamines may affect the spinal reflexes changing the pattern of the nervous inflow to the spinal cord. The study of the reflexes after barrage of the impulses arising from the structures located in the injection circuit will throw some light on the mechanism of the action of the amines.

I. Effects on single cellular elements

The data reported in the preceeding sections have been obtained in the course of experiments in which 5-HT reached the CNS through the blood stream, or was applied into the cerebral ventricles or to the exposed cerebral cortex. This section will deal with: I. experiments in which the action of 5-HT and other indolealkylamines on neurones was examined introducing the amines into the extracellular environment and observing the effects upon extracellularly recorded action potentials, and II. experiments in which the action of the amines on brain cells (glia cells and neurones) was studied applying the drug to cultures of nervous tissue "in vitro".

I. Single neurones

Curtis and Koizumi (1961) studied the effect of 5-HT on the spontaneous and synaptically evoked discharges of neurones of mesencephalic reticular formation and inferior colliculi in decerebrated cats. The extracellular fluid surrounding neurones was reached by multibarrel electrodes. One of the barrels contained a saturated aqueous solution of 5-HT creatinine sulphate. The amine was ejected as a cation from the electrode orifice electrophoretically by currents of about 50—250 nA. No change in cellular activity was observed during and after 5-HT application.

The suspicion that 5-HT might not reach a local concentration sufficient to cause a detectable effect is weakened by the fact that amine applied by lower currents (10 to 40 nA) to neurones of the lateral geniculate nucleus greatly affected the synaptic firing of the neurones (Curtis and Davis 1962). 5-HT blocked the post-synaptic spike potentials produced by stimulation of the optic nerve fibres (orthodromic excitation) but failed to influence those produced by stimulation of the optic radiation fibres (antidromic excitation) and those induced by L-glutamic acid electrophoretically applied. When the effect of 5-HT upon potentials generated by groups of cells (focal potentials) was studied, the observations made upon single cells were confirmed. The amine depressed the orthodromically evoked post-synaptic focal potentials, but was without action upon those generated antidromically. The rate of recovery of the focal potentials, following a depression of 40 to 60% was in the order of 15 to 60 sec. These results suggest that 5-HT does not alter the membrane conductance of geniculate neurones; the amine could affect synaptic transmission by reducing the release of transmitter from the presynaptic terminals or by blocking subsynaptic receptors specialised for combination with the excitatory transmitter.

The amines listed below had the same effect as 5-HT upon the synaptic transmission in the lateral geniculate nucleus of the cat: tryptamine, 4-HT, 6-HT, 7-HT, 4-methoxytryptamine, 5-methoxytryptamine, N,N-dimethyltryptamine, N,N-diethyltryptamine, psilocin, bufotenine, psilocybin, 6-hydroxy-N,N-dimethyltryptamine, 7-hydroxy-N,N-dimethyltryptamine, α-methyltryptamine, 4-hydroxy-α-methyltryptamine, 1-benzyl-2-methyl-5-methoxytryptamine (BAS), melatonin and 4,α-dimethyltryptamine. All the drugs, except 4-HT and 7-HT, were less potent that 5-HT, melatonin and 4,α-dimethyltryptamine being the less active (CURTIS and DAVIS 1962).

KRNJEVIĆ and PHILLIS (1963a) studied the action of 5-HT on single neurones of the cerebral cortex of the cat. The amine at low concentrations lowered the frequency of discharge evoked by the application of glutamate ions as well as that evoked by afferent impulses (orthodromic excitation), but failed to prevent the antidromic excitation of single Betz cells. At relatively higher concentrations it produced paroxysmal cellular discharge, lasting for several seconds after the application and followed by depression of the responsiveness.

KRNJEVIĆ and PHILLIS (1963b) tested a number of derivatives of tryptamine and tryptophan on cortical neurones. 4-HT, 6-HT, tryptamine and tryptophan were as active as 5-HT in inhibiting cellular activity, whereas 7-HT was less active. 4-HTP, 5-HTP, 6-HTP were less active than the parents amines. N,N-dimethyltryptamine, N,N-diethyltryptamine, 4-methoxytryptamine, 5-methoxytryptamine, psilocin, bufotenine, 6-hydroxy-N,N-dimethyltryptamine were less active than 5-HT. Melatonin had no clear action.

CURTIS et al. (1961) applied 5-HT into the environment of interneurones in cat spinal cord. The amine failed to affect the neuronic activity even though it was applied by currents as large as 200 nA. Tryptamine and α-methyltryptamine behaved like 5-HT (CURTIS 1962).

Although the same technique was employed in the above reported investigations, the results differ in important respects. This lends to believe that neurones in various regions of the brain respond in different way to indolealkylamines.

II. Brain cells cultured "in vitro"

BENITEZ et al. (1955) first described 5-HT effect on brain cells of humans and rats cultured "in vitro". 5-HT (2 μg/ml) transformed the spontaneous pulsating movements of the oligodendroglia into a tetanic contraction but was inactive on astrocytes which do not contract spontaneously. NAKAZAWA (1960) confirmed these observations. GEIGER (1957, 1958) briefly reported that 5-HT changed the structure of cortical neurones cultured "in vitro". At concentrations of 0.5—2 μg/ml it induced repetitive pumping movements of the perikarya of the neurones and changed the pattern of movements in the synaptic areas.

J. Effects on sympathetic ganglia

I. 5-Hydroxytryptamine

Robertson (1954) was the first to observe that 5-HT stimulated the perfused superior cervical ganglion of the cat, but it was Trendelenburg (1956) (see also Trendelenburg 1958, 1959) who extensively studied the ganglionic effects of the amine. 5-HT was injected through the lingual artery into the blood supply of the superior cervical ganglion. As the external and internal carotid arteries were occluded, the drug reached the ganglion but not the nictitating membrane. Preganglionic fibres were sectioned. In the most sensitive preparations 0.43 to 4.3 μg of 5-HT caused a contraction of the nictitating membrane. The ganglionic origin of the effect was definitively demonstrated by the fact that it was abolished crushing the ganglion. Hexamethonium failed to block the 5-HT stimulating action; nicotine and cocaine blocked it. Low doses (0.0043—0.43 μg) which did not stimulate the ganglion by themselves, potentiated the response of the nictitating membrane to submaximal preganglionic stimulation: 0.43 μg increased the response to nearly maximum height. Even in large quantities (43 μg) the amine never produced ganglionic paralysis, nor did it potentiate the response to supramaximal stimulation of the preganglionic fibres. The potentiating action was not due to a lowering of the threshold of the fibres to electrical stimulation. This was demonstrated in experiments in which the cervical sympathetic chain was split longitudinally and a portion of the preganglionic fibres was stimulated supramaximally. Under these conditions 5-HT had the usual effect. The potentiation of ganglionic transmission was reduced by cocaine but not by atropine and mepyramine. In experiments on the perfused ganglion Trendelenburg (1956b) demonstrated that 5-HT also potentiated the ganglionic response to acetylcholine, nicotine, carbaminoylcholine, choline and potassium chloride. Vasoconstriction was not responsible for the potentiation. The potentiation of the ganglionic transmission was smaller on the perfused ganglion than on that with normal blood supply. 5-HT differed from nicotine and nicotine-like substances in that it potentiated and never depressed the ganglionic response to preganglionic and to chemical stimulation. Histamine and pilocarpine behaved as 5-HT.

Recording the action potentials of the postganglionic fibres, Trendelenburg (1957) demonstrated that 5-HT (like pilocarpine and histamine) potentiated the ganglionic transmission of the impulses travelling on both groups of fibres of the cervical sympathetic chain: the fast-conducting S 1 fibres innervating the nictitating membrane and the slow-conducting S 2 fibres innervating the blood vessels. 5-HT (4.3—8.6 μg) was injected into the central end of the cut lingual artery during occlusion of the external carotid artery. Potentiation occurred 5—15 sec after injection and lasted for about 2—3 min. 5-HT did not once inhibit the ganglionic transmission nor affect the postganglionic response to a supramaximal preganglionic stimulation.

Gertner and Romano (1961) reported that 5-HT had only a slight potentiating effect on the ganglionic transmission through the perfused superior cervical ganglion of the cat. This is in agreement with Trendelenburg's observation that the perfused ganglion is much less sensitive to 5-HT than that with normal blood supply.

Hertzler (1961a, 1961b) studied the effect of 5-HT on the transmission through the stellate ganglion of the rat. The isolated ganglion with a portion of the preganglionic thoracic sympathetic chain and of the postganglionic cervical sympathetic trunk were maintained in a moist chamber and intermittently immersed in physiological saline. 5-HT was added to the saline. Postganglionic responses evoked by submaximal preganglionic stimulation were recorded. 5-HT (0.21—27 μg/ml) applied for 30 sec increased the amplitude and lowered the threshold of the postganglionic response. After contact with a 2.15 μg/ml solution the effect lasted about 20 min. The response of S 2 slow-conducting fibres was more sensitive to 5-HT than that of S 1 fast-conducting fibres. In the intact animal 5-HT (8.6 μg i.v.) had the same effect.

Gyermek and Bindler (1962b) studied the effects of the amine on the inferior mesenteric ganglion of the cat. Postganglionic activity was recorded from small bundles of fibres or single fibres of hypogastric nerve cut distally to the ganglion. Close intrarterial injection of 5-HT (0.54—4.3 μg) produced a marked increase in postganglionic spontaneous activity, leaving the preganglionic activity unchanged. The effect started 3—7 sec after the injection. Preganglionic fibres transection knocked out spontaneous postganglionic activity, but not that produced by 5-HT.

To sum up: 5-HT stimulates the sympathetic ganglia and causes facilitation of ganglionic transmission. The stimulating action of 5-HT is abolished by depolarizing agents but not by competitive ganglionic blocking substances. This leads us to conclude that the amine acts on the ganglionic cells and that it attaches itself to receptors different from the acetylcholine receptors.

Gertner et al. (1957, 1959) dosed the 5-HT content of the effluent from the perfused superior cervical ganglion of cats. No measurable 5-HT was present in the perfusate at rest and during preganglionic supramaximal stimulation. The addition of iproniazid (200 μg/ml) to the perfusion liquid resulted in an immediate but partial depression of ganglionic transmission (nictitating membrane recording). No 5-HT appeared in the perfusate up to 2 hrs from the beginning of the perfusion with iproniazid. After this period 5-HT began to appear and continued to do so until the end of the experiment (at the rate of about 10 mμ/min). Preganglionic stimulation did not accelerate the appearance of 5-HT nor did it increase its content in the effluent. The addition of iproniazid (200 μg/ml) and 5-HTP (22 μg/ml) to the perfusion liquid resulted in a depression of transmission equal to that produced by iproniazid alone. In this case the 5-HT appeared in the perfusate within 5 min from the beginning of the perfusion, but preganglionic stimulation did not influence the 5-HT release. The significance of these findings must await further experimental results. It must be noted that the use of supramaximal stimuli precluded the possibility to evidentiate a facilitation of the transmission by 5-HT released.

II. Other indolealkylamines

Gyermek and Bindler (1962a) (see also Gyermek et al. 1962) evaluated the ganglionic stimulating activity of a series of indolealkylamines on the inferior mesenteric ganglion of cats; the discharge of the postganglionic fibres was taken as a index of the stimulating actions. The drugs were injected into the cannulated inferior mesenteric artery close to the ganglion. 5-HT (0.43—2.15 μg), N-methyl-5-hydroxytryptamine (2.5—10 μg), bufotenine hydrogenoxalate (1.2—5 μg), bufotenine iodide (0.3—1.2 μg), N,N-dimethyltryptamine (80—1000 μg) and N,N,N-trimethyltryptamine iodide (5—10 μg) caused stimulation of the ganglion. The action of N-methyl-5-hydroxytryptamine, as that of 5-HT, was blocked by 5-hydroxy-3-indoleacetamidine (an anti-5-HT) but not by hexamethonium. The action of the other amines was blocked by hexamethonium. The substances listed below were inactive up to doses of 80 μg or more: N,N-dipropyl-5-hydroxytryptamine HCl, 5-hydroxy-α-methyltryptamine dipicrate, 5-methoxy-α-methyltryptamine HCl, 5-methoxytryptamine, 5-benzyloxygramine, tryptamine HCl, N,N-diethyltryptamine ,N,N-dipropyltryptamine HCl, 6-hydroxytryptamine creatinine sulfate, N,N-dimethyl-6-hydroxytryptamine, 7-benzyloxygramine, 4-hydroxytryptamine oxalate, psilocin, pislocybin.

GERTNER and ROMANO (1961) briefly reported that tryptamine (10 μg/ml) blocked the ganglionic transmission when perfused through the superior cervical ganglion of the cat. MATTHEWS et al. (1961) (see also MATTHEWS 1963) observed that DL-α-ethyltryptamine, a MAO inhibitor, intravenously injected at a dose of 10 mg/kg caused partial depression of the transmission through the inferior mesenteric ganglion in the cat. Recovery occurred in 60—80 min.

K. Effects on cutaneous sensory endings

The action of 5-HT on the peripheral receptors must be particularly borne in mind in interpreting the central effects of the amine peripherally administered. In fact, amine injected into the blood flow does not reach the CNS only but also peripheral structures with central connections. It is quite likely that afferent discharges play an important part in producing some of the 5-HT central effects (for instance, the block of the patellar reflex). The data concerning the effects of indolealkylamines on the cutaneous nerve endings will be reviewed in this section. The effects on the receptors of the autonomic nervous system will be reviewed in other chapters.

ARMSTRONG et al. (1952, 1953) observed that the application of 5-HT creatinine sulphate in low concentrations (down to 10 ng/ml) to the exposed base of the cantharidin blister in humans caused pain. Tryptamine had the same action as 5-HT, but was more than 10 times weaker than the latter. Tryptophan was inactive even when applied in concentrations up to $1:10^3$. The pain arose 10 to 45 sec after 5-HT or tryptamine application and lasted for a few minutes. Further applications developped a refractory state. Using the blister area technique ARMSTRONG (1958) defined the pain-producing potency of a number of tryptamines. 4-HT, 6-HT and bufotenine were respectively 5,25 and 50 times less active than 5-HT. α,α-dimethyltryptamine, β,β-dimethyltryptamine and N,N-dimethyltryptamine were more than 2000 times weaker than 5-HT. ARMSTRONG et al. (1957) demonstrated that 5-HT could not be identified with the substance responsible for the pain-producing activity of plasma and exudates.

There is convincing evidence that, in animals, close arterial injection of 5-HT activates cutaneous afferent fibres. DOUGLAS and RITCHIE (1957) reported that 5-HT (20 μg) intrarterially injected evoked a powerful long-lasting discharge in non-myelinated afferent fibres in the cat's saphenous nerve. The same fibres also fired in response to gentle mechanical stimulation of the skin and to acetylcholine injection. FJALLBRANT and IGGO (1959, 1961) found that 5-HT (4—40 μg) injected into the saphenous artery evoked an intermittent low-frequency discharge in some fibres in a multifibre-strand of cat's saphenous nerve. The discharge began within 20 sec and persisted for several minutes. Recording from single-unit preparations the AA. found that the amine (1—20 μg) excited myelinated fibres from slow adapting mechanoreceptors and non-myelinated fibres from mechano- and thermo-receptors. Following 5-HT injection the response of the units to mechanical and thermal stimuli passed through a cycle of enhancement and depression. VAN GELDER (1962) injected 5-HT close arterially into a region of the skin of the rat and recorded impulses from a small branch of the saphenous nerve innervating the perfused area. The normal blood supply to the skin was blocked during the injection and during the 2 min which followed it. 5-HT

(1.8 μg) produced a sensory discharge lasting at least 2 min and intervalled by a brief period of diminished activity.

GUZMAN et al. (1962) injected 5-HT into many arteries in dogs and cats under chloralose anaesthesia. The injections were made through catheters tied into collaterals. The injection of 10.7—86 μg of 5-HT into each one of the arteries listed below evoked vocalisation, hypertension and hyperpnea, three symptoms considered by the AA. suggestive of pain: femoral, brachial, splenic, gastric, superior mesenteric and pulmonar. The amine appeared to be less effective when injected into the left coronary artery and into the internal carotid artery. Sectioning the sciatic nerve prevented the response to femoral injection.

From the data reported above it is clear that 5-HT when applied to the exposed base of a blister in humans or when intrarterially injected in animals evokes afferent discharges. The minutiae of the mechanism whereby 5-HT excites sensory nerve endings remain open to investigation.

L. Effects on the central nervous system of lower animals

HORRIDGE (1961) studied the action of 5-HT on the transmission through the cerebral ganglion of the clam *Mya*. A single shock to the cerebro-visceral connective (preganglionic stimulation) evoked a burst of impulses in the postganglionic fibres (anterior pallial nerve) which brought about the retraction of the mantle and the closure of the shell. 5-HT applied to the ganglion at a concentration of 10^{-5} caused a spontaneous discharge of motor impulses and slightly prolonged the duration of the burst induced by preganglionic stimulation.

GERSCHENFELD and TAUC (1961) studied the action of 5-HT on the neurons of the abdominal ganglion of the mollusc *Aplysia depilans* (intracellular recordings). The amine, added to the perfusion fluid, excited the cells having only inhibitory input (H cells) as well as those having only excitatory input (D cells), but its effects was more than ten times more intense on the latter. Furthermore the amine inhibited the H cells by exciting inhibitory interneurons.

SALÀNKI (1963) reported that the application of 5-HT on the cerebral ganglia of fresh-water mussels (*Anodonta cygnea*) provoked at 10^{-6} the relaxation of the contracted posterior adductor muscle and at 10^{-5}—10^{-4} a long lasting activity of the muscle.

References

ANDERSON, E. G., and D. D. BONNYCASTLE: A study of the central depressant action of pentobarbital, phenobarbital and diethyl ether in relationship to increases in brain 5-hydroxytryptamine. J. Pharmacol. exp. Ther. **130**, 138—143 (1960).

— S. D. MARKOWITZ and D. D. BONNYCASTLE: Brain 5-hydroxytryptamine and anticonvulsant activity. J. Pharmacol. exp. Ther. **136**, 179—182 (1962).

ANGELUCCI, L.: Experiments with perfused frog's spinal cord. Brit. J. Pharmacol. **11**, 161—170 (1956).

ANTONELLI, A. R., G. BERTACCINI and P. MANTEGAZZINI: Relationship between mesencephalic-hypothalamic concentration of 5-hydroxytryptamine and cortical electrical activity of cats. J. Neurochem. **8**, 157—158 (1961).

APRISON, M. H., and C. B. FERSTER: Behavioral effects of 5-hydroxytryptophan. Experientia (Basel) **16**, 159—160 (1960).

— — Neurochemical correlates of behavior. I. Quantitative measurement of the behavioral effects of the serotonin precursor, 5-hydroxytryptophan. J. Pharmacol. exp. Ther. **131**, 100—107 (1961a).

— — Neurochemical correlates of behavior. II. Correlation of brain monoamine oxidase activity with behavioral changes after iproniazid and 5-hydroxytryptophan administration. J. Neurochem. **6**, 350—357 (1961b).

Aprison, M, H., and C, B. Ferster: Serotonin and behavior. In: J. Wortis, Ed., Recent advances in biological psychiatry, vol. III, p. 151—162. New York: Grune & Stratton 1961 (c).
Armstrong, D.: The relation of pain production by tryptamines to their chemical structure. In: G. P. Lewis, Ed., 5-Hydroxytryptamine, p. 140—142. London: Pergamon Press 1958.
— R. M. L. Dry, C. A. Keele, and J. W. Markham: Pain-producing actions of tryptamine and 5-hydroxytryptamine. J. Physiol. (Lond.) **117**, 70—71 P (1952).
— — — — Observations on chemical excitants of cutaneous pain in man. J. Physiol. (Lond.) **120**, 326—351 (1953).
— J. B. Jepson, C. A. Keele and J. W. Stewart: Pain-producing substance in human inflammatory exsudates and plasma. J. Physiol. (Lond.) **135**, 350—357 (1957).
Aston, R., and H. Cullumbine: The effects of combinations of ataraxics with hypnotics, LSD and iproniazid in the mouse. Arch. int. Pharmacodyn. **126**, 219—227 (1960).
Barucci, M.: Some effects of 5-hydroxytryptamine on the central nervous system of the rabbit [in Italian]. Rass. Studi psichiat. **45**, 893—898 (1956).
Batini, C., G. Moruzzi, M. Palestini, G. F. Rossi and A. Zanchetti: Effects of complete pontine transection on the sleep-wakefulness rhythm: the midpontine pretrigeminal preparation. Arch. ital. Biol. **97**, 1—12 (1959a).
— M. Palestini, G. F. Rossi and A. Zanchetti: EEG activation patterns in the midpontine pretrigeminal cat following sensory deafferentation. Arch. ital. Biol. **97**, 26—32 (1959b).
Benitez, H. H., M. R. Murray and D. W. Wooley: Effects of serotonin and its antagonists upon oligodendroglia in vitro. Anat. Rec. **121**, 446 (1955).
Bertaccini, G.: Effect of convulsant treatment on the 5-hydroxytryptamine content of brain and other tissues of the rat. J. Neurochem. **4**, 217—222 (1959).
Bianchi, C.: Reserpine and serotonin in experimental convulsions. Nature (Lond.) **179**, 202—203 (1957).
Bogdanski, D. F., H. Weissbach and S. Udenfriend: Pharmacological effects of 5-hydroxytryptophan, the precursor of serotonin. Fed. Proc. **15**, 402 (1956).
— — — Pharmacological studies with the serotonin precursor, 5-hydroxytryptophan. J. Pharmacol. exp. Ther. **122**, 182—194 (1958).
Bonamini, F., and L. Garello: Catatonia induced by injection of 5-hydroxytryptamine into the cisterna magna of dogs [in Italian]. Sist. nerv. 8, 157—166 (1956).
Bonnycastle, D. D., M. F. Bonnycastle, and E. G. Anderson: The effect of a number of central depressant drugs upon brain 5-hydroxytryptamine levels in the rat. J. Pharmacol. exp. Ther. **135**, 17—20 (1962).
— N. J. Giarman, and M. K. Paasonen: Anticonvulsant compounds and 5-hydroxytryptamine in rat brain. Brit. J. Pharmacol. **12**, 228—231 (1957).
— M. K. Paasonen, and N. J. Giarman: Diphenylhydantoin and brain-levels of 5-hydroxytryptamine. Nature (Lond.) **178**, 990—991 (1956).
Bradley, P. B.: The effects of 5-hydroxytryptamine on the electrical activity of the brain and on behaviour in the conscious cat. In: G. P. Lewis, Ed., 5-Hydroxytryptamine, p. 214—220. London: Pergamon Press 1958.
—, and A. J. Hance: The effects of intraventricular injections of d-lysergic acid diethylamide (LSD 25) and 5-hydroxytryptamine (serotonin) on the electrical activity of the brain of the conscious cat. J. Physiol. (Lond.) **132**, 50—51 P (1956).
Brodey, J. F., W. G. Steiner, and H. E. Himwich: An electrographic study of psilocin and 4-methyl-α-methyl tryptamine (MP-809). J. Pharmacol. exp. Ther. **140**, 8—18 (1963).
Brodie, B. A., P. A. Shore, and A. Pletscher: Serotonin-releasing activity limited to rauwolfia alkaloids with tranquilizing action. Science **123**, 992—993 (1956).
Brown, B. B.: Lysergic acid diethylamide antagonism of certain drugs. Ann. N.Y. Acad. Sci. **66**, 677—685 (1957).
— CNS drugs actions and interactions in mice. Arch. int. Pharmacodyn. **128**, 391—414 (1960).
Brunaud, M., et G. Siou: Action de substances psycotropes, chez le rat, sur un état d'agressivité provoquée. In: P. B. Bradley, P. Deniker and C. Radouco-Thomas, Ed., Neuropsychopharmacology, p. 282—286. London: Elsevier 1959.
Carels, G.: Dépression par la sérotonine de la transmission monosynaptique dans la moelle isolée de la grenouille. Arch. int. Pharmacodyn. **138**, 326—328 (1962).
Cerletti, A.: Pharmacology of psilocybin. In: P. B. Bradley, P. Deniker and C. Radouco-Thomas, Ed., Neuro-psychopharmacology, p. 291—294. London: Elsevier 1959.
Chessin, M., B. Dubnick, E. R. Kramer, and C. C. Scott: Modifications of pharmacology of reserpine and serotonin by iproniazid. Fed. Proc. **15**, 409 (1956).
— E. R. Kramer, and C. C. Scott: Modifications of the pharmacology of reserpine and serotonin by iproniazid. J. Pharmacol. exp. Ther. **199**, 453—460 (1957).

CHRISTIANSEN, A., R. BAUM, and P. N. WITT: Changes in spider webs brought about by mescaline, psilocybin and an increase in body weight. J. Pharmacol. exp. Ther. **136**, 31—37 (1962).
COOK, L., and E. WEIDLEY: Behavioral effects of some psychopharmacological agents. Ann. N.Y. Acad. Sci. **66**, 740—752 (1957).
CORDEAU, J. P., and M. MANCIA: Effect of unilateral chronic lesions of the midbrain on the electrocortical activity of the cat. Arch. ital. Biol. **96**, 374—399 (1958).
CORREALE, P.: Action of 5-HT on blood pressure and clotting-time in rats [in Italian]. Arch. int. Pharmacodyn. **97**, 106—114 (1954).
COSTA, E., and M. H. APRISON: Fate of serotonin perfused through an isolated brain with intact nervous connections. Fed. Proc. **16**, 25 (1957).
— — Distribution of intracarotidly injected serotonin in the brain. Amer. J. Physiol. **192**, 95—100 (1958).
— W. A. HIMWICH, and H. E. HIMWICH: Effects of injections of bufotenine into various arterial sites. In: P. B. BRADLEY, P. DENIKER and C. RADOUCO-THOMAS, Ed., Neuropsychopharmacology, p. 299—303. London: Elsevier 1959.
— G. R. PSCHEIDT, W. G. VAN METER, and H. E. HIMWICH: Brain concentrations of biogenic amines and EEG patterns of rabbits. J. Pharmacol. exp. Ther. **130**, 81—88 (1960).
—, and F. RINALDI: Biochemical and electroencefalographic changes in the brain of rabbits injected with 5-hydroxytryptophan (influence of chlorpromazine premedication). Amer. J. Physiol. **194**, 214—220 (1958).
CREPAX, P., and F. INFANTELLINA: Action of 5-hydroxytryptamine on the electrical activity of the cerebral cortex of the cat [in Italian]. Arch. Sci. biol. **41**, 207—232 (1957).
CRONHEIM, G. E., and J. T. GOURZIS: Cardiovascular and behavioral effects of serotonin and related substances in dogs without and with reserpine premedication. J. Pharmacol. exp. Ther. **130**, 444—449 (1960).
CROSSLAND, J., and J. MITCHELL: The effect on the electrical activity of the cerebellum of a substance present in cerebellar extracts. J. Physiol. (Lond.) **132**, 391—405 (1956).
CURTIS, D. R.: Action of 3-hydroxytryptamine and some tryptamine derivatives on spinal neurones. Nature (Lond.) **194**, 292 (1962).
—, and R. DAVIS: Pharmacological studies upon neurones of the lateral geniculate nucleus of the cat. Brit. J. Pharmacol. **18**, 217—246 (1962).
— J. C. ECCLES, and R. M. ECCLES: Pharmacological studies on reflexes. Amer. J. Physiol. **183**, 606 (1955).
—, and K. KOIZUMI: Chemical transmitter substances in brain stem of cat. J. Neurophysiol. **24**, 80—90 (1961).
—, J. W. PHILLIS, and J. C. WATKINS: Cholinergic and non cholinergic transmission in the mammalian spinal cord. J. Physiol. (Lond.) **158**, 296—323 (1961).
DANDIYA, P. C., and E. A. SELLERS: Mechanism of the hypnosis prolongation action of 5-hydroxytryptamine and some sympathomimetic amines. Arch. int. Pharmacodyn. **130**, 32—41 (1961).
DELAY, J., J. THUILLIER, H. NAKAJIMA et M. C. DURANDIN: Action de la psilocybine sur le comportement des souris normales et des souris I.D.P.N. Comparaison avec les monoéthylamide (LAE) et diéthylamide (LSD 25) de l'acide lysergique. C. R. Soc. Biol. (Paris) **153**, 244—248 (1959).
DOLCE, G., and L. GARELLO: The catalepsy induced by serotonin in rana esculenta: experimental technique [in Italian]. Boll. Soc. ital. Biol. sper. **32**, 441—443 (1956).
DOMER, F. R., and W. FELDBERG: Tremor in cats: the effect of administration of drugs into the cerebral ventricles. Brit. J. Pharmacol. **15**, 578—587 (1960a).
— — Abolition and initiation of tremor by drugs injected into the cerebral ventricles of cats. J. Physiol. (Lond.) **154**, 34—35P (1960b).
—, and V. G. LONGO: Effect of 5-hydroxytryptophan on the cerebral electrical activity of the rabbit. Arch. int. Pharmacodyn. **136**, 204—218 (1962).
DOUGLAS, W. W., and J. M. RITCHIE: Discharges in non-medullated afferent fibres in the cat's saphenous nerve in response to touch and to drugs. J. Physiol. (Lond.) **139**, 9—10P (1957).
EDERY, H., and G. SCHATZBERG-PORATH: Some biological properties of two fluoro-derivatives of tryptamine. Experientia (Basel) **16**, 200 (1960).
EFRON, D. H., and G. L. GESSA: Failure of ethanol and barbiturates to alter brain monoamine content. Arch. int. Pharmacodyn. **142**, 111—116 (1963).
ERSPAMER, V.: 5-HT and 5-methoxytryptamine. Toxicity. Action on the diuresis, the blood pressure and some smooth muscles [in Italian]. Ric. Sci. **22**, 694—702 (1952).
— Recent research in the field of 5-hydroxytryptamine and related indolealkylamines. In: E. JUCKER, Ed., Progress in drug research, vol. III, p. 151—367. Basel: Birkhäuser 1961.

ERSPAMER, V., A. GLÄSSER, and P. MANTEGAZZINI: Pharmacological actions of 4-hydroxytryptamine and 4-hydroxytryptophan. Experientia (Basel) **16**, 505—506 (1960a).
— — B. M. NOBILI, and C. PASINI: The fate of 4-hydroxytryptophan in the rat organism. Experientia (Basel) **16**, 506—507 (1960b).
— — C. PASINI, and G. STOPPANI: In vitro decarboxylation of tryptophans by mammalian decarboxylase. Nature (Lond.) **189**, 483 (1961).
EVARTS, E. V.: Some effects of bufotenine and lysergic acid diethylamide on the monkey. Neurol. Psychiat. (Chic.) **75**, 49—53 (1956).
— Effects of a series of indoles on synaptic transmission in the lateral geniculate nucleus of the cat. In: H. H. PENNES, Ed., Psychopharmacology, p. 173—194. New Uork: A Hoeber-Harper Book 1958.
— W. LANDAU, W. FREYGANG, and W. H. MARSHALL: Some effects of lysergic acid diethylamide and bufotenine on electrical activity in the cat's visual system. Amer. J. Physiol. **182**, 594—598 (1955).
FABING, H. D., and J. R. HAWKINS: Intravenous bufotenine injection in human being. Science **123**, 886—887 (1956).
FASTIER, F. N.: Prolongation of hypnosis by 5-hydroxytryptamine (serotonin). Experientia (Basel) **12**, 351 (1956).
— R. N. SPEDEN, and H. WAAL: Prolongation of chloral hydrate sleeping time by 5-hydroxytryptamine and by certain other drugs. Brit. J. Pharmacol. **12**, 251—256 (1957).
FELDBERG, W., and S. L. SHERWOOD: Injection of drugs into the lateral ventricle of the cat. J. Physiol. (Lond.) **123**, 148—167 (1954).
FERRO MILONE, F., and G. GOMIRATO: Observations on the effects of serotonin (5-HT) on the central nervous system [in Italian]. G. Psichiat. Neuropat. **3**, 449—462 (1956).
FJALLBRANT, N., and A. IGGO: Cutaneous afferent fibres and pain-producing chemicals. J. Physiol. (Lond.) **145**, 28—29 P (1959).
— — The effect of histamine, 5-hydroxytryptamine and acetylcholine on cutaneous afferent fibres. J. Physiol. (Lond.) **156**, 578—590 (1961).
FLORU, R., A. COSTIN, M. STERESCU-VOLANSCHI, and I. OPESCU: On the central interrelation between the serotonin and some psychotropic drugs. XXI. Internat. Congr. of Physiological Sciences. Abstr. Comm. 94—95 (1959).
FÖLDES, I., u. E. KOMLÓS: Die Wirkung von Serotonin (5-hydroxytryptamin) auf den Gasstoffwechsel und die Körpertemperaturen weißer Ratten. Arch. int. Pharmacodyn. **120**, 121—129 (1959).
FORNAROLI, P., and M. KOLLER: 5-Hydroxytryptamine and barbiturates [in Italian]. Farmaco, Ed. sci. **9**, 546—547 (1954).
— — Interaction between 5-hydroxytryptamine and CNS depressants [in Italian]. Farmaco, Ed. sci. **10**, 984—990 (1955).
FRESIA, P., E. GENOVESE, R. KATO, and L. VALZELLI: 5-HT content in different areas of the CNS in dogs after electroshock [in Italian]. Boll. Soc. ital. Biol. sper. **34**, 1397—1399 (1958).
— — A. VALSECCHI, and L. VALZELLI: Changes of 5-HT content in the brain of different animal species after electroshock [in Italian]. Boll. Soc. ital. Biol. sper. **33**, 888—890 (1957).
FUHRMAN, F. A.: The effect of body temperature on the duration of barbiturate anesthesia in mice. Science **105**, 387—388 (1957).
GADDUM, J. H., and M. VOGT: Some central actions of 5-hydroxytryptamine and various antagonists. Brit. J. Pharmacol. **11**, 175—179 (1956).
GAL, E. M., and P. A. DREWES: Levels of serotonin during convulsions and the effect of reserpine. Nature (Lond.) **189**, 234 (1961).
GANGLOFF, H., and M. MONNIER: Topic action of reserpine, serotonin and chlorpromazine on the unanesthetized rabbit's brain. Helv. physiol. pharmacol. Acta **15**, 83—104 (1957).
GARATTINI, S., R. KATO, L. LAMESTA, and L. VALZELLI: Electroshock, brain serotonin and barbiturate narcosis. Experientia (Basel) **16**, 156—157 (1960).
— A. VALSECCHI, and L. VALZELLI: Variations in encephalic and intestinal serotonin after electrical shock. Experientia (Basel) **13**, 330—331 (1957).
—, and L. VALZELLI: Serotonin and electroshock. In: S. GARATTINI and V. GHETTI, Ed., Psycotropic drugs, p. 428—436. London: Elsevier 1957.
GEIGER, R. S.: Effect of lysergic acid diethylamide (LSD 25) and serotonin on adult cortical brain cells in tissue culture. Fed. Proc. **16**, 44—54 (1957).
— Effects of metrazol, serotonin and schizophrenic sera on adult brain cells in tissue culture (motion picture). Fed. Proc. **17**, 52 (1958).
GELDER, N. M. VAN: Effects on sensory nerves of injecting 5-hydroxytryptamine into the skin. Nature (London) **195**, 185—186 (1962).

GERSCHENFELD, G. A., and L. TAUC: Pharmacological specificities of neurones in an elementary central nervous system. Nature (Lond.) **189**, 924—925 (1961).
GERTNER, S. B., M. K. PAASONEN, and N. J. GIARMAN: Presence of 5-hydroxytryptamine (serotonin) in perfusate from sympathetic ganglia. Fed. Proc. **16**, 299 (1957).
— — — Studies concerning the presence of 5-hydroxytryptamine (serotonin) in the perfusate from the superior cervical ganglion. J. Pharmacol. exp. Ther. **127**, 268—275 (1959).
—, and A. ROMANO: The effect of various amines on transmission through the superior cervical ganglion of the cat. Biochem. Pharmacol. 8, 19—20 (1961).
GESSNER, P. K., P. A. KHAIRALLAH, W. M. MCISAAC, and I. H. PAGE: The relationship between the metabolic fate and pharmacological actions of serotonin, bufotenine and psilocybin. J. Pharmacol. exp. Ther. **130**, 126—133 (1960).
— W. M. MCISAAC, and I. H. PAGE: Pharmacological actions of some methoxyindolealkylamines. Nature (Lond.) **190**, 179—180 (1961).
GLÄSSER, A., and P. MANTEGAZZINI: Action of 5-hydroxytryptamine and 5-hydroxytryptophan on the cortical electrical activity of the midpontine pretrigeminal preparation of the cat with and without mesencephalic hemisection. Arch. ital. Biol. **98**, 351—366 (1960a).
— — The action of 5-hydroxytryptamine and 5-hydroxytryptophan on the cortical electrical activity of the "midpontine pretrigeminal preparation". Experientia (Basel) **16**, 213—214 (1960b).
GRANDJEAN, E., u. K. BÄTTIG: Die Wirkung von Serotonin (5-Hydroxytryptamin) auf eine konditionierte Fluchtreaktion der Ratte. Helv. physiol. pharmacol. Acta **15**, 366—370 (1957).
GREEN, H., and J. L. SAWYER: Correlation of tryptamine-induced convulsions in rats with brain tryptamine concentration. Proc. Soc. exp. Biol. (N.Y.) **104**, 153—155 (1960).
GREIG, M. E., P. H. SEAY, and W. A. FREYBURGER: The pharmacology of etryptamine. J. Neuropsychiat. **1**, S131—S135 (1961).
— R. A. WALK, and A. J. GIBBONS: The effect of three tryptamine derivatives on serotonin metabolism in vitro and in vivo. J. Pharmacol. exp. Ther. **127**, 110—115 (1959).
GURSEY, D., and R. E. OLSON: Depression of serotonin and norepinephrine levels in brain stem of rabbit by ethanol. Proc. Soc. exp. Biol. (N.Y.) **104**, 280—281 (1960).
GUTH, P. S., and M. A. SPIRTES: An interaction in the central nervous system between serotonin and lysergic acid derivatives. In: P. B. BRADLEY, P. DENIKER, and C. RADOUCO-THOMAS, Ed., Neuro-psychopharmacology, p. 319—323. London: Elsevier 1959.
GUZMAN, F., C. BRAUN, and R. K. S. LIM: Visceral pain and pseudoaffective response to intra-arterial injection of bradykinin and other algesic agents. Arch. int. Pharmacodyn. **136**, 353—384 (1962).
GYERMEK, L., and E. BINDLER: Action of indole alkylamines and amidines on the inferior mesenteric ganglion of the cat. J. Pharmacol. exp. Ther. **138**, 159—164 (1962a).
— — Blockade of the ganglionic stimulant action of 5-hydroxytryptamine. J. Pharmacol. exp. Ther. **135**, 344—348 (1962b).
— — and L. SOFFER: Ganglionic stimulation by ω-N-methyl-derivatives of 5-hydroxytryptamine (5-HT). Fed. Proc. **21**, 335 (1962).
HÄGGENDAL, J., and M. LINDQVIST: Ineffectiveness of ethanol on noradrenaline, dopamine or 5-hydroxytryptamine levels in brain. Acta pharmacol. (Kbh.) **18**, 278—280 (1961).
HALEY, T. J.: 5-Hydroxytryptamine antagonism by lysergic acid diethylamide after intracerebral injection in conscious mice. J. Amer. pharm. Ass., sci. Ed. **47**, 428—430 (1957a).
— Intracerebral injection of psychotomimetic and psychotherapentic drugs into conscious mice. Acta pharmacol. (Kbh.) **13**, 107—112 (1957b).
HART, E. R., T. W. LANGFITT, and A. S. MARAZZI: Influence of certain indoles on cerebral synaptic transmission. Fed. Proc. **15**, 88 (1956).
HARVEY, J. A., A. HELLER, and R. Y. MOORE: The effect of unilateral and bilateral medial forebrain bundle lesions on brain serotonin. J. Pharmacol. exp. Ther. **140**, 103—110 (1963).
HELLER, A., J. A. HARVEY, and R. Y. MOORE: A demonstration of fall in brain serotonin following central nervous system lesions in the rat. Biochem. Pharmacol. **11**, 859—866 (1962).
HERTZLER, E. C.: 5-Hydroxytryptamine and transmission in sympathetic ganglia. Brit. J. Pharmacol. **17**, 406—413 (1961a).
— Serotonin and transmission in sympathetic ganglia. Fed. Proc. **20**, 317 (1961b).
HESS, S. M., and W. DOEPFNER: Behavioral effects and brain amine content in rats. Arch. int. Pharmacodyn. **134**, 89—99 (1961).
— B. G. REDFIELD, and S. UDENFRIEND: The effect of monoamine oxidase inhibitors and tryptophan on the tryptamine content of animal tissues and urine. J. Pharmacol. exp. Ther. **127**, 178—181 (1959).

HIMWICH, H. E., E. COSTA, and W. A. HIMWICH: Behavioral responses of dogs to bufotenine reaching the brain either by the vertebral artery or internal carotid artery. Fed. Proc. **18**, 402 (1959).

HIMWICH, W. A., and E. COSTA: Behavioral changes associated with changes in concentrations of brain serotonin. Fed. Proc. **19**, 838—845 (1960).

HOFFMAN, R. A.: Effect of and interaction between tranquillizers, serotonin and lysergic acid diethylmamide on the body temperature of pigeons. Amer. J. Physiol. **195**, 751—754 (1958a).

— Temperature response of the rat to action and interaction of chlorpromazine, reserpine and serotonin. Amer. J. Physiol. **195**, 755—758 (1958b).

— Influence of adrenal gland on hypothermic response of the rat to chlorpromazine, reserpine and serotonin. Amer. J. Physiol. **196**, 876—880 (1959).

HOLTZ, P., H. BALZER, E. WESTERMANN u. E. WEZLER: Beeinflussung der Evipannarcose durch Reserpin, Iproniazid und biogene Amine. Naunyn-Schmiedebergs Arch. exp. Path. Pharmak. **231**, 333—348 (1957).

HORITA, A., and J. H. GOGERTY: The pyretogenic effect of 5-hydroxytryptophan and its comparison with that of LSD. J. Pharmacol. exp. Ther. **122**, 195—200 (1958).

HORRIDGE, G. A.: The centrally determined sequence of impulses initiated from a ganglion in the clam Mya. J. Physiol. (Lond.) **155**, 320—336 (1961).

JOHN, E. R., B. M. WENZEL, and R. D. TSCHIRGI: Differential effects on various conditioned responses in cats caused by intraventricular and intramuscular injections of reserpine and other substances. J. Pharmacol. exp. Ther. **123**, 193—205 (1958).

JORI, A., A. VALSECCHI, and L. VALZELLI: Convulsions and cerebral serotonin [in Italian]. Boll. Soc. Ital. Biol. sper. **33**, 921—924 (1957).

KÄRKI, N. T., and M. K. PAASONEN: The influence of iproniazid and raunescine on the penetration of 5-hydroxytryptamine into brain tissue from circulation. Acta pharmacol. (Kbh.) **16**, 20—27 (1959).

KATO, R.: An antagonism between 3-4-dioxyphenylalanine (DOPA) and 5-hydroxytryptophan (5-HTP). Experientia (Basel) **15**, 324—325 (1959).

—, and L. VALZELLI: Cortisone and cerebral 5-hydroxytryptamine [in Italian]. Boll. Soc. ital. Biol. sper. **34**, 1402—1404 (1958).

KISSEL, J. W., and E. F. DOMINO: Effects of serotonin, adrenergic, and adrenergic blocking agents on spinal cord reflexes before and after blood pressure stabilization. J. Pharmacol. exp. Ther. **119**, 157—158 (1957).

— — The effects of some possible neurohumoral agents on spinal cord reflexes. J. Pharmacol. exp. Ther. **125**, 168—177 (1959).

KOBINGER, W.: Beeinflussung der Cardiazolkrampfschwelle durch veränderten 5-Hydroxytryptamingehalt des Zentralnervensystems Naunyn-Schmiedebergs Arch. exp. Path. Pharmak. **233**, 559—566 (1958).

— Differentiation between the sedative actions of 5-hydroxytryptamine and reserpine in mice by means of two stimulating substances. Acta pharmacol. (Kbh.) **14**, 138—147 (1958a).

KOELLA, W. P., J. R. SMYTHIES, and D. M. BULL: Factors involved in the effect of serotonin on the evoked electrocortical potentials. Science **129**, 1231 (1959).

— — — and C. K. LEVY: Physiological fractionation of the effect of serotonin on evoked potentials. Amer. J. Physiol. **198**, 205—212 (1960).

KRNJEVIĆ, K., and J. W. PHILLIS: Iontophoretic studies of neurones in the mammalian cerebral cortex. J. Physiol. (Lond.) **165**, 274—304 (1963a).

— — Actions of certain amines on cerebral cortical neurones. Brit. J. Pharmacol. **20**, 471—490 (1963b).

LESSIN, A. W., and M. W. PARKES: The relation between sedation and body temperature in the mouse. Brit. J. Pharmacol. **12**, 245—250 (1957).

— — The effects of reserpine and other agents upon leptazol convulsions in mice. Brit. J. Pharmacol. **14**, 108—111 (1959).

LÉVY, J., et E. MICHEL-BER: Hypothèse sur les mécanismes d'action des inhibiteurs de la monoamino-oxidase au niveau du système nerveux central. C. R. Acad. Sci. (Paris) **250**, 415—417 (1960).

LEWIS, G. P.: 5-Hydroxytryptamine. J. Pharm. Pharmacol. **10**, 529—540 (1958).

LITTLE, K. D., V. DI STEFANO, and D. E. LEARY: LSD and serotonin effects on spinal reflexes in the cat. J. Pharmacol. exp. Ther. **119**, 161 (1957).

MAHLER, D. J., and F. L. HUMOLLER: Effect of lysergic acid diethylamide and bufotenine on performance of trained rats. Proc. Soc. exp. Biol. (N.Y.) **102**, 697—701 (1959).

— — and A. L. DUNN: Comparison of effects of lysergic acid diethylamide and bufotenine on performance of trained rats. Fed. Proc. **17**, 103 (1958).

MALCOLM, J. L.: Effects of 5-hydroxytryptamine on evoked responses in the brain of anesthetized cats. In: G. P. LEWIS, Ed., 5-Hydroxytryptamine, p. 221—228. London: Pergamon Press 1958.
MANTEGAZZINI, P.: Observations on the action of high doses of 5-HT on the CNS [in Italian]. Boll. Soc. ital. Biol. sper. **32**, 839—841 (1956).
— Action of 5-hydroxytryptamine on the cortical activity of the "encéphale isolé" of the cat. Naturwissenschaften **44**, 41 (1957a).
— Action de la 5-hydroxytryptamine (entéramine) et de l'acéthylcholine sur le tracé electroencéphalographique du chat. Arch. int. Pharmacodyn. **112**, 199—211 (1957b).
— G. DEFFENU, and A. R. ANTONIELLI: Effects of 5-HT on the patellar reflex in spinal cats. (To be published.)
MARAZZI, A. S.: The effects of certain drugs on cerebral synapses. Ann. N.Y. Acad. Sci. **66**, 496—507 (1957).
—, and E. R. HART: Relationship of hallucinogens to adrenergic cerebral neurohumors. Science **121**, 365—367 (1955).
MATTHEWS, R. J.: Further studies on the neuropharmacological effects of etryptamine acetate. Arch. int. Pharmacodyn. **142**, 90—110 (1963).
— B. J. ROBERTS, and P. K. ADKINS: Neuropharmacological studies on dl-alpha-ethyltryptamine acetate. J. Neuropsychiat. **1**, S 151—S 158 (1961).
MAXWELL, D. R.: The activity of some adrenaline antagonists in tests for tranquillizing action. In: P. B. BRADLEY, P. DENIKER, and C. RADOUCO-THOMAS ,Ed. ,Neuropsychopharmacology, p. 365—373. London: Elsevier 1959.
MCISAAC, W. M., and I. H. PAGE: The metabolism of serotonin (5-hydroxytryptamine). J. biol. Chem. **234**, 858—864 (1959).
METER, W. G. VAN, G. F. AYALA, E. COSTA, and H. E. HIMWICH: Biochemical and EEG changes caused by α-methyltryptamine (IT 403). Fed. Proc. **19**, 265 (1960).
MONNIER, M.: Action de la psilocybine sur le cerveau du lapin. Experientia (Basel) **15**, 321—323 (1959).
— Actions électro-physiologiques des stimulants du système nerveux central. I. Système adrénergiques, cholinergiques et neurohumeurs sérotoniques. Arch. int. Pharmacodyn. **124**, 281—301 (1960).
—, et P. KRUPP: Classification électro-physiologiques des stimulants du système nerveux central. II. Action des stimulants hallucinogènes, psychotoniques, analeptiques sur les mécanismes d'éveil e de détente. Arch. int. Pharmacodyn. **127**, 337—360 (1960).
—, et R. TISSOT: Action de la réserpine et de ses médiateurs (5-hydroxytryptophan-sérotonine et DOPA-noradrénaline) sur le comportement et le cerveau du lapin. Helv. physiol. pharmacol. Acta **16**, 255—267 (1958).
NAKAZAWA, T.: Effects of chlorpromazine and serotinin on the contractility of oligodendrocytes. Tex. Rep. Biol. Med. **18**, 52—65 (1960).
OCHS, S., H. BOOKER, and M. H. APRISON: Serotonin on direct cortical responses. Physiologist **3**, 121 (1960).
OLDS, J., and M. E. OLDS: Positive reinforcement produced by stimulating hypothalamus with iproniazid and other compounds. Science **127**, 1175—1176 (1958).
PENNEFATHER, J. N., and R. H. THORP: The influence of β-tetrahydronaphthylamine and a derivative on the central effects of 5-hydroxytryptamine, reserpine and iproniazid. J. Pharm. Pharmacol. **10**, 249—252 (1958).
PIERRE, R., et J. CAHN: Essais d'anesthésie prolongée par la 5-hydroxytryptamine. C. R. Soc. Biol. (Paris) **149**, 1406—1407 (1955).
PLETSCHER, A., F. A. STEINER, and A. VOELKER: Discussion. In: P. B. BRADLEY, P. DENIKER, and C. RADOUCO-THOMAS, Ed., Neuropsychopharmacology, p. 138—144. London: Elsevier 1959.
PROCKOP, D. J., P. A. SHORE, and B. B. BRODIE: Anticonvulsant properties of monoamine oxidase inhibitors. Ann. N.Y. Acad. Sci. **80**, 643—650 (1959).
RECH, R. H., and E. F. DOMINO: Effects of various drugs on activity of the neuronally isolated cerebral cortex. Exp. Neurol **2**, 364—378 (1960).
REVZIN, A. M., and E. COSTA: The effects of monoamine oxidase substrates on evoked potentials. Fed. Proc. **19**, 265 (1960).
ROBERTSON, P. A.: Potentiation of 5-hydroxytryptamine by the true-cholinesterase inhibitor 284C51. J. Physiol. (Lond.) **125**, 37P—38P (1954).
RODRIGUEZ, J. M., E. R. HART, and A. S. MARAZZI: The lack of carotid sinus or carotid body effect in cerebral synaptic inhibition by serotonin. Fed. Proc. **20**, 333 (1961).
ROTHBALLER, A. B.: The effect of phenylephrine, methamphetamine, cocaine and serotonin upon the adrenaline-sensitive component of the reticular activating system. Electroenceph. clin. Neurophysiol. **9**, 409—417 (1957).

SACCHI, U., F. BONAMINI, G. DOLCE, and L. GARELLO: LSD 25 and catalepsy induced by 5-hydroxytryptamine in the dog [in Italian]. Boll. Soc. ital. Biol. sper. **31**, 665—667 (1955a).
— — L. GARELLO, and G. DOLCE: Studies on the cataleptic action of 5-HT injected into the cerebral ventricles or into the arachnoid spaces in the dog [in Italian]. Boll. Soc. ital. Biol. sper. **32**, 179—182 (1956).
— L. GARELLO, G. DOLCE, and F. BONAMINI: Cataleptic action of 5-hydroxytryptamine injected into the cisterna magna of the dog [in Italian]. Boll. Soc. ital. Biol. sper. **31**, 663—665 (1955b).
—, and G. GIANNIOTTI: Inhibition of motor activity after 5-HT in "Carassius auratus" [in Italian]. Boll. Soc. ital. Biol. sper. **32**, 175—177 (1956a).
— — LSD 25—5-HT antagonism on the motility of "Carassius auratus" [in Italian]. Boll. Soc. ital. Biol. sper. **32**, 177—179 (1956b).
SAÏ-HALÂSZ, A., and E. ENDRÖCZY: The effect of tryptamine derivatives on the behaviour of dogs during brain-stem stimulation. In: P. B. BRADLEY, P. DENIKER, and C. RADOUCO-THOMAS, Ed., Neuro-psychopharmacology, p. 405—407. London: Elsevier 1959.
SALÁNKI, J.: The effect of serotonin and catecholamines on the nervous control of periodic activity in fresh-water mussel (*Anodonta cygnea*). Comp. Biochem. Physiol. **8**, 163—171 (1963).
SALMOIRAGHI, G. C., and I. H. PAGE: Effects of LSD 25, BOL 148, bufotenine, mescaline and ibogaine on the potentiation of hexobarbital hypnosis produced by serotonin and reserpine. J. Pharmacol. exp. Ther. **120**, 20—25 (1957).
— — and J. W. MCCUBBIN: Cardiovascular and respiratory response to intravenous serotonin in rats. J. Pharmacol. exp. Ther. **118**, 477—481 (1956a).
— L. SOLLERO, and I. H. PAGE: Blockade by brom-lysergic-acid-diethylamide (BOL) of the potentiating action of serotonin and reserpine on hexobarbital hypnosis. J. Pharmacol. exp. Ther. **117**, 166—168 (1956b).
SCHAIN, R. J.: Some effects of a monoamine oxidase inhibitor upon changes produced by centrally administered amines. Brit. J. Pharmacol. **17**, 261—266 (1961).
SCHANBERG, S. M., and N. J. GIARMAN: Drug-induced alterations in the subcellular distribution of 5-hydroxytryptamine in rat's brain. Biochem. Pharmacol. **11**, 187—194 (1962).
SCHAUMANN, W.: Beeinflussung der analgetischen Wirkung des Morphins durch Reserpin. Naunyn-Schmiedebergs Arch. exp. Path. Pharmak. **235**, 1—9 (1958).
SCHWARZ, B. E., K. G. WAKIM, R. G. BLICKFORD, and F. R. LICHTENFELD: Behavioral and electroencephalographic effects of hallucinogenic drugs. Arch. Neurol. Psychiat. (Chic.) **75**, 83—90 (1956).
SHORE, P. A., A. PLETSCHER, E. G. TOMICH, A. CARLSSON, R. KUNTZMAN, and B. B. BRODIE: Role of brain serotonin in reserpine action. Ann. N.Y. Acad. Sci. **66**, 609—615 (1957).
— S. L. SILVER, and B. B. BRODIE: Interaction of serotonin and lysergic acid diethylamide (LSD) in the central nervous system. Experientia (Basel) **11**, 272—273 (1955).
SIGG, E. B., G. CAPRIO, and J. A. SCHNEIDER: Synergism of amines and antagonism of reserpine to morphine analgesia. Proc. Soc. exp. Biol. (N.Y.) **97**, 97—100 (1958).
SLATER, I. H., K. H. DAVIS, D. E. LEARY, and E. S. BOYD: The action of serotonin and lysergic acid diethylamide on spinal reflexes. J. Pharmacol. exp. Ther. **113**, 48—49 (1955).
SMYTHIES, J. R., D. M. BULL, and W. P. KOELLA: Factors involved in the effect of serotonin on the evoked electrocortical potentials. Fed. Proc. **18**, 446 (1959).
STEIN, L.: Self-selected brain stimulation reward thresholds modified by drugs. Fed. Proc. **19**, 264 (1960).
STEINER, F. A., B. PELLMONT u. A. PLETSCHER: Beeinflussung einer bedingten Fluchtreaktion durch Harmala-Alkaloide und Monoamine-Vorstufen. Helv. physiol. pharmacol. Acta **17**, C 43—C 44 (1959).
STEFANO, V. DI, D. E. LEARY, and I. FELDMAN: Effect of serotonin on cerebral oxygen tension and evoked electrical activity in the cerebral cortex. Fed. Proc. **15**, 417—418 (1956).
TAESCHLER, M., and A. CERLETTI: Some observations on the interaction of reserpine and LSD. J. Pharmacol. exp. Ther. **120**, 179—183 (1957).
TEDESCHI, D. H., R. E. TEDESCHI, and E. J. FELLOWS: The effects of tryptamine on the central nervous system, including pharmacological procedure for the evaluation of iproniazid-like drugs. J. Pharmacol. exp. Ther. **126**, 223—232 (1959a).
— — — A pharmacological procedure for the evaluation in vivo of inhibitors of monoaminooxidase; observations on the neuropharmacological effects of tryptamine hydrochloride. Fed. Proc. **18**, 450 (1959b).
TOH, C. C.: Effects of temperature on the 5-hydroxytryptamine (serotonin) content of the tissues. J. Physiol. (Lond.) **151**, 410—415 (1960).
TRENDELENBURG, U.: The action of 5-hydroxytryptamine on the nictitating membrane and on the superior cervical ganglion of the cat. Brit. J. Pharmacol. **11**, 74—80 (1956a).

TRENDELENBURG, U.: Modification of transmission through the superior cervical ganglion of the cat. J. Physiol. (Lond.) **132**, 529—541 (1956b).
— The action of histamine, pilocarpine and 5-hydroxytryptamine on transmission through the superior cervical ganglion. J. Physiol. (Lond.) **135**, 66—72 (1957).
— The 5-hydroxytryptamine receptors of the cat's superior cervical ganglion. In: G. P. LEWIS, Ed., 5-Hydroxytryptamine, p. 136—139. London: Pergamon Press 1958.
— Non-nicotinic ganglion-stimulating substances. Fed. Proc. **18**, 1001—1005 (1959).
TRIPOD, J., A. STUDER et R. MEIER: Essai de différenciation expérimentale d'une série d'inhibiteurs du système nerveux central. Arch. int. Pharmacodyn. **112**, 319—341 (1957).
TROUT, D. L.: Interaction of serotonin and lysergic acid diethylamide in the siamese fighting fish. J. Pharmacol. exp. Ther. **121**, 130—135 (1957).
UDENFRIEND, S., D. F. BOGDANSKI, and H. WEISSBACH: Increase in tissue serotonin by administration of its precursor, 5-hydroxytryptophan. Fed. Proc. **15**, 493 (1956).
— H. WEISSBACH, and D. F. BOGDANSKI: Increase in tissue serotonin following administration of its precursor 5-hydroxytryptophan. J. biol. Chem. **224**, 803—810 (1957a).
— — — Biochemical findings relating to the action of serotonin. Ann. N.Y. Acad. Sci. **66**, 602—608 (1957d).
VANE, J. R., H. O. J. COLLIER, S. J. CORNE, E. MARLEY, and P. B. BRADLEY: Tryptamine receptors in the central nervous system. Nature (Lond.) **191**, 1068—1069 (1961).
WEIDMANN, H., u. A. CERLETTI: Die Wirkung von D-Lysergsäure-diethylamid und 5-Hydroxytryptamin (Serotonin) auf spinale Reflexe der Katze. Helv. physiol. pharmacol. Acta **15**, 376—383 (1957).
— — Zur pharmakodynamischen Differenzierung der 4-Oxyindolderivate Psilocybin und Psilocin im Vergleich mit 5-Oxyindolkörpern (Serotonin, Bufotenin). Helv. physiol. pharmacol. Acta **17**, C 46—C 48 (1959).
— — Studies on psilocybin and related compounds. I. Communication: Structure/activity relationship of oxyindole derivatives with regard to their effect on the knee jerk of spinal cats. Helv. physiol. pharmacol. Acta **18**, 174—182 (1960).
— M. TAESCHLER u. H. KONZETT: Zur Pharmakologie von Psilocybin, einem Wirkstoff aus Psilocybe mexicana Heim. Experientia (Basel) **14**, 378—379 (1958).
WEST, G. B.: Studies on 5-hydroxytryptamine and 5-hydroxytryptophan. J. Pharm. Pharmacol. **10**, 92T—97T (1958).
WINTER, C. A., and L. FLATAKER: Effects of lysergic acid diethylamide upon performance of trained rats. Proc. Soc. exp. Biol. (N.Y.) **92**, 285—289 (1956).
WITT, P. N.: Effects of psilocybin on web-building behavior of spiders. Pharmacologist **2**, 63 (1960).
WOOLEY, D. W., and E. SHAW: A biochemical and pharmacological suggestion about certain mental disorders. Proc. nat. Acad. Sci. (Wash.) **40**, 228—231 (1954).
YEN, C. Y., R. L. STANGER, and N. MILLMAN: Ataractic suppression of isolation-induced aggressive behavior. Arch. int. Pharmacodyn. **123**, 179—185 (1959).
ZANOWIAK, P., and M. J. RODMAN: A study of LSD-Serotonin central interaction. J. Amer. pharm. Ass., sci. Ed. **48**, 165—168 (1959).

Chapter 10

Drugs which antagonize 5-hydroxytryptamine and related indolealkylamines

By

Laszlo Gyermek

A. Introduction

Many concepts of drug antagonism in the last few decades have undergone significant change but certain principles of the subject are basically the same as laid down in the fundamental work of Clark published in 1937 on the pages of this handbook. The phenomenon of drug antagonism is certainly a complex one in which many factors participate. Its nature depends not only on the type of drug but more significantly on the biological system employed. In addition to the living substrate, the factors of its environment and time patterns are of major importance. Considering these factors the problem of drugs which antagonize 5-hydroxytryptamine (5-HT) and related indolealkylamines must also be realized as being rather complex. One escape from this problem would be to follow the trend of radical simplification which neglects most of the factors mentioned and deal with the drug-substrate complex on a purely mechanistic basis. This approach is certainly useful for the understanding of some basic underlying mechanisms which are biophysical and physicochemical in nature and are indeed more amenable to scientific analysis. Confronted, however, by a system such as the mammalian organism the solving of problems of drug antagonisms on a theoretical basis is nearly impossible. Accordingly, two trends of extremes are detected in the works published on this subject: First, the theoretical, with analyzing efforts, and a second, the practical aimed at data collecting. The first approach so far has not been able to develop new drugs, the second was often criticized as being nonscientific. The only possible way today is still to compromise and utilize both approaches. The information offered on these pages is a result of such a compromise utilizing the results of both types of research approaches.

With the discovery of 5-HT the biologic significance of indole compounds became more widely recognized than before. Many efforts were made to explore the pharmacological actions of 5-HT and to describe its possible physiologic and pathologic role. The necessity of developing compounds which would counteract its biologic actions also emerged as a logical sequence of this research. When 5-HT as a widely occurring and potent biogenic amine was added about fifteen years ago to the list of known, important biogenic amines it was soon subjected to a focus of interest which was perhaps not fully deserved, e.g., it turned out that besides the potent pharmacologic actions of exogenous 5-HT the endogenous amine in mammals does not play many well defined physiologic or pathologic roles. With the increasing knowledge of the biochemistry of indole compounds, indolealkylamines other than 5-HT are emerging, the existence of which may eventually better explain certain biologic phenomena, so far believed but not proved to be connected to 5-HT. This possibility was rightly recognized by the editor by proposing the above title for this review. The aim of the reviewer is therefore to cover, besides the overwhelming percentage of work on 5-HT antagonists, a few studies dealing with the problem of pharmacological antagonism of other indolealkylamines. At the present the major importance of antagonists of 5-HT seems to be that some of them may be used as indispensible tools for defining and analyzing the physiologic and pathologic role of biogenic amines of the indole type. With the expanding horizon of the biologically active catechol and indole amines there is a necessity of finding selective, thus characteristic antagonists for every biologically occurring indole compound. Antagonists which fulfill the rigid criteria of a high degree of selectivity thus can be of immense value in analyzing the effects of indolealkylamines in various organisms. The significance of the existing classes of 5-HT antagonists as possible therapeutic agents in view of their shortcomings certainly seems to be of lesser importance today.

It is recognized that the gap between the hypothetical function of drug receptor systems and the behavior of drugs in living systems is very marked. Drug antagonism throughout this review will be considered more or less in the classical sense as being a phenomenon which results from an interference between two drug molecules exercised on a specific biological substrate which usually is called the receptor. By the adoption of the commonly known drug-receptor complex theory as the basis of drug antagonisms certain assumptions have to be made without really knowing whether these are correct or not. Thus it must be presumed that the antagonist:

1. Will not react directly with the agonist,
2. May or may not act irreversibly with the receptor,
3. Will not interfere with the formation or metabolism of the agent,
4. Will interfere only with the biologic reactions mediated by the agonist,
5. Will perform the above role by substituting the agonist at a certain step of biologic reactions related to an effect.

The specific nature of the antagonist is based on the assumption that it has similar or higher affinity to a certain receptor or stage of biochemical reaction than the agonist; however, unlike in the case of agonist the process of interacting of the antagonist with the receptor does not produce a pharmacologic response (i.e. there is a lack of intrinsic activity with the antagonist). The antagonist, however, may also exhibit the characteristics of an intrinsic activity which is masked by inhibitory properties. In this latter case the interaction of the drug, antagonist, and receptor is becoming more complex and could not be characterized easily by the conventional competitive drug-antagonist receptor complex interactions of the first kinetic-order type.

B. Reviews of antagonists of 5-HT

Reviews available to date on this topic offer information collected with somewhat different aims since the subject was approached by the individual reviewers from different angles. The general pharmacologic and cardiovascular aspects were first summarized ten years ago by GADDUM (1954) followed by another survey by the same reviewer dealing mostly with studies on isolated organs (GADDUM 1957). The most extensively investigated group of compounds, the lysergic acid derivatives, where the main focus of interest of comprehensive articles by GADDUM (1957a) and ROTHLIN (1957a, b). The structure and action of indole derivatives was the major subject of a shorter review by VERCELLONE and ASERO (1954). A most detailed pharmacological description of 5-HT by PAGE (1958) also devoted a full chapter to its antagonists. The first comprehensive compilation of data and literature with chemical classification of the antagonists, a detailed description of their pharmacological actions on isolated organs and cardiovascular preparations was published by JACOB (1960) with over one hundred references. The main emphasis was placed on summarizing all the available information on testing methods, classes of compounds with quantitative data on potency, nature of 5-HT receptors and possible clinical uses in the review of GYERMEK (1961a). This was followed by another survey introducing the class of peripheral neurotropic antagonists of 5-HT (GYERMEK 1962b). Pharmacological as well as clinical aspects were outlined in the recent less extensive summarizing articles of the subject (CHODERA 1962, MARTINEZ 1962 and NEUMAN 1963).

C. General description of 5-HT antagonists

The classes of agents which are recognized so far as being potent in antagonizing one or another characteristic pharmacological action of 5-HT are entirely different in their chemical structure. In contrast, compounds which block the peripheral actions of some other biogenic amines, e.g., ACH possess certain defined common molecular features. Furthermore, some structural characteristics of ACH blocking molecules can be associated to a specific blockade at certain different cholinergic (i.e., ganglionic, postganglionic-parasympathetic or neuromuscular) receptor types. The great majority of potent antihistaminic agents belongs to a single structural type, i.e., substituted ethylene diamines. These examples illustrate the close association of a certain agonist molecule to a given type of antagonist. In contrast, blocking agents of 5-HT belong to several different classes of organic compounds (i.e., indolealkylamines, lysergic acid derivatives, beta haloethylamines and phenothiazines). The structural difference of the blocking molecules of 5-HT is somewhat similar to the situation existing with antagonists of epinephrine. These also are highly different chemically (i.e., benzodioxanes, beta haloethylamines, substituted ethylenediamines, ergot and yohimbin type alkaloids). The existence of several classes of blocking agents to sympathomimetic amines and 5-HT and the fact that often members of the same class of blocking agents are effective against both types of biogenic amines raises the suspicion that the tissue receptor types of these amines might also be somewhat similar. More direct evidence of this came from recent studies of MANSOUR (1957) and INNES (1962) suggesting that d-amphetamine, a member of the sympathomimetic amine family acts on 5-HT receptors and thus should rather be considered to be a 5-HT-like agent. Overlap in the substrate specificity of the metabolizing enzymes of these two classes of agents (i.e., amino oxidase and O-methyl transferase) also suggests that 5-HT and sympathomimetic amines may be fairly close in their basic mechanism of action. The catalyzing effect of 5-HT on the formation of cyclic adenosine 3,5-phosphate and on phosphorylase activity which is similar to the effect of epinephrine in other organisms (MANSOUR et al. 1960) seems to substantiate this hypothesis further. Predominant tissue specificity to one type of amine does not necessarily contradict the theory that basic biochemical mechanisms in the action of sympathomimetic amines and indolealkylamines might be similar in nature.

1. Relations of 5-HT and its antagonists to the "specific" tissue receptors

Characterization of those reactive sites of the tissues which exhibit specific sensitivity to 5-HT has been attempted in several studies. Although a variety of methods and approaches utilizing structural analogues, antagonists and inactivating enzyme-inhibitors of 5-HT were employed, it is still difficult to draw uniform conclusions with regard to the exact nature of 5-HT receptors. Some of the findings are of importance to the extent that they offer guidance for future investigations. It seems justified to accept the existence of tissue receptors which preferentially react to 5-HT as compared to other physiologically occurring neurohumoral agents. Studies comparing the pharmacological actions of 5-HT in vivo and in vitro with that of agents like epinephrine, norepinephrine, ACH, histamine and some physiologically potent peptides indicated that 5-HT has characteristic actions which differ from those of the compounds mentioned (Page 1954, 1958; Meier et al. 1957; Brownlee and Johnson 1963). The difference in the actions of these agents as detected in the whole animal, however, only suggests but does not prove the possible existence of pharmacologically distinct receptor sites for 5-HT. The question as to whether a certain proportion of receptors sensitive to neurotransmitter substances other than 5-HT might be activated indirectly by this agent is pertinent and certainly cannot be answered by ultilizing the whole animal as the test object. The question which arises concerning the selectivity of tissue receptors to 5-HT as compared to other indolealkylamines will be discussed later. For the reasons mentioned most of the studies investigating the nature of 5-HT receptors employed two isolated organs: the rat uterus and the guinea pig ileum. In an isolated organ system which often responds to various drugs with a simple and fairly uniform reaction (i.e., contraction, change in firing rate, secretory response) differentiation of the hypothetical receptor sites can usually be obtained by the application of "selective" blocking agents. This approach was therefore extensively used in the exploration of 5-HT receptors.

It was first shown on the guinea pig ileum that 5-HT acts on receptors distinguishable from those which are stimulated by ACH, histamine and bradykinin (Rocha e Silva et al. 1953). Systematic testing of a number of antagonists on different organs (Gaddum and Hameed 1954) led to the assumption that even in a simple, isolated organ like a piece of gut more than one 5-HT receptor type exists. Successively Gaddum and Picarelli (1957) found that the guinea pig ileum contains two types of 5-HT receptors. Differentiation between them was made by the use of different antagonists. The findings indicated that one type of receptor of the guinea pig ileum is a nervous element (*M*-receptor) which is stimulated by 5-HT and blocked by morphine, methadone, atropine and cocaine. The other receptor is located in the smooth muscle (*D* receptors). This latter one, besides being sensitive to 5-HT, was blocked by dibenzyline, ergot derivatives, and 5-benzyl-oxygramine. While in the case of the "*D*" receptors a more "direct" action on the contractile elements is assumed, the tissue response to stimulation of "*M*" receptors may involve more intermediate steps, including the participation of other receptors. That indeed this may be the case is indicated by more recent studies on 5-HT receptors in the guinea pig ileum:

A. Harry (1963) found that the circular muscle strip of the gut shows a characteristic high degree of potentiation of ACH and 5-HT effects by inhibition of cholinesterase. Results obtained on this preparation by using blocking agents of different types, e.g., procaine, botulinum toxin, morphine and hemicholinium demonstrated that 5-HT acts on the intramural nerve plexuses by releasing ACH which was suggested earlier (Moussatche and Pereira 1957). Histamine and nicotine produce a similar release of ACH but the receptor types in the nervous network of the gut for these latter two stimulants are different. The existence of specific sites for 5-HT is indicated by:

1. Specific desensitization by 5-HT itself,
2. Lack of blockade by hexamethonium.

These findings in the autonomic nervous plexus of the guinea pig ileum seem to parallel those indicating the specific nature of 5-HT receptors in autonomic ganglia (TRENDELENBURG 1956, 1957; BINDLER and GYERMEK 1961; GYERMEK and BINDLER 1962; GYERMEK, BINDLER, and SOFFER 1962).

B. BROWNLEE and JOHNSON (1963) in a detailed study using six different stimulant agents (ACH, 5-HT, nicotine, DMPP, choline phenyl ether and histamine) twelve antagonists and a cholinesterase inhibitor showed that most of these compounds including 5-HT were antagonized by hyoscine and procaine and potentiated by a cholinesterase inhibiting agent. The effect of 5-HT was not blocked by its typical antagonists: LSD, BOL and phenoxybenamine or by competitively acting ganglionic blocking agents. It was, however, suppressed by using larger doses of 5-HT and by depolarization type of blocking agents (e.g., nicotine and DMPP). These findings indicate beyond doubt that 5-HT acts on specific receptors at the intramural parasympathetic ganglion cells. These receptors are not "nicotine-like" and also differ from the muscular "D" receptors. Recent results concerning the action of LSD and BOL on the "*D*" receptors and the specific nature of the morphine effect on the "*M*" receptors are somewhat in conflict with those of GADDUM and PICARELLI (1957) and of BARLOW and KHAN (1959). It was found in these studies that lysergic acid derivatives are fairly ineffective on the guinea pig ileum and that morphine has much less specific effect on this test organ than suggested before (LEWIS 1960). Nevertheless the theory of more than one 5-HT receptor in the guinea pig ileum cannot be rejected on the above grounds. In view of the results obtained by morphine on sympathetic ganglia (TRENDELENBURG 1957, GYERMEK and BINDLER 1962) showing a definite and a specific blocking action of this agent against 5-HT it must be concluded that the difficulty in separating the various sites of actions of 5-HT on the guinea pig ileum lies in the technical problems inherent in a nerve-muscle preparation.

C. DAY and VANE (1963) also found that on the guinea pig ileum 5-HT falls into the same category of stimulant agents as nicotine, TMA, and DMPP which elicit their action through stimulating cholinergic nerve fibers. Their findings with morphine and phenoxybenzamine indicate the difficulty of achieving a distinct separation of "*M*" and "*D*" receptors in the guinea pig ileum as both receptors contribute to the observed response. An attempt was made to clarify to what extent these different receptors are responsible for the normal response of the ileum. The results showed that the nervous receptors makes the major contribution to the effect.

Based on the findings outlined above, it seems that in organs like the guinea pig ileum where both nervous and smooth muscle elements sensitive to 5-HT occur, a "priming" effect on nervous receptors is necessary to obtain a high degree of responsiveness of muscular receptors. Similar observations were made on the dog bladder (GYERMEK 1962) where two effects of 5-HT could be distinguished: a fast twitch-like response which was due to the stimulation of nervous receptors, and a slower contraction as a result of stimulating the muscular receptors. The second component was more dependent on the first one than vice versa.

On the heart of the mollusc, Venus mescenaria 5-HT has two distinct effects. In low concentrations it produces a positive inotropic effect whereas in high concentration there is a large increase of the muscle tone (GREENBERG 1961). BOL is effective only in antagonizing the effect of moderate doses. Large doses of 5-HT produce tachyphylaxis and also render the tissue insensitive to related indolealkylamines, e.g., tryptamine and bufotenin. These indole compounds and 5-hydroxy-α-methyltryptamine in turn desensitize the heart to 5-HT. The desensitizing effect is not shown against catecholamines, indicating common receptor sites for the above indole compounds differing from those of catecholamines. Further studies on the heart of *Venus mercenaria* (chosen for its high sensitivity to 5-HT and because 5-HT is a neurotransmitter substance in molluscan hearts), indicated that not only 5-HT and some indolealkylamines but tyramine and phenylethylamine also act on the same receptors. This finding and the observation that certain indoles (those lacking an alkylamine side chain at C3) are incative suggest that the indole nucleus is not necessary for a 5-HT-like action in the mollusc. (This finding seems to accord with observations on other 5-HT receptors such as the neural receptors in autonomic ganglia and afferent nerve endings, in which a 5-HT-like effect can be obtained with aromatic guanidines and the effect of both types of stimulants can be blocked by guanidine derivatives and certain anti-5-HT agents (Fastier et al. 1959; Bevan and Verity 1961; Gyermek 1964a, b). Besides the high sensitivity and adequate selectivity of the Venus receptors to 5-HT the absence of monoamineoxydase in this tissue offered another advantage for drug-receptor studies. While tryptamine and several N-alkylated tryptamines were found to be about 5—10 times less potent than 5-HT, bufotenine proved to be approximately 30 times more effective than 5-HT on the molar basis indicating a higher degree of conformity of the venus heart receptor to bufotenine than in the majority of mammalian receptors, where the optimal structure seems to be 5-HT.

Lysergic acid diethylamide produces 5-HT-like effects in the molluscan heart in minute concentrations, markedly surpassing the efficacy of 5-HT, therefore, the structural features including aspects of the steric orientation of pharmacophore groups were studied in detail and suggestions were made in regard to the optimal steric configurations for a 5-HT-like activity (Greenberg 1961). The use of LSD as a model for 5-HT in this tissue seemed justified because of the favorably rigid nature of the lysergic acid part of the molecule. It is, however, impossible to draw conclusions insofar as the conformity of this stable steric structure with that of a hypothetical configuration of the flexible indolealkylamines is concerned (the hypothetical optimal configuration representing the active form of the molecule is assumed to exist in certain percentage of population of different steric forms). A major criticism against this portion of the study of Greenberg (1960) is that it disregarded the existence of an important functional group (diethylamide moiety) in the LSD molecule which group unfortunately is quite freely rotating. Whatever conclusions can be deduced from the structural configuration of flexible 5-HT-like molecules and LSD-like molecules (which thus prove eventually to be only semi-rigid) the findings will probably be relevant only to molluscan receptors where LSD is stimulatory in nature. It must be noted, however, that fairly small structural changes convert the stimulant type of lysergic acid derivatives into a blocking type of agent. Thus compounds with substituents at the C 1 and 2 atoms of the lysergic acid (methysergid, BOL) possess only blocking properties. (Wright et al. 1962) indicating that in the molluscan organ these substitutions markedly influence the "intrinsic activity" and probably leave the "affinity" to the receptors unchanged.

2. Relations of 5-HT and its antagonists to other biological sites reacting with 5-HT

In spite of the many studies on the characteristics of antagonism of 5-HT which occur at the pharmacologically active sites between 5-HT and its blocking agents relatively few data are available on the binding of the compounds to these receptors. Chlorpromazine (CPZ) was shown to interfere with the uptake of labelled 5-HT in the lung of the guinea pig. It similarly blocked the uptake of 5-HT in the uterine and intestinal tissue (MARIANI and VERTUA 1960, 1961). Since such an effect was not found in other organs it seems that competition between the two agents occurred at receptor-like binding sites. More information is available on the displacement of 5-HT by blocking agents which also alter its active transport at a nonreceptor type of storage site, the blood platelets. Both tryptamine and 5-HT were taken up by human platelets and tryptamine inhibited the uptake of 5-HT. Agents like imipramine, cocaine and CPZ were also potent in interfering with the binding of 5-HT to the platelets (STACEY 1960). Except for CPZ these agents were shown to potentiate certain actions of 5-HT (GYERMEK and POSSEMATO 1960, SOFFER and GYERMEK 1961). On the other hand, compounds competing less vigorously with 5-HT at the platelets (i.e., DHE, LSD and CPZ) are known as 5-HT antagonists (STACEY 1960). In addition to the potent compounds mentioned, another study investigated ibogaine, α-methyl-tryptamine, harmaline, amphetamine and some MAO inhibitors (LONG and LESSIN 1962). These agents were also found to inhibit the active transport of 5-HT into the platelets. Here, again, most of these compounds are known pharmacologically either as potentiators or inhibitors of 5-HT. Furthermore, among the compounds found inactive in interfering with 5-HT uptake, hardly any is known as a sensitizing or blocking agent for 5-HT. Imipramine also depleted the 5-HT content of human platelets in vivo. Iproniazide produced an opposite effect, a marked increase in the amount of 5-HT which in turn is inhibited by imipramine (MARSHALL et al. 1960). The observation (COSTA cit. by MARSHALL et al. 1960) that imipramine increases brain 5-HT in the rabbit may indicate that the amount of 5HT displacement from peripheral storage sites is taken up by the brain. Chlorpromazine and chloroprothixine, two potent antagonists of 5-HT, were found to interfere with the release of 5-HT (and norepinephrine) by reserpine in the brain and with the increase of 5-HT levels following 5-HTP and MAO inhibitors. This effect is conceivably brought about by some influence on the penetration of 5-HT into storage organelles (GEY and PLETSCHER 1961).

The interesting studies of VANE (1959) and BARLOW (1961) on peripheral organ receptors utilized structural analogs of 5-HT as well as 5-HT antagonist and MAO enzyme inbibitors. It was shown that the differential character of blocking actions with BOL and indole-type antagonists against 5-HT and tryptamine may be ascribed (1) to a selective interference with the transport of tryptamine through cell membranes assuming similar intracellular receptors for tryptamine and 5-HT, or (2) to different receptors for these two amines (BARLOW 1961). Employing analogues of 5-HT, VANE (1959) distinguished three different types of agents: (1) those like 5-HT having a certain affinity for tissue receptors (rat stomach) and monoamineoxidase (MAO) (the action of this group could not be potentiated in the isolated organ preparation by MAO inhibition); (2) those similar to 5-methyltryptamine exhibiting certain affinity for the tissue receptors and for MAO (however, the actions of this group could be potentiated in the isolated organ by MAO inhibitors); (3) those like 5-hydroxy-1-methyltryptamine which showed affinity for the tissue receptors only and not for MAO.

These observations suggest that the tissue receptors for 5-HT are separated from the intracellular enzyme receptors. Some of the compounds, such as tryptamine, penetrate into the cells and can be attacked there by MAO, but some, like 5-HT, cannot penetrate into the cells. Studies on the dissociation constants of the pharmacophore groups of 5-HT and on the partition coefficients of tryptamine and 5-HT showed that 5-HT did not penetrate into the lipid phase, whereas tryptamine did. The demonstration of the different types of 5-HT tissue receptors and MAO receptors is of great importance in comparing 5-HT with norepinephrine because it has been suggested that the tissue receptors for norepinephrine are also responsible for its enzymatic destruction. Besides the identity of tissue receptors and enzyme receptors for norepinephrine, the identity of certain tissue receptors sensitive to 5-HT and sympathomimetic amines is still an open question. In contrast to several studies which indicated that 5-HT acts on specific receptor types distinguishable from those of ACH, histamine and sympathomimetic amines, MANSOUR (1957) found in the liver fluke that 5-HT and amphetamine are indistinguishable in their actions and INNES (1962) demonstrated that on the cat spleen 5-HT and epinephrine act on the same receptor. This conclusion was based on a thorough study using antagonists such as phenoxybenzamine, BOL and DHE which blocked both amines. Epinephrine overdosage protected the tissue from the blocking effect of phenoxybenzamine against 5-HT and vice versa. Cross tachyphylaxis was also demonstrated between 5-HT, epinephrine and tyramine. The situation is somewhat complicated by the possible existence of a dual action of 5-HT on this organ, e.g., a major action resulting in release of norepinephrine and a minor one directly effecting the epinephrine receptors. Based on the failure of morphine and atropine to inhibit 5-HT on this preparation the above study also indicates that the cat spleen has no "*M*" receptors. Results obtained with the other antagonists suggest that the receptors of this preparation, although resembling those of the "*D*" receptors of the guinea pig ileum, due to their sensitivity to epinephrine, are not specific to 5-HT. Phentolamine blockade and iproniazid potentiation to 5-HT observed in rat blood pressure experiments suggest an adrenergic mechanism in the action of 5-HT (BELESLIN and VARAGIĆ 1960) which seems in accord with the findings of INNES (1962) in the cat.

It is unknown whether an interference found at inactivating enzyme receptors will influence the tissue receptors and storage sites of 5-HT in vivo. Thus practically no prediction can be made as far as the over-all effect on 5-HT receptors of a certain agent is concerned. The above examples serve the purpose of indicating that the binding to an inactivating enzyme surface may be coupled with a high affinity to tissue receptors and storage sites. In case of such a multiple affinity to different receptor sites, the over-all effect could be the product of (1) the different time-effect relationships at different receptors; (2) the number and distribution of the various types of sites. Thus it seems to be pertinent to consider that the distribution of a certain agent between true and pseudo receptors (binding sites) and inactivating enzyme surfaces will determine whether it can be classified as a 5-HT antagonist or potentiator when tested in the whole animal or on an organ which contains all the above-mentioned sites.

Even if a blocking agent interferes with the agonist at only one receptor type two effects may take place: (1) competition with the agonist for unoccupied receptor sites resulting in interference with its fixation to the receptor; and (2) attacking the occupied sites which result in replacement and release of the agonist molecules from those sites (WOOLLEY and EDELMAN 1958). Thus a possibility for a very variable state and lack of equilibrium between agonist and antago nistic molecules can be expected in many systems due to the possibility of shifts of 5-HT from one receptor to another. Such a redistribution of an amine like 5-HT in different compartments of the organism in vivo may be the explanation for the differences which exist in the interfering effect between CPZ (classified as a receptor blocking agent) with iproniazid (classified as an enzyme inhibitor) as reflected in 5-HT levels in the brain in vitro as compared to in vivo (HORNYKIEWICZ et al.). The finding that LSD increases 5-HT levels of many organs (SANKAR et al. 1961) indicates that this is most likely due to an interference with its enzymatic inactivation and that the effect of LSD as measured in changes of 5-HT levels is due to this influence rather than to a competition with 5-HT uptake at receptor or storage sites which would ordinarily lead to a depletion of 5-HT content. Time differences in the binding of 5-HT to different sites as influenced by imipramine can be the explanation for the findings that this agent in contrast to isolated organs first inhibits, later potentiates the blood pressure increasing effect of 5-HT and produces exclusively potentiation of 5-HT effects on certain receptors (i.e., the nictitating membrane of the cat) SABELLI and SINAY 1960. (GYERMEK and POSSEMATO 1960, SOFFER and GYERMEK 1961). Since it is unknown how the antagonistic effect on a tissue receptor of 5-HT should be weighed against the interference with 5-HT on a storage site or inactivating enzyme surface of the same species the significance of isolated organ studies as far as the predictability of the over-all in vivo effect of an agent is negligible.

3. Relations of indolealkylamines other than 5-HT to the 5-HT receptors

The studies of BARLOW and KHAN (1959a, b, c), VANE (1959), BERTACCINI and ZAMBONI (1961) on smooth muscle receptors and of GYERMEK and BINDLER (1962b) on ganglionic receptors using a series of indolealkylamines indicated that 5-HT is so far the most potent indolealkylamine on a majority of peripheral 5-HT receptors. Alkylation on the terminal N-atom of indolealkylamines in most cases significantly reduces the 5-HT-like potency on the smooth muscle receptors. In addition, in the case of bufotenine and bufotenidine, a different type of action has to be considered because of the refractoriness of these agents to a specific 5-HT antagonist, methysergid (SOLLERO and KURTZ 1962). On the nervous receptors, parallel with a decrease of the 5-HT-like response a cholinergic type of stimulant action appears with N-methylation. This applies to tertiary amines (i.e., N,N-dimethyltryptamine and bufotenine) and especially to the corresponding methyl-quaternary derivatives. Of the N-methylated derivatives of tryptamine and 5-HT: N-methyltryptamine, N-methyl-5-OH tryptamine, N,N-dimethyltryptamine and bufotenin (N,N-dimethyl 5-OH tryptamine) may perhaps have biological significance in the mammalian organism. In addition to the suggestion that end products of an altered indole metabolism may play a role in symptoms of schizophrenia (BUSCAINO 1960, SPRINCE 1961), AXELROD (1962) demonstrated that N-methylation of tryptamine and 5-HT takes place in the lung tissue of the rabbit. One characteristic feature of the N-alkylated tryptamine and 5-HT derivatives is their hallucinogenic property. Thus the possibility that hallucinogenic indolealkylamines are formed in the human organism must be kept in mind and the receptors for these and similar available amines have to be analyzed and possibly classified pharmacologically. Two other structural transformation processes of physiologically occurring indolealkylamines have recently been recognized: (a) the enzymatic O-methylation of 5-HT whereby 5-methoxytryptamine and its N-acetyl derivative melatonin is formed (WURTMAN et al. 1963); and (b) 6-hydroxylation of indolealklyamines (AXELROD and SZARA 1959). The physiologic role of 5-methoxytryptamine is unknown. On the peripheral smooth muscle receptors of 5-HT it is fairly potent (BARLOW and KHAN 1959, GESSNER et al. 1961), but on the nervous receptors sensitive to 5-HT it shows only negligible potency (GYERMEK and BINDLER 1962b). On the other hand, it is capable of altering the conditioned behavior of animals (GESSNER et al. 1961). Two derivatives of 5-methoxytryptamine may have physiologic significance. The first is the N-acetyl derivative or melatonin. It is quite inert pharmacologically on the smooth muscle (GESSNER et al. 1961, BERTACCINI and ZAMBONI 1961) and ganglionic receptors of 5-HT (GYERMEK 1964c). Recently, however, it was shown that melatonin has a significant action on the CNS in influencing the epithalamopituitary system and may participate in the transmission of optical influences to the gonadotropic-pituitary mechanism. Its significance at least in certain mammalian species with light sensitive gonadal regulatory mechanisms seems to be important (WURTMAN et al. 1963). The second derivative is the N,N-dimethyl analogue of 5-methoxytryptamine which exhibits marked behavioral effects on animals and also stimulates peripheral 5-HT receptors (GESSNER et al. 1962). The known 6-hydroxy derivatives of tryptamine and related indolealkylamines are uniformly inactive in the conventional peripheral tissue preparations (GYERMEK 1964c) thus it seems that the process of 6-hydroxylation can rather be considered as leading to peripherally inactive metabolites than the 5-O methylation which leads to some peripherally as well as centrally active derivatives. Few of the peripherally inactive 6-OH indole derivatives, however, are potent behaviorally (SZARA 1962, SZARA et al. 1962) indicating a clear separation of the structural requirements for CNS and peripheral organ receptors.

The pharmacologic nature of the receptors influenced by these latter groups of compounds in the brain is completely unknown. The existing examples indicate that peripheral receptors which are influenced by these indolealkylamines cannot be taken as "model" systems for the hypothetical CNS receptors. Consequently the elucidation of drug antagonistic interactions between the few indolealkylamines occurring biologically (and perhaps the ones which may occur but for which evidence is not yet available) and certain specific antagonists can be of great value provided the proper test preparations are used. The nature of the receptors influenced by these compounds as compared to 5-HT receptors remains a fundamental problem and deserves attention. The need for adequate and relatively simple neurophysiologic and behavioral methods is obvious. In our present stage of knowledge, as mentioned at the outset, two kinds of approaches, both representing extremes, are applicable to the problems of biological antagonists of 5-HT. (1) Analysis of the simplest possible isolated systems which are still biologically responsive, with the aim of exploring the nature of interaction between the agents and the receptor. The information thus obtained may be valid: (a) only at a given receptor system, or (b) at other receptors also but possibly only if these can be treated as separate functional entities; (2) observation of the overall effect of the drug on a possibly intact unmedicated animal. In the case of 5-HT antagonists both of the above-mentioned different investigational approaches can be utilized, considering the many organs systems which are vigorously responsive to 5-HT and its antagonists as compared to several other classes of drugs which often can be tested only in the whole animal. As information accumulates, possibilities for thoroughly exploring systems of intermediate complexity with a number of various types of mutually interacting receptors and organelles may become available.

D. Methods

1. Critical considerations of methods for assessing blocking action to 5-HT and related indolealkylamines

Many, but certainly not all, technical aspects of these methods were outlined in a previous review (GYERMEK 1961a).

Most of the methods available today are listed below with references and certain comments which the reviewer felt would be of assistance in selecting suitable procedures from those listed. The use of appropriate methods would not only facilitate the interpretation of data concerning a certain compound but would also be of great help in comparing different classes of antagonists based on their spectrum of actions. At the present, only very superficial information is available on these aspects. In vitro methods generally offer the advantage of being fairly simple, many times reproducible and also suited for determining certain quantitative relations of drug antagonism. They may yield information on the surmountable of nonsurmountable nature of the blockade, onset and duration of action not much influenced by adsorption, transport and metabolic factors. The in vivo methods enable one to determine the value of a given antagonist which prevents certain pharmacologic effects in animals or which antagonize symptoms of 5-HT in which it is pathologically implicated. The information to be obtained, however, will most likely be applicable only to the same species and to similar experimental or pathologic conditions. The test preparations many times are entirely inadequate to explore the antagonistic agents beyond determining potency and approximately classifying the compund as far as the type of action is concerned. Questions regarding the site and mode of action can hardly be approached and certainly cannot be answered by using the whole animal as the only test object.

The term "selectivity of blockade" is obviously relative and its validity is usually restricted to certain groups of drug combinations. Furthermore, this term is necessarily based on results obtained by certain assay methods, the limitations of which have to be recognized. An isolated organ system such as the rat uterus permits one the comparison of blocking potencies of a drug against agents like ACH, oxytocin, histamine and 5-HT. The guinea pig ileum is suitable for differentiating between anticholinergic, antihistaminic and anti-5-HT effects. To accurately resolve the problem of the type of action is complicated using this organ because of the presence of at least two different receptor types for ACH as well as 5-HT. It is therefore obvious that the spectrum and degree of specificity of an anti-5-HT agent will largely depend on the test organ used and on the number and nature of challenging agents (agonists) employed. Ergot derivatives, for example, show high selectivity to 5-HT when tested on the uterus against 5-HT and ACH; such selectivity, however, cannot be demonstrated using a test organ, which besides anti-5-HT potency, measures efficacy against epinephrine. Many groups of drugs are known with only a limited degree of selectivity to 5-HT (i.e. many anti-histamines which exhibit a fair degree of potency against 5-HT and histamine but also have a weak effect against epinephrine). Other groups show practically no sign of selectivity at all, e.g., aromatic beta-haloethylamines, of the sympatholytic class which possess anti-epinephrine, antihistamine and anti-5-HT potencies at a similar dose level. Selectivity of a compound observed in an organ system of a certain species is possibly not applicable to another species. Since this field is largely unexplored, extrapolation of the data from one to another species seems to be unwarranted.

A major inherent methodological difficulty with antagonists of 5-HT as well as with many other blocking agents is the lack of availability of properly functioning isolated receptor systems. The use of isolated organs cannot overcome this difficulty, even if the preparation is taken from a very primitive organism, because too many interfering factors influence the entirely hypothetical basic steps of drug antagonism which are oversimplified rather than characterized by the following two schemes:

a) $A + X = AX \rightarrow$ effect,

b) $A + B + X = BX + A \rightarrow$ no effect

where A is the agonist B is the antagonist and X is the receptor because:

1. The association of A and B to X is usually not a linear function and is also reversible.

2. X, while reacting with either A or B is by its nature liable to morphologic changes.

It is felt that although the nature of drug-receptor interactions can be approximated by mathematical treatments, these will remain approximations serving to help understand the phenomena but will not solve many problems of drug-receptor interactions. Concerning the group of 5-HT antagonists it should also be realized that:

1. 5-HT often has a dual action, e.g., stimulation and, especially in higher concentration, self-blockade;
2. 5-HT shows the phenomenon of tachyphylaxis. This results in a self-blocking effect by applying a series of doses which seem exclusively stimulant at the beginning of application.
3. There are 5-HT antagonists which, in addition to their primarily blocking action, are stimulants either at the "same" receptor sites where 5-HT acts or "pseudo receptors" of 5-HT, the stimulation of which may somehow interfere with the action of 5-HT.

While an abundance of methods exists for measuring in vitro or in vivo the effects of exogenous indolealkylamines there is a definite shortage of those procedures which can adequately analyze actions of 5-HT and of endogenously occurring indolealkylamines in the CNS. Manipulations for obtaining effects on the brain of supposedly endogenous 5-HT by administering one of its precursors 5-HTP and interfering whit its deamination by MAO inhibitors is worth mentioning but should be looked upon critically. To produce an exclusively 5-HT mediated action by utilizing a precursor of 5-HT or employing an agent which releases endogenous 5-HT from its binding sites is questionable. Formation of other metabolites may produce interference in the first case and a shift of 5-HT from receptor to receptor and an exchange of 5-HT with similar but not identical amines storage sites may present difficulties in the second condition.

2. Methods for testing anti-5-HT action

I. Isolated organs

Heart of different molluscs[1,2,3,4,5] Goldfish-intestine[6]	High sensitivity to 5-HT. Some LSD derivatives cannot be tested because of their intensive stimulant action. Methysergid is highly potent
Rat stomach fundus[7,8,9] Rat ileum[10] Rat colon[11,12,13] Rat uterus[7,14,15,16,17,18,19,20,21,22,23,24] Rat kidney (perfused)[17,25,26] Guinea pig ileum, circular muscle strip[27]	Of the rat preparations the stomach and the uterus are the most sensitive. For practical purposes the uterus is recommended which was used so far most exclusively among the isolated organ preparations. On the kidney preparation information on LSD derivatives is available only.
Guinea pig ileum[15,22,28,29,30,31,32,33,34,35,36,37,38,39,40] Guinea pig colon[41] Guinea pig lung (perfused)[42,43,44] Guinea pig auricle[10,45]	Sensitivity to 5-HT and to the antagonists is generally not too high. The ileum preparation can be used to distinguish between two different (i.e. muscular "D" and nervous "M") receptor types. Peristaltic reflex actions of 5-HT can also be studied.
Rabbit ileum[23,46,47,48] Rabbit auricle[10,49,45,50] Rabbit heart[51] Rabbit ear (perfused)[50,52,53,54] Rabbit hindleg (perfused)[55]	Except the rabbit auricle which is suitable to distinguish between direct and indirect (i.e. catecholamine-mediation) effects these preparations are not extensively used.
Cat atria[45] Cat lung (perfused)[56] Cat hingleg (perfused)[57] Cat renal vessels (perfused)[57] Cat pulmonary vessels (perfused)[57]	Adequate information on the usefulness and characteristics of these preparations are lacking. Only ergot and LSD derivatives were studied.
Dog hindleg (perfused)[57]	Only LSD was used as antagonist.

Isolated artery rings (sheep)[58,59,60] Aneural smooth muscle preparation of chick amnion[61]	Fairly sensitive preparation used almost exclusively for analyzing action of indole type of antagonists. Lack of nervous elements may help in characterizing "purely" muscular receptors.
Fowl caecum[62]	Variable sensitivity to 5-HT.
II. In vivo preparations	
Liver fluke, contraction[63] Mussels-metabolic rate[64]	Not only 5-HT but amphetamine and LSD are also stimulant. BOL antagonizes all.
Chicken BP[65]	Selective stimulation by 5-HT. BOL is inhibiting
Mouse behavioral changes on intraventricular injection[66]	The vasodepressor and pressor effects can be analyzed separately.
Mouse, antagonism of the 5-HT-induced narcosis potentiation[17,67,68,69,70,71,72,73] Mouse depression of spontaneous motility[74] Mouse, antagonism against HT toxicity[75,76] Mouse, brain edema produced by 5-HT[77] Mouse, action in pregnancy and placental vessels[78] Mouse, paw edema[79,80]	5-HT induced narcosis potentiation is not necessarily occurring at the CNS. The intraventricular injection technique may be of greater usefulness. The other mouse methods are less explored. The paw edema test can be useful for testing species differences vs. the rat or other species.
Rat, conditioned behavioral response; depression of[81,82] Rat, antidiuretic action[1,19,83,84,85,86,87] Rat, BP[88,89,90] Rat, ulcer of the stomach[91,92,93] Rat, defecation[85] Rat, paw edema[11,94,95,96,97,98,99] Rat, skin capillary permeability[100,101,102]	In view of the adequate information available on the paw edema and antidiuretic tests, these methods are useful in routine studies for obtaining data on in vivo efficacy.
Guinea pig bronchospasm[13,103,104,105,106,107,108] Rabbit BP[65,109]	A suitable in vivo method for distinguishing between bronchospasms produced by 5-HT and other agents.
Rabbit, peristaltic reflex[45,110] Cat, spinal, BP[21,111,112]	May offer supplemental information in addition to the isolated guinea pig method.
Cat, BP under ganglionic blockade[21,65,113,114] Cat, intrathoracic receptors[115]	The ganglionically blocked cat is suitable for obtaining preliminary information on antagonism of vascular effects.
Cat, superior cervical ganglion-nictitating membrane preparation[116,117,118,119] Cat, inferior mesenteric ganglion preparation[120,121,122,123]	The ganglionic preparations are suitable for analyzing action on peripheral nervous receptors. Intraarterial administration allows the use of minute quantities without systemic effects.
Cat transcallosal pathway preparation chlorpromazine restores depression[124] Cat, behavioral and EEG changes on intraventricular injection[125,126,127,128]	The intraventricular injection technique for behavioral studies can be of great value.
Dog, BP[19,24,59,65,106,129,130,131,132] Dog cardiopulmonary reflex[133,134] Dog, pulmonary BP [155]	Ganglionically blocked dogs are preferable for the blood pressure test. Recommended only for obtaining orientative data.
Dog, urinary bladder (in situ)[85,135] Dog, gut villi (in situ)[136]	The study of cardiopulmonary reflex and bladder actions are suitable for testing efficacy on peripheral nervous receptors.
Man, intradermal tests[137,138]	Information so far is limited.
III. Indirect methods	
Mouse, antagonism against 5-HTP-induced defecation[139]	An exclusive effect of 5-HT after 5-HTP administration cannot be ascertained, but even so the narcosis potentiation test with 5-HTP seems to be preferable to the similar test employing 5-HT.
Mouse, antagonism against reserpine-induced narcosis potentiation[68,72,140] Mouse, cat, dog antagonism against 5-HTP-induced excitement in iproniazid treated animals[141,142]	Comparative studies with tryptamine and centrally active other indolealkylamines are also possible.

Mouse, rat and rabbit, antagonism against the excitement produced by reserpine plus iproniazid[141,143]
Guinea pig and monkey, allergic encephalomyelitis[144]
Mouse enaphylaxis and lethal toxic action [145,146,147,148]
Rat, experimental inflammation[149]
Rats, 5-HTP and tryptamine convulsion[150]
Mouse behavioral and reflex responses to tryptamine derivatives[151,152]
Mouse antagonism of 5-HTP toxicity[153]
Cat, spinal reflexes, tryptamine[154]

Due to the differences in the techniques used, most of the indirect methods utilizing releasing agents, precursors and enzyme inhibitors of 5-HT should be evaluated individually according to the specific nature of the problem presented.

References. [1] ERSPAMER (1952b). — [2] GADDUM and PAASONEN (1955). — [3] GREENBERG (1960a). — [4] WELSH (1953, 1954). — [5] WRIGHT et al. (1962). — [6] GADDUM and SZERB (1961). — [7] BARLOW and KHAN (1959a, 1959b). — [8] BARTLET (1962). — [9] VANE (1957, 1959). — [10] LÉVY and MICHEL-BER (1956). — [11] BENDITT and ROWLEY (1956). — [12] BERGER et al. (1957). — [13] JAQUES et al. (1956). — [14] ARNOLD and HOFMAN (1957). — [15] BERDE et al. (1956). — [16] BERTACCINI and ZAMBONI (1961). — [17] CERLETTI and KONZETT (1956). — [18] COSTA (1956). — [19] ERSPAMER (1952a). — [20] GADDUM (1953, 1954). — [21] GYERMEK et al. (1956). — [22] KIMURA et al. (1960). — [23] SOLLERO et al. (1956). — [24] STONE et al. (1961). — [25] PASSOW et al. (1960). — [26] ROTHLIN (1957a). — [27] HARRY (1963). — [28] ADLER and ALBERT (1963). — [29] BARLOW and KHAN (1959c). — [30] BELESLIN and VARAGIĆ (1958). — [31] BROWNLEE and JOHNSON (1963). — [32] DAY and VANE (1963). — [33] DOMENJOZ and THEOBALD (1959). — [34] GADDUM and PICARELLI (1957). — [35] GINZEL (1957). — [36] SCHWARZ et al. (1956). — [37] KOSHINO (1961). — [38] RAPPORT and KOELLE (1952). — [39] ROCHA E SILVA et al. (1953). — [40] RUMMEL (1961). — [41] QUADBECK and RÖHM (1954). — [42] BHATTACHARYA (1955). — [43] KING (1957). — [44] STORMORKEN (1959). — [45] TRENDELENBURG (1960). — [46] MARCZYNSKI and VETULANI (1961). — [47] SINHA and WEST (1953). — [48] TRIPOD (1957). — [49] MAGISTRETTI and VALZELLI (1955). — [50] YOON (1960). — [51] JACOB and POITE-BEVIERRE (1960). — [52] GADDUM (1957b). — [53] GADDUM and HAMEED (1954). — [54] SAVINI (1956). — [55] MEIER et al. (1957). — [56] GADDUM et al. (1953). — [57] GINZEL and KOTTEGODA (1953). — [58] REID and RAND (1951, 1952). — [59] SHAW and WOOLLEY (1953, 1956). — [60] WOOLLEY and SHAW (1953). — [61] FERGUSON (1957). — [62] CLEUGH et al. (1961). — [63] MANSOUR (1957). — [64] MOORE et al. (1961). — [65] BUÑAG and WALASZEK (1962, 1963). — [66] HALEY (1957). — [67] GARATTINI and VALZELLI (1955). — [68] GYERMEK (1964c). — [69] ROTHLIN (1957c). — [70] SALMOIRAGHI and PAGE (1957). — [71] SHORE et al. (1955). — [72] TAESCHLER (1956). — [73] ZANOWIAK and RODMAN (1959). — [74] BROWN (1957). — [75] FANCHAMPS et al. (1960). — [76] TRAPOLD et al. (1960). — [77] BULLE (1957). — [78] POULSON and ROBSON (1963). — [79] WEIS (1963). — [80] NORTHOVER and SUBRAMANIAN (1962). — [81] COOK and WEIDLEY (1957). — [82] SOLLERO and KURTZ (1962). — [83] DASGUPTA (1957). — [84] DE CARO (1963). — [85] ERSPAMER (1953b, 1955). — [86] GARATTINI and VALZELLI (1956b). — [87] VAN ARMAN (1956). — [88] BELESLIN and VARAGIĆ (1960). — [89] DEL GRECO et al. (1956). — [90] SALMOIRAGHI et al. (1957). — [91] CAHEN et al. (1963). — [92] WILHELMI (1957). — [93] WILHELMI and SCHINDLER (1959). — [94] DOEPFNER and CERLETTI (1958). — [95] FRANCHIMONT et al. (1961b). — [96] KELEMEN (1957). — [97] MÖRSDORF and BODE (1959). — [98] PARRATT and WEST (1956). — [99] VOGEL and MAREK (1961). — [100] GÖZSY and KÁTO (1961). — [101] HALPERN et al. (1959). — [102] LIACOPOULOS et al. (1957). — [103] HERXHEIMER (1956). — [104] HOLGATE and WARNER (1960). — [105] KONZETT (1956). — [106] REUSE (1958). — [107] SICUTERI et al. (1960). — [108] ZICHA and BREGULLA (1962). — [109] JACOB and CUGURRA (1960). — [110] HUKUHARA et al. (1960). — [111] SALMOIRAGHI et al. (1957). — [112] WEIDMANN and CERLETTI (1957). — [113] SCHNEIDER and YONKMAN (1954). — [114] WIRTH et al. (1959). — [115] BEVAN and VERITY (1961). — [116] LECOMTE (1955). — [117] SCHAEPPI (1963). — [118] SIGG et al. (1963). — [119] TRENDELENBURG (1956, 1957). — [120] BINDLER and GYERMEK (1961). — [121] GYERMEK (1961b). — [122] GYERMEK and BINDLER (1962a, 1962b). — [123] GYERMEK et al. (1962). — [124] MARAZZI (1960). — [125] BRADLEY and HANCE (1956). — [126] BRADLEY and KEY (1959). — [127] HANCE and BRADLEY (1956). — [128] SCHWARZ et al. (1956). — [129] CERLETTI and WEIDMANN (1962). — [130] JACOB and MICHAUD (1962). — [131] PAGE and MCCUBBIN (1953). — [132] SCHMID et al. (1959). — [133] GYERMEK (1964a). — [134] MEDAKOVIĆ (1958). — [135] GYERMEK (1960, 1962). — [136] LUDÁNY et al. (1959). — [137] BALESTRA (1962). — [138] KALZ and FEKETE (1961). — [139] WOOLLEY (1957, 1958). — [140] CERLETTI and ROTHLIN (1955). — [141] CHESSIN et al. (1957). — [142] FRANCO-BROWDERS et al. (1958). — [143] SHORE and BRODIE (1957). — [144] O'BRIEN et al. (1962). — [145] GANLEY (1962). — [146] GELFAND and WEST (1961). — [147] HALBERT et al. (1963). — [148] HALBERT et al. (1963). — [149] UDA (1960). — [150] TEDESCHI et al. (1961a, 1961b). — [151] CORNE et al. (1963). — [152] VANE et al. (1961). — [153] KARJA et al. (1961). [154] MARLEY and VANE (1963). — [155] ROSE and LAZARO (1958).

E. Classes of anti-5-HT drugs

Name of class	Subgroups	Biological characteristics
Ergot alkaloids and related compounds	Natural and hydrogenated alkaloids	High potency and selectivity in certain isolated organs (CERLETTI and DOEPFNER 1958). Predominant action on the muscular "*D*" receptors (GADDUM and PICARELLI 1957). Some (i.e. ergotamine) but not all of them are highly potent in vivo (PAGE 1958, SALMOIRAGHI et al. 1957). Anti-5-HT action is unrelated to adrenolytic action. Ergonovine group is the most, ergotamine group the least potent (CERLETTI and DOEPFNER 1958). For peripheral effects see ERSPAMER (1953b), FINGL and GADDUM (1953), GADDUM and HAMEED (1954), GINZEL and KOTTEGODA (1953), SAVINI (1956), WOOLLEY and SHAW (1963). For CNS effects see CAHN et al. (1956), GADDUM and VOGT (1956), SNOW et al. (1956), YUI and TAKEO (1958).
	Lysergic acid derivatives	
	1. LSD	Outstanding potency on isolated organs, i.e. rat uterus (CERLETTI and DOEPFNER 1958, CERLETTI and KONZETT 1956, FANCHAMPS et al. 1960, SAVINI 1956, STONE et al. 1961, TRAPOLD et al. 1960), and perfused rabbit ear (GADDUM et al. 1955, MEIER et al. 1957, SAVINI 1956). On molluscan preparations and in minute doses stimulates 5-HT receptors (COSTA 1956). Also sensitizes certain peripheral nervous receptors to 5-HT (GYERMEK and SUMI 1963, VALDECASAS et al. 1956). Extremely potent hallucinogenic agent. This effect is not related to the peripheral anti-5-HT efficacy (CHODERA 1962, PAGE 1958). Inhibits certain CNS effects elicited by 5-HT in animals (DOEPFNER and CERLETTI 1958, GADDUM and VOGT 1956, ROTHLIN 1957a, SALMOIRAGHI and PAGE 1957, TAESCHLER 1956). It is weak or ineffective on peripheral nervous receptors of 5-HT (GYERMEK and BINDLER 1962a, ZAKUSOV 1962). For peripheral effects see also BHATTACHARYA (1955), BINDLER and GYERMEK (1961), CASENTINI and GALLI (1956), CERLETTI and BERDE (1955), CIMA and FRESCHI (1957), COSTA (1956), DOEPFNER and CERLETTI (1958), FINK (1956), GADDUM (1953, 1957b), GADDUM et al. (1953, 1955), GADDUM and PAASONEN (1955), HERXHEIMER (1956), KING (1957), KONZETT (1956), LÉVY and MICHEL-BER (1956), LUDÁNY et al. (1959), MAGISTRETTI and VALZELLI (1955), MÖRSDORF and BODE (1959), SCOTT and STONE (1959), SNOW et al. (1956), TRENDELENBURG (1960), WILHELMI (1957). For CNS effect see BRADLEY and HANCE (1956), BROWN (1957), CAHN et al. (1956), CERLETTI and ROTHLIN (1955), GADDUM (1957a), GADDUM and VOGT (1956), GARATTINI and VALZELLI (1956a), GYERMEK (1964c), HALEY (1957), PENNEFEATHER and THORP (1958), RODNIGHT and MCILWAIN (1956), ROTHLIN (1957a, 1957b), SACCHI et al. (1955), SALMOIRAGHI and PAGE (1957), SHORE et al. (1955), SLATER et al. (1955), TAESCHLER (1956), TROUT (1957), ZANOWIAK and RODMAN (1959).
	2. 2-bromo-LSD	It is sometimes more active then LSD on peripheral 5-HT receptors (BELESLIN and VARAGIĆ 1958, CERLETTI and KONZETT 1956, ROTHLIN 1957a, SALMOIRAGHI and PAGE 1957, TAESCHLER 1956). Not hallu-

Name of class	Subgroups	Biological characteristics
		cinogenic and also inactive in certain animal-CNS tests (Cerletti and Konzett 1956, Cerletti and Rothlin 1955, Taeschler 1956). For peripheral effects see also Del Greco et al. (1956), Doepfner and Cerletti (1957, 1958), Parratt and West (1956, 1958), Rose and Lazaro (1958), Salmoiraghi et al. (1957), Savini (1956), Snow et al. (1956). For CNS effects see Cerletti and Rothlin (1955), Gaddum and Vogt (1956), Gyermek (1964c), Moussatche and Pereira (1957), Rothlin (1957a), Salmoiraghi et al. (1957).
	3. 1-methyl-d-lysergic acid butanolamide UML-491	Very potent in peripheral, muscular receptors of 5-HT (Cerletti and Doepfner 1958, Fanchamps et al. 1960, Rothlin 1957b, Votava and Lamplova 1959) and in few in vivo tests (Doepfner and Cerletti 1958, Fanchamps et al. 1960). Lacks CNS effects (Gallant et al. 1963).
	4. Other lysergic acid derivatives	Many of them are potent peripheral antagonists (Cerletti and Doepfner 1958, Fanchamps et al. 1960, Rothlin 1957b, Votava and Lamplová 1959, Votava et al. 1958). Some of them are centrally active or hallucinogenic (Cerletti and Doepfner 1958, Rothlin 1957a).
Indole compounds	a) Derivatives of indole	Most potent compounds: 2-methyl-3-ethyl-5-dimethyl amino indole (medmain) and its methyl derivative (methylmedmain) (Shaw and Woolley 1954), but even these are inferior in potency to many ergot derivatives. Ineffective in man as hypotensive agents (Iversen and Bull 1953). See also Erspamer (1953a), Gaddum et al. (1955), Iversen and Bull (1953), Kopf and Møeller Nielsen (1959), Quadbeck (1954), Shaw and Woolley (1954), Wilhelmi and Schindler (1959), Woolley (1959), Woolley and Shaw (1957a).
	b) Derivatives of gramine	Most potent members: 2-methyl-5-halo gramines and 5-benzyloxygramine (Erspamer 1955, Quadbeck 1954, Vercellone and Asero 1954, Ehrhart and Henning 1961, Salmoiraghi and Page 1957, Shaw and Woolley 1957a).
	c) Derivatives of tryptamine (indolealkylamines)	Tryptamine itself is antagonistic to 5-HT (Gaddum 1953, Vane 1957). Best known derivatives are: BAS (1-benzyl-2-methyl-5-methoxy-tryptamine), BAS phenol (1-benzyl-2-methyl-5-hydroxytryptamine) (Barlow and Khan 1959a, Shaw and Woolley 1956, Stormorken 1959, Stone et al. 1961), BAB (1-benzyl-dimethyl-bufotenine) (Shaw and Woolley 1956, Woolley 1958) and 1-(p-methoxybenzyl)-2-methyl-5-hydroxytryptamine (Stone et al. 1961). Show hypotensive effects on dogs and on humans (Wilkins 1956, Wilkins and Hollander 1957). See also Erspamer (1953a), Gaddum et al. (1955), Jacob and Cugurra (1960), Murelli et al. (1960), Rinaldi (1958), Rudy et al. (1958), Schneckloth et al. (1957), Shaw and Woolley (1956, 1957b), Shore et al. (1955), Sletzinger et al. (1957), Stormorken (1959), Strandmann et al. (1963), Woolley (1959), Merck & Co. (1961).
	d) Quaternary ammonium salts of N,N-dialkyltryptamines	Neurotropic 5-HT antagonists of peripheral receptors Low potency on muscular receptors (Gyermek 1964a).

Name of class	Subgroups	Biological characteristics
	e) Indoleacetamidines	Neurotropic 5-HT antagonists on peripheral receptors (Gyermek 1961b, 1962).
	f) Derivatives of carbazole	6-N-phenyl-carboxamidino-1,2,3,4-tetrahydrocarbazole is quite active in vivo. Some behavioral effects in dogs (Shaw and Woolley 1957a).
	g) Derivatives of harmine	Alkaloids of the harmine group besides exhibiting weak anti-5-HT actions possess MAO inhibitory properties (Gyermek 1964c). Some of the alkaloids show marked central effects in man. See Erspamer (1953a), Shaw and Woolley (1953), Woolley and Shaw (1957b), Sigg et al. 1964.
Antihistaminic agents	Substituted ethylendiamines	Moderate to marked potency in isolated organs but usually only moderate efficacy in vivo (Doepfner and Cerletti 1957, Herxheimer 1956, Parratt and West 1958). Antihistaminic vs. anti-5-HT potencies vary markedly. See Calì and Cordova (1956), Domenjoz and Theobald (1959), Gyermek (1953), Rapport and Koelle (1952), Schmid et al. (1959).
Phenotiazines	a) Chlorpromazine	It is very potent in vitro (Benditt and Rowley 1956, Gyermek 1955, Gyermek et al. 1956); in vivo efficacy varies. Anti-5-HT and psychosedative effects seem to parallel each other (Courvoisier et al. 1957, Tedeschi et al. 1961a). Effective against symptoms in carcinoid syndrome (Sjoerdsma et al. 1957, Snow et al. 1956). For peripheral effects see Berger et al. (1957), Domenjoz and Theobald (1959), Garattini and Valzelli (1955), Lecomte (1955), Meier et al. (1957), Niaussat et al. (1961). For CNS effects see Cahn et al. (1956), Chessin et al. (1957), Costa and Rinaldi (1958), Franco-Browders et al. (1958), Herxheimer (1955).
	b) Other phenotiazines	Sometimes show high potency. Specificity is moderate (Doepfner and Cerletti 1957, 1958; Domenjoz and Theobald 1959, Gyermek 1964a, Gyermek et al. 1956, Haley et al. 1959, Meier et al. 1957, Parratt and West 1958, Schmid et al. 1959, Sollero et al. 1956, Wielding 1958, Wirth et al. 1959). Low efficacy on peripheral nervous receptors (Gyermek 1964c).
Antidepressants	Iminodibenzyl Iminostilbene Dibenzothiazepine derivatives	Peripheral anti-5-HT effects are similar to that of potent phenotiazines. CNS effects are different. Some effects of 5-HT are potentiated (Domenjoz and Theobald 1959, Hoffman 1958, Mörsdorf and Bode 1959, Wilhelmi 1957, Gyermek and Possemato 1960, Sigg et al. 1963, Soffer and Gyermek 1961).
Adrenolytic and hypotensive agents	Dibenamine Dibenzyline and analogues	Highly potent on isolated organs (Erspamer 1953b, Fingl and Gaddum 1953, Bhattacharya 1955, Gaddum and Hameed 1954, Gaddum et al. 1955, Gaddum and Picarelli 1957, Meier et al. 1957, Vane 1957). Low specificity (Fingl and Gaddum 1953, Furchgott 1955, Gaddum 1957b), irreversible or slowly reversible action (Gaddum et al. 1955). Predominantly affect the "*D*" receptors (Gaddum and Picarelli 1957), weak on the peripheral nervous receptors (Gyermek and Bindler 1962a). For in vivo effects see also Erspamer (1952b, 1953b), Freyburger et al. (1952), Gaddum et al. (1953), McCawley et al. (1952), Smith and Smith (1955), van Arman (1956). For CNS effects see Chessin et al. (1957) and Walaszek and Abood (1957).
	Yohimbine	Fairly potent but not very selective (Gaddum et al. 1955, Lévy and Michel-Ber 1956, Meier et al. 1957, Woolley and Shaw 1953). Weak potency in vivo.

Name of class	subgroups	Biological characteristics
	Phentolamine	Low selectivity and low potency (BHATTACHARYA 1955, BOCK et al. 1957, MAGISTRETTI and VALZELLI 1955, MEIER et al. 1957, NAERS and SCHANCHE 1956, PAGE and MCCUBBIN 1953).
	Tolazolidine	GINZEL and KOTTEGODA (1953).
	Azapetine	LÉVY and MICHEL-BER (1956).
	Piperoxane	ERSPAMER (1953a), FINGL and GADDUM (1953), GADDUM and HAMEED (1954), GRETTE (1957), PAGE and MCCUBBIN (1953).
	Reserpine	Low potency in isolated organs (BERGER et al. 1957, CASENTINI and GALLI 1956, COSTA 1956, MEIER et al. 1957). Variable in vivo efficacy (BULLE 1957, GARATTINI and VALZELLI 1956a, MEIER et al. 1957, PARRATT and WEST 1956, SCHNEIDER and RINEHART 1956, WILHELMI 1957). Inhibits 5-HT sensitive chemoreceptores (ZAKUSOV 1963).
	Hydrazinophthalazine	Low potency, nonspecific blocking action (ERSPAMER 1952a, MEIER et al. 1957, NAERS and SKRAMSTAD 1954).
	Ganglionic blocking agents	Inactive (ERSPAMER 1952a, FERGUSON 1957, LEVY and MICHEL-BER 1956, WESTERMANN 1958).
Atropine and atropin-like drugs		On certain neuromuscular preparations (i.e. guinea pig ileum) very effective (ROBERTSON 1953, ROCHA E SILVA et al. 1953). Besides the "*M*" receptors, cholinergic receptors might also be involved (CAMBRIDGE and HOLGATE 1955, RAPPORT and KOELLE 1952). Much lower potency on purely muscular receptor organs (GADDUM and PICCARELLI 1957). Weak action on peripheral nervous preparations (BINDLER and GYERMEK 1961, GYERMEK 1960, GYERMEK and BINDLER 1962a, TRENDELENBURG 1957). For in vitro effects see also BHATTACHARYA (1955), FERGUSON (1957), GADDUM and HAMEED (1954), GADDUM et al. (1955), LÉVY and MICHEL-BER (1956), ROBERTSON (1953), NIR et al. (1956). For in vivo effects see BINDLER and GYERMEK (1961), GYERMEK and BINDLER (1962a), CAHN et al. (1956), HOLGATE and WARNER (1960), KONZETT (1956), LUDÁNY et al. (1959), MCCAWLEY et al. (1952), WESTERMANN (1958), WILHELMI (1955).
Local anesthetics	Procaine	No significant action at the muscular 5-HT receptors. Effective on some nervous receptors and against reflex actions of 5-HT (BINDLER and GYERMEK 1961, FRAHM 1957, GYERMEK and BINDLER 1962a, GYERMEK and POSSEMATO 1960, LEVY and MICHEL-BER 1956, PAGE and MCCUBBIN 1953, REID and RAND 1951, SCHNEIDER and YONKMAN 1954, SINHA and WEST 1953, THEOBALD, and DOMENJOZ 1958, TRENDELENBURG 1956, WESTERMANN 1958).
Morphine type analgesics	Morphine	Highly potent on nerve-muscle and peripheral nervous preparations ("*M*" receptors of the guinea pig ileum, autonomic ganglia) (BINDLER and GYERMEK 1961, GADDUM 1957b, GYERMEK 1962a, 1962b, MEDAKOVIĆ 1958, TRENDELENBURG 1957). Inactive on muscular preparations (GADDUM 1957a, MEDAKOVIĆ 1958, SAVINI 1956, TRIPOD 1957).
	Morphine derivatives	Some of these are highly potent in mice against 5-HT (GADDUM and PICARELLI 1957, KING 1957, MEDAKOVIĆ 1958).
Sympathomimetic amines		These are probably nonspecific antagonists but may have physiologic significance counteracting effects of 5-HT. Isoproterenol is the most effective (CASENTINI

Name of class	subgroups	Biological characteristics
		and GALLI 1956, GARATTINI and VALZELLI 1956a, JAQUES et al. 1956). Antagonism in isolated organs: BHATTACHARYA (1955), GALLANT et al. (1963), VANE (1957), WOOLLEY (1957). Antagonism in vivo: ERSPAMER (1952b), JAQUES et al. (1956), LÉVY and MICHEL-BER (1956), PARRATT and WEST (1958).
Arylguanidines and biguanides		Neurotrop antagonists on peripheral receptors; sometimes marked 5-HT-like stimulant actions are present (GYERMEK 1964b).

F. Neurotropic antagonists of 5-HT

A search for neurotropic antagonists of 5-HT seems indicated for the following reasons:

1. Incomplete knowledge on the spectrum of action of many 5-HT antagonists. This became obvious when certain well known antagonists were investigated in different biologic preparations and a relative lack of efficacy to peripheral nervous receptors of 5-HT was observed.

2. The uncertain role of 5-HT in influencing the functions of the CNS.

3. The need to establish a closer correlation between certain mental effects and 5-HT.

Consequently it is felt that the development of antagonists which offer considerable selectivity at certain nervous receptors of 5-HT can be of great help in defining the role of 5-HT on nervous tissue and, in addition, may lead to therapeutic agents effective in the neuropathologic syndromes produced by this amine or by related indole compounds. The first pharmacologically useful data on nervous receptors distinguishable from those obtained on smooth muscles came from the studies of COMROE et al. (1953) and GADDUM and PICARELLI (1957). The first group observed the antagonistic action of 2-methyl, 3-ethyl 5-amino indole on 5-HT induced cardiorespiratory reflexes in the cat, which was, however, fairly weak. The second group described nervous receptors in the guinea pig ileum which were markedly influenced by drugs such as cocaine and morphine. These agents were the first ones described as neurotropic 5-HT antagonists. Their blocking effects against 5-HT, however, are usually overshadowed by a wide spectrum of other pharmacologic effects. In addition to the guinea pig ileum, other preparations have been introduced to test the efficacy and type of action of antagonists at peripheral nervous receptors. After establishing the marked stimulant action of 5-HT on the autonomic ganglia (i.e., superior cervical ganglion, inferior mesenteric ganglion of the cat, and coeliac ganglion of the rat) (ROBERTSON 1954 cited by TRENDELENBURG 1956, TRENDELENBURG 1956, HERTLZER 1961, GYERMEK and BINDER 1962a), the inferior mesenteric ganglion preparation of the cat has been used for the analysis of several classes of neurotropic antagonists of 5-HT. When the usefulness of another in vivo preparation detecting the action of 5-HT on pelvic ganglia of the dog (GYERMEK 1961) became established this preparation was also included in the study of this class of blocking agents. Besides autonomic ganglia chemoreceptors of the carotid body, aortic arc, and certain receptors of the afferent vagus and pelvic nerves are also highly sensitive to 5-HT. Although studies of these latter nervous receptors in establishing the characteristics of neurotropic 5-HT antagonists are also indicated only a few agents were studied recording afferent nerve activity or cardiovascular and respiratory reflex actions as influenced by 5-HT and by its antagonists (COMROE et al. 1953;

FASTIER et al. 1959; GYERMEK 1961 b, 1964 a, b; GYERMEK and SUMI 1963; ZAKUSOV 1962). Utilizing the above preparations several classes of agents became known as fairly selective and potent inhibitors of peripheral nervous receptors of 5-HT. These neurotropic "B" type of 5-HT antagonists are distinguished from the musculotropic "*A*" type of antagonists (GYERMEK 1962 b). The neurotropic group besides cocaine and morphine includes three groups of agents: a) indole-acetamidines; b) quarternary indolealkyl ammonium compounds; c) guanidines. The following common characteristics are ascribed to these classes of agents:

1. High potency against stimulation of nervous receptors by 5-HT and relatively low potency against cholinergenic stimulation.

2. Stimulant actions of varying degree before blockade ensues. This stimulant action is either 5-HT-like as in the case of indoleacetamidines (GYERMEK 1961 b) and guanidines (GYERMEK 1964 b) or similar to a cholinergenic type of ganglion stimulation as in the case of indolealkylammonium derivatives (GYERMEK 1964 a).

The most important compound of the indoleacetamidine group was 5-hydroxy indole-3-acetamidine, a compound first reported as having 5-HT-like stimulant properties on the dog (WOOLLEY and SHAW 1957 a). On IV administration to the dog it stimulated respiration and raised the blood pressure but also inhibited the pressor reflex and respiratory stimulant action of 5-HT. In turn, however, 5-HT did not influence the 5-HT-like stimulant actions of 5-hydroxy indoleacetamidine. It blocked the stimulant actions of 5-HT on different ganglionic preparations of the dog and cat in the dose range of 1—20 μg. Only slight ganglionic stimulation has been noted on the inferior mesenteric ganglion preparation. 5-hydroxy-3-indoleacetamidine was at least 20 times more potent than either LSD or BOL, cocaine and morphine against the ganglionic stimulant action of 5-HT. In addition, it was more effective than BOL inhibiting the reflex respiratory stimulation of 5-HT, but its blocking action on the rat uterus was much inferior to commonly known musculotropic 5-HT blocking agents (i.e. blocking agents of the "*A*" type).

Removal of the hydroxy group from 5-hydroxy-3-indoleacidamide and/or substitutions on the primary amine group by alkyl or cycloalkyl groups resulted in a decline of neurotropic anti-5-HT activity (GYERMEK 1964 c).

In the class of quarternary indole alkylammonium compounds the indolealkylamine moiety was combined with aralkyl quarternary ammonium radicals which were known to yield high potency on cholinergic ganglionic receptors (GYERMEK and NÁDOR 1957). It was expected that by this structural modification the tertiary ω-dialkylaminoalkyl indole bases used (e.g. bufotenine, dimethyltryptamine) in the quarternary salt form would become more effective on peripheral 5-HT sensitive nervous receptors. Introduction of different, substituted benzyl groups with the formation of the corresponding quarternary indolealkylammonium salts indeed resulted in few extremely potent compounds with predominantly blocking action at the 5-HT sensitive ganglionic receptors and enteroceptors of afferent autonomic nerves. Accordingly, the stimulant effect of 5-HT on the inferior mesenteric ganglion of the cat and on the pelvic ganglia of the dog, carotid chemoreceptors of the afferent pelvic nerves were blocked by the most potent members of the series in the 1—10 μg/kg dose range. Peak blocking activity was observed with meta-substituted benzyl quarternary compounds (i.e. m-chloro-benzyl bufoteninium bromide). This compound so far exhibits the highest potency on the 5-HT sensitive receptors of the autonomic nervous system. One mole of this agent is capable of antagonizing 10—50 moles of 5-HT. It also showed considerable selectivity in its ganglionic blocking action. Doses 4—30 times higher than those effective against 5-HT were not effective against cholinergic type of ganglion-stimulation. The relative potencies of this group of agents on 5-HT sensitive ganglionic receptors are indicated in Table 5b. The compounds were relatively inactive on the rat uterus preparation. In spite of their selectivity of 5-HT blocking action this group of compounds is not free of a certain affinity to cholinergic receptors of autonomic ganglia. Some of them showed a "nicotinic" type of stimulant action. It remains to be determined whether this affinity to cholinergic receptors, manifested in a stimulant but hardly any cholinergic ganglionic blocking action, plays any role in the 5-HT blocking action. It is interesting to note that other compounds which are powerful inhibitors of the peripheral nervous receptors of 5-HT also exhibit stimulant properties. Unlike the quarternary indolealkylamine compounds in the groups of indole acetamidines and arylguanidines this stimulant action seems to be at the 5-HT receptors. Nevertheless, there is no direct relationship between the degree of stimulation and blockade. Thus it seems that the blockade is not a consequence of the preceeding stimulant action. CNS and behavioral effects have not yet been investigated with these classes of 5-HT antagonists because of the paralyzing action on neuromuscular synapses of the quarternary ammonium indole derivatives observed in mice and rats and because of their possibly poor penetration rate into the CNS. This class of compounds thus seems to deserve only theoretical interest. The third group of agents with marked blocking action in nervous receptors of 5-HT belongs to a class of guanidine derivatives. The similarities in the cardiovascular and respiratory reflex actions of 5-HT and guanidines (Fastier 1962) indicated that further exploration of their ganglionic and possible 5-HT blocking actions might be of value. Therefore, a few aromatic guanidine and biguanide derivatives have been studied with respect to their actions on 5-HT sensitive nervous receptors. Actions on autonomic ganglia, cardiovascular and respiratory reflexes and smooth muscles were investigated and several similarities between the ganglionic and reflex stimulant actions of 5-HT and guanidines (i.e. phenyldiguanide, benzylguanidine, 2-Naphthylguanidine, 2-Anthrylguanidine, 2-Anthrylbiguanidine, 2-Acridylbiguanide) have been established: 1. the stimulant actions of these guanidines on the nervous receptors studied were not blocked by cholinergic ganglionic' blockade (i.e. hexamethonium) but were abolished by the neurotropic blocking 5-HT agents such as m-chlorbenzyl bufoteninium bromide and 5-hydroxy-3-indoleacetamidine; 2. there was about equal efficacy of ganglionic blocking guanidines (i.e. 2-anthrylguanidine) found against 5-HT and phenyldiguanide and a lack of potency against cholinergic ganglion-stimulation; 3. participation of the same receptor type in the ganglionic actions of 5-HT and guanidines (i.e. phenyldiguanide) was also indicated in cross tachyphylaxis experiments. Based on the similarity of the stimulant action at peripheral nervous receptors of 5-HT and certain guanidines it is not surprising to find that few compounds of the guanidine type were outstanding blocking agents of the nervous receptors of 5-HT, e.g., 2-anthrylguanidine besides stimulating characteristics markedly inhibited the autonomic reflex actions of 5-HT and the 5-HT produced ganglionic stimulation. Another compound, 2-acridylbiguanide, however, although less potent than the former one, showed a considerable degree of separation of potencies between the 5-HT-like stimulant and blocking actions. Few of them also showed some degree of blockade at the muscular "*D*" receptors on the rat uterus, thus their specificity for the neural receptors is not as high as in the case of the indoleacetamidine and quarternary indolealkylammonium type of blocking agents. The relative potencies of this class of agents are shown in Table 18.

The structural resemblance between certain amidine derivatives (i.e., phenyldiguanide and 2-naphthylguanidine) and 5-HT has been discussed by Fastier

(1962) in connection with their stimulant action on nervous receptors eliciting chemoreflexes. It is obvious that several structural factors are involved in satisfying the criteria of a suitable "fit" of molecules to these receptors.

In conclusion, it can be stated that a satisfactory degree of potency and certain selectivity to neural receptors of 5-HT as compared to muscular receptors of 5-HT and to other neural receptors has been established with three classes of neurotropic antagonists. However, numerous unsolved problems still exist with these agents. Regarding the mechanism of action the possible role of the observed different types of stimulant properties awaits for elucidation. There is a lack of information on the efficacy of these agents in the CNS when given alone or in influencing the effects of centrally acting indole compounds. In the group of potent quaternary ammonium type agents the possible low degree of entry into the CSN and the presence of neuromuscular side effects are marked limiting factors. Provided the cardiovascular type of side effects of agents such as 5-hydroxyindoleacetamidine and 2-anthrylguanidine can be minimized or eliminated, agents similar to these could be used as valuable tools for investigating mental effects in connection with blockade of 5-HT at peripheral or central 5-HT receptors. These compounds might also serve as a guide for developing additional classes of neurotropic blocking agents for 5-HT and related indolealkylamines.

The marked difference in the stimulant potencies of tryptamine and 5-HT (GYERMEK and BINDLER 1962b) and in the blocking potencies on nervous receptors of indoleacetamidine and quarternary indolealkylammonuim compounds as compared to their more potent 5-hydroxy analogues indicates that among the required structural factors the presence of the 5-hydroxy group of the indole ring has major importance.

G. Actions of antagonists of 5-HT on the CNS

Some of the most intriguing new aspects of psychopharmacology and behavioral sciences derive from the observation that many of the drugs which antagonize 5-HT also produce marked symptoms in the CNS. The correlation between 5-HT and CNS effects has been recognized lately and eventually led to stimulating but at the same time oversimplifying and sometimes even misleading theories. The claims that a) schizophrenia is due to a "lack" of 5-HT in the brain (WOOLLEY and SHAW 1957b); and b) 5-HT is a neurotransmitter substance with exclusively depressant role in synaptic transmission (MARAZZI and HART 1955, MARAZZI 1959) and the suggestion that 5-HT and norepinephrine two oppositely acting neurohumors of the brain are responsible for a great deal of its functioning (BRODIE and SHORE 1957) would be examples of these interesting but debatable theories (ROTHLIN 1957c, BUSCAINO 1960, CROSSLAND 1960). Concerning the theory of two antagonistically operating neurotransmitter substances of the brain: norepinephrine and 5-HT, the reviewer feels that it was based too great an extent on pharmacological findings utilizing the whole animal as test object and on "specific" blocking agents as pharmacologic tools (COSTA et al. 1962). The extremely complex situation concerning the coexistence of various receptors in the organism as outlined before indicates that it is not justified to consider CPZ a selective norepinephrine blocking agent and LSD and imipramine as 5-HT blocking agents because no evidence for such a selective blocking action especially for the brain tissue is available. These studies, therefore, offer only the suggestion and not the proof for considering 5-HT as a central neurotransmitter agent. As our knowledge stands at present one can only assume the possibility for correlations which may exist in a very broad sense between the frequent CNS effects observed and a certain interference (not necessarily antagonism) with 5-HT in the brain. The following is a list of aspects which have to be considered before any evaluation of the problem regarding 5-HT antagonism versus CNS effects is attempted: 1. the CNS effects observed with antagonists of 5-HT are quite varied. Some of the potent antagonists of 5-HT are hallucinogenic, others are tranquilizers, anti-depressants or narcotic analgesics. This varied list of CNS effects obviously cannot be explained on the basis of a certain competition with a single neurohumor especially since the interference between these agents and 5-HT has been observed mostly in organs which have nothing to do with higher nervous function; 2. CNS effects observed with drugs which mainly antagonize peripheral actions of 5-HT are only assumed but not proved to be due to an interference with 5-HT in the brain tissue. Unfortunately, the question about the efficacy of an agent in the CNS cannot easily be answered, because a) exogenously administered 5-HT does not penetrate into the brain; b) 5-HT many times does not produce significant changes when injected into the brain, or the effects do not resemble those which are observed after the administration of its precursor 5-HTP. (This precursor was often given either alone or in combination with enzyme inhibitors aiming at the protection of the endogenously formed 5-HT); 3. it is very difficult to duplicate the effects produced by 5-HT injected into the brain with those elicited by 5-HT releasing agents (i.e. reserpine). One complication arises from the possibility of the release of more than a single neurally active amine by the releasing agent. In the case of enzyme inhibitors an interference with the metabolism of amines other than 5-HT has also to be encountered. In addition, it is not known whether depletion of storage sites and the resulting lack of 5-HT at certain sites is responsible for the CNS effects observed with releasing agents. There is, for example, a possibility of a concomitant resaturation of these 5-HT binding sites by related amines. How this phenomena would contribute to the pharmacological effect of a releasing agent is entirely unknown. Without going into further details, therefore, it seems clear that a comparison between the effects of intracerebrally injected 5-HT and that of 5-HT releasing agents and MAO inhibitors can hardly be made. Consequently, it can be anticipated that the action of a 5-HT antagonist in the CNS will be different against exogenously administered 5-HT and endogenously released and/or potentiated 5-HT (or other amines). It is mainly because of these considerations that results reported in the literature on the effects of 5-HT antagonists utilizing the so-called indirect effects of 5-HT (evoked by releasing agents and precursors) have to be evaluated separately from those employing 5-HT and with a great deal of reservation. Other considerations to be kept in mind in connection with the behavioral effects of indolealkylamines are: the possibility of vascular effects influencing certain parts of the brain. Unfortunately, little is known about the effect of these agents on brain vessels and about the criteria of their pharmacologic blockade. It is likely, however, that the hallucinogenic N-alkylated indoles would not act by the same mechanism as does 5-HT; a peculiar contracting effect of 5-HT observed on the glial cells might also be implicated in its behavioral effects (Wooley and Shaw 1957b).

1. Summary of the actions of antagonists on CNS effects produced by 5-HT

An antagonism between 5-HT and mescaline but not between 5-HT and LSD has been in the behavioral action of fish (colisa lalia) (Saxena et al. 1962). In mice, 5-HT given intraventricularly produced excitatory actions followed by stupor. Lysergic acid diethylamide and some of its derivatives were potent preventing these actions (HALEY 1957). In rats, cats, and dogs 5-HT in large doses produced catalepsy and depression. These effects were antagonized by LSD (SACCHI et al. 1955, GADDUM and VOGT 1956, BROWN 1957). The conditioned pole climbing response of rats, which is depressed by 5-HT, could be restored by LSD (COOK and WEIDLEY 1957). 5-Hydroxytryptamine in large doses potentiates the effect of different hypnotic drugs (e.g., hexobarbital, pentobarbital, ethanol) probably by a central mechanism, and LSD is capable of antagonizing this narcosis-potentiating effect (SHORE et al. 1955, GARATTINI and VALZELLI 1956a, TAESCHLER 1956, SALMOIRAGHI and PAGE 1957). In contrast to the above data, when EEG and behavioral changes in cats were studied with 5-HT and LSD, no antagonism has been found between these agents (SCHWARZ et al. 1956). The results obtained were rather suggestive of a synergism between LSD and 5-HT (BRADLEY and HANCE 1956). The presence or absence of antagonism in EEG experiments, however, seems to depend largely on the regional differences of the brain because observing the electrical activity changes in the amygdala and basal ganglia of the cat opposite actions of 5-HT and LSD have been observed (SAWYER see GADDUM 1957a). On intraventricular injection of cats, 5-HT produces low amplitude activity in many subcortical areas. LSD pretreatment changes the 5-HT response in the amygdala. LSD and 5-HT produced seizure-like activity in the midbrain (GUNN 1960). Very interesting and also fundamental studies on indolealkylamines and certain 5-HT antagonists were done in the cat's brain with the use of direct iontophoretic application of substances through micropipettes (CURTIS and DAVIS 1962, KRNJEVIC and PHILLIS 1963). While 5-HT in general has been proved to be a depressant agent to cortical neuronal activity (driven by l-glutamate) dopamine surpassed it in this capacity. LSD derivatives also showed a depressant action which, however, was slower developing and longer lasting. Interestingly, 6-OH tryptamine was more potent than 5-HT; LSD was unable to antagonize the depressant effect of 5-HT. In view of MARAZZI's (1960) findings indicating that CPZ counteracts the depressant action of 5-HT on trans-callosal pathways it is unfortunate that this agent was not tested with the micro-pipette technique on cortical neurones. The finding that N-alkylation diminishes the depressant action of primary indolealkylamines suggests that this cortical neuronal depressant action per se would not be involved in the hallucinogenic activity of indoles. In addition, this study indicates that indolealkylamines cannot be considered as neurotransmitter substances for cortical neurones. Negative results with iontophoretically applied indolealkylamines has been obtained in brain stem neurones (CURTIS and KOIZUMI 1961) and in the spinal cord (CURTIS 1962). For the neurones of the lateral geniculate nucleus of the cat, however, CURTIS and DAVIS (1962) suggested that the depressant action of 5-HT and related indolealkylamines might be part of a physiologically occurring inhibitory function. Although peripherally active 5-HT antagonists (i.e. BOL, methysergid, harmaline, CPZ, dibenamine and phentolamine) did not alter the 5-HT-induced neuronal inhibition, the authors forwarded the hypothesis that the behaviorally active LDS and related indole compounds may interfere with a central neurotransmitter which could either be 5-HT or a similar but yet unrecognized indole derivative operating at certain synapses of the CSN.

Findings with BOL and LSD in cats in combination with 5-HT indicate that the relative degree of competition between these compounds determines the type of CNS action which develops (GUTH and SPIRTES 1959). In spite of its potent peripheral anti-5-HT action and efficacy in antagonizing the potentiation by 5-HT of hexobarbital narcosis (SALMOIRAGHI et al. 1957) BOL is frequently inactive in other tests measuring its action on the CNS. The depressant action of 5-HT on cats, for example, is not antagonized by BOL but only by LSD (Gaddum and Vogt 1956). The length of reserpine-hexobarbital narcosis was also unaffected by it (Cerletti and Rothlin 1955, Gyermek 1964c). An opposite effect, however, was also reported (Salmoiraghi et al. 1957). Among other lysergic acid derivatives acetyl-lysergic acid diethylamide an as potent anti-5-HT agent as LSD in vitro and in vivo (Cerletti and Konzett 1956, Haley 1957) also produced psychic effects in man similar to that of LSD (Rothlin 1957a). 1-Methyl lysergic acid diethylamide exhibited a potency two hundred times that of LSD in antagonizing the 5-HT-potentiated hexobarbital hypnosis (Cerletti and Doepfner 1958). 1-Methyl-d-lysergic acid butanolamide was also considerably more potent than LSD in this respect (Fanchamps et al. 1960), but in the human it was ineffective in producing behavioral changes. The fever-producing action of 1-methyl LSD was weaker than that of LSD (Cerletti and Doepfner 1958). Some of the phenothiazines were tested against 5-HT-induced narcosis-potentiation in the mouse. No significant antagonism with CPZ, promethazine (Gyermek 1964c) or diathazine (Cahn et al. 1956, Gyermek 1964c) could be demonstrated. It is difficult to estimate the anti-5-HT action of agents like CPZ in such a test because of the intensive narcosis-potentiation induced by CPZ itself. CPZ inhibits the O_2 uptake of the rat brain in vitro and there is no interference between 5-HT and CPZ in this respect (Starbuck and Heim 1959). Treatment of rats with phenothiazines or phenothiazines plus 5-HT and exposed to electro and acoustic shocks did not indicate significant reaction differences between the two groups. Again, it is difficult to interpret these data since 5-HT alone in the dose used did not seem to influence the reactivity of the animals (Venulet 1961). On the cat CPZ counteracts the inhibition of the transcallosal pathways by 5-HT (Marazzi 1960) but does not alter 5-HT-induced EEG changes (Yu et al. 1962). 5-HT induced flaccidity and diminution of initiative in monkeys inhibited the CPZ effects and increased reserpine effects (Baruk et al. 1962). Atropine may interfere with some of the actions of 5-HT in the CNS. This is indicated by the finding that it is capable of antagonizing the 5-HT plus pentothal-induced narcosis in rats (Cahn et al. 1956) and that atropine and mephenazine antagonize the cataleptic effect of 5-HT plus bulbocapnine treatment of mice (Buchel et al. 1960). In spite of its moderately weak anti-5-HT action in vitro, harmine was highly potent in antagonizing the potentiation of narcosis produced by reserpine (Gyermek 1964c). Harmine, like bromo LSD, illustrates that anti-HT action and the action against the potentiated hypnosis produced by reserpine are phenomena not necessarily related to each other. Studies of the influence of morphine on the central effects of 5-HT (Gaddum and Vogt 1956) are in accordance with the theory that it acts at certain 5-HT-sensitive nervous receptors. On the other hand, experiments attempting to prevent fixation of 5-HT to brain mitochondria by morphine and LSD showed no effect (Walaszek and Abood 1957). That Dibenamine may influence certain central nervous receptors sensitive to 5-HT is suggested by the observation that it can inhibit fixation of 5-HT to the brain cell particles (Walaszek and Abood 1957). The potentiating effect of 5-HT on hexobarbital anesthesia in mice could be reversed by levarterenol, as well as by dopamine. The analeptic effect of injections of 5-HT into the hindbrain could also be abolished by simultaneous injection of these agents (Schmidt et al. 1961). It is unfortunate that there are no more data available to demonstrate the actions of catecholamines against 5-HT on the CNS. Thus, the very intriguing question of a possible functional interaction between catecholamines and 5-HT in the CNS remains largely unanswered at present.

2. Influence of antagonists on CNS effects produced by 5-HT precursors and releasing agents

These agents were used to overcome the difficulty of the limited penetration of 5-HT into the brain. Usually 5-HTP used as precursor agent. The most frequently employed releasing agent is reserpine. Antagonists of the effects produced by both agents were studied extensively. In the group of lysergic acid derivatives, LSD was the most potent agent in antagonizing the reserpine-hexobarbital narcosis potentiation, whereas BOL which did not share the hallucinogenic property of LSD, was inactive (CERLETTI and KONZETT 1956, CERLETTI and ROTHLIN 1955, WOOLLEY 1959). Methysergid, LSD and ergotamine prevent mice from the toxic effects of 5-HTP. Although the pyrogenic action of 5-HTP was also prevented by methysergid it is unknown as to what extent the peripheral anti-5-HT effect of this agent contributes to the over-all protective effect (KARJA et al. 1961). A detailed study (CORNE et al. 1963) analyzed the protective action of a fairly large number of agents against 5-HTP induced CNS effects in the mouse. The observed effects of 5-HTP are assumed to be due to 5-HT because MAO inhibitors potentiate and inhibition of decarboxylation reduces the actions of 5-HTP. Among the agents effective against the central actions of supposedly endogenous 5-HT were: etonitazene (an analgesic), chlorprothixine CPZ (tranquilizers) and cyproheptadine (a peripheral 5-HT antagonist). Since the behaviorally very potent LSD was considerably less effective than cyproheptadine which shows no significant psychic effects the correlation between a central 5-HT inhibition and CNS effects in the mouse does not seem to be established. This study nevertheless revealed some interesting relationships between CNS effects, peripheral and central 5-HT antagonism. Studies so far have not investigated the crucial questions as to whether the interference with 5-HT of these drugs develops because of their 1. antagonism to 5-HT on CNS receptors; 2. interference with the permeability of storage organelles to 5-HT and/or norepinephrine; 3. interference with binding and transport of 5-HT. In another study chlorpromazine and chlorprothixine counteracted the following alterations of monoamine metabolism in rat brain: 1. increase in 5-HT and 3-hydroxytyramine content caused by MAO inhibitors; and 2. depletion of 5-HT, norepinephrine and 3-hydroxytyramine due to reserpine. Imipramine and amitriptyline caused no similar alteractions (GEY and PLETSCHER 1961). Of course there is a possibility that an agent may interfere with more than one process related to 5-HT as is the case with N-methyltryptamine, which, besides being an antagonist of convulsive actions of tryptamine and effective in blocking MAO in rats, does not inhibit 5-HTP-induced convulsions (TEDESCHI et al. 1962). A number of phenothiazines has been found to be effective antagonizing certain CNS actions of tryptamine and 5-HTP on the rat and in general a correlation between these actions and the behavioral effects of these phenothiazines (conditioned escape responses, catalepsy and locomotor activity tests) has been detected (TEDESCHI et al. 1961a). The most active 5-HTP and tryptamine antagonists in the phenothiazine group were perphenazine and triflupromazine. Behaviorally trifluoperazine and perphenazine were the most effective. There was a close correlation between anti-5-HT, anti-tryptamine and behavioral effects in a group of the less effective agents (TEDESCHI et al. 1961a, b). Among the peripherally highly potent phenothiazines CPZ did not change the amount of 5-HT in the tissues of rabbits after 5-HTP administration, however, it blocked the behavioral (SHAW and WOOLLEY 1957a) and EEG changes (COSTA and RINALDI 1958) produced by 5-HTP. α-methyl DOPA (a decarboxylase inhibitor) and CPZ in the rabbit delay the occurrence of EEG signs (flattening of cortical waves and rhinencephalic high frequency discharges) following 5-HTP administration. The already developed rhinencephalic discharges were not influenced, however, by agents like LSD (DOMER and LONGO 1962). Likewise, CPZ proved to be highly potent in preventing the iproniazid-reserpine-induced excitation of mice, rats, and rabbits (CHESSIN et al. 1957, FRANCO-BROWDERS et al. 1958, SHAW and WOOLLEY 1957a). Dibenamine did not block the CNS excitation produced by combined iproniazid-reserpine treatment in mice (CHESSIN et al. 1957). It is difficult to determine in case of a varied spectrum of action of an agent as to which should be taken as the predominant one especially when a compound is tested in the whole animal (TEDESCHI et al. 1962). As it could be anticipated not only typical anti-5-HT drugs but also some CNS depressants found inactive against 5-HT in peripheral organ receptors (i.e. barbiturates) interfere with some central actions of 5-HT (i.e. the spinal reflex actions). Some anesthetics (i.e. chloralose, hydroxydione) are markedly less potent in this respect (MARLEY and VANE 1963). The anti-5-HT action of barbiturates seems to be nonspecific.

H. Effects on the CNS of indolealkylamines related to 5-HT

So far information on phenomena elicited either by 5-HT or by its precursors on the CNS and certain effects of 5-HT antagonists on these phenomena has been outlined. The possible biological occurrence of indolealkylamines other than 5-HT as discussed earlier in connection with peripheral receptors necessitates a short survey of the CNS actions of indole derivatives which are structurally related to the biologically occurring indoles and those which can be considered to be of interest either as psychoactive drugs or pharmacologic tools in the exploration of CNS effects. The agonistic or antagonistic actions are not easily separable but there is also an overlap in the use of these agents, 5-HT and its precursors. These facts have to be realized when one consults the available data.

In addition to the well known CNS stimulant and convulsive effects of tryptamine and 5-HTP on hippocampal neurones, stimulant and inhibitory action of tryptamine and an inhibiting action of 5-HTP has been detected. The inhibitory effect of these indolealkylamines on these neurones resembles that of LSD (DE BARAN et al. 1963).

Methyltryptamine (probably α-methyltryptamine) exhibits tranquilizing and depressant effects on the mouse, monkey and man. It is ineffective in the rabbit. Combination with chlorpromazine intensifies the depressant effect (FU and HSU 1960). DL-α-ethyltryptamine is known to be a powerful CNS stimulant (MATTHEWS 1963). Its actions against 5-HT are unexplored. Part of the CNS effects of N,N-diethyltryptamine (i.e. diminution of spontaneous motor activity) is counteracted by reserpine, chlorpromazine and iproniazid (PFEIFER et al. 1961). 5-methoxy-N-methyltryptamine produces synchronization of hippocampal and desyncronization of cortical EEG activity in rabbits, later cortical spindles occur. It counteracts CPZ-induced EEG changes in rabbits but bufotenine is more effective. 5-methoxy-N-methyltryptamine also partially antagonizes the depression of conditioned responses produced by CPZ in rats. (MARCZYNSKI and VETULANI 1960). Melatonin in fairly low doses produces a gradually deepening depression on the rabbit (SUPNIEWSKI et al. 1960). A catatonic action of structurally related 5-methoxytryptamine is noted in rats injected intraventricularly (MICHAUX 1962). 5-Methoxy-N,N-dimethyltryptamine also deserves attention as a behaviorally potent indolealkylamine (GESSNER and PAGE 1962). Its effect on the performance of trained rats is more intense than with other commonly known indolealkylamines. Psylocin and 4-methyl-α-methyltryptamine show an alerting effect on rabbit EEG. Transections of the brain stem indicate that the two agents act at different levels. It is suggested that the slight changes in brain 5-HT levels following these amines would not account for the EEG effects observed (BRODEY et al. 1963). Psylocibin, a weak peripheral antagonist of 5-HT (CERLETTI 1959, GYERMEK and BINDLER 1962a), is about 100 times less potent than LSD producing behavioral effects (i.e. dreamy state, anxiety, visual effects) (HOLLISTER 1961). It was demonstrated that 6-hydroxylation may qualitatively alter the type of central nervous activity of N-alkyl tryptamine derivatives (SZARA et al. 1962). Since the degree of 6-hydroxylation of the hallucinogenic N,N-diethyltryptamine varies considerably from species to species extrapolation of the behavioral data on hallucinogenic indolealkylamines seems difficult. The mechanism of action of this type of an agent is likely to be an interference with the metabolism of 5-HT in the brain (SZARA 1962). This may well happen through competition with 5-HT receptor and/or enzyme surfaces in the CNS. A marked degree of interference with 5-HT in the group of hallucinogenic N-alkylated indoles and their 6-hydroxylated derivatives, however, could not be demonstrated in peripheral 5-HT receptors (GYERMEK 1964c). 10-methoxyarmalan, a proposed metabolite of melatonin, exhibits marked antagonistic properties to 5-HT and also causes behavioral alterations in conditioned rats (MCISAAC et al. 1961). Some of the 5-aza-indole derivatives are strong convulsants (ADLER and ALBERT 1963).

A correlation between the cerebral stimulant and depressant actions and peripheral actions on 5-HT receptors in this class of compounds could not be established. The results obtained with BOL and with 1-methyl-d-lysergic acid butanolamide which blocked some behavioral, electrophysiologic and spinal reflex actions of centrally active 5-methoxy-derivatives suggest that these indoles act on common receptor sites in the CNS which resemble those of tryptamine. (Some studies on peripheral receptors indicate the same (BUÑAG and WALASZEK 1962). However, there seems to be no direct evidence indicating that these receptor sites are identical in the CNS with the 5-HT receptors (VANE et al. 1961).

I. Action of 5-HT antagonists in inflammatory and anaphylactic processes

Although the role of 5-HT in inflammatory and allergic diseases was discussed repeatedly it still seems to be obscure. A relatively large number of animal and human experiments were performed utilizing different antagonists in order to clarify the role of 5-HT in the above-mentioned disease entities and offer therapeutic action in symptoms which were thought to develop through the possible participation of 5-HT. In some of the animal experiments the edema formation on the rat's paw produced by 5-HT and other inflammatory agents was utilized. While CPZ and some other phenothiazines were potent against the 5-HT-induced local edema, diethazine with a lower in vitro anti-HT potency showed no protective effect (GIÃO and RICO 1962). Although LSD and ergotamine inhibited primarily the 5-HT-produced edema, they were also effective against edemas resulting from tryptamine, 48/80, ovalbumin, dextran, hyaluronidase and kaolin administration (VOGEL and MARCH 1961). 5-HT, dextrane and hyaluronidase-induced reactions were also favorably responding to dibenamine but less favorably to neoantergan (UDA 1960). Based on these results it seems to be possible that 5-HT plays a role in the above-listed edematic reactions. Data on mice with formaline-induced edema seem to indicate that it releases 5-HT in this species and that 5-HT at least contributes to the edema formation. Consequently stronger inhibition of the 5-HT edema than that produced by formaldehyde has been observed by agents like yohimbine, phentolamine and thenalidine (NORTHOVER and SUBRAMANIAN

1962). Other reactions to 5-HT, e.g., edema formation in the skin, changes in capillary permeability as indicated by the spread of dyes and anaphylactic reactions were also studied on mice and rats. Selective inhibition of the 5-HT effects on the skin by RP 8647 (diazo-9-) dimethylamino-3'-methyl-2'-propyl)-10 phenothiazine has been observed while other phenothiazines inhibited the effect of other edema-producing agents (i.e. histamine, 48/80, polymyxin (Gözsy and Kato 1961). 5-HT, dextran and 48/80 produced skin edema and anaphylactic shock symptoms were inhibited by lysergic acid propanol amide and butanol-amide without influencing histamine edema and toxicity (Gelfand and West 1961). ECG signs of anaphylactic shock can be mimicked by 5-HT administration andbe minimized by CPZ which antagonizes 5-HT and by urethane which possibly inhibits 5-HT release (Mariani et al. 1961). In contrast to other species (i.e. dog, guinea pig) in mice the anaphylactic reactions are mediated through histamine and 5-HT release. Therefore, compounds which exhibit antihistamine as well as anti-5-HT properties offer full protection against anaphylactic shock whereas agents with either antihistaminic (i.e. mepyramine) or anti-5-HT (i.e. LSD) potency show complete protection only when given in combination (Halpern et al. 1963). Similar results were obtained in another study with anaphylactic reactions and lethal burns on mice. Cyproheptadine with antihistamine and anti-5-HT potencies showed full protective action while other agents were less effective (Ganley 1962). In the rat cutaneous anaphylaxis is protected by antihistamines rather than by anti-5-HT agents (Craps and Inderbitzin 1961). On the other hand, the anaphylactoid reaction produced by egg white is more sensitive to chlorpromazine and BOL than to antihistamines (Beach and Steinetz 1961). Results with 5-HT depleting agents are conflicting with the theory that 5-HT plays a significant role in the egg white produced reaction. The streptolysin "O" induced toxicity in mice is also favorably influenced by anti-5-HT agents, e.g. methysergid and BOL (Halbert et al. 1963). That 5-HT may participate in certain forms of cutaneous allergy is indicated by the following: a) A more marked antagonistic action of cyproheptadine to dermal reaction of intracutaneous 5-HT than to that of histamine; b) different behavior of other blocking agents (Balestra 1962); c) the positive effect of cyproheptadine against various other capillary damaging agents (i.e., histamine, histamine releasers and trypsin (Kalz and Fekete 1961). The few results obtained by using the rat granuloma pouch technique with the administration of 5-HT and its antagonists are inadequate either to determine the role of 5-HT in this model-inflammatory system or to obtain satisfactory answer to the question of efficacy of anti-5-HT agents. Methysergid showed some anti-inflammatory action against the croton oil induced granuloma reaction, but exogenous 5-HT itself also produced a reduction of granuloma pouch. The action of 5-HT on the exoserosis in the pouch is opposite that of methysergid (Zileli et al. 1962). It is noteworthy that cortisol, with a chemical structure atypical for anti-5-HT agents, showed a specific antagonistic action in the mouse paw edema test (Weis 1963) and that it also exhibited marked protective effect against the impaired resistance to 5-HT on adrenalectomized mice. Less marked protection was offered on these adrenalectomized animals against the toxic effects of histamine, endotoxine and anaphylactic shock (Higginbotham 1962).

K. Clinical applications of antagonists of 5-HT

The carcinoid syndrome is the only disease entity with a proven pathologic disturbance of 5-HT metabolism. The carcinoid tumor tissue contains and releases abnormal amounts of 5-HT and several clinical symptoms in this disease are the obvious result of its oversecretion. The pathogenesis, clinical aspects, and therapeutic approaches are thoroughly reviewed by LEMBECK (1961). Treatment of the symptoms may consist of a) utilizing antagonists of 5-HT; b) reducing the amount of precursors of 5-HT by limiting tryptophan intake; and c) interfering with the synthesis of 5-HT. Of the antagonists of 5-HT only a few have proved to be effective in suppressing the symptoms. Ergotamine LSD, BOL, methysergid and the antihistamines were ineffective against the flushing attacks characteristic of the disease (LANZ 1960, SJOERDSMA et al. 1957, SNOW et al. 1955). Although methysergid did not interfere with the appearance of the increased amount of 5-HT metabolite: 5-hydroxyindolic acetic acid in the urine it inhibited the gastrointestinal symptoms (i.e. oesophageal stricture (JENSEN 1963) and diarrhea (LANZ 1960). Chlorpromazine seemed to be the most effective agent with beneficial effects against most of the symptoms and also in suppressing 5-indoleacetic acid excretion (COLE and BERTINO 1956, SJOERDSMA et al. 1957, LEMBECK 1961). The participation of 5-HT as a pathological factor in other diseases (e.g. migraine and other different types of vascular headaches, inflammatory, allergic, and anaphylactic syndromes, abnormal vascular reactions in pulmonary embolism, phlebothrombosis and REYNAUD's disease) is also suspected. Certain manifestations of mental diseases, epilepsy and some endocrine disorders may also be connected to abnormal amounts or the altered metabolism of 5-HT (NEUMAN 1963). In the field of vascular headaches several studies reported beneficial effects from anti-5-HT agents especially from methysergid (OSTFIELD 1960, SICUTERI 1960, DALESSIO 1962, ABBOTT 1962, DOMINGUEZ et al. 1962). Atypical types of migraine (i.e. Horton syndrome) usually showed the best response (BERGOUIGNAN and SEILHEAN 1960).

Several animal studies indicate a possible role of 5-HT in inflammatory and allergic manifestations consequently the efficacy of anti-5-HT agents in human cutaneous allergy was tested in few studies. The increased capillary permeability and over-all cutaneous reactions to intradermal application of irritant agents, including histamine and 5-HT were effectively antagonized by cyproheptadine (KATZ and FEKETE 1961, BALESTRA 1962). In spite of the favorable effects which cyproheptadine in allergic skin reactions and pruritic conditions (JENSEN 1960, KAMINSKY and ASRILANT 1960, MALLEN and CUEVA 1961) the efficacy of "pure" anti-5-HT agents against endogenous allergic skin manifestations is still questionable (JENSEN 1960, PINSKER and THAYER 1963). The antiphlogistic action of several blocking agents of 5-HT against different types of inflammation producing agents in animal edema tests was discussed before. The specific anti-5-HT action of cortisol in the mouse paw edema test (WEIS 1963), the restoration of the normal sensitivity to 5-HT of adrenalectomized mice by hydrocortisone (HIGGINBOTHAM 1962), and the interference of hydrocortisone with 5-hydroxy indoleacetic acid excretion in patients (VACCAREZZA and BOCHI 1964) suggest that in the case of cortison-like agents for the treatment of certain inflammatory and allergic symptoms an anti-5-HT effect may participate in the over-all action of the drug. Only a few attempts have been made exploring this possibility. Patients with rheumatoid arthritis were tested in regard to their sensitivity to 5-HT and its antagonists (SCHERBEL and HARRISON 1959) and the intraarticular administration of methysergid has also been utilized (MÉRIEL et al. 1960). An anti-inflammatory action against the ocular manifestations of BASEDOW's disease has been reported with methysergid (LINQUETTE et al. 1962).

From the considerations based on animal experiments and discussed before it is not surprising that in clinical studies no correlation has been found between anti-5-HT and psychic actions. To illustrate this lack of correlation the following table is presented (from GADDUM 1957a).

	Anti-5-HT effects rat uterus	Schizoid changes	Excitement
LSD	+	+	+
BOL	+	0	0
Ergometrine	+	0	+
Mescaline	0	+	—
Morphine	0	+	+
B-tetrahydro-naphtylamine	0	—	+

In addition to the compounds listed in the table, BAS produced certain central effects, e.g., convulsive-like nonspreading electric discharges in the hypothalamus of the rabbit, but it did not influence human EEG patterns (RINALDI 1958). When given continuously (IV or orally), it showed mild tranquilizing effects (BENASSI 1958, RUDY et al. 1958) and reduced the cardiovascular and respiratory effects of 5-HT in patients, but antihistaminic agents with a very low anti-HT action were also found as effective (HOLLANDER et al. 1957). Although LSD and CPZ, perhaps the two best known psychopharmacologic agents, are outstandingly potent inhibitors of many actions of 5-HT, they not only antagonize the action of 5-HT but also may interfere with its uptake (GEY and PLETSCHER 1961) and metabolism. Thus LSD and CPZ were both shown to decrease the urinary excretion of 5-HT and its metabolite 5-indoleacetic acid (COLE and BERTINO 1956, RODNIGHT and MCILWAIN 1956, SANO et al. 1957). Chlorpromazine is also known to interfere with the N-methylation of 5-HT (AXELROD 1962). The efficacy of CPZ in clinical studies stands opposite to the lack of behavioral efficacy of methysergid (FANCHAMPS et al. 1960) and cyproheptadine (BODI et al. 1960). The observation that methysergid potentiates model psychosis produced by N,N-dimethyltryptamine (SAI-HALASZ 1962) and the lack of correlation found between the peripheral anti-5-HT and CNS effects indicate that the blocking action to 5-HT of most of these agents observed in animal organs is probably a very distinctly separable phenomenon from those which are connected to indolealkylamine receptor mechanisms and behavioral effects in the brain.

L. Biological data of the available antagonists of 5-HT

(Tables 1 trough 19)

Column
I. Isolated rat uterus
II. Other mammalian isolated organs
III. Nonmammalian isolated organs
IV. Nervous preparations
V. In vivo experiments
VI. Notes

Crosses in column 1. Approximate potencies obtained on the isolated uterus.
++++ = > 50% LSD
+++ = 50 > 10% LSD
++ = 10 > 1% LSD
+ = 1 > 0.1% LSD

Table 1. *Ergot derivatives*

Compound	I	II	III	IV, V, VI
Ergotamine	++ [1]	2, 3	4, 5	
Dihydroergotamine	+++ [1, 6]	6, 2, 7, 3	8, 4, 9, 10	
Ergosine	++ [1]			
Dihydroergosine	++ [1]			
Ergocornine	++ [1]			
Dihydroergocornine	++ [1, 11]			

Table 1 (Continued)

Compound	I	II	III	IV, V, VI
Ergocristine	++ [1]			
Dihydroergocristine	++ [1,11]			
Ergokryptine	++ [1]			
Dihydroergokryptine	++ [1]			
Ergonovine	+++ [1,12]	2, 13	8	
Dihydroergonovine	+++ [1]			
Methylergonovine	++++ [1]			
Dihydroergonovine	++++ [1]		14	

References to Table 1. [1] CERLETTI and DOEPFNER (1958). — [2] GADDUM and HAMEED (1954). — [3] MEIER et al. (1957). — [4] DOEPFNER and CERLETTI (1957). — [5] VOGEL and MAREK (1961). — [6] ERSPAMER (1953b). — [7] GREEFF et al. (1959). — [8] BUÑAG and WALASZEK (1962). — [9] FREYBURGER et al. (1952). — [10] OUTSCHOORN and JACOB (1960). — [11] GADDUM et al. (1955). — [12] GADDUM and PICARELLI (1957). — [13] SAVINI (1956). — [14] TAKEO (1962).

Table 2. *Lysergic acid derivatives*

Compound	I	II	III	IV, V, VI
d-lysergic acid amide	++ [1]			
d-lysergic acid methylamide	++ [1]			
d-lysergic acid ethylamide	+++ [1,2]		1	[3] IV
d-lysergic acid isopropylamide . . .	+++ [1,2]			
d-lysergic acid butylamide	+++ [1,2]			
d-lysergic acid amylamide	++++ [1]			
d-lysergic acid propylamide	+++ [2]			
d-lysergic acid cyclopropylamide . .	++++ [4]	4	5	
d-lysergic acid cyclobutylamide . .	++++ [2,4]	4	5	
d-lysergic acid cyclopentylamide . .	++++ [2,4]	4	5	
d-lysergic acid cyclohexylamide . .	++++ [2,4]	4	5	
d-lysergic acid cycloheptylamide . .	++++ [2,4]	4		
d-lysergic acid propanolamide . . .			1	[3] IV
d-lysergic acid butanolamide			1*	[3] IV
di-hydro d-lysergic acid butanolamide			1	
1-methyl, d-lysergic acid ethylamide			1	
1-methyl, d-lysergic acid propanolamide			1*, 6, 7, 8	
1-methyl-d-lysergic acid butanolamide (UML 491) (methysergid) .	++++ [9,8]	10, 11	12, 13, 14, 1*, 15, 16, 17, 6, 18, 19, 8, 21, 22, 23, 24, 25	[10] IV, [20,3] **
d-lysergic acid dimethylamide . . .	+++ [1,2]		26	
d-lysergic acid dipropylamide . . .	+++			
d-lysergic acid diisopropylamide . .	+++			
d-lysergic acid dibutylamide . . .	+++			
d-lysergic acid piperidide	++			
d-lysergic acid morpholide	++ [1,2] +++ [27]			
d-lysergic acid pyrrolidide	++ [1,2]			
d-lysergic acid pyrrolinide	++ [1,2]			
d-lysergic acid diethylamide (LSD) .	++++ 28, 29, 30, 31	32, 29, 33, 34, 35, 36, 31, 37, 38	12, 13, 16, 6, 39, 8, 40, 41, 42, 43, 44, 45, 24, 46, 47	[49] V
1-lysergic acid diethylamide	+ [2]			
d-isolysergic acid diethylamide . . .	+ [2]			
1-isolysergic acid diethylamide . .	+ [2]			
Dihydro LSD	+ [2]		26	
Lumi LSD	+ [2]			
Acetyl LSD	++++ [2]			[3] IV
1-methyl LSD	++++ [1]		16	[3] IV
1-oxymethyl LSD	+++ [1]			

Table 2 (Continued)

Compound	I	II	III	IV, V, VI
1-carbanilido LSD	++[1]			
2-bromo LSD	++++ 49, 2, 31	49, 2, 50, 36, 31, 51	12, 13, 52, 15, 26, 39, 41, 53, 24	48, 24*** V 54, 55, 3
2-iodo LSD	++++[1]			
2-dimethylaminomethyl LSD . . .	+++[1]			
8-methyl LSD	+++[1]			
1-methyl, 2-bromo-LSD		16, 26		

* More active than LSD. ** Inactive. *** Ineffective.

References to Table 2. [1] Cerletti and Doepfner (1958). — [2] Cerletti and Konzett (1956). — [3] Wright et al. (1962). — [4] Votava et al. (1962). — [5] Voltava and Lamplova (1959). — [6] Flückinger and Salzmann (1961). — [7] Gelfand and West (1961). — [8] Gyermek et al. (1962). — [9] Fanchamps et al. (1960). — [10] Day and Vane (1963). — [11] Sollero and Kurtz (1962). — [12] Berde et al. (1956). — [13] Buñag and Walaszek (1963). — [14] Buñag and Walaszek (1963). — [15] Chodera (1963). — [16] de Caro (1963). — [17] Eble (1963). — [18] Franchimont et al. (1961a). — [19] Franchimont et al. (1961b). — [20] Gaddum and Szerb (1961). — [21] Karja et al. (1961). — [22] Karlsberg et al. (1962). — [23] Poulson and Robson (1963). — [24] Sicuteri et al. (1960). — [25] Trapold et al. (1960). — [26] Doepfner and Cerletti (1958). — [27] Gogerty and Dille (1957). — [28] Costa (1956). — [29] Gaddum and Hameed (1954). — [30] Gaddum et al. (1955). — [31] Sollero et al. (1956). — [32] Barlow (1961). — [33] Gaddum and Vogt (1956). — [34] Meier et al. (1957). — [35] Passow et al. (1960). — [36] Savini (1956). — [37] Trendelenburg (1960). — [38] Woolley (1957b). — [39] Guth and Spirtes (1959). — [40] Halpern et al. (1963). — [41] Holgate and Warner (1960). — [42] Kroeger and Lucco (1960). — [43] O'Brien et al. (1962). — [44] Outschoorn and Jacob (1960). — [45] Schmitt and Schmitt (1959). — [46] Vogel and Marek (1961). — [47] Wilhelmi and Schindler (1959). — [48] Brownlee and Johnson (1963). — [49] Barlow andKhan (1959a). — [50] King (1957). — [51] Vane (1957). — [52] Chodera (1962). — [53] Parratt and West (1956). — [54] Mansour (1957). — [55] Moore et al. (1961).

Table 3. *Indole derivatives*

Compound	I	II	III	IV, V, VI
Indole	1	2		
1-methylindole	1			
2-methylindole		2		
3-methylindole		2		
4-methylindole	1			
4-indole carboxylic acid diethylamide	3 *			
5-methylindole	1	2		
5-fluoroindole		2		
5-hydroxyindole	1 **			
5-aminoindole		4		
5-methylaminoindole		4		
5-dimethylaminoindole		4		
6-methylindole	1			
6-hydroxyindole	1 **			
5-hydroxy, 2-β aminoethyl indole			5	
2-methyl, 5-fluoro indole.		2		
2-methyl, 5-chloro indole		2		
2-methyl, 5-bromo indole		2		
2-methyl, 5-methoxy-indole		2		
3-methyl, 5-fluoro-indole.		2		
3-ethyl, 5-aminoindole		6		
N-methyl indolyl-2-(methyl)amine		7		
2-methyl, 3-ethyl-4-nitroindole	1			
2-methyl, 3-ethyl-7-nitroindole	1			
2-methyl, 3-ethyl-4-aminoindole	1			
2-methyl, 3-ethyl-7-aminoindole	1, 8	4, 6	9	
2-methyl, 3-ethyl-5-aminoindole		4	10	

Table 3 (Continued)

Compound	I	II	III	IV, V, VI
2-methyl, 3-ethyl-5-methylaminoindole	8	4		
2-methyl, 3-ethyl-5-dimethylaminoindole (Medmain)	4,8	4		
2-methyl, 3-ethyl-5-trimethylammonium indole cloride		4		
2-methyl, 3-(β-hydroxyethyl) 5-dimethylamino indole		4		
2-methyl, 3-(β-chloroethyl) 5-dimethylamino-indole		4		
2-methyl, 3-ethyl, 5-(N-pyrrolidyl) indole . . .		4		
2,3-dimethyl, 4-nitro indole	1			
2,3-dimethyl, 6-nitro indole	1			
2,3-dimethyl, 7-nitro indole	1 **			
2,3-dimethyl, 4-amino indole	1 **			
2,3-dimethyl, 5-amino indole		2		
2,3-dimethyl, 6-amino indole	1			
2,3-dimethyl, 7-amino indole	1			
2,3-dimethyl, 5-fluoro indole		2		
2-phenyl, 3,5-dinitro indole	1			
1,2-dimethyl, 3-ethyl, 5-dimethylaminoindole (methyl medmain)	8	4		
2-methyl, 3-ethyl, 5-dimethylamino, 7-chloro-indole		4		
4-4′dicyano-3,3′ diindolyl methane	3 ***			
3-diethylaminomethylindole	8			
1-phenyl-3-(N-piperidino)-methyl indole	11			
1-phenyl, 3β-(N-dimethylamino)-propyl indole .	11			
1-phenyl, 3-(N-piperidino)-propyl indole	11	4		
2-methyl, 3-piperidyl-methyl, 5-chloroindole . .	4,8			
N-butyl, 4-chloroindolyl 2-(methyl) amine . . .	7	7		
N-ethyl 1-methyl indolyl 2-(methyl) amine . . .	7	7		
N-methyl 5-methoxy-indolyl 2-(methyl) amine .	7	7		
N-butyl 5-chloro indolyl 2-(methyl) amine . . .	7	7		
5-hydroxyindole alkylamines			12	
5-acyloxyindole alkylamines				
5-alkoxyindole alkylamines				
5-benzyloxyindole alkylamines				

* Several other 4-substituted indoles reported. ** Ineffective. *** Several other 4-substituted bis-indoles were reported.

References to Table 3. [1] GADDUM et al. (1955). — [2] QUADBECK and RÖHM (1954). — [3] HARRIS and UHLE (1960). — [4] SHAW and WOOLLEY (1954). — [5] WILHELMI and SCHINDLER (1959). — [6] SHAW and WOOLLEY (1953). — [7] BERTACCINI and ZAMBONI (1961). — [8] ERSPAMER (1955). — [9] ERSPAMER (1953a). — [10] COMORE et al. (1953). — [11] KOPF and MØELLER NIELSEN (1959). — [12] STRANDTMANN et al. (1963).

Table 4. *Gramine derivatives*

Compound	I	II	III	IV, V, VI
Gramine	1, 2, 3	2,4, 5	6	
1-methylgramine	3			
2-methylgramine	1,6	5		
4-carbomethoxygramine	7 *			
4-methylgramine	3			
5-methylgramine	3	5		
6-methylgramine				[4] IV
5-fluorogramine		5		
5-chlorogramine		5		
5-benzyloxygramine	8, 3	8, 9		
6-benzyloxygramine	3			[4] IV

Table 4a. (Continued)

Compound	I	II	III	IV, V, VI
2-methyl, 5-nitro gramine	1			
2-methyl, 5-amino gramine.	1			
2-methyl, 5-fluoro gramine		5	1	
2-methyl, 5-chloro gramine.	1	5		
2-methyl, 5-bromo gramine	1	5		
2-methyl, 5-metoxy gramine		5		
2-methyl, 7-chloro gramine.	1			
2,5-dimethyl gramine		5		
5,6-dimethyl gramine	1			

* Several other 4-substituted gramines are reported.

References to Table 4. [1] ERSPAMER (1955). — [2] GADDUM and HAMEED (1954). — [3] GADDUM et al. (1955). — [4] GADDUM and PAASONEN (1955). — [5] QUADBECK and RÖHM (1954). — [6] ERSPAMER (1953a). — [7] HARRIS and UHLE (1960). — [8] BARLOW and KHAN (1959a). — [9] GADDUM and VOGT (1956).

Table 5a. *Tryptamine derivatives*

Compound	I	II	III	IV, V, VI
Tryptamine	1	2, 3		4, 5, 6
1-methyltryptamine	7			
2-methyltryptamine	7			
4-methyltryptamine	7			
5-methyltryptamine	7			
5-methoxytryptamine				[26] IV
6-methyltryptamine	7			
7-methyltryptamine	7			
α-methyltryptamine	7			
α-ethyltryptamine			8	
N-methyltryptamine	8			
N-isopropyltryptamine	7, 9		8	
5-methoxytryptophanol	13			
α,α-dimethyltryptamine	7			
N,N-dimethyltryptamine	1, 7, 9	9, 10	8	
N,N-diethyltryptamine	9, 11	9		
N,N-dipropyltryptamine		9		
N,N-dibutyltryptamine	9	9		
5-hydroxy α-methyltryptamine				[6] IV
5-methyl, α-methyl tryptamine	9	9		
N,N-dimethyl, 5-hydroxytryptamine (Bufotenine)	7			[6] IV
N,N-dibutyl, 5-hydroxytryptamine	9, 12 *			
2-methyl, 5-hydroxytryptamine	13			
2-methyl, 5-methoxytryptamine	13			
1-benzyl, 5-methoxytryptamine.	13			
1-benzyl, 2-methyl-5-methoxytryptamine (BAS)	14	15, 16	17, 18	
1-phenyl, 2-methyl 5-methoxytryptamine . . .	9	9		
1,2-dimethyl, 5-methoxytryptamine	13			
1,5-dimethyl bufotenine	13			
1-benzyl, 2,5-dimethyl bufotenine (BAB) . . .	19	15	13, 19	
1-benzyl 2-methyl 5-hydroxytryptamine . . .			25	
1-(p-methoxybenzyl)-2-methyl-5-hydroxytrypt-amine HCl (Hydroxindasol)	14 *		14	[20] VI *
N,N-dimethyl 2-methyl tryptamine		10		
N,N-dimethyl 4-hydroxytryptamine (psylocin) .	21	21		
N,N-dimethyl 4-hydroxy tryptamine O-phosphate (Psylocybin)	21, 22	21		
5-Benzyloxy, 3(2-dimethylaminoethyl) indole .	1, 9	9, 10		
5-Benzyloxy, 3(2-diethylaminoethyl) indole . .	12			
5-Benzyloxy, 3(2-dipropylaminoethyl) indole . .		12		
5-Benzyloxy, 3(2-di-isopropylaminoethyl) indole	12			

Table 5a. (Continued)

Compound	I	II	III	IV, V, VI
5-Benzyloxy, 3(2-morpholinoethyl)-indole . . .	12			
5-Benzyloxy, 3(2-aminopropyl) indole	12			
5-Benzyloxy, 3(2-aminoethyl) indole	9	9		
3-β-N-(1,2,3,4 tetrahydroisoquinolyl) ethyl indole				
3β-N(1,2,3,4 tetrahydroisoquinolyl) ethyl, 5-aminoindole				
N-methyl indolyl 3-(β-hydroxyethyl) amine . .	9	9		
N,N-dimethyl indolyl 3-(β-hydroxy-ethyl) amine	9	9		
N,N-dimethyl, 5-hydroxy indolyl 3-(β-hydroxy-ethyl) amine	9	9		
N,N-dimethyl, 1-phenylethyl-5-methoxy tryptamine		23	23	
1,10-decamethylene bis 1-benzyl-2-benzyl 2-methyl tryptamine derivatives		21		

* And other related 1-aralkyltryptamines.

References to Table 5. [1] Barlow and Khan (1959a). — [2] Gaddum (1953). — [3] Vane (1957). — [4] Cleugh et al. (1961). — [5] Gaddum and Szerb (1961). — [6] Greenberg (1960a). — [7] Gaddum et al. (1955). — [8] Erspamer (1953a). — [9] Bertaccini and Zamboni (1961). — [10] Barlow (1961). — [11] Arnold and Hofman (1957). — [12] Barlow and Khan (1959b). — [13] Shaw and Woolley (1956). — [14] Stone et al. (1961). — [15] Stormorken (1959). — [16] Jacob and Poite-Bevierre (1960). — [17] Konzett (1956). — [18] Outschoorn (1960). — [19] Shaw and Wooлle y(1956). — [20] Ginzel and Kottegoda (1953). — [21] Woolley and Campbell (1962). — [22] Cerletti (1959). — [23] Julia et al. (1960). — [24] Wolley (1959). — [25] Shore et al. (1955). [26] Gyermek and Bindler (1962b).

Table 5b. *Quaternary indolealkylammonium compounds*

	MED*
N-(benzyl)-N,N-dimethyl β-(3-indolyl-ethyl)-ammonium bromide	30
N-(o-xylyl)-N,N-dimethyl β(3-indolyl-ethyl)-ammonium bromide . .	80
N-(o-chlorbenzyl) N,N-dimethyl β-3-(indolyl-ethyl)-ammonium bromide . . .	50
N-(m-xylyl) N,N-dimethyl β-(3-indolyl-ethyl)-ammonium bromide	20
N-(m-nitrobenzyl) N,N-dimethyl β-(3-indolyl ethyl) ammonium bromide. . .	20
N-(m-chlorbenzyl) N,N-dimethyl β-(3-indolyl-ethyl)-ammonium bromide . .	7
N-(m-chlorbenzyl) N,N-diethyl β-(3-indolyl-ethyl)-ammonium bromide . . .	80
N-(p-xylyl) N,N-dimethyl β-(3-indolyl ethyl)-ammonium bromide.	80
N-(p-bromobenzyl) N,N-dimethyl β-(3-indolyl-ethyl)-ammonium bromide . .	20
N-(benzyl)-N,N-dimethyl β-(5-hydroxy 3-indolyl-ethyl)-ammonium bromide .	4.2
N-(m-xylyl) N,N-dimethyl β-(5-hydroxy 3-indolyl-ethyl)-ammonium bromide	8.3
N-(m-chlorbenzyl) N,N-dimethyl β-(5-hydroxy 3-indolethyl-ammonium bromide	0.66

*MED: Minimal effective blocking doses in μg/kg against 5-HT on the inferior mesenteric ganglion preparation of the cat. Gyermek (1964a).

Table 6. *Carbazol derviatives*

Compound	I	II	III	IV, V, VI
1-nitro carbazole	1			
2-nitro carbazole	1			
3-nitro carbazole	1			
4-nitro carbazole	1			
1-amino carbazole	1			
2-amino carbazole	1			
3-amino carbazole	1			
1,2,3,4-tetrahydro carbazole	1	2		
5-nitro, 1,2,3,4-tetrahydrocarbazole	1			
7-nitro, 1,2,3,4-tetrahydrocarbazole	1			
6-nitro, 1,2,3,4-tetrahydrocarbazole	1			
5-amino, 1,2,3,4-tetrahydrocarbazole	1			

Table 6 (Continued)

Compound	I	II	III	IV, V, VI
6-amino, 1,2,3,4-tetrahydrocarbazole	1	2		
7-amino, 1,2,3,4-tetrahydrocarbazole	1			
8-amino, 1,2,3,4-tetrahydrocarbazole	1			
6-carboxamidino, 1,2,3,4-tetrahydro carbazole	2	2		
6-N-phenylcarboxamidino, 1,2,3,4-tetrahydro-carbazole	2	2		
6-aminomethyl-1,2,3,4-tetrahydro carbazole		2		
6-N,N-dimethylaminomethyl, 1,2,3,4-tetrahydro carbazole	2	2		
9-benzyl, 6.N,N-dimethylaminomethyl, 1,2,3,4-tetrahydrocarbazole	2			

References to Table 6. [1] Gaddum et al. (1955). — [2] Shaw and Woolley (1957a).

Table 7. *Carboline derivatives*

Compound	I	II	III	IV, V, VI
Harmane	1, 9	2		
Harmine	1, 3, 4	5		[6] IV
Harmaline	1, 3, 4			[7] V *
Harmalol	1			
Harmol	1			
Tetrahydroharmane	8			
6-aminoharmane		2		
10-methoxyharmalan	+ + + [4]	4	4	
3-trimethoxybenzamido methyl harmane and other 3-substituted harmane derivatives	9			[9] V

* Inactive.

References to Table 7. [1] Erspamer (1953a). — [2] Shaw and Woolley (1953). — [3] Harris and Uhle (1960). — [4] McIsaac et al. (1961). — [5] Woolley and Shaw (1957b). — [6] Mansour (1957). — [7] Curtis and Davis (1962). — [8] Gaddum et al. (1955). — [9] Sigg et al. (1964).

Table 8. *Antihistamines*

Compound	I	II	III	IV, V, VI
Antazoline	1		2, 3	
Bayer 1219			3	
Diphenhydramine	+ + [1, 4]	5	6, 7	
Mepazine			3	
Phenindamine	+ + [1, 2]		3	
Pipadrol	8			
Pyrilamine	+ + [1, 9]	10, 11	12	
Synopen (Synpen)			3	
Thenophenopiperidine	+ + + [1]	13	3, 14	
Tripelennamine	+ + [1]	5, 15	2, 3, 15	
4-Benzylanilino-1-methylpiperidine			2	
N-phenyl-N-benzyl-4-amino-1-methyl-piperidine [Soventol (R)]			3	
Thenalidine			16, 17	
Mepyramine			7, 18	
Chlorcyclizine	+ + + [19]	19	19	
Homochlorcyclizine	+ + + [19] *	19	19	

* 24 related compounds are also reported.

References to Table 8. [1] Doepfner and Cerletti (1957). — [2] Doepfner and Cerletti (1958). — [3] Schmid et al. (1959). — [4] Gaddum and Paasonen (1955). — [5] Rapport and Koelle (1952). — [6] Eble (1963). — [7] Holgate and Warner (1960). — [8] Costa (1956). — [9] Gaddum and Hameed (1954). — [10] Grette (1957). — [11] Bhattacharya (1955). — [12] Herxheimer (1955). — [13] King (1957). — [14] Konzett (1956). — [15] Meier et al. (1957). — [16] Nikodijevic and Vanov (1960). — [17] Northover and Subramanian (1962). — [18] Halpern et al. (1963). — [19] Kimura et al. (1960).

Table 9. *Phenothiazines and related compounds*

Compound		I	II	III	IV, V, VI
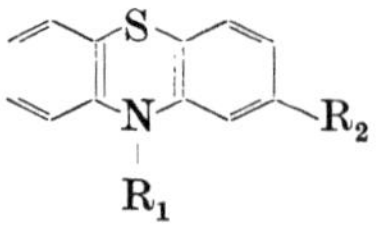					
R_1	R_2				
—$(CH_2)_3$—$N(Me)_2$ Chlorpromazine (Cpz)	Cl	+++[1] ++++[2,3,4]	4, 5, 6, 7, 8	1, 4, 8, 9, 10, 11, 12, 13, 14, 15, 16, 17, 18	19 * V 20, 21
—$(CH_2)_2$—$N(Et)_2$ Diethazine	H	++[1] 3			
—$(CH_2)_3$—N N—Me Taxilan (P-725)	H	++[22]		22	
—$(CH_2)_3$—N N—Me Prochlorperazine	Cl		10		
—CH_2—CH—$N(Me)_2$ CH_3 Promethazine	H	++++[1,3]	8, 10, 23	1, 13, 17, 18, 24, 25	
R_1	R_2				
—$(CH_2)_3$—$N(Me)_2$ Promazine	H		10		
—CO—CH—$N(Me)_2$ CH_3 Secergan (R)	H		26		
—CH_2—CH—$\overset{+}{N}(Me)_3$ CH_3 Thiazinamium	H		10		
—COO—$(CH_2)_2$—$N(Et)_2$	H		27		
—CH_2—CH—CH_2—$N(Me)_2$ CH_3 Trimeprazine	H	28		28, 29	
—$(CH_2)_3$—$N(Me)_2$	$COCH_3$		30		
—$(CH_2)_3$—$N(Me)_2$	COC_2H_5		30		
—$(CH_2)_3$—$N(Me)_2$	COC_3H_7		30		
—$(CH_2)_3$—N N—ME	$COCH_3$		30		
Acetylpromazine		4	31		
Valeroylpromazine			31		
(Diazo-9-)-dimethylamino-3′-methyl-2′-propyl)-10-phenothiazine (RP 6847)		32		24	
Levomepromazine					
R_1	R_2				
—$(CH_2$ —N	H	++[33]			

Table 9. (Continued)

Compound	I	II	III	IV, V, VI
—$(CH_2)_3$—N(ring) OH** Cl or Br	++++[33]			
—CH_2—CH_2—$CH_2N(Me)_2$ CH_3 RP-4627			34	
—CH_2—CH_2—CH_2N(ring) H RP-4670			34	
—CH_2—CH—$CH_2N(Me)_2$ CH_3O CH_3 RP-7044			*** 34	
—$(CH_2)_3$—N N—Me CF_3 Trifluoperazine			35	
—$(CH_2)_2$— N(ring) SCH_3 CH_3 Mellaril (R)		36		
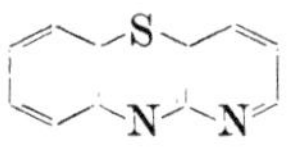 R_1				
—CH_2—CH—$N(Me)_2$ CH_3 D-201			17	
—$(CH_2)_3$—$N(Me)_2$			17	

* Inactive. ** Cis or trans. *** More effective than CPZ.

References to Table 9. [1] DOEPFNER and CERLETTI (1957). — [2] COSTA (1956). — [3] GYERMEK et al. (1956). — [4] VENULET (1961). — [5] BENDITT and ROWLEY (1956). — [6] BERGER et al. (1957). — [7] KING (1957). — [8] MEIER et al. (1957). — [9] DASGUPTA (1957). — [10] DOMENJOZ and THEOBALD (1959). — [11] GANLEY (1962). — [12] GINZEL (1957). — [13] HALPERN et al. (1963). — [14] MARIANI and VERTUA (1960). — [15] MÖRSDORF and BODE (1959). — [16] NIAUSSAT et al. (1961). — [17] SCHMID et al. (1959). — [18] WILHELMI (1957). — [19] CURTIS and DAVIS (1962). — [20] MARAZZI (1960). — [21] YU et al. (1962). — [22] NIESCHULZ et al. (1958). — [23] BHATTACHARYA (1955). — [24] GÖZSY and KATO (1961). — [25] PARRATT and WEST (1956). — [26] WIELDING (1958). [27] WIEDLING (1959). — [28] STONE et al. (1961). — [29] SICUTERI et al. (1960). — [30] WIRTH et al. (1959). — [31] RUMMEL (1961). — [32] COURVOISIER et al. (1962). — [33] WYLIE (1959). — [34] PARRATT and WEST (1958). — [35] TEDESCHI et al. (1959). — [36] HALEY et al. (1959).

Table 10. *Dibenzothiazepine derivatives*

Compound	I	II	III	IV, V, VI
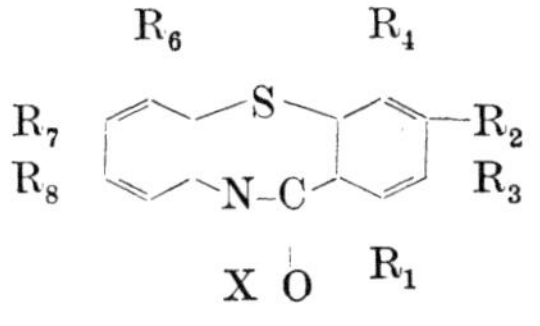				

Table 9. (Continued)

Compound		I	II	III	IV, V, VI
X	$R_8{=}CH_3$				
$—CH_2—CH_2—N(Me)_2$	$R_8{=}CH_3$		1*	1 △	
$—CH_2—CH_2—N(Et)_2$	$R_8{=}CH_3$		1	1	
$—CH_2—CH_2—CH_2—N(Me)_2$	$R_8{=}CH_3$		1	1	
$—CH_2—CH(CH_3)—N(Me)_2$	$R_8{=}CH_3$		1		
$—CH_2—CH_2—N\langle\rangle N—Me$ (piperazine)	$R_8{=}CH_3$		1		
$—CH_2—CH_2—N(Me)_2$	$R_2{=}Cl$		1	1	
$—CH_2—CH_2—N(Me)_2$	$R_6{=}Cl$		1		
$—CH_2—CH_2—N(Me)_2$	$R_2{=}CH_3$		1		
$—CH_2—CH_2—N(Me)_2$	—		1		
$—CH_2—CH_2—N(Me)_2$	$R_2, R_8{=}CH_3$		1		
$—CH_2—CH_2—N(Me)_2$	$R_7, R_8{=}CH_3$		1		
$—CH_2—CH_2—N(Me)_2$	$R_8{=}CH_3O$		1	1 △	

* Guinea pig ileum. △ Guinea pig bronchospasm.

References to Table 10. [1] JAQUES et al. (1959).

Table 11. *Iminodibenzyl and iminostilbene derivatives*

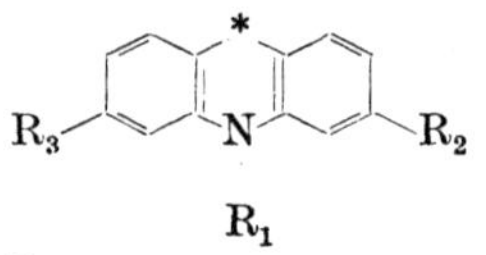

Compound R_1	R_2	R_3	*	I	II	III	IV, V, VI
$—CH_2—CH_2—N(Et)_2$	H	H	$—CH_2—CH_2$		1*		
$—CH_2—CH_2—CH_2—N(Me)_2$	H	H			1*	1, 2, 3	
$—CH(CH_3)—CH_2—N(Me)_2$	H	H			1		
$—CH_2—CH(CH_3)—N(Me)_2$	H	H			1*		
$—CH_2—CH(CH_3)—N(Me)_3$	H	H			1*		
$—CH_2—CH_2—CH_2—N(Me)_2$	Cl	Cl			1		
$—CH_2—CH_2—N(Et)_2$	H	H	$—CH{=}CH—$		1*		
$—CH_2—CH_2—CH_2—N(Me)_2$	H	H			1*		
$—CH_2—CH(CH_3)—N(Me)_2$	H	H			1*		
$—CH_2—CH_2—CH_2—N(Me)_2$	Cl	Cl			1*		
$—(CH_2)_3—N\langle\rangle N—CH_3$ (piperazine)	Cl	Cl			1		

* More potent than CPZ.

References to Table 11. [1] DOMENJOZ and THEOBALD (1959). — [2] MÖRSDORF and BODE (1959). — [3] SABELLI and SINAY (1960).

Table 12. *Other compounds related to phenothiazines*

Compound	I	II	III	IV, V, VI
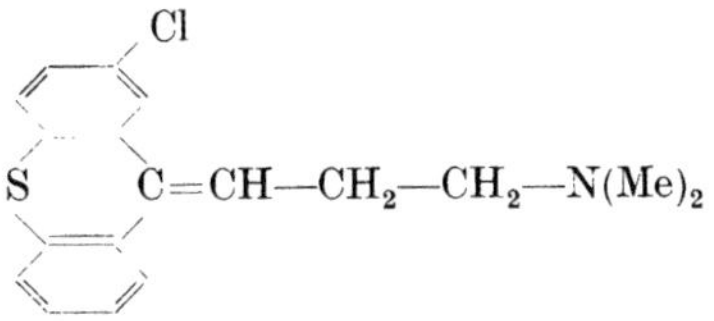 Chlorprothixine		1 *		
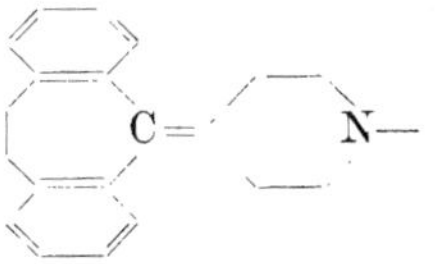 Cyproheptadine [8] ***	+ + + + [2] **		2, 3, 4, 5, 6, 7	

* More potent than CPZ. ** More potent than LSD. *** Structurally similar dibenzo-cycloheptane derivatives

References to Table 12. [1] NIELSEN and NEUHOLD (1959). — [2] STONE et al. (1961). — [3] BENASSI (1958). — [4] GANLEY (1962). — [5] KALZ and FEKETE (1961). — [6] NORTHOVER and SUBRAMANIAN (1962). — [7] POULSEN and ROBSON (1963). — [8] Geigy A.G. (1962).

Table 13. *Adrenolytic and hypotensive drugs*

Compound	I	II	III	IV, V, VI
Dibenamine	+ + + [1]	2, 3, 4, 5	5, 6, 7, 8	[9] V *
Dibenzyline		10, 11, 12, 13		[13] VI [14] V
1-Hydrazinophtalazine	15, 16	2, 5	5	
Phentolamine		2	17, 19	[9] V *
Piperoxane	4	4		
Reserpine	20	5, 21	5, 18, 22, 23, 24	[9] V *
Yohimbine		5, 25, 26	5, 18, 27	[28] IV

* Inactive.

References to Table 13. [1] GADDUM et al. (1955). — [2] BHATTACHARYA (1955). — [3] FURCHGOTT (1955). — [4] GADDUM and HAMEED (1954). — [5] MEIER et al. (1957). — [6] ERSPAMER (1953b). — [7] OUTSCHOORN and JACOB (1960). — [8] TEDESCHI et al. (1961b). — [9] CURTIS and DAVIS (1962). — [10] DAY and VANE (1963). — [11] GADDUM and VOGT (1956). — [12] VANE (1957). [13] YOON (1960). — [14] BROWNLEE and JOHNSON (1963). — [15] ERSPAMER (1952a). — [16] NAERS and SKRAMSTAD (1954). — [17] BELESLIN and VARAGIĆ (1960). — [18] NORTHOVER and SUBRAMANIAN (1962). — [19] SCHAEPPI (1963). — [20] COSTA (1956). — [21] BERGER et al. (1957). — [22] CERLETTI and WEIDMANN (1962). — [23] KROEGER and LUCCO (1960). — [24] WILHELMI (1957). — [25] WOOLLEY and SHAW (1953). — [26] WOOLLEY and SHAW (1957b). — [27] FREYBURGER et al. (1952). — [28] MANSOUR (1957).

Table 14. *Atropine and atropine-like drugs; spasmolytics*

Compound	I	II	III	IV, V, VI
Atropine	1, 2	1, 3, 4, 5, 6, 7, 8	7, 9, 10, 11	
Benactyzine		12, 13		
Hyoscine		14, 18		[15] IV [16] V
Oxyphenonium		7	7	
Papaverine		7	7	
2-diethylaminoethyl-diphenylacetate HCl (Trasentine (R)		7	7	
1-(diethylamino), 3-diphenyl, 3-oxy-propane methoidide		6, 17		

Table 14. (Continued)

Compound	I	II	III	IV, V, VI
1-(N-pyrrolidino), 3-phenyl, 3-cyclohexyl, 3-oxypropane HCl		6		
1-(N-pyrrolidino), 3-phenyl, 3-cyclohexyl, 3-oxypropane methoiodide		6		
1-(N-piperidino), 3-diphenyl, 3-oxypropane HBr		6		

References to Table 14. [1] GADDUM and HAMEED (1954). — [2] GADDUM et al. (1955). — [3] BERGER et al. (1957). — [4] BHATTACHARYA (1955). — [5] CAMBRIDGE and HOLGATE (1955). — [6] GARATTINI and VALZELLI (1956a). — [7] MEIER et al. (1957). — [8] RAPPORT and KOELLE (1952). — [9] FREYBURGER et al. (1952). — [10] HOLGATE and WARNER (1960). — [11] WILHELMI (1957). — [12] ROBERTSON (1953). — [13] SINHA and WEST (1953). — [14] VANE (1957). — [15] BARLOW and KHAN (1957a). — [16] BROWNLEE and JOHNSON (1963). — [17] GARVEN (1956). — [18] DAY and VANE (1963).

Table 15. *Local anaesthetics*

Compound	I	II	III	IV, V, VI
Amylocain	1	1		
Cocaine	1	1, 2, 3, 4	2, 5, 6	
Dibucaine	1	1, 2, 7	2	
Lidocaine	1	1		
Procaine	1	1, 2, 7, 8, 9	2, 5, 10, 11, 12	13 V
Tetracain	1	1	10	
Amethocain			12	
Cinchocain			12	
Cocaine diethylamide	14			

References to Table 15. [1] SINHA and WEST (1953). — [2] MEIER et al. (1957). — [3] ROCHA E SILVA et al. (1953). — [4] TRENDELENBURG (1960). — [5] CERLETTI and ROTHLIN (1955). — [6] TRENDELENBURG (1956). — [7] JAQUES et al. (1956). — [8] GADDUM and VOGT (1956). — [9] HARRY (1963). — [10] FRAHM (1957). — [11] KROEGER and LUCCO (1960). — [12] NORTHOVER and SUBRAMANIAN (1962). — [13] BROWNLEE and JOHNSON (1963). — [14] JORDAN et al. (1958).

Table 16. *Morphine type analgesics*

Compound	I	II	III	IV, V, VI
Aethylmorphine		1		
Codeine		1		
Dihydromorphinone		1		
Methadone		1		
Morphine		1, 2, 3, 4, 5	6	7 V
Pethidine				

References to Table 16. [1] MEDAKOVIĆ (1958). — [2] DAY and VANE (1963). — [3] GADDUM and VOGT (1956). — [4] HARRY (1963). — [5] TRENDELENBURG (1960). — [6] TRENDELENBURG (1957). — [7] MEDAKOVIĆ (1958).

Table 17. *Sympathomimetic amines*

Compound	I	II	III	IV, V, VI
Adrenochrome	1			
Amphetamine		2	2	
Desoxyephedrine		2	2	
Dopamine				3 IV
Ephedrine		2	2	
Epinephrine		2, 4, 5	2	
Isopropylnorepinephrine		2, 4, 5	2, 6, 7	
Norepinephrine		2, 5	2, 8	

Table 17 (Continued)

Compound	I	II	III	IV, V, VI
3,4-dichloroisopropyl norepinephrine			9	
2,4-dichloro phenoxyethylamine . .	10			
2,4,6-trichloro phenoxyethylamine .	10			
4-methoxy phenoxyethylamine. . .	10			
2,6-dimethoxy phenoxyethylamine .	10			
3,4,5-trimethoxy phenoxyethylamine	10			

References to Table 17. [1] GADDUM et al. (1955). — [2] JAQUES et al. (1956). — [3] MANSOUR (1957). — [4] BHATTACHARYA (1955). — [5] VANE (1957). — [6] BELESLIN and VARAGIĆ (1960). — [7] FRAHM (1957). — [8] SCHMIDT (1963). — [9] OUTSCHOORN and JACOB (1960). — [10] WOOLLEY (1957).

Table 18. *Guanidine derivatives*

Compound	I	II	III	IV, V, VI
Phenyldiguanide				12 *
Benzylguanidine				55 *
Phenoxypropylguanidine		1		
2-Naphthylguanidine				5 * [2] V
2-Anthrylguanidine				1.6 *
2-Anthrylbiguanide				15 *
2-Acridylbiguanide				10 *

* Minimal effective blocking doses in μg/kg against 5-HT on the inferior mesenteric ganglion preparation of the cat. [3]

References to Table 18. [1] BARTLET (1962). — [2] BEVAN and VERITY (1961). — [3] GYERMEK (1964b).

Table 19. *Miscellaneous compounds*

Acetylcholine	1
Acetylsalicylic acid	2
Aescin (saponin from Aesculus hippocastanum) . . .	3
Aminopyrine	2
Azacyclonol	4
Benzo (b) thiophenes	5
Bulbocapnine	6
Caramiphen	1, 7
Cinchophen	2
Cortisone acetate	2, 8
DMPP	9
Gamma-amino-butyric acid	10, 11
Gamma-aminobutyrylcholine	12
Guaiazulene	13
Hemicholinium	14
Heparin	15
Hexamethonium	16
Hydroxyzine	17
Hydroxyphenylbutazone	18
Indazoles.	19
Iproniazid	20
Kallikrein	1
Laburnum extract	21
Marplan, monodral (penthienate)	22
Nicotine	9, 23, 24
Parabromdylamine	25
Phenazone (antipyrine)	2
Phenylbutazone.	2, 18
Prednisolone derivatives	26
Progesterone, prolactin.	27

Table 19 (continued)

p-chloro α-(2-dimethylaminoethoxy) benzyl pyridine	28
Quinine	2, 8
Sodium salicylate	2, 29
TEA	16
Tetrahydrobenz (cd) indoles	30
Tetrazotized diorthoanisidine	31
Theophylline	7
Tyramine	1
TM 10	24

References to Table 19. [1] MEIER et al. (1957). — [2] THEOBALD and DOMENJOZ (1958). — [3] VOGEL and MARCH (1962). — [4] COSTA (1956). — [5] LEWIS et al. (1953). — [6] WALASZEK and CHAPMAN (1962). — [7] JAQUES et al. (1956). — [8] WEIS (1963). — [9] BROWNLEE and JOHNSON (1963). — [10] HERXHEIMER (1956). — [11] KOSHINO (1961). — [12] GRYGLEWSKI (1963). — [13] UDA (1960). — [14] HARRY (1963). — [15] SMITH and SMITH (1955). — [16] HUKUHARA et al. (1960). — [17] REUSE (1958). — [18] ZICHA and BREGULLA (1963). — [19] STRANDTMANN et al. (1963). — [20] ZAKUSOV (1963). — [21] CAHEN et al. (1961). — [22] BALESTRA (1962). — [23] JACOB and MICHAUD (1962). — [24] TRENDELENBURG (1960). — [25] BUÑAG and WALASZEK (1962). — [26] ZICHA et al. (1960). — [27] POULSON and ROBSON (1963). — [28] CAHEN et al. (1963). — [29] KELEMEN (1957). — [30] HARRIS and UHLE (1960). — [31] CATO and CAFRUNY (1960).

M. Conclusions

A large number of chemically unrelated compounds interfere with the biological actions of 5-HT and other similar indolealkylamines. To establish valid concepts on their mode of action is difficult at the present level of understanding, when even the exact site of interaction between the antagonist and 5-HT is often unknown. Antagonists, however, can still be of value as pharmacological tools exploring receptors of 5-HT and analyzing drug-receptor interactions; and as possible therapeutic agents in syndromes where 5-HT is implicated in the pathologic mechanism.

The different pharmacological behavior of muscular and peripheral nervous receptors and of storage sites for 5-HT has been stressed. It seems justified to assume that other receptor types of indolealkylamines which are largely unexplored (e.g. in the CNS) will be found to be pharmacologically different from those mentioned. Based on the structural differences existing between the various classes of musculotropic and neurotropic antagonists and 5-HT releasing agents it is anticipated that characteristic differences in the optimal molecular structures for stimulating the indolealkylamine-sensitive receptors could be established and their nature better understood. The existence of a variety of receptors, storage sites and inactivating enzyme surfaces indicate that a complex competition occurs between these sites for structurally related biogenic amines. Additional knowledge on the biochemistry of indole compounds, the nature of drug receptor interactions and methods for integrating findings derived from simple systems into more organized patterns are needed before additional questions can be raised in regard to the biological actions and importance of this class of pharmacologic agents.

References

[1] ABBOTT, K. H.: A new antiserotonin compound, UML-491 in the treatment of headache. Dis. nerv. Syst. **23**, 579—583 (1962).

[2] ADLER, T. K., and A. ALBERT: The biological and physical properties of the azaindoles. J. Med. Chem. **6**, 480—483 (1963).

[3] ARNOLD, O. H., u. G. HOFMAN: Zur Psychopathologie des Dimethyl-traptamine. Wien. Z. Nervenheilk. **13**, 438 (1957).

[4] AXELROD, J.: The enzymatic N-methylation of serotonin and other amines. J. Pharmacol. exp. Ther. **138**, 28—33 (1962).
[5] BALESTRA, E. F.: Changes in (dermal reactions to) histamine and serotonin produced by various drugs. Sem. méd. **120**, 498—500 (1962).
[6] BARLOW, R. B.: Effects on amine oxidase of substances which antagonize 5-hydroxytryptamine more than tryptamine on the rat fundus strip. Brit. J. Pharmacol. **16**, 153—162 (1961).
[7] —, and I. KHAN: Actions of some analogues of tryptamine on the isolated rat uterus and on the isolated rat fundus strip preparation. Brit. J. Pharmacol. **14**, 99—107 (1959a).
[8] — — Actions of some analogues of 5-hydroxytryptamine on the isolated rat uterus and the rat fundus strip preparations. Brit. J. Pharmacol. **14**, 265—272 (1959b).
[9] — — The use of the guinea-pig ileum preparation for the testing the activity of substances which imitate or antagonize the actions of 5-hydroxytryptamine and tryptamine. Brit. J. Pharmacol. **14**, 553—558 (1959).
[10] BARTLET, A. L.: Some cocaine-like actions of 3-phenoxypropylguanide . Brit. J. Pharmacol. **18**, 475—489 (1962).
[11] BARUK, H., J. LAUNAY, BERGES, and R. PERLES: Action experimentale de la serotonine sur le comportement psychomoteur du Singe. Antagonisme et synergie avec les neuroleptiques et le L.S.D. 25. In: HENRI BARUK and JACQUES LAUNAY (eds.). Annales Moreau de Tours, vol. I, Current memoires in psychopharmacology, p. 275—290. Paris: Presse Univ. France 1962.
[12] BEACH, V. L., and B. G. STEINETZ: Quantitative measurement of Evans blue space in tissue of the rat; influence of 5-hydroxytryptamine antagonists and phenelzine on experimental inflammation. J. Pharmacol. exp. Ther. **131**, 400—408 (1961).
[13] BELESLIN, D., and V. VARAGIĆ: The effect of noradrenaline on the blood pressure response to 5-hydroxytryptamine in rat. Arch. int. Pharmacodyn. **128**, 100—111 (1960).
[14] — — The effect of cooling and of 5-hydroxytryptamine on the peristaltic reflex of the isolated guinea pig ileum. Brit. J. Pharmacol. **13**, 266—270 (1958).
[15] BENASSI, P.: Clinical experience with the pharmacodynamic action of BAS an antimetabolite of serotonin. [Ital.] Riv. sper. Freniat. **82**, 266—270 (1958).
[16] BENDITT, E. P., and D. A. ROWLEY: Antagonism of 5-hydroxytryptamine by chlorpromazine. Science **123**, 24 (1956).
[17] BERDE, B., W. DOEPFNER u. A. CERLETTI: Über die Wirkungsdauer einiger Serotoninantagonisten. Helv. physiol. pharmacol. Acta **18**, 537—544 (1956).
[18] BERGER, F. M., G. L. CAMPBELL, C. D. HENDLEY, B. J. LUNDWIG, and T. D. LYNES: The action of transquilizers on brain potentials and serotonin. Ann. N.Y. Acad .Sci. **66**, 686—699 (1957).
[19] BERGOUIGNAN, M., et A. SEILHEAN: La place des anti-serotonines dans le traitement des migraines et des cephalees vaso-motorices. Presse méd. **68**, 2176—2178 (1960).
[20] BERTACCINI, G., and P. ZAMBONI: The relative potency of 5-hydroxytryptamine like substances. Arch. int. Pharmacodyn. **133**, 138—156 (1961).
[21] BEVAN, J. A., and M. VERITY: Action of lobeline on intrathoracic receptors: a comparison with phenyldiguanide, serotonin and veratridine. J. Pharmacol. exp. Ther. **132**, 42—49 (1961).
[22] BHATTACHARYA, B. K.: A pharmacological study on the effect of 5-hydroxytryptamine and its antagonists on the bronchial musculature. Arch. int. Pharmacodyn. **103**, 357—369 (1955).
[23] BINDLER, E., and L. GYERMEK: Influence of 5-HT antagonists on the ganglionic stimulant action of 5-HT and DMPP. Fed. Proc. **20**, 319 (1961).
[24] BOCK, K. H., H. DENGLER, H. M. KUHN u. K. MATTHES: Die Wirkung von 5-hydroxytryptamin auf Blutdruck, Haut- und Muskeldurchblutung des Menschen. Naunyn-Schmiedebergs Arch. exp. Path. Pharmak. **230**, 257—273 (1957).
[25] BODI, T., P. E. SIEGLER, M. GERSCHENFELD, E. B. BROWN, and J. H. NODINE: Clinical evaluation of a new antihistamin (cyproheptadine). Fed. Proc. **19**, 195 (1960).
[26] BRADLEY, P. B., and A. J. HANCE: The effects of intraventricular injections of d-LSD and 5-hydroxytryptamine on the electrical activity of the brain of the conscious cat. J. Physiol. (Lond.) **132**, 50 (1956).
[27] —, and B. J. KEY: A comparative study on the effects of drugs on the arousal system of the brain. Brit. J. Pharmacol. **14**, 340—349 (1959).
[28] BRODEY, J. F., WM. G. STEINER, and HAROLD E. HIMWICH: An electrographic study of psilocin and 4-methyl-alpha-methyltryptamine (MP-809-Sandoz). J. Pharmacol. exp. Ther. **140**, 8—18 (1963).
[29] BRODIE, B. B., and P. A. SHORE: A concept for a role of serotonin and norepinephrine as chemical mediators in the brain. Ann. N.Y. Acad. Sci. **66**, 631—642 (1957).

[30] Brown, B. B.: Lysergic acid diethylamide antagonism of certain drugs. Ann. N.Y. Acad. Sci. **66**, 677—685 (1957).
[31] Brownlee, G., and E. S. Johnson: The site of the 5-hydroxytryptamine receptors on the intramural nervous plexus of the guinea pig isolated ileum. Brit. J. Pharmacol. **21**, 306—322 (1963).
[32] Buchel, L., J. Lévy, and O. Tanguy: Influence of serotonin and dl-5-hydroxytryptophane upon experimental sleep with or without iproniazid. Agressologie **1**, 389—396 (1960) [French].
[33] Bulle, P. H.: Effects of reserpine and chlorpromazine in prevention of cerebral edema and reversible cell damage. Proc. Soc. exp. Biol. (N.Y.) **94**, 553—556 (1957).
[34] Buñag, R. D., and E. J. Walaszek: Differential antagonism by BAS-phenol (1-benzyl-2-methyl-5-hydroxytryptamine) of responses to the indolealkylamines. J. Pharmacol. exp. Ther. **136**, 59—67 (1962).
[35] — — Blockade of depressor responses to serotonin and tryptamine by lysergic acid derivatives in the chicken. Arch. int. Pharmacodyn. **135**, 142—151 (1962).
[36] — — The latent vasopressor effect of serotonin in the chicken. Arch. int. Pharmacodyn. **143**, 108—118 (1963).
[37] Buscaino, G. A.: Serotonin and psychiatry. Symposium IVth Giornata della Settimana Medica Fiorentina 1960, p. 123—150.
[38] Cahen, R., J. Nadaud, and S. Aubron: New antagonists of 5-hydroxytryptamine (HT). Biochem. Pharmacol. 8, 1, 34 (1961).
[39] — — M. Sautai, D. Bonnet, and F. Bouche: Pharmacology of p-chloro-alpha-(2-dimethylaminoethoxy) benzylpyridine. II. Peripheral anti-serotonin activity. Ann. pharm. franç. **21**, 123—131 (1963).
[40] Cahn, J., G. Georges et R. Pierre: Essais d'anesthésie prolongée par la 5-hydroxytryptamine (séronine) et contrôlée par des drouges à action neurovégétative. II. Etude chez. le rat. C. R. Soc. Biol. (Paris) **150**, 162—164 (1956).
[41] Calì, G., and C. Cordova: Influences of synthetic antihistamines on the rate of gastric secretion by 5-hydroxytryptamine. [Ital.] Rass. Fisiopat. clin. ter. **28**, 1072—1085 (1956).
[42] Cambridge, G. W., and A. J. Holgate: Superfusion as a method for the study of drug antagonism. Brit. J. Pharmacol. **10**, 326—335 (1955).
[43] Canal, N., and A. Ornesi: Serotonin as a hyperthermal agent. Atti Accad. med. lombarda **16**, 64—69 (1961).
[44] Casentini, S., and G. Galli: Serotonin and antiserotonins and gastric motility. Boll. Soc. ital. Biol. sper. **32**, 1640—1642 (1956).
[45] Cato, J., and E. J. Cafruny: Effects of tetrazotized diorthoanisidine on depressor response to 5-hydroxytryptamine in the rabbit. Proc. Soc. exp. Biol. (N.Y.) **104**, 103—105 (1960).
[46] Cerletti, A.: Pharmacology of psilocybin. Proc. intern. Congr. Neuro-Pharm. 1st Rome 1959, p. 291—294.
[47] —, u. B. Berde: Die Wirkung von d-Lysergsäure-diäthylamid (LSD-25) and 5-Oxytryptamin auf die Chromatophoren von Poecilia reticulatus. Experientia (Basel) **11**, 312—313 (1955).
[48] —, and W. Doepfner: Comparative study on the serotonin antagonism of hydrazides of lysergic acid and of ergot alkaloids. J. Pharmacol. exp. Ther. **122**, 124—136 (1958).
[49] —, u. H. Konzett: Spezifische Hemmung von 5-Oxytryptamin-Effekten durch Lysergsäurediäthylamid und ähnliche Körper. Naunyn-Schmiedebergs Arch. exp. Path. Pharmak. **228**, 146—148 (1956).
[50] —, and E. Rothlin: Role of 5-hydroxytryptamine in mental diseases and its antagonism to lysergic acid derivatives. Nature (Lond.) **176**, 785—786 (1955).
[51] —, u. H. Weidmann: Untersuchungen zur Differenzierung des vasokonstriktorischen Effektes von Serotonin. Arch. int. Pharmacodyn. **139**, 177—186 (1962).
[52] Chessin, M., E. R. Kramer, and C. C. Scott: Modification of the pharmacology of reserpine and serotonin by iproniazid. J. Pharmacol. exp. Ther. **119**, 453—460 (1957).
[53] Chodera, A.: Anti-serotonin compounds. Polski Tyg. lek. **17**, 1797—1800 (1962).
[54] — Blockade of 5-hydroxytryptamine antidiuresis in rats by 2-bromolysergic acid diethylamide tartrate and 1-methyl-lysergic acid butanol-amide. J. Pharm. Pharmacol. **15**, 386—389 (1963).
[55] Cima, G., and C. Freschi: Action of serotonin and its antagonists on the isolated uterus (Ital.) Boll. Soc. ital. Biol. sper. **33**, 867—869 (1957).
[56] Clark, A. J.: General pharmacology, vol. 4 of Heffter, Heubner and Schüller, Handbuch der experimentellen Pharmakologie. Berlin: Springer 1937.
[57] Cleugh, J., J. H. Gaddum, P. Holton, and E. Leach: Essay of substance *P* on the fowl rectal caecum. Brit. J. Pharmacol. **17**, 144—158 (1961).

[58] Cole, J. W., and G. G. Bertino: Effect of chlorpromazine on excretion of 5-hydroxy-indoleacetic acid in a patient with malignant carcinoid. Proc. Soc. exp. Biol. (N.Y.) **93**, 100—102 (1956).
[59] Comroe jr., J. H., B. van Lingen, R. C. Stroud, and A. Roncoroni: Reflex and direct cardiopulmonary effects of 5-OH-5-tryptamine (serotonin) their possible role in pulmonary embolism and coronary thrombosis. J. Physiol. (Lond.) **173**, 379—386 (1953).
[60] Cook, L., and E. Weidley: Behavioral effects of some psychopharmacological agents. Ann. N.Y. Acad. Sci. **66**, 740—752 (1957).
[61] Corne, S. J., R. W. Pickering, and B. T. Warner: A method for assessing the effects of drugs on the central actions of 5-hydroxytryptamine. Brit. J. Pharmacol. **20**, 106—120 (1963).
[62] Costa, E.: Effects of hallucinogenic and tranquillizing drugs on serotonin evoked uterine contractions. Proc. soc. exp. Biol. (N.Y.) **91**, 39—41 (1956).
[63] — G. L. Gessa, C. W. Hirsch, R. Kuntzman, and B. B. Brodie: On current status of serotonin as a brain neurohormone and on action of reserpine-like drugs. Ann. N.Y. Acad. Sci. **96**, 118—130 (1942).
[64] —, and F. Rinaldi: Biochemical and EEG changes in the brain of rabbits injected with 5-hydroxytryptophane (influence of chlorpromazine premedication). Amer. J. Physiol. **194**, 214—220 (1958).
[65] Courvoisier, S., R. Ducrot et L. Lulou: Nouveaux aspects expérimentaux de l'activité central des dérives de la phénothiazine. Psychotropic drugs ed. by S. Garattini and V. Ghetti, p. 373—391. Amsterdam: Elsevier Publ. Co. 1957.
[66] — — — et O. Leau: Propriétés pharmacologiques générales d'un nouveau dérive de la phénothiazine doué d'activité antihistaminique et antiallergique puissante, la dioxo-9-(dimethylamino-3′-methyl-2′-propyl)-10-phenothiazine. Arch. int. Pharmacodyn. **135**, 364—375 (1962).
[67] Craps, L., and Th. Inderbitzin: Anaphylactoid and anaphylactic cutaneous exoserosis in the rat. Int. Arch. Allergy **18**, 268—285 (1961).
[68] Crossland, J.: Chemical transmission in the central nervous system. J. Parm. Pharmacol. **12**, 1—36 (1960).
[69] Curtis, D. R.: Action of 3-hydroxytyramine and some tryptamine derivatives on spinal neurones. Nature (Lond.) **194**, 292 (1962).
[70] —, and R. Davis: Pharmacological studies upon neurones of the lateral geniculate nucleus of the cat. Brit. J. Pharmacol. **18**, 217—246 (1962).
[71] —, and K. Koizumi: Chemical transmitter substances in the brain stem of the cat. J. Neurophysiol. **24**, 80—90 (1961).
[72] Dalessio, D. J.: Migraine headache. Serotonin and serotonin antagonism. J. Amer. med Ass. **181**, 318—321 (1962).
[73] Dasgupta, S. R.: Effect of chlorpromazine on antidiuresis provoked by 5-hydroxy-tryptamine. Arch. int. Pharmacodyn. **112**, 264—271 (1957).
[74] Day, M., and J. R. Vane: An analysis of the direct and indirect actions of drugs on the isolated guinea pig ileum. Brit. J. Pharmacol. **20**, 150—170 (1963).
[75] De Baran, L., G. Gogolak, V. G. Longo, and Ch. Stumpf: Action of tryptamine on the electrical activity of single hippocampal neurons. J. Pharmacol. exp. Ther. **139**, 337—344 (1963).
[76] De Caro, G.: Antagonistic action of several lysergic acid derivatives on antidiuresis induced by 5-hydroxytryptamine. Arch. int. Pharmacodyn. **14**, 54—61 (1963).
[77] Del Greco, F., G. M. C. Masson, and A. C. Corcoran: Renal and arterial effects of serotonin in the anesthetized rat. Amer. J. Physiol. **187**, 509—514 (1956).
[78] Delay, J., et J. Thuillier: Dualité d'action du diéthylamide de l'acide lysergique sur la contraction utérine provoqueé par la 5-hydroxytryptamine (serotonine). C. R. Soc. biol. (Paris) **150**, 1335—1336 (1956).
[79] Doepfner, W., u. A. Cerletti: Über den Serotonin-Antagonismus einiger Antihistaminika unter Berücksichtigung ihrer chemischen Struktur. Int. Arch. Allergy **10**, 348—354 (1957).
[80] — — Comparison of lysergic acid derivatives and antihistamines as inhibitors of the edema provoked in the rat's paw by serotonin. Int. Arch. Allergy **12**, 89—97 (1958).
[81] Domenjoz, R., and W. Theobald: Pharmakologie des Tofranil (N-(3-Dimethyl-amino-propyl)-iminodibenzyl-Hydrochlorid). Arch. int. Pharmacodyn. **120**, 450—488 (1959).
[82] Domer, F. R., and V. G. Longo: Effect of 5-hydroxytryptophan on the cerebral electrical activity of the rabbit. Arch. int. Pharmacodyn. **136**, 204—218 (1962).
[83] Dominguez-Lazaro, A. R., A. Sastre-Castillo, J. Perez-Guerrero, and J. L. Calleja-Canelas: UML-491 (1-methyl-D-lysergic acid butanolamide) in the prevention and treatment of migraine and other types of headaches. Rev. clin. esp. **87**, 273—277 (1962).

[84] Eble, J. N.: An analysis of the reversal of the tryptamine depressor effect in the chicken by diphenhydramine and tranylcypromine. J. Pharmacol. exp. Ther. **140**, 243—248 (1963).

[85] Ehrhart, G., and I. Henning: 1-Benzylgramine derivatives with serotonin antagonism. Arch. Pharm. **294**, 550—555 (1961).

[86] Erspamer, V.: Observations on alleged serotonin-(enteramine)-like nature of cerebral pressor substance of Taylor, Page and Cocoran. Arch. intern. Med. **90**, 505—512 (1952).

[87] — Modification of the actions of enteramine by sympathomimetic and sympatholytic agents. Ric. Sci. **22**, 694—702 (1952).

[88] — The enteramine-like action of certain indolealkylamines, 2-methyl-3-ethyl-5-amino-indole and of alkaloids of the harmine group. Ric. Sci. **23**, 1203—1207 (1953).

[89] — Pharmacological studies on enteramine (5-hydroxytryptamine). IX. Influences of sympathomimetic and sympatholytic drugs on the physiological and pharmacological actions of enteramine. Arch. int. Pharmacodyn. **93**, 293—316 (1953).

[90] — Gramine derivatives antagonistic to 5-hydroxytryptamine. Science **121**, 369—370 (1955).

[91] Fanchamps, A., W. Doepfner, H. Weidmann u. A. Cerletti: Pharmakologische Charakterisierung von Deseril, einem Serotonin-Antagonisten. Schweiz. med. Wschr. **90**, 1040—1046 (1960).

[92] Fastier, F. N.: Structure activity relationships of amidine derivatives. Pharmacol. Rev. **14**,37—90 (1962).

[93] — M. A. McDowell, and H. Waal: Pharmacological properties of phenyldiguanide and other amidine derivatives in relation to those of 5-hydroxytryptamine. Brit. J. Pharmacol. **14**, 527—535 (1959).

[94] Ferguson, J.: Action of serotonin on motility of aneural smooth muscle. Fed. Proc. **16**, 37 (1957).

[95] Fingl, E., and J. H. Gaddum: Hydroxytryptamine blockade by dihydroergotamine in vitro. Fed. Proc. **12**, 320 (1953).

[96] Fink, M. A.: Anaphylaxis in the mouse: Possible relation of the Schultz-Dale reaction to serotonin release. Proc. Soc. exp. Biol. (N.Y.) **92**, 673—675 (1956).

[97] Flückiger, E., and R. Salzmann: Serotoninantagonismus an der Placenta. Experientia (Basel) **17**, 131 (1961).

[98] Frahm, M.: Beeinflussung der Meerschweinchenatmung durch 5-Hydroxytryptamine. Naunyn-Schmiedebergs Arch. exp. Path. Pharmak. **232**, 286—287 (1957).

[99] Franchimont, P., H. van Cauwenberg, and J. Lecomte: Action of serotonin and one of its inhibitors (UML-491) on development of granulation tissue reactions in the rat. C. R. Soc. Biol. (Paris) **155**, 432—435 (1961).

[100] — J. Lecomte, and H. van Cauwenberg: Influence of serotonin and one of its antagonists on development of local edematous reactions provoked by various agents in the rat. C. R. Soc. Biol. (Paris) **155**, 180—184 (1961).

[101] Franco-Browders, S., G. M. S. Masson, and A. C. Corcoran: Pharmacologic characterization of reserpine responses in rats treated with Iproniazid. Proc. Soc. exp. Biol. (N.Y.) **97**, 778—780 (1958).

[102] Freyburger, W. A., B. E. Graham, M. M. Rapport, P. H. Seay, W. M. Govier, O. F. Swoap, and M. J. van der Brook: The pharmacology of 5-hydroxy tryptamine (Serotonin). J. Pharmacol. exp. Ther. **105**, 80—86 (1952).

[103] Fu, Ch. Ch., and Hsu, Ch. T.: Studies on the tranquilizing effect of methyltryptamine. Tai-wan-i-hsueh-hui tsa-chih. **59**, 296—301 (1960).

[104] Furchgott, R. F.: Dibenamine blockade in strips of rabbit aorta and its use in differentiating receptors. J. Pharmacol. exp. Ther. **111**, 265—284 (1955).

[105] Gaddum, J. H.: Antagonism between LSD and 5-hydroxytryptamine. J. Physiol. (Lond.) **121**, 15 (1953).

[106] — Tryptamine receptors. J. Physiol. (Lond.) **119**, 363—368 (1953).

[107] — Drugs antagonistic to 5-hydroxytryptamine. In: Ciba Symposium on Hypertension, p. 75—77. London: Churchill Ltd. 1954.

[108] — Serotonin LSD interactions. Ann. N.Y. Acad. Sci. **66**, 643—648 (1957 a).

[109] — Drugs which antagonize the actions of 5-hydroxytryptamine on peripheral tissues. In: 5-hydroxytryptamine, ed. by G. P. Lewis, p. 195—205. New York: Pergamon Press 1957 b.

[110] —, and K. A. Hameed: Drugs which antagonize 5-hydroxytryptamine. Brit. J. Pharmacol. **9**, 240—248 (1954).

[111] — — D. E. Hathaway, and F. F. Stephens: Quantitative studies of antagonists for 5-hydroxytryptamine. Quart. J. exp. Physiol. **40**, 49—74 (1955).

[112] GADDUM, J. H,, C. O. HEBB, A. SILVER, and A. A. B. SWAN: 5-Hydroxytryptamine. Pharmacological action and destruction in perfused lungs. Quart. J. exp. Physiol. **38**, 255—262 (1953).

[113] —, and M. K. PAASONEN: The use of some Molluscan hearts for the estimation of 5-hydroxytryptamine. Brit. J. Pharmacol. **10**, 474—483 (1955).

[114] —, and Z. P. PICARELLI: Two kinds of tryptamine receptor. Brit. J. Pharmacol. **12**, 323—328 (1957).

[115] —, and J. C. SZERB: Essay of substance *P* on goldfish intestine in a microbath. Brit. J. Pharmacol. **7**, 451—463 (1961).

[116] —, and M. VOGT: Some central actions of 5-hydroxytryptamine, tryptamine and various antagonists. Brit. J. Pharmacol. **11**, 175—179 (1956).

[117] GALLANT, D. M., M. P. BISHOP, C. A. STEELE, and C. D. NOBLIN: The relationship between serotonin antagonism and tranquilizing activity. Amer. J. Psychiat. **119**, 882 (1963).

[118] GANLEY, O. H.: Protective effect of cyproheptadine, a new antihistamine antiserotonin compound on lethal burns in the mouse. Arch. int. Pharmacodyn. **138**, 125—132 (1962).

[119] GARATTINI, S., and L. VALZELLI: Antagonism of serotonin by chlorpromazine from one side and by reserpine on the other (Ital.). Boll. Soc. ital. Biol. sper. **31**, 1648—1652 (1955).

[120] — — Substances interfering with the narcosis-potentiating activity of serotonin (Ital.). Boll. Soc. ital. Biol. sper. **32**, 292—295 (1956a).

[121a] — — Substances interfering with the antidiuretic action of serotonin (Ital.). Boll. Soc. ital. Biol. sper. **32**, 295—299 (1956b).

[121] GARVEN, J. D.: Pharmacological blocking actions of atropine and certain atropine-like compounds. J. Pharm. Pharmacol. **8**, 256—263 (1956).

[122] GELFAND, M. D., and G. B. WEST: Hydroxybutypropylamide and hydroxylamide of 1-methyllysergic acid. Int. Arch. Allergy **18**, 286—291 (1961).

[123] GESSNER, P. K., W. M. MCISAAC, and I. H. PAGE: Pharmacological actions of some methoxyindolealkylamines. Nature (Lond.) **190**, 179—180 (1961).

[124] —, and I. H. PAGE: Behavioral effects of 5-methoxy-N, N-dimethyltryptamine and other tryptamines and lysergic acid diethylamide (LSD-25). Amer. J. Physiol. **203**, 167—172 (1962).

[125] GEY, K. F., and A. PLETSCHER: Influence of chlorpromazine and chlorprothixene on cerebral metabolism of 5-hydroxytryptamine, noradrenaline, and dopamine. J. Pharmacol. exp. Ther. **133**, 18—24 (1961).

[126] GIÃO, J. M., and T. RICO: Action of some phenothiazine derivatives on the edema provoked by serotonin in the rat. C. R. Acad. Sci. (Paris) **156**, 207—209 (1962).

[126a] GINZEL, K. H.: Die Wirkung von 5-OH Tryptaminen und Antagonisten auf das peristaltische Reflex. Naunyn-Schmiedebergs Arch. exp. Path Pharmak. **232**, 287—288 (1957).

[127] —, and S. R. KOTTEGODA: A study of the vascular actions of 5-hydrcxytryptamine, tryptamine, adrenaline, and nor-adrenaline. Quart. J. exp. Physiol. **38**, 225—231 (1953).

[128] GOGERTY, J. H., and J. M. DILLE: Pharmacology of d-lysergic acid morpholide (LSM). J. Pharmacol. exp. Ther. **120**, 340—348 (1957).

[129] GÖZSY, B., and L. KÁTÓ: Factors other than histamine affecting capillary permeability. Int. Arch. Allergy **19**, 168—177 (1961).

[130] GREEFF, K., B. G. BENFEY u. A. BOKELMANN: Anaphylaktische Reaktionen am isolierten Herzvorhofpräparat des Meerschweinchens und ihre Beeinflussung durch Antihistaminica, B.O.L., Dihydroergotamine und Reserpin. Naunyn-Schmiedebergs Arch. exp. Path. Pharmak. **236**, 421—434 (1959).

[131] GREENBERG, M. J.: The responses of the venus heart to catechol amines and high concentrations of 5-hydroxytryptamine. Brit. J. Pharmacol. **15**, 365—374 (1960a).

[132] — Structure activity relationship of tryptamine analogues on the heart of venus mercenaria. Brit. J. Pharmacol. **15**, 375—388 (1960b).

[133] GRETTE, K.: Determination of 5-hydroxytryptamine on the isolated, perfused pig ear. Acta pharmacol. (Kbh.) **13**, 177—183 (1957).

[134] GRYGLEWSKI, R.: The antiserotonin properties of γ-aminobutyrylcholine. Bull. Acad. pol. Sci., Ser. Sci. Biol. II, 51—52 (1963).

[134a] GUNN, C. G.: Some CNS electrophysiologic effects of serotonin and lysergic acid diethylamide. Psychiat. Res. Rep. Amer. psychiat. Ass. **12**, 194—203 (1960).

[135] GUTH, P. S., and M. A. SPIRTES: Interaction in the central nervous system between serotonin and lysergic acid derivatives. Proc. intern. Congr. Neuro-Pharm. Ist, Rome 1958, p. 319—323 (1959).

[136] GYERMEK, L.: Beiträge zur Pharmakologie vom Tryptamin, Tyramin und Phenylethylamin. Acta physiol. Acad. Sci. hung. **4**, 323—332 (1953).
[137] — Chlorpromazine: A serotonin antagonist? Lancet **1955 II**, 274.
[138] — The action of 5-hydroxytryptamine on the urinary bladder of the dog. Pharmacologist **2**, 89 (1960).
[139] — 5-Hydroxytryptamine antagonists. Pharmacol. Rev. **13**, 399—439 (1961).
[140] — 5-Hydroxy-3-indoleacetamidine: a new type of blocking agent against 5-hydroxytryptamine. Nature (Lond.) **192**, 465 (1961b).
[141] — Action of 5-hydroxytryptamine on the urinary bladder of the dog. Arch. int. Pharmacodyn. **137**, 137—144 (1962b).
[142] — Antagonists of 5-hydroxytryptamine. Proceedings of the I.U.P.S. XXII. Int. Congr., Leiden 1962b. Excerpta med. (Amst.) I/1, 28—36 (1962).
[143] — A new class of 5-hydroxytryptamine antagonists. J. Med. Chem. **7**, 280—284 (1964a).
[144] — Action of guanidine derivatives on autonomic ganglia. Arch. int. Pharmacodyn. **150**, 570—581 (1964b).
[145] — Unpublished observations (1964c).
[146] —, and E. BINDLER: Blockade of the ganglionic stimulant action of 5-hydroxytryptamine. J. Pharmacol. exp. Ther. **135**, 344—348 (1962a).
[147] — — Action of indole alkylamines and amidines on the inferior mesenteric ganglion of the cat. J. Pharmacol. exp. Ther. **138**, 159—164 (1962b).
[148] — — and L. SOFFER: Ganglionic stimulation by ω-N-methyl derivatives of 5-hydroxytryptamine (5-HT). Fed. Proc. **21**, 335 (1962).
[149] — G. LAZAR, and Z. CSAK: The antiserotonin action of chlorpromazine and some other phenothiazine derivatives. Arch. int. Pharmacodyn. **107**, 62—74 (1956).
[150] —, and K. NÁDOR: The pharmacology of tropane compounds in relation of their steric structure. J. Pharm. Pharmacol. **9**, 209 (1957).
[151] —, and C. POSSEMATO: Potentiation of 5-hydroxytryptamine by imipramine. Med. exp. (Basel) **3**, 225—229 (1960).
[152] —, and T. SUMI: Potentiating actions of indolealkylamines and lysergic acid diethylamide on reflexes elicited by 5-hydroxytryptamine. Proc. Soc. exp. Biol. (N.Y.) **114**, 436—439 (1963).
[153] HALBERT, S. A., R. BIRCHER, and E. DAHL: Studies on the mechanism of the lethal toxic action of streptolysin "O" and the protection by certain antiserotonin drugs. J. Lab. clin. Med. **61**, 437—452 (1963).
[154] HALEY, T. J.: 5-Hydroxytryptamine antagonism by LSD after intracerebral injection in conscious mice. J. Amer. pharm. Ass., sci. Ed. **46**, 428—430 (1957).
[155] — A. M. FLESHER, K. RAYMOND, N. KOMESU, and P. WILLIAMS: A pharmacologic study of Mellaril, 2-methyl-mercapto 10-(2-(N-methyl-2-piperidyl)-ethyl) phenothiazine HCl. Toxicol. appl. Pharmacol. **1**, 377—383 (1959).
[156] HALPERN, B. N., P. LIACOPOULOS et M. LIACOPOULOS-BRIOT: Recherches sur les substances exogènes et endogènes agissant sur la permeabilité capillaire et leur antagonistes. Arch. int. Pharmacodyn. **119**, 56—101 (1959).
[157] — T. NEVEU, and S. SPECTOR: On the nature of the chemical mediators involved in anaphylactic reactions in mice. Brit. J. Pharmacol. **20**, 389—398 (1963).
[158] HANCE, A. J., and P. B. BRADLEY: The effect of intraventricular injections of drugs on the electrical activity of the brain of the conscious cat. Abstr. XXth Int. Physiol. Congr. p. 391—393, Brussels 1956.
[159] HARRIS, L. S., and F. L. UHLE: Four substituted indoles as antagonists to 5-hydroxytryptamine and to the veratrine response. J. Pharmacol. exp. Ther. **128**, 358—262 (1960).
[160] HARRY, J.: The action of drugs on the circular muscle strip from the guinea pig isolated ileum. Brit. J. Pharmacol. **20**, 399—417 (1963).
[161] HERTZLER, E. C.: 5-hydroxytryptamine and transmission in sympathetic ganglia. Brit. J. Pharmacol. **17**, 406—413 (1961).
[162] HERXHEIMER, H.: The 5-hydroxytryptamine shock in the guinea pig. J. Physiol. (Lond.) **128**, 435 (1955).
[163] — Bronchoconstrictor agents and their antagonists in the intact guinea pig. Arch. int. Pharmacodyn. **106**, 371—380 (1956).
[164] HIGGINBOTHAM, R. D.: Influence of adrenalectomy and cortisol on resistance of mice to histamine, serotonin, anaphylactic and endotoxin shocks. J. Allergy **33**, 35—44 (1962).
[165] HOBBIGER, F.: Antagonism by aminobutyric acid to the actions of 5-hydroxy-tryptamine and nicotine on isolated organs. J. Physiol. (Lond.) **144**, 349—360 (1958).
[165a] HOFFMAN, R. A.: Temperature responses of the rat to action and interaction of chlorpromazine, reserpine and serotonin. Amer. J. Physiol. **195**, 755—758 (1958).

[166] HOLGATE, J. A., and B. T. WARNER: Evaluation of antagonists of histamine, 5-hydroxytryptamine and acetylcholine in the guinea pig. Brit. J. Pharmacol. **15**, 561—566 (1960).

[167] HOLLANDER, W., A. L. MICHELSON, and R. W. WILKINS: Serotonin and antiserotonines. I. Their circulatory, respiratory, and renal effects in man. Circulation **16**, 246—262 (1957).

[168] HOLLISTER, L. E.: Clinical, biochemical and physiological effects of psilocybin. Arch. int. Pharmacodyn. **130**, 42—52 (1961).

[169] HORNYKIEWICZ, O., H. EHRINGER u. K. LECHNER: Beeinflussung der Iproniazidwirkung auf die Katecholamine und das 5-Hydroxytryptamin des Rattenhirnes durch Chlorpromazin. Naunyn-Schmiedebergs Arch. exp. Path. Pharmak. **241**, 198 (1961).

[170] HUKUHARA, T., S. NAKAYAMA, and R. NAUBA: The effects of 5-hydroxytryptamine upon the intestinal motility, especially with respect to the intestinal mucosal intrinsic reflex. Jap. Physiol. **10**, 420—426 (1960).

[171] INNES, I. R.: Action of 5-hydroxytryptamine on adrenaline receptors. Brit. J. Pharmacol. **19**, 427—441 (1962).

[172] IVERSEN, M., and B. BULL: The effect of 2,3-dimethyl-5-aminoidole on blood perssure. Acta pharmacol. (Kbh.) **9**, 253—254 (1953).

[173] JACOB, J.: Antagonists to the peripheral action of 5-hydroxytryptamine. Actualités Pharmacol. **13**, 131—160 (1960).

[174] —, et F. CUGURRA: Actions de la benzyl-1 diméthyl-2,5 sérotonine (B.A.S.) sur les effets tensionnels de la sérotonine et sur l'activité cardiaque chez le chien et chez le lapin. Arch. int. Pharmacodyn. **123**, 362—376 (1960).

[175] —, et G. MICHAUD: Effets de la 5-hydroxytryptamine et de la nicotine sur les hypertensions provoquées par la 5-hydroxytryptamine, la nicotine, la tryptamine et l'acétaldehyde. Arch. int. Pharmacodyn. **140**, 92 (1962).

[176] —, et M. POITE-BEVIERRE: Actions de la serotonine et de la benzyl-1 dimethyl-2, 5 Serotonine sur le ceur isolé de lapin. Arch. int. Pharmacodyn. **127**, 11—26 (1960).

[177] JAQUES, R., H. J. BEIN, and R. MEIER: 5-Hydroxytryptamine antagonists with special reference to the importance of sympathomimetic amines and isopropylnoradrenaline. Helv. physiol. pharmacol. Acta **14**, 269—278 (1956).

[178] — A. ROSSI, E. URECH, H. J. BEIN u. K. HOFFMANN: Über Dibenzothiazepinderivate und ihre pharmakologische Wirkung. Helv. chim. Acta **42**, 1265—1278 (1959).

[179] JENSEN, K.: The effect of antiserotonin (cyproheptadine) and antihistamine on cutaneous allergy. Acta allerg. (Kbh.) **15**, 293—305 (1960).

[180] — Serotonin-producing tumors. A case treated with serotonin antagonists. Nord. Med. **69**, 601—605 (1963).

[181] JORDAN, S. E., A. LASSLO, H. L. LIVINGSTON, H. ALPERIN, and A. GERSING: Comparative pharmacology of cocaine and the diethylamide derivative of cocaine. Arch. int. Pharmacodyn. **115**, 452—473 (1958).

[182] JULIA, M., J. IGOLEN, M. FELIX et J. JACOB: Sur quelques tryptamines substituées et leurs proprietés pharmacologiques. C. R. Acad. Sci. (Paris) **250**, 1741—1743 (1960).

[183] KATZ, P., and Z. FEKETE: Capillary permeability using coomassie blue as indicator. J. invest. Derm. **36**, 37—46 (1961).

[184] KAMINSKY, A., and M. ASRILANT: Therapeutic activity of a new antiserotonin preparation in dermatology. [Spanish.] Día méd. **32**, 1970—1973 (1960).

[185] KARJA, J., N. T. KÄRKI, and E. TALA: Inhibition by methysergid of 5-hydroxytryptophan toxicity to mice. Acta pharmacol. (Kbh.) **18**, 255—262 (1961).

[186] KARLSBERG, F., J. E. ADAMS, and H. W. ELLIOTT: Inhibition and reversal of serotonin induced cerebral vasospasm. Surg. Forum **13**, 425—427 (1962).

[187] KELEMEN, E.: The inhibition by sodium salicylate of oedema of the hind paw of the rat induced by 5-hydroxytryptamine. Brit. J. Pharmacol. **12**, 28—29 (1957).

[188] KIMURA, E. T., P. R. YOUNG, and R. K. RICHARDS: Pharmacologic properties of N-p-chloro-benzhydryl-N′-methyl homopiperazine dihydrochloride (Homochlorcyclizine; SA-97), a serotonin antagonist. J. Allergy **31**, 237—247 (1960).

[189] KING, T. O.: The antagonism of 5-hydroxytryptamine pneumoconstriction. Arch. int. Pharmacodyn. **110**, 71—76 (1957).

[190] KONZETT, H.: The effects of 5-hydroxytryptamine and its antagonists on tidal air. Brit. J. Pharmacol. **11**, 289—294 (1956).

[191] KOPF, R., u. I. MØELLER NIELSEN: Pharmakologische Eigenschaften einiger Phenylindolderivaten. Arch. int. Pharmacodyn. **119**, 119—132 (1959).

[192] KOSHINO, F.: Antagonistic action of γ-aminobutyric acid and its derivatives against acetylcholine, 5-hydroxytryptamine, nicotine, and histamine on guinea pig ileum. Nippon Seirigaku Zasshi **23**, 161—169 (1961).

[193] KRNJEVIC, K., and J. W. PHILLIS: Actions of certain amines on cerebral cortical neurones. Brit. J. Pharmacol. **20**, 471—490 (1963).

[194] KROEGER, D. C., and L. J. LUCCO: Serotonin-induced apnea. J. Amer. pharm. Ass., sci. Ed. **49**, 170—175 (1960).

[195] LANZ, R.: Beobachtungen bei einem Karzinoidsyndrom. Schweiz. med. Wschr. **90**, 1046—1048 (1960).

[196] LECOMTE, J.: 5-Hydroxytryptamine et membrane nictitante du chat. Arch. int. Pharmacodyn. **100**, 457—465 (1955).

[197] LEMBECK, F.: Serotonin and the carcinoid syndrome. Gastroenterologia (Basel) **95**, 189—208 (1961).

[198] LÉVY, J., et E. MICHEL-BER: Contribution à l'action pharmacologique exercée par la sérotonine sur quelques organes isolés (intestin et oreillette). J. Physiol. (Paris) **48**, 1051—1084 (1956).

[199] LEWIS, G. P.: The inhibition by morphine of the action of smooth muscle stimulants on the guinea pig ileum. Brit. J. Pharmacol. **15**, 425—431 (1960).

[200] LEWIS, J. J., M. MARTIN-SMITH, T. C. MUIR, S. N. NANJAPPA, and S. T. REID: Benzo(b) thiophene derivatives. IV. The preparation and pharmacological activity of compounds related to serotonin and gramine. J. Med. Chem. **6**, 711—716 (1963).

[200a] LIACOPOULOS, P., B. N. HALPERN et M. LIACOPOULOS-BRIOT: Modalités de l'inhibition des effects de l'histamine, des substances histamine-liberatrices et de la 5-hydroxytryptamine sur la permeabilité capillaire par leurs antagonistes. C. R. Acad. Sci. (Paris) **151**, 1661—1666 (1957).

[201] LINQUETTE, M., P. FOSSATI, J. P. MAY, and H. LEBRUN: Action of an antiserotonin substance on the ocular manifestations of BASEDOW's diseases. Ann. Endocr. (Paris) **23**, 457—464 (1962).

[202] LONG, R. F., and A. W. LESSIN: Inhibition of 5-hydroxytryptamine uptake by platelet in vivo. Biochem. J. **82**, 4P—5P (1962).

[203] LUDÁNY, G., T. GÁTI, ST. SZABÓ u. J. HIDEG: 5-Hydroxytryptamine (Enteramin, Serotonin), und die Darmzottbewegung. Arch. int. Pharmacodyn. **118**, 62—69 (1959).

[204] MAGISTRETTI, M., and L. VALZELLI: Investigation of the inotropic action of serotonin on isolated hearts and auricles (Ital.). Boll. Soc. ital. Biol. sper. **31**, 1035—1037 (1955).

[205] MALLEN, M. S., and J. CUEVA: The rise of psychopharmacologic drugs in the treatment of allergic manifestations. [Spanish.] Alergia (Méx,) **8**, 3—8 (1961).

[206] MANSOUR, T. E.: The effect of lysergic acid diethylamide, 5-hydroxytryptamine and related compounds on the liver fluke, fasciola hepatica. Brit. J. Pharmacol. **12**, 406 (1957).

[207] — E. W. SUTHERLAND, T. W. RALL, and E. BUEDING: The effect of serotonin (5-hydroxytryptamine) on the formation of adenosine 3′, 5′-phosphate by tissue particles from the liver fluke, Fasciola hepatica. J. biol. Chem. **235**, 466—470 (1960).

[208] MARAZZI, A. S., and E. R. HART: Relationship of hallucinogens to adrenergic cerebral neurohumors. Science **121**, 365—367 (1955).

[209] — Comparison of natural cerebral synaptic inhibitors. Inhibition of the nervous system and gamma-amino-butyric-acid. Proc. intern. Symp. Duarte, California, 1959, p. 531—539. Pergamon 1960.

[210] MARCZYNSKI, T., and J. VETULANI: Further investigations on the pharmacological properties of 5-methoxy-N-methyltryptamine. Diss. pharm. (Kraków) **12**, 67—84 (1960).

[211] — — The effect of bufotenin and serotonin on some autonomic reflexes of the circulatory system and peristaltic activity of the intestine. Diss. pharm. (Kraków) **13**, 11—25 (1961).

[212] MARIANI, L., A. MORTARI, and G. SIOLI: Electrocardiographic modifications in anaphylactic shock in the guinea pig: intervention of serotonin and protective activity of chlorpromazine and ethylurethane. Mal. Cardiov. **2**, 577—590 (1961).

[213] —, and R. VERTUA: Electivity of the antagonism between chlorpromazine and serotonin in the lung. [Ital.] Ric. sci. **30**, 1552—1555 (1960).

[214] — — Modification of the in vitro and in vivo binding of labeled serotonin in the presence of chlorpromazine. [Ital.] Minerva nucl. **5**, 90—93 (1961).

[215] MARLEY, E., and J. R. VANE: Tryptamine receptors in the central nervous system; effects of anesthetics. Nature (Lond.) **188**, 441—444 (1963).

[217] MAROIS, M.: Serotonine et accouchement. C. R. Acad. Sci. (Paris) **154**, 1200—1203 (1960).

[218] MARTINEZ, A. M. V.: Antiserotoninas. [Spanish.] Medicina (Madr.) **30**, 411—428 (1962).

[219] MATTHEWS, R. S.: The neuropharmacological effects of etryptamine (diethyltryptamine acetate). Arch. int. Pharmacodyn. **142**, 90—110 (1963).

[220] McCawley, E. L., P. E. Leveque, and H. L. H. Dick: Certain actions of serotonin (5-hydroxytryptamine creatinine sulfate) on cardiac rhythm. J. Pharmacol. exp. Ther. **106**, 406 (1961).
[221] McIsaac, W. M., P. A. Khairallah, and I. H. Page: 10-Methoxyharmalan, a potent serotonin antagonist which affects conditioned behavior. Science **134**, 674—675 (1961).
[222] Medaković, M.: Action of 5-hydroxytryptamine on the respiration of the dog and its interaction with morphine. Acta med. iugos. **12**, 193—304 (1958).
[223] — Comparisons of antagonistic potencies of morphine-like analgesics towards 5-hydroxytryptamine on the guinea pig ileum. Arch. int. Pharmacodyn. **114**, 201—209 (1958).
[224] Meier, R., J. Tripod et E. Wirz: Classification d'une série d'antagonistes de la sérotonine et analyse de ses points d'attaque vasculaires périfériques. Arch. int. Pharmacodyn. **109**, 55—77 (1957).
[225] Mériel, P., R. Ruffié, A. Fournié, Ch. Ayrolles et P. Cuq: Utilisation d'une antiserotonine (UML-491) en injections intra-articulaires. Rev. Rhum. **27**, 149—155 (1960).
[226] Michaux, R.: Catatonic action of 5-methoxytryptamine. Life Sci. **1**, 617—619 (1962).
[227] Moore, K. E., A. S. Milton, and R. E. Gosselin: Effect of 5-hydroxytryptamine on the respiration of excised lamellibranch gill. Brit. J. Pharmacol. **17**, 278—285 (1961).
[228] Mörsdorf, K., u. H. H. Bode: Zur Beeinflussung der permeabilitätssteigernden Wirkung des Serotonins durch verschiedenartige Pharmaka. Arch. int. Pharmacodyn. **118**, 292—297 (1959).
[229] Moussatche, H., and N. Alvares Pereira: Release of ACTH by 5-hydroxytryptamine. Acta physiol. lat.-amer. **7**, 71—75 (1957).
[230] Murelli, B., A. Valsecchi, and L. Valzelli: On the activity of the antiserotonin molecule: the 1,1 benzyl-2-methyl-5-methoxytryptamine (BAS) on some isolated organs and on the diuresis. [Ital.] Boll. Soc. ital. Biol. sper. **33**, 859—863 (1957).
[231] Naers, K., and S. Schanche: Effect of regitine on 5-hydroxytryptamine in rabbit serum. Acta pharmacol. (Kbh.) **12**, 406—410 (1956).
[232] —, and K. H. Skramstad: The action of 1-hydrazinophthalazine (hydralazine, apresoline) and the relationship between hydralazine and 5-hydroxytryptamine (enteramine, serotonin). Acta pharmacol. (Kbh.) **10**, 178—198 (1954).
[233] Neuman, M.: Serotonin and anti-serotonins. Concours. méd. **85**, 2187—2196 (1963).
[234] Niaussat, P., J. Drouet, and J. Berthou: Influence of 5-hydroxytryptamine used at pharmacologic doses in the normal or experimentally diabetic rabbit. Med. exp. (Basel) **4**, 197—206 (1961).
[235] Nielsen, I. M., and K. Neuhold: The comparative pharmacology and toxicology of the trans isomer of 2-chloro-9-(3′-dimethylaminopropylidene) thiaxanthen. Acta pharmacol. (Kbh.) **15**, 335—355 (1959).
[235a] Nieschulz, O., J. Hoffmann u. K. Popendiker: Pharmacologische Untersuchungen über N-Methylpiperazinyl-N′-propyl-phenothiazin. Arzneimittel-Forsch. **8**, 199—210 (1958).
[236] Nikodijevic, B., and S. Vanov: The influence of thenalidine on reserpine- and serotonin-induced gastric ulcers in rats. Experientia (Basel) **16**, 464 (1960).
[237] Nir, I., O. Peczenik, and E. Weissenberg: Influence of anticholinergic drugs on actions of cholinesters, histamine and serotonin. Abstr. XXth Int. Physiol. Congr., p. 680—681, Brussels 1956.
[238] Northover, B. J., and G. Subramanian: A study of possible mediators of inflammatory reactions in the mouse foot. Brit. J. Pharmacol. **18**, 346—355 (1962).
[239] O'Brien, D. J., W. F. Hughes, and J. Newberne: Influence of lysergic acid diethylamide on experimental allergic encephalomyelitis. Proc. Soc. exp. Biol. (N.Y.) **111**, 490—493 (1962).
[240] Ostfield, A. M.: Migraine headache, its physiology and biochemistry. J. Amer. med. Ass. **174**, 1188—1190 (1960).
[241] Outschoorn, A. S., and J. Jacob: A study of antagonists of 5-hydroxytryptamine and catechol amines on the rat's blood pressure. Brit. J. Pharmacol. **15**, 131—139 (1960).
[242] Page, I. H.: Serotonin (5-hydroxytryptamine); the last four years. Physiol. Rev. **38**, 277—335 (1958).
[242a] —, and J. W. McCubbin: Modification of vascular response to serotonin by drugs. Amer. J. Physiol. **174**, 436—444 (1953).
[243] Parratt, J. R., and G. B. West: Inhibition of oedema production in the rat. J. Physiol. (Lond.) **135**, 24—25 (1956).
[243a] — — Inhibition by various substances of oedema formation in the hind paw of the rat induced by 5-hydroxytryptamine, histamine, dextran, eggwhite and compound 48/80. Brit. J. Pharmacol. **13**, 65—70 (1958).

[244] PASSOW, H., H. SCHNIEWIND, and C. WEISS: The action of 5-hydroxytryptamine on the vascular system of isolated rat kidneys. Naunyn-Schmiedebergs Arch. exp. Path. Pharmak. **240**, 179—286 (1960).
[245] PENNEFEATHER, I. N., and R. H. THORP: The influence of beta-tetrahydronaphthylamine and a derivative on the central effects of 5-hydroxytryptamine, reserpine, and iproniazid. J. Pharm. Pharmacol. **10**, 249—252 (1958).
[246] PFEIFER, A. K., E. SATORY, and I. PATAKY: Effect of tranquilizing drugs on the pharmacological actions of diethyltryptamine. Acta physiol. Acad. Sci. hung. **19**, 225—233 (1961).
[247] PINSKER, W., and K. H. THAYER: Treatment of allergic conditions with methysergide (1-methyl-D-lysergic acid butanolamide bimaleate), a new antiserotonin drug. A pilot study. Ann. Allergy **21**, 200—205 (1963).
[248] POULSON, E., and J. M. ROBSON: Prevention by antagonists of the toxic action of 5-hydroxytryptamine on pregnancy. Brit. J. Pharmacol. **21**, 150—154 (1963).
[249] QUADBECK, G., u. E. RÖHM: Über substituierte Gramine als wirksame Serotonin-Antagonisten. Hoppe-Seylers Z. physiol. Chem. **297**, 229—237 (1954).
[250] RAPPORT, M. M., and G. B. KOELLE: The action of antihistaminics and atropine in blocking the spasmogenic activity of serotonin on the guinea pig ileum. Arch. int. Pharmacodyn. **92**, 464—470 (1952).
[251] REID, G., and M. RAND: Physiological actions of the partially purified serum vasoconstrictor (serotonin). Aust. J. exp. Biol. med. Sci. **29**, 401—415 (1951).
[252] — — Pharmacological actions of synthetic 5-hydroxytryptamine (serotonin, thrombocytin). Nature (Lond.) **169**, 801—802 (1952).
[253] REUSE, J. J.: Pharmacological properties of hydroxyzine. Arch. int. Pharmacodyn. **114**, 471—474 (1958).
[254] RINALDI, F.: The effects of two antiserotonin substances BAS and BAB and of bufotenin on the spontaneous electrical activity of the brain. J. nerv. ment. Dis. **126**, 272—283 (1958).
[255] ROBERTSON, P. A.: An antagonism of 5-hydroxytryptamine by atropine. J. Physiol. (Lond.) **121**, 54 (1953).
[256] ROCHA E. SILVA, M., J. R. VALLE, and Z. P. PICARELLI: A pharmacological analysis of the mode of action of serotonin upon the guinea pig ileum. Brit. J. Pharmacol. **8**, 378—388 (1953).
[257] RODNIGHT, R., and H. MCILWAIN: Serotonin, LSD and mental status. Brit. med. J. **1956 I**, 108.
[258] ROSE, J. C., and E. J. LAZARO: Pulmonary vascular responses to serotonin and effects of certain serotonin antagonists. Circulat. Res. **6**, 283—288 (1958).
[259] ROTHLIN, E.: Pharmacology of lysergic acid diethylamide (LSD) and some of its related compounds. In: Psychotropic drugs, ed. by S. GARATTINI and V. GHETTI, p. 36—47. Amsterdam: Elsevier Press 1957a.
[260] — Lysergic acid diethylamide and related substances. Ann. N.Y. Acad. Sci. **66**, 668—676 (1957b).
[261] — Pharmacology of lysergic acid diethylamide and some of its related compounds. J. Pharm. Pharmacol. **9**, 569—587 (1957c).
[262] RUDY, L. H., E. COSTA, F. RINALDI, and H. E HIMWICH: Clinical evaluation of BAS (benzyl analogue of serotonin) a tranquilizing drug. J. nerv. ment. Dis. **126**, 284—293 (1958).
[263] RUMMEL, W.: Comparative study of the antagonistic properties of phenothiazine derivatives against serotonin, adrenaline, and histamine in the terminal ileum of the guinea pig. Med. exp. (Basel) **4**, 126—134 (1961).
[264] SABELLI, H. C., and I. SINAY: Pressor effects of adrenergic agents and serotonin after administration of imipramine. Arzneimittel-Forsch. **10**, 935—936 (1960).
[265] SACCHI, U., F. BONAMINI, G. DOLCE, and L. GARELLO: Lysergic acid diethylamide and 5-hydroxytryptamine induced catalepsy in the dog. [Ital.] Boll. Soc. ital. Biol. sper. **31**, 665—667 (1955).
[266] SAI-HALÂSZ, A.: Effect of antiserotonin on the experimental psychosis induced by dimethyltryptamine. Experientia (Basel) **18**, 137—138 (1962).
267] SALMOIRAGHI, G. C., J. W. MCCUBBIN, and I. H. PAGE: Effects of d-lysergic acid diethylamide and its bromo derivative on cardiovascular responses to serotonin and on arterial pressure. J. Pharmacol. exp. Ther. **119**, 240—247 (1957).
[268] —, and I. H. PAGE: Effects of LSD-25, BOL-148, bufotenine, mescaline and ibogaine on the potentiation of hexobarbital hypnosis produced by serotonine and reserpine. J. Pharmacol. exp. Ther. **120**, 20—25 (1957).
[269] SANO, I., Y. KAKIMOTO u. T. OKAMOTO: Der Einfluß von Phenothiazinderivaten auf den Serotoninabbau. Nervenarzt **28**, 363—364 (1957).

[270] SAVINI, E. C.: The antagonism between 5-hydroxytryptamine and certain derivatives of lysergic acid. Brit. J. Pharmacol. **11**, 313—317 (1956).
[271] SAXENA, A., B. K. BHATTACHARYA, and B. MUKERJI: Behavioural studies in fish with mescaline, LSD, and thiopropazate and their interactions with serotonin and dopa. Arch. int. Pharmacodyn. **140**, 327—335 (1962).
[272] SCHAEPPI, U.: Comparison of serotonin with directly or indirectly acting compounds in their effect on the nictitating membrane of spinal cats. J. Pharmacol. exp. Ther. **139**, 330—336 (1963).
[273] SCHERBEL, A. L., and J. W. HARRISON: Response to serotonin and its antagonists with rheumatoid arthritis and related diseases. Angiology **10**, 29—33 (1959).
[274] SCHLICHTEGROLL, A. v.: Zur Pharmakologie verschiedener Thiophenylpyridylaminderivate. Arzneimittel-Forsch. **7**, 237—252 (1957).
[275] SCHMID, E., L. ZICHA, F. SCHEIFFARTH u. O. BUTTNER: Untersuchungen über den Antagonismus von antihistaminen gegen Serotonin. Arzneimittel-Forsch. **9**, 474—476 (1959).
[276] SCHMIDT, J.: Die Beeinflussung des Serotonin-Ödems der Rattenpfote durch Noradrenalin und Adrenalin. Acta biol. med. germ. **10**, 194—196 (1963).
[277] —, u. H. MATTHIES: Über einen zentralen Serotonin-Noradrenalin-Antagonismus. Acta biol. Med. germ. **7**, 107—109 (1961).
[278] SCHMITT, H., et H. SCHMITT: Sur les effects hypertenseurs de la reserpine aprés certains sympathicomimetiques. Arch. int. Pharmacodyn. **120**, 251—262 (1959).
[279] SCHNECKLOTH, R. E., I. H. PAGE, F. DELGRECO, and A. C. CORCORAN: Effects of serotonin antagonists in normal subjects and patients with carcinoid tumours. Circulation **16**, 523—532 (1957).
[280] SCHNEIDER, J. A., and R. K. RINEHART: Circulatory interactions of serotonin and reserpine in dogs. Arch. int. Pharmacodyn. **105**, 253—268 (1956).
[281] —, and F. F. YONKMAN: Species differences in the respiratory and cardiovascular response to serotonin (5-hydroxytryptamine). J. Pharmacol. exp. Ther. **111**, 84—98 (1954).
[282] SCHWARZ, B. E., K. G. WAKIM, R. G. BLICKFORD, and F. R. LICHTENFELD: Behavioral and electroencephalographic effects of hallucinogenic drugs. Arch. Neurol. Psychiat. (Chic.) **75**, 83—90 (1956).
[283] SCOTT, K. G., and R. S. STONE: The anti-tumor action of lysergic acid derivatives and their serotonin-blocking effect as reflected by the I^{131} distribution in rats. Cancer Res. **19**, 783—787 (1959).
[284] SHAW, E., and D. W. WOOLLEY: Yohimbine and ergot alkaloids as naturally occurring antimetabolites of serotonin. J. biol. Chem. **203**, 979—989 (1953).
[285] — — Pharmacological properties of some antimetabolites of serotonin having unusually high activity on isolated tissues. J. Pharmacol. exp. Ther. **111**, 43—53 (1954).
[286] — — Benzyldimethylbufotenin, a powerful antimetabolite of serotonin. Proc. Soc. exp. Biol. (N.Y.) **93**, 217—220 (1956).
[287] — — Methylserotonines as potent metabolites of serotonin active both in vitro and in vivo. J. Pharmacol. exp. Ther. **116**, 164—176 (1956).
[288] — — Indole carboxamidines and aminomethylindoles as metabolites of serotonin. J. Amer. chem. Soc. **79**, 3561—3564 (1957a).
[289] — — Synthesis and demonstration of antiserotonin activity of 1-benzyl-2-methyl-5-hydroxytryptamine (BAS-phenol). Proc. Soc. exp. Biol. (N.Y.) **96**, 439—442 (1957b).
[290] SHORE, P. A., and B. B. BRODIE: LSD-like effects elicited by reserpine in rabbits pretreated with iproniazid. Proc. Soc. exp. Biol. (N.Y.) **94**, 433—354 (1957).
[291] — S. L. SILVER, and B. B. BRODIE: Interaction of serotonin and LSD in the CNS. Experientia (Basel) **11**, 272—273 (1955).
[292] SICUTERI, F.: Premier essai therapeutique de la migraine par une substance antiserotoninique. Acta allerg. (Kbh.), Suppl. **7**, 128—135 (1960).
[293] — G. FRANCHI, and S. MICHELACCI: Inhibition by lysergic acid derivatives of bronchospasm induced in guinea pigs by serotonin aerosol. Med. exp. (Basel) **3**, 89—94 (1960).
[294a] SIGG, E. B., L. GYERMEK, R. T. HILL and H. C. Y. YEN: Neuropharmacology of some harmane derivatives. Arch. int. Pharmacodyn. **149**, 164—176 (1964).
[294] — L. SOFFER, and L. GYERMEK: Influence of imipramine and related psychoactive agents on the effect of 5-hydroxytryptamine and catecholamines on the cat nictitating membrane. J. Pharmacol. exp. Ther. **142**, 13—20 (1963).
[295] SINHA, Y. K., and G. B. WEST: The antagonism between local anesthetic drugs and 5-hydroxytryptamine. J. Pharm. Pharmacol. **5**, 370—374 (1953).
[296] SANKAR, D. V. S., D. SANKAR, E. PHIPPS, and E. GOLD: Effect of administration of lysergic acid diethylamide on serotonin levels in the body. Nature (Lond.) **191**, 499—500 (1961).

[297] SJOERDSMA, A., H. WEISSBACH, L. L. TERRY, and S. UDENFRIEND: Further observations on patients with malignant carcinoid. Amer. J. Med. **23**, 5—15 (1957).
[298] SLATER, I. H., K. H. DAVIS, D. E. LEARY, and E. BOYD: The action of serotonin and LSD on spinal reflexes. J. Pharmacol. exp. Ther. **113**, 48 (1955).
[299] SLETZINGER, M., W. V. RUYLE, and W. A. GAINES: Tryptamine derivatives. Appl. Feb. 8, 1957. U.S. Patent 2,995,566.
[300] SMITH, G., and A. N. SMITH: The role of serotonin in experimental pulmonary embolism. Surg. Gynec. Obstet. **101**, 691—700 (1955).
[301] SNOW, P. J. D., J. E. LENNARD-JONES, G. CURZON, and R. S. STACEY: Humoral effects of metastasing carcinoid tumors. Lancet **1965 II**, 1004—1009.
[302] SOFFER, L., and L. GYERMEK: The interaction of imipramine, its derivatives and phenothiazines with 5-HT, epinephrine and norepinephrine. Fed. Proc. **20**, 396 (1961).
[303] SOLLERO, L., and G. S. KURTZ: Blocking of the action of substances related to tryptamine on smooth muscle by 1-methyllysergic acid butanolamide (UML-491), Hospital (Rio de J.) **62**, 9—11 (1962).
[304] — I. H. PAGE, and G. C. SALMOIRAGHI: Bromo LSD: a highly potent serotonin antagonist. J. Pharmacol. exp. Ther. **117**, 10—15 (1956).
[305] SPIES, T. D., and R. E. STONE: Effect of serotonin on blood pressure and lack of effect of antimetabolite. J. Amer. med. Ass. **150**, 1599—1600 (1952).
[306] SPRINCE, H.: Indole metabolism in mental illness. Clin. Chem. **7**, 203—230 (1961).
[307] STACEY, R. S.: Uptake of 5-hydroxytryptamine by platelets. Brit. J. Pharmacol. **16**, 284—295 (1961).
[308] STARBUCK, C., and H. C. HEIM: Some in vitro effects of chlorpromazine, LSD and 5-hydroxytryptamine of rat brain. J. Amer. pharm. Ass., sci. Ed. **48**, 251—254 (1959).
[309] STONE, C. A., H. C. WENGER, C. T. LUDDEN, J. M. STAVORSKI, and A. C. ROSS: Antiserotonin-antihistaminic properties of cyproheptadine. J. Pharmacol. exp. Ther. **131**, 73—84 (1961).
[310] STORMORKEN, H.: The antiserotonin effect of the benzyl analog of bufotenin (BAB) and the benzyl analog of serotonin (BAS) in the isolated guinea pig lung. Arch. int. Pharmacodyn. **119**, 232—237 (1959).
[311] STRANDTMANN, M. v., M. P. COHEN, and J. SHAVEL jr.: Acyltryptamines. II. Synthesis of acyltryptamines, indazoles and azepinoindoles from the acylpenylhydrazones of 2,3-piperidinedione. J. Med. Chem. **6**, 719—725 (1963).
[312] SUPNIEWSKI, J. V., T. MARCZYNSKI, and S. MISZTAL: Biological properties of melatonin (5-methoxy-N-acetyltryptamine). Bull. Acad. pol. Sci., Ser. Sci. Biol. 8, 483—487 (1960).
[313] SZARA, S.: Behavioral correlates of 6-hydroxylation and the effect of psychotropic tryptamine derivatives on brain serotonin levels. Proc. Vth Internat. Neurochem. Symp. 1962, p. 425—432.
[314] —, and J. AXELROD: Hydroxylation and N-demethylation of N.N-dimethyltryptamine. Experientia (Basel) **15**, 216—217 (1959).
[315] — E. HEARST, and F. PUTNEY: Metabolism and behavioral action of psychotropic tryptamine homologues. Int. J. Neuropharm. **1**, 111—117 (1962).
[316] TAESCHLER, M.: Serotonin blocking effect and some central actions of lysergic acid derivatives. Abstr. XXth Int. Congr. Physiol., p. 873—874, Brussels 1956.
[317] TAKEO, Y.: Pharmacological studies on clavine-type alkaloids. II. The effect of clavine-type alkaloids on the cardiovascular system and several organs and the interaction between them and 5-HT action. Folia pharmacol. jap. **58**, 417—425 (1962).
[318] TEDESCHI, D. H., R. E. TEDESCHI, L. COOK, P. A. MATTIS, and E. J. FELLOWS: The neuropharmacology of trifluoperazine: a potent psychotherapeutic agent. Arch. int. Pharmacodyn. **122**, 129—143 (1959).
[319] — — and E. J. FELLOWS: Central (nervous system) serotonin antagonist activity of a number of phenothiazines. Arch. int. Pharmacodyn. **132**, 172—179 (1961a).
[320] — — — Interaction of neuroleptics with serotonin in the central nervous system. Rev. canad. Biol. **20**, 209—214 (1961b).
[321] — — P. J. FOWLER, H. GREEN, and E. J. FELLOWS: N-methyl-alpha-methyltryptamine a potent monoamine oxidase inhibitor and tryptamine antagonist. Biochem. Pharmacol. **11**, 481—485 (1962).
[322] THEOBALD, W., u. R. DOMENJOZ: Das Serotonin-Ödem der Ratte und seine Beeinflussung durch Antiphlogistica. Arzneimittel-Forsch. **8**, 18—19 (1958).
[323] THOMPSON, J. W.: Studies on the responses of the isolated nictitating membrane of the cat. J. Physiol. (Lond.) **141**, 46—72 (1958).
[324] TRAPOLD, J. H., R. MULFORD, and D. GROHMAN: Pharmacological and cardiovascular effects of 1-methyl lysergic acid butanolamide bimaleinate; a potent antiserotonin compound. Fed. Proc. **19**, 87 (1960).

[325] TRENDELENBURG, U.: The action of 5-hydroxytryptamine on the nictitating membrane and on the superior cervical ganglion of the cat. Brit. J. Pharmacol. **11**, 74—80 (1956).
[326] — The action of morphine on the superior cervical ganglion and on the nictitating membrane of the cat. Brit. J. Pharmacol. **12**, 79—85 (1957).
[327] — The action of histamine and 5-hydroxytryptamine on isolated mammalian atria. J. Pharmacol. exp. Ther. **130**, 450—460 (1960).
[328] TRIPOD, J.: Charactérisation générale des effets pharmacodynamiques de substances psychotropiques. In: Psychotropic drugs, ed. by S. GARATTINI and V. GHETTI, p. 437. Amsterdam: Elsevier Publ. Co. 1957.
[329] TROUT, D. L.: Interaction of serotonin and LSD in the siamese fighting fish. J. Pharmacol. exp. Ther. **121**, 130—135 (1957).
[330] UDA, T.: The mode of inhibiting action of guaiazulene and some other antiinflammatory agents on anaphylactoid edemas. Nippon Yakurigaku Zasshi **56**, 1151—1163 (1960).
[331] VACCAREZZA, J. R., and A. BOCHI: Effect of corticotropin and cortisol on urinary excretion of metabolites of serotonin (5-HIAA) in normal subjects and respiratory allergic patients. Ann. Allergy **22**, 12—19 (1964).
[332] VALDECASAS, F. G., F. CALVET, E. CUENCA u. J. A. SALVA: Die potenzierende Wirkung verschiedener psychoaktiver Substanzen auf Adrenalin und Serotonin. Arzneimittel-Forsch. **6**, 594—596 (1956).
[333] VAN ARMAN, C. G.: The antidiuretic effect of 5-hydroxytryptamine in the rat as influenced by dibenamine. Arch. int. Pharmacodyn. **108**, 356—365 (1956).
[334] VANE, J. R.: A sensitive method for the assay of 5-hydroxytryptamine. Brit. J. Pharmacol. **12**, 344—349 (1957).
[335] — The relative activities of some tryptamine analogues on the isolated rat stomach strip preparation. Brit. J. Pharmacol. **14**, 87—98 (1959).
[336] — H. O. J. COLLIER, S. J. CORNE, E. MARLEY, and P. B. BRADLEY: Tryptamine receptors in the central nervous system. Nature (Lond.) **191**, 1068—1069 (1961).
[337] VENULET, J.: Correlation of the antiserotonin and depressor activities of some phenothiazine derivatives. Acta physiol. pol. **12**, 281—290 (1961).
[338] VERCELLONE, A., and B. ASERO: 5-hydroxytryptamine (enteramine, serotonin) a possibly new hormone. II. Farmaco, Ed. sci. **9**, 629—641 (1954).
[339] VOGEL, G., and M. L. MAREK: Inhibition of rat-paw edema of various origins by serotonin antagonists. Arzneimittel-Forsch. **11**, 1051—1054 (1961).
[340] —, u. M. L. MAREK: Zur Pharmakologie einiger Saponine. Arzneimittel-Forsch. **12**, 815—825 (1962).
[341] VOTAVA, Z., and J. LAMPLOVÁ: Antiserotonin effect of derivatives of d-lysergic acid (cycloalkylamides, LSD, ergometrine) and chlorpromazine in rats. [Czech.] Activ. nerv. sup. (Praha) **1**, 269—275 (1959).
[342] —, I. PODVALOVÁ, and M. SEMONSKÝ: Studies on the pharmacology of d-lysergic acid cycloalkylamides. Arch. int. Pharmacodyn. **115**, 114—130 (1958).
[343] WALASZEK, E. J., and L. G. ABOOD: Fixation of 5-hydroxytryptamine by brain mitochondria. Fed. Proc. **16**, 133 (1957).
[344] —, and J. E. CHAPMAN: Bulbocapnine: an adrenergic and serotonin blocking agent. J. Pharmacol. exp. Ther. **138**, 285—290 (1962).
[345] WEIDMANN, H., u. A. CERLETTI: Untersuchungen über die pressorische Wirkung des 5-Hydroxytryptamin (Serotonin). Arch. int. Pharmacodyn. **111**, 98—107 (1957).
[346] WEIS, J.: Investigations on some experimental inflammations in mouse paws. Med. exp. (Basel) **8**, 1—11 (1963).
[347] WELSH, J. H.: Excitation of the heart of Venus mercenaria. Naunyn-Schmiedebergs Arch. exp. Path. Pharmak. **219**, 23—29 (1953).
[348] — Marine invertebrate preparations useful in the bioassay of acetylcholine and 5-hydroxytryptamine. Nature (Lond.) **173**, 955—956 (1954).
[349] WESTERMANN, E.: Über die Wirkung von 5-hydroxytryptamine (Serotonin) auf die Atmung. Naunyn-Schmiedebergs Arch. exp. Path. Pharmak. **233**, 518—530 (1958).
[349a] WIELDING, S.: Pharmacological and toxicological studies on beta-diethylaminoethyl phenothiazine-10-carboxylate hydrochloride (Transergan), a new spasmolytic and anti-Parkinsonism agent. Acta pharmacol. (Kbh.) **13**, 59—79 (1957).
[350] — Secergan, a quaternary phenothiazine compound having anticholinergic and ganglion-blocking actions. Acta pharmacol. (Kbh.) **14**, 112—129 (1958).
[351] WILHELMI, G.: Ulcerogenic effect of 5-hydroxytryptamine on rat stomach and influence of various drugs. Helv. physiol. pharmacol. Acta **15**, 83 (1957).
[352] —, u. W. SCHINDLER: Über die gastrotrope Wirkung von 5-Hydroxytryptamin, seiner Vorstufen und der entsprechenden Isomeren bei der Ratte. Naunyn-Schmiedebergs Arch. exp. Path. Pharmak. **236**, 49—51 (1959).

[353] WILKINS, R. W.: Serotonin, antiserotonins and hypertension. New Engl. J. Med. **255**, 115—118 (1956).
[354] —, and W. HOLLANDER: Serotonin and antiserotonines. II. Clinical studies especially in essential hypertension with the benzyl analogue of serotonin (BAS) Circulation **16**, 256—262 (1957).
[355] WIRTH, W., R. GOSSWALD, u. W. VATER: Zur Pharmakologie acylierter Phenothiazin-Derivate. Arch. int. Pharmacodyn. **123**, 78—114 (1959).
[356] WOOLLEY, D. W.: Probable evolutionary relationship of serotonin and indoleacetic acid, and some practical consequences therefrom. Nature (Lond.) **180**, 630—633 (1957).
[357] — Convenient method for assay in vivo of antimetabolites of serotonin. Proc. Soc. exp. Biol. (N.Y.) **98**, 367—370 (1958).
[358] — Highly potent antimetabolites of serotonin with little serotonin-like action. Biochem. Pharmacol. **3**, 51—59 (1959).
[359] —, and N. K. CAMPBELL: Serotonin-like and antiserotonin properties of psilocybin and psilocin. Science **136**, 777—778 (1962).
[360] —, and P. M. EDELMAN: Displacement of serotonin from tissue by a specific antimetabolite. Science **127**, 281—282 (1958).
[361] —, and E. SHAW: Yohimbine and ergotoxin as naturally occurring antimetabolities of serotonin. Fed. Proc. **12**, 292 (1953).
[362] — — Differentiation between receptors for serotonin and tryptamine by means of the exquisite specificity of antimetabolites. J. Pharmacol. exp. Ther. **121**, 13—17 (1957a).
[363] — — Evidence for the participation of serotonin in mental processes. Ann. N.Y. Acad. Sci. **66**, 649—667 (1957b).
[364] WRIGHT, A. M., M. MOORHEAD, and J. H. WELSH: Actions of derivatives of lysergic acid on the heart of venus mercenaris. Brit. J. Pharmacol. **18**, 440—450 (1962).
[365] WURTMAN, R. J., J. AXELROD, and L. S. PHILLIPS: Melatonin synthesis in the pineal gland: Control. by light. Science **142**, 1071—1073 (1963).
[366] WYLIE, D. W.: Pharmacology of some stereoisomers of hydroxytropane derivatives of phenothiazine. J. Pharmacol. exp. Ther. **127**, 276—280 (1959).
[367] YOON, S. R.: Phenoxybenzamine as an antagonist of 5-hydroxytryptamine. Kor. med. J. **12**, 67—72 (1960).
[368] YU, R., I. YUCHENOK, and L. A. NAZAROV: Relation of serotonin to central adrenoreceptive and cholinoreceptive systems in the mechanism of electroencephalogram activation. Dokl. Akad. Nauk SSSR **146**, 1237—1240 (1962).
[369] YUI, T., and Y. TAKEO: Neuropharmacological studies on a new series of ergot alkaloids. Jap. J. Pharmacol. **7**, 157—161 (1958).
[370] ZAKUSOV, V. V.: Principles of pharmacological influences on coronary chemoreflexes. Arch. int. Pharmacodyn. **140**, 646—655 (1962).
[371] — Some serotonin antagonists. Farmakol. i Toksikol. **26**, 131—138 (1963).
[372] ZANOWIAK, P., and M. J. RODMAN: A study of LSD-serotonin central interaction. J. Amer. Pharm. Ass., sci. Ed. **48**, 165—168 (1959).
[373] ZICHA, L., F. SCHEIFFARTH, H. KOSCHERA, E. SCHMID u. N. GRAF: Vergleichende Untersuchungen mit neueren Corticoid-Derivaten am Histamin- und Serotonin-Asthma des Meerschweinchens. Arzneimittel-Forsch. **10**, 728—731 (1960).
[374] —, and B. BREGULLA: Comparative studies on the antagonistic effects of phenylbutazone and hydroxyphenylbutazone toward histamine, serotonin, and acetylcholine. Arzneimittel-Forsch. **12**, 474—477 (1962).
[375] ZILELI, T., L. F. CHAPMAN, and H. G. WOLFF: Anti-inflammatory action of UML-491 (1-methyl-D-lysergic acid butanolamide dimaleate) demonstrated by the granuloma pouch technique in rats. Arch. int. Pharmacodyn. **136**, 463 —464 (1962).
[376] GEIGY, J. R., A-G.: Amines derived from dibenzocycloheptane. Belg. pat. **615**, 025, September 13, 1962.
[377] Merck & Co., Inc.: Tryptamine Compounds. British pat. 859,223, January 18, 1961.

Chapter 11

Drugs which block the storage of 5-hydroxytryptamine and related amines*

By

Arvid Carlsson

With 38 Figures

I. Introduction

In 1955 Shore, Brodie and coworkers (Shore, Silver and Brodie 1955, Pletscher, Shore and Brodie 1955) discovered that reserpine caused a marked decrease in the concentration of 5-hydroxytryptamine (5-HT) in tissues and a concomitant rise in the urinary excretion of the 5-HT metabolite 5-hydroxyindoleacetic acid. The deep physiological significance of this discovery became even more evident when reserpine soon afterwards was found to affect tissue catecholamines in a similar manner, an effect leading to block of adrenergic transmission mechanisms (Carlsson and Hillarp 1956a, Bertler, Carlsson and Rosengren 1956). Since then numerous papers have appeared, in which the effects of *Rauwolfia* alkaloids and a group of similarly acting benzoquinolizines (Pletscher, Besendorf and Bächtold 1958) have been further analyzed. Particular interest has been focussed on the mechanism of action on the abovementioned amines and on the relationship between this action and the various pharmacological effects of *Rauwolfia* alkaloids and benzoquinolizines. It is the aim of the present Chapter to review and discuss the pertinent literature dealing with these fundamental problems rather than to review in detail the enormous literature on the pharmacology of these agents.

II. Reserpine

A. Chemistry and metabolism

The alkaloid reserpine occurs in the tropical plant *Rauwolfia serpentina* and a number of related plants. In India the root of *Rauwolfia serpentina* has been used for a long time for treatment of *inter alia* hypertension and various nervous disorders. Reserpine was identified by Müller, Schlittler and Bein (1952) and has become the most important *Rauwolfia* alkaloid. It is a colourless crystalline powder almost insoluble in water but soluble in solutions of organic acids, *e.g.* acetic, ascorbic or citric acid. It can also be dissolved in a mixed solvent such as citric acid, benzyl alcohol, polyethylene glycol and water. Solvents containing

* The work done in the reviewer's laboratory which is described in this chapter was supported largely by research grants from the United States Air Force, monitored by the European Office, Office of Aerospace Research (Grant No. AF-EOAR 63—14), and from the Swedish State Medical Research Council.

mineral salts should be avoided as they precipitate reserpine immediately. For pharmacological experiments lyophilized reserpine phosphate is available. This salt may be readily dissolved in 5 per cent glucose (or distilled water); a 0.5 per cent solution of reserpine can thus be easily obtained.

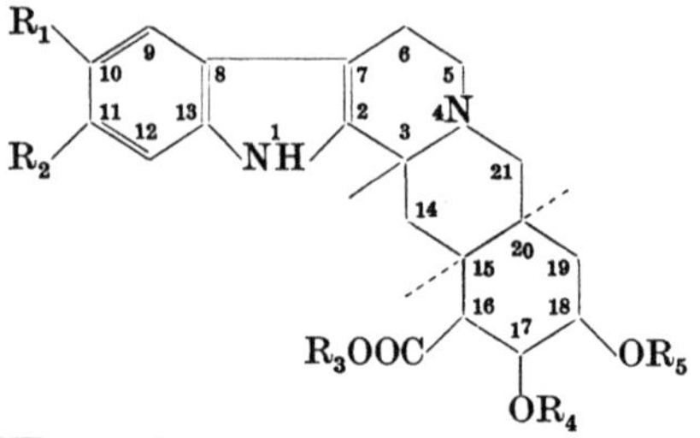

	R_1	R_2	R_3	R_4	R_5
Reserpine Isoreserpine[1]	H	OCH_3	CH_3	CH_3	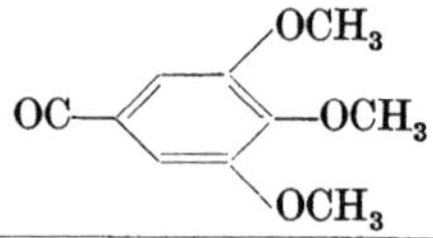
Reserpic acid	H	OCH_3	H	CH_3	H
Methyl reserpate	H	OCH_3	CH_3	CH_3	H
Rescinnamine	H	OCH_3	CH_3	CH_3	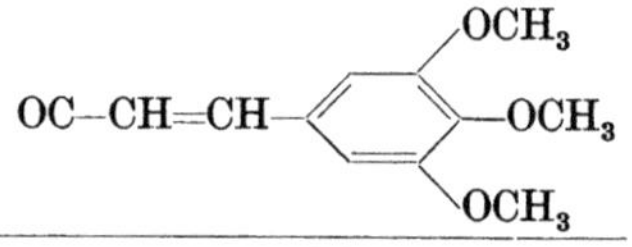
Syrosingopine	H	OCH_3	CH_3	CH_3	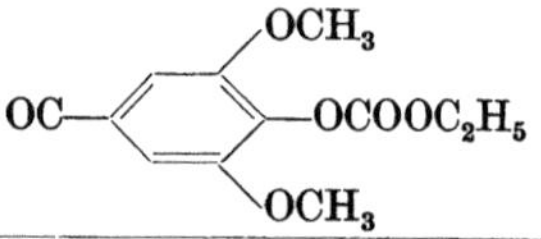
Deserpidine	H	H	CH_3	CH_3	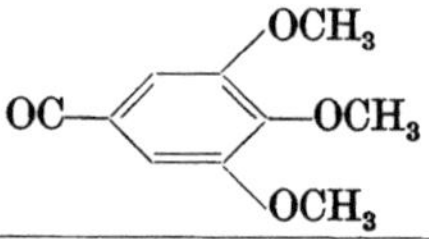
Raunescine Isoraunescine[1]	H	H	CH_3	H	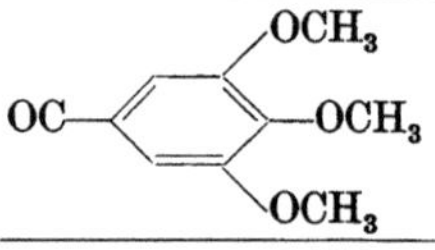
10-Methoxydeserpidine	OCH_3	H	CH_3	CH_3	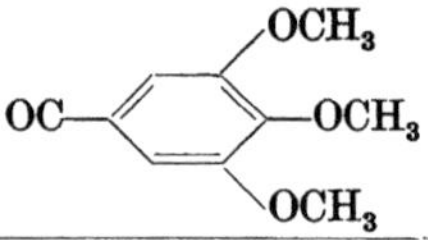
Methyl 18-epireserpate methylether[2] (Su-9064)	H	OCH_3	CH_3	CH_3	CH_3

[1] 3-Iso; [2] 18-Epi.

Fig. 1. Chemical constitution of reserpine and related compounds

The chemical structure of reserpine and a number of related natural and semisynthetic alkaloids are shown in Fig. 1. The molecular weight of reserpine is 609.

For details of the botany, pharmacognosy and chemistry of *Rauwolfia*, see WOODSON et al. (1957), SAXTON (1960), and SCHLITTLER, DRUEY and MARXER (1962).

Reserpine is an ester which is easily hydrolyzed, *in vitro* as well as *in vivo*, to form methyl reserpate and trimethoxybenzoate (DHAR, KOHLI and SRIVASTAVA 1955, GLAZKO et al. 1956, SHEPPARD, LUCAS and TSIEN 1955, SHEPPARD et al. 1957, PLUMMER, SHEPPARD and SCHULERT 1957). In rats this hydrolysis takes place to a much larger extent after oral than after parenteral administration, which may be referable to the high hydrolyzing activity of the intestinal mucosa *in vitro* (GLAZKO et al. 1956). The intestinal hydrolysis takes place to a smaller extent in monkeys and seems to be even less important in dogs.

The presence of reserpic acid in urine after administration of reserpine to rats indicates that splitting of the other ester linkage of the reserpine molecule may also take place (DHAR et al. 1955). Using isotope technique SHEPPARD et al. (1957) detected fairly extensive splitting of the 4-methoxy carbon from the trimethoxybenzoate portion of reserpine (in rats 24 per cent in 6 hours) under formation of carbon dioxide, syringoyl methyl reserpate, and syringic acid.

All the known metabolites of reserpine are less active than reserpine itself. Together with the fact that reserpine in low concentration is active on isolated structures such as platelets and adrenal medullary granules this indicates that the major effects of reserpine are not mediated by any metabolite.

A major fraction of reserpine is metabolized within a few hours (NUMEROF, GORDON and KELLY 1955). Using a fluorometric technique HESS, SHORE and BRODIE (1956) observed that reserpine, administered intravenously as a single large dose to rabbits, readily entered the brain, reaching a maximal level within 15 minutes, when it was considerably higher than in plasma. It rapidly disappeared from the brain and was almost undetectable in about 4 hours (Fig. 2). It was virtually absent from the body within 13 hours. On the other hand, the central effects of reserpine lasted about 48 hours and were considered to be temporally related to a decrease in brain 5-HT. (However, this decrease lasted considerably longer.) On this basis the concept has been advanced that reserpine is a "hit and run" drug, whose actions persist long after the drug has disappeared. Using a sensitive tracer technique, however, PLUMMER et al. (1957) observed that even after a relatively low dose of reserpine, 0.1 mg/kg, given subcutaneously to guinea pigs, reserpine can be detected in brain in a concentration of 0.007 μg/g up to at least 48 hours after injection. This concentration may be sufficient to explain the persistent effects of reserpine. Needless to say, the presence or absence of reserpine in the brain does not permit any conclusions as to whether the drug acts *via* its effects on amines or by some other mechanism.

B. Effects on monoamine levels in tissues

a) Effects of a single dose or short-term treatment

Reserpine causes a decrease of the *5-HT* concentration in various tissues. The time course of the effect of a single large dose given to rabbits (5 mg/kg intravenously) is illustrated in Fig. 2 (brain), 3 (intestine), and 4 (blood). Minimum values are reached after about 1 hour in brain, and 16 hours in blood (platelets). Recovery is slow and requires at least a week in all tissues. It is also seen that the disappearance is less complete in the intestine than in the other tissues. The difference between tissues is further illustrated by the dose-response curves (Fig. 5 to 7). The intestine requires larger doses than brain and platelets for a maximum response.

These observations of BRODIE's laboratory have been confirmed and extended by numerous investigators. Thus among the extracerebral tissues the *platelets* of rats (ERSPAMER 1956a), guinea pigs (SHORE et al. 1956), pigeons (ERSPAMER 1956b), and man (1 mg intramuscularly) (HARDISTY, INGRAM and STACEY 1956) seem to behave essentially as described above. In man recovery is remarkably slow and may require more than 3 weeks. The *spleen* 5-HT appears to behave essentially as platelet 5-HT, as might be expected (ERSPAMER 1956a and c). The relative resistance of the *gastro-intestinal tract* (enterochromaffin system) has been confirmed (WAALKES et al. 1957). In this organ species differences are particularly marked. Rats and certain lower vertebrates (PICCINELLI 1958, ERSPAMER 1956a, KÄRKI and PAASONEN 1959) appear to be much more resistant than rabbits, guinea-pigs (BENDITT and WONG 1957, WAALKES, COBURN and TERRY 1959) and hens (ERSPAMER 1956b). Within the gastro-intestinal tract, differences between various sections have been observed: the 5-HT of the fundus of the rabbit stomach could hardly be affected by the drug, while the prepyloric part of the stomach appeared to be as sensitive as the small intestine (ZBINDEN, PLETSCHER and STUDER 1957a, PLETSCHER 1957a). The *lung* also shows species differences, the rabbit being more sensitive than the rat (WAALKES, COBURN and TERRY 1959). This may in part be related to the fact that some of the tissue 5-HT of the latter species (and the mouse) occurs in *mast cells*, which are almost completely resistant to reserpine (BHATTACHARYA and LEWIS 1956, ERSPAMER 1956a, PARRATT and WEST 1957, CASS, MARSHALL and RILEY 1958, FIORE-DONATI and MOLTKE 1960, MORAN and WESTERHOLM 1963).

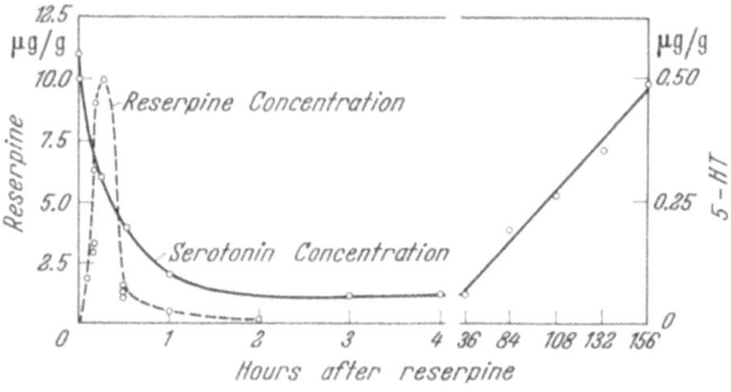

Fig. 2. Brain levels of reserpine and 5-HT after the intravenous administration of 5 mg/kg reserpine to rabbits. (From HESS, SHORE and BRODIE 1956.)

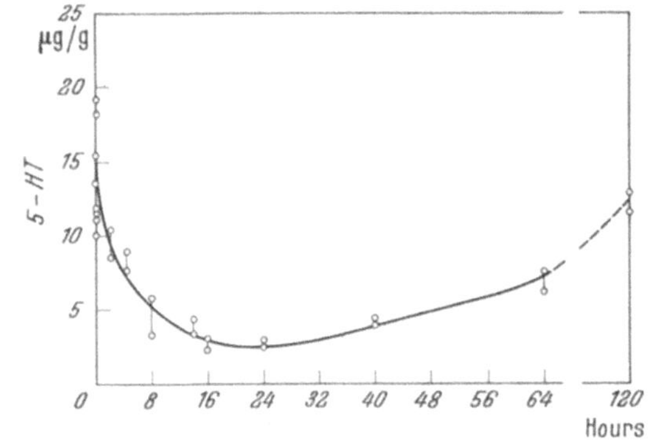

Fig. 3. Level of 5-HT in small intestine of rabbits after the intraperitoneal administration of 5 mg/kg reserpine. (From PLETSCHER, SHORE and BRODIE 1955.)

The effect of reserpine on *brain* 5-HT has been confirmed in several species: monkey (PSCHEIDT and HIMWICH 1963), dog (PAASONEN and VOGT 1956), cat (QUINN and BRODIE 1961), guinea pig (ORLANS and BRODIE 1960, WAALKES, COBURN and TERRY 1959), rat and mouse (ERSPAMER 1956a, HOLTZ, BALZER and WESTERMANN 1957, BARTLET 1960), frogs and fish (BRODIE and BOGDANSKI 1963, PSCHEIDT 1964). Certain quantitative species differences exist. Again rats and mice are relatively resistant to the drug and require as much as 5 times higher doses than rabbits for the same degree of depletion. Also frogs and fish are relatively resistant.

In molluscs reserpine causes depletion of 5-HT from ganglia and peripheral nerves (PICCINELLI 1958, BERTACCINI 1960, DAHL et al. 1962).

The indolealkylamines of the amphibian skin *(Discoglossus pictus, Rana esculenta, Bufo bufo)* show no significant change even after large daily doses of reserpine, 10 to 20 mg/kg for 3 to 6 days (LIEBECQ-HUTTER and BACQ 1958, LIEBECQ-HUTTER, RENSON and FISCHER 1959, PICCINELLI 1958). This is true also of the posterior salivary glands of octopoda (single intracardiac injection of 5 to 10 mg/kg reserpine (PICCINELLI 1958).

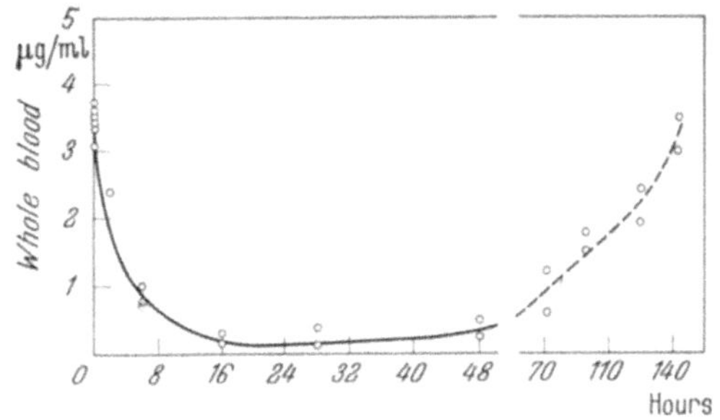

Fig. 4. Level of 5-HT in rabbit whole blood after the intravenous administration of 5 mg/kg reserpine. (From SHORE et al. 1956.)

Reserpine has been found to cause depletion of *catecholamines* from all tissues investigated: adrenals (CARLSSON and HILLARP 1956a, HOLZBAUER and VOGT 1956), heart and other tissues containing sympathetic nerves (BERTLER, CARLSSON and ROSENGREN 1956, BURN and RAND 1957, MUSCHOLL and VOGT 1958, HIGUCHI 1962) and brain (HOLZBAUER and VOGT 1956, CARLSSON et al. 1957, BRODIE et al. 1957a). Also the dopamine of brain is brought to disappear almost completely (CARLSSON et al. 1958, BERTLER 1961). Like 5-HT, the catecholamines in different locations show considerable variations in sensitivity (CARLSSON et al. 1957). The adrenergic nerves of the heart are very sensitive. In the hearts of rabbits a significant drop in

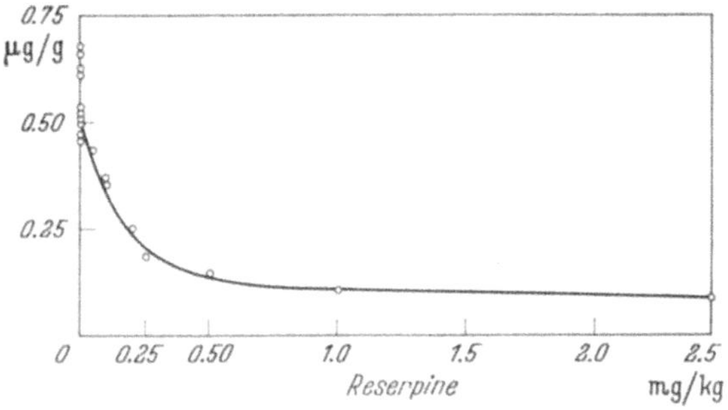

Fig. 5. Brain level of 5-HT four hours after various intravenous doses of reserpine. (From PLETSCHER, SHORE and BRODIE 1956).

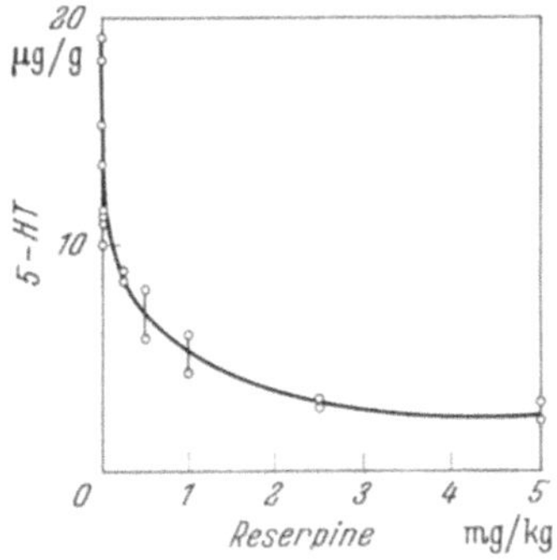

Fig. 6. Level of 5-HT in small intestine 16 hours after the intraperitoneal injection of various doses of reserpine. (From PLETSCHER, SHORE and BRODIE 1955.)

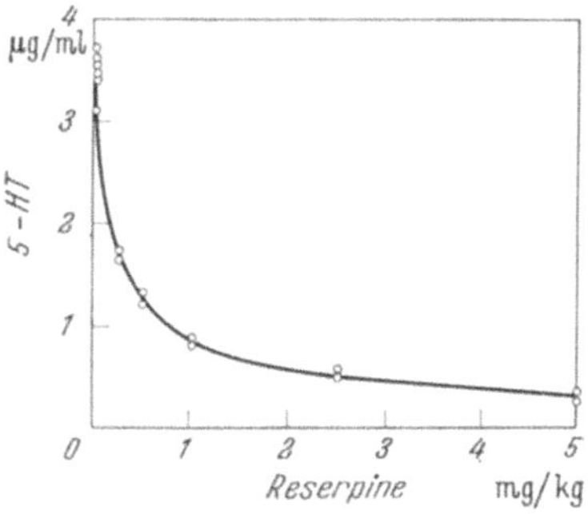

Fig. 7. Level of 5-HT in rabbit whole blood 16 hours after various intravenous doses of reserpine. (From SHORE et al. 1956.)

noradrenaline is observed after an intravenous dose of 5 μg/kg. The heart of the cat, however, does not differ much from the brain with respect to the sensitivity of the noradrenaline level to reserpine (unpublished data of this laboratory). The adrenals are relatively resistant: in rabbits 0.5 mg/kg intravenously was required for a 50% drop in adrenaline (Fig. 8). The brain occupies an intermediate

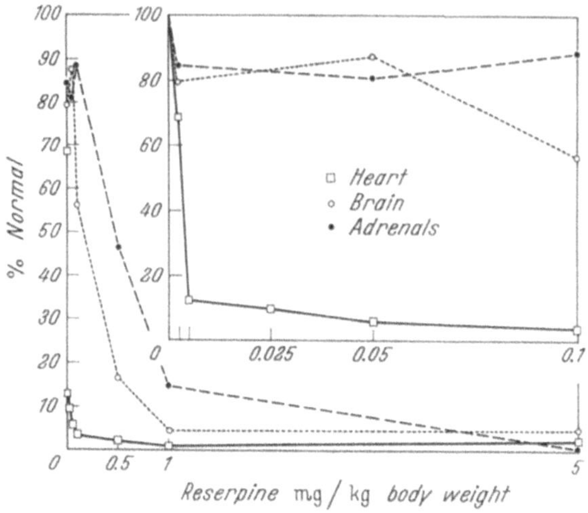

Fig. 8. Catecholamine (noradrenaline + adrenaline) levels in rabbit tissues 16 hours after various intravenous doses of reserpine. (From CARLSSON et al. 1957.)

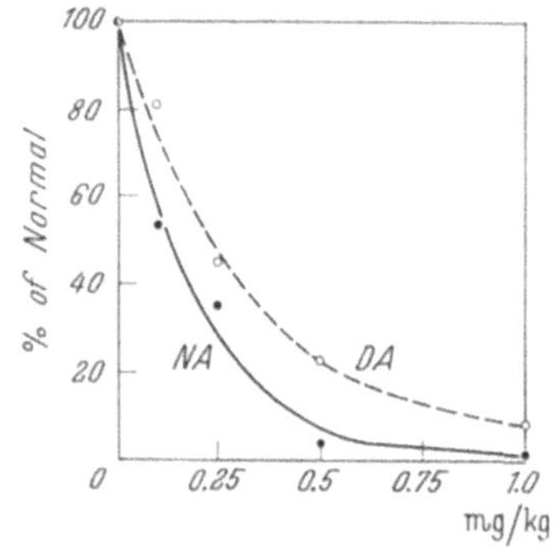

Fig. 9. Noradrenaline (NA) and dopamine (DA) in rabbit brain 16 hours after various intravenous doses of reserpine. (From BERTLER 1961.)

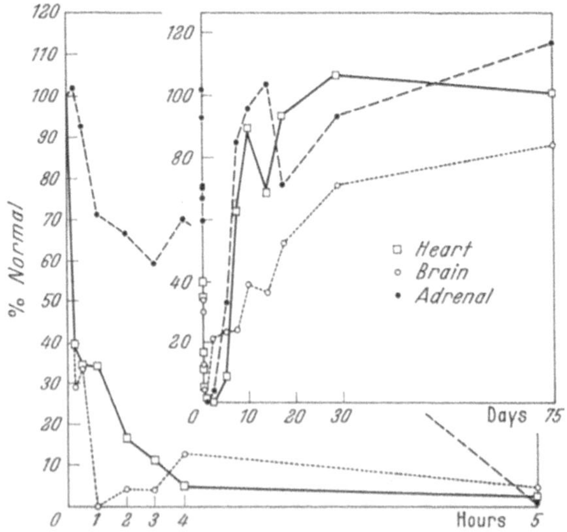

Fig. 10. Catecholamines (noradrenaline + adrenaline) in rabbit tissues after 5 mg/kg reserpine intravenously. (From CARLSSON et al. 1957).

position, the corresponding dose being 0.1 mg/kg for noradrenaline and 0.25 mg/kg for dopamine (Fig. 9). The dopamine-containing chromaffin cells of ruminants are relatively resistant to reserpine (BERTLER 1961).

The time course also differs in different locations (Figs. 10 and 11). In brain the most rapid fall took place: after 5 mg per kg intravenously less than 20 minutes were required for a 50 per cent decrease in noradrenaline, the corresponding interval after 1 mg/kg being 30 to 60 minutes (BERTLER 1961). The dopamine in brain dropped even more rapidly, reaching the 50 per cent level 10 to 20 minutes after 1 mg/kg intravenously. In the heart the noradrenaline reached the 50 per cent level about as rapidly as in the brain, but the maximum response was reached earlier in the brain than in the heart (about 1 and 4 hours, respectively, after 5 mg/kg). In the adrenals depletion took place even more slowly. The 50 per cent level had not yet been reached 4 hours after 5 mg/kg; after 16 hours depletion was virtually complete.

The restoration of catecholamine levels to normal values after a single dose of reserpine (0.2 to 5 mg/kg to rabbits) required about four weeks in the heart and adrenals and possibly more in brain (Figs. 10 and 12; CARLSSON et al. 1957, HÄGGENDAL and LINDQVIST 1964). In contrast SHORE and BRODIE (1957a) found that recovery of noradrenaline and 5-HT in rabbit brain required about one week. This discrepancy exists also with respect to 5-HT, which according to HÄGGENDAL and LINDQVIST (1964) requires several weeks for fuller covery. According to QUINN and BRODIE

(1961) the monoamines of cat brain require several weeks for full recovery after a single large dose of reserpine (4 mg/kg). According to SHORE and BRODIE (1957a) the entire course of time and doseresponse curves of 5-HT and noradrenaline in rabbit brain are strikingly similar and, in fact, superimposable. On the other hand, HÄGGENDAL and LINDQVIST (unpublished observations) found clearcut differences between 5-HT, noradrenaline, and dopamine in rabbit brain after 1 mg/kg of the drug, 5-HT levels being highest initially. These various discrepancies are possibly due to differences in experimental conditions, *e.g.* age, strain, diet etc. During recovery from a single dose of reserpine a transient rise in noradrenaline preceding the

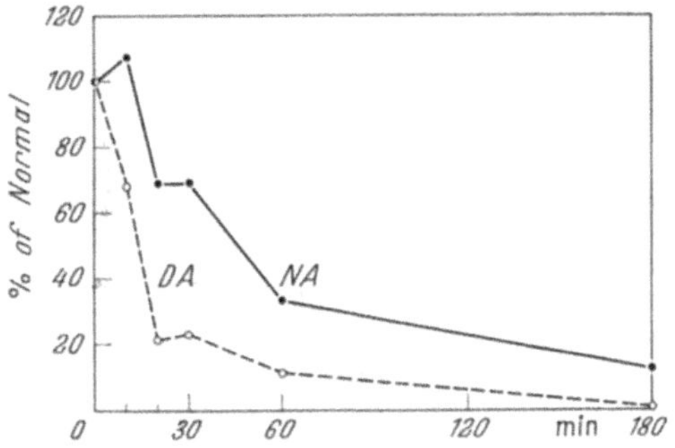

Fig. 11. Noradrenaline (NA) and dopamine (DA) in rabbit brain after 1 mg/kg reserpine intravenously. (From BERTLER 1961.)

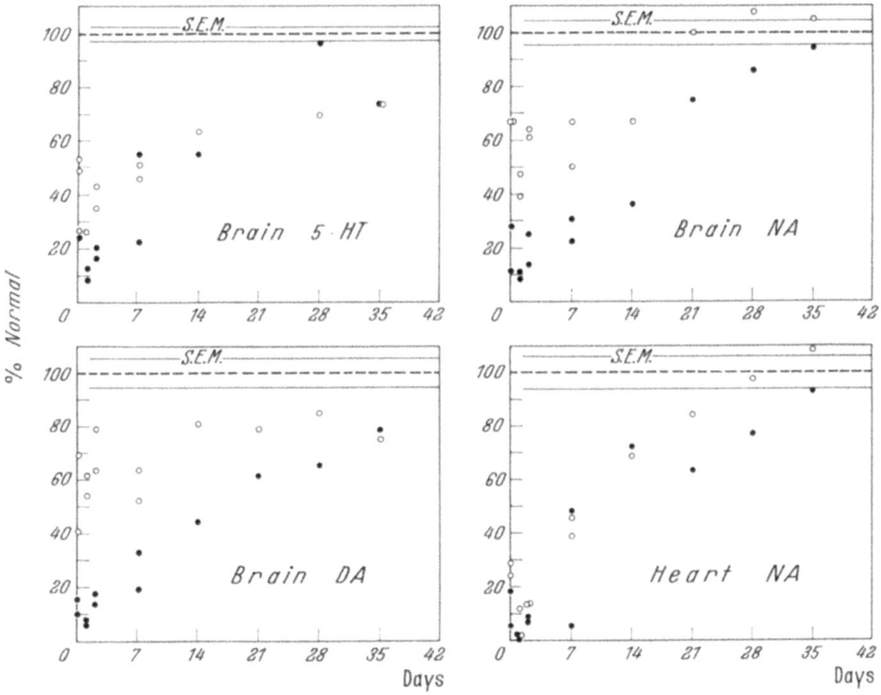

Fig. 12. Noradrenaline (NA) in brain and heart, dopamine (DA) and 5-HT in brain after a single subcutaneous injection of reserpine, 0.2 mg/kg (circles) and 1.0 mg/kg (dots) to rabbits. (From HÄGGENDAL and LINDQVIST 1964.)

adrenaline recovery, has been observed in cat adrenals (CALLINGHAM and MANN 1962).

Using a new histochemical technique (FALCK 1962, 1963) the noradrenaline of adrenergic neurons (cell bodies and nerve terminals) has been visualized. Neurons containing noradrenaline and 5-HT have been detected in the hypothalamus and other parts of the central nervous system. Depletion of catechol-

Table 1. *Effect of drugs on catecholamines and 5-HT in hypothalamic area of the rat, as observed histochemically*

Unless otherwise indicated the fluorescence was greenish, corresponding to catecholamines, and located in nerve fibers. Greenish fluorescence occurred also in neuronal cell bodies, *i.e.* in the arcuate nuclei and in the mesencephalon. The greenish fluorescence probably represents mainly noradrenaline, except in certain areas with diffuse greenish fluorescence and in the median eminence, where *inter alia* persistence after treatment with α-methyl metatyrosine suggests that dopamine is present. The yellow fluorescence, which persists after treatment with metatyrosine and α-methyl metatyrosine, in all probability represents 5-HT.

Note the marked differences in the response to reserpine both with respect to dosage and time course; compare, for example, the preoptic region with the supraoptic nuclei. There is also a marked difference in the response of nerve fibers and of cell bodies.

The injections of reserpine were made subcutaneously. (Compiled from Carlsson, Falck and Hillarp 1962).

Treatment	Preoptic region	Supra-optic nuclei	Para-ventr. nuclei	Peri-ventr. nuclei	Median eminence	Arcuate nuclei (bodies)	Mesenceph. (bodies)	Yellow fluor.	Diffuse green. fl.	Vasomotor nerves
Reserpine 24 hours										
5 mg/kg	—	—	—	—	—	+	+	—	—	—
1.5 mg/kg	+	—	+	+	+	+	++	+	+	—
0.5 mg/kg	+	—	+	+	+	+	++	+	+	—
0.15 mg/kg	++	+	++	++	+	+	+++	++	++	+
Reserpine 5 mg/kg										
2 hours	+++	+	++	++	(+)	+	+	+	+	++
4 hours	++	—	+	+	—	—	—	(+)	(+)	(+)
8 hours	(+)	—	—	—	—	—	—	—	—	—
24 hours	—	—	—	—	—	+	+	—	—	—
48 hours	—	—	—	—	—	+	+	—	—	—
72 hours	(+)	—	—	—	+	++	++	—	—	—
120 hours	+	+	+	+	+	+++	+++	+	+	+
M-tyrosine	—	—	—	—	(+)	(+)	(+)	+++	(+)	—
α-methyl m-tyrosine 400 mg/kg	—	—	—	—	+	(+)	(+)	+++	+	—
Reserpine + Nialamide	—	—	—	—	—	(+)	(+)			

Fluorescence +++ normal; ++ reduced; + faint; (+) very faint or absent; — absent.

amines by this drug is not uniform with respect to rate of onset and sensitivity but varies in different areas, *e.g.* in the hypothalamus (Carlsson, Falck and Hillarp 1962, Table 1). This complicates the interpretation of reserpine-induced changes in monoamine levels in the whole brain or in gross parts of the brain. Future attempts to correlate monoamine levels with functional changes caused by reserpine will therefore probably often require the combined chemical and histochemical approach.

In molluscs the histochemical technique has been utilized for visualization of 5-hydroxytryptamine and dopamine in separate neurons (cell bodies and nerve terminals). Both monoamines are brought to disappear by treatment with reserpine (Dahl et al. 1962).

b) Effects of long-term treatment

Comparably few investigations have dealt with the long-term effects of small daily doses of reserpine on monoamine levels, not withstanding the fact that this type of treatment comes closer to the clinical use of the drug. It is clear, however, that the action of the drug is strongly cumulative. Almost complete depletion of platelet 5-HT has thus been observed within one or two weeks of treatment with as little as 0.010 to 0.015 mg/kg/day both in animals and in man (HAVERBACK et al. 1956, 1957, ERSPAMER 1956c). For depletion of intestine and brain 5-HT larger doses are required. In dogs DE SCHAEPDRYVER (1960) observed that 0.007 mg/kg/day intramuscularly caused a decrease in tissue noradrenaline (adrenals, heart, liver, and spleen) to about one-fourth in one week; further depletion was observed after another week's treatment. There was

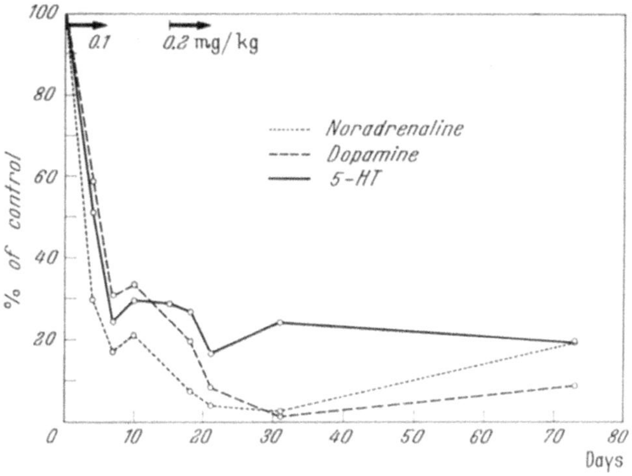

Fig. 13. Monoamines in rabbit brain during long-term subcutaneous administration of reserpine. (From HÄGGENDAL and LINDQVIST 1963.)

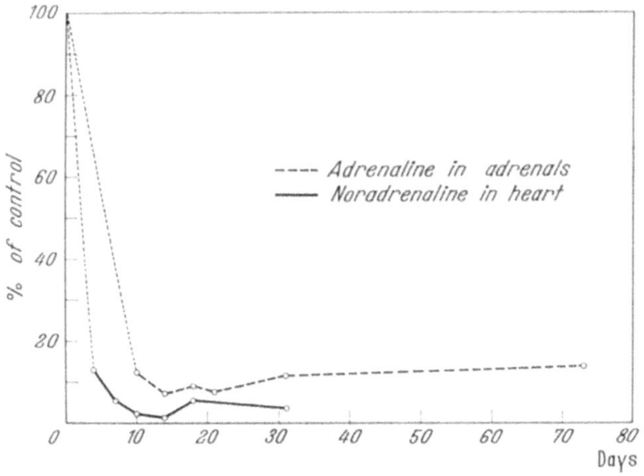

Fig. 14. Catecholamines in rabbit heart and adrenals during long-term subcutaneous administration of reserpine. (From HÄGGENDAL and LINDQVIST 1963.)

a considerable decrease also of the adrenaline of the adrenal medulla. In rabbits treated with 0.1 to 0.2 mg/kg/day subcutaneously the brain monoamines (5-HT, noradrenaline, and dopamine) dropped to very low levels within one or two weeks (Fig. 13; HÄGGENDAL and LINDQVIST 1963). This was true also of the heart and adrenal medullary catecholamines (Fig. 14). Similar results were obtained in mice treated with 0.08 mg/kg/day subcutaneously (MARKIEWICZ 1963). However, in this investigation on mice, the monoamine levels after one to two weeks of continuous decrease showed a more or less distinct tendency to restoration in spite of continued treatment with the drug. This was particularly true of the adrenal medullary amines which reached almost normal values after 2 to 3 months' treatment. In man a decrease in myocardial noradrenaline following reserpine treatment has been observed (CHIDSEY et al. 1963).

In their chronically treated rabbits HÄGGENDAL and LINDQVIST (1963, 1964) made a detailed study of the time course of the brain monoamine levels during the 24 hours following the daily injection of 0.2 mg/kg subcutaneously (Fig 15). The levels of all the three monoamines dropped from their initial low values to minimum values within a few hours and started to rise after about 12 hours in order to reach the preinjection level at 24 hours. This time curve differs from that observed in animals receiving the same dose of reserpine for the first time. Here the amine levels are lower after 24 than after 4 hours. In both categories of animals the degree of response to the drug (sedation, eye symptoms, posture, etc.) appears to parallel the time course of the amine levels of the chronically treated animals. In other words, it appears that the chronic treatment has disclosed small labile monoamine fractions which are closely correlated with function. Normally this fraction is too small to influence notably the total monoamine levels. The relationship betwe en this fraction and the labile fraction into which isotope-labelled noradrenaline is primarily incorporated, will be discussed in later sections of this Chapter.

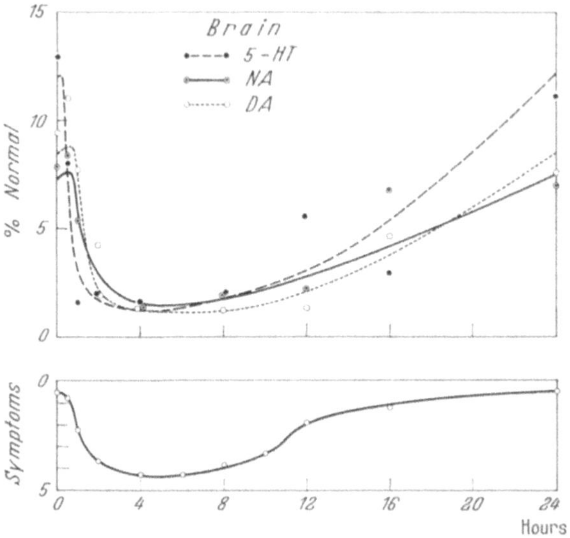

Fig. 15. Changes in behaviour and monoamine levels during the 24 hours following the daily subcutaneous injection in rabbits on long-term treatment with reserpine (0.2 mg/kg/day). Upper graph: levels of noradrenaline (NA), dopamine (DA), and 5-HT in per cent of normal. Lower graph: four symptoms of reserpine action: sedation (decreased motor activity and lowered responsiveness to stimuli), changes in posture, miosis and ptosis, were each valued according to a point scale ranging between 0 (no symptoms) and 5 (very strong symptoms). The mean values obtained are given in the graph. (From HÄGGENDAL and LINDQVIST 1964.)

C. Effects on monoamines in body fluids and on their metabolites in body fluids and tissues

In their first study on the action of reserpine on 5-HT metabolism, SHORE, SILVER and BRODIE (1955) demonstrated that the administration of a single large dose of reserpine (3 mg/kg intraperitoneally) to dogs resulted in a severalfold increase in urinary 5-hydroxyindoleacetic acid (5-HIAA) lasting 8 hours or more (Fig. 16). These observations were soon confirmed and extended in experiments on rats (ERSPAMER 1956a), dogs (ERSPAMER and CICERI 1957), rabbits (FISCHER and LECOMTE 1956), and man (SANO et al. 1957, TODRICK, DICK and TAIT 1958, VALCOURT 1959). The depletion of tissue 5-HT is due to increased release and metabolism rather than decreased formation of 5-HT. After the initial response has vanished, continued administration of reserpine leaves the urinary 5-HIAA excretion unchanged (Fig. 16; ERSPAMER and CICERI 1957, STACEY 1959). The question arises whether the 5-HT released by reserpine reaches the extracellular space and the blood stream in unchanged or metabolized form. *In-vitro* experiments have shown that reserpine is capable of releasing 5-HT in unchanged form from platelets if oxidation is prevented *e.g.* by excluding oxygen from the system (Carlsson, Shore and Brodie 1957), but it seems doubtful if this holds true *in vivo*. In all probability monoamine oxidase is present in the monoamine storing cells. Most of the 5-HT released from the storage granules may thus be metabolized before it leaves the cell. Data showing an increase in 5-HT in plasma following administration of a reserpine-like drug (Kärki and Paasonen 1960) should be interpreted with caution, since release of 5-HT from platelets may occur after removing the blood from the circulation. It should be noted that reserpine does not cause any conspicuous 5-HT-like actions concomitantly with 5-HT release. Any 5-HT being released in unchanged state is therefore in all probability rapidly metabolized.

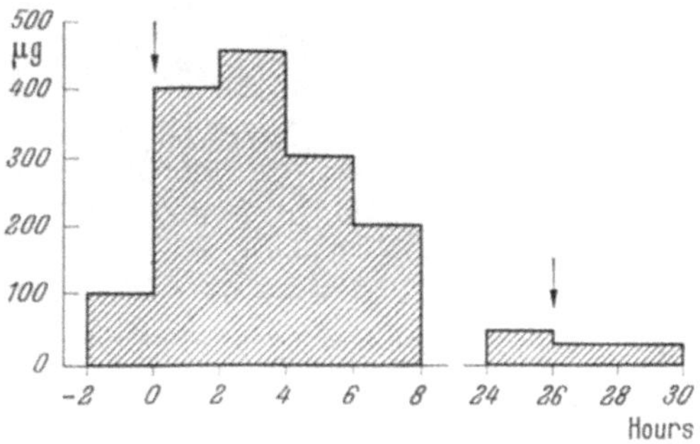

Fig. 16. Effect of reserpine on urinary excretion of 5-hydroxyindoleacetic acid in the dog. Arrows depicts times at which reserpine, 3 mg/kg, was injected intraperitoneally. Note that an increase occurred only after the first injection. (From Shore, Silver and Brodie 1955.)

Reserpine has been found to increase the urinary excretion of the catecholamine metabolite 3-methoxy-4-hydroxymandelic acid in man (McDonald and Weise 1962). The adrenaline (but not noradrenaline) level in plasma (Muscholl and Vogt 1957) and urine (Carlsson et al. 1957, Pscheidt, Brune and Himwich 1961, Bickel, Carpi and Bovet 1961) is increased by a single dose of reserpine, but this seems to be due to an indirect action on the adrenal medulla (Kroneberg and Schümann 1958). Although there is no doubt that reserpine has a direct action on the adrenal medulla, the alkaloid also stimulates this organ indirectly, *via* the splanchnic nerves (see Section II Gg). — It appears to be mainly under conditions with a low or absent sympathetic nerve activity and/or a high catecholamine sensitivity that reserpine causes signs of catecholamine release from adrenergic neurons (blood pressure rise etc.), *e.g.* in spinal dogs (Maxwell et al. 1956, Schneider and Rinehart 1956), in an isolated organ such as the dog heart (Paasonen and Krayer 1958), after ganglion blockade (Maxwell et al. 1957, Beck, Falcon and Domino 1957, Domino and Rech 1957), and after cocaine sensitization (Horita 1958). In coronary sinus blood of dogs Harrison et al. (1963) were unable to detect any consistent increase in noradrenaline concentration in spite of a decrease in heart noradrenaline following the intravenous administration of reserpine (3 mg/kg).

When depletion of catecholamines from the adrenergic nerves has reached a high degree, nerve stimulation no longer results in release of the adrenergic transmitter (Figs. 17 and 29; Bertler, Carlsson and Rosengren 1956, Carlsson et al. 1957, Bertler et al. 1958, Muscholl and Vogt 1958, Gaffney, Chidsey and Braunwald 1963). Long-term treatment of patients with reserpine results in low urinary catecholamine levels (Gaddum, Krivoy and Laverty 1958, Carlsson, Boje Rasmussen and Kristjansen 1959, Brune, Pscheidt and Himwich 1963).

In rabbit brain reserpine causes an increase in the level of 5-HIAA concomitantly with 5-HT depletion (Ashcroft and Sharman 1962, Roos and Werdinius 1962). Remarkably enough, the 5-HIAA level remained elevated for about 24 hours (Fig. 18; Andén, Roos and Werdinius 1963). These data do not merely seem to reflect release of 5-HT but possibly also mirror changes in the functional activity of hydroxytryptaminergic neurons.

In rabbit brain reserpine has been found to cause an increase in the dopamine metabolites 3,4-dihydroxyphenylacetic acid (ANDÉN, ROOS and WERDINIUS

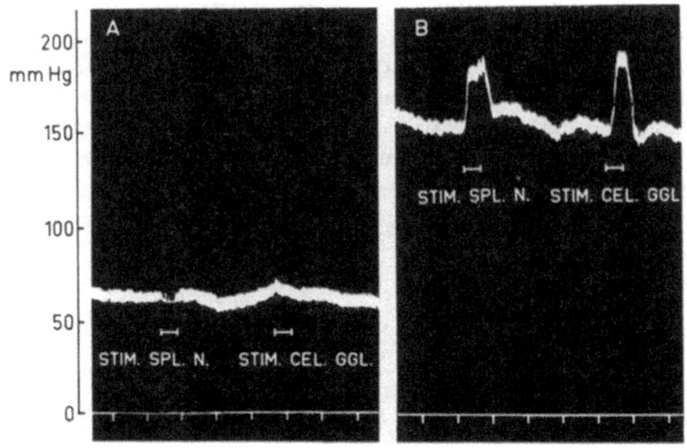

Fig. 17. The blood pressure responses to electrical stimulation of the left splanchnic nerve and celiac ganglion, as observed in (A) a reserpine-treated and (B) a control cat. In A reserpine was injected subcutaneously in a dose of 7 mg/kg 16 hours before the experiment. The cats were anesthetized with nembutal (30 mg/kg intraperitoneally). Both adrenals were removed. The arterial pressure was recorded *via* a cannula in the right carotid artery. The left major splanchnic nerve and celiac ganglion were prepared, and the nerve was divided. The distal stump of the nerve and the ganglion were stimulated, using a square-wave electronic stimulator (10 pulses per second; pulse width 10 milliseconds; 8 V). Each stimulation lasted 30 seconds. Upper record: arterial blood pressure. Lower record: time in minutes. (From CARLSSON et al. 1957.)

1963) and its 3-O-methylated derivative homovanillic acid (Fig. 19). The increase in the former acid precedes the increase in the latter, indicating that the dopamine released by reserpine is metabolized mainly by monoamine oxidase

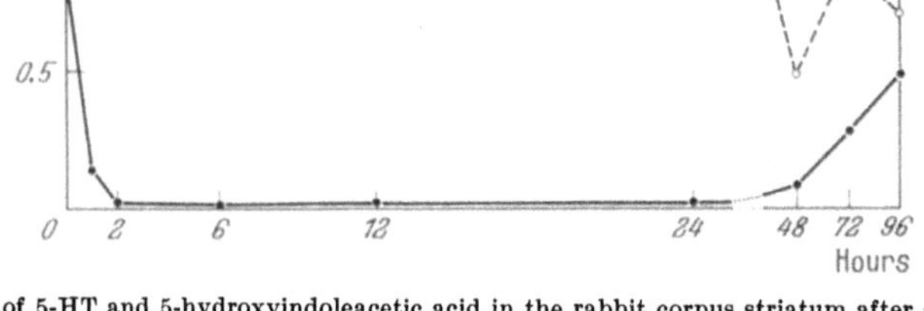

Fig. 18. Levels of 5-HT and 5-hydroxyindoleacetic acid in the rabbit corpus striatum after a single intravenous injection of reserpine (2 to 5 mg/kg). (From ANDÉN, ROOS and WERDINIUS 1963.)

(ANDÉN, ROOS and WERDINIUS 1964). This view is further supported by the observation that reserpine causes a marked decrease in the level of normetanephrine and methoxytyramine in rabbit brain (HÄGGENDAL 1963). This decrease took place within 4 hours after the subcutaneous injection of reserpine (0.2 mg/kg), when the noradrenaline and dopamine levels were moderately reduced. Reserpine thus appears to cause an increase in the availability of catecholamines for monoamine oxidase and a decrease in the availability of these amines for catechol-O-methyl transferase. Since the former enzyme seems to be mainly involved in the metabolism of intracellular and the latter of extracellular catecholamines (SPECTOR et al. 1960, CARLSSON, LINDQVIST and MAGNUSSON 1960, CARLSSON 1960, CARLSSON and HILLARP 1962, CARLSSON 1963a, POTTER and AXELROD 1963), the data support the view (CARLSSON et al. 1957) that the release and degradation of monoamines by monoamine oxidase following reserpine administration essentially take place intracellularly.

KOPIN and GORDON (1962, 1963) studied the urinary excretion of labelled metabolites in rats which had received tritium-labelled noradrenaline or normetanephrine. On the basis of certain assumptions the amounts of labelled noradrenaline and normetanephrine released from the tissues into the circulation were calculated. It was concluded that reserpine depletes tissues of catecholamines by metabolism within the tissue, predominantly by deamination, while tyramine in very large doses released bound catecholamines directly into the circulation.

In man a single dose of reserpine has been found to cause a temporary increase in the urinary excretion of homovanillic acid, suggesting release of a dopamine store. The amount of the acid excreted was too large to be accounted for by the store of dopamine in the brain. The data thus suggest the presence of a so far undetected store of dopamine outside the brain (WILLIAMS 1962).

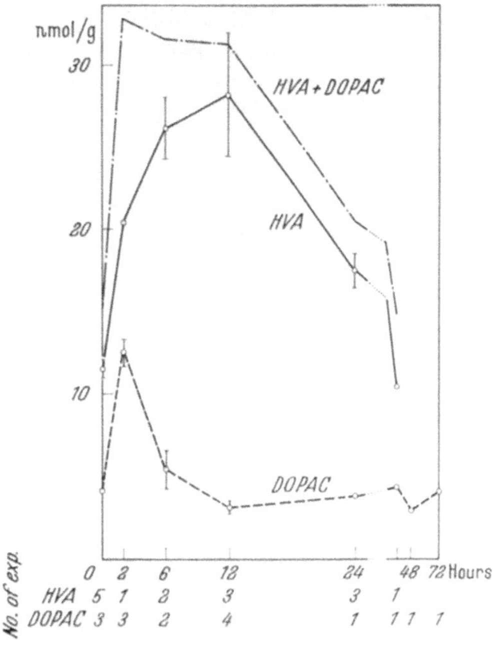

Fig. 19. Levels of 3,4-dihydroxyphenylacetic acid (DOPAC) and homovanillic acid (HVA) in the rabbit corpus striatum after a single intravenous injection of reserpine (1 mg/kg). (From ANDÉN, ROOS and WERDINIUS 1964.)

D. Effects on uptake of monoamines

a) In-vitro experiments

Experiments on isolated systems have contributed greatly to the understanding of the mode of action of reserpine. The alkaloid was first found to release 5-HT from isolated platelets (CARLSSON, SHORE and BRODIE 1957). The release takes place slowly, 50 per cent in 4 hours at 37° C (Fig. 20). Release was brought about by as little as 0.06 μg reserpine per ml incubation fluid (10^{-7} M), maximum rate being reached at about 0.3 μg per ml (Fig. 21). Among several drugs studied only *Rauwolfia* alkaloids with tranquillizing properties were active (Table 4, Section III). The reserpine stereoisomer 3-isoreserpine was practically inactive, as it is *in vivo*. Reserpine caused almost no release at an incubation temperature of 2° C. The release was not a simple mole-for-mole displacement, since one molecule of reserpine was calculated to cause release of hundreds of molecules of 5-HT. Further *in-vitro* studies (BRODIE et al. 1957b, HUGHES, SHORE and BRODIE 1958, HUGHES and BRODIE 1959) revealed that reserpine inhibited the uptake of 5-HT or catecholamines from the suspension fluid. This blockade appeared to set in almost instantaneously following addition of reserpine in a fairly high concentration to the suspension fluid (1 μg/ml). It was concluded that the primary action of reserpine is to block the uptake of amines by the platelets; normally a leakage of amine occurs which is balanced by the uptake. When the uptake is blocked, the leakage results in a slow loss of amine. SANO, KAKIMOTO and TANIGUCHI (1958) have data indicating that the uptake of 5-HT by platelets which is blocked by reserpine is ATP dependent. The uptake of 5-HT by platelets was later shown to be partly inhibited by ouabain and digitoxin (10^{-5} M) and by fluoride, but not by 2,4-dinitrophenol (WEISSBACH, REDFIELD and TITUS 1960). It was stimulated by potassium and phosphate. These data suggest that a variety of mechanisms may be involved even in an apparently simple *in-vitro* system such as a platelet suspension. Several points of attack have to be considered, such as specific amine-storing granules, cytoplasmic enzymes, and the cell membrane. As to reserpine, HUGHES and BRODIE (1959) suggested that it acts on a "pump" mechanism at the cell boundary, because they were unable to detect a 5-HT complex after disruption of the platelets. However, this does not exclude the possibility that 5-HT in the platelets, like the catecholamines in the adrenal medullary granules (CARLSSON and HILLARP 1958), occurs in a complex, which is split immediately after disruption of the platelets.

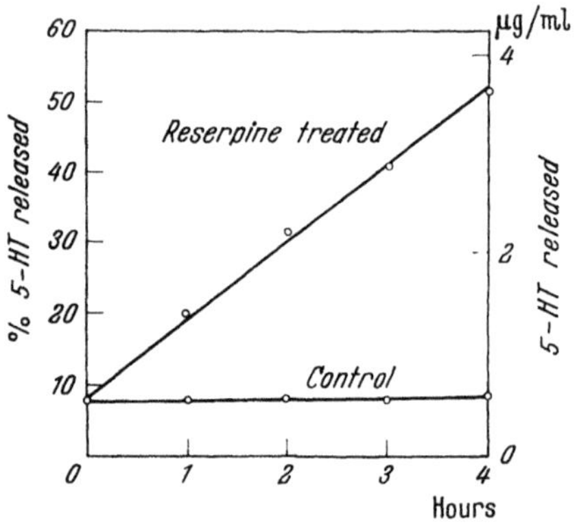

Fig. 20. Release of 5-HT from rabbit platelets incubated with reserpine (1 μg/ml). (From CARLSSON, SHORE and BRODIE 1957.)

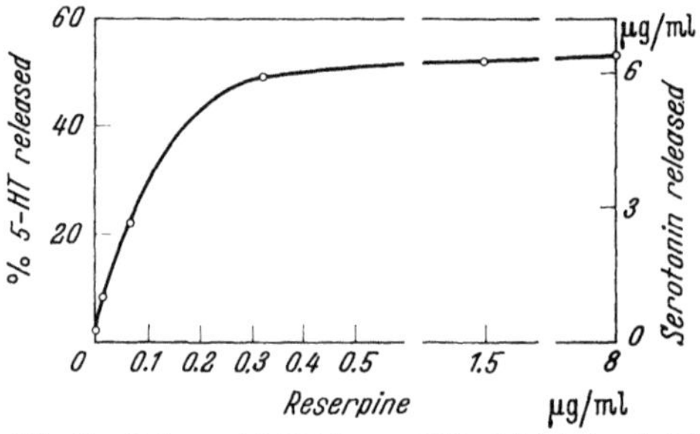

Fig. 21. Release of 5-HT from rabbit platelets incubated for 4 hours with various concentrations of reserpine. (From CARLSSON, SHORE and BRODIE 1957.)

Recently an effect of reserpine on isolated storage granules was demonstrated (KIRSHNER 1962a and b, CARLSSON, HILLARP and WALDECK 1962, 1963). Adrenal medullary granules are capable of taking up amines such as adrenaline, noradrenaline, dopamine, and 5-HT, when these are present in low concentrations in the incubation medium, provided that adenosine triphosphate (ATP) and Mg (or Mn) ions have been added to the medium (Fig. 22). This Mg^{++}-ATP dependent mechanism is blocked by low concentrations of reserpine (4×10^{-8} M), the concentration curve being remarkably similar to that obtained in the platelet experiments described above (CARLSSON, SHORE and BRODIE 1957). Again 3-isoreserpine was found much less active. Among several drugs tested some were active but reserpine was unique in being active in such low concentrations. Among active inhibitors of the storage mechanism the following may be mentioned (CARLSSON, HILLARP and WALDECK 1963): chlorpromazine, haloperidol, several α- and β-adrenergic blocking agents, and all SH reagents tested. Ouabain and sodium fluoride were inactive (*cf.* the results with platelets mentioned above). TM 10 (choline 2:6 xylyl other bromide), bretylium tosylate, and guanethidine were likewise inactive.

As mentioned above the storage mechanism has been suggested to function as a pump across a membrane (HUGHES and BRODIE 1959). In so far as the adrenal medullary granules are concerned this possibility seems unlikely, since catecholamines added to the suspension medium at 0° C appear to move freely in an out across the granule membrane and to have access to the major part of the granule water without exchanging rapidly with the preexisting catecholamines (CARLSSON and HILLARP 1958, HILLARP 1959, KIRSHNER, personal communication). The labelled amines taken up by the MgATP-dependent mechanism are not released from granules kept for several days at 0° C. It must be assumed, then, that the MgATP-dependent uptake is brought about by the incorporation of the amine into a storage complex. Two possibilities have to be considered here (*cf.* HILLARP 1960a): 1. incorporation into a large pool of amines bound together with ATP, and 2. incorporation into a smaller, loosely bound pool which does not contain ATP. The fact that ATP is taken up in much smaller than equivalent amounts, suggests that the amines are primarily incorporated in the latter pool. We thus have to consider the possibility that reserpine by blocking the uptake mechanism primarily causes depletion of a small but physiologically important pool of easily available amine. Evidence in favour of this view is now accumulating.

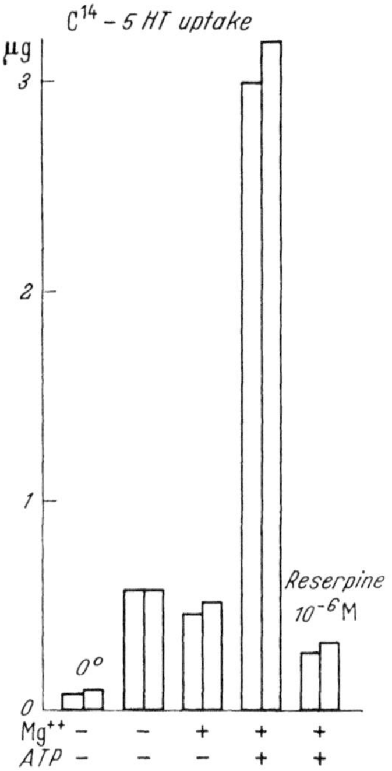

Fig. 22. Uptake of C^{14}-labelled 5-HT by bovine adrenal medullary granules, incubated for 30 minutes with or without adenosine triphosphate (ATP; 0.0025 M) $MgCl_2$ (0.0025 M), and reserpine (10^{-6} M). Buffer: glycylglycine pH 7.3. Concentration of 5-HT added to medium 5 μg/ml. Incubation temperature 31° C (except when 0° is indicated). (From CARLSSON, HILLARP and WALDECK 1963.)

Although the effect of reserpine on the uptake mechanism, once it had developed, was irreversible, it could be counteracted by the simultaneous addition of catecholamines (CARLSSON, HILLARP and WALDECK 1963). The phenomenon has been analyzed by JONASSON, ROSENGREN and WALDECK (1964) according to LINEWEAVER and BURK (Fig. 23). The analysis indicates that catecholamines and reserpine compete for the same sites in the uptake mechanism. These results afford an explanation of the preventive action of monoamine oxidase inhibitors on monoamine depletion by reserpine: inhibition of the enzyme results in intracellular accumulation of monoamines which then compete with reserpine for the receptor sites (Fig. 38).

According to KIRSHNER (1962b) the conversion of dopamine to noradrenaline is inhibited as a consequence of the blockade of the uptake mechanism; normally the conversion takes place in the granules. It will be interesting to see if reserpine inhibits the step dopamine-noradrenaline also *in vivo*. Data in favour of this view have been reported by KRONEBERG and SCHÜMANN (1958, 1960).

LUNDBORG (1963) has studied the Mg^{++}-ATP-dependent storage function of granules isolated from rabbits treated with a large dose of reserpine (2 to 5 mg/kg). The storage function was found to be blocked 12 and 24 hours after the injection, when the animals were sedated, but was restored to normal already after 48 hours. At this interval the animals are no longer sedated, but the catecholamine content of the adrenal medulla and other tissues is still very low (Fig. 24). The pharmacological actions of reserpine thus appear to be more closely correlated to the storage function than to the amine content of the stores. Further evidence in favour of this view will be given below.

Studies on the action of reserpine on granules isolated from the splenic nerve have yielded interesting results (EULER and LISHAJKO 1960, 1961a, b, c, 1962).

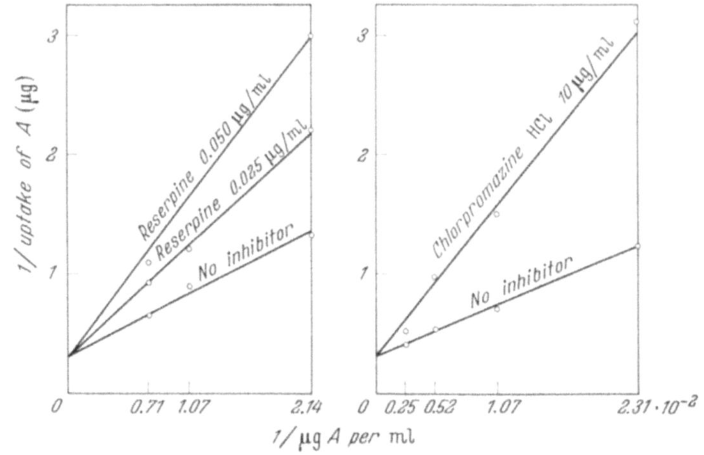

Fig. 23. Lineweaver-Burk plots indicating competitive inhibition by reserpine and chlorpromazine of *in-vitro* uptake of adrenaline (A) by bovine adrenal medullary granules. (From JONASSON, ROSENGREN and WALDECK 1964.)

In these granules, unlike the adrenal medullary granules, a rapid release takes place spontaneously. This release is blocked by low concentrations, enhanced by very high concentrations of reserpine. Recently these authors discovered a

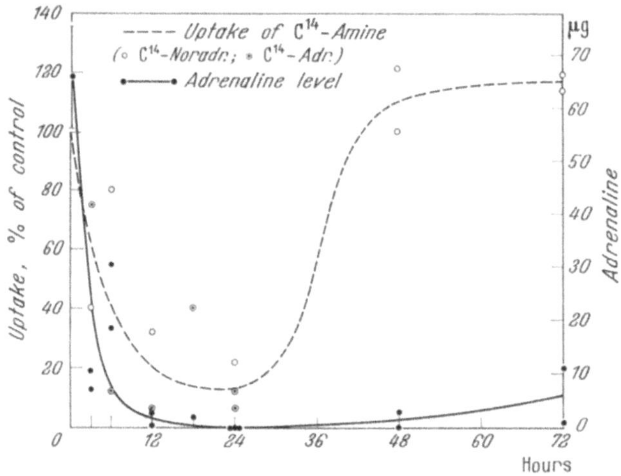

Fig. 24. Adrenaline level in adrenal medulla and *in-vitro* uptake of C^{14}-labelled catecholamines by adrenal medullary granules at various intervals after the intravenous injection of reserpine (5 mg/kg) to rabbits. (From LUNDBORG 1963.)

MgATP-dependent uptake of noradrenaline by these granules. The uptake was blocked by low concentrations of reserpine (EULER and LISHAJKO 1963). This is strong support for the view that the storage mechanisms of adrenal medullary granules and adrenergic nerve granules are fundamentally similar.

DENGLER et al. (1961a and b, 1962) and WILSON, MURRAY and TITUS (1962) have studied the uptake of tritiated noradrenaline and adrenaline by slices of brain and other tissues. When low amine concentrations were used, the uptake was blocked by reserpine, ouabain, and dinitrophenol. The tissue slices thus resemble the platelets more than the adrenal medullary granules, supporting the view that at least two mechanisms are at work in whole cells, one operating at the cell membrane and sensitive to ouabain and dinitrophenol, the other operating in the storage granules and sensitive to reserpine. Common to the different types of preparations appears to be that a major part of the preexistent store does not exchange rapidly with the exogenous amines and that a reserpine-insensitive uptake occurs at high amine concentrations in the incubation medium.

b) In-vivo experiments

Tissues of intact animals are capable of taking up catecholamines from the blood plasma. This uptake is blocked by reserpine. Thus MUSCHOLL (1960) observed that infusion of 20 μg of noradrenaline to rats caused an increase in heart noradrenaline from 0.6 to 1.0 μg/g. In rats treated with reserpine (5 mg/kg 20 hours previously or 2.5 mg/kg/day for two days preceding the experiment, intraperitoneally or subcutaneously) this infusion caused no significant increase in heart noradrenaline; it remained at the very low pre-infusion level (0.006 to 0.025 μg/g). In similar experiments CROUT, MUSKUS and TRENDELENBURG (1962), working on guinea-pig atria, observed a very slight increase. Using radioactive noradrenaline HERTTING, AXELROD and WHITBY (1961) made similar observations in cats. Two doses of reserpine, each 3 mg/kg, given intraperitoneally 24 and 2 hours before the experiment, almost completely blocked the uptake of intravenously administered H^3-noradrenaline by heart, spleen, liver, and adrenal gland. Similar results have been obtained in mice (CARLSSON, CORRODI and WALDECK 1963).

In rats the time course of this blockade has been studied following a large single dose of reserpine (10 mg/kg intraperitoneally) (ANDÉN, MAGNUSSON and WALDECK 1964). Virtually complete blockade of the uptake of H^3-noradrenaline by the heart was observed between 3 and 30 hours after the injection. Partial recovery of the uptake took place between 30 and 72 hours after the injection. During this period the noradrenaline remained virtually at zero level; it started to rise 96 hours after the injection. In the same rats the response to electrical stimulation of the cervical sympathetic (protrusion of the eye, dilatation of the pupil) was followed. Between 3 and 30 hours after the injection of reserpine no response was observed. Partial recovery was found at 48 hours and full recovery at 72 hours following the injection. These data support the view that the adrenergic transmission mechanism is dependent upon the ability of the storage mechanism to incorporate noradrenaline into a small labile fraction. Presumably this incorporation is necessary in order to make the noradrenaline available for transmission.

BERTLER, HILLARP and ROSENGREN (1960a, 1961) injected L-DOPA (100 mg/kg intravenously) to rabbits and examined the intracellular distribution of the amines formed in the adrenal medulla. Dopamine and noradrenaline were rapidly formed and incorporated into the adrenal medullary granules. (Unlike their precursor they did not easily penetrate through the adrenal medullary cell membranes.) The incorporation into the granules was blocked by reserpine (5 mg/kg 20 hours before the experiments) in accordance with the more recent *in-vitro* observations quoted above. Again in agreement with the *in-vitro* findings, it was observed that the adrenal medullary granules are able to store not only catecholamines but also 5-HT (formed after injection of 5-hydroxytryptophan), thus demonstrating the limited specificity of the storage mechanism. Carlsson, Jonasson and Rosengren (1963) observed that the storage mechanism, when studied in this way, was almost completely restored in 48 hours, when the adrenal medullary amine levels were still very low (Fig. 25). The data are in agreement with the *in-vitro* observations of Lundborg (1963) and give additional support to the view that the uptake mechanism is functionally more important than the amine levels.

The concept that two different mechanisms cooperate in the uptake and accumulation of amines in the adrenergic nerve endings (Carlsson, Hillarp and Waldeck 1963), has received strong support through data recently obtained by means of the histochemical fluorescence technique. Adrenergic nerve endings of the rat iris deprived of their transmitter by pretreatment with reserpine, are still able to take up and concentrate noradrenaline from the surrounding tissue fluid. The intraneuronal distribution of noradrenaline thus taken up differs from the normal distribution in being apparently unrelated to the distribution of storage granules. Additional evidence that the noradrenaline in these reserpine-treated animals is not taken up by the granules is supplied by the fact that the amine appears to be entirely unprotected from the action of monoamine oxidase. The reserpine-resistent uptake mechanism which appears to be located in the cell membrane, is blocked by cocaine and imipramine (Hamberger et al. 1964, Hillarp and Malmfors 1964 and unpublished data; cf. Andén, Carlsson and Waldeck 1963).

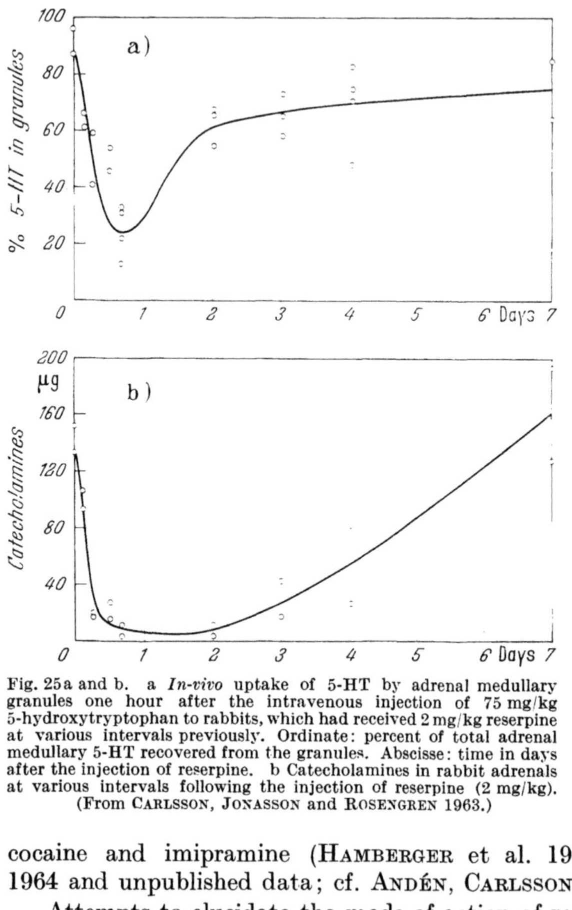

Fig. 25a and b. a *In-vivo* uptake of 5-HT by adrenal medullary granules one hour after the intravenous injection of 75 mg/kg 5-hydroxytryptophan to rabbits, which had received 2 mg/kg reserpine at various intervals previously. Ordinate: percent of total adrenal medullary 5-HT recovered from the granules. Abscisse: time in days after the injection of reserpine. b Catecholamines in rabbit adrenals at various intervals following the injection of reserpine (2 mg/kg). (From Carlsson, Jonasson and Rosengren 1963.)

Attempts to elucidate the mode of action of reserpine by studying the distribution of monoamines in homogenates of tissues containing adrenergic and/or hydroxytryptaminergic neurons have yielded inconclusive results (Weil-Malherbe and Bone 1957, Weil-Malherbe, Posner and Bowles 1961, Giarman and Schanberg 1958, 1961, 1962, Giarman 1963, Green, Sawyer and Erickson 1959, Green and Sawyer 1960, 1962, Bertler, Hillarp and Rosengren 1960b). The reason for this seems to be largely technical. For example, homogenization of brain tissue and subsequent centrifugation does not yield a uniform monoamine-containing fraction of granules as in the adrenal medulla. A considerable part of the monoamines occurs in pinched-off nerve endings (Whittaker 1964, De Robertis 1964). Needless to say, the interpretation of reserpine-induced changes in "intracellular distribution" studied by this technique is difficult. Recent technical improvements will possibly result in more conclusive data.

E. Miscellaneous biochemical actions

There can be little doubt that reserpine has a profound direct influence not only on peripheral adrenergic transmission but also on various monoaminergic mechanisms in the central nervous system. Such effects may be expected to lead to a variety of secondary physiological and biochemical actions. The question arises whether reserpine, in addition to these secondary actions, may produce effects which are unrelated to the actions on the monoamines. As the physiology of monoaminergic mechanisms is largely unknown, this question is difficult to answer. It seems at present doubtful if any of the biochemical actions of reserpine which will be briefly described below, are primary actions of the drug.

a) Adenosine phosphates

The main part of the catecholamines of the adrenal medulla is stored in granules together with an equivalent amount of adenosine triphosphate (ATP). In addition, some adenosine diphosphate (ADP) and adenosine monophosphate (AMP) occur in the storage granules (see HILLARP 1960b). Administration of reserpine brings about a decrease in adrenal medullary amines and a concomitant fall in ATP, ADP, and AMP (SCHÜMANN 1958, KIRPEKAR, GOODLAD and LEWIS 1958, HILLARP 1960b, BURACK, WEINER and HAGEN 1960). Similar changes are induced by stimulation of the adrenal medulla *via* the secretory nerves (CARLSSON and HILLARP 1956b, CARLSSON, HILLARP and HÖKFELT 1957). The action of reserpine on the adrenal medulla is partly dependent on an intact nerve supply, and it seems probable that reserpine actually causes an increased impulse flow through the secretory nerves (see Section II Gg). Whether reserpine causes a decrease in adrenal medullary ATP, ADP, or AMP apart from this indirect effect, is not known.

In isolated adrenal medullary granules the uptake of catecholamines from the incubation medium requires the presence of ATP. However, the uptake of ATP by the granules is considerably smaller than the amine uptake. Furthermore, reserpine completely blocked the amine incorporation but inhibited the uptake of ATP only about 30 per cent (CARLSSON, HILLARP and WALDECK 1963). These data lend no support to the view that reserpine has a primary effect on the interaction between ATP and the storage granules but do not exclude this possibility. The problem merits further investigation.

KIRPEKAR and LEWIS (1959, see also KAUL and LEWIS 1963) found that reserpine given to rats in a dose of 5 mg/kg lowered ATP and raised the ADP levels of the brain and liver. In mice given the same dose of reserpine BALZER, HOLTZ and PALM (1961b) found a slight increase in brain ATP, ADP, and AMP. In the platelets of reserpine-treated patients BORN, INGRAM and STACEY (1958) found a decrease in 5-HT but no corresponding fall in ATP. — Certain *in-vitro* effects of reserpine on mitochondria have been described, but the concentrations of reserpine have been very large (10^{-4} M) (ABOOD and ROMANCHEK 1957, KIRPEKAR and LEWIS 1960). — In rats a stimulating action of reserpine (0.5 mg/kg/day for 5 days) on brain ATP formation from labelled acetate has been observed (AHLBAUM and MILCH 1962).

b) Carbohydrates etc.

The glycogen content and turnover in the brain, liver, skeletal muscle, and heart of mice are increased following treatment with reserpine (5 mg/kg) (BALZER,

HOLTZ and PALM 1961b, BALZER and PALM 1962). Similar observations have been made in rats (MÁTHÉ, KASSAY and HUNKÁR 1961). The percentage of phosphorylase *a* in the heart, and possibly in the brain has been found to decrease after one week's treatment with reserpine (1 mg/kg/day) (BELFORD and FEINLEIB 1961). Concerning the effect of reserpine on the blood sugar, see Section II F c.

The nicotinamide-induced elevation of diphosphopyridine nucleotide in the liver was prolonged by treating rats with reserpine (BURTON et al. 1958). The response was not modified by pretreatment with iproniazid. Tetrabenazine was inactive (RANDALL, ATKINSON and ILIEV 1960). The effect is possibly mediated through the hypophysis (QUINN, REID and GREENGARD 1962, GREENGARD and QUINN 1962).

c) γ-Aminobutyric acid

A moderate decrease in the level of this amino acid in brain has been observed after treatment of mice with 5 mg/kg reserpine. The effect is prevented by iproniazid. It is possibly involved in the action of the drug on the electroshock seizure threshold (see Section II F a) (BALZER, HOLTZ and PALM 1961a, PALM, BALZER and HOLTZ 1961). The penetration of the amino acid into the mouse brain is retarded by reserpine (5 mg/kg) (BALZER and PALM 1962). Hypothermia may possibly be involved; chlorpromazine-induced hypothermia has been found to inhibit the penetration of dopa and tryptamine into the brain (PLETSCHER, GEY and KUNZ 1964). Also the penetration of barbital into the brain has been observed to be retarded in reserpine-treated mice, possibly a consequence of hypothermia (CHILD, SUTHERLAND and TOMICH 1961).

The uptake of another amino acid, *i.e.* S^{35}-methionine, in the hippocampal region has been reported to be reduced by reserpine (MACLEAN 1955).

d) Histamine

Reserpine has been found to produce a decrease in histamine in the blood, lung and intestine of the rabbit and the lung of the guinea pig, but no significant decrease was found in the brain (WAALKES and WEISSBACH 1956, WAALKES, COBURN and TERRY 1959). In the rat stomach both histamine and 5-HT were reduced by reserpine, 5 mg/kg intraperitoneally (KIM and SHORE 1963).

e) Acetylcholine

In dogs reserpine has been found to cause an increase in the acetylcholine levels of the heart, ileum, hypothalamus and other parts of the brain except the hippocampus (MALHOTRA and PUNDLIK 1959, MALHOTRA and DAS 1962). The effect is at least partly indirect (MALHOTRA and PRASAD 1963).

f) Lipids

In adrenal demedullated rats the mobilization of free fatty acids produced by cold exposure is prevented by reserpine, 0.2 mg/kg intravenously; the effect is probably a consequence of "chemical sympathectomy" (GILGEN et al. 1962).

F. Survey of pharmacology of reserpine

A detailed discussion of the pharmacological actions of reserpine is beyond the scope of the present chapter. A brief survey only will be given. Several excellent reviews of the extensive literature in this field are available.

For detailed discussions of the pharmacology of reserpine and related drugs, the reader is referred to the following articles.

General surveys of the pharmacology of reserpine: PLUMMER et al. (1954), BEIN (1956), SCHNEIDER (1957), KOHLI and MUKERJI (1961), DOMINO (1962a), LEWIS (1963).

Pharmacology of the central nervous system: KILLAM and KILLAM (1960), E. K. KILLAM (1962), UHR and MILLER (1960), DEWS and MORSE (1961), DOMINO (1962b), TOMAN (1963), ROSS and CARR (1962).

Cardiovascular pharmacology: COTTEN and MORAN (1961), GREEN (1962), FAWAZ (1963).

Pharmacology of the autonomic nervous system: VOLLE (1963).

Endocrine pharmacology: GAUNT, CHART and RENZI (1963).

All the actions of reserpine are slow in onset, maximum being reached after several hours, and long lasting. In rodents symptoms usually last two to three days, in other species longer, for example in cats about seven days. In all species the gross symptoms disappear long before the monoamine levels have returned to normal. However, not all the symptoms last equally long. For example, in mice treated with 2 mg/kg intraperitoneally sedation and hypothermia lasted about two days, reduction of pentylenetetrazol survival time about seven days (LESSIN and PARKES 1959).

a) Effects on behaviour and various brain functions

Reserpine induces a characteristic state of tranquillity which can reach the stage of sleep but not that of anesthesia (Figs. 26 and 27). The individual can be aroused by external stimuli, if sufficiently strong, but after cessation of the stimulus tranquillity soon returns. Spontaneous as well as induced motility may be inhibited with but little loss of motor coordination, which is in marked contrast to the action of classical sedatives such as the barbiturates. The animals can be placed in unusual positions, in which they remain (catalepsy). Both avoidance behaviour and food-rewarded responses are depressed by particularly low doses of reserpine, which do not effect escape reactions. Larger doses have a markedly depressant effect on food intake. Respiratory movements may be somewhat inhibited.

Neurophysiological techniques have so far failed to localize precisely the tranquillizing action of reserpine. The "reticular activating system" is not depressed; it may even be stimulated by the drug (RINALDI and HIMWICH 1955).

Reserpine interferes with so-called extrapyramidal motor functions. In man the *extrapyramidal actions* form a picture which comes very close to parkinsonism, with hypokinesia, muscle rigidity, and tremors. Conversely, reserpine may exert a favourable action on hyperkinetic conditions such as HUNTINGTON'S chorea.

The extrapyramidal actions of reserpine are of particular interest in view of the following facts. 1. About 80 per cent of the dopamine of brain is located in the corpus striatum and substantia nigra. 2. The dopamine level of brain is reduced by reserpine. 3. The central effects of reserpine are counteracted by increasing the dopamine level in the brain (by injection of L-3,4-dihydroxyphenyn alanine or DOPA). 4. In clinical cases of parkinsonism the dopamine level in brail- has been found very low. 5. Administration of DOPA to patients suffering from parkinsonism has a favourable influence on the symptoms (for review, see BIRKMAYER and HORNYKIEWICZ 1962, BARBEAU, SOURKES and MURPHY 1962, CARLSSON 1964b).

In reserpine-treated animals equivalents of parkinsonian symptoms are observed, *e.g.* akinesia, signs of general flexor dominance including a characteristic hunched back posture, muscle rigidity, and tremors. In rats these symptoms are accompanied by an increased activity of the *alpha* motoneurons and a decreased activity of the *gamma* motoneurons (STEG 1964). These changes were efficiently reversed by L-DOPA (100 mg/kg intravenously) and DL-5-hydroxytryptophan (200 mg/kg intravenously; ROOS and STEG 1964).

Reserpine causes ***hypothermia*** of complex origin. Centrally and peripherally induced vascular changes may be involved; inhibition of the thyroid

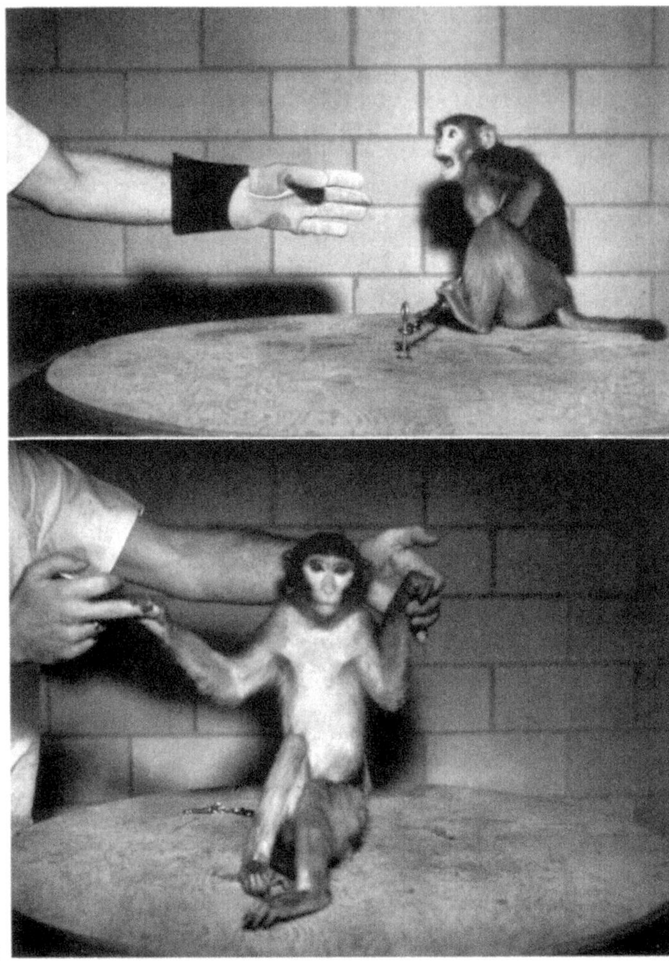

a

b

Fig. 26a and b. a Untreated monkey showing normal aggressive attitude to the presence of people. b Same monkey demonstrating loss of fear and aggressiveness two hours after an intravenous injection of 1 mg/kg reserpine. (From PLUMMER et al. 1954.) Courtesy of the N.Y. Academy of Sciences.

gland may contribute (TAYLOR and FREGLY 1962). The hypothermia may in turn induce severe cardiovascular changes. For example, in cats kept at room temperature hypothermia easily develops following treatment with reserpine. In such animals severe circulatory failure with unresponsiveness to the pressor effect of catecholamines and even anatomical changes in the heart have been observed (ZAIMIS 1961, WITHRINGTON and ZAIMIS 1961). ZAIMIS has suggested that these changes are due to a direct action of reserpine on the heart. No such effect has been demonstrated, however, except in concentrations which are above those necessary for influencing the adrenergic system (NAYLOR 1963). —

These observations emphasize the importance of keeping in mind the possibility of secondary changes induced by hypothermia in reserpine-treated animals. Whenever such changes may be involved, care should be taken to avoid hypothermia by keeping the animals in a warm environment. At a high environmental temperature, however, an increase in body temperature may be produced by reserpine (see Bein 1956).

A well-known effect of reserpine is the *prolongation of the anesthesia* induced by various agents, *e.g.* barbiturates and ethanol. The effect is seen also after low doses of the alkaloid which do not alone produce very profound central depression, but hypothermia may contribute to the effect (Lessin and Parkes 1957). — The penetration of barbital into the brain was found to be retarded in mice given 2 mg/kg reserpine, possibly a consequence of hypothermia (Child, Sutherland and Tomich 1961).

Reserpine *potentiates the action of several convulsants*, *e.g.* pentylenetetrazole, coffeine and camphor, and *lowers the threshold for the electrical induction of seizures* (for review, see Lewis 1963). The effects of anticonvulsants, *e.g.* phenytoin, phenacetamide and carboanhydrase inhibitors, are antagonized. The anticonvulsant effect of a carbonanhydrase inhibitor, which had been blocked by reserpine, tetrabenazine or α-methyl DOPA, could be restored by monoamine oxidase inhibitors and DOPA, but not by tryptophan or 5-hydroxytryptophan, suggesting that catecholamines are involved (Gray, Rauh and Shanahan 1963; *cf.* Section II G c). On the other hand, the reduction by reserpine

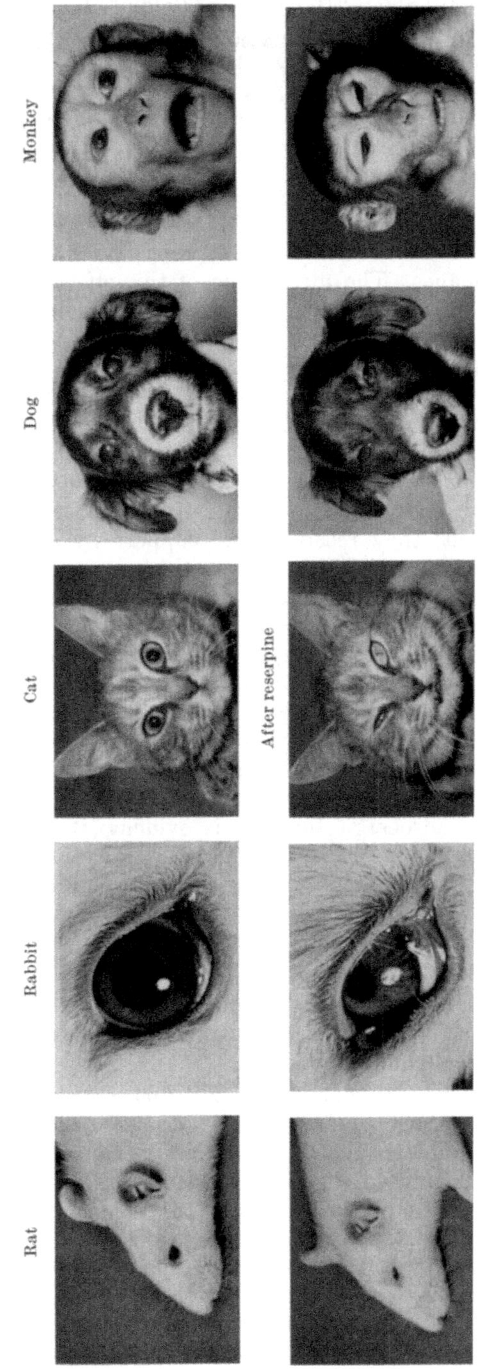

Fig. 27. The effect of reserpine on facial expression, eyes, pupils and nictitating membranes of five different species of animals. In the rat, ptosis is the most pronounced sign of drug effect. Marked miosis and relaxation of the nictitating membrane are portrayed in the rabbit eye and in the cat. The dog and the monkey show general quiescence in their facial expression after reserpine. Salivation is visible on the lower lip of the monkey. (From Schneider 1957.)

(2 mg/kg) and tetrabenazine (75 mg/kg) of the pentylenetetrazole survival time in mice was antagonized by the combination iproniazid-5-hydroxytryptophan, not by the combination iproniazid-DOPA, indicating that 5-HT rather catecholamines play a part in pentylenetetrazole sensitivity (LESSIN and PARKES 1959). PROCKOP, SHORE and BRODIE (1959) observed that neither of the amino acids, given in large doses to normal and reserpine-treated rats, influenced the response to electroshock.

b) Effects on the autonomic nervous system

The picture produced by reserpine is that of general parasympathetic predominance. The mechanism of this effect is complex. At first it was believed that the effect was entirely central in origin (see BEIN 1956). Later it was found that reserpine causes depletion of the adrenergic transmitter, leading to inhibition of adrenergic nervous activity (see Section II C). It seems to be a favoured view today that the effect of the drug on the adrenergic nervous system is entirely peripheral in origin. In support of this view the observation is often quoted that in the cervical sympathetic trunk of reserpine-treated cats the centrifugal flow of impulses is not decreased but possibly even increased (IGGO and VOGT 1960). Although the interpretation of such observations on mixed nerve trunks are difficult, they receive some support by earlier work (McQUEEN, DOYLE and SMIRK 1954, 1955), in which the vascular tone of the perfused innervated but otherwise isolated hind limb of the rabbit was studied. Systemic injection of reserpine caused a fall in blood pressure but a vasoconstriction in the perfused limb. When reserpine was injected into the perfusion fluid, vasodilation quickly developed in the limb. There is some evidence, however, that the action of reserpine on the adrenergic nervous system is not entirely peripheral in origin. Inhibition of adrenergic nervous activity resulting in, for example, relaxation of the nictitating membrane, narrowing of the palpebral fissure, and depression of the carotid occlusion reflex has been found to set in before any decrease in the peripheral adrenergic function is evident (BEIN 1955, SCHNEIDER 1955, BHARGAVA and BORISON 1955). Furthermore, injection of reserpine in a dose of as little as 10 μg in the lateral ventricle of cats may result in a number of typical effects, *e.g.* relaxation of the nictitating membrane and narrowing of the palpebral fissure, and these effects may set in first at the side of injection (DASGUPTA and HALEY 1957, BEIN 1957).

It would thus appear that reserpine causes depression of adrenergic nervous activity by combined central and peripheral effects and that the peripheral effects dominate.

In man de la LANDE et al. (1960; see also PARKS et al. 1961, PARKS, SKINNER and WHELAN 1961) observed that infusion of reserpine (50 μg/minute during 10 minutes) into the brachial artery caused marked dilatation of the skin vessels on the infused side. This commenced after a latent period of 10—20 minutes and lasted about 24 hours. In patients who had received 2—4 mg reserpine orally for 3 weeks no such response to intraarterial infusion of reserpine was observed. At the peak of reserpine-induced vasodilatation there was no interference with reflex vasoconstriction produced by application of ice to the head and neck. Immediately after sympathectomy the local effect of reserpine was absent. It gradually became re-established over a period of 6—12 weeks. The authors make the interesting suggestion (see WHELAN and SKINNER 1963) that the local action of reserpine is due to depletion of a peripheral store. This store is depleted also by sympathetic denervation. The return of responsiveness to reserpine was not believed to be due to re-innervation, since large doses of ephedrine had no effect, but was suggested to be due to replenishment of an independent store. The last-mentioned point appears to require further clarification.

According to COSTA et al. (1961) reserpine facilitates *transmission in sympathetic ganglia*, whereas monoamine oxidase inhibitors have the opposite action. The results are of particular interest in view of the existence of adrenergic nerve terminals innervating sympathetic ganglion cells (FALCK 1962). Unfortunately, the results of COSTA et al. could not be confirmed by REINERT (1963), who presented data suggesting that the changes observed by COSTA et al. were induced by dehydration.

Reserpine has profound actions on the *gastrointestinal tract*, with increased gastric secretion, formation of peptic ulcers, and increased gastrointestinal motility. The mechanisms underlying these actions have not been fully elucidated (see BEIN 1956, BÜLBRING and CREMA 1959, ERSPAMER 1961, HAVERBACK and WIRTSCHAFTLER 1962). Of particular interest is the early work of PLUMMER, BARRETT and RUTLEDGE (1955), showing that in dogs the increased motor activity of the intestine caused by reserpine (1 mg/kg intravenously) persisted after vagotomy and transection of the spinal cord at the sixth cervical segment but was inhibited by ganglion blocking and anticholinergic agents. It was suggested that reserpine acted by stimulating parasympathetic ganglia. In a study on the effect of reserpine on gastric secretion a similar conclusion was reached (BARRETT et al. 1955, see however, CASTIAU and REUSE 1962, SCHAPIRO and WOODWARD 1961). In this connection it is of interest to note that the ganglion cells of the intestinal wall receive an adrenergic innervation (FALCK 1963). As this innervation is probably inhibitory, its blockade by reserpine should lead to stimulation of intestinal motor activity. — On the isolated intestine reserpine ($> 1\ \mu$g/ml) is inhibitory.

Reserpine causes a general increase in parasympathetic tone. For example, in rabbits reserpine has been observed to induce miosis persisting after sympathetic denervation, lacrimation and salivation (BOGDANSKI, SULSER and BRODIE 1961). In intact animals the miosis induced by reserpine is a consequence of 3 independent actions, 1. blockade of adrenergic innervation, 2. increased parasympathetic tone, and 3. enhancement of the light reflex, which also includes active closure of the eyelids, retraction of the eyeball etc. The third effect is of interest in view of the presence of dopamine-containing neurons in the retina, which are sensitive to reserpine (MALMFORS 1963, HÄGGENDAL and MALMFORS 1963).

c) Endocrine effects

Space does not permit a detailed review of the extensive literature in this field (for reviews, see GAUNT, CHART and RENZI 1961, 1963, DOMINO 1962a, KOHLI and MUKERJI 1961). In view of the accumulation of monoamines in the median eminence as well as in hypothalamic nuclei with established endocrine functions, *e.g.* the supraoptic and hypothalamic nuclei, and the effect of reserpine on these monoamines (CARLSSON, FALCK and HILLARP 1962), endocrinological effects of reserpine are to be expected. No doubt such effects exist, but the data so far obtained are often contradictory and inconclusive. In particular, it is not seldom difficult to decide whether the changes observed are specific or caused by changes such as hypothermia, inanition, and "stress".

Reserpine initially stimulates and later inhibits *ACTH* release, possibly via an action on the hypothalamus (GAUNT et al. 1954, WELLS, BRIGGS and MUNSON 1956, HERTTING and HORNYKIEWICZ 1957, KITAY et al. 1959, SAFFRON and VOGT 1960, WESTERMANN, MAICKEL and BRODIE 1961, MAICKEL, WESTERMANN and BRODIE 1962). The inhibitory effect of reserpine on the *thyroid* may be related to reduced food intake (see KOHLI and MUKERJI 1961, PREMACHANDRA 1961, YAMAZAKI, SLINGERLAND and NOGUCHI 1961). The mechanism of the inhibitory action of the drug on the *gonads* is uncertain; it is possibly mediated by inhibition of the release of follicle-stimulating hormones. Perhaps the most striking effect of reserpine on the endocrine system is *stimulation of prolactin secretion* from the anterior pituitary, resulting in mammary growth and lactation (MEITES 1958, DESCLIN 1958, BENSON 1958, 1960, MEITES et al. 1959).

In ovariectomized, oestrogen-primed rabbits KANEMATSU, HILLIARD and SAWYER (1963) observed that prolactin secretion could be induced either by reserpine (0.5 mg/kg intravenously) or by a discrete electrolytic lesion in the basal tuberal hypothalamus. After such a lesion reserpine had lost its action on prolactin secretion. KANEMATSU and SAWYER (1963) were able to produce prolactin secretion by implanting minute amounts of solid reserpine phosphate into the posterior median eminence or the basal tuberal area of the hypothalamus. It appears that reserpine stimulates prolactin secretion by blocking an inhibitory mechanism in this region.

In rats stimulation (GAUNT et al. 1954, GABE, TUCHMANN-DUPLESSIS and MERCIER-PAROT 1961) as well as inhibition (HOLEĆEK et al. 1957) by reserpine of the secretion of *antidiuretic* hormone has been reported. From histological data on hares MILINE et al. (1957) conclude that reserpine stimulates the supraoptic and para-ventricular nuclei. According to KHAZAN et al. (1962) release of 5-HT rather than ADH is involved in the antidiuretic action of reserpine.

In *Rana* frogs KHAZAN and SULMAN (1961) observed a melanophore-dispersing effect of reserpine, suggested to be due to enhanced secretion of *melanocyte-stimulating hormone.*

Reserpine (5 mg/kg intravenously) causes a rise in *blood sugar* in rabbits. The response is abolished by adrenalectomy or hexamethonium (TAKETOMO et al. 1957, *cf.* RUTISHAUSER 1963). Similarly an initial increase in metabolic rate observed in reserpine-treated rats was prevented by adrenalectomy or dibenzyline (JOHNSON and SELLERS 1961). Injection of deserpidine into the pancreatico-duodenal artery of dogs causes release of a hyperglycemic agent, probably glucagon and not 5-HT or catecholamines (GALANSINO et al. 1963). A compound behaving histochemically as 5-HT has been detected in insular cells; it is brought to disappear partly by reserpine (FALCK and HELLMAN 1963).

In the *pineal gland* BERTLER, FALCK and OWMAN (1963), using histochemical as well as analytical techniques, were able to detect 5-HT in the parenchymal cells and in the pineal sympathetic nerves. In rats treatment with reserpine, like cervical sympathectomy, caused a 50 per cent decrease in the 5-HT of the gland and the disappearance of fluorescent nerves. The remaining 5-HT, like the parenchymal fluorescence, proved refractory towards even intense reserpine treatment.

In the parenchymal cells of rat pineal glands dense granules have been observed by means of the electron microscope (PELLEGRINO DE IRALDI and DE ROBERTIS 1961, see also DE ROBERTIS 1962). The dense granules were found to disappear within 2 hours following treatment with reserpine (5 mg/kg intraperitoneally). Recovery took place between 2 and 7 days after the injection. The time curve was similar to that of 5-HT and noradrenaline in rabbit brain, as observed by SHORE and BRODIE (see Section II Ba). In the light of the above-mentioned data of BERTLER et al. the interpretation of these electron-microscopic observations must await further studies.

Catecholamines persisting after reserpine treatment have been detected histochemically and analytically in the pituitary of cats (unpublished data of HILLARP, HÄGGENDAL and coworkers).

d) Cumulation and tolerance

Plummer et al. (1954) observed that when a daily dose of 25 μg/kg orally or 15 to 20 μg/kg intravenously was given to dogs, mild sedation appeared after 5 to 7 days, increased in intensity over a period of a few weeks, and reached a steady state which persisted with continuous administration of the drug for 10 months. No evidence of tolerance was observed. Häggendal and Lindqvist (1963, 1964) observed a cumulative response in rabbits given 100 to 200 μg/kg/day subcutaneously. After about two weeks the rabbits showed a certain degree of adaptation which was particularly evident 24 hours after each daily dose. The tissue monoamines remained low during this period of adaptation (see Section IIBb). In mice given 0.08 mg/kg/day subcutaneously cumulation followed by adaptation, with return of spontaneous motility, appetite, and increase in body weight, has also been observed (Markiewicz 1963). During the period of adaptation the adrenal medullary catecholamines were gradually restored towards normal, while the monoamines of brain and heart remained at low levels, with at most a slight tendency to recover. Since the decrease in adrenal medullary amines is partly centrally mediated, their recovery may be secondary to the functional recovery of the brain. This recovery, in spite of persistently low monoamine levels, may be due to recovery of the storage mechanism — which may occur without any increase in amine levels (see Section IID) — and/or to increased sensitivity according to the "law of denervation". Further investigations are needed to elucidate this point.

The observations of Khazan, Sulman and Winnik (1961) may form part of the adaptation phenomenon. They observed that in rats given reserpine in a dose of 0.01 mg/kg/day for 10 days the adrenal glands showed 30 to 50 per cent hypertrophy, while after 40 days' continuous treatment there was almost no hypertrophy. Data on adrenal ascorbic acid depletion (rats) and urinary steroids (man) gave additional support to the view that the stimulating action of reserpine on the pituitary-adrenal cortex axis was transitory in spite of continued treatment with the drug.

G. Interaction between reserpine and other drugs and factors

a) Tetrabenazine

A number of synthetic bensoquinolizines, among which tetrabenazine has been studied particularly extensively, exert biochemical and pharmacological effects very similar to those of reserpine but have a shorter duration of action (see Section IV). Pretreatment of rabbits with tetrabenazine (50 mg/kg 15 minutes before) appears to protect the animals against reserpine (1 mg/kg); the duration of sedation will be as short as if tetrabenazine alone had been given (Quinn, Shore and Brodie 1959). Similarly, the duration of 5-HT depletion in brain was found to be shortened, while no statistically significant effect on noradrenaline depletion was detected. Similar observations on rabbits and mice have been made in the present laboratory, except that the protective action of tetrabenazine against reserpine was about equally strong on brain 5-HT, noradrenaline, and dopamine (unpublished data). The results support the assumption that tetrabenazine and reserpine compete for the same receptor sites.

Also the release by reserpine of ACTH is inhibited by pretreatment with tetrabenazine (Eechaute, Lacroix and Leusen 1962).

b) Monoamine oxidase inhibitors

The interaction between reserpine and the monoamine oxidase (MAO) inhibitors is complex. It depends *inter alia* on the order in which the two drugs are given (Brodie, Pletscher and Shore 1956, Pletscher 1956, Besendorf and Pletscher 1956, Carlsson et al. 1957, and unpublished observations of this laboratory; review on MAO: Pletscher, Gey and Zeller 1960).

If the MAO inhibitor is given first, the sedative action of reserpine may not only be prevented but even reversed, with excitation and signs of increased sympathetic activity (piloerection, exophtalmus, hypertension etc.). If large doses of the drugs are given and the interval between the two injections is not too short (at least two hours), excitation may reach extreme degrees and may end in fatal hyperthermia.

When the dose of reserpine is moderate, the animals may survive the excitation which gradually wears off without being followed by any sedation or any

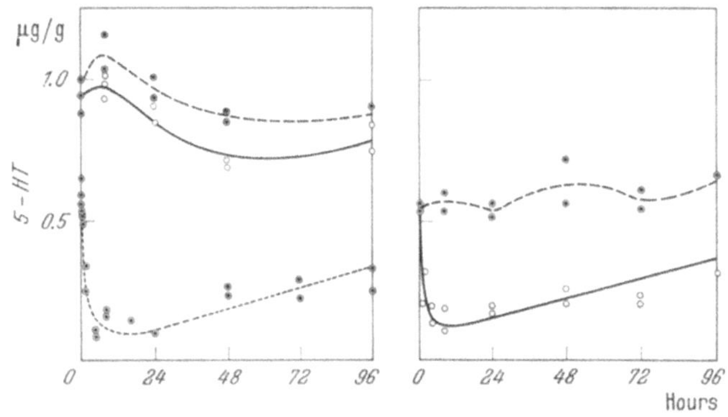

Fig. 28. Level of 5-HT in rat brain after the administration of reserpine alone and after pretreatment with the monoamine oxidase inhibitor iproniazid (left). For comparison the corresponding data on isoniazid, which does not inhibit monoamine oxidase, are shown (right). Ordinate: 5-HT in brain, µg/g. Abscisse: time in hours. ⊙———⊙ 100 mg/kg iproniazid (or isoniazid) subcutaneously 16 hours before 0 time; ⊙------⊙ 3 mg/kg reserpine intraperitoneally at 0 time; ○——○ 3 mg/kg reserpine intraperitoneally at 0 time, 16 hours after 100 mg/kg iproniazid (or isoniazid) subcutaneously. (From Pletscher, Gey and Zeller 1960.)

other of the characteristic actions of reserpine. If the dose of MAO inhibitor has been low or the interval between administration of the two drugs short (less than one hour), the excitation following reserpine administration may be short or even absent; it may be followed by the characteristic reserpine sedation.

The MAO inhibitors also cause partial prevention of the depletion by reserpine of 5-HT (Fig. 28; Brodie, Pletscher and Shore 1956, Pletscher 1956) and catecholamines (Carlsson et al. 1957). The degree of prevention varies according to dose and time interval as indicated above. There are also differences between tissues. For example, prevention of noradrenaline depletion is by far more complete in brain than in heart (Table 2). In brain 5-HT depletion appears to be more easily prevented than catecholamine depletion. In general, a correlation between biochemical and behavioural prevention appears to exist.

The picture of reserpine reversal comes fairly close to that caused by monoamine precursors (5-hydroxytryptophan and DOPA) and may therefore be due to an excess of free monoamines caused by the simultaneous block of monoamine breakdown and storage. In addition, there is histochemical evidence that the depletion of monoamine stores by reserpine is partially prevented by MAO inhibitors (Zbinden, Pletscher and Studer 1957b, Zbinden and Studer 1958). This is possibly due to competition of excess free monoamines with reserpine for receptor sites of the storage mechanisms, in analogy with the competition between the benzoquinolizines and reserpine. In fact, a large dose of 5-HT appears to prevent depletion of 5-HT stores by reserpine (Erspamer 1956a).

Table 2. *Prevention by iproniazid of catecholamine disappearance after reserpine* (From CARLSSON et al. 1957)

	No. of animals	Behaviour of animals	Catechol amines		
			Heart[1] μg/g	Brain[1] μg/g	Adrenals[2] μg/2 glands
1. Control	7	Normal	1.59 ± 0.135	0.24 ± 0.025	110 ± 16.6
2. Iproniazid (100 mg/kg), 22 h .	5	Normal	1.34 ± 0.198	0.25 ± 0.041	142 ± 25.0
3. Reserpine (1 mg/kg), 16 h . .	4	Tranquillized	0.01 ± 0.005	0.01 ± 0.004	16 ± 3.0
4. Iproniazid + Reserpine, 6+16 h .	5	Not tranquillized, initially restless	0.21 ± 0.051	0.14 ± 0.020	97 ± 10.4
			(4–3: $P < 0.01$)	(4–3: $P < 0.001$)	(4–3: $P < 0.001$)

[1] Noradrenaline; [2] Adrenaline.

Direct evidence of a competition between monoamines and reserpine for the uptake mechanism of storage granules has now been obtained (see Section II D a).

AXELROD, HERTTING and PATRICK (1961) observed that MAO inhibitors reduce the rate of disappearance of labelled catecholamines from tissue stores and therefore proposed that MAO inhibitors inhibit release of catecholamines from the stores. As a more likely alternative, their data may be interpreted to show that inhibition of the MAO of the storage cell increases the life span of intracellular monoamines by preventing their oxidative deamination.

If the MAO inhibitor is given after the monoamine stores have been depleted by reserpine, the effect is less dramatic (BESENDORF and PLETSCHER 1956, SHORE and BRODIE 1957 b). Again the outcome is largely dependent upon the doses used. In mice and rabbits a large dose of reserpine has been found to retard considerably the accumulation of 5-HT and especially catecholamines as well as their 3-O-methyl metabolites in brain caused by the MAO inhibitor nialamide (CARLSSON, LINDQVIST and MAGNUSSON 1960, BERTLER 1961). After a moderate dose of reserpine (1 mg per kg to rabbits intravenously) this retardation was less pronounced (BERTLER 1961). Only after this lower dose did a significant accumulation of catecholamines occur, whereas toxic levels of 5-HT, resulting in tremors and convulsions, finally were reached even when a large dose of reserpine had been given (25 mg per kg intraperitoneally) to mice. The MAO inhibitor was able to restore the sedative action of reserpine only in those cases where an increase in catecholamines took place. The antagonistic effect, which developed in the course of a few hours, thus seemed to be related to accumulation of catecholamines rather than 5-HT. A similar conclusion has been reached by STEIN and RAY (1960), who studied behavioural effects of MAO inhibitors on rats chronically treated with reserpine, and recently by SPECTOR, HIRSCH and BRODIE (1963) on the basis of experiments with the MAO inhibitor MO 911. These authors consider that free noradrenaline rather than dopamine and 5-HT is responsible for the counteraction by MO 911 of the reserpine effect.

Not all MAO inhibitors are ideal tools for studies of this kind. For example, tranylcypromine has been shown to cause release of noradrenaline in brain (CARLSSON, LINDQVIST and MAGNUSSON 1960). If such "side effects" are not taken into account erroneous conclusions may be drawn. — The problem of the relative role of different monoamines in the antagonism of reserpine effects by MAO inhibitors cannot be regarded as definitely solved. Further investigation is required.

The ability of MAO inhibitors to restore behaviour and monoamine levels in reserpine-treated animals is considerably enhanced, if hypothermia is prevented by keeping the animals in a warm environment (unpublished data of the present laboratory).

c) Monoamine analogs and precursors

A drug causing "chemical sympathectomy" might be expected to increase the sensitivity to injected catecholamines and to decrease sensitivity to an indirectly

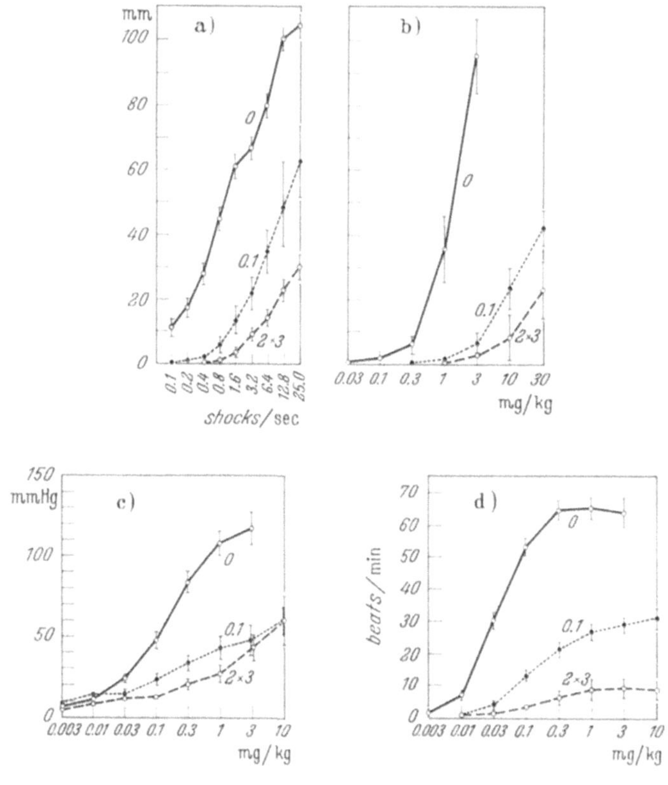

Fig. 29a—d. Effect of pretreatment with reserpine on response to tyramine. Spinal cats. Shown are the mean response of the nictitating membrane (in mm on drum) to continuous supramaximal preganglionic stimulation applied at increasing rates of stimulation (a) and dose-response curves for intravenously injected tyramine obtained on the nictitating membrane (b), blood pressure (c) and heart rate (d). Given are the mean values and their standard errors. 0 = untreated control preparations; 0.1 = 24 hours after pretreatment with 0.1 mg/kg reserpine intraperitoneally (10 experiments). 2 × 3 = after pretreatment with 3 mg/kg reserpine given 48 and 24 hours prior to experiment (10 preparations). (From TRENDELENBURG 1961.)

acting sympathomimetic such as tyramine. The former effect was observed very early by BEIN (1953), the latter by CARLSSON et al. (1957). These observations have been confirmed by numerous other investigators and been studied in particular detail by *e.g.* BURN and RAND (1958) and TRENDELENBURG (1961, 1963, Fig. 29). According to the latter author, the two effects can be separated experimentally and therefore are caused by different mechanisms. However, both phenomena may well be consequences of one and the same primary effect of reserpine, *i.e.* blockade of the adrenergic storage mechanism (see Section IID). In man a decrease in the vascular responses to tyramine has been observed after reserpine treatment (0.25 to 1 mg orally for two weeks), whereas the responses to noradrenaline remained unchanged (ABBOUD and ECKSTEIN 1964).

In reserpine-treated animals the function of the adrenergic nerves may be temporarily restored by infusion of noradrenaline or one of its precursors. For a certain period after the infusion stimulation of the nerves or injection of tyramine results in typical responses (vasoconstriction etc.; BURN and RAND 1958, 1960, 1962, ROSELL and SEDVALL 1961). As to the response to stimulation of noradrenergic nerves, DE SCHAEPDRYVER et al. (1963) and GAFFNEY, CHIDSEY and BRAUNWALD (1963) report, however, that in reserpine-treated dogs no restoration occurred after infusion of noradrenaline. At first it was believed that the noradrenaline infusion resulted in replenishment of the transmitter stores, but as pointed out by MUSCHOLL (1960; *cf.* KUSCHINSKY et al. 1960) this cannot be the explanation, because the uptake of amines by the stores is blocked by reserpine. It appears that the effect of tyramine exists during and for a very short time after the infusion of noradrenaline and therefore depends on the existence of a very mobile pool of noradrenaline (NASMYTH 1962, SMITH 1963). This pool is probably located in or close to the adrenergic nerve endings since infusion of noradrenaline is unable to restore the effect of tyramine after postganglionic denervation (BURN and RAND 1960). The exact localization of this pool and the mechanism by which it is affected by tyramine are unknown. Possibly tyramine blocks the entry of noradrenaline into nerve endings and/or storage granules (*cf.* FARRANT 1963 ,FURCHGOTT and KIRPEKAR 1963).

During the initial stage of reserpine action the pressor response to tyramine and similar drugs is potentiated (NASMYTH 1962, ROSS et al. 1963, WALASZEK and BURFORD 1963). As the tyramine response is potentiated by infusion of noradrenaline or adrenaline, this effect may possibly be due to the increased level of adrenaline in blood plasma released from the adrenal medulla during the early stage of reserpine effect (see Section II C). The observation that reserpine also after pretreatment with iproniazid augments the pressor response to tyramine (WALASZEK and BURFORD 1963) may possibly be related to the release of noradrenaline from nerve endings, which seems to take place after administration of this drug combination. In this case the adrenal medulla probably is not involved since the adrenal medullary secretion caused by reserpine is prevented by iproniazid (KRONEBERG and SCHÜMANN 1960).

To what extent monoamines interfere with the central effects of reserpine cannot be studied directly, because the monoamines do not readily penetrate the blood-brain barrier. It is possible to circumvent this difficulty, however. The physiological precursors 5-hydroxytryptophan (5-HTP) (UDENFRIEND, WEISSBACH and BOGDANSKI 1957) and 3,4-dihydroxyphenylalanine (DOPA) (CARLSSON, LINDQVIST and MAGNUSSON 1957) are able to penetrate into brain, where they undergo decarboxylation to form 5-HT and dopamine respectively. In this way central effects are produced, which beyond any doubt are caused by the monoamines: the effects are prevented by decarboxylase inhibitors and potentiated by MAO and (in the case of DOPA) COMT[1] inhibitors. The precursors *per se* appear to be fairly inert from the pharmacological point of view. Using these precursors it has been shown that the accumulation of dopamine (from DOPA) in the brains of reserpine-treated animals is accompanied by marked alleviation of the reserpine syndrome (Fig. 30; CARLSSON, LINDQVIST and MAGNUSSON 1957, EVERETT and TOMAN 1959, BLASCHKO and CHRUŚCIEL 1960, SMITH and DEWS 1962). This is true not only of the gross motor disturbances but also of the blockade of conditioned avoidance behaviour (Fig. 31; SEIDEN and CARLSSON 1963a and b, and unpublished observations). The antagonistic effect of DOPA

[1] COMT = catechol-O-methyl transferase, *i.e.* one of the enzymes responsible for the metabolic degradation of catecholamines.

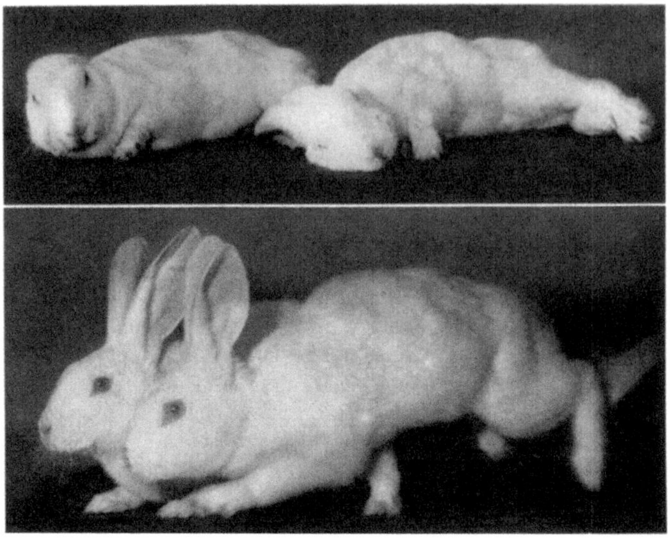

a

b

Fig. 30a and b. a Rabbits treated with reserpine (5 mg/kg intravenously). b Same rabbits 15 minutes after DL-DOPA (200 mg/kg intravenously). The effects of reserpine are no longer visible. (From CARLSSON, A.: Zur Frage der Wirkungsweise einiger Psychopharmaka, Psychiat. Neurol. **140**, 220—222, 1960.)

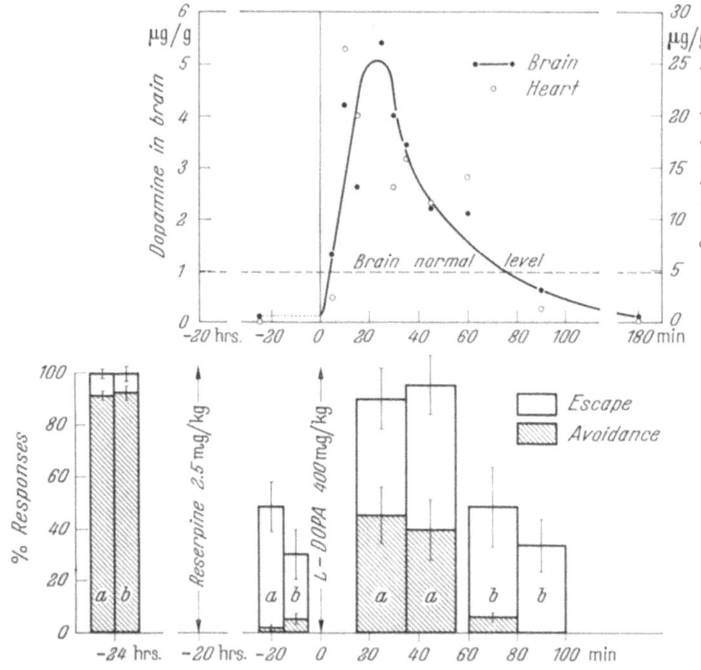

Fig. 31. Effect of L-DOPA on brain and heart dopamine (above) and on a conditioned avoidance reaction (shuttle box; below) in reserpine-treated mice. Explanation: 24 hours before 0 time the animals showed about 90 per cent avoidance response; 20 hours before 0 time reserpine (2.5 mg/kg intraperitoneally) was injected; 20 minutes before 0 time the avoidance response had decreased to a few per cent, while escape reactions to the shock stimulus were less affected. At 0 time L-DOPA (400 mg/kg intraperitoneally) was given. Between 15 and 55 minutes after the injection, when the tissue dopamine levels were much increased, the avoidance reactions were partially restored. Between 60 and 100 minutes after the injection, when the dopamine levels had decreased, the avoidance reactions had almost disappeared. — a and b are separate experiments. Vertical lines: standard error of the mean. Experiment a: $n = 7$; experiment b: $n = 6$. (From SEIDEN and CARLSSON 1963b.)

has been observed in mice, rats, rabbits, cats, monkeys, and also in man (DEGKWITZ et al. 1960). In rats, admittedly, DOPA is sometimes ineffective. It is noteworthy that DOPA is capable of restoring the normal pattern of behaviour characteristic of the species or individual. We are thus not merely dealing with an unspecific excitatory effect.

The dopamine formed from DOPA is partly converted into noradrenaline, whose accumulation is easily detectable if a MAO inhibitor has been given prior to the DOPA. The question arises whether the central effects are referable to dopamine, or noradrenaline, or both. With MAO intact the accumulation of noradrenaline following DOPA administration to reserpine-treated animals is hardly detectable. If noradrenaline alone were responsible for the central actions of DOPA, it must therefore be assumed to be extremely active. Experiments in this laboratory with 3,4-dihydroxyphenylserine (DOPS), a (probably unphysiological) precursor which on decarboxylation yields noradrenaline directly, have thrown light on this problem (CARLSSON and CORRODI, unpublished observations, see CARLSSON 1963a). It has been shown that DOPS is capable of counteracting the sedative effect of reserpine provided that MAO has been inhibited. The amounts of noradrenaline which have to accumulate in order to create the effect are low but detectable. From this it can be inferred that the ability of DOPA to counteract the effect of reserpine is mainly referable to the dopamine formed. However, it is not possible from this to draw any conclusions about the relative importance of dopamine and noradrenaline for the central actions of reserpine. The possibility should be kept in mind that dopamine can activate not only its own receptors but also those of noradrenaline, and *vice versa*. For further discussion of this problem, see Section VI.

Another DOPA analog, *i.e.* m-tyrosine, is capable of antagonizing the sedative effect of reserpine (BLASCHKO and CHRUŚCIEL 1960). The effect is presumably mediated by the decarboxylation product m-tyramine.

If a methyl group is introduced on the α-carbon of the side chain of DOPA and m-tyrosine, α-methyl DOPA and α-methyl metatyrosine (α-MMT), respectively, are obtained. These analogs are decarboxylated at a much lower rate than their parent compounds and consequently they are less efficient as reserpine antagonists. However, their decarboxylation products are resistant towards MAO, and therefore fairly large concentrations may finally be built up (CARLSSON and LINDQVIST 1962). In fact, it has been observed in our laboratory (unpublished experiments on mice and rabbits) that the sedative effect of reserpine may be partly counteracted by pretreatment with α-methyl DOPA or α-MMT. Analogous results have been obtained by NEČINA (1962), who observed that α-methyl DOPA (400 mg/kg intraperitoneally 2 hours before reserpine, 5 mg/kg intraperitoneally), given to rats and mice, prevented the following actions of reserpine: catalepsy, ptosis, decrease of seizure threshold of pentylenetetrazol, adrenal cholesterol and ascorbic acid. On the other hand, BRODIE and coworkers (GESSA et al. 1962) report that the effect of reserpine is not modified by α-MMT pretreatment.

Among the sympathomimetic amines certain compounds, *e.g.* amphetamine and ephedrine, penetrate easily into the brain. These compounds lack hydroxyl groups on the benzene ring and therefore belong to the so-called indirectly acting sympathomimetic amines (see above). Like tyramine they might therefore be expected to be inactive in reserpine-treated animals. According to BURN and RAND (1958, 1962) this is true of the pressor effect of amphetamine and ephedrine in spinal cats. On the other hand, FURCHGOTT (1960) has made observations suggesting that in arterial strips amphetamine activates adrenergic receptors by a direct action. This seems to hold true also for the central action of amphetamine.

In any event it persists after treatment with reserpine. In fact, amphetamine and a number of related drugs are fairly potent reserpine antagonists (EVERETT and TOMAN 1959, PLUMMER, MAXWELL and EARL 1957).

While there is thus evidence that activation of catecholamine receptors in brain leads to restoration of some of the major central disturbances caused by reserpine, it is remarkable to find that this is not true of activation of 5-HT receptors. Accumulation of 5-HT brought about by injection of 5-HTP does not lead to any conspicuous alleviation of the reserpine syndrome (CARLSSON, LINDQVIST and MAGNUSSON 1957, EVERETT and TOMAN 1959). There is no evidence of blockade of 5-HT receptors in reserpine-treated animals: the symptoms (tremors, extension of limbs etc.) brought about by 5-HT accumulation are seen also after reserpine treatment.

These precursor data like those obtained with MAO inhibitors (see under b above), support the view that lack of dopamine and/or noradrenaline play a role in the central actions of reserpine. In favour of an involvement also of 5-HT, it may be recalled that certain central actions of reserpine are counteracted by 5-HTP (see Section II F a).

d) Other agents

The ability of the well-known antidepressant agent *imipramine* to counteract certain effects of reserpine seems to have been observed first by GARATTINI and by HIMWICH (see DOMENJOZ and THEOBALD 1959). The antagonism is observed both when imipramine is given before and after reserpine and includes the following reserpine effects: sedation, potentiation of effects of hypnotics, ptosis, miosis, and diarrhea (DOMENJOZ and THEOBALD 1959, GARATTINI and VALZELLI 1962, SULSER, BICKEL and BRODIE 1962) and according to IZQUIERDO, COUSSIO and KAUMAN (1962), hypotension. The effects on amine levels are unaffected, however. The effect of the benzoquinolizine Ro-4-1284 is also counteracted (SULSER et al., *l.c.*).

The monomethyl analog of imipramine, *desmethylimipramine*, is an even more potent reserpine and benzoquinolizine antagonist than its parent compound. In fact, pretreatment with desmethylimipramine not only inhibits but reverses the sedative effect of reserpine and Ro-4-1284. Furthermore, its action sets in more rapidly. Desmethylimipramine is a metabolite of imipramine and may well be the mediator of the antireserpine activity (SULSER et al., *l.c.*). Whether this is true also of the antidepressant activity, remains to be demonstrated; the clinical trials reported so far do not seem to answer this question conclusively. It should be kept in mind that also amphetamine, which is a poor antidepressant, is capable of reversing the sedative action of reserpine.

Amitriptyline, an antidepressant closely related to imipramine, and *desmethylamitriptyline* also show antireserpine activity (GARATTINI et al. 1962).

Large doses of *chlorpromazine* have been shown to partially prevent the effects of reserpine — and also the effects of monoamine oxidase inhibitors — on the brain monoamine levels (EHRINGER, HORNYKIEWICZ and LECHNER 1960, PLETSCHER and GEY 1962). It appears that these effects are at least partly due to the hypothermia caused by large doses of chlorpromazine (COSTA, GESSA and BRODIE 1962, PLETSCHER, GEY and KUNZ 1963).

In small doses *chlorpromazine* and *haloperidol* cause an increase in the concentration of catecholamine metabolites in brain (CARLSSON and LINDQVIST 1963, ANDÉN, ROOS and WERDINIUS 1964). The effects are possibly due to compensatory activation of monoaminergic neurons following blockade of monoamine receptors.

Bretylium and *cocaine* have been shown to interfere with the depletion of noradrenaline by reserpine (CALLINGHAM and CASS 1962, HERTTING, AXELROD and PATRICK 1962, POTTER and AXELROD 1963). Whether 5-HT is affected in similar manner does not seem to have been investigated.

e) Exposure to high and low temperatures

LESSIN and PARKES (1957) reported that in mice exposed to temperatures of 32° C or more reserpine no longer caused sedation. According to GARATTINI and VALZELLI (1958) previous exposure of rats to heat (37° C) or cold (0° C) abolished the sedation as well as depression of brain 5-HT level caused by reserpine. SULSER and BRODIE (1960) and BRODIE et al. (1960) made similar observations in rats exposed to cold (+4° C). They also reported that exposure to cold failed to prevent the reserpine-induced depression of brain noradrenaline, while the action on 5-HT was prevented. This was taken to indicate that sedation was related to 5-HT rather than noradrenaline. Certain workers have failed to reproduce these experiments (WERDINIUS 1962, LAVERTY 1963, *cf.* also KNOLL and KNOLL 1961, NEČINA and KREJČI 1961). GREENGARD and QUINN (1962) observed that cold exposure prevented the sedative action of reserpine (5 mg/kg) in rats. The effect on liver diphosphopyridine nucleotide was also prevented (see Section IIEb).

f) Diet

The effect of reserpine on tryptophan-deficient rats has been studied (GAL, DREWES and BARRACLOUGH 1961). After 6 weeks on the deficient diet 5-HT in brain was 70 per cent below normal. A single dose of 5 mg/kg of reserpine caused sedation and 80 per cent mortality. After 8 days on the deficient diet the same dose of reserpine caused a persistent depletion of 5-HT. The 5-HT levels remained 75, 75, 70, and 60 per cent lower than normal in brain, spleen, blood, and small intestine, respectively. A second injection of reserpine (1—2 mg/kg) on the twenty-third day caused sedation in deficient as well as control rats. By means of a monoamine oxidase inhibitor it was demonstrated that the rate of synthesis of 5-HT was markedly inhibited in the brains of the tryptophan-deficient rats. These data are hard to reconcile with the hypothesis of BRODIE and coworkers (see BRODIE, SPECTOR and SHORE 1959) that reserpine acts by causing an increased level of free and active 5-HT.

g) Functional activity and rate of turnover

As pointed out in Section IID, the primary action of reserpine appears to be inhibition of amine uptake by the storage granules. The decrease in tissue amine levels following reserpine administration would then be due to spontaneous or functionally induced (*e.g.* by nerve activity) release from the storage granules, and the considerable differences in the rate of disappearance of amines from various tissues would reflect differences in rates of release. If no release at all took place, the tissue might mistakenly be considered to be resistant to reserpine (*cf.* Fig. 38).

The available data do not exclude the possibility that the picture outlined above is correct. As pointed out by BERTLER (1961), there seems to be a general correlation between turnover rates and rates of disappearance of amines after reserpine administration. For example, the monoamines of brain have a high turnover rate and disappear rapidly, while the catecholamines of the adrenal medulla and the 5-HT of the intestine have a slow turnover rate and disappear slowly. In the adrenal medulla the disappearance is slowed down even more if the flow of impulses through the secretory nerves is inhibited by ganglionic blockade (hexamethonium 10 mg/kg intraperitoneally to rats) (MIRKIN 1961) or disrupted by denervation or transection of the spinal cord (HOLZBAUER and VOGT 1956, KRONEBERG and SCHÜMANN 1957, CARLSSON et al. 1957, BRODIE et al. 1957a). In fact, there has been some discussion whether reserpine has any direct effect at all on the adrenal medulla, since in certain species and under certain conditions the effect on the decentralized adrenal medulla is not easy to detect. However, several workers have succeeded in clearly demonstrating such an action (KRONEBERG and SCHÜMANN 1957, 1958, 1959, 1960, MIRKIN 1958, CALLINGHAM and MANN 1958). Furthermore, the inhibitory effect of reserpine on the uptake of catecholamines by the adrenal medullary granules *in vivo* persists after transection of the spinal cord at the sixth cervical segment (rabbits) (BERTLER, HILLARP and ROSENGREN 1961). Final proof of the direct effect is provided by the effect of low concentrations of reserpine on the uptake mechanism *in vitro* (see Section II Da).

While these observations on the adrenal medulla support the view that reserpine has little or no direct action on the release of monoamines, data on other tissues present a somewhat different picture. KÄRKI, PAASONEN and VANHAKARTANO (1959) observed that ganglionic blockade by pentolonium inhibited the action of reserpine (5 mg/kg intraperitoneally) on the noradrenaline of the rat heart and intestine to a certain extent. Similar results were reported by HERTTING, POTTER and AXELROD (1962). KIRPEKAR, CERVONI and FURCHGOTT (1962), on the other hand, found that decentralization did not interfere with the action of reserpine (1 mg/kg intraperitoneally) on the noradrenaline content of the nictitating membranes or superior sympathetic ganglia of the cat. In rats WEINER, PERKINS and SIDMAN (1962) observed that postganglionic denervation slowed, but did not block the noradrenaline-depleting action of reserpine (5 mg/kg) on the nerve endings of brown adipose tissue. Spinal section (rabbits) had little effect on the ability of reserpine to deplete the heart of noradrenaline (BRODIE et al. 1957a). ROSELL and SEDVALL (1962) observed that the blockade of responsiveness of sympathetic vasoconstrictor nerves caused by reserpine was counteracted by decentralization and promoted by high-frequency stimulation.

Comparison of the adrenal medulla with the various adrenergically innervated tissues shows that although in both cases the effect of reserpine on catecholamine levels is inhibited by disruption of the flow of nerve impulses from the central nervous system, the effect on the latter tissues is comparably slight. Returning to the model outlined above this would mean that the amine release from adrenergic nerve granules, in contrast to adrenal medullary granules, occurred at a relatively high rate even in the absence of nerve activity.

In this connection it is interesting to note that the spontaneous amine release *in vitro* from adrenergic nerve granules appears to be much more rapid than from adrenal medullary granules, possibly owing to the difference in size (for references, see Section II Da).

III. Other Rauwolfia alkaloids

Several natural and semisynthetic analogs of reserpine have been studied, permitting certain conclusions on structure-activity relationships (see Fig. 1). The high structural specificity of reserpine is illustrated by the fact that *3-iso-reserpine* is about 100 times less active than reserpine (Tables 3 and 4). Removal of the methoxy group in ring A results in 11-desmethoxyreserpine or *deserpidine*, the activity of which is quantitatively and qualitatively almost indistinguishable from that of reserpine (SCHNEIDER et al. 1955). Minor alterations in the benzoic acid moiety can be made without any considerable change in activity. For example, *rescinnamine* is somewhat less potent than reserpine. Particular interest has been focussed on a number of compounds which have been reported to cause a weaker central than peripheral action. The compound most extensively studied so far is *syrosingopine*. PLUMMER et al. (1959) reported that this compound given to dogs was equipotent with reserpine as regards the hypotensive response but considerably less potent with respect to sedative effect in dogs and mice and prolongation of hexobarbital sleeping time in mice. In dogs syrosingopine was slightly less active than reserpine in increasing gastric hydrochloric acid secretion and much less active in producing diarrhea. ORLANS, FINGER and BRODIE (1960, cf. GARATTINI et al. 1959, 1960) made similar observations and found that the responsiveness of the peripheral sympathetic system, as studied by means of a ganglionic stimulant (tetramethylammonium bromide) or by electrical stimulation of the celiac ganglion, was reduced by syrosingopine (0.5 mg per kg intravenously 24 hours prior to the experiment). The same dose was found to reduce the heart noradrenaline more than the brain noradrenaline and 5-HT. No comparable data on the effect of reserpine on tissue monoamines in dogs seem to be available. In rabbits ORLANS et al. (1959) observed that

Table 3. *5-HT in rabbit brain 4 hours after the intravenous administration of various Rauwolfia alkaloids*
(From BRODIE, B. B.: Storage and release of 5-hydroxytryptamine. In: G. P. LEWIS, Ed., 5-Hydroxytryptamine, p. 64—83. London: Pergamon Press 1958.)

Alkaloid	Dose (mg/kg)	Sedative action	HT concentration (μg/g)
None	—	—	0.57
Reserpine	2	Active	0.06
Deserpidine (recanescine)	2	Active	0.09
Rescinnamine	2	Active	0.10
Methyl reserpate syringate	3	Active	0.06
Raunescine	5	Active	0.07
11-Desmethoxyreserpine	2	Active	0.15
Methyl reserpate acetoacetate	3	Slightly active	0.34
*Iso*reserpine	2	Inactive	0.48
*Iso*raunescine	5	Inactive	0.47
Methyl reserpate	2	Inactive	0.44
Reserpic acid	2	Inactive	0.52
Reserpinine	2	Inactive	0.49
Serpentine	2	Inactive	0.45
Ajmaline	2	Inactive	0.44
Ajmalicine	2	Inactive	0.55

Table 4. *Release of 5-HT from rabbit platelets incubated with various drugs for 4 hours*
(From CARLSSON, SHORE and BRODIE 1957.)

Drug	Conc. of drug μg/ml	Serotonin released per cent of total[1]
Reserpine	1—2	47, 37, 39, 36, 47, 45
Deserpidine (recanescine)	1—2	38, 37
Rescinnamine	1—2	37, 37
Raunescine	1—2	37, 41
11-Desmethoxyreserpine	2	39
Methyl reserpate syringate	2	47
Methyl reserpate acetoacetate	2	18
Methyl reserpate	2	8
Isoraunescine	1	6
Isoreserpine	1—2	0, 0
Reserpinine	2	0
Ajmaline	2	0
Reserpic acid	2	0
Chlorpromazine	20	5
Azacyclonol	20	2
Phenobarbital	20	0
Lysergic acid diethylamide	20	0
48/80	1	0

[1] Figures represent release caused solely by drug action; that is total per cent released less the small release (averaging 6 per cent) that occurred spontaneously in the control platelet suspension preparation.

reserpine and syrosingopine were about equipotent in reducing heart noradrenaline whereas syrosingopine was clearly less potent in reducing brain stem noradrenaline and 5-HT levels. In monkeys and rats (TRČKA, DLABAČ and VANEČEK (personal communication) were unable to detect any significant difference between syrosingopine and reserpine as regards the relation of sedative and hypotensive actions.

Table 5. *Potencies of reserpine-type alkaloids in relation to reserpine, as observed by various methods*

Alkaloid	LIEBMAN et al. (1962)[1]	INNES et al. (1958)[2]	MUSKUS (1962)[3]	PAASONEN and KRAYER (1959)[4]	KRONEBERG and SCHÜMANN (1957)[5]	ORLANS et al. (1960)	PAASONEN and DEWS (1958)[9]	BRODIE et al. (1960)[10]	BEIN (1956)	SCHNEIDER et al. (1955)
Reserpine . . .	1.00	1	1.00	1	1	1	1	1	1	1
Deserpidine . .	1.21	1			1					1[13] 0.71[14] 0.97[15]
Rescinamine . .	0.7	< 1			< 0.5				0.33[11] 0.25[12]	
Raunescine . .	0.44	< 1	0.23	< 1			< 1	< 0.4		
Syrosingopine .	0.27		0.25			1[6] 0.12[7] < 0.10[8]				
Isoraunescine .	0.05	< 1	0.02	0.05			< 0.1			
Dimethylamino-benzoyl-methyl reserpate (Su 5171). . .			0.12							

[1] Response of normal dog heart-lung preparation to challenging dose of reserpine-type alkaloid. Relative potency as computed from dose-response curves.

[2] Response of normal dog heart-lung preparation to challenging dose of reserpine-type alkaloid.

[3] Response of guinea-pig atria to tyramine 24 hr. after treatment.

[4] Depletion (determined by bioassay) of catecholamines of rat heart

[5] Depletion (determined by fluorimetric method) of catecholamines of rabbit adrenal medulla.

[6] Depletion (determined by fluorimetric method) of norepinephrine of rabbit heart.

[7] Depletion (determined by fluorimetric method) of norepinephrine of rabbit brain.

[8] Central effects in rabbits (elicitation of miosis and lowering of threshold of blink reflex).

[9] Behavioural changes in pigeons.

[10] Depletion (determined by fluorimetric method) of norepinephrine and 5-HT of rat brain.

[11] Depletion (method not indicated) of 5-HT from rabbit brain.

[12] Inhibition of stimulation by caffeine of CNS of mice.

[13] Tranquillization, miosis, slowing of heart rate, drop in body temperature, diarrhea, relaxation of nictitating membrane and stimulation of gastric secretion in different species (dog, cat, rabbit and monkey).

[14] Emesis in pigeon.

[15] Acute toxicity in rat.

Indirect methods, such as the response (increase in heart rate) of the heart-lung preparation to a challenging dose of reserpine, have also been employed to assess the relative potencies of various reserpine-type alkaloids. Data obtained by means of various methods are compiled in Table 5. According to data obtained by indirect methods syrosingopine is clearly less potent than reserpine in its action on the heart. Syrosingopine and reserpine have been found approximately equipotent in potentiating the vasopressor responses to phenetylamine and tyramine (Ross et al. 1963).

In man syrosingopine, given orally, has been found much less effective than reserpine as a hypotensive agent (see SHELBURNE and ORGAIN 1963). Whether this is due to poor absorption or some other cause, remains to be established.

Other compounds which have been reported to cause predominantly peripheral effects are *10-methoxy deserpidine* (PETERFALVI and JEQUIER 1960), *β-diethylaminoethyl reserpine* (BUZAS and RÉGNIER 1960), and *isobutyl serpentinate* (VAN PROOSDIJ-HERTZEMA, AKKERMAN and DE JONGH 1959, GARATTINI et al. 1961). — Species differences exist, however. SANAN and VOGT (1962) thus observed that 10-methoxy deserpidine *(methoserpidine)* in a dose of 12 mg/kg given to rabbits lowered the noradrenaline content of sympathetic ganglia but not that of brain; no sedation was observed. On the other hand, in cats doses of 0.5 to 12 mg/kg lowered the noradrenaline of ganglia and brain alike and caused sedation. In fact, a similar difference between rabbits and cats exists in the response to reserpine (see Section II Ba).

On the other hand, reserpine derivatives with predominantly central effects have been prepared. Examples are *dimethylaminobenzoyl-methyl-reserpate* (Su 5171) (BRODIE et al. 1960, GARATTINI et al. 1959, 1960), *methyl-18-epireserpate methyl ether* (Su 9064) (ROBISON et al. 1961, CUENCA et al. 1961, BARRET, RUTLEDGE and PLUMMER 1961, BARRETT et al. 1962), and *10-chlorodeserpidine* (VELLUZ, PETERFALVI and JEQUIER 1958). Su 9064 and related ethers showed an onset of action in minutes rather than hours and a short duration of action. No diarrhea was observed in dogs given sedative doses. Gastric secretion was but slightly stimulated.

The data of PAULSEN and HESS (1963) raise some doubt as to the predominantly central action of Su 9064. In guinea-pigs a dose of 5 mg/kg intraperitoneally lowered noradrenaline in heart almost completely, at least as much as noradrenaline and dopamine in brain.

As mentioned in Section II Da, the affinity of 5-HT for the storage mechanism of adrenal medullary granules is higher than that of the catecholamines. It is therefore not surprising that in general 5-HT tends to be less affected than the catecholamines by the reserpine type of drugs (see Section II B and IV). According to BRODIE et al. (1960) this is particularly true of dimethylaminobenzoyl methylreserpate (Su 5171). Small doses of the drug were found to depress the brain noradrenaline level in rabbits by 50 per cent and the 5-HT level by about 15 per cent. The animals were not sedated. Higher doses which depressed 5-HT by 50 per cent and noradrenaline still more caused sedation. This was considered to indicate that sedation was caused by release of 5-HT. KÄRKI and PAASONEN (1959) observed that *raunescine* in doses which depress noradrenaline but not 5-HT in brain has a sedative effect in rats. BRODIE et al. (1960) were unable to confirm this. They found that various sedative doses of raunescine lowered noradrenaline and 5-HT alike.

The endocrine pharmacology of several methyl reserpate derivatives has been described (GAUNT, RENZI and CHART 1962).

FURNESS and PLUMMER (1961) have described the reserpine-like action of *methyl-O-(2-tetrahydropyranyl) reserpate* (Su 7064). Its onset and duration of action are shorter than those of reserpine. The sedative action of the compound can be reversed by treatment with a MAO inhibitor.

IV. Tetrabenazine and other benzoquinolizines

In 1958 it was discovered that certain synthetic benzoquinolizine derivatives cause reserpine-like sedation and depress 5-HT and noradrenaline in brain

(PLETSCHER, BESENDORF and BÄCHTOLD 1958, PLETSCHER, BESENDORF and GEY 1959, PLETSCHER, BROSSI and GEY 1962, PLETSCHER et al. 1962, QUINN, SHORE and BRODIE 1959).

A. Chemistry and metabolism

The basic ring system is 1,2,3,4,6,7-hexahydro-11 b*H*-benzo[a]quinolizine. The formula of tetrabenazine (Ro 1-9569), *i.e.* the most extensively studied member of the group, is shown in Fig. 32. Its molecular weight is 317. Other compounds of interest are Ro 4-1284 and benzquinamide, also shown in Fig. 32.

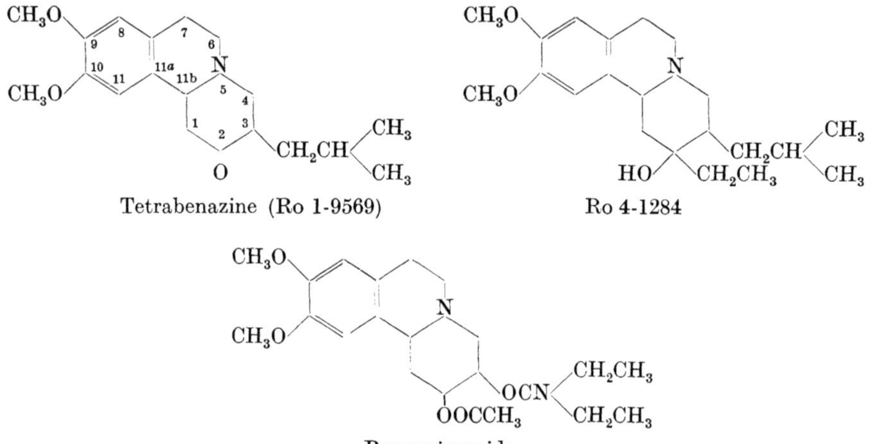

Fig. 32. Chemical constitution of some benzoquinolizines

The benzoquinolizines have a short duration of action. The half life of tetrabenazine in rodents is of the order of a few hours (QUINN, SHORE and BRODIE 1959, SCHWARTZ et al. 1960). Like reserpine, tetrabenazine has a high affinity for body fat. Most of the compound is metabolized in the body. Several metabolites have been detected, but only a few of them have been identified (PLETSCHER, BROSSI and GEY 1962). The elimination of tetrabenazine is rapid also in man (STUMPF, GRAUL and HUNDESHAGEN 1961).

B. Effects on monoamine metabolism

In *brain*, several members of the benzoquinolizine group cause a decrease in monoamine levels (Figs. 33 and 34). The decrease is not so marked as after the administration of reserpine, and larger doses are required. Maximal depression of the amines occurs more rapidly than after reserpine, and the effects last much shorter. As seen in Figs. 33 and 34, benzoquinolizines differ widely in duration and intensity of action. The structural specificity of these compounds seems to be high. For example, an isomer of Ro 4-1284, in which the ethyl and isobutyl groups have changed places, has no effect on brain 5-HT (PLETSCHER et al. 1962). The effect of benzquinamide on the brain monoamines is relatively weak. It is possibly mediated by the more active deacetylated metabolite (WEISSMAN and FINGER 1962).

Like many members of the *Rauwolfia* group the benzoquinolizines are generally less active in causing reduction of 5-HT than catecholamine levels in brain (*cf.* Figs. 33 and 34). In fact, benzquinamide in a dose of 100 mg/kg intraperitoneally to mice was found to leave 5-HT unaffected, while reducing the noradrenaline and dopamine levels to half or less (CARLSSON and LINDQVIST, unpublished observations). In rats, on the other hand, a decrease in both 5-HT and noradrenaline after benzquinamide (50 mg/kg intraperitoneally) has been reported (WEISSMAN and FINGER 1962).

In analogy with observations on reserpine, the tetrabenazine-induced depression of brain monoamines may be partially prevented by monoamine oxidase inhibitors (PLETSCHER, BESENDORF and BÄCHTOLD 1958). Whether this is true also of the benzquinamide-induced amine depletion remains to be established. Preliminary observations in this laboratory suggest that the phenomenon is less striking after benzquinamide than after reserpine.

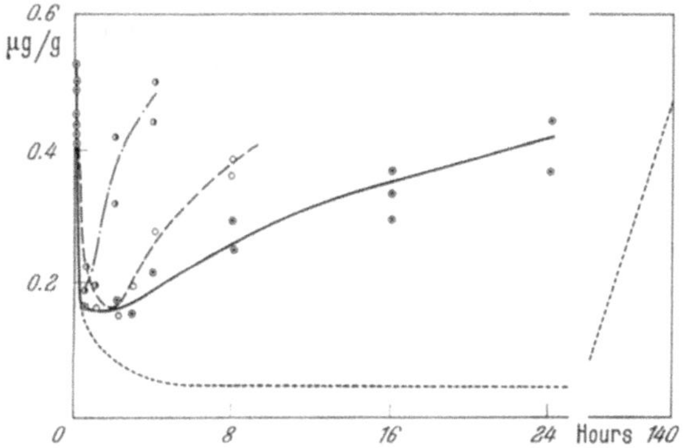

Fig. 33. Levels of 5-HT in rabbit brain after the intravenous administration of benzoquinolizines and reserpine. Ordinate: µg/g. Abscisse: time in hours. Curves: ——— tetrabenazine, 40 mg/kg; ––– Ro 1-9571, 30 mg/kg; –·–·– Ro 1-9288, 30 mg/kg; ···· reserpine, 2 mg/kg. (From PLETSCHER, BESENDORF and BÄCHTOLD 1958.)

The interaction between tetrabenazine and reserpine has been described above (Section II Ga).

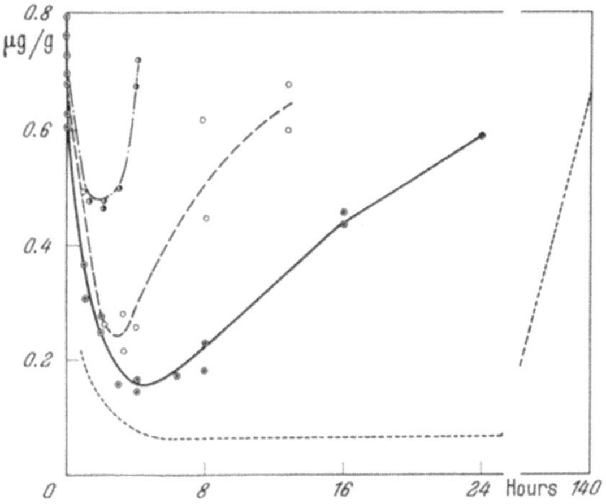

Fig. 34. Levels of noradrenaline in rabbit brain stem after the intravenous administration of benzoquinolizines and reserpine. Explanation: see text of Fig. 33. (From PLETSCHER, BESENDORF and BÄCHTOLD 1958.)

In *extracerebral tissues*, the effect of benzoquinolizines on monoamine levels is generally less pronounced than in brain. Thus, in rabbits and guinea pigs high doses of tetrabenazine do not affect the 5-HT levels of platelets and small intestine markedly. In rabbits the noradrenaline level of heart was found to be largely unaffected (QUINN, SHORE and BRODIE 1959), while a 50 per cent decrease has been observed in guinea-pigs (SCHWARTZ et al. 1960, Fig. 35). In guinea-pigs Ro 4-1284 has a weaker effect on heart noradrenaline than on brain noradrenaline and dopamine (PAULSEN and HESS 1963). In the adrenals of rabbits large doses of tetrabenazine cause a moderate decrease in catecholamines (QUINN, SHORE and BRODIE 1959, SCHWARTZ et al. 1960).

In vitro tetrabenazine, like reserpine, causes release of platelet 5-HT (6×10^{-5} M) (PAASONEN and PLETSCHER 1959) and blockade of the specific storage mechanism of adrenal medullary granules (5×10^{-6} M) (CARLSSON, HILLARP and WALDECK 1963). The reason why the effect of the benzoquinolizines on extracerebral tissues *in vivo* is so weak compared to the action on brain, is obscure. It should be noted that in extracerebral tissues the depletion of monoamines by reserpine takes place more slowly than in brain. The possibility that the short duration of action of the benzoquinolizines is a contributory factor, appears to merit consideration.

In rabbits tetrabenazine, like reserpine, causes a fairly marked increase in urinary 5-hydroxyindoleacetic acid (PLETSCHER 1957b). This suggests that a certain depletion even of the major 5-HT stores of the body takes place, *i.e.* in the enterochromaffin system, and is thus somewhat contradictory to the lack of effect on the 5-HT of the small intestine. This problem merits further investigation.

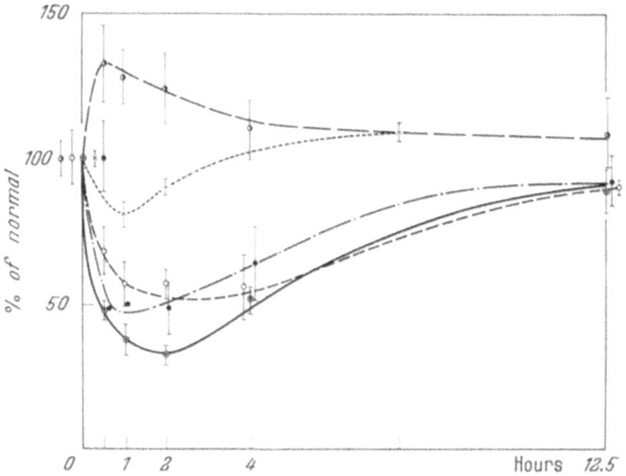

Fig. 35. Effect of tetrabenazine on tissue monoamine levels in guinea pigs and on whole-blood 5-HT in rabbits. Abscisse: hours after 20 mg/kg tetrabenazine intraperitoneally (guinea pigs) or intravenously (rabbits); ordinate: monoamine level in per cent of controls. Curves: —·—·— 5-HT in brain; —— noradrenaline in brain stem; – – – noradrenaline in heart; – – – 5-HT in small intestine; ···· 5-HT in whole blood. Mean values ± standard error of four experiments are given. (From SCHWARTZ et al. 1960.)

C. Pharmacology

Tetrabenazine and other benzoquinolizines which lower brain monoamines influence the *central nervous system* in a reserpine-like manner. Depression of spontaneous and induced locomotor activity, and of conditioned avoidance reactions are thus observed (PLETSCHER, BROSSI and GEY 1962, CAHN and HEROLD 1960, LEUSEN 1960, LEUSEN, LACROIX and DEMEESTER 1959, QUINN, SHORE and BRODIE 1959). Other central actions are the typical hunched back posture, prolongation of ethanol and barbiturate anesthesia, hypothermia, enhancement of the convulsant effect of pentylenetetrazole, and various autonomic effects, *e.g.* miosis, lacrimation, and increased responsiveness of pupils and eyelids to light (Figs. 36 and 37).

The effects of monoamine-depleting benzoquinolizines on the central nervous system is counteracted or reversed by monoamine oxidase inhibitors (Fig. 9 of Chapter 12; p. 632 PLETSCHER et al. 1958, PLETSCHER, BROSSI and GEY 1962).

In all these respects tetrabenazine and related benzoquinolizines resemble reserpine. The most important differences are lower potency and shorter duration of action.

A number of benzoquinolizines seem to cause central depression by a different mechanism. For example, the isomer of Ro 4-1284 mentioned above, which was found not to influence brain 5-HT, caused reduction of spontaneous motor activity and prolongation of ethanol anesthesia in mice. The dose required for these effects was about 50 mg/kg intraperitoneally as compared with 5 mg/kg for the monoamine-reducing isomer Ro 4-1284. Further, only the latter type of compound caused the characteristic hunch-back posture and exhibited the phenomenon of reversal by monoamine oxidase inhibitors (PLETSCHER et al. 1962). Benzquinamide seems to occupy an intermediate position. It causes decrease in brain monoamines (see above) but may produce central depression in doses which are inactive in this respect. Of particular interest is the selective disruption of conditioned avoidance behaviour by low doses of benzquinamide. This effect is only partially counteracted by monoamine oxidase inhibitors (WEISSMAN and FINGER 1962). Effective doses are 15 mg/kg intraperitoneally in rats and 1 mg/kg orally in rhesus monkeys. In both species the dose had to be raised severalfold (to 50 and 5 mg/kg, respectively) in order to produce amine depletion and reserpine-like symptoms (salivation, lacrimation, diarrhea, miosis, ptosis, and deep sedation).

The *cardiovascular system* is influenced less by tetrabenazine than by reserpine. In anesthetized dogs and cats 10—20 mg/kg intravenously are only moderately hypotensive. Similarly, the effect of tetrabenazine on the *gastro-intestinal tract* seems to be weaker than that of reserpine, although stimulation of intestinal peristalsis and gastric secretion have been observed (PLETSCHER, BROSSI and GEY 1962a).

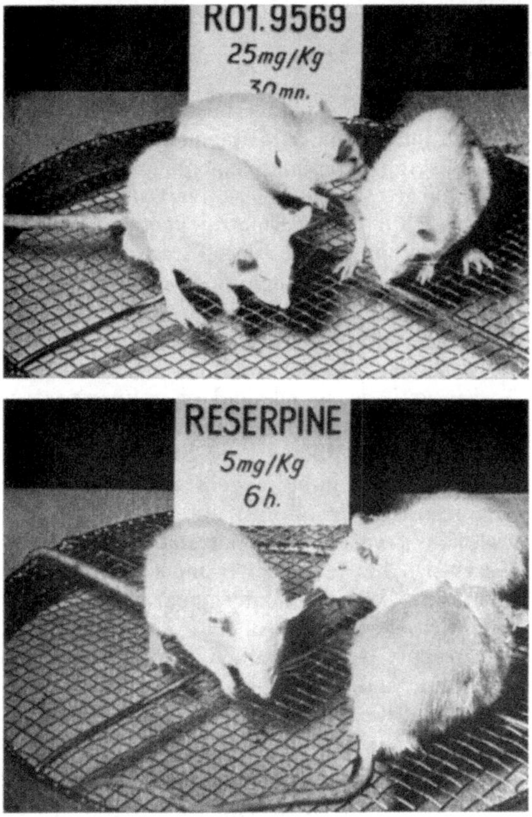

Fig. 36a and b. Mice treated with tetrabenazine (a) and reserpine (b). (From CAHN and HEROLD 1960.)

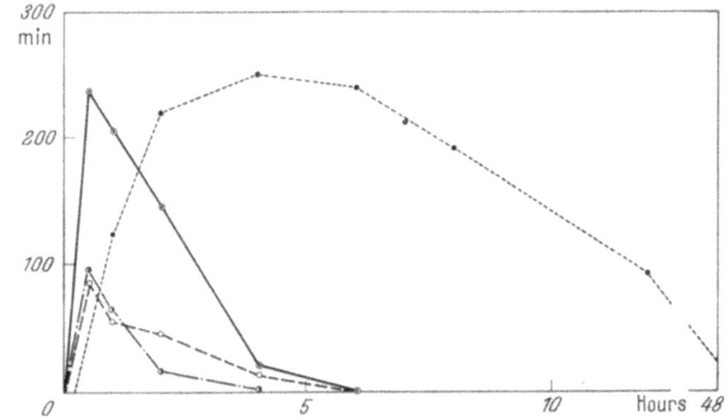

Fig. 37. Prolongation of ethanol anesthesia by benzoquinolizines and reserpine in mice. Abscisse: interval in hours between the subcutaneous injection of the compounds and the intraperitoneal injection of ethanol (4 g/kg). Ordinate: sleeping time in minutes. Curves: for explanation, see text of Fig. 33. (From PLETSCHER, BESENDORF and BÄCHTOLD 1958.)

In psychiatry tetrabenazine has proved qualitatively similar to reserpine, both with respect to therapeutic actions and side effects, although the latter are possibly less severe (for references, see PLETSCHER, BROSSI and GEY 1962a).

V. Other agents

Several agents reduce tissue levels of catecholamines by various mechanisms without influencing 5-HT levels to the same extent. This seems to be the case with several sympathomimetic agents, *e.g.* adrenaline, metaraminol, and tyramine, and amino acids which are converted into sympathomimetic agents in the body, *e.g.* α-methyl dopa, α-methyl metatyrosine, and metatyrosine. Other examples are guanethidine and related compounds (see SHORE 1962, CARLSSON 1964a). Whether 6-hydroxy-dopamine has an effect on catecholamines only or if it also reduces 5-HT levels, is not yet known (PORTER et al. 1963). Since this Chapter deals primarily with drugs which affect 5-HT storage, these agents will not be discussed here (*cf.* Section VI).

Vincamin is an alkaloid of unknown structure but probably containing an indole ring. It has been found to produce reserpine-like effects on behaviour and on amine levels (GÖRÖG and SZPORNY 1961, SZPORNY and GÖRÖG 1962).

Triethyltin has been reported to cause a decrease in noradrenaline and 5-HT levels in rat brain (MOORE and BRODY 1961). Peripheral tissues were unaffected with the exception of the adrenal medulla, in which a decrease in adrenaline was observed. This decrease was blocked by section of the spinal cord or pretreatment with a ganglionic blocking agent. After a dose of 5 mg/kg the effect on amine levels lasted several days.

A report (GURSEY and OLSON 1960) that ethanol causes a decrease in noradrenaline and 5-HT in rabbit brain could not be confirmed (HÄGGENDAL and LINDQVIST 1961).

VI. Concluding remarks on the functional significance of the effect of reserpine-like drugs on tissue monoamines

A causal relationship between the effects of reserpine on a monoamine and on functional activity has been established beyond any doubt only in the case of *adrenergic neurons*. Doses of reserpine which cause depletion of the transmitter noradrenaline also produce blockade of adrenergic transmission: stimulation of the nerves no longer results in release of transmitter or in response of the effector cells. The functional disturbance does not set in until severe depletion of the transmitter has taken place. There thus seems to be a good correlation between the degree of noradrenaline depletion and blockade of transmission. However, functional recovery sets in when the noradrenaline levels are still very low. Equally striking is the fact that the adrenergic nerves still function normally after displacement of some 97 per cent of the transmitter by analogs of much lower pharmacological activity, such as metaraminol and d-adrenaline (ANDÉN and MAGNUSSON 1963). It would thus appear that the store of transmitter is not essential for function — with the exception of a very small fraction, which perhaps should not be looked upon as a true store — and that the blockade of transmission brought about by reserpine cannot be explained merely by the reduced noradrenaline level. Some additional action which reserpine does not share with transmitter analogs such as metaraminol and d-adrenaline, must be sought. This action appears to be the blockade of the uptake mechanism in the storage granules. This effect shows a more rapid recovery than the amine levels and seems to be more closely correlated to the transmission blockade. The available data suggest that the storage granules have a dual action, a) to function as a transmitter store, and b) to make newly formed transmitter available for release by nerve activity. Only the latter function appears to be essential under normal conditions. It is directly dependent on the specific, reserpine-sensitive uptake mechanism. When this mechanism is blocked by reserpine, transmission can still take place at the expense of the store. When the store has been depleted — which is only partly a consequence of release by nerve activity, a major fraction being destroyed intracellularly by monoamine oxidase — transmitter is no longer available for release by nerve activity, and the transmission mechanism is blocked. When recovery of the uptake mechanism in the storage granules sets in, newly formed transmitter is again made available for release by nerve activity, and the transmission mechanism can recover before the store is replenished.

It may be concluded from the above that effects on the uptake mechanism of the storage granules should be recorded, if possible, whenever attempts are made to analyze the mode of action of reserpine-like drugs. Such data are likely to yield more information of functional importance than can be gained merely by following amine levels. But more accurate knowledge of dose and time relationships as regards the effect of reserpine on amine levels, particularly the low, functionally critical levels, is also desirable. From the data available it appears that newly formed amine is taken up by the storage granules and incorporated in a small labile fraction which does not seem to contain adenosine triphosphate (ATP). The exact size of this fraction is unknown. In the adrenal medullary granules some 10 to 20 per cent of the catecholamines occur in the ATP-free pool (Hillarp 1960a). Probably a much smaller fraction is sufficient for maintaining normal function. Studies of the uptake of labelled amines by adrenal medullary granules *in vitro* and *in vivo* and by adrenergically innervated tissues *in vivo* at various time intervals after reserpine administration have yielded results which are in fairly good agreement, suggesting that *in vivo* data on uptake by tissues may serve as indicator of the specific uptake by the adrenergic nerve granules. A close quantitative comparison between the uptake mechanism and the functional efficiency of the adrenal medulla as well as the adrenergic nerve endings would be desirable. The available data strongly suggest that a correlation exists.

So far it has been possible to study the functional effect of reserpine-like drugs only on *peripheral adrenergic neurons*. Recent histochemical studies show that in the central nervous system noradrenaline-containing neurons exist, with the same general appearance and intracellular distribution of noradrenaline as the peripheral adrenergic neurons. There can be little doubt that we are dealing with true *adrenergic neurons in the central nervous system*. The majority of these neurons originate in various brain stem areas and give rise to different pathways terminating *e.g.* in the hypothalamus, thalamus, cerebral cortex (particularly those parts belonging to the limbic system), cerebellum, brain stem, and spinal cord (Dahlström and Fuxe 1964, Fuxe 1964b, Carlsson et al. 1964). These neurons, like the peripheral adrenergic neurons, are deprived of their transmitter by reserpine. There is no reason to doubt that this deprivation is followed by blockade of transmission also in the central adrenergic neurons. It has been postulated that such blockade does not take place, since the sympathetic centers appear to remain active after treatment with reserpine (Brodie and Costa 1962). However, there is no reason why *adrenergic* neurons should be identified with *sympathetic* centers. Adrenergic (as well as hydroxytryptaminergic) pathways innervate the spinal sympathetic centers in the intermediolateral nucleus. The localization of the pathways and their cell bodies suggests that they are inhibitory. Disruption of such pathways should lead to an increased flow of impulses through the peripheral sympathetic pathways. This might explain some observations along this line by IGGO and VOGT (1960), as well as the nerve-dependent discharge of adrenal medullary hormones caused by reserpine.

There is thus no reason to reject the possibility that some of the central actions of reserpine are due to blockade of central adrenergic neurons. Indirect evidence in support of this possibility is provided by the fact that reintroduction of noradrenaline in brain (through administration of 3,4-dihydroxyphenylserine, or DOPS, after inhibition of monoamine oxidase) counteracts the sedative effect of reserpine. However, reintroduction of dopamine (through administration of 3,4-dihydroxyphenylalanine, or DOPA) has a similar effect. As is well known, the distribution of dopamine in brain differs from that of noradrenaline, indicating that the two catecholamines occur in different cells. Histochemical investigations in combination with chemical analyses have shown that dopamine occurs in at least three different neuronal systems within the central nervous system: a) a pathway originating in the substantia nigra (where the cell bodies are located) and ascending through the internal capsule to the caudate nucleus-putamen; the parkinsonian symptoms after reserpine treatment are probably at least partly due to blockade of transmission at these nerve endings, just as clinical cases of parkinsonism are probably due to destruction of these neurons (ANDÉN et al. 1964a, FUXE, HÖKFELT and NILSSON 1964); b) a pathway originating in the arcuate nucleus of the hypothalamus and terminating at the primary capillary plexus of the hypophyseal portal system (FUXE 1963, 1964); blockade of this pathway may explain some of the effects of reserpine on the anterior lobe of the pituitary; c) retinal neurons, which may be involved in the increased light sensitivity induced by reserpine (HÄGGENDAL and MALMFORS 1963). — Preliminary data suggest that other dopamine pathways exist.

Histochemical data show that 5-HT occurs in neurons in the central nervous system. The intracellular distribution is very similar to that of noradrenaline in noradrenergic neurons. Since electrical stimulation of the axons results in release and increased synthesis of 5-HT, there can be little doubt that we are dealing with true *hydroxytryptaminergic neurons* (ANDÉN et al. 1964b). Such neurons originate in the lower brain stem and terminate in various parts of the brain and spinal cord. They innervate, for example, the spinal sympathetic centers in the intermediolateral nucleus, where they probably have an inhibitory action (ANDÉN, CARLSSON and HILLARP 1964); this may be the site of paradoxical actions of reserpine and MAO inhibitors on blood pressure. It has been suggested that reserpine causes an increase in free and active 5-HT in the brain and that 5-HT has an excitatory influence on the parasympathetic system, which would explain the stimulant action of reserpine on this system (BOGDANSKI, SULSER and BRODIE 1961). Since reserpine appears to have the same fundamental action on catecholamines and 5-HT, *i.e.* blockade of the storage mechanism, it seems likely, however, that the drug affects the different transmitter mechanisms in the same direction. Reserpine causes blockade of adrenergic transmission, and it is thus reasonable to assume that it has a similar action, if any, on hydroxytryptaminergic transmission. The stimulation of the parasympathetic system by reserpine may be explained by disruption of inhibitory hydroxytryptaminergic and/or noradrenergic transmission in parasympathetic nuclei of the brain stem and the spinal cord (DAHLSTRÖM et al. 1964 and FUXE, unpublished data). However, adrenergic nerve endings have been observed also in certain parasympathetic ganglia. The possibility that reserpine causes an increase in parasympathetic tone by blocking an inhibitory adrenergic mechanism in parasympathetic ganglia, therefore cannot be excluded. In fact, data indicating an action of reserpine on parasympathetic ganglia have been reported (PLUMMER, BARRETT and RUTLEDGE 1955, BARRETT et al. 1955). In addition, the possible disruption of inhibitory transmission mechanisms in supramedullar centers has to be taken into account.

For several reasons great caution should be exercised in attempts to *correlate behaviour directly with tissue amine levels*. The monoamines occur in neurons belonging to many different functional systems which show marked differences in the sensitivity of reserpine. This is true, for example, of the noradrenergic nerve endings in different areas of the hypothalamus (CARLSSON, FALCK and HILLARP 1962, see Table 1). It seems reasonable to assume that a considerable part of the monoamines belongs to functional systems of the brain which are not directly involved in behavioural mechanisms. The fact that storage granules contain different pools further complicates the picture. In fact, experiments in this laboratory show that no direct correlation exists between the amine levels in brain and the central action of reserpine. In rabbits the sedation caused by a single intravenous dose of reserpine (0.2 mg/kg) is stronger after 4 than 24 hours, but the amine levels are lower at the later interval (HÄGGENDAL and LINDQVIST 1963, 1964). Repeated daily injections of this dose cause severe depletion of the amines but — after a month's treatment — only transient sedation lasting some 12 hours after each injection. A close examination revealed, however, that in these chronically treated animals with low amine levels a fairly close correlation between amine levels in brain and central actions of reserpine seems to exist. For example, the amine levels were found to be significantly lower at the time of maximum sedation, about 6 hours, than at longer intervals, *e.g.* 24 hours after the last injection. It appears that this chronic treatment has disclosed a small labile, functionally essential amine fraction. The phenomenon certainly merits further analysis and should be studied also with histochemical technique. Another line of investigation that may throw light on the functional significance of the brain monoamines, will be to study the uptake mechanism of the storage granules, in analogy with the work already started on peripheral adrenergic neurons. Here labelled precursors (DOPA and 5-hydroxytryptophan) may prove useful. It seems reasonable to suggest that the mobile fraction disclosed in the experiments of HÄGGENDAL and LINDQVIST, is identical with the fraction into which labelled monoamines are primarily incorporated.

The DOPA analog α-methyl metatyrosine (α-MMT) has been claimed to permit *functional differentiation between the different monoamines in brain* (GESSA et al. 1962, COSTA and BRODIE 1962). Thus α-MMT has been found to cause nearly complete depletion of brain noradrenaline while leaving the 5-HT unaffected; no sedation was observed. Subsequent injection of reserpine caused depletion of 5-HT and sedation. It was concluded that sedation was due to depletion of 5-HT rather than noradrenaline. It was not taken into account, however, that α-MMT causes depletion of noradrenaline also in peripheral adrenergic neurons *without impairing transmission*. There is no reason for believing that central adrenergic neurons should behave differently. Furthermore, other workers have observed that the sedative action of reserpine is partially counteracted by pretreatment with α-MMT (NEČINA 1962, CARLSSON and LINDQVIST, unpublished observations; see Section II Gc).

Attempts to differentiate between the functions of the different brain monoamines have also been made by utilizing the somewhat stronger effect of many reserpine-like drugs on the catecholamines than on 5-HT. It has thus been stated that low doses of such drugs do not cause sedation when noradrenaline has decreased to 50 per cent and 5-HT is almost unaffected. Higher doses which cause a 50 per cent decrease in 5-HT and a more pronounced decrease in noradrenaline caused sedation. This has been taken as evidence that sedation is caused by 5-HT rather than noradrenaline depletion. Alternatively, one might interpret the data to mean that sedation is correlated to a more than 50 per cent decrease in noradrenaline. Only with the advent of a reserpine-like drug with clearcut selectivity in its action on the different monoamines will such differentiation prove fruitful. No such drug is available as yet.

The discovery of a group of *benzoquinolizines* with reserpine-like effects on both brain monoamines and behaviour has strengthened the view that a causal relationship exists between the two effects. This is further supported by the fact that also the biochemical and central depressant effects of the benzoquinolizine group can be counteracted by pretreatment with monoamine oxidase inhibitors. Of great interest is also the observation that the effects of reserpine can be prevented by pretreatment with a benzoquinolizine, indicating that the two types of drugs compete for the same receptors. The chief differences between the two groups of drugs appear to be a) that the benzoquinolizines have a lower affinity for the receptors, which requires higher dosage and results in shorter duration of action, and b) that the activity of the benzoquinolizines is more selectively located in the *central* nervous system.

The observations on benzoquinolizines, like the reserpine data discussed earlier, clearly show that there is no direct correlation between monoamine levels in brain and behaviour. Particularly striking is the fact that the central effects of *e.g.* tetrabenazine set in almost immediately following intravenous injection (QUINN et al. 1959). Data on monoamine levels in brain during this initial stage do not seem available, but a close parallelism between these and the onset of central depression does not seem probable. This might suggest that the pharmacological actions of tetrabenazine are partly unrelated to its effect on monoamine metabolism. To a certain extent this possibility is supported by the fact that certain benzoquinolizines cause central depression without reducing monoamine levels. However, in view of the existence of different monoamine pools a direct causal relationship is by no means excluded.

To summarize the functional significance of the effects of reserpine and reserpine-like drugs on brain monoamines, the fundamental action probably consists in disruption of their neurotransmitter functions. These neurotransmitters occur in neurons belonging to widely different functional systems and operating at various levels of integration. From our present knowledge of these systems it is understandable that reserpine can exert such a great variety of central actions as, for example, on light sensitivity, parasympathetic and adrenal impulse flow, hypothalamic control of the pituitary, spinal and supraspinal ("extrapyramidal") control of the motoneurons, conditioned reactions, alertness, and emotional activity. However, although in some cases suggestive evidence exists, it is hardly possible as yet to define with certainty the role of the different transmitters and pathways for any particular action of reserpine.

There seems hardly to exist a sufficient basis for attempting to analyze the functional significance of the effect of reserpine-like drugs on *monoamine stores in cells of non-neuronal origin, e.g.* the 5-HT of platelets and entero-chromaffin cells. For a critical discussion of these problems, the reader is referred to ERSPAMER (1961). Suffice it here to state that depletion of platelet 5-HT in man or animals by reserpine has not resulted in any disturbance in blood coagulation or hemostasis (SHORE, PLETSCHER and BRODIE 1956, SHORE et al. 1956, WEINER and UDENFRIEND 1957, HUTCHISON, STARK and CHAPMAN 1959), and that it has not yet been possible to demonstrate effects of reserpine on the gastrointestinal tract, which are clearly referable to depletion of the 5-HT of entero-chromaffin cells. These cells seem to be fairly resistant to reserpine-like drugs; blockade of adrenergic mechanisms and stimulation of the parasympathetic system are therefore likely to dominate the picture after low doses of these drugs.

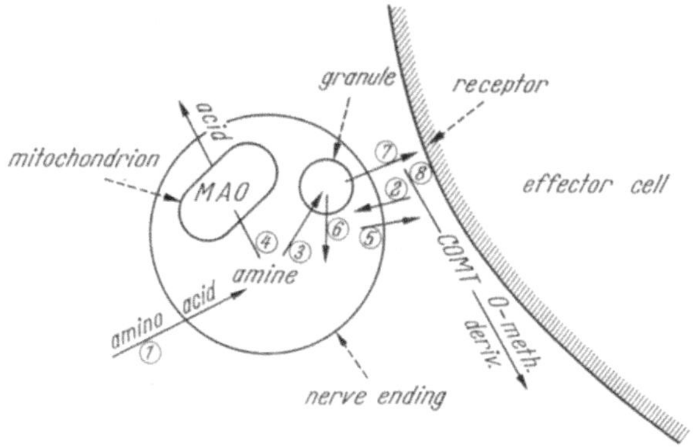

Treatment \ Arrow no.	①	②	③	④	⑤	⑥	⑦	⑧	gran.
None	N	N	N	N	N	N	N	N	
Reserpine, early stage	N	N	MR*	I	I	N?	N	I?	
Reserpine, full effect	N	MR	MR*	N	N	MR	MR	MR	
Reserpine, early recovery	N	N	N	N	N	MR	N	N	
MAO inhibitor	N	N	I	MR*	I	N?	N	I?	
MAO inhibitor + Reserpine	N	N	R*	MR*	MI	N?	N	I	

Fig. 38. Hypothetical model of monoaminergic transmission unit illustrating the effect of reserpine. Explanation: (1) The normal supply of transmitter is derived from a precursor amino acid (tryptophan or tyrosine) which is hydroxylated on the ring and decarboxylated, in the nerve ending. (2) Some of the transmitter present in the extracellular space may be taken up and re-utilized by the nerve ending. From the cytoplasmic sap the amine may (3) enter the granules, where it is incorporated primarily in a labile fraction, (4) enter the mitochondria, where it may undergo oxidative deamination by monoamine oxidase (MAO); it will finally leave the cell as an acid metabolite; some MAO may also occur in the cytoplasm outside the mitochondria; (5) enter the extracellular space (probably a minor process normally). The amine of the granules may occur in a labile (circles) and a stable form (dots). Quantitatively, the latter dominates under normal conditions. In adrenergic and noradrenergic transmission units the hydroxylation of dopamine also takes place in the granules. (6) From the granules amine may leak out in the cytoplasm; this process seems to be of minor importance in the adrenal medulla. (7) The release by nerve activity seems to occur through an action on the granules; the function of the granules is not simply that of a store replacing cytoplasmic amine released into the extracellular space by the nerve impulse, because transmission depends on the efficiency of the granules to incorporate amines and may proceed even in the virtual absence of stored transmitter. (8) After release into the extracellular space amine (in the case of catecholamines only) becomes available for catechol-O-methyl transferase (COMT). — Besides interfering with the monoamine metabolism directly, drugs may influence the impulse flow and metabolism of the neurons through actions on other neurons. Below the impulse flow of the neuron under consideration is assumed to remain normal.

Early stage of reserpine action

The primary action of reserpine is to block the incorporation of cytoplasmic amine into the labile granule fraction (3). As a consequence, amine accumulates in the cytoplasm, leading to increased oxidative deamination (4) and increased leakage into the extracellular space (5). Under certain conditions this leakage may be of sufficient magnitude to cause activation of receptors with hypertension, tachycardia etc. (see Section II C). During the early stage of reserpine action transmitter is still present in the granules and thus available for release by nerve activity (7).

Fully developed reserpine action

The granules are now empty, and newly formed amine cannot be taken up by the granules. Consequently amine is no more available for release by the nerve impulse (7), and transmission is blocked. As a consequence, less catecholamine is available for O-methylation by COMT (8).

Early recovery from the action of reserpine

When the incorporation of cytoplasmic amine into the labile granule fraction (3) recovers, transmission is restored, even though the amine store, particularly the stable fraction, remains almost fully depleted for some time. Sensitization according to the law of denervation may contribute to the recovery of transmission in the early stage. Transmission may therefore function normally before the nerve-induced release (and O-methylation) has become fully normalized.

Effect of MAO inhibition

Amine accumulates in the cytoplasm and granules. If a high degree of MAO inhibition persists after the storage capacity of the granules has been maximally utilized, leakage into the extracellular space (5) becomes sufficiently high to activate receptors and to cause excessive O-methylation, but this ultimate stage of MAO inhibition need not be reached in order to produce the interference with reserpine described below.

Effect of reserpine after MAO inhibition

Inhibition of the incorporation into the labile granule fraction, preceded by MAO inhibition, leads to excessive amine accumulation in the cytoplasm and leakage into the extracellular space with activation of amine receptors. At the same time the combination of reserpine with active sites of the storage mechanism is partially inhibited through the competitive action of cytoplasmic amine. Full depletion of the stores is thus prevented.

N = Normal; *I* = Increased; *MI* = Much increased; *R* = Reduced; *MR* = Much Reduced;
* Primary site of action of reserpine or *MAO* inhibitor.

Fig. 38 shows a hypothetical model of a monoaminergic transmission unit with an attempt to illustrate how the reserpine type of agents interfere with the various processes going on in this unit. The Figure with the accompanying description is presented as a working hypothesis, subject to modification as new data become available.

References[1]

Abboud, F. M., and J. W. Eckstein: Effects of small oral doses of reserpine on vascular responses to tyramine and norepinephrine in man. Circulation **29**, 219—223 (1964).

Abood, L. G., and K. L. Romanchek: The chemical constitution and biochemical effects of psychotherapeutic and structurally related agents. Ann. N.Y. Acad. Sci. **66**, 812—825 (1957).

Ahlbaum, H. G., and L. J. Milch: The effect of central nervous system drugs on the incorporation of radioactive carbon into brain adenosine triphosphate (ATP). Ann. N.Y. Acad. Sci. **96**, 190—198 (1962).

Andén, N.-E., A. Carlsson, A. Dahlström, K. Fuxe, N.-Å. Hillarp, and K. Larsson: Demonstration and mapping out of nigro-neostriatal dopamine neurons. Life Sci. **3**, 523—530 (1964a).

— — and N.-Å. Hillarp: Inhibition by 5-hydroxytryptophan of insulininduced adrenaline depletion. Acta pharmacol. (Kbh.) **21**, 183—186 (1964).

— — — and T. Magnusson: 5-Hydroxytryptamine release by nerve stimulation of the spinal cord. Life Sci. **3**, 473—478 (1964b).

— — and B. Waldeck: Reserpine-resistent uptake mechanisms of noradrenaline in tissues. Life Sci. **2**, 889—894 (1963).

— and T. Magnusson: Functional effect of noradrenaline depletion by α-methyl meta-tyrosine, metaraminol and d-adrenaline. Paper read at Second Internat. Pharmacological Meeting, August 20—23, 1963, Prague, Czeckoslovakia.

— — and B. Waldeck: Correlation between noradrenaline uptake and adrenergic nerve function after reserpine treatment. Life Sci. **3**, 19—25 (1964).

— B.-E. Roos, and B. Werdinius: 3,4-Dihydroxyphenylacetic acid in rabbit corpus striatum normally and after reserpine treatment. Life Sci. **2**, 319—325 (1963).

— — — Effects of chlorpromazine, haloperidol and reserpine on the levels of phenolic acids in rabbit corpus striatum. Life Sci. **3**, 149—158 (1964).

Ashcroft, G. W., and D. F. Sharman: Drug-induced changes in the concentration of 5-OR indolyl compounds in cerebrospinal fluid and caudate nucleus. Brit. J. Pharmacol. **19**, 153—160 (1962).

Axelrod, J., G. Hertting, and R. W. Patrick: Inhibition of H^3-norepinephrine release by monoamine oxidase inhibitors. J. Pharmacol. exp. Ther. **134**, 325—328 (1961).

Balzer, H., P. Holtz u. D. Palm: Reserpin und γ-Aminobuttersäuregehalt des Gehirns. Experientia (Basel) **17**, 38—40 (1961a).

— — — Reserpin und Glykogengehalt der Organe. Experientia (Basel) **17**, 304—305 (1961b).

—, u. D. Palm: Über den Mechanismus der Wirkung des Reserpins auf den Glykogengehalt der Organe. Naunyn-Schmiedebergs Arch. exp. Path. Pharmak. **243**, 65—84 (1962).

Barbeau, A., T. L. Sourkes et G. F. Murphy: Les catécholamines dans la maladie de Parkinson. In: J. de Ajuriaguerra, Ed., Monoamines et système nerveux central. Symposium Bel-Air, Geneva 1961, p. 247—262. Geneva: Georg & Co. 1962.

Barrett, W. E., A. J. Plummer, A. E. Earl, and B. Rogie: Effect of reserpine on gastric secretion of the dog. J. Pharmacol. exp. Ther. **113**, 3 (1955).

— — R. A. Rutledge, and R. Weiss: A pharmacological investigation of an ether of methyl epireserpate. J. Pharmacol. exp. Ther. **138**, 78—81 (1962).

— R. Rutledge, and A. J. Plummer: Pharmacology of SU-2064, an ether of methyl epireserpate. Fed. Proc. **20** (Part 1), 393 (1961).

Bartlet, A. L.: The 5-hydroxytryptamine content of mouse brain and whole mice after treatment with some drugs affecting the central nervous system. Brit. J. Pharmacol. **15**, 140—146 (1960).

Beck, L., L. Y. Falcon, and E. F. Domino: Hemodynamic responses to reserpine in unanesthetized dogs immobilized with neuromuscular blocking agents. J. Pharmacol. exp. Ther. **119**, 133 (1957).

[1] When the number of authors is more than three, the first author's name followed by "et al." is given in the text.

BEIN, H. J.: Zur Pharmakologie des Reserpin, eines neuen Alkaloids, aus *Rauwolfia Serpentina* BENTH. Experientia (Basel) **9**, 107—110 (1953).
— Significance of selected central mechanisms for the analysis of the action of reserpine. Ann. N.Y. Acad. Sci. **61**, Art. 1, 4—16 (1955).
— The pharmacology of Rauwolfia. Pharmacol. Rev. **8**, 435—483 (1956).
— Effects of reserpine on the functional strata of the nervous system. In: S. GARATTINI and V. GHETTI, Eds., Psychotropic Drugs, p. 325—331. Amsterdam: Elsevier Publ. Co. 1957.
BELFORD, J., and M. R. FEINLEIB: Phosphorylase activity in heart and brain after reserpine, iproniazid and other drugs affecting the central nervous system. Biochem. Pharmacol. **6**, 189—194 (1961).
BENDITT, E. P., and R. L. WONG: Concentration of 5-hydroxytryptamine in mammalian enterochromaffin cells and its release by reserpine. J. exp. Med. **105**, 509—520 (1957).
BENSON, G. K.: Effect of reserpine on mammary gland involution, and on other organs in the rat. Proc. Soc. exp. Biol. (N.Y.) **99**, 550—553 (1958).
— Effects of tranquilizing drugs on mammary involution in the rat. Proc. Soc. exp. Biol. (N.Y.) **103**, 132—137 (1960).
BERTACCINI, G. (1960): Quoted from ERSPAMER 1961.
BERTLER, Å.: Effect of reserpine on the storage of catecholamines in brain and other tissues. Acta physiol. scand. **51**, 75—83 (1961).
— A. CARLSSON, M. LINDQVIST, and T. MAGNUSSON: On the catechol amine levels in blood plasma after stimulation of the sympatho-adrenal system. Experientia (Basel) **14**, 184 (1958).
— —, and E. ROSENGREN: Release by reserpine of catecholamines from rabbits' hearts. Naturwissenschaften **22**, 521 (1956).
— B. FALCK, and CHR. OWMAN: Cellular localization of 5-hydroxytryptamine in the rat pineal gland. Kgl. Fysiogr. Sällsk. Lund Förh. **33**, No 2, 13—16 (1963).
— N.-Å. HILLARP, and E. ROSENGREN: Storage of new-formed catecholamines in the adrenal medulla. Experientia (Basel) **16**, 419 (1960a).
— — — "Bound" and "free" catecholamines in the brain. Acta physiol. scand. **50**, 113—118 (1960b).
— — — Effect of reserpine on the storage of new-formed catecholamines in the adrenal medulla. Acta physiol. scand. **52**, 44—48 (1961).
BESENDORF, H., u. A. PLETSCHER: Beeinflussung zentraler Wirkungen von Reserpin und 5-Hydroxytryptamin durch Isonicotinsäurehydrazide. Helv. physiol. pharmacol. Acta **14**, 383—390 (1956).
BHARGAVA, K. P., and H. L. BORISON: Effects of Rauwolfia alkaloids on hypothalamic, medullary and spinal vasoregulatory systems. J. Pharmacol. exp. Ther. **115**, 464—479 (1955).
BHATTACHARYA, B. K., and G. P. LEWIS: The effects of reserpine and compound 48/80 or the release of amines from the mast cells of rats. Brit. J. Pharmacol. **11**, 411—416 (1956).
BICKEL, M. H., A. CARPI, and D. BOVET: Action of reserpine and monoamine oxidase inhibitors on the urinary excretion of catecholamines in the rat. Helv. physiol. pharmacol. Acta **19**, 279—284 (1961).
BIRKMAYER, W., u. O. HORNYKIEWICZ: Der L-Dioxyphenylalanin (= L-DOPA)-Effekt beim Parkinson-Syndrom des Menschen: Zur Pathogenese und Behandlung der Parkinson-Akinese. Arch. Psychiat. Nervenkr. **203**, 560—574 (1962).
BLASCHKO, H., and T. L. CHRUŚCIEL: The decarboxylation of amino acids related to tyrosine and their awakening action in mice. J. Physiol. (Lond.) **151**, 272—284 (1960).
BOGDANSKI, D. F., F. SULSER, and B. B. BRODIE: Comparative action of reserpine, tetrabenazine and chlorpromazine on central parasympathetic activity: effects on pupillary size and lacrimation in rabbit and salivation in dogs. J. Pharmacol. exp. Ther. **132**, 176—182 (1961).
BORN, G. V. R., G. I. C. INGRAM, and R. S. STACEY: The relationship between 5-hydroxy-tryptamine and adenosine triphosphate in blood platelets. Brit. J. Pharmacol. **13**, 62—64 (1958).
BRODIE, B. B., and F. BOGDANSKI: Drug action and brain monoamines in lower vertebrates. Internat. symposium on problems of the brain. Held in Galesburg, Illinois, March 1 to 3, 1963; to be published in Progress in Brain Research.
—, and E. COSTA: Some current views on brain monoamines. In: J. DE AJURIAGUERRA, Ed., Monoamines et système nerveux central. Symposium Bel-Air, Geneva 1961, p. 13—49. Geneva: Georg & Co. 1962.
— K. F. FINGER, F. B. ORLANS, G. P. QUINN, and F. SULSER: Evidence that tranquilizing action of reserpine is associated with change in brain serotonin and not in brain norepinephrine. J. Pharmacol. exp. Ther. **129**, 250—256 (1960).
— J. S. OLIN, R. KUNTZMAN, and P. A. SHORE: Possible interrelationship between release of brain norepinephrine and serotonin by reserpine. Science **125**, 1293—1294 (1957a).

BRODIE, B. B., A. PLETSCHER, and P. A. SHORE: Possible role of serotonin in brain function. J. Pharmacol. exp. Ther. **116**, 9 (1956).
— S. SPECTOR, and P. A. SHORE: Interaction of drugs with norepinephrine in the brain. Pharmacol. Rev. **11**, 548—564 (1959).
— E. G. TOMICH, R. KUNTZMAN, and P. A. SHORE: On the mechanism of action of reserpine: effect of reserpine on capacity of tissues to bind serotonin. J. Pharmacol. exp. Ther. **119**, 461—467 (1957b).
BRUNE, G., G. R. PSCHEIDT, and H. E. HIMWICH: Different responses of urinary tryptamine and of total catecholamines during treatment with reserpine and isocarboxazid in schizophrenic patients. Intern. J. Neuropharmacol. **2**, 17—24 (1963).
BÜLBRING, E., and A. CREMA: The action of 5-hydroxytryptamine, 5-hydroxytryptophan and reserpine on intestinal peristalsis in anaesthetized guinea-pigs. J. Physiol. (Lond.) **146**, 29—53 (1959).
BURACK, W. R., N. WEINER, and P. B. HAGEN: The effect of reserpine on the catecholamine and adenine nucleotide contents of adrenal gland. J. Pharmacol. exp. Ther. **130**, 245—250 (1960).
BURN, J. H., and M. J. RAND: Reserpine and noradrenaline in artery walls. Lancet **1957 II**, 1097.
— — The action of sympathomimetic amines in animals treated with reserpine. J. Physiol. (Lond.) **144**, 314—336 (1958).
— — The effect of precursors of noradrenaline on the response to tyramine and sympathetic stimulation. Brit. J. Pharmacol. **15**, 47—55 (1960).
— — A new interpretation of the adrenergic nerve fiber. In: S. GARATTINI and P. A. SHORE, Eds. Advanc. Pharmacol. **1**, 2—30 (1962).
BURTON, R. M., N. O. KAPLAN, A. GOLDIN, M. LEITENBERG, S. R. HUMPHREYS, and M. A. SODD: Effect of reserpine and promazine on diphosphopyridine nucleotide synthesis in liver. Science **127**, 30—32 (1958).
BUZAS, A., et G. RÉGNIER: Aminoalcoyl-l réserpines. C. R. Acad. Sci. (Paris) **250**, 1340—1342 (1960).
CAHN, J., et M. HEROLD: Étude pharmacologique du Ro 1-9569 (Tétrabenazine). Psychiat. Neurol. (Basel) **140**, 210—215 (1960).
CALLINGHAM, B. A., and R. CASS: The effects of bretylium and cocaine on noradrenaline depletion. J. Pharm. Pharmacol. **14**, 385—389 (1962).
—, and M. MANN: Replacement of adrenaline and noradrenaline in the innervated and denervated adrenal gland, following depletion with reserpine. Nature (Lond.) **182**, 1020—1021 (1958).
— — Depletion and replacement of the adrenaline and noradrenaline contents of the rat adrenal gland, following treatment with reserpine. Brit. J. Pharmacol. **18**, 138—149 (1962).
CARLSSON, A.: Discussion remark in: J. R. VANE, G. E. W. WOLSTENHOLME, and M. O'CONNOR, Eds., Ciba Symposium on Adrenergic Mechanisms, p. 558. London: J. & A. Churchill 1960.
— Functional significance of drug-induced changes in brain monoamine levels. Symposium on "Binding Sites of Brain Biogenic Amines", held at Galesburg, Illinois, March 1963; Progress in Brain Research **8**, 9—27 (1964a).
— Evidence for a role of dopamine in extrapyramidal functions. Acta neuroveg. (Wien) **26**, 484—493 (1964b).
— E. BOJE RASMUSSEN, and P. KRISTJANSEN: The urinary excretion of adrenaline and noradrenaline by schizophrenic patients during reserpine treatment. J. Neurochem. **4**, 318—320 (1959).
— H. CORRODI u. B. WALDECK: α-Substituierte Dopacetamide als Hemmer der Catechol-O-methyl-transferase und der enzymatischen Hydroxylierung aromatischer Aminosäuren. In den Catecholaminmetabolismus eingreifende Substanzen. 2. Mitt. Helv. chim. Acta **46**, 2271—2285 (1963).
— B. FALCK, K. FUXE, and N.-Å. HILLARP: Cellular localization of monoamines in the spinal cord. Acta physiol. scand. **60**, 112—119 (1964).
— —, and N.-Å. HILLARP: Cellular localization of brain monoamines. Acta physiol. scand. **56** (Suppl. 196), 1—27 (1962).
—, and N.-Å. HILLARP: Release of adrenaline from the adrenal medulla of rabbits produced by reserpine. Kgl. Fysiogr. Sällsk. Lund Förh. **26**, No 8 (1956a).
— — Release of adenosine triphosphate along with adrenaline and noradrenaline following stimulation of the adrenal medulla. Acta physiol. scand. **37**, 235—239 (1956b).
— — On the state of the catechol amines of the adrenal medullary granules. Acta physiol. scand. **44**, 163—169 (1958).

CARLSSON, A., and N,-Å, HILLARP: Formation of phenolic acids in brain after administration of 3,4-dihydroxyphenylalanine. Acta physiol. scand. **55**, 95—100 (1962).

— —, and B. HÖKFELT: The concomitant release of adenosine triphosphate and catechol amines from the adrenal medulla. J. biol. Chem. **227**, 243—252 (1957).

— —, and B. WALDECK: A Mg^{++}-ATP-dependent storage mechanism in the amine granules of the adrenal medulla. Med. exp. (Basel) **6**, 47—53 (1962).

— — — Analysis of the Mg^{++}-ATP dependent storage mechanism in the amine granules of the adrenal medulla. Acta physiol. scand. **59** (Suppl. 215), 1—38 (1963).

— J. JONASSON, and E. ROSENGREN: Time correlation between the effects of reserpine on behaviour and storage mechanism for arylalkylamines. Acta physiol. scand. **59**, 474—477 (1963).

—, and M. LINDQVIST: In-vivo decarboxylation of α-methyl DOPA and α-methyl metatyrosine. Acta physiol. scand. **54**, 87—94 (1962).

— — Effect of chlorpromazine and haloperidol on the formation of 3-methoxytyramine and normetanephrine in mouse brain. Acta pharmacol. (Kbh.) **20**, 140—144 (1963).

— —, and T. MAGNUSSON: 3,4-Dihydroxyphenylalanine and 5-hydroxytryptophan as reserpine antagonists. Nature (Lond.) **180**, 1200 (1957).

— — — On the biochemistry and possible functions of dopamine and noradrenaline in brain. In: J. R. VANE, G. E. W. WOLSTENHOLME and M. O'CONNOR, Eds. Ciba Symposium on Adrenergic Mechanisms, p. 434—439. London: J. & A. Churchill 1960.

— — —, and B. WALDECK: On the presence of 3-hydroxytyramine in brain. Science **127**, 471 (1958).

— E. ROSENGREN, Å. BERTLER, and J. NILSSON: Effect of reserpine on the metabolism of catecholamines. In: S. GARATTINI and V. GHETTI, Eds., Psychotropic drugs, p. 363—372. Amsterdam: Elsevier Publ. Co. 1957.

— P. A. SHORE, and B. B. BRODIE: Release of serotonin from blood platelets by reserpine *in vitro*. J. Pharmacol exp. Ther. **120**, 334—339 (1957).

CASS, R., P. B. MARSHALL, and J. F. RILEY: 5-Hydroxytryptamine and histamine in mast cells of the mouse and rat. J. Physiol. (Lond.) **141**, 510—519 (1958).

CASTIAU, J., et J. J. REUSE: Contribution à l'étude de la sécrétion gastrique postréserpinique. Arch. int. Pharmacodyn. **135**, 489—491 (1962).

CHIDSEY, C. A., E. BRAUNWALD, A. G. MORROW, and D. T. MASON: Myocardial norepinephrine concentration in man. Effects of reserpine and of congestive heart failure. New Engl. J. Med. **269**, 653—658 (1963).

CHILD, J. J., P. SUTHERLAND, and E. G. TOMICH: Some effects of reserpine on barbitone anesthesia in mice. Biochem. Pharmacol. **6**, 252—256 (1961).

COSTA, E.: The neurochemical transducer concept-units in nervous system that synthesize, store and release monoamines in receptor sites. Symposium on "Binding Sites of Brain Biogenic Amines", held at Galesburg, Illinois, March 1963; Progress in Brain Research **8**, 168—185 (1964).

— G. L. GESSA, and B. B. BRODIE: Influence of hypothermia on chlorpromazine induced changes in brain amine levels. Life Sci. No 7, 315—319 (1962).

— A. M. REVZIN, R. KUNTZMAN, S. SPECTOR, and B. B. BRODIE: Role for ganglionic norepinephrine in sympathetic synaptic transmission. Science **133**, 1822—1823 (1961).

COTTEN, M. DE V., and N. C. MORAN: Cardiovascular pharmacology. Ann. Rev. Pharmacol. **1**, 261—286 (1961).

CROUT, J. R., A. J. MUSKUS, and U. TRENDELENBURG: Effect of tyramine on isolated guineapig atria in relation to their noradrenaline stores. Brit. J. Pharmacol. **18**, 600—611 (1962).

CUENCA, E., E. COSTA, R. KUNTZMAN, and B. B. BRODIE: The methyl ether of methyl reserpate; a prototype of reversible short-acting tranquilizing agents. Med. exp. (Basel) **5**, 20—24 (1961).

DAHL, E., B. FALCK, M. LINDQVIST, and C. v. MECKLENBURG: Monoamines in mollusc neurons. Kgl. fysiogr. Sällsk. Lund Förh. **32**, No 8, 89—91 (1962).

DAHLSTRÖM, A., and K. FUXE: Existence of monoamine-containing neurons in the central nervous system. I. Demonstration of monoamines in the cell bodies of brain stem neurons. Acta physiol. scand. **62**, Suppl. 232, 1—55 (1964).

— — N.-Å. HILLARP, and T. MALMFORS: Adrenergic mechanisms in the pupillary lightreflex path. Acta physiol. scand. **62**, 119—124 (1964).

DASGUPTA, S. R., and T. J. HALEY: Intraventricular administration of reserpine and its metabolites to conscious cats. Brit. J. Pharmacol. **12**, 529—531 (1957).

DEGKWITZ, R., R. FROWEIN, C. KULENKAMPFF u. U. MOHS: Über die Wirkungen des L-dopa beim Menschen und deren Beeinflussung durch Reserpin, Chlorpromazin, Iproniazid und Vitamin B_6. Klin. Wschr. **38**, 120—123 (1960).

DENGLER, H. J., I. A. MICHAELSON, H. E. SPIEGEL, and E. O. TITUS: The uptake of labeled norepinephrine by isolated brain and other tissues of the cat. Intern. J. Neuropharmacol. **1**, 23—38 (1962).
— H. E. SPIEGEL, and E. O. TITUS: Uptake of tritium-labeled norepinephrine in brain and other tissues of cat *in vitro*. Science **133**, 1072—1073 (1961a).
— — — Effects of drugs on uptake of isotopic norepinephrine by cat tissues. Nature (Lond.) **191**, 816—817 (1961b).
DE IRALDI, A. P., and E. DE ROBERTIS: Action of reserpine on the submicroscopic morphology of the pineal gland. Experientia (Basel) **17**, 122—124 (1961).
DESCLIN, L.: Influence de la réserpine sur la glande mammaire du rat normal, du rat hypophysectomisé ou du rat hypophysectomisé porteur d'une greffe hypophysaire dans la capsule du rein. C. R. Soc. Biol. (Paris) **151**, 1774—1776 (1958).
DEWS, P. B., and W. H. MORSE: Behavioral pharmacology. Ann. Rev. Pharmacol. **1**, 145—174 (1961).
DHAR, M. M., J. D. KOHLI, and S. K. SRIVASTAVA: Studies on the metabolism of reserpine. I. Identification of metabolites. J. Sci. Ind. Res. **14** C, 179—181 (1955).
DOMENJOZ, R., u. W. THEOBALD: Zur Pharmakologie des Tofranil® (N-(3-Dimethylaminopropyl)-iminodibenzyl-hydrochlorid). Arch. int. Pharmacodyn. **120**, 450—489 (1959).
DOMINO, E. F.: Human pharmacology of tranquilizing drugs. Clin. Pharmacol. Ther. **3**, 599—664 (1962a).
— Sites of action of some central nervous system depressants. Ann. Rev. Pharmacol. **2**, 215—250 (1962b).
—, and R. H. RECH: Observations on the initial hypertensive response to reserpine. J. Pharmacol. exp. Ther. **121**, 171—182 (1957).
EECHAUTE, W., E. LACROIX et I. LEUSEN: Effet inhibiteur de la tétrabénazine sur l'influence corticosurrénalienne de la réserpine. Experientia (Basel) **18**, 233—234 (1962).
EHRINGER, H., O. HORNYKIEWICZ u. K. LECHNER: Die Wirkung des Chlorpromazins auf den Katecholamin- und 5-Hydroxytryptaminstoffwechsel im Gehirn der Ratte. Naunyn-Schmiedebergs Arch. exp. Path. Pharmak. **239**, 507—519 (1960).
ERSPAMER, V.: Observations on the 5-hydroxytryptamine (enteramine) release caused by reserpine in the rat. Experientia (Basel) **12**, 63—64 (1956a).
— Wirkung des Reserpins auf den 5-Hydroxytryptamin-(Enteramin)-Gehalt des Serums, der Milz des Darmtraktes und des Gehirns beim Huhn. Naturwissenschaften **43**, 61—62 (1956b).
— Release of 5-hydroxytryptamine by reserpine. Lancet **1956 I** c, 511.
— Recent research in the field of 5-hydroxytryptamine and related indolealkylamines. Fortschr. Arzneimittelforsch. **3**, 151—367 (1961).
—, and C. CICERI: Action of reserpine on the 5-hydroxytryptamine (enteramine) biosynthesis and metabolism in dogs and rats. Experientia (Basel) **13**, 87—88 (1957).
EULER, U. S. v., and F. LISHAJKO: Effect of reserpine on the release of noradrenaline from transmitter granules in adrenergic nerves. Science **132**, 351—352 (1960).
— — Noradrenaline release from isolated nerve granules. Acta physiol. scand. **51**, 193—203 (1961a).
— — Effect of reserpine on the release of catecholamines from isolated nerve and chromaffin cell granules. Acta physiol. scand. **52**, 137—145 (1961b).
— — Effect of some drugs on noradrenaline release from nerve granules. Biochem. Pharmacol. **8**, 62 (1961c).
— — Effect of some drugs on the release of noradrenaline from isolated nerve granules. Biochem. Pharmacol. **9**, 77—84 (1962).
— — Effect of adenine nucleotides on catecholamine release and uptake in isolated adrenergic nerve granules. Acta physiol. scand. (1963, in press).
EVERETT, G. M., and J. E. P. TOMAN: Mode of action of Rauwolfia alkaloids and motor activity. Biol. Psychiat. **2**, 75—81 (1959).
FALCK, B.: Observations on the possibilities of the cellular localization of monoamines by a fluorescence method. Acta physiol. scand. **56** (Suppl. 197), 1—25 (1962).
— Cellular localization of monoamines. Symposium on "Binding Sites of Brain Biogenic Amines", held at Galesburg, Illinois, March 1963; Progress in Brain Research 8, 28—44 (1964).
—, and B. HELLMAN: Evidence for the presence of biogenic amines in pancreatic islets. Experientia (Basel) **19**, 139 (1963).
FARRANT, J.: Interactions between cocaine, tyramine and noradrenaline at the noradrenaline store. Brit. J. Pharmacol. **20**, 540—549 (1963).
FAWAZ, G.: Cardiovascular pharmacology. Ann. Rev. Pharmacol. **3**, 57—90 (1963).
FIORE-DONATI, L., and E. MOLTKE: Effect of reserpine, 5-hydroxytryptamine and polymyxin B on mast cells and or tensile strength of healing wounds. Acta endocr. (Kbh.) **34**, 430—436 (1960).

FISCHER, P., et J. LECOMTE: Choc anaphylactique chez le lapin traité par réserpine. C. R. Soc. Biol. (Paris) **150**, 1026—1028 (1956).

FURCHGOTT, R. F.: Discussion remark. In: J. R. VANE, G. E. W. WOLSTENHOLME and M. O'CONNOR, Eds., Ciba Symposium on Adrenergic Mechanisms, p. 584. London: J. & A. Churchill Ltd. 1960.

—, and S. M. KIRPEKAR: Competition between β-haloalkylamines and norepinephrine for sites in cardiac muscle. In: B. UVNÄS Ed., First International Pharmacological Meeting, vol. 7, Modern concepts in the relationship between structure and pharmacological activity, p. 339—350. Oxford: Pergamon Press 1963.

FURNESS, P., and A. J. PLUMMER: Reversal of depressant activity of methyl O-(2-tetrahydropyranyl) reserpate by monoamine oxidase inhibitors. Fed. Proc. **20** (Part 1), 394 (1961).

FUXE, K.: Cellular localization of monoamines in the median eminence and in the infundibular stem of some mammals. Acta physiol. scand. **58**, 383—384 (1963).

— Cellular localization of monoamines in the median eminence and the infundibular stem of some mammals. Z. Zellforsch. **61**, 710—724 (1964).

— T. HÖKFELT, and O. NILSSON: Observations on the cellular localization of dopamine in the caudate nucleus of the rat. Z. Zellforsch. **63**, 701—706 (1964).

GABE, M., H. TUCHMANN-DUPLESSIS et L. MERCIER-PAROT: Influence de la réserpine sur la neurosécrétion hypothalamo-hypophysaire du rat albinos. C. R. Acad. Sci. (Paris) **252**, 1857—1859 (1961).

GADDUM, J. H., W. A. KRIVOY, and G. LAVERTY: The action of reserpine on the excretion of adrenaline and noradrenaline. J. Neurochem. **2**, 249—253 (1958).

GAFFNEY, TH. E., CH. A. CHIDSEY, and E. BRAUNWALD: Study of the relationship between the neurotransmitter store and adrenergic nerve block induced by reserpine and guanethidine. Circulat. Res. **12**, 264—268 (1963).

GAL, E. M., P. A. DREWES, and C. A. BARRACLOUGH: Effect of reserpine and the metabolism of serotonin in tryptophan deficient rats. Biochem. Pharmacol. **8**, 32 (1961).

GALANSINO, G., R. LITTA-MODIGNANI, F. BERLINGER, D. BILLINGER, and P. P. FOÁ: Studies on the release of serotonin and catecholamines in the pancreato-duodenal area. Proc. Soc. exp. Biol. (N.Y.) **112**, 542—544 (1963).

GARATTINI, S., A. GIACHETTI, A. JORI, L. PIERI, and L. VALZELLI: Effect of imipramine, amitriptyline and their monomethyl derivatives on reserpine activity. J. Pharm. Pharmacol. **14**, 509—514 (1962).

— R. KATO, and L. VALZELLI: Effect of reserpine analogues on tissue serotonin. Experientia (Basel) **16**, 120 (1960).

— L. LAMESTA, A. MORTARI, and L. VALZELLI: Pharmacological and biochemical effects of some reserpine derivatives. J. Pharm. Pharmacol. **13**, 548—564 (1961).

— A. MORTARI, A. VALSECCHI, and L. VALZELLI: Reserpine derivatives with specific hypotensive or sedative activity. Nature (Lond.) **183**, 1273—1274 (1959).

—, and L. VALZELLI: Researches on the mechanism of reserpine sedative action. Science **128**, 1278—1279 (1958).

— — Biochemistry and pharmacology of serotonin in the central nervous system. In: J. DE AJURIAGUERRA, Ed., Monoamines et système nerveux central, p. 59—88. Genève: George & Co. 1962.

GAUNT, R., J. J. CHART, and A. A. RENZI: Endocrine Pharmacology. Science **133**, 613–621 (1961).

— — — Interactions of drugs with endocrines. Ann. Rev. Pharmacol. **3**, 109—128 (1963).

— A. A. RENZI, N. ANTONCHAK, G. J. MILLER, and M. GILMAN: Endocrine aspects of the pharmacology of reserpine. Ann. N.Y. Acad. Sci. **59**, 22—35 (1954).

— —, and J. J. CHART: Endocrine pharmacology of methyl reserpate derivatives. Endocrinology **71**, 527—535 (1962).

GESSA, G. L., E. COSTA, R. KUNTZMAN, and B. B. BRODIE: Evidence that the loss of brain catecholamine stores due to blockade of storage does not cause sedation. Life Sci. No 11, 605—616 (1962).

GIARMAN, N. J.: Drug-induced changes in sub-cellular distribution of serotonin in brain. Symposium on "Binding Sites of Brain Biogenic Amines, held at Galesburg, Illinois, March 1963; to be published in Progress in Brain Research.

—, and S. M. SCHANBERG: The intracellular distribution of 5-hydroxytryptamine (HT; serotonin) in the rat's brain. Biochem. Pharmacol. **1**, 301—306 (1958).

— — Drug-induced alterations in the intracellular distribution of 5-hydroxytryptamine in rat's brain. Biochem. Pharmacol. **8**, 6 (1961).

— — Drug-induced alterations of the subcellular distribution of 5-hydroxytryptamine (serotonin) in rat's brain. Biochem. Pharmacol. **9**, 93—96 (1962).

GILGEN, A., R. P. MAICKEL, O. NIKODIJEVIC, and B. B. BRODIE: Essential role of catecholamines in the mobilization of free fatty acids and glucose after exposure to cold. Life Sci. No 12, 709—715 (1962).

GLAZKO, A. J., W. A. DILL, L. M. WOLF, and A. KAZENKO: Studies on the metabolism of reserpine. J. Pharmacol. exp. Ther. **118**, 377—387 (1956).
GÖRÖG, P., and L. SZPORNY: Effect of vincamin on the noradrenaline content of rat tissue. Biochem. Pharmacol. 8, 259—262 (1961).
GRAY, W. D., CH. E. RAUH, and R. W. SHANAHAN: The mechanism of the antagonistic action of reserpine on the anticonvulsant effect of inhibitors of carbonic anhydrase. J. Pharmacol. exp. Ther. **139**, 350—360 (1963).
GREEN, A. F.: Antihypertensive drugs. In: S. GARATTINI and P. A. SHORE, Eds. Advanc. Pharmac. **1**, 162—228 (1962).
GREEN, H., and J. SAWYER: Intracellular distribution of norepinephrine in rat brain. I. Effect of reserpine and the monoamine oxidase inhibitors, trans-2-phenylcyclopropylamine and isonicotinyl-2-isopropyl hydrazine. J. Pharmacol. exp. Ther. **129**, 243—249 (1960).
— — Intracellular distribution of serotonin in rat brain. I. Effect of reserpine and the monoamine oxidase inhibitors, tranylcypromine and iproniazid. Arch. int. Pharmacodyn. **135**, 426—441 (1962).
— —, and R. ERICKSON: Intracellular distribution of noradrenaline in rat brain. Pharmacol. Soc. Meet. Coral Gables. Florida 1959.
GREENGARD, P., and G. P. QUINN: Metabolic effects of tranquilizers and hypophysectomy. In: D. V. SIVA SANKAR, Ed. Some biological aspects of schizophrenic behavior. Ann. N.Y. Acad. Sci. **96**, Art. 1, 179—184 (1962).
GURSEY, D., and R. E. OLSON: Depression of serotonin and norepinephrine levels in brain stem of rabbit by ethanol. Proc. Soc. exp. Biol. (N.Y.) **104**, 280—281 (1960).
HÄGGENDAL, J.: The presence of O-methylated noradrenaline (normetanephrine) in normal brain tissue. Acta physiol. scand. **59**, 261—268 (1963).
—, and M. LINDQVIST: Ineffectiveness of ethanol on noradrenaline, dopamine or 5-hydroxytryptamine levels in brain. Acta pharmacol. (Kbh.) **18**, 278—280 (1961).
— — Behaviour and monoamine levels during long-term administration of reserpine to rabbits. Acta physiol. scand. **57**, 431—436 (1963).
— — Disclosure of labile monoamine fractions in brain and their correlation to behaviour. Acta physiol. scand. **60**, 351—357 (1964).
—, and T. MALMFORS: Evidence of dopamine-containing neurons in the retina of rabbits. Acta physiol. scand. **59**, 295—296 (1963).
HAMBERGER, B., T. MALMFORS, K.-A. NORBERG, and CH. SACHS: Uptake and accumulation of catecholamines in peripheral adrenergic neurons of reserpinized animals, studied with a histochemical method. Biochem. Pharmacol. **13**, 841—844 (1964).
HARDISTY, R. M., G. I. C. INGRAM, and R. S. STACEY: Reserpine and human platelet 5-hydroxytryptamine. Experientia (Basel) **12**, 424—425 (1956).
HARRISON, D. C., CH. A. CHIDSEY, R. GOLDMAN, and E. BRAUNWALD: Relationship between the release and tissue depletion of norepinephrine from the heart by guanethidine and reserpine. Circulat. Res. **12**, 256—263 (1963).
HAVERBACK, B. J., F. T. DUTSCHER, P. A. SHORE, E. G. TOMICH, L. L. TERRY, and B. B. BRODIE: Serotonin changes in platelets and brain induced by small daily doses of reserpine. New Engl. J. Med. **256**, 343—345 (1957).
— P. A. SHORE, E. G. TOMICH, and B. B. BRODIE: Cumulative effect of small doses of reserpine on serotonin in man. Fed. Proc. **15**, 434—435 (1956).
—, and S. K. WIRTSCHAFTLER: The gastrointestinal tract and naturally occurring pharmacologically active amines. In: S. GARATTINI and P. A. SHORE, Eds. Advanc. Pharmac. **1**, 309—347 (1962).
HERTTING, G., J. AXELROD, and R. W. PATRICK: Actions of bretylium and guanethidine on the uptake and release of ^{3}H-noradrenaline. Brit. J. Pharmacol. 18, 161—166 (1962).
— —, and L. G. WHITBY: Effect of drugs on the uptake and metabolism of H^3-norepinephrine. J. Pharmacol. exp. Ther. **134**, 146—153 (1961).
—, u. O. HORNYKIEWICZ: Beeinflussung der durch Reserpin hervorgerufenen Nebennierenrinden-hypertrophie durch Cortison. Acta endocr. (Kbh.) **26**, 204—208 (1957).
— L. T. POTTER, and J. AXELROD: Effect of decentralization and ganglionic blocking agents on the spontaneous release of H^3-norepinephrine. J. Pharmacol. exp. Ther. **136**, 289—292 (1962).
HESS, S. M., P. A. SHORE, and B. B. BRODIE: Persistence of reserpine action after the disappearance of drug from brain: effect on serotonin. J. Pharmacol. exp. Ther. **118**, 84—89 (1956).
HIGUCHI, H.: Effects of intravenous and intracarotid administration of reserpine on catecholamine contents of the brain, heart and adrenal gland in rabbit. Jap. J. Pharmacol. **12**, 34—47 (1962).
HILLARP, N.-Å.: Further observations on the state of the catecholamines stored in the adrenal medullary granules. Acta physiol. scand. **47**, 271—279 (1959).

HILLARP, N,-Å.: Different pools of catecholamines stored in the adrenal medulla. Acta physiol. scand. **50**, 8—22 (1960a).
— Effect of reserpine on the adrenal medulla of sheep. Acta physiol. scand. **49**, 376—382 (1960b).
—, and T. MALMFORS: Reserpine and cocaine blocking of uptake and storage mechanisms in adrenergic nerves. Life Sci. **3**, 703—708 (1964).
HOLEČEK, V., V. SCHREIBER, and V. KMENTOVÁ: The influence of serpasil on the secretion of antidiuretic hormone. Čas., Lék. čes. **96**, 1060—1062 (1957).
HOLTZ, P., H. BALZER u. E. WESTERMANN: Die Beeinflussung der Reserpinwirkung auf das Nebennierenmark durch Hemmung der Monoaminoxidase. Naunyn-Schmiedebergs Arch. exp. Path. Pharmak. **231**, 361—372 (1957).
HOLZBAUER, M., and M. VOGT: Depression by reserpine of the noradrenaline concentration in the hypothalamus of the cat. J. Neurochem. **1**, 8—11 (1956).
HORITA, A.: A vasopressor response to reserpine in the cocainized dog. J. Pharmacol. exp. Ther. **122**, 474—479 (1958).
HUGHES, F. B., and B. B. BRODIE: The mechanism of serotonin and catecholamine uptake by platelets. J. Pharmacol. exp. Ther. **127**, 96—102 (1959).
— P. A. SHORE, and B. B. BRODIE: Serotonin storage mechanism and its interaction with reserpine. Experientia (Basel) **14**, 178 (1958).
HUTCHISON, H. E., J. M. STARK, and J. A. CHAPMAN: Platelet serotonin and normal haemostasis. J. clin. Path. **12**, 265—267 (1959).
IGGO, A., and M. VOGT: Preganglionic sympathetic activity in normal and reserpine-treated cats. J. Physiol. (Lond.) **150**, 114—133 (1960).
INNES, I. R., O. KRAYER, and D. R. WAUD: The action of Rauwolfia alkaloids on the heart rate and on the functional refractory period of atrioventricular transmission in the heart-lung preparation of the dog. J. Pharmacol. exp. Ther. **124**, 324—332 (1958).
IZQUIERDO, J. A., J. D. COUSSIO, and A. J. KAUMANN: Effect of imipramine on the pressor responses to the afferent vagal stimulation of reserpinized dogs. Arch. int. Pharmacodyn. **135**, 303—310 (1962).
JOHNSON, G. E., and E. A. SELLERS: The effect of reserpine on the metabolic rate of rats. Canad. J. Biochem. **39**, 279—285 (1961).
JONASSON, J., E. ROSENGREN, and B. WALDECK: Effects of some pharmacologically active amines on the uptake of arylalkylamines by adrenal medullary granules. Acta physiol. scand. **60**, 136—140 (1964).
KANEMATSU, S., J. HILLIARD, and C. H. SAWYER: Effect of reserpine on pituitary prolactin content and its hypothalamic site of action in the rabbit. Acta endocr. (Kbh.) **44**, 467—477 (1963).
—, and C. H. SAWYER: Effects of intrahypothalamic implants of reserpine on lactation and pituitary prolactin content in the rabbit. Proc. Soc. exp. Biol. (N.Y.) **113**, 967—969 (1963).
KÄRKI, N. T., and M. K. PAASONEN: Selective depletion of noradrenaline and 5-hydroxytryptamine from rat brain and intestine by Rauwolfia alkaloids. J. Neurochem. **3**, 352—357 (1959).
— — Presence of 5-hydroxytryptamine after raunescine in blood plasma *in vivo*. Nature (Lond.) **185**, 109 (1960).
— —, and P. A. VANHAKARTANO: The influence of pentolonium, isoraunescine and yohimbine on the noradrenaline depleting action of reserpine. Acta pharmacol. (Kbh.) **16**, 13—19 (1959).
KAUL, C. L., and J. J. LEWIS: The effects of reserpine and some related compounds upon the levels of adenine nucleotides, creatine phosphate and inorganic phosphate in the rat brain *in vivo*. J. Pharmacol. exp. Ther. **140**, 111—116 (1963).
KHAZAN, N., J. ADIR, Y. PFEIFER, and F. G. SULMAN: Mechanism of antidiuretic action of reserpine. Proc. Soc. exp. Biol. (N.Y.) **109**, 32—35 (1962).
— and F. G. SULMAN: Melanophore-dispersing activity of reserpine in Rana frogs. Proc. Soc. exp. Biol. (N.Y.) **107**, 282—284 (1961).
— —, and H. Z. WINNIK: Activity of pituitary-adrenal cortex axis during acute and chronic reserpine treatment. Proc. Soc. exp. Biol. (N.Y.) **106**, 579—581 (1961).
KILLAM, E. K.: Drug action on the brain-stem reticular formation. Pharmacol. Rev. **14**, 175—223 (1962).
KILLAM, K. F., and E. K. KILLAM: Central action of chlorpromazine and reserpine. In: H. A. ABRAHAMSON, Ed., Neuropharmacology, Transactions of the Vth Conference, p. 131—198. New York: Josiah Macy, Jr. Foundation 1960.
KIM, K. S., and P. A. SHORE: Production of gastric lesions in the rat by insulin and reserpine: effect on gastric histamine and serotonin. Fed. Proc. **22**, 276 (1963).

KIRPEKAR, S. M., P. CERVONI, and R. F. FURCHGOTT: Catecholamine content of the cat nictitating membrane following procedures sensitizing it to norepinephrine. J. Pharmacol. exp. Ther. **135**, 180—190 (1962).
— G. A. J. GOODLAD, and J. J. LEWIS: Reserpine depletion of adenosine triphosphate from the rat suprarenal medulla. Biochem. Pharmacol. **1**, 232—233 (1958).
—, and J. J. LEWIS: Some effects of reserpine and hydrallazine upon tissue respiration and the concentration of adenosine nucleotides in certain tissues. Brit. J. Pharmacol. **14**, 40—45 (1959).
— — Effects of reserpine, chlorpromazine and sodium salicylate on the enzymic activity of rat liver. Brit. J. Pharmacol. **15**, 175—180 (1960).
KIRSHNER, N.: Uptake of catecholamines by a particulate fraction of the adrenal medulla. Science **135**, 107—108 (1962a).
— Uptake of catecholamines by a particulate fraction of the adrenal medulla. J. biol. Chem. **237**, 2311—2317 (1962b).
KITAY, J. I., D. A. HOLUB, and J. W. JAILER: "Inhibition" of pituitary ACTH release after administration of reserpine or epinephrine. Endocrinology **65**, 548—554 (1959).
KNOLL, J., and B. KNOLL: Reserpine: modification of its tranquilizer effect and analysis of its central node of action. Arch. int. Pharmacodyn. **133**, 310—326 (1961).
KOHLI, J. D., and B. MUKERJI: Reserpine & Rauwolfia alkaloids — recent pharmacological studies. J. Sci. Ind. Res. **20** A, 69—87 (1961).
KOPIN, I. J., and E. K. GORDON: Metabolism of norepinephrine-H^3 released by tyramine and reserpine. J. Pharmacol. exp. Ther. **138**, 351—359 (1962).
— — Metabolism of administered and drug-released norepinephrine-7-H^3 in the rat. J. Pharmacol. exp. Ther. **140**, 207—216 (1963).
KRONEBERG, G., u. H. J. SCHÜMANN: Die Wirkung des Reserpins auf den Hormongehalt des Nebennierenmarks. Naunyn-Schmiedebergs Arch. exp. Path. Pharmak. **231**, 349—360 (1957).
— — Adrenalinsekretion und Adrenalinverarmung der Kaninchennebennieren nach Reserpin. Naunyn-Schmiedebergs Arch. exp. Path. Pharmak. **234**, 133—146 (1958).
— — Über die Bedeutung der Innervation für die Adrenalinsynthese im Nebennierenmark. Experientia (Basel) **15**, 234 (1959).
— — Der Einfluß von Iproniacid auf die durch Reserpin gesteigerte Sekretion des Kaninchennebennierenmarks. Naunyn-Schmiedebergs Arch. exp. Path. Pharmak. **239**, 29—34 (1960).
KUSCHINSKY, G., R. LINDMAR, H. LÜLLMANN u. E. MUSCHOLL: Der Einfluß von Reserpin auf die Wirkung der „Neuro-Sympathomimetika". Naunyn Schmiedebergs Arch. exp. Path. Pharmak. **240**, 242—252 (1960).
LA LANDE, I. S. DE, V. J. PARKS, A. G. SANDISON, S. L. SKINNER, and R. F. WHELAN: The peripheral dilator action of reserpine in man. Aust. J. exp. Biol. med. Sci. **38**, 313—320 (1960).
LAVERTY, R.: The influence of cold environmental temperature and histamine treatment on the effect of reserpine in the rat. J. Neurochem. **10**, 151—154 (1963).
LESSIN, A. W., and M. W. PARKES: The relation between sedation and body temperature in the mouse. Brit. J. Pharmacol. **12**, 245—250 (1957).
— — The effects of reserpine and other agents upon leptazol convulsions in mice. Brit. J. Pharmacol. **14**, 108—111 (1959).
LEUSEN, I.: Monoamin-Freisetzer und Monoaminoxydase-Hemmer. Psychiat. et Neurol. (Basel) **140**, 154—164 (1960).
— E. LACROIX et G. DEMEESTER: Quelques propriétés pharmacodynamiques de la tétrabénazine, substance libératrice de sérotonine. Arch. int. Pharmacodyn. **119**, 225—231 (1959).
LEWIS, J. J.: Rauwolfia derivatives. In: W. S. ROOT and F. G. HOFMANN, Eds., Physiological Pharmacology. A comprehensive treatise, vol. I. The nervous system — Part A. p. 479—536. New York: Academic Press 1963.
LIEBECQ-HUTTER, S., and Z. M. BACQ: Disappearance of 5-hydroxytryptamine in the granulations of the glands of the skin of *Discoglossus pictus* and of *Rana temporaria* after injection of reserpine. Experientia (Basel) **14**, 180—181 (1958).
— J. F. RENSON et P. FISCHER: Action de la réserpine sur la teneur en 5-hydroxytryptamine des tissus de *Discoglossus pictus*. Arch. int. Physiol. **67**, 144—147 (1959).
LIEBMAN, J., A. J. MUSKUS, and O. R. WAUD: The depletion of norepinephrine stores in the heart of the dog by reserpine-type alkaloids. J. Pharmacol. exp. Ther. **136**, 75—79 (1962).
LUNDBORG, P.: Storage function and amine levels of the adrenal medullary granules at various intervals after reserpine treatment. Experientia (Basel) **19**, 479 (1963).
MACLEAN, P. D.: Hippocampal studies: Their possible bearing on neuropsychiatry. Arch. Neurol. Psychiat. (Chic.) **74**, 219—220 (1955).

MAGNUSSON, T., and E. ROSENGREN: Catecholamines of the spinal cord normally and after transection. Experientia (Basel) **19**, 229—230 (1963).
MAICKEL, R. P., E. O. WESTERMANN, and B. B. BRODIE: Effects of reserpine and cold-exposure on pituitary adrenocortical function in rats. J. Pharmacol. exp. Ther. **134**, 167—175 (1962).
MALHOTRA, C. L., and P. K. DAS: Effect of reserpine on the acetylcholine content of the heart, the ileum and the hypothalamus of the dog. Brit. J. Pharmacol. **18**, 190—193 (1962).
—, and K. PRASAD: The effect of intra(cerebro)ventricular reserpine on the acetylcholine content of the heart, ileum and hypothalamus of the dog. Brit. J. Pharmacol. **21**, 355—360 (1963).
—, and P. G. PUNDLIK: The effect of reserpine on the acetyl choline content of different areas of the nervous system of the dog. Brit. J. Pharmacol. **14**, 46—47 (1959).
MALMFORS, T.: Evidence of adrenergic neurons with synaptic terminals in the retina of rats demonstrated with fluorescence and electron microscopy. Acta physiol. scand. **58**, 99—100 (1963).
MARKIEWICZ, L.: Biochemical and functional effects of long-term administration of reserpine in mice. Acta physiol. scand. **58**, 376—380 (1963).
MATHÉ, V., GY. KASSAY u. K. HUNKÁR: Die Wirkung des Reserpins auf den Gehalt des Rattengehirns an gesamtreduzierenden Stoffen und Glykogen. Z. ges. exp. Med. **134**, 249—253 (1961).
MAXWELL, R. A., A. J. PLUMMER, M. W. OSBORNE, and S. D. ROSS: Evidence for a peripheral action of reserpine. J. Pharmacol. exp. Ther. **116**, 42 (1956).
— S. D. ROSS, A. J. PLUMMER, and E. B. SIGG: A peripheral action of reserpine. J. Pharmacol. exp. Ther. **119**, 69—77 (1957).
McDONALD, R. K., and V. K. WEISE: The effect of certain psychotropic drugs on the urinary excretion of 3-methoxy-4-hydroxymandelic acid in man. J. Pharmacol. exp. Ther. **136**, 26—30 (1962).
McQUEEN, E. G., A. E. DOYLE, and F. H. SMIRK: Mechanism of hypotensive action of reserpine, an alkaloid of *Rauwolfia serpentina*. Nature (Lond.) **174**, 1015 (1954).
— — — The circulatory effects of reserpine. Circulation **11**, 161—169 (1955).
MEITES, J.: Effect of reserpine on prolactin content of rabbit pituitary. Proc. Soc. exp. Biol. (N.Y.) **97**, 742—744 (1958).
— C. S. NICOLL, and P. R. TALWALKER: Effect of reserpine and serotonin on milk secretion and mammary growth in the rat. Proc. Soc. exp. Biol. (N.Y.) **101**, 563—565 (1959).
MILINE, R., P. STERN, E. SERSTNEV et M. MUHIBIC: Effet de la réserpine et de la réserpine associée au luminal sur le complexe hypothalamo-hypophysaire. In: S. GARATTINI and V. GHETTI, Eds., Psychotropic Drugs, p. 332—349. Amsterdam: Elsevier Publ. Co. 1957.
MIRKIN, B. L.: Catechol amine depletion in the rat's denervated adrenal gland following chronic administration of reserpine. Nature (Lond.) **182**, 113—114 (1958).
— The effect of synaptic blocking agents on reserpine-induced alterations in adrenal medullary and urinary catecholamine levels. J. Pharmacol. exp. Ther. **133**, 34—40 (1961).
MOORE, K. E., and T. M. BRODY: The effect of triethyltin on tissue amines. J. Pharmacol. exp. Ther. **132**, 6—12 (1961).
MORAN, N. C., and B. WESTERHOLM: The influence of reserpine on 5-hydroxytryptamine and histamine content of rat mast cells and of some rat tissues. Acta physiol. scand. **58**, 20—29 (1963).
MÜLLER, J. M., E. SCHLITTLER u. H. J. BEIN: Reserpin, der sedative Wirkstoff aus *Rauwolfia serpentina* BENTH. Experientia (Basel) **8**, 338 (1952).
MUSCHOLL, E.: Die Hemmung der Noradrenalin-Aufnahme des Herzens durch Reserpin und die Wirkung von Tyramin. Naunyn-Schmiedebergs Arch. exp. Path. Pharmak. **240**, 234—241 (1960).
—, and M. VOGT: Concentration of adrenaline in plasma of rabbits treated with reserpine. Brit. J. Pharmacol. **12**, 532—535 (1957).
— — The action of reserpine on the peripheral sympathetic system. J. Physiol. (Lond.) **141**, 132—155 (1958).
MUSKUS, A. J.: Effect of pretreatment with reserpine and reserpine analogs on the response of isolated guinea-pig atria to tyramine. J. Pharmacol. exp. Ther. **138**, 296—300 (1962).
NASMYTH, P. A.: An investigation of the action of tyramine and its interrelationship with the effects of other sympathomimetic amines. Brit. J. Pharmacol. **18**, 65—75 (1962).
NAYLER, W. G.: A direct effect of reserpine on ventricular contractility. J. Pharmacol. exp. Ther. **139**, 222—229 (1963).
NEČINA, J.: Antagonism between α-methyl DOPA and reserpine. Life Sci. **1**, 301—303 (1962).
—, and I. KREJČI: On the role of serotonin and catecholamines in relation to some effects of reserpine. Biochem. Pharmacol. **8**, 35 (1961).

NUMEROF, P., M. GORDON, and J. M. KELLY: The metabolism of reserpine. I. Studies in the mouse with C^{14}-labeled reserpine. J. Pharmacol. exp. Ther. **115**, 427—431 (1955).

ORLANS, F. B. H., and B. B. BRODIE: A suggested effect on levels of catecholamine in brain produced by small doses of reserpine. Nature (Lond.) **187**, 1034—1035 (1960).

— K. F. FINGER, and B. B. BRODIE: Pharmacological consequences of the selective release of peripheral norepinephrine by syrosingopine (SU 3118). J. Pharmacol. exp. Ther. **128**, 131—139 (1960).

PAASONEN, M. K., and P. B. DEWS: Effects of raunescine and isoraunescine on behaviour and on the 5-hydroxytryptamine and noradrenaline contents of brain. Brit. J. Pharmacol. **13**, 84—88 (1958).

—, and O. KRAYER: The release of norepinephrine from the mammalian heart by reserpine. J. Pharmacol. exp. Ther. **123**, 153—160 (1958).

— — The content of noradrenaline and adrenaline in the rat heart after administration of Rauwolfia alkaloids. Experientia (Basel) **15**, 75—76 (1959).

—, and A. PLETSCHER: Increase of free 5-hydroxytryptamine in blood plasma by reserpine and a benzoquinolizine derivative. Experientia (Basel) **15**, 477 (1959).

—, and M. VOGT: The effect of drugs on the amounts of substance P and 5-hydroxytryptamine in mammalian brain. J. Physiol. (Lond.) **131**, 617—626 (1956).

PALM, D., H. BALZER u. P. HOLTZ: Reserpin und γ-Aminobuttersäuregehalt des Gehirns. Naunyn-Schmiedebergs Arch. exp. Path. Pharmak. **241**, 190—191 (1961).

PARKS, V. J., A. G. SANDISON, S. L. SKINNER, and R. F. WHELAN: The mechanism of the vasodilator action of reserpine in man. Clin. Sci. **20**, 289—295 (1961).

— S. L. SKINNER, and R. F. WHELAN: Mechanisms in the return of vascular tone following sympathectomy in man. Circulat. Res. **9**, 1026—1033 (1961).

PARRATT, J. R., and G. B. WEST: Release of 5-hydroxytryptamine and histamine from tissues of the rat. J. Physiol. (Lond.) **137**, 179—192 (1957).

PAULSEN, E. C., and S. M. HESS: The rate of synthesis of catecholamines following depletion in guinea pig brain and heart. J. Neurochem. **10**, 453—459 (1963).

PETERFALVI, M., et R. JEQUIER: La 10-methoxy deserpidine. Étude pharmacologique. Arch. int. Pharmacodyn. **124**, 237—254 (1960).

PICCINELLI, D.: Effect of reserpine on indole-alkylamine and phenylalkylamine levels in tissues of lower vertebrates and molluscs. Arch. int. Pharmacodyn. **117**, 452—459 (1958).

PLETSCHER, A.: Beeinflussung des 5-Hydroxytryptamin-Stoffwechsels im Gehirn durch Isonikotinsäurehydrazide. Experientia (Basel) **12**, 479—480 (1956).

— Topographical difference of the behaviour of 5-hydroxytryptamine in the gastric mucosa after reserpine administration. In: G. P. LEWIS, Ed., 5-Hydroxytryptamine, p. 84—85. London: Pergamon Press 1957a.

— Release of 5-hydroxytryptamine by benzoquinolizine derivatives with sedative action. Science **126**, 507 (1957b).

— Alterations of monoamine metabolism caused by drugs acting on the central nervous system. In: N. S. KLINE, Ed., Psychopharmacology frontiers, p. 395—401. Boston: Little, Brown & Co. 1959.

— H. BESENDORF u. H. P. BÄCHTOLD: Benzo[a]chinolizine, eine neue Körperklasse mit Wirkung auf den 5-Hydroxytryptamin- und Noradrenalin-Stoffwechsel des Gehirns. Naunyn-Schmiedebergs Arch. exp. Path. Pharmak. **232**, 499—507 (1958).

— —, and K. F. GEY: Depression of norepinephrine and 5-hydroxytryptamine in the brain by benzoquinolizine derivatives. Science **129**, 844 (1959).

— — F. A. STEINER, and K. F. GEY: The effect of 2-hydroxy-benzoquinolizines on cerebral 5-hydroxytryptamine, spontaneous locomotor activity, and ethanol hypnosis in mice. Med. exp. (Basel) **7**, 15—20 (1962).

— A. BROSSI, and K. F. GEY: Benzoquinolizine derivatives: a new class of monoamine decreasing drugs with psychotropic action. Int. Rev. Neurobiol. **4**, 275—306 (1962).

—, and K. F. GEY: Interference with the permeation of aromatic monoamines and amino acids in brain by chlorpromazine and chlorprothixene. In: W. D. M. PATON and P. LINDGREN, Eds., Proc. of the First Intern. Pharmacol. Meeting, vol. 8. Pharmacological analysis of central nervous action, p. 75—84. Oxford: Pergamon Press 1962.

— —, and E. KUNZ: Accumulation of exogenous monoamines in brain *in vivo* and its alteration by drugs. Symposium on "Binding Sites of Brain Biogenic Amines", held at Galesburg, Illinois, March 1963; Progress in Brain Research 8, 45—52 (1964).

— — u. P. ZELLER: Monoaminoxidase-Hemmer. Biochemie, Chemie, Pharmakologie, Klinik. Fortschr. Arzneimittelforsch. **2**, 417—590 (1960).

— P. A. SHORE, and B. B. BRODIE: Serotonin release as a possible mechanism of reserpine action. Science **122**, 374—375 (1955).

PLETSCHER, A., P. A. SHORE, and B. B, BRODIE: Serotonin as a mediator of reserpine action in brain. J. Pharmacol. exp. Ther. **116**, 84—89 (1956).
PLUMMER, A. J., W. E. BARRETT, R. A. MAXWELL, D. FINOCCHIO, R. A. LUCAS, and A. E. EARL: Hypotensive properties of syrosingopine, SU-3118, an ester of methyl reserpate. Arch. int. Pharmacodyn. **119**, 245—257 (1959).
— —, and R. RUTLEDGE: The action of reserpine on the motility of the digestive tract. Amer. J. dig. Dis. **22**, 337—342 (1955).
— A. EARL, J. A. SCHNEIDER, J. TRAPOLD, and W. E. BARRETT: Pharmacology of *Rauwolfia* alkaloids, including reserpine. Ann. N.Y. Acad. Sci. **59**, 8—21 (1954).
— R. A. MAXWELL, and A. E. EARL: The influence of Ritalin (methylphenidate) on the behavioral and circulatory effects of reserpine. Schweiz. med. Wschr. **14** (Suppl.), 370—372 (1957).
— H. SHEPPARD, and A. R. SCHULERT: The metabolism of reserpine. In: S. GARATTINI and V. GHETTI, Eds., Psychotropic Drugs, p. 350—362 Amsterdam: Elsevier Publ. Co. 1957.
PORTER, C. C., J. A. TOTARO, and C. A. STONE: Effect of 6-hydroxydopamine and some other compounds on the concentration of norepinephrine in the hearts of mice. J. Pharmacol. exp. Ther. **140**, 308—316 (1963).
POTTER, L. T., and J. AXELROD: Studies on the storage of norepinephrine and the effect of drugs. J. Pharmacol. exp. Ther. **140**, 199—206 (1963).
PREMACHANDRA, B. N.: Reserpine and thyroid function in the fowl. Biochem. Pharmacol. **8**, 104 (1961).
PROCKOP, D. J., P. A. SHORE, and B. B. BRODIE: Anticonvulsant properties of monoamine oxidase inhibitors. Ann. N.Y. Acad. Sci. **80**, 643—651 (1959).
PROOSDIJ-HERTZEMA, E. G. VAN, A. M. AKKERMAN, and D. K. DE JONGH: A new hypotensive agent derived from serpentine. Arch. int. Pharmacodyn. **123**, 168—178 (1959).
PSCHEIDT, G. R.: Effects of reserpine and isocarboxazid in the frog. International Symposium on Problems of the Brain, held in Galesburg, Illinois, March 1 to 3, 1963.
— G. W. BRUNE, and H. E. HIMWICH: Uniform response of biogenic amines to psychotropic drugs in selected schizophrenic patients. Fed. Proc. **20**, 305 (1961).
—, and H. E. HIMWICH: Reserpine, monoamine oxidase inhibitors, and distribution of biogenic amines in monkey brain. Biochem. Pharmacol. **12**, 65—71 (1963).
QUINN, G. P., and B. B. BRODIE: Effect of chlorpromazine and reserpine on the central actions of morphine in the cat. Med. exp. (Basel) **4**, 349—355 (1961).
— M. B. REID, and P. GREENGARD: Effect of tranquilizers and hypophysectomy on the response of liver DPN to nicotinamide administration. Fed. Proc. **21**, 419 (1962).
— P. A. SHORE, and B. B. BRODIE: Biochemical and pharmacological studies of Ro 1-9569 (tetrabenazine), a non-indole tranquilizing agent with reserpine-like effects. J. Pharmacol. exp. Ther. **127**, 103—109 (1959).
RANDALL, L. O., N. ATKINSON, and V. ILIEV: The effect of psychostimulants and psychodepressants on DPN synthesis in the liver. Arch. int. Pharmacodyn. **129**, 434—437 (1960).
REIMERT, H.: Role and origin of noradrenaline in the superior cervical ganglion. J. Physiol. (Lond.) **167**, 18—29 (1963).
RINALDI, F., and H. E. HIMWICH: A comparison of effects of reserpine and some barbiturates on the electrical activity of cortical and subcortical structures in the brain of rabbits. Ann. N.Y. Acad. Sci. **61**, 27—35 (1955).
ROBERTIS, E. DE: Contribution of electronmicroscopy to neuropharmacological problems. Biochem. Pharmacol. **9**, 49—60 (1962).
— Electron microscope and chemical study of binding sites of brain biogenic amines. Symposium on "Binding Sites of Brain Biogenic Amines", held at Galesburg, Illinois, March 1963; Progress in Brain Research 8, 118—136 (1964).
ROBISON, M. M., R. A. LUCAS, H. B. MACPHILLARMY, W. E. BARRETT, and A. J. PLUMMER: Rauwolfia alkaloids. XXXV. Potent, fast-acting sedatives derived from methyl reserpate. Experientia (Basel) **17**, 14—15 (1961).
ROOS, B.-E., and G. STEG: The effect of L-3,4-dihydroxyphenylalanine and DL-5-hydroxytryptophan on rigidity and tremor induced by reserpine, chlorpromazine and phenoxybenzamine. Life Sci. **3**, 351—360 (1964).
—, and B. WERDINIUS: Effect of reserpine on the level of 5-hydroxyindoleacetic acid in brain. Life Sci. No 3, 105—107 (1962).
ROSELL, S., and G. SEDVALL: Restoration of vasoconstrictor effects in reserpinized cats. Acta physiol. scand. **53**, 174—184 (1961).
— — The rate of disappearance of vasoconstrictor responses to sympathetic chain stimulation after reserpine treatment. Acta physiol. scand. **56**, 306—314 (1962).
ROSS, CH. A., H. C. WENGER, C. T. LUDDEN, and C. A. STONE: Selective potentiation of sympathomimetic amines by reserpine, syrosingopine and 2,6-xylylcholine ether bromide (TM-10) in the dog. Arch. int. Pharmacodyn. **142**, 141—151 (1963).

ROSS, S., and C. J. CARR: Behavioural pharmacology. In: E. S. E. HAFEZ, Ed., The Behaviour of Domestic Animals, p. 181—200. London: Baillière, Tindall & Co. 1962.

RUTISHAUSER, M.: Beeinflussung des Kohlenhydratstoffwechsels des Rattenhirns durch Psychopharmaka mit sedativer Wirkung. Naunyn-Schmiedebergs Arch. exp. Path. Pharmak. **245**, 396—413 (1963).

SAFFRON, M., and M. VOGT: Depletion of pituitary corticotrophin by reserpine and by a nitrogen mustard. Brit. J. Pharmacol. **15**, 165—169 (1960).

SANAN, S., and M. VOGT: Effect of drugs on the noradrenaline content of brain and peripheral tissues and its significance. Brit. J. Pharmacol. **18**, 109—127 (1962).

SANO, I., Y. KAKIMOTO, T. OKAMOTO, H. NAKAJIMA u. Y. KUDO: Über 5-Oxyindolessigsäure-Ausscheidung im Urin von Schizophrenen mit Berücksichtigung des Einflusses von Chlorpromazin und Reserpin auf den Serotoninstoffwechsel. Schweiz. med. Wschr. **87**, 214—217 (1957).

— —, and K. TANIGUCHI: Binding and transport of serotonin in rabbit blood platelets and action of reserpine. Amer. J. Physiol. **195**, 495—498 (1958).

SAXTON, J. E.: The indole alkaloids. In: R. H. F. MANSKE, Ed., The alkaloids. Chemistry and physiology, vol. VII, p. 4—200. New York: Academic Press 1960.

SCHAEPDRYVER, A. F. DE: Hypertensive responses in reserpinized dogs. Arch. int. Pharmacodyn. **124**, 45—52 (1960).

— M. BOGAERT, A. L. DELANNOIS, A. L. BERNARD, and P. BERNARD: Peripheral noradrenergic reactivity. Arch. int. Pharmacodyn. **142**, 243—259 (1963).

SCHAPIRO, H., and E. R. WOODWARD: The mechanism of action of reserpine on gastric secretion. Fed. Proc. **20**, 248 (1961).

SCHLITTLER, E., J. DRUEY, and A. MARXER: Antihypertensive agents. Fortschr. Arzneimittelforsch. **4**, 295—352 (1962).

SCHNEIDER, J. A.: Further characterization of central effects of reserpine (Serpasil), Amer. J. Physiol. **181**, 64—68 (1955).

— The pharmacology of Rauwolfia. In: R. E. WOODSON jr., H. W. YOUNGKEN, E. SCHLITTLER and J. A. SCHNEIDER. *Rauwolfia:* Botany, Pharmacognosy, Chemistry and Pharmacology, p. 109—144. Boston: Little, Brown & Co. 1957.

— A. J. PLUMMER, A. E. EARL, W. E. BARRETT, R. RINEHART, and R. C. DIBBLE: Pharmacological studies with deserpidine, a new alkaloid from Rauwolfia canescens. J. Pharmacol. exp. Ther. **114**, 10—13 (1955).

—, and R. K. RINEHART: Circulatory interactions of serotonin and reserpine (Serpasil) in dogs. Arch. int. Pharmacodyn. **105**, 253—268 (1956).

SCHÜMANN, H. J.: Die Wirkung von Insulin und Reserpin auf den Adrenalin- und ATP-Gehalt der chromaffinen Granula des Nebennierenmarks. Naunyn-Schmiedebergs Arch. exp. Path. Pharmak. **233**, 237—249 (1958).

SCHWARTZ, D. E., A. PLETSCHER, K. F. GEY u. J. RIEDER: Biologische Verteilung eines Benzochinolizinderivates und dessen Wirkung auf den 5-Hydroxytryptamin- und Noradrenalin-Gehalt der Gewebe. Helv. physiol. pharmacol. Acta **18**, 10—16 (1960).

SEIDEN, L. S., and A. CARLSSON: Temporary and partial antagonism by L-DOPA of reserpine-induced suppression of a conditioned avoidance response. Psychopharmacologia (Berl.) **4**, 418—423 (1963).

— — Brain and heart catecholamine levels after L-DOPA administration in reserpine treated mice: correlations with conditioned avoidance response. Psychopharmacologia (Berl.) **5**, 178—181 (1964).

SHELBURNE, P. F., and E. S. ORGAIN: Comparison of syrosyngopine and reserpine in the treatment of ambulatory hypertensive patients. Amer. J. med. Sci. **245**, 304—310 (1963).

SHEPPARD, H., R. A. LUCAS, and W. H. TSIEN: The metabolism of reserpine-C^{14}. Arch. int. Pharmacodyn. **103**, 256—269 (1955).

— W. H. TSIEN, E. B. SIGG, R. A. LUCAS, and A. J. PLUMMER: The metabolism of reserpine-C^{14}. III. C^{14}-concentration vs. time in the brains and other tissues of rats and guinea pigs. Arch. int. Pharmacodyn. **113**, 160—168 (1957).

SHORE, P. A.: Release of serotonin and catecholamines by drugs. Pharmacol. Rev. **14**, 531—550 (1962).

—, and B. B. BRODIE: Influence of various drugs on serotonin and norepinephrine in brain. In: S. GARATTINI and V. GHETTI, Eds., Psychotropic Drugs, p. 423—427, Amsterdam: Elsevier Publ. Co. 1957a.

— — LSD-like effects elicited by reserpine in rabbits pretreated with iproniazid. Proc. Soc. exp. Biol. (N.Y.) **94**, 433—435 (1957b).

— A. PLETSCHER, and B. B. BRODIE: Release of platelet serotonin by reserpine — effect on hemostasis. J. Pharmacol. exp. Ther. **116**, 51—52 (1956).

— — E. G. TOMICH, R. KUNTZMAN, and B. B. BRODIE: Release of blood platelet serotonin by reserpine and lack of effect on bleeding time. J. Pharmacol. exp. Ther. **117**, 232—236 (1956).

SHORE. P. A., S. L. SILVER, and B. B. BRODIE: Interaction of reserpine, serotonin, and lysergic acid diethylamide in brain. Science **122**, 284—285 (1955).

SMITH, C. B., and P. B. DEWS: Antagonism of locomotor suppressant effects of reserpine in mice. Psychopharmacologia (Berl.) **3**, 55—59 (1962).

SMITH, E. R.: The effect of norepinephrine infusions upon some responses of reserpine-treated spinal cats to tyramine. J. Pharmacol. exp. Ther. **139**, 321—329 (1963).

SPECTOR, S., C. W. HIRSCH, and B. B. BRODIE: Association of behavioural effects of pargyline, a non-hydrazide MAO inhibitor, with increase in brain norepinephrine. Intern. J. Neuropharmacol. **2**, 81—93 (1963).

— R. KUNTZMAN, P. A. SHORE, and B. B. BRODIE: Evidence for release of brain amines by reserpine in presence of monoamine oxidase inhibitors: implication of monoamine oxidase in norepinephrine metabolism in brain. J. Pharmacol. exp. Ther. **130**, 256—261 (1960).

STACEY, R. S.: 5-Hydroxytryptamine and other pharmacologically active substances in the central nervous system. Acta physiol. pharmacol. neerl. **8**, 222—239 (1959).

STEG, G.: Efferent muscle innervation and rigidity. Acta physiol. scand. **61**, Suppl. 225, 1—53 (1964).

STEIN, L., and O. S. RAY: Accelerated recovery from reserpine depression by monoamine oxidase inhibitors. Nature (Lond.) **188**, 1199—1200 (1960).

STUMPF, W., E. H. GRAUL u. H. HUNDESHAGEN: Experimentelle Untersuchungen zur Pharmakologie des mit ^{3}H-markierten Tetrabenazins. Arzneimittel-Forsch. **11**, 47—49 (1961).

SULSER, F., M. H. BICKEL, and B. B. BRODIE: On mechanism of the anti-depressant action of imipramine. In: W. D. M. PATON and P. LINDGREN Eds., Proc. of the First Intern. Pharmacol. Meeting, vol. 8, Pharmacological analysis of central nervous action, p. 123—129. Oxford: Pergamon Press 1962.

—, and B. B. BRODIE: Is reserpine tranquilization linked to change in brain serotonin or brain norepinephrine? Science **131**, 1440—1441 (1960).

SZPORNY, L., and P. GÖRÖG: The effect of vincamine on the blood pressure of the rat. Arch. int. Pharmacodyn. **138**, 451—461 (1962).

TAKETOMO, Y., P. A. SHORE, E. G. TOMICH, R. KUNTZMAN, and B. B. BRODIE: Studies on the mechanism of reserpine-induced epinephrine release and hyperglycemia. J. Pharmacol. exp. Ther. **119**, 188 (1957).

TAYLOR jr. R. E., and M. J. FREGLY: Effect of reserpine on body temperature regulation of the rat. J. Pharmacol. exp. Ther. **138**, 200—207 (1962).

TODRICK, H., M. DICK, and A. C. TAIT: Effect of reserpine in therapeutic dosage on excretion of 5-hydroxyindoleacetic acid. Brit. med. J. **1958 I**, 496—499.

TOMAN, J. E. P.: Some aspects of central nervous pharmacology. Ann. Rev. Pharmacol. **3**, 153—184 (1963).

TRENDELENBURG, U.: Modification of the effect of tyramine by various agents and procedures. J. Pharmacol. exp. Ther. **134**, 8—17 (1961).

— Supersensitivity and subsensitivity to sympathomimetic amines. Pharmacol. Rev. **15**, 225—276 (1963).

UDENFRIEND, S., H. WEISSBACH, and D. F. BOGDANSKI: Increase in tissue serotonin following administration of its precursor 5-hydroxytryptophan. J. biol. Chem. **224**, 803—810 (1957).

UHR, L., and J. G. MILLER (Eds.): Drugs and behavior. New York: John Wiley & Sons, Inc 1960.

VALCOURT, A. J.: Excretion of 5-hydroxyindoleacetic acid in mental patients. Arch. Neurol. Psychiat. (Chic.) **81**, 292—298 (1959).

VELLUZ, L., M. PETERFALVI, and R. JEQUIER: Separation of reserpine effects. C. R. Acad. Sci. (Paris) **247**, 1905—1907 (1958).

VOLLE, R. L.: Pharmacology of the autonomic nervous system. Ann. Rev. Pharmacol. **3**, 129—152 (1963).

WAALKES, T. P., H. COBURN, and L. L. TERRY: The effect of reserpine on histamine and serotonin. J. Allergy **30**, 408—414 (1959).

—, and H. WEISSBACH: In vivo release of histamine from rabbit blood by reserpine. Proc. Soc. exp. Biol. (N.Y.) **93**, 394—396 (1956).

— — J. BOZICEVICH, and S. UDENFRIEND: Further studies on release of serotonin and histamine during anaphylaxis in the rabbit. Proc. exp. Biol. (N.Y.) **95**, 479—482 (1957).

WALASZEK, E. J., and H. BURFORD: Modification of the vasopressor effect of tryptamine and tyramine by reserpine. Arch. int. Pharmacodyn. **143**, 543—549 (1963).

WEIL-MALHERBE, H., and A. D. BONE: Intracellular distribution of catecholamines in the brain. Nature (Lond.) **180**, 1050—1051 (1957).

— H. S. POSNER, and G. R. BOWLES: Changes in the concentration and intracellular distribution of brain catecholamines: the effects of reserpine, β-phenylisopropylhydrazine. pyrogallol, and 3,4-dihydroxyphenylalanine, alone and in combination. J. Pharmacol. exp. Ther. **132**, 278—286 (1961).

WEINER, M., and S. UDENFRIEND: Relation of platelet serotonin to disturbances of clotting and hemostasis. Circulation **15**, 353—357 (1957).

— M. PERKINS, and R. L. SIDMAN: Effect of reserpine on noradrenaline content of innervated and denervated brown adipose tissue of the rat. Nature (Lond.) **193**, 137—138 (1962).

WEISSBACH, H., B. G. REDFIELD, and E. TITUS: Effect of cardiac glycosides and inorganic ions on binding of serotonin by platelets. Nature (Lond.) **185**, 99—100 (1960).

WEISSMAN, A., and K. F. FINGER: Effects of benzquinamide on avoidance behaviour and brain amine levels. Biochem. Pharmacol. **11**, 871—880 (1962).

WELLS, H., N. BRIGGS, and P. L. MUNSON: The inhibitory effect of reserpine on ACTH secretion in response to stressful stimuli. Endocrinology **59**, 571—579 (1956).

WERDINIUS, B.: Effect of temperature on the action of reserpine. Acta pharmacol. (Kbh.) **19**, 43—46 (1962).

WESTERMANN, E., R. P. MAICKEL u. B. B. BRODIE: Untersuchungen über den Mechanismus einer Reserpinwirkung auf die Hypophyse. Naunyn-Schmiedebergs Arch. exp. Path. Pharmak. **241**, 189—190 (1961).

WHELAN, R. F., and S. L. SKINNER: Autonomic transmitter mechanisms. In Peripheral Circulation in Man. Brit. med. Bull. **19**, 120—124 (1963).

WHITTAKER, V. P.: Investigations on the storage sites of biogenic amines in the central nervous system. Symposium on "Binding Sites of Brain Biogenic Amines", held at Galesburg, Illinois, March 1963; Progress in Brain Research 8, 90—117 (1964).

WILLIAMS, C. M.: The effect of reserpine on dopamine metabolism in humans. J. Neurochem. **9**, 335—336 (1962).

WILSON, C. W. M., A. W. MURRAY and E. TITUS: Effects of reserpine on uptake of adrenaline in brain and certain areas outside the blood-brain barrier. J. Pharmacol. exp. Ther. **135**, 11—16 (1962).

WITHRINGTON, P., and E. ZAIMIS: The reserpine-treated cat. Brit. J. Pharmacol. **17**, 390—391 (1961).

WOODSON jr. R. E., H. W. YOUNGKEN, E. SCHLITTLER, and J. A. SCHNEIDER: Rauwolfia. Botany, pharmacognosy, chemistry and pharmacology. Boston: Little, Brown & Co. 1957.

YAMAZAKI, E., D. W. SLINGERLAND, and A. NOGUCHI: The effect of reserpine on thyroxine degradation and thyrotrophin secretion. Acta endocr. (Kbh.) **36**, 319—326 (1961).

ZAIMIS, E.: The reserpine-induced circulatory failure. Nature (Lond.) **192**, 521—523 (1961).

ZBINDEN, G., A. PLETSCHER u. A. STUDER: Regionäre Unterschiede der Reserpinwirkung auf enterochromaffine Zellen und 5-Hydroxytryptamin-Gehalt im Magendarmtrakt. Schweiz. med. Wschr. **87**, 629—630 (1957a).

— — — Hemmung der Reserpin-bedingten 5-Hydroxytryptamin-Freisetzung im enterochromaffinen System durch Isopropyl-isonicotinsäurehydrazid. Klin. Wschr. **33**, 565—567 (1957b).

—, u. A. STUDER: Histochemische Untersuchungen über den Einfluß von Iproniazid (Marsilid) auf die durch Reserpin erzeugte Freisetzung von Adrenalin und Noradrenalin aus dem Nebennierenmark. Experientia (Basel) **14**, 201 (1958).

Chapter 12

Inhibitors of monoamine oxidase and decarboxylase of aromatic amino acids

By

A. PLETSCHER, K. F. GEY and W. P. BURKARD

With 13 Figures

I. Introduction

In recent years it has become evident that pharmacological interference with the metabolism of monoamines might be of therapeutic value in certain diseases. Inhibition of the enzymes responsible for the formation and degradation of biogenic monoamines has been an approach for creating new drugs. So far inhibitors of monoamine oxidase (MAO) and decarboxylase of aromatic L-amino acids (DCA), enzymes involved in the degradation and formation respectively of monoamines, have got therapeutic importance. This development is closely connected with the research on the metabolism of aromatic amines which progresses rapidly.

The first potent inhibitor of MAO used in human therapy was iproniazid. This derivative of hydrazine had originally been developed for the treatment of tuberculosis, but on the basis of clinical observations by KLINE (LOOMER et al. 1958; SAUNDERS et al. 1957) as well as by CESARMAN (CESARMANN 1957) it was introduced in 1957 for the therapy of mental depression and angina pectoris. Contrary to other psychotropic drugs, a biochemical mechanism of iproniazid was already known since ZELLER (ZELLER and BARSKY 1952; ZELLER et al. 1952a; ZELLER et al. 1952b; ZELLER et al. 1952c) had shown in 1952 that the drug potently inhibited MAO. These observations constituted the basis for a rapid development in the field of MAO inhibitors. At present, several MAO inhibitors, hydrazines and nonhydrazines, are in therapeutic use.

With the progressing knowledge of the metabolism of monoamines, attempts have also been made to inhibit their formation. The first inhibitor of DCA introduced in 1962 for the therapy of arterial hypertension was α-methyl-3,4-dihydroxyphenylalanine (α-methyldopa). This compound was shown in 1954 by SOURKES (SOURKES 1954a) to inhibit DCA. This α-alkylated amino acid stimulated further research, although its main effect in hypertension may not be due to inhibition of DCA. Other more potent and specific inhibitors have been developed; none has, however, been introduced in human therapy.

A survey of a fast developing field, such as inhibitors of MAO and DCA, is, of course, rather problematic. The present review is mainly concerned with those inhibitors of MAO and DCA which have a potent effect in vivo. Thereby attempts are made to correlate biochemical and pharmacodynamic effects[1].

[1] The literature was reviewed systematically until October 1962 and partially until July 1964.

II. Monoamine oxidase[1]

A. Biochemistry of the enzyme

Oxidative deamination of primary amines in vivo, in situ, and in vitro has been reported about 80 years ago (EWINS and LAIDLAW 1910/11, 1913; GUGGENHEIM and LÖFFLER 1916; MINKOWSKY 1883; MOSSO 1890; SCHMIEDEBERG 1881). An enzyme responsible for this reaction was first described as tyramine oxidase in 1928 (M. L. C. BERNHEIM 1931; HARE 1928) and subsequently found to correspond to an enzyme oxidizing aliphatic amines and epinephrine (BHAGVAT et al. 1939; BLASCHKO et al. 1937a, 1937b, 1937c; H. I. KOHN 1937; PUGH and QUASTEL 1937a, 1937b; RICHTER 1937). In order to differentiate this enzyme from diamine oxidase (DAO) (EC 1.4.3.6), the term monoamine oxidase (MAO) (ZELLER 1938) has been used. Several reviews on MAO have been published previously (BLASCHKO 1952, 1963; DAVISON 1958c; PLETSCHER et al. 1960c; ZELLER 1942).

1. Reaction formula

Amine oxidases transform the terminal amino-alkyl group of primary or secondary amines into a carbonyl group according to the general equation:

$$R{-}CH_2{-}N^+H_3 + O_2 + H_2O \rightarrow R{-}CHO + N^+H_4 + H_2O_2 \qquad (I)$$

The net balance of this formula has been proved with numerous amines (AEBI 1962; AEBI et al. 1962b; M. L. C. BERNHEIM 1931; CREASEY 1956; FELLMAN 1959a; GOLDSTEIN et al. 1960c; HARE 1928; KOBAYASHI and SCHAYER 1955; H. I. KOHN 1937; KOPIN 1960; KOPIN and AXELROD 1960; LEEPER et al. 1958; LUSCHINSKY and SINGHER 1948; PHILPOT 1937; PUGH and QUASTEL 1937b; RICHTER 1937; WEISSBACH et al. 1957d; ZELLER 1940a).

Since H_2O_2 is decomposed (e.g. by catalase) (CREASEY 1956) to H_2O and $^1/_2\ O_2$, the following overall reaction results:

$$R{-}CH_2{-}N^+H_3 + {}^1/_2\,O_2 \rightarrow R{-}CHO + N^+H_4 \qquad (II)$$

With regard to formula I, amine oxidases belong to the two-electrone transfer oxidases (H. S. MASON 1957a, 1957b):

$$O_2 + 2e^- \rightleftharpoons O_2^{--}\ [= H_2O_2] \qquad (III)$$

Accordingly, amines are probably transformed into imino compounds which undergo immediate hydrolysis (M. L. C. BERNHEIM 1931; BLASCHKO 1952; RICHTER 1937; T. E. SMITH et al. 1962):

$$R{-}CH_2{-}N^+H_3 + O_2 \rightarrow R{-}CH{=}N^+H_2 + H_2O_2 \qquad (IV)$$

$$R{-}CH = N^+H_2 + H_2O \rightarrow R{-}CHO + N^+H_4 \qquad (V)$$

2. Differentiation

Amine oxidases can only in part be classified according to their substrates. Thus, monoamine oxidases deaminate aliphatic and aromatic monoamines as well as some long-chain alkylene diamines, derivatives of ethylene diamine, histamine, etc. On the other hand, diamine oxidases deaminate, besides their typical substrates, i.e. the short-chained diamines, also some monoamines (BLANKSMA 1962; BLASCHKO 1952, 1963; BLASCHKO and DUTHIE 1945b; BLASCHKO and HAWKINS 1950; BLASCHKO and HIMMS 1955; FOUTS 1954; FOUTS et al. 1957; KOBAYASHI 1957; MANN and SMITHIES 1955a, 1955b; SATAKE et al. 1953; ZELLER et al. 1956b, 1957a). Because of this lack of substrate specificity, both classes of amine oxidases can be better distinguished by their inhibitors. Monoamine oxidases are relatively resistant to some carbonyl reagents (e.g. semicarbazide, isoniazid, aminoguanidine) and to cyanide, but are inhibited by octanol. Diamine oxidases are inhibited by the carbonyl reagents mentioned above, but not by octanol (BLASCHKO 1956; BLASCHKO et al. 1959; BURKARD et al. 1962a; DAVISON 1958c; LAZANAS and ZELLER 1958; ZELLER 1956a, 1959; ZELLER et al. 1940, 1958b, 1959).

The group of monamine oxidases consists of the typical monoamine oxidase (MAO) (to which this review mainly refers) and of amphetamine oxidase, whereas the group of diamine oxidases contains the typical diamine oxidase (DAO), spermine or benzylamine oxidase of blood plasma, methylamine oxidase, and mezcaline oxidase (ZELLER et al. 1959).

[1] Official name according to the Enzyme Commission (Int. Union Biochem. 1961): Monoamine: O_2 oxidoreductase (deaminating); EC 1.4.3.4.

3. Substrates

Substrates of the classical MAO have been found among primary and secondary alkyl-, aralkyl-, indolyl-, and imidazolyl-amines (ALLES and HEEGARDS 1943; BARLOW et al. 1955; BARSKY 1958; F. BERNHEIM and M. L. C. BERNHEIM 1938; BEYER 1943; BEYER and MORRISON 1945; BHAGVAT et al. 1939; BLANKSMA 1962; BLASCHKO 1952, 1963; BLASCHKO and CHRUŚCIEL 1959; BLASCHKO and DUTHIE 1945a, b; BLASCHKO and HAWKINS 1950; BLASCHKO et al. 1937a; ERSPAMER et al. 1960a; HEIM 1950a; KANAOKA et al. 1961; KISHI et al. 1957; H. I. KOHN 1937; PUGH and QUASTEL 1937a, 1937b; RANDALL 1946; RANDALL and BAGDON 1958; SNYDER and OBERST 1946; WERLE and ROEWER 1952; ZELLER 1963a; ZELLER et al. 1958b, 1959). The best substrate hitherto known is meta-iodobenzylamine (ZELLER 1963a, b). The relative rate of deamination of some physiological amines by MAO may be approximated as follows (ALLES and HEEGARDS 1943; F. BERNHEIM and M. L. C. BERNHEIM 1938; BLASCHKO 1952; BLASCHKO and PHILPOT 1953; BLASCHKO et al. 1937a; DAVISON 1958b; FREYBURGER et al. 1952; GOVIER et al. 1953; HEEGARD and ALLES 1943; HOPE and SMITH 1960; KALIMAN 1961; KOBAYASHI 1957; KOBAYASHI and SCHAYER 1955; H. I. KOHN 1937; LINDELL and WESTLING 1957; LUSCHINSKY and SINGHER 1948; MANN and QUASTEL 1940; PUGH and QUASTEL 1937a, 1937b; RANDALL 1946; RICHTER 1937; SJOERDSMA et al. 1955; THOMPSON and TICKNER 1951; VANE 1959; WEINER 1960; WEISSBACH et al. 1957d, 1960b; ZELLER et al. 1955a, 1956, 1958b, 1959):

High (100—66%) 3-hydroxytyramine (dopamine), tyramine.

Medium (65—34%) 3-methoxytyramine, tryptamine, 5-hydroxytryptamine (5-HT), isoamylamine (and similar alkylamines).

Low ($<33\%$) metanephrine (3-O-methylepinephrine), normetanephrine (3-O-methylnorepinephrine), epinephrine, norepinephrine (NE), phenylethanolamine, octopamine (4-hydroxyphenylethanolamine), phenylethylamine, kynuramine, N-methylhistamine and in some species also histamine.

This classification is, however, limited by many exceptions, since the extent of deamination varies greatly according to the source of the enzyme (organ, species) and to the method of tissue preparation (ALLES and HEEGARD 1943; BHAGVAT et al. 1939; BLASCHKO and PHILPOT 1953; BLASCHKO et al. 1937a; HOPE and SMITH 1960; LUSCHINSKY and SINGHER 1948; SJOERDSMA et al. 1955; WEINER 1960). With regard to the human brain, for instance, dialyzed total homogenate shows a relative order of substrate deamination similar to that given above, whereas mitochondria oxidize isoamylamine to the greatest extent (WEINER 1960). Tertiary monoamines (e.g. hordenine) are poorly deaminated, quarternary amines not at all. Oxidation of secondary and tertiary monoamines results in the formation of alkylamine instead of ammonia (ALLES and HEEGARDS 1943; F. BERNHEIM and M. L. C. BERNHEIM 1938; BEYER 1943; BLASCHKO et al. 1937a; ERSPAMER et al. 1960a; EWINS and LAIDLAW 1910/11; H. I. KOHN 1937; RANDALL 1946; RICHTER 1937; SNYDER et al. 1946).

Stereospecificity of various MAO preparations has been demonstrated using epinephrine, phenylethanolamine, and tyramine asymmetrically labelled with deuterium. Thereby, the natural R- respectively D(-)-isomeres are preferentially oxidized (BELLEAU and BURBA 1960; BELLEAU and MORAN 1962, 1963; BELLEAU et al. 1960, 1961; BIEL et al. 1959a; BLASCHKO and PRATESI 1959; BLASCHKO et al. 1937b; PRATESI and BLASCHKO 1959; ZELLER et al. 1957c).

4. Tissue distribution

MAO occurs widely in mammalian tissues, which show approximately the following activity of the enzyme (ARMIN et al. 1953; BARLOW 1961; BARSKY 1958; F. BERNHEIM and M. L. C. BERNHEIM 1945; BERNHEIMER et al. 1962; BIRKHÄUSER 1940, 1941; BLASCHKO 1952, 1963; BLASCHKO et al. 1937a, 1937b; BOGDANSKI et al. 1957; BURN and ROBINSON 1952; DAVISON et al. 1957; DAVISON and SANDLER 1956; EPPS 1945; GANROT et al. 1962b; GIARMAN and DAY 1959; HAGEN and WEINER 1959; HOLTZ et al. 1938b; HOPE and SMITH 1960; IISALO 1962; IISALO and PEKKARINEN 1954; KALIMAN 1961; KOELLE 1959; KOELLE and VALK 1954; KRISHNA et al. 1961; LANGEMANN 1944, 1951; LANGEMANN et al. 1943; LEVINE and SJOERDSMA 1962b, 1963a; LOVENBERG et al. 1962a; LUSCHINSKY and SINGHER 1948; D. R. MAXWELL et al. 1961; OTSUKA and KOBAYASHI 1964; PAASONEN 1961a; PAASONEN and KIVALO 1962; PAASONEN et al. 1964; PEKKARINEN et al. 1958; PHILPOT 1937; PLETSCHER et al. 1960c; PUGH and QUASTEL 1937a; RICHTER and TINGEY 1939; J. ROBINSON 1952; SCHAPIRA 1945; SJOERDSMA et al. 1955; SKILLEN et al. 1962; STOCK and WESTERMANN 1962a; STRÖMBLAD 1959a, 1959b; THOMPSON 1952; THOMPSON and TICKNER 1949, 1951; UDENFRIEND et al. 1958b; VANE 1959; WAALKES and COBURN 1958; WEINER 1959; WERLE and MENNICKEN 1938; WERLE and PECHMANN 1948/49; WERLE and ROEWER 1952; WEST 1958a; ZELLER and JOËL 1941; ZELLER et al. 1956b):

High (approx. 1600—400 μl O_2/g tissue/h): liver, sympathetic ganglia, salivary glands, kidney.

Moderate (approx. 400—75 µl O_2/g/h): large arteries, intestine, spleen, lung, skeletal muscle, uterus, brain, iris-ciliary body, optic nerve, adrenal medulla, placenta.

Low (< 75 µl O_2/g/h): heart, extraocular muscle, retina, cornea, lens, pituitary, thyreoidea, pancreas, adipose tissue, testis, blood.

MAO activity of tumors has been found equal to that of the corresponding normal tissue or lower (BIRKHÄUSER 1940; BÜLBRING 1953; DAVISON and SANDLER 1956; HAGEN 1959; LANGEMANN 1944; SARKAR et al. 1960b; STARR et al. 1962).

Marked species differences exist concerning the absolute and relative activity of MAO in various tissues. Men seem to differ from animals by a much higher MAO activity in heart and jejunal mucosa and a relatively lower activity in sympathetic ganglia (GANROT et al. 1962b; LEVINE and SJOERDSMA 1962b; WEINER 1961).

MAO activity within one organ may vary markedly according to the anatomical structure (BLASCHKO 1952; DAVISON 1958c; LANGEMANN 1944). The brain, for instance, shows high activity in the hypothalamus, thalamus, several parts of the limbic system, the caudate nucleus, mesencephalon, pons, and about three times lower values in the cortex, subcortex and cerebellum. Furthermore, MAO is present in nerve cells and capillary walls, but not in glial cells or nerve fibers. This has been shown biochemically (APRISON et al. 1964; BERNHEIMER and HORNYKIEWICZ 1962; BIRKHÄUSER 1940, 1941; BOGDANSKI et al. 1957; GANROT et al. 1962b; LEVINE and SJOERDSMA 1962a; WEINER 1961) and by histochemical techniques (ARIOKA and TANIMUKAI 1957; ARVY 1960, 1961; BLASCHKO and HELLMANN 1953; EDER 1957; FRANCIS 1953; GLENNER et al. 1957; KOELLE and VALK 1954; MICHOTTE and DE VAHIA 1958; MUSTAKALLIO et al. 1961; SHIMUZU et al. 1959; B. SMITH 1962; YASUDA 1962; WATARI 1958; WATTENBERG 1959; WOHLRAB 1960, 1961).

Within the cell, MAO is predominantly (up to 75%) bound to the particulate fraction, mainly to mitochondria, whereas the remainder is contained in the microsomal fraction (BARSKY 1958; BAUDHIN et al. 1964; COTZIAS and DOLE 1951b; DUVE et al. 1960; HAWKINS 1952a; LORES ARNAIZ et al. 1962; OSWALD and STRITTMATTER 1963; WEINER 1959, 1961; ZELLER et al. 1955a). In certain tissues (e.g. guinea pig liver), some MAO has also been found in the supernatant (BLASCHKO and DUTHIE 1945a; WEISSBACH et al. 1957d), but this might result from lytic changes of the mitochondria (OSWALD and STRITTMATTER 1963). The particulate bound MAO seems to be a true mitochondrial enzyme and not related to synaptic membranes or vesicles of nerve endings (LORES ARNAIZ et al. 1962).

5. Purification and properties

The enzyme shows great stability at a physiological pH if bound to mitochondria (ALLES and HEEGARDS 1943; BLASCHKO et al. 1937b; DAVISON 1958c; GIORDANO et al. 1960a; WESTLEY and SEIDEN 1962). The latter can be solubilized to some extent (BARSKY 1958; BLASCHKO 1952; COQ and BARON 1964; COTZIAS et al. 1954; GORKIN et al. 1963; KOBAYASHI and SCHAYER 1955; SAKOMOTO et al. 1963; SOURKES and LAGNADO 1957a, 1957b; SOURKES et al. 1955; VEREVKINA et al. 1964; WERLE and HENNIG 1960; WESTLEY and SEIDEN 1962; ZELLER et al. 1955a, 1958b; ZILE and LARDY 1959). Complete disorganization of the mitochondria, however, inactivates MAO. Therefore, purification has not increased the activity of the mitochondrial enzyme by more than a factor 20 to 300 (ALLES and HEEGARDS 1943; BARBATO and ABOOD 1963; BLASCHKO et al. 1937b; BORN et al. 1958; GANROT and ROSENGREN 1962; GORKIN 1959; HARE 1928; E. S. HARRIS 1960; SAKOMOTO et al. 1963; SEIDEN and WESTLEY 1962; WEISSBACH et al. 1957d; WESTLEY and SEIDEN 1962).

It has not been ascertained whether MAO is homogenous or heterogenous. The fact that deamination is not additive if several substrates are present simulataneously (BLASCHKO 1952; BLASCHKO et al. 1937a; KOBAYASHI and SCHAYER 1955; H. I. KOHN 1937; PUGH and QUASTEL 1937b) may be an argument in favour of homogeneity. Marked species- and organ-dependent differences in the substrate pattern of MAO as well as other kinetic observations, however, indicate that MAO can be separated into various types each with preference for special substrates (homologuous enzymes or isoenzymes). Thereby, it has not been distinguished wether various specific monoamine oxidases are associated in different proportions or whether different protein moieties cause various degrees of steric hindrance of the hydrocarbon residue of certain substrates. (ALLES and HEEGARD 1943; BARBATO and ABOOD 1963; BARLOW 1961; F. BERNHEIM and M. L. C. BERNHEIM 1938; BLANKSMA 1962; CHODERA et al. 1964; GORKIN 1963, 1964b; HAGEN 1959; HAGEN and WEINER 1959; HARDEGG 1961; HARDEGG and HEILBRONN 1961; HOPE and SMITH 1960; LONG 1962a, 1962b; MCCARMAN 1961; OSWALD and STRITTMATTER 1963; RANDALL 1946; SARKAR and ZELLER 1961; SARKAR et al. 1960b; SATAKE 1955; WEINER 1960; WERLE and ROEWER 1952; ZELLER 1961, 1963a, 1963b, 1963d; ZELLER and FOUTS 1963). Recently, fractionation of liver mitochondria succeeded in a partial separation of at least two different monoamine oxidases (GORKIN 1963, pers. comm.).

The activity of MAO increases with oxygen tension (AEBI et al. 1962b; F. BERNHEIM and M. L. C. BERNHEIM 1938, 1945; IISALO and PEKKARINEN 1958; H. I. KOHN 1937; NOVICK 1961a, 1961b; PHILPOT 1937) and depends also on the functional state of mitochondria. Thus, swollen mitochondria of liver with impairment of pyruvate oxidation and of oxidative phosphorylation were found to have a higher activity of the enzyme than intact mitochondria (AEBI 1962; AEBI et al. 1963). This may be related to the finding that high concentrations of 5'(pyro)-triphosphate of adenosine (ATP) or adenosinemonophosphate inhibit MAO (STÜTTGEN et al. 1961).

Optimal substrate concentrations are of the order of 10^{-2} to 10^{-3} M (BLASCHKO et al. 1937a; COTZIAS and DOLE 1951a; HOPE and SMITH 1960; KOBAYASHI and SCHAYER 1955; H.I. KOHN 1937; LAGNADO and SOURKES 1956b; WEISSBACH et al. 1957d). With a MICHAELIS-MENTON constant of about 10^{-3} for tyramine and 5-HT (DAVISON 1957; A. L. GREEN 1964; OSWALD and STRITTMATTER 1963; ZELLER 1963a), MAO has a moderate substrate affinity.

The optimal pH varies markedly according to the source, purity and pretreatment of the preparation as well as to the substrate (ALLES and HEEGARD 1943; M. L. C. BERNHEIM 1931; BLASCHKO et al. 1937b; HARE 1928; E. S. HARRIS 1960; HOPE and SMITH 1960; WERLE and MENNICKEN 1938; YOUDIM and SOURKES 1964). Washed mitochondria, for instance, show maximal deamination of tyramine at pH = 7.2—7.3 (MALAFAYA-BAPTISTA et al. 1957), but of 5-HT at pH = 8.1 or even higher (HOPE and SMITH 1960; HORITA 1962a; WEISSBACH et al. 1957d). The redox potential of MAO seems to range between —0.23 and +0.195 V (PHILPOT 1937; PLETSCHER et al. 1960c).

MAO requires free sulfhydril groups (AGIN 1959; BARBATO and ABOOD 1963; FRIEDENWALD and HERRMANN 1942; LAGNADO and SOURKES 1956b, 1956c; MANUKHIN 1958; OKUMURA 1960; SINGER and BARBON 1945), whereas dialyzable cofactors could not be detected (BLASCHKO et al. 1937b; PUGH and QUASTEL 1937b). The hypothesis that MAO is a flavoprotein remains to be proven, but deficiency of riboflavine might decrease the de novo synthesis of this enzyme (ALLEGRETTI and VUKADINOVIČ 1950; BELLEAU and MORAN 1963; BERNSOHN and LOZAITYTE 1958; HAWKINS 1952b; LAGNADO 1958; LAGNADO and SOURKES 1956a, 1956c, 1958; SOURKES 1958; SOURKES and D'IORIO 1963; WISEMAN and SOURKES 1961; WISEMAN-DISTLER and SOURKES 1963; YOUDIM and SOURKES 1964). The involvement of pyridoxal-5'-phosphate is unlikely (BERNSOHN and LOZAITYTE 1958; LAGNADO 1958; PHILLIPS et al. 1962). MAO might be a copper enzyme, because chelating agents (e.g. ethylenediaminetetraacetic acid, 8-hydroxyquinoline, o-phenanthroline) have been found by some investigators to induce an inhibition partially reversible by bivalent cations. The latter may be without action or even inhibit the enzyme (BARBATO and ABOOD 1963; GORKIN 1959; A. L. GREEN 1964; LAGNADO and SOURKES 1956b; OGAWA and KUROSAWA 1963; OKUMURA 1960).

MAO resists inactivation by cyanide, arsenite, CO, hydrazine, semicarbazide, isoniazide, hydroxylamine, monoiodoacetate, thiourea, fluoride, malonate, etc. (BARSKY 1958; M. L. C. BERNHEIM 1931; BLASCHKO 1952; BLASCHKO et al. 1937b; CREASEY 1956; M. L. C. HARE 1928; E. S. HARRIS 1960; H. I. KOHN 1937; OKUMURA 1960; PHILPOT 1937; PUGH and QUASTEL 1937b; WERLE and MENNICKEN 1938).

6. Active center and reaction mechanism

Comparisons of optically active substrates (BELLEAU and MORAN 1963; see also above) and inhibitors (BERNSTEIN et al. 1959; BIEL et al. 1959a; BLASCHKO and PRATESI 1959; BLASCHKO and STRÖMBLAD 1960; GRANA and LILLA 1959; HOPE and SMITH 1960; OZAKI et al. 1960; PLETSCHER and GEY 1958b; PRATESI and BLASCHKO 1959; R. E. TEDESCHI et al. 1959b) indicate that MAO shows absolute R-stereospecificity. It might be assumed that at first the amino group of the substrate and its α-carbon (respectively the polarizable C=N bond) is firmly attached to the active site of MAO. If the properties of the bound compound allow an electrophilic attack on the amino group, an α-CH bond is presumably weakened. In consequence, an α-hydrogen might form a long and weak bond with a special acceptor of the enzyme which subsequently splits off this α-hydrogen in the form of a proton or radical. The second α-hydrogen is certainly of importance for oxidation of the substrate, but presumably not for its binding, since substitution (e.g. alkylation in amphetamine or phenylcypromine) produces inhibitors which are not deaminated by MAO. The β-hydrogen is also of importance for the oxidation of the substrate, possibly because in the transition state the α,β-carbon-carbon bond of the substrate acquires a double bond character. Thereby, the α- and β-carbons might approach the trigonal state (BARSKY 1958; BARSKY et al. 1959; BELLEAU and BURBA 1960; BELLEAU and MORAN 1962, 1963; BELLEAU et al. 1960, 1961; DAVISON 1957; FOUTS et al. 1957; MCGRATH and HORITA 1962; SARKAR et al. 1960a; T. E. SMITH et al. 1962; ZELLER 1963d; ZELLER and SARKAR 1960, 1962; ZELLER et al. 1957a, 1958a, 1959, 1960, 1962;

ZIRKLE et al. 1962). The structure of the hydrocarbon residue of substrates (and inhibitors) seems also to determine whether an amine is either attached to the active center without subsequent deamination (dystopic complex) or attached as well as degradated (eutopic complex) (ZELLER 1963a, 1963b). Such changes in structure might cause steric hindrance, i.e. affect the interaction of the hydrocarbon residue with nonspecific sites of the active center. Thus, the hydrocarbon residue of substrates (and inhibitors) might be bound to the enzyme by VAN DER WAALS forces (SARKAR et al. 1960a; ZELLER 1960; ZELLER and SARKAR 1962; ZELLER et al. 1960; ZIRKLE et al. 1962). Thereby, these forces possibly operate maximally if the substrates (and inhibitors respectively) were able to approach planarity when attached to the complementary surface of the MAO center (ZIRKLE et al. 1962).

7. Determination

Direct measurement of MAO activity *in vitro* is carried out in total homogenates or preferentially in the mitochondrial fraction (BLASCHKO 1952; CREASEY 1956; DAVISON 1958c; GEY and PLETSCHER 1961b; GIORDANO et al. 1960a). Various principles may be used (PLETSCHER et al. 1960c; SOEP 1962):

a) Disappearance of substrate

by biological (GADDUM 1959; HOLTZ et al. 1938b; WERLE and MENNICKEN 1938), spectrophotometrical (HORITA 1958b, 1959; NACHMIAS 1960; SJOERDSMA et al. 1955; SOEP 1962; SOURKES et al. 1955; UDENFRIEND et al. 1958a; WEISSBACH et al. 1960b; ZILE and LARDY 1959), and spectrophotofluorometrical methods (BOGDANSKI et al. 1956; HORITA 1959; KUNTZMAN et al. 1961b; OZAKI et al. 1960; SJOERDSMA et al. 1955; WEISSBACH et al. 1960b; ZILE and LARDY 1959).

b) Reduction of electrone acceptors

(e.g. tetrazolium salts) due to amine dehydrogenation or aldehyde oxidation (A. L. GREEN and HAUGHTON 1960; LAGNADO and SOURKES 1956a, 1956c; PLETSCHER et al. 1960c; SOURKES 1958; SOURKES and LAGNADO 1957a, 1957b; WEISSBACH et al. 1957c).

c) Oxygen consumption

provided that unspecific oxygen uptake is prevented (BARSKY 1958; M. L. C. BERNHEIM 1931; BEYER 1943; BLASCHKO 1952; BLASCHKO et al. 1937a; COTZIAS and GREENOUGH 1958, 1959; CREASEY 1956; DAVISON 1957, 1958c; GEY and PLETSCHER 1961b; GIORDANO et al. 1960a; A. L. GREEN 1962; HARDEGG and HEILBRONN 1961; HORITA 1962a; KOBAYASHI and SCHAYER 1955; H. I. KOHN 1937; LUSCHINSKY and SINGHER 1948; PUGH and QUASTEL 1937b; UDENFRIEND et al. 1953; ZELLER et al. 1955a).

d) Ammonia formation

(COTZIAS and DOLE 1951a, 1951b, 1952; COTZIAS and GREENOUGH 1958, 1959; CONWAY 1957; H. I. KOHN 1937; LUSCHINSKY and SINGHER 1948; RICHTER 1937; SOEP 1962; ZELLER 1940b; ZELLER et al. 1962).

e) Peroxyde formation

(AEBI 1962; AEBI et al. 1962a, 1962b; M. L. C. HARE 1928; HEIM 1950b; H. I. KOHN 1937; PHILPOT 1937; PUGH and QUASTEL 1937b; ZELLER 1940a, 1941b).

f) Formation of aldehyde

directly by spectrophotometry (BRUSOVA et al. 1963; GORKIN et al. 1963, 1964a; TABOR et al. 1955; ZELLER 1964), extraction (McCAMAN 1961; OTSUKA and KOBAYASHI 1964), or trapping of the aldehyde (A. L. GREEN 1962; A. L. GREEN and HAUGHTON 1960, 1961; I. J. STERN et al. 1961); indirectly by reduction of diphosphopyridine nucleotide (DPN) in the presence of aldehyde dehydrogenase (LOVENBERG et al. 1961, 1962a; WEISSBACH et al. 1957d).

g) Accumulation of a carboxylic acid

(e.g. indolacetic acid) subsequent to aldehyde formation (e.g. from tryptamine) (LEVINE and SJOERDSMA 1962b, 1963b; LOVENBERG et al. 1961, 1962a; WURTMAN and AXELROD 1963a).

h) Formation of dark pigments

e.g. from 5-HT (SWETT et al. 1963; WYKES et al. 1959; ZELLER et al. 1962).

The methods mostly used are manometry as well as extraction and spectrophotofluorometric determination of 5-HT. An elegant procedure consists in direct spectrophotometric measurement of kynuramine deamination (SOEP 1962; WEISSBACH et al. 1960b). Each method has principal or technical advantages and disadvantages; in consequence, measurements with more than one procedure are desirable.

Indirect estimation of decreased MAO activity *in vivo* may be carried out according to the following principles:

— Enhancement of the monoamine increase in several tissues (especially in brain) subsequent to injection of the corresponding aromatic amino acid, e.g. the 5-HT accumulation induced by 5-hydroxytryptophan (5-HTP) (GEY and PLETSCHER 1960a; HESS et al 1959c; UDENFRIEND et al. 1957a, 1957d);

— Enhancement of monoamine accumulation in extracerebral tissues (e.g. heart) following injection of monoamines metabolized mainly by MAO, e.g. 5-HT, tryptamine (HESS et al. 1959b; PLETSCHER and GEY 1961a; PLETSCHER et al. 1960a, 1960c; WEISSBACH et al. 1959, 1961a);

— Increased urinary elimination of exogenous or endogenous monoamines preferentially metabolized by MAO, e.g. tyramine, tryptamine, etc. (JEPSON et al. 1960; LEVINE and SJOERDSMA 1963a, 1963b; OATES and ZALTZMAN 1959; RESNICK et al. 1960b; SCHAYER 1953b; SCHAYER et al. 1954; SJOERDSMA et al. 1959a, 1959c, 1959d, 1960a; TABOR et al. 1954; D. H. TEDESCHI et al. 1959b; UDENFRIEND 1959a);

— Increase of endogenous monoamines in tissues (especially brain) and urine, e.g. phenylethylamine, meta-tyramine, 3-hydroxyethanolamine, tryptamine, 5-HT (CREDNER et al. 1962; E. J. DAVIS and ROPP 1960; JEPSON et al. 1960; OATES and ZALTZMAN 1959; PLETSCHER et al. 1960c; SJOERDSMA et al. 1959b, 1959c, 1959d; S. SPECTOR et al. 1958b; UDENFRIEND et al. 1957d);

— Decrease of metabolites of endogenous monoamines in tissues (brain, etc.) and urine, e.g. of 5-hydroxyindoleacetic acid and phenolcarbonic acids (J. A. ANDERSON et al. 1958; CARLSSON and HILLARP 1962; CORNE and GRAHAM 1957; HESS et al. 1959c; JEPSON et al. 1960; LEVINE and SJOERDSMA 1963b; MCISAAC and PAGE 1959; NAKAI 1958; ROOS 1962; ROSENGREN 1960b; SJOERDSMA et al. 1958, 1959a, 1960a; STUDNITZ 1959a; TABACHNIK and RUBIN 1959; TABOR et al. 1960; D. H. TEDESCHI et al. 1959b; TICKNER 1951; WEISSBACH et al. 1958).

8. Physiological role

MAO seems to inactivate the monoamines released from a pool with a slow turnover which presumably represents the major part of the stored and thus of the total monoamines in tissues, such as heart and brain. Monoamines belonging to a pool with a fast turnover, however, undergo O-methylation prior to oxidative deamination. This is also true for exogenous catecholamines which are mainly metabolized in the liver. Alternative routes for the metabolism of monoamines (including O-methylated catecholamines) are the conjugation with sulfuric or glucuronic acid and the formation of N-derivatives (AXELROD 1959b; CARLSSON and WALDECK 1963; CHIDSEY and HARRISON 1963; CROUT et al. 1960, 1961; DAVISON 1958c; DAY and GREEN 1962b; GEY and PLETSCHER 1960c; N. D. GOLDBERG and SHIDEMAN 1962; H. GREEN 1962; HERTTING and AXELROD 1961; HERTTING and LABROSSE 1962; HERTTING et al. 1962; HORITA 1962a; IISALO 1962; KEGLEVIĆ et al. 1959; KOPIN 1964; KOPIN and GORDON 1963; KOPIN et al. 1961, 1962; LABROSSE et al. 1961; MCGOODALL et al. 1959; MCISAAC and PAGE 1959; MASAMI et al. 1962; PLETSCHER et al. 1960c; POTTER and AXELROD 1963; ROSENGREN 1960b; SCHAEPDRYVER and KIRSHNER 1960, 1961a; SHORE 1962; UDENFRIEND 1959b; WEINER 1964; WHITBY et al. 1961).

The products of oxidative deamination, e.g. the aldehydes and the corresponding alcohols and carboxylic acids, may have physiological effects of their own. H_2O_2, also formed in this reaction, is either decomposed by catalase or used for oxidations, e.g. of formate (AEBI et al. 1962a). The role of ammonia split off by MAO has not been investigated.

MAO activity, at least as measured in vitro, is very high in comparison to the normal content and turnover of monoamines in the organs (GEY and PLETSCHER 1961b; RICHTER et al. 1941). Therefore, it seems doubtful whether the activity of MAO controls the total monoamine content under physiological conditions. This doubt is supported by the following facts: The monoamine content in brain and other tissues does not parallel the activity of MAO but rather that of other enzymes, e.g. DCA (BERTLER and ROSENGREN 1959b; BOGDANSKI et al. 1957; DALGLIESH and DUTTON 1947; KÄRKI et al. 1962; KLINGMAN et al. 1964; KUNTZMAN et al. 1961b; SANDLER and WEST 1958; WEST 1958a); monoamines accumulate in brain and other tissues only after extensive (at least 85%) MAO inhibition (CHESSIN et al. 1959; DUBNICK et al. 1962b; GEY and PLETSCHER 1959a, 1961b, 1961c; H. GREEN and ERICKSON 1962; WURTMAN and AXELROD 1963b) (Fig. 4).

Variations of MAO activity have been found in different organs, e.g. with age (BIRKHÄUSER 1940; BURKARD et al. 1961; EPPS 1945; GEY et al. 1964; NACHMIAS 1960; NOVICK

1961a; SCHWEPPE et al. 1951; ZELLER 1962; ZELLER et al. 1940), with regard to different sexes after thyroxine administration (NOVICK 1961a, 1961b; SKILLEN et al. 1961; ZELLER 1959; ZILE 1960; ZILE and LARDY 1959), by deficiency of thiamine (BAL and DREWES 1961; MELTZER 1961a), or pyridoxine (PHILLIPS et al. 1962); by sleep depreviation (NIKAIDO 1961), thyreoidectomy (ZELLER 1959), sexual steroids (PAVLIN and ŽUPANČIČ 1956; WURTMAN and AXELROD 1963b), anaphylactic shock (ARAI 1963), toxemia of pregnancy (LINDBERG and WESTLING 1962; LUSCHINSKY 1950; SANDLER and COVENEY 1962). It has not been ascertained whether these variations are related to still unknown activation/inhibition mechanisms or to changes in enzyme synthesis. The latter is possible since the half-life time of the enzyme appears to be less than 3 days (ZELLER 1964).

B. Monoamine oxidase inhibitors[1]

1. Chemical classification

MAO is inhibited by numerous compounds which belong to various chemical classes and show different pharmacological actions, e.g. central stimulation, sedation, anesthetic, anticonvulsive, and antihistaminic properties. Most inhibitors act only in vitro; compounds active in vivo, however, must not necessarily affect the enzyme in vitro. The following substances have been shown to inhibit MAO:

Alcohols and aldehydes, e.g. octanol, thymol, but also ethanol and acetaldehyde (BLASCHKO et al. 1937a, 1937b, 1937c; COTZIAS and GREENOUGH 1960; FOUTS et al. 1957; HEIM 1947, 1950b; HOLTZ et al. 1938a; MAYNARD and SCHENKER 1962; ROSENFELD 1960; TOWNE 1964; USDIN and USDIN 1961; WARTBURG and AEBI 1960; WERLE and MENNICKEN 1938; ZELLER 1959; ZELLER et al. 1958b). Alcohols are typical MAO inhibitors not affecting DAO.

α-Alkylated aralkylamines, e.g. amphetamine, ephedrine (BHAGVAT et al. 1939; BLASCHKO 1938, 1940; BLASCHKO and STRÖMBLAD 1960; B. G. BROWN and HEY 1956; EULER and HELLNER-BJÖRKMAN 1955; FELDSTEIN et al. 1959; FELLOWS and BERNHEIM 1950; FUJIMURA and OHATA 1958; A. L. GREEN 1964; HAUSCHILD 1941; HEEGARD and ALLES 1943; HEIM 1947; IISALO 1962; MAASS and NIMMO 1959; MANN and QUASTEL 1939, 1940; MCCOUBREY 1959; ORZECHOWSKI 1941; OZAKI et al. 1960; PARMAR and NICKERSON 1961; PHILPOT 1940; PLETSCHER and GEY 1959; PRATESI and BLASCHKO 1959; RICHTER and TINGEY 1939; SNYDER and OBERST 1946; SYMUL 1947, 1957; VINCENT and SEGONZAC 1960), *α-alkylated indolyl alkylamines*, e.g. α-methyltryptamine and its N-methylderivative, α-ethyltryptamine, and *tertiary N-alkyl derivatives*, e.g. hordenine and N-dimethylaminoethylindol (BARLOW 1961; FRETER et al. 1958; GOVIER et al. 1953; GREIG and GIBBONS 1962; GREIG et al. 1959, 1961a, 1961b; HESTER et al. 1964; HUSZTI and BORSY 1964; METER et al. 1960; PFEIFER et al. 1961; SATORY et al. 1961; D. H. TEDESCHI et al. 1962; VANE 1959; VINCENT and SEGONZAC 1960; WOOLLEY and EDELMAN 1958). These compounds presumably have a high affinity for MAO, but they can hardly be deaminated because of the α-alkyl residue (BEYER 1943, 1946; BEYER and MORRISON 1945; BEYER and SHAPIRO 1945; BLASCHKO and HAWKINS 1950; BLASCHKO et al. 1937a; K. K. CHEN et al. 1929; S. C. HARRIS et al. 1947; HEEGARD and ALLES 1943; RICHTER 1938; SNYDER et al. 1946; SORIANO 1958). In vivo, short and weak MAO inhibition has been demonstrated for α-alkylated aralkylamines (PLETSCHER and GEY 1959) and α-alkylated indolylalkylamines mainly by indirect procedures (GEY and PLETSCHER 1962; GREIG and GIBBONS 1962; GREIG et al. 1959, 1961a, 1961b; HESTER et al. 1964; LESSIN 1959a). It is, however, doubtful whether MAO inhibition is of importance for the pharmacological action of these compounds (GEY and PLETSCHER 1962; GRANA and

[1] This topic has been reviewed several times (BIEL et al. 1964; BLASCHKO 1963; PLETSCHER et al. 1960c; PSCHEIDT 1964; SOURKES and D'IORIO 1963; ZELLER 1963d; ZELLER and FOUTS 1963; ZIRKLE and KAISER 1964).

LILLA 1959; GREIG and GIBBONS 1962; McGEER et al. 1960; PARKES et al. 1962a, 1962b; SCHOOT et al. 1962). These α-alkylated compounds are rapidly excreted in the urine; their metabolism includes hydroxylation, conjugation, and deamination (AXELROD 1954, 1959c; BEYER and SKINNER 1940; EBERTS 1961; EBERTS and DANIELS 1962; PINSON et al. 1961b, 1962a; SZARA 1961).

Aryl ethers of choline, e.g. para-tolyl choline ether (BARSKY 1958; B. G. BROWN and HEY 1952, 1956; CORNE and GRAHAM 1957; KOBAYASHI and SCHAYER 1955; OZAKI et al. 1960; SCHAYER et al. 1955; USDIN and USDIN 1961). In vitro they cause moderate competitive inhibition of MAO. In vivo they inhibit the enzyme in intestine (DAVISON 1957; SCHAYER et al. 1954), but not in brain and liver (CORNE and GRAHAM 1957; EULER and HELLNER-BJÖRKMAN 1955; PLETSCHER and GEY 1959); they also reduce the oxidation of some exogenous monoamines (GRIESEMER and WELLS 1956; SCHAYER 1953b; SCHAYER et al. 1954, 1955).

Harmane derivatives, e.g. harmaline (OZAKI et al. 1960; PLETSCHER and GEY 1959; PLETSCHER et al. 1959a; SJOERDSMA et al. 1959a; TAYLOR et al. 1960a; TUNG 1960b; TUNG et al. 1960a; UDENFRIEND et al. 1958b; VINCENT and SEGONZAC 1960). These are strong and reversible MAO inhibitors in vitro (TUNG et al. 1960a). In vivo they cause MAO inhibition of short duration, i.e. of a few hours (PLETSCHER et al. 1959a; UDENFRIEND et al. 1958b). Hydrogenation to tetrahydroharmine, dealkylation (e.g. to harmol) or methylation of the pyridine ring reduces MAO inhibition. Harmaline is metabolized to harmine, harmalol, and harminic acid (FLURY 1911).

N-Alkyl tertiary and quarternary nitrogen derivatives and carbonium compounds, e.g. neostigmine, pyridine-aldoxime dodecyliodide and bretylium. They may induce strong, in some cases irreversible MAO inhibition in vitro, but no or only moderate inhibition in vivo (DVORNIK et al. 1963; KUNTZMAN and JACOBSON 1963; MELTZER 1961a, 1961b, 1962; PANT et al. 1964a, 1964b; USDIN and USDIN 1961; VINCENT et al. 1962).

Aralkylguanidines, mono- and polyamidines (e.g. pentamidine), *stilbamidines, biguanides, mono- and dithiourea derivatives* (AXELROD 1957; F. BERNHEIM 1943; BLASCHKO and DUTHIE 1945a, 1945b; BLASCHKO and HIMMS 1955; CHRUŚCIEL 1962; DAVISON 1958b; DVORNIK et al. 1963; FASTIER and HAWKINS 1951; GESSA et al. 1962c; KADZIELAWA 1962; KUNTZMAN and JACOBSON 1963a, 1963b; M. MEYER 1960; SCHULER and MEYER 1955). Guanidine derivatives are strong but reversible and competitive inhibitors with weak action in vivo (DVORNIK et al. 1963; KUNTZMAN and JACOBSON 1963a, 1963b). The other compounds have an irreversible, but moderate action in vitro. In vivo pentamidine inhibits MAO in liver, but not in brain (BAXTER and ROBERTS 1958; DAVISON 1958a; PLETSCHER and GEY 1959).

Methylene blue (EHRINGER et al. 1961; GOVIER et al. 1946; IMAIZUMI et al. 1959; JAKUBOVIČ and NEČINA 1963; PHILPOT 1937, 1940; THOMPSON and TICKNER 1951; WERLE and ROEWER 1952). Its action in vitro is moderate, in vivo short and incomplete.

Myristicin, a terpene-like nitrogen-free compound, seems to inhibit MAO moderately in vivo (TRUITT et al. 1963).

Other substances. Quite a number of compounds have been described to inhibit MAO in vitro, e.g. derivatives of *aminoalkane* (BLASCHKO 1952; HEEGARD and ALLES 1943), *dialkylamino alkyl derivatives* (BOSE and VIJAYVARGYA 1960; BROWN and HEY 1956; ERNSTING et al. 1962; HEIM 1950a, 1950b; IMAIZUMI et al. 1959; ORZECHOWSKI 1941; OZAKI et al. 1960; PHILPOT 1940; PLETSCHER and GEY 1959; POLONOVSKI et al. 1953; SCHAUMANN and KURBJUWEIT 1961; SCHULER and WIEDEMANN 1935; SJOERDSMA et al. 1959a; TICKNER 1951; USDIN and

USDIN 1961; VITEK and RYSANEK 1960), *urea* (BHAGVAT et al. 1939; GIORDANO et al. 1962; HEIM 1947; MANUKHIN 1958; PHILPOT 1937; ZELLER 1941 a), *urethane* (BLASCHKO et al. 1937 b; KOHN 1937), *carbon disulfide* (MAGISTRETTI and PEIRONE 1961), and possibly *azides* (OKUMURA 1960; WERLE and MENNICKEN 1938; WERLE and ROEWER 1952); *hydroquinone* and *polyphenols* (A. L. GREEN 1964); derivatives of *pyridine* (NANTKA-NAMIRSKI et al. 1963), of *piperidine* (SZPORNY and GÖRÖG 1961; VINCENT and SEGONZAC 1960; WERLE and PECHMANN 1948/49), of *piperazine* (USDIN and USDIN 1961), of *isoquinoline* (USDIN and USDIN 1961), of *indazole* (MINATOYA 1963), of *carbazol* (OZAKI et al. 1960), of *carboline* (NANTKA-NAMIRSKI et al. 1963; OZAKI et al. 1960), of *oxazine* (McCOLL and RICE 1960;

Table 1. *MAO inhibitors with long duration of action in vivo*

Chemical class	Examples
a) Hydrazine derivatives	Iproniazid (Marsilid) 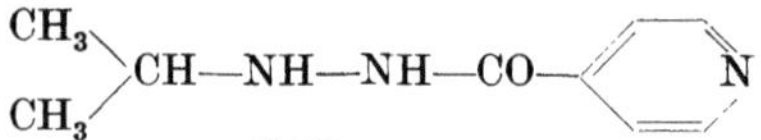 Phenelzine (Nardil) 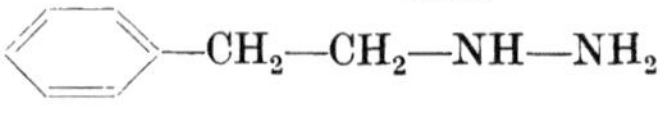
b) Arylcycloalkylamines	Tranylcypromine (Parnate) 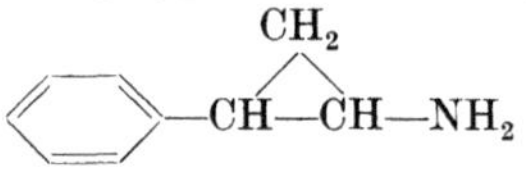
c) N-Benzyl-N-methyl-propargylamine	Pargyline (Eutonyl) 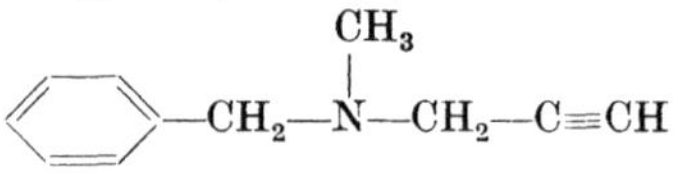
d) 2-Methyl-3-piperidinopyrazine	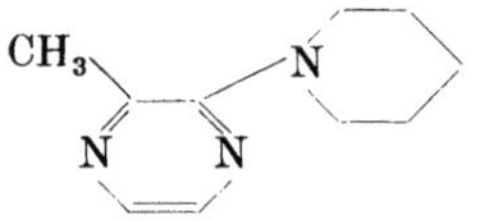

F. A. SMITH et al. 1961; USDIN and USDIN 1961), of *1:2:4-triazol* (JACKSON et al. 1962), of *tetrazole* (USDIN and USDIN 1961); *phenanthroline* (BARBATO and ABOOD 1961), *proflavine* (GORKIN et al. 1964 b), *xanthines* (CAHN 1960; VINCENT and SEGONZAC 1960; ZELLER 1941 a), *quinine* and *quinidine* (IIDA 1958; VINCENT and SEGONZAC 1960), *nicotine* (WERLE and PECHMANN 1948/49; WERLE and PESCHEL 1949), *chlortetracycline* (OKUDA and OKADA 1956), *alkaloids of Ergot* (HEIM 1947) and *Rauwolfia* (BOSE and VIJAYVARGYA 1960), *hydrazinophthalazines* (KUBIKOWSKI and WYSOKOWSKI 1963; PERRY et al. 1955; SCHULER and MEYER 1955; WERLE et al. 1955), *phenothiazines* and *similar compounds* (BOSE and VIJAYVARGYA 1960; GEY and PLETSCHER 1961 a; GORKIN 1959; JACOBI et al. 1961; KIVALO et al. 1961; NAKAJIMA 1959 b; OZAKI et al. 1960; D. SCHWARTZ et al. 1963; USDIN and USDIN 1961), *atebrine* (ALLEGRETTI and VUKADINOVIČ 1950; LAGNADO and SOURKES 1956 a; YODIM and SOURKES 1964), and various *unidentified compounds* (FRIEDENWALD and HERRMANN 1942; ZELLER 1941 a). As far as investigated, these substances have in general no or only little effect on MAO in vivo.

The present review is mainly concerned with irreversible (long acting) MAO inhibitors which have a strong effect in vivo and which may be used in the therapy of human disease. The following four types of compounds belong into this category (Table 1).

a) Hydrazine derivatives

with the general formula

$$R—NH—NH—R'$$

In order to get activity in vitro, at least one hydrogen of the hydrazine moiety has to remain free (Barsky et al. 1959; Davison 1957; McGrath and Horita 1962; Zeller and Sarkar 1962; Zeller et al. 1955a, 1955b) and one residue (R) must be an alkyl- or aralkyl group, whereas R′ may represent H, an alkyl, aralkyl, or acyl residue. Corresponding hydroxylamines are no MAO inhibitors (Major and Ohly 1961). Iproniazid is the first compound of this group which has been shown by E. A. Zeller, 1952, to inhibit MAO in vitro and in vivo[1] (Barsky et al. 1959; Zeller and Barsky 1952; Zeller et al. 1952a, 1952c). The following MAO inhibitors have mainly been used in human therapy (Crowther et al. 1962; Jenni and Pletscher 1962):

N[1]-isonicotinoyl-N[2]-isopropylhydrazine

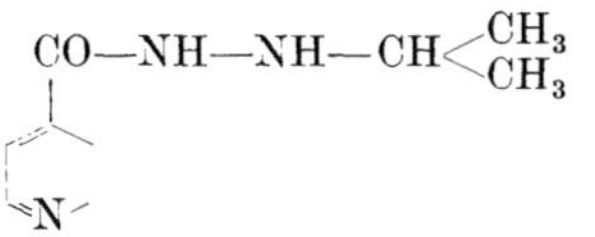

Iproniazid (Marsilid)

N[1]-(5-methyl-3-isoxazolylcarbonyl)-N[2]-benzylhydrazine

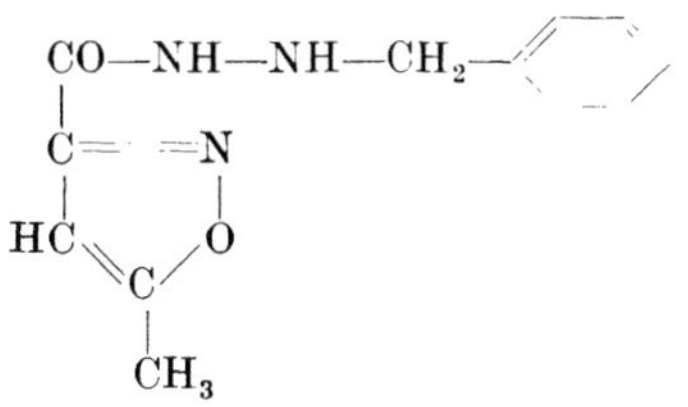

Isocarboxazid (Marplan)

N[1]-isonicotinoyl-N[2]-[β-(N-benzylcarbamoyl)-ethyl]-hydrazine

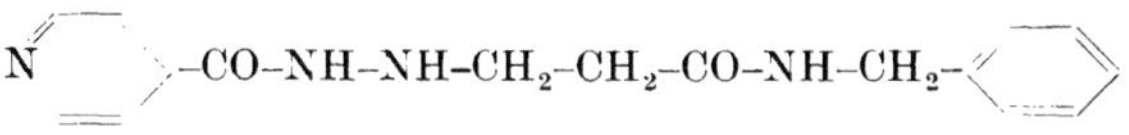

Nialamide (Niamid)

N[1]-pivaloyl-N[2]-benzylhydrazine

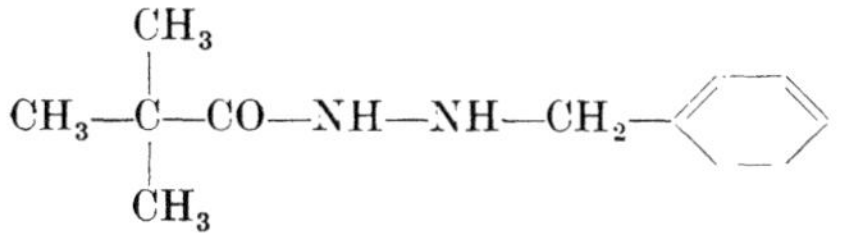

Pivazid (Tersavid)

phenylethylhydrazine

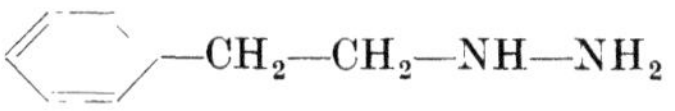

Phenelzine (Nardil)

phenylisopropylhydrazine

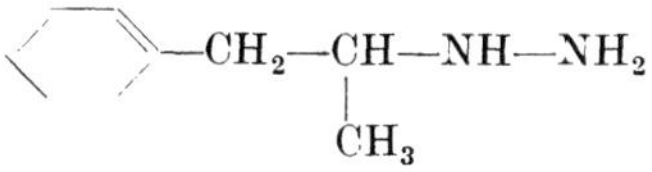

Pheniprazine (Catron)

α-methylbenzylhydrazine

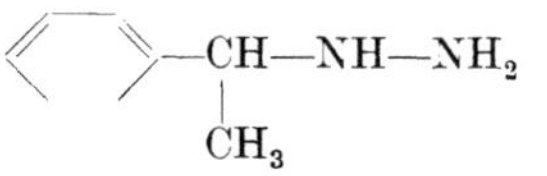

Mebamazine (Actomol)

α) Monoalkyl-, monoaryl-, and monoaralkyl-hydrazines. In the series of *alkylhydrazines* of the general formula

$$CH_3—(CH_2)n—NH—NH_2$$

---

[1] In this chapter MAO inhibition in vivo means either reduction of MAO activity as measured in vitro after pretreatment of intact animals or monoamine accumulation in brain or pharmacodynamic changes related to MAO inhibition (e.g. the potentiation of exogenous dopa, reversal of the effect of monoamine releasers).

derivatives with $n = 2$—4 are most effective in vivo. Branching of the alkyl residue may enhance the inhibition, e.g. isopropylhydrazine is superior to n-propylhydrazine. Basic substitution of the alkyl residue partly yields very potent compounds, e.g. $(CH_3)_2N$—$(CH_2)_2$—$CH(CH_3)$—NH—NH_2, whereas hydroxyl or carboxyl groups reduce the inhibitory potency (BLANKSMA 1962; EBNÖTHER et al. 1959; GEY and PLETSCHER, unpubl.; HAAS and APPEL 1962; JUCKER 1959) (Table 2).

Table 2. *Doses of hydrazine derivatives causing 100% increase of the content of 5-hydroxytryptamine in rat brain*

Hydrazine derivatives	ED_{100}*
Isopropylhydrazine	0.09
N^1,N^2-Diisopropylhydrazine	0.04
Benzylhydrazine	0.20
β-Phenylisopropylhydrazine (1)	0.04
N^1-Isonicotinoyl-N^2-isopropylhydrazine (2)	0.52
N^1-Acetyl-N^1,N^2-diisopropylhydrazine	0.04
N^1,N^2-Diisopropylsemicarbazide	0.075
N^1-Picolinoyl-N^2-benzylhydrazine	0.075
N^1-(5-Methyl-3-isoxazolylcarbonyl)-N^2-benzylhydrazine (3)	0.085
N^1-Pivaloyl-N^2-benzylhydrazine (4)	0.36
N^1-DL-Seryl-N^2-isopropylhydrazine	0.20
N^1-L-Alanyl-N^2-isopropylhydrazine	0.14

* ED_{100} = dose of the hydrazine derivative in mmoles/kg i.p. causing 100% increase of the 5-hydroxytryptamine content in brain after 16 hours. The ED_{100} was calculated on the basis of dose response curves. Spectrophotofluorimetric determination of 5-hydroxytryptamine (PLETSCHER et al. 1960).

(1) Pheniprazine (Catron)
(2) Iproniazid (Marsilid)
(3) Isocarboxazid (Marplan)
(4) Pivazid (Tersavid)

Arylhydrazines, such as phenylhydrazine, are weak MAO inhibitors in vitro (ARAI 1960; BARSKY 1958; F. BERNHEIM 1940; BIEL et al. 1958; OKUMURA 1960) and practically inactive in vivo (BIEL et al. 1959b, 1959c; GEY and PLETSCHER, unpubl.). By para-methylation, however, e.g. of phenylhydrazine, MAO inhibition is increased in vitro and in vivo (ARAI 1960). Sulfamidophenylhydrazine derivatives have a weak inhibitor potency in vitro and in vivo (LESPAGNOL et al. 1964).

In the series of *phenylalkylhydrazines* with the general formula

$$C_6H_5\text{—}(CH_2)_n\text{—}NH\text{—}NH_2$$

the compounds with $n = 1$—2 are most potent in vitro and in vivo. Monoalkylation, preferably with a methyl group on the α-carbon, or arylation of the side chain increases, but hydroxylation decreases the inhibition in vitro and in vivo. Alkylation of the side chain might also determine the degree of MAO inhibition in different tissues. Introduction of O, NH or S between the aryl group and the side chain might slightly reduce the potency (BARSKY et al. 1959; BIEL et al. 1958, 1959b, 1959c; BLOOM 1963; BRODIE et al. 1958b; CHESSIN et al. 1959; CROWTHER et al. 1962; DRAIN et al. 1963; GEY and PLETSCHER, unpubl.; GOGERTY and HORITA 1959; HORITA 1958b; JORI et al. 1963; MCGRATH and HORITA 1962; RUDZIK and MILLER 1963; SPINKS and YOUNG 1961; ZELLER et al. 1959) (Table 2).

Aralkylhydrazines, e.g. pheniprazine, are more active than the corresponding alkylhydrazines, e.g. isopropylhydrazine (BIEL et al. 1959c; GEY et al., unpubl.;

RANDALL et al., unpubl.). Nuclear substitution, e.g. by halogen, hydroxyl-, alkyl-, alkoxy- or aromatic groups, hydrogenation of the benzene ring either increases or reduces MAO inhibition in vitro and in vivo (F. E. ANDERSON et al. 1962; BIEL et al. 1959c, 1961; GARDNER et al. 1961; A. L. GREEN 1962, 1964; McGRATH and HORITA 1962; PLETSCHER and GEY, unpubl.; SCHUMANN et al. 1961; ZELLER 1963c). Replacement of the phenyl residue by *heterocyclic rings* substantially diminishes the inhibitory effect in vitro and in vivo (BIEL et al. 1959b, 1959c; CARISSIMI 1958; CROWTHER et al. 1962; A. L. GREEN 1962; ZELLER 1960).

β) Dialkyl-, diaralkyl-, and alkyl-aralkyl-hydrazines.

$$R{-}NH{-}NH{-}R'$$
$$\genfrac{}{}{0pt}{}{R}{R'}{>}N{-}NH_2$$
$$[R \text{ and } R' = \text{alkyl or aralkyl}]$$

In vitro N^1,N^2-disubstituted hydrazines are weak inhibitors of the enzyme (BIEL et al. 1959c; CARBON et al. 1958; GEY and PLETSCHER, unpubl.; A. L. GREEN 1964; WEIKEL and SALMON 1962). In vivo they may be either less, equally or more potent than the corresponding monosubstituted compounds. Often they show a special preference for brain (BIEL et al. 1959c; CHESSIN et al. 1959; HOFFMANN et al. 1962; PLETSCHER and GEY, unpubl.; PLETSCHER et al. 1960c). N^1,N^1-Dialkyl derivatives show more or less potency than monoalkylhydrazines (BIEL et al. 1959c; CROWTHER et al. 1962; A. L. GREEN 1964; PLETSCHER and GEY, unpubl.; PLETSCHER et al. 1960c). Among some heterocyclic compounds N^1-benzyl-N^1-(1,4-benzodioxane-2-ylmethyl) hydrazine was found to be very active (BIGNAMI et al. 1962; BOVET-NITTI et al. 1961) (Table 2).

γ) Hydrazones with the general formula

$$R{-}HN{-}N{=}C{<}\genfrac{}{}{0pt}{}{R'}{R''}$$

Hydrazones of aralkyl aldehydes, e.g. benzaldehyde-hydrazone, have no action (CHESSIN et al. 1959). Hydrazones of alkylhydrazines are no or weak inhibitors in vitro (BARSKY et al. 1959; CANAL et al. 1958; DAVISON 1957; HEILBRONN 1960; OZAKI et al. 1960); in vivo they may, however, be as potent as the corresponding hydrazines, presumably due to hydrolysis in the intact animal (PLETSCHER et al. 1960c).

δ) N-Acylated alkyl- and aralkylhydrazines.

$$\underset{}{R{-}C{-}O{-}}\underset{R'}{N}{-}\underset{R''}{N}{-}R''' \quad \text{or} \quad R{-}C{-}O{-}\underset{R''}{N}{-}\underset{R'''}{N}{-}C{-}O{-}R'$$

N-Acetylation decreases MAO inhibition in vitro, but on long-term incubation of total tissue homogenate the potency of N-acyl derivatives increases probably owing to hydrolysis of the acylhydrazine bond. In vivo the activity of acetylated hydrazines may be higher than in vitro and seems to be proportional to the rate of deacetylation (F. E. ANDERSON et al. 1962; CROWTHER et al. 1962; A. L. GREEN 1962; HEIM and DIEMER 1960; PLETSCHER et al. 1960c; M. A. SCHWARTZ 1962; WESTLEY and SEIDEN 1962). The velocity of hydrolysis in vivo and in part the tissue distribution seem to be determined by the character of the acyl moiety. The potency of derivatives with identical acyl residues varies according to the structure of the alkyl- or aralkyl group. Potent in vitro and in vivo inhibition of MAO is exerted by alkyl- or aralkylhydrazines acylated with saturated and unsaturated aliphatic, araliphatic, cycloaliphatic acids, amino acids, and their

N-acyl derivatives, peptides, hydroxy-, alkoxy-, alkylmercaptoacids, sulfonic acids, pyridinecarboxylic acids (e.g. isonicotinic acid), pyrazinecarboxylic, isoxazolecarboxylic, furancarboxylic, thiophenecarboxylic acids, carbamic acids (semicarbazides), thiocarbamic acids (thiosemicarbazides) and dihydrazides of dicarboxylic acids partly with additional substitution by alkyl, alkoxy, hydroxy, amino, nitro, halogen groups (Biel et al. 1959c; Cahn et al. 1961a; Canal et al. 1958; Chessin et al. 1959; Crowther et al. 1962; Dat-Xuong et al. 1962; Finkelstein et al. 1963; Gardner et al. 1960, 1961, 1962; Gey et al., unpubl.; Jori et al. 1963; Kaminski et al. 1964; Libermann and Denis 1961; Logemann et al. 1960; Naranjo and Palacios 1961; Ogawa et al. 1964; Pletscher and Gey 1958b; Pletscher et al. 1960c; Randall et al., unpubl.; Rooney et al. 1962; Rowe et al. 1959b; Smuszkovicz and Greig 1961; Zbinden et al. 1960; P. Zeller et al. 1959). N^1,N^2-Diacylhydrazines with or without an alkyl residue do not affect MAO in vivo (Gey and Pletscher, unpubl.) (Table 2).

ε) Cyclic hydrazines, e.g. 1,2,3,4-tetrahydrophthalazine and certain phenyldiaziridines, may be very effective MAO inhibitors in vitro and in vivo (Paget and Davis 1964; Zbinden et al. 1960).

b) 2-Phenylcyclopropylamine and derivatives

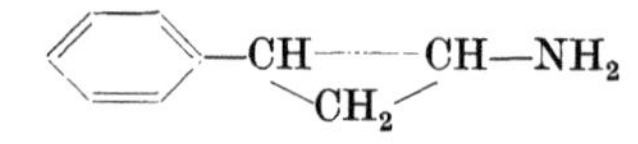

tranylcypromine (Parnate)

These are the most potent in vitro inhibitors of MAO hitherto found (Sarkar et al. 1960a; Tedeschi et al. 1960a). In vivo they are also very active; the action appears faster than that of hydrazine derivatives, but is of similar duration (Costa 1959; Gey et al., unpubl.; H. Green and Erickson 1960, 1962; Maass and Nimmo 1959; Tedeschi et al. 1959b). The cis- and trans-forms have about the same potency, the cis-isomer being slightly more potent (Zeller and Sarkar 1962; Zirkle et al. 1962). The (—)-isomere inhibits MAO somewhat more than the (+)-isomere (Belleau and Moran 1963). Systematic comparisons show that the structural requirements for potent in vivo inhibition of MAO are:

— a cyclopropane ring,
— an amino group attached directly to the cyclopropane ring,
— a β-substituent containing an aromatic moiety.

In this group of compounds the α-hydrogen may be replaced by alkyl- or aryl groups with only a moderate reduction of inhibitory activity (Belleau and Moran 1963; Sarkar et al. 1960a; Zeller 1960; Zeller and Sarkar 1962; Zirkle et al. 1962). N-Benzyl-N-cyclopropyl-ethylcarbamate is a very potent MAO inhibitor in vivo, but not in vitro (Everett and Wiegand 1961).

c) N-Benzyl-N-methyl-propargylamine and derivatives

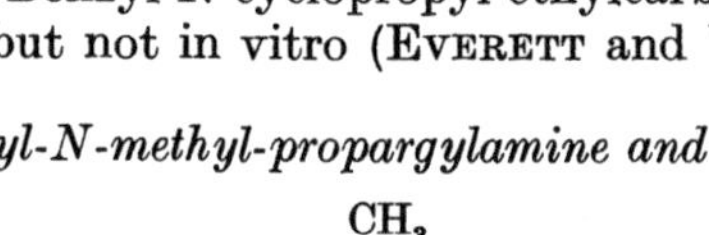

pargyline (Eutonyl)

These compounds induce strong and irreversible MAO inhibition in vitro and have a long-lasting marked effect in vivo (Everett et al. 1963; Swett et al. 1963; Taylor et al. 1960a, 1960b).

The triple bond is essential for MAO inhibition and must be in β-position to the nitrogen. The nitrogen has to remain free, may be incorporated into a heterocycle, or substituted by a methyl group. The benzene residue is the least specific part of the molecule and might even be omitted (McLean and Chen 1963).

Halogenation, methylation, and aryl substitution of the phenyl residue, however, increase the potency, whereas substitution by longer aliphatic chains, hydroxy-, aminoalkyl-, alkoxy groups, or hydrogenation as well as replacement of the phenyl residue by heterocycles have a weakening effect. The methylene group between the nitrogen and phenyl group may be replaced without loss of potency by chains up to 3 C-atoms. A derivative superior to pargyline in vivo, but inactive in vitro, is Mo 1255.

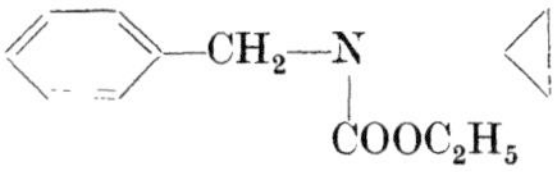

Mo 1255

d) 2-Methyl-3-piperidinopyrazine

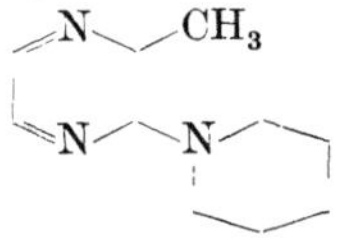

In vivo, this inhibitor has a very potent, long-lasting action on brain MAO probably due to an oxidized metabolite (DUBNICK et al. 1962c, 1963; GYLYS et al. 1963).

MAO inhibition in vivo by methylpiperidinopyrazines requires a single alkyl group (methyl or ethyl) on the pyrazine residue adjacent to the piperidine.

Halogenation of the pyrazine nucleus, formation of pyrazine-N-oxides, and replacement of the latter by quinoxaline abolishes MAO inhibition, whereas the piperidine residue may be transformed into a N-oxide or replaced without marked changes of potency by other cyclic amino groups or even by an acyclic tertiary amino group.

2. Distribution and metabolism in tissues

a) Hydrazines

α) Distribution and excretion. In animals the concentration of *iproniazid* in blood and tissues is maximal one hour after injection. The inhibitor penetrates into the brain in measurable amounts within 1—5 minutes following i.v. administration. Excretion is almost complete within 24 hours (HESS and WEISSBACH 1958; HESS et al. 1958; KOECHLIN and ILIEV 1959; NAIR 1959; NAIR et al. 1960, 1962). *Isocarboxazid* and *nialamide* behave similarly to iproniazid (SCHNEIDER et al. 1959; M. A. SCHWARTZ 1960). In humans the turnover of orally administered iproniazid and isocarboxazide is somewhat slower than in animals; within 24 hours only about 50—60% are recovered in the urine (KOECHLIN et al. 1962). *Phenelzine* has been reported to accumulate more in the mesencephalon than in the cortical and bulbar regions of the guinea pig brain (ZARA and BELSANTI 1961); it seems to enter the brain more rapidly than iproniazid (HOROWITZ 1960).

β) Metabolism. In the brain in vivo as well as in brain slices, but not in mitochondria, the uptake of iproniazid is faster than the development of MAO inhibition (GLUCKMAN and HOROWITZ 1959). Acylhydrazines need an aerobic preincubation for 15—20 minutes for maximal MAO inhibition even with mitochondria, whereas aralkylhydrazines require oxygen, but not as much as their acyl derivatives (DAVISON 1957; A. L. GREEN 1962, 1964; HARDEGG and HEILBRONN 1961; NICKERSON and PARMAR 1960; M. A. SCHWARTZ 1962; SEIDEN and WESTLEY 1963; SMITH et al. 1964; TAYLOR et al. 1960a; ZELLER 1961; ZELLER et al. 1955a). MAO inhibition in vivo persists for a longer time than unchanged iproniazid or isonicotinic acid can be detected in the tissues (HESS et al. 1958; NAIR

1959; NAIR et al. 1960). This suggests that iproniazid has to be transformed into a compound representing the *actual inhibitor* (HEIM and DIEMER 1960; PLETSCHER 1958b). Indeed the isopropylhydrazine moiety is the essential part of the iproniazid molecule (BARSKY et al. 1959; ZELLER et al. 1955b) and represents the active metabolite in vivo (KOECHLIN 1959; ROTH and RIEDER 1964). Recent in vitro-studies demonstrate that the actual inhibitor is a volatile compound, i.e. isopropylhydrazine or an oxidized product derived from isopropylhydrazine respectively. The formation of the actual inhibitor requires an electron acceptor, e.g. oxygen or under anaerobic conditions tetrazolium salts (DAVISON 1957; A. L. GREEN 1964; KORY and MINGIOLI 1964; M. A. SCHWARTZ 1962; SEIDEN and WESTLEY 1962, 1963; SMITH et al. 1964; ZELLER 1955a; ZELLER and SARKAR 1962). Cyanide or thiourea increase the formation of the actual inhibitor and possibly its attachment to the active center of MAO (BARBATO and ABOOD 1963; DAVISON 1957; A. L. GREEN 1964; SMITH et al. 1964). Cupric ions also catalyze this reaction (EBERSON and PERSSON 1962; A. L. GREEN 1964). The formation of the actual inhibitor may occur nonenzymatically, but is possibly enhanced by tissue constituents, e.g. porphyrine derivatives or chymotrypsin (ALBERT and REES 1955; BEAVAN and WHITE 1954; KORY and MINGIOLI 1964; KRÜGER-THIEMER 1955; LONG, unpubl.; LUTWACK et al. 1957; SEIDEN and WESTLEY 1963; SMITH et al. 1964). Based on studies on the cupric ion-catalyzed autoxidation of MAO inhibitors with hydrazine moiety, it has also been proposed that one electron of the hydrazine could be transferred to MAO followed by oxidation of the hydrazine radical by molecular oxygen (EBERSON and PERSSON 1962).

It is very likely that other MAO inhibitors with acylhydrazine structure undergo corresponding transformations. Thus, the actual inhibitor of isocarboxazid is probably benzylhydrazine or a more highly oxidized metabolite (KORY and MINGIOLI 1964; ROTH and RIEDER 1964; M. A. SCHWARTZ 1962; SMITH et al. 1964).

Besides hydrolysis of the acylhydrazine bond, the metabolism of hydrazides also includes cleavage of the alkyl or aralkyl substituent, although the first reaction is probably of major quantitative importance.

Iproniazid is metabolized to isonicotinic acid, isopropylhydrazine, and to a small extend to isoniazid. Isonicotinic acid appears mostly in the urine and has also been detected in brain. Isopropylhydrazine is mainly oxidized to CO_2, but it also forms hydrazones with physiological keto compounds (HESS et al. 1958; HORITA 1962a; KOECHLIN and ILIEV 1959; KOECHLIN et al. 1962; NAIR 1959, 1962; RITTER et al. 1952; ROTH and RIEDER 1964; RUBIN et al. 1952; SEYDEN and WESTLEY 1963; SMITH et al. 1964). The further metabolism of isoniazid includes N-acetylation (main pathway), formation of hydrazones with α-keto acids, or hydrolysis to isonicotinic acid (CHALMERS 1962; PETERS 1960; ZAMBONI and DEFRANCESCHI 1954).

Isocarboxazid yields benzylhydrazine as the major metabolite in blood and tissues. Benzylhydrazine is probably oxidized to benzoate which appears in the urine as hippurate. In vitro isocarboxazid undergoes rapid hydrolysis into benzylhydrazine which actually seems to be the inhibitor (KOECHLIN et al. 1962; ROTH and RIEDER 1964; M. A. SCHWARTZ 1960, 1961a, 1961b, 1962).

Nialamide probably follows the two pathways indicated for iproniazid, but in addition the amide bond in the alkyl side chain is split (PINSON et al. 1962).

Sulfonic acid aralkylhydrazides have been reported to yield metabolites similar to the corresponding acyl-aralkylhydrazines (ROONEY et al. 1962).

The metabolism of *unacylated alkyl- and aralkylhydrazines* has not been investigated thus far. In analogy to the fate of phenylhydrazine (MCISAAC et al.

1958) it may be concluded that aralkylhydrazines are hydroxylated in para-position and also form hydrazones with physiological α-keto acids (HORITA and MATSUMOTO 1962). In any case, the metabolism of aralkylhydrazines, e.g. pheniprazine, proceeds in vitro and in vivo more rapidly than that of acylated hydrazines, e.g. iproniazid (HORITA 1963b).

b) Other compounds

Tranylcypromine does not seem to be altered by MAO in vitro (BELLEAU and MORAN 1962). In the rat in vivo, however, the main part of the compound is metabolized within 24 hours, i.e. by cleavage of the cyclopropane ring resulting in urinary excretion of hippurate and of 4 metabolites of minor quantitative importance. A considerable portion of tranylcypromine is excreted unchanged in the urine (ALLEVA 1963).

Pargyline, after oral administration, reaches a maximal concentration in blood and tissues within 1—2 hours followed by a slow decline over 48 hours. The inhibitor is excreted partly unchanged and partly metabolized (TAYLOR and KRAUSE 1962). In tissue homogenates, pargyline does not seem to be rapidly metabolized (HORITA 1963b).

2-Methyl-3-piperidinopyrazine has to be transformed into an oxidized derivative in order to inhibit MAO. In vitro, this transformation may be catalyzed by the unspecific oxidase of liver microsomes. In vivo, the actual inhibitor, which does not seem to be an N-oxide or a product with an opened piperidine ring, probably undergoes further metabolism. After i.v. injection, 80% of the drug is excreted in the urine within 24 hours (BLUM et al. 1964; DUBNICK et al. 1962c, 1963).

3. Effect on monoamine oxidase

a) Hydrazine derivatives

In vitro hydrazine derivatives inhibit MAO of numerous tissues to a comparable degree (BARSKY 1958; CANAL et al. 1958; CORNE and GRAHAM 1957; DAVISON 1956, 1958a, 1958b; FINGER 1960; FUNDERBURK et al. 1962; GRIESEMER and WELLS 1956; HORITA 1958b, 1962a; IISALO 1957, 1962; KRISHNA et al. 1961; MAXWELL et al. 1961; NAKAI 1958; PEPEU et al. 1961; SCHIATTI 1960; SHORE et al. 1957; SJOERDSMA et al. 1955; ZELLER et al. 1952c, 1955a). The extent of inhibition in tissue slices and cell fractions, e.g. mitochondria and microsomes, is similar, whereas total homogenates are less susceptible to some hydrazine derivatives, e.g. iproniazid. This might be due either to unidentified factors protecting MAO, to side reactions between the inhibitor and some tissue components, or to metabolic inactivation of the inhibitor in total homogenates (BARSKY 1958; GLUCKMAN et al. 1958; A. L. GREEN 1962; HORITA 1963a, 1963b; HORITA and MATSUMOTO 1962; ZELLER et al. 1955a). The inhibition of mitochondrial MAO is only slightly influenced by the functional state of the mitochondria (AEBI 1962; AEBI et al. 1962b). MAO inhibition by hydrazides, e.g. iproniazid, isocarboxazid, and nialamide, becomes maximal only after aerobic preincubation in the absence of substrates for about 15—20 minutes (see above). This progression must be attributed to the formation of free isopropyl- or benzylhydrazines and oxidized metabolites respectively, which in the case of iproniazid and isocarboxazid seem to be the actual MAO inhibitors. Although the inhibition of MAO by iproniazid is at least a bimolecular reaction, its kinetics are of first order (DAVISON 1957; A. L. GREEN 1962; HARDEGG and HEILBRONN 1961), probably because iproniazid is much in excess of the enzyme (WEBB 1963). With iproniazid and isopropylhydrazine respectively an inhibition rate of $1{,}7 \times 10^3$ and $1{,}6 \times 10^4$ liters $mole^{-1}$ $minutes^{-1}$ as well as an overall enthalpy of activation of about 30 and 26 kcal/mole was determined (DAVISON 1957). This corresponds to a very high increase of entropy (WEBB 1963) which could explain the irreversibility of MAO inhibition (see below). Since, however, MAO inhibition by iproniazid and isopropylhydrazine is certainly not a monomolecular reaction (see above), it remains uncertain whether formation of the actual inhibitor or its attachment to the enzyme is mainly responsible for the change of entropy.

MAO inhibition by hydrazine derivatives with or without acyl residue has been found by most investigators to be competitive with the substrate as long as the inhibition is not fully established (ARAI 1960; DAVISON 1957; GLUCKMAN and MARAZZI 1958; A. L. GREEN 1962; NICKERSON and PARMAR 1960; SEIDEN and WESTLEY 1962; SMITH et al. 1964; TUNG et al. 1960; ZELLER et al. 1955a). Correspondingly, the rate of formation of the enzyme-inhibitor-complex depends on the affinity of the substrate used (HARDEGG and HEILBRONN 1961). The dissociation constant for the complex MAO-iproniazid is about $2 \cdot 10^{-4}$. Therefore, the affinity of iproniazid for the enzyme is about 15 times stronger than that of a good substrate such as tyramine (DAVISON 1957). Once the inhibition of MAO has been established, it seems to be uncompetitive with the substrate (SEIDEN and WESTLEY 1962, 1963) and is almost irreversible by dialysis, by washing of the mitochondria, or by urea treatment (ARAI 1960; BARSKY 1958; DAVISON 1957; GLUCKMAN and MARAZZI 1958; A. L. GREEN 1962; SMITH et al. 1964; VIOLLIER et al. 1953; ZELLER et al. 1955a). At 37°C the oxidative deamination of substrates with different affinity, e.g. 5-HT, tyramine, norepinephrine (NE), epinephrine, normetanephrine, isoamylamine, is inhibited to a similar degree (BARSKY 1958; GEY and PLETSCHER, unpubl.; HARDEGG 1961; HOPE and SMITH 1960; KOBAYASHI and SCHAYER 1955; SJOERDSMA et al. 1955; SEPCTOR et al. 1960d; TABACHNICK 1959; UDENFRIEND and WEISSBACH 1958).

The question how MAO inhibitors interfere with the enzyme has not been fully elucidated. The actual inhibitor with hydrazine structure presumably combines with the active center of the enzyme because of its structural resemblance to monoamines. Hydrazine derivatives may be considered to be pseudoamines, since the isosteric residues —NH— and —CH_2— behave very similarly in various chemical and physical respects. The hydrazines, in contrast to the substrates, might be irreversibly bound to the electrophilic site of MAO (presumably covalent bond). Hydrazine derivatives do not require a free α-hydrogen for interaction with MAO (BARSKY et al. 1959; BELLEAU and MORAN 1963; DAVISON 1957; DAVISON and SANDLER 1958; A. L. GREEN 1964; ZELLER 1960, 1963d; ZELLER and FOUTS 1963; ZELLER et al. 1952b, 1955a). No oxygen is required for the attachment of the actual inhibitor to MAO (KORY and MINGIOLI 1964; A. L. GREEN 1964; SMITH et al. 1964).

In vivo, MAO inhibition by hydrazine derivatives has been demonstrated in numerous tissues, e.g. brain, sympathetic ganglia, liver, heart, spleen (APRISON and FERSTER 1961; BARSKY 1958; CORNE and GRAHAM 1957; DAVISON 1958a, 1958b; DAVISON et al. 1957; FINGER 1960; GRIESEMER et al. 1953; HESS et al. 1958; HEIM and DIEMER 1960; IISALO 1962; KAMIJO et al. 1956; LEVINE 1962; LOTLIKAR and MCCUTCHEON 1961; MCGRATH and HORITA 1962; NARANJO and PALACIOS 1961; OZAKI et al. 1960; RANDALL and BAGDON 1959; RANDALL et al., unpubl.; SCHNEIDER et al. 1959; SJOERDSMA et al. 1955; VIOLLIER et al. 1953; WEISSBACH et al. 1957a; WITT et al. 1961; ZELLER et al. 1952a, 1955a). After large single doses of the inhibitors the reduction of enzyme activity persists for several days or weeks (BURKARD et al. 1960; DAVISON et al. 1957; HESS et al. 1958; HORITA 1958a; RANDALL and BAGDON 1959; WITT et al. 1961; ZELLER et al. 1955a) and outlasts by far the presence of the unchanged inhibitor in blood and tissues (HESS et al. 1958; HORITA and CHINN 1964; NAIR 1959; NAIR et al. 1960). MAO inhibition in vivo may vary according to the type of tissue and the route of administration of the inhibitor. Hydrazides, e.g. iproniazid and nialamide, given parenterally or orally inhibit MAO in liver and kidney faster and more markedly, but for a shorter period than in brain. In consequence, 1—2 weeks after a single administration of the inhibitors, MAO is practically no longer affected in liver, but still markedly inhibited in brain (BARSKY 1958; CANAL et al. 1958; DAVISON 1958b; DAVISON et al. 1957; FINGER 1960; FOLKERTH and APRISON 1962; GOGERTY and HORITA 1959; HEIM and DIEMER 1960; HESS et al. 1958; HOPE and SMITH 1960; HORITA 1959, 1961; RANDALL et al., unpubl.; SPECTOR et al. 1960d; TAYLOR and KRAUSE 1962; TAYLOR et al. 1960a; WEIKEL and SALMON 1962). Thereby, the inhibition in midbrain, medulla, pons, and cerebral hemispheres outlasts that in cerebellum (FOLKERTH and APRISON 1962). By the parenteral route, single doses of aralkylhydrazines, e.g. pheniprazine and phenelzine, inhibit MAO in brain more markedly than in liver, but on oral administration they show the opposite pattern, i.e. they behave in general similarly to hydrazides like iproniazid, nialamide, isocarboxazid (GOGERTY and HORITA 1960; HORITA 1959, 1960, 1961; HORITA and MCGRATH 1960b; HORITA and PARKER 1958; KAMINSKI et al. 1964; MCGRATH and HORITA 1962). Since the restitution of MAO activity is probably due to de novo formation of the enzyme, the above differences in the time course might indicate a lower turnover of MAO in brain than in other organs. Behavioural changes caused by MAO inhibitors of the hydrazine type rather parallel the reduction of MAO activity in brain than that in liver (APRISON and FERSTER 1961; HEISE and BOFF 1960; HESS and DÖPFNER 1961).

Some hydrazine derivatives have been described which on oral administration inhibit MAO in brain at least as much as in liver, e.g. an acylderivative of N^1,N^2-diisopropylhydrazine (GEY and PLETSCHER, unpubl.), N-aralkylhydrazines (JORI et al. 1963), and N^1-benzyl-N^1-(1,4-benzodioxan-2-ylmethyl-hydrazine (BOVET-NITTI et al. 1961). Repeated administration of MAO inhibitors of the hydrazine type in therapeutic doses, e.g. iproniazid and Ro 4-2637[1], reduces the enzyme activity more markedly in brain than in liver and kidney of animals (HOPE and SMITH 1960; SMUSZKOVICZ and GREIG 1961) as well as of humans (BERNHEIMER et al. 1962; GANROT et al. 1962b). Therapeutic doses of hydrazine derivatives inhibit MAO in several regions of the human brain up to 100% (BERNHEIMER et al. 1962; GANROT et al. 1962b).

Preexposition of MAO in vitro and in vivo to reversible inhibitors like amphetamine (PARMAR and NICKERSON 1961) or harmane derivatives (HORITA and CHINN 1964; HORITA and MCGRATH 1960a; LONG, unpubl.) prevents the action of irreversible inhibitors with hydrazine structure. This indicates that the reversible inhibitors and the hydrazines compete for the same active site of MAO. Once inhibited by a hydrazine compound, e.g. pheniprazine, MAO can no longer bind other hydrazine derivatives, e.g. iproniazid or its metabolites (SMITH et al. 1964).

b) *Phenylcyclopropylamine*

In vitro, this compound reduces MAO activity more markedly than inhibitors of the other classes. The inhibition is either competitive or uncompetitive according to the substrate, almost irreversible, maximal without aerobic preincubation,

[1] Ro 4-2637 = para-toluene sulfonic acid N^1-benzylhydrazide.

and independent from cyanide. MAO of different tissues is inhibited to a varying degree (BARBATO and ABOOD 1961, 1963; BELLEAU and MORAN 1962, 1963; GEY et al., unpubl.; H. GREEN and ERICKSON 1960; MAASS and NIMMO 1959; D. R. MAXWELL et al. 1961; SARKAR et al. 1960a; D. H. TEDESCHI et al. 1960a; R. E. TEDESCHI et al. 1959b; ZELLER 1961, 1963a; ZELLER and SARKAR 1962; ZELLER et al. 1962). It can be assumed that tranylcypromine is bound to the active site of MAO, because its steric and electronic properties are very similar to those of the intermediary forms of the monoamines during oxidation (BELLEAU and MORAN 1962, 1963; BELLEAU et al. 1961; SARKAR et al. 1960a; ZELLER and SARKAR 1962).

In vivo, a single oral or parenteral dose of tranylcypromine strongly inhibits MAO in brain already after 1 hour. This inhibition lasts for about 15 hours (H. GREEN and ERICKSON 1960; SARKAR et al. 1960a). In liver the effect is less pronounced and of shorter duration (HORITA 1960; SARKAR et al. 1960).

Preexposition of MAO with tranylcypromine only slightly reduces MAO inhibition by hydrazine compounds (SMITH et al. 1964). This and the competition between tranylcypromine and some substrates (see above) suggest that the complex between MAO and tranylcypromine may be reversed by compounds with a higher affinity for the active site of the enzyme. Preexposition of MAO in vivo to reversible inhibitors like harmaline and harmine does not prevent the action of tranylcypromine (HORITA and MCGRATH 1960a), since the latter presumably persists in the tissue longer than the harmane derivatives (HORITA and CHINN 1964).

c) N-Benzyl-N-methyl-propargylamine and derivatives

In vitro, this drug reduces MAO activity slightly more than iproniazid and pheniprazine. The inhibition, similarly to iproniazid, is not reversed by washing and maximal only after preincubation (SWETT et al. 1963; TAYLOR et al. 1960a; ZELLER 1963a). It is conceivable that the acetylene linkage of pargyline reacts with sulfhydryl groups essential for MAO (BELLEAU and MORAN 1963).

In vivo, single oral doses inhibit MAO in liver slightly more than in brain within the first hours; 1—5 days after oral or intraperitoneal administration, the degree of inhibition in brain, heart, and liver is similar but higher than in the stomach and jejunum (LEVINE and SJOERDSMA 1963a). The subsequent restoration of MAO activity in brain and heart proceeds at a slower rate than in the other tissues (TAYLOR et al. 1960a, 1960b); LEVINE and SJOERDSMA 1963). The enzyme activity of other tissues is also reduced, e.g. in sympathetic ganglia (LEVINE 1962). Far lower doses are required to produce significant reduction of MAO activity in man than in animals (LEVINE and SJOERDSMA 1962a, 1963a). One oral or parenteral application of 50—100 mg to hypertensive patients results in marked inhibition of MAO activity (87—95%) in jejunal mucosa with complete recovery within 7—9 days (LEVINE and SJOERDSMA 1962a, 1963).

Preexposition of MAO with pargyline does not prevent the attachment of iproniazid, i.e. of its inhibitory metabolite, to the enzyme (SMITH et al. 1964).

d) 2-Methyl-3-piperidinopyrazine

In vitro, 2-methyl-3-piperidinopyrazine has a rather weak action on MAO if it is not oxidized to the actual inhibitor. The latter competes with the substrates for MAO.

In vivo, the compound has a rapid onset and a long duration of action on MAO resembling the more effective aralkylhydrazines. Thereby, MAO of brain is inhibited more markedly and for a longer period of time than MAO of liver. On oral administration the pyrazine derivative is more potent than after intravenous injection.

Preexposition of intact mice to harmaline prevents the MAO inhibition due to 2-methyl-3-piperidinopyrazine (DUBNICK et al. 1962c, 1963).

4. Effects on other enzyme systems

Several enzymes are influenced by MAO inhibitors of the hydrazine type. Interference seems, however, to be dependent on the structure of the hydrazine moiety. Thus, hydrazines not inhibiting MAO (e.g. isoniazid, semicarbazide) are also effective, and MAO inhibitors without the hydrazine residue are inactive. Up to now, no enzyme system besides MAO has been found to be related to the therapeutic effects of MAO inhibitors.

a) Other amine oxidases

α) Amphetamine oxidase. Amphetamine oxidase (oxidase of non-terminal amines: triphosphopyridine nucleotide-dependent unspecific oxidase of microsomes) deaminates α-alkylated aralkylamines which cause competitive and reversible inhibition of MAO in vitro; furthermore, the enzyme acts on several classes of drugs, e.g. barbiturates, aminopyrine, acetanilide (AXELROD 1955, 1959c; BRODIE et al. 1958a; GAUDETTE and BRODIE 1959; ZELLER et al. 1958a). MAO inhibitors with hydrazine structure reduce the activity of amphetamine oxidase slightly in vitro (EBERHOLST et al. 1958; FOUTS and BRODIE 1955, 1956; SERRONE and FUJIMOTO 1960); in vivo short and weak inhibition is followed by an activation (SCHOTT and CLARK 1952; STOCK and WESTERMANN 1962a; WESTERMANN and STOCK 1962).

The alteration of this oxidative system might at least in part be responsible for the enhancement of drug effects (e.g. amphetamine excitation) by MAO inhibitors of the hydrazine type (ARRIGONI-MARTELLI et al. 1958; BIANCHI and DAVID 1960; DANDIYA et al. 1959; GAUDETTE and COATNEY 1961; JACOB and ECHINARD-GARIN 1961; SHEE 1960). Furthermore, the biphasic effect on the enzyme possibly explains why barbiturate narcosis is initially enhanced and subsequently diminished (see below). Some MAO inhibitors of the non-hydrazine type have no effect on amphetamine oxidase in vivo (STOCK and WESTERMANN 1962a; WESTERMANN and STOCK 1962). Other typical inhibitors of amphetamine oxidase, e.g. SKF-525A, lack the pharmacological effects of MAO inhibitors (AXELROD et al. 1954; BUCHEL and STURTZ-MOURY 1957; COOPER et al. 1954; FOUTS and BRODIE 1955; LA DU et al. 1955).

β) Diamine oxidases (EC 1.4.3.6) (BAKER and CHAYKIN 1960; BLASCHKO 1952, 1962; BUFFONI and BLASCHKO 1963; BURKARD et al. 1962a, 1963; FOUTS et al. 1957; KAPELLER-ADLER and KRAEL 1931; KAPELLER-ADLER and MACFARLANE 1963; R. KOHN 1931; MCEWEN and COHEN 1963; PLETSCHER et al. 1960c; POHL 1893; PUGH and QUASTEL 1937a, 1937b; SCHIEVELBEIN and WERLE 1957; TABOR et al. 1964; WERNER and SEILER 1963; YAMADA and YASUNOBU 1962a, 1962b, 1962c, 1963; YAMADA et al. 1963, 1964; ZELLER 1940a, 1942, 1951, 1956b; ZELLER et al. 1956a, 1958b, 1963c).

In vitro, hydrazine derivatives with and without MAO inhibition reduce the activity of the classical diamine oxidase (DAO) (ARAI 1960; BARSKY et al. 1959; BLASCHKO et al. 1959; BURKARD et al. 1960; DALY et al. 1962; GEY et al. 1960; HEILBRONN 1960; HOLMSTEDT and THAM 1959; KOBAYASHI and OKUYAMA 1962;

LINDAHL et al. 1957; SCHULER and MEYER 1955; SHORE and COHN 1960; TABACHNIK 1959; UDENFRIEND et al. 1958b; WATON 1956; ZELLER et al. 1952c, 1955b, 1957a), of spermine oxidase (EC 1.5.3.3) (BARSKY 1958; BLASCHKO 1962; BLASCHKO et al. 1959; TABOR et al. 1954), of mezcaline oxidase (ARAI 1960; BARSKY 1958; DALY et al. 1962; TABACHNIK 1960; ZELLER et al. 1958b) and of methylamine oxidase (WERNER and SEILER 1963). *In vivo* iproniazid and similar hydrazides, regardless of their effect on MAO, inhibit mezcaline oxidase, methylamine oxidase, and the classical DAO. The activity of the latter may even be

Table 3. *Comparison of diamine oxidase and monoamine oxidase inhibition in cat kidney by various compounds*

Inhibitor	Diamine oxidase		Monoamine oxidase	
	ED_{50} in µmoles/kg	number of cats	ED_{50} in µmoles/kg	number of cats
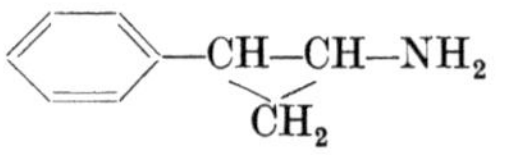 cis-trans-phenylcyclopropylamine	*>168*	1	*3,6* (1.8—7.0)	11
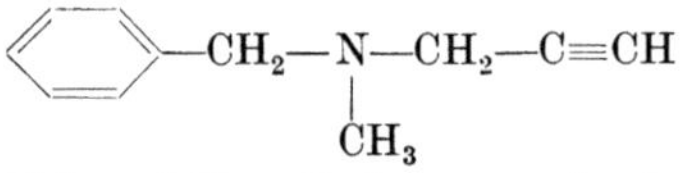 N-benzyl-N-methyl-propargylamine	*450* (360—1450)	16	*16* (15—19)	20
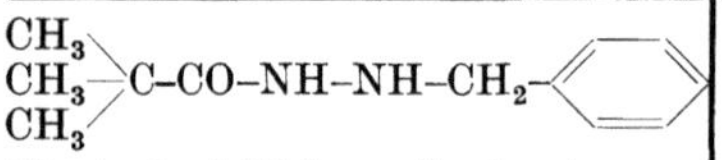 N^1-pivaloyl-N^2-benzylhydrazine	*20* (15—29)	20	*2.6* (1.0—5.6)	10
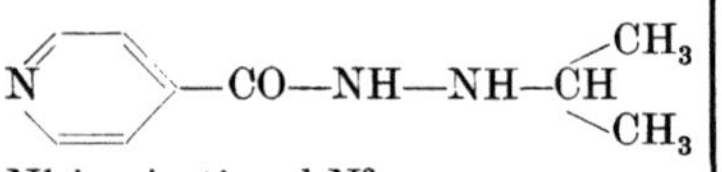 N^1-isonicotinoyl-N^2-isopropylhydrazine	*3.5* (2.5—4.9)	8	*6.9* (5.0—9.9)	8
$H_2N—NH—C(=NH)—NH_2$ aminoguanidine	*0.4* (0.2—0.6)	12	> *560*	2

The activity of the enzymes was measured 16 hours after i.p. administration of the inhibitors. Each inhibitor was compared to a group of untreated animals (4—6) sacrificed simultaneously. The degree of inhibition is expressed by the ED_{50} (dose of the drug causing 50% inhibition); fiducial limits in parentheses (BURKARD et al. 1962a).

more reduced than that of MAO (BURKARD et al. 1960, 1962a; E. J. DAVIS and ROPP 1960; FRIEDHOFF and GOLDSTEIN 1962; GEY et al. 1960, 1963; SCHIEVELBEIN and WERLE 1957; SHORE and COHN 1960; WERNER and SEILER 1963; WERNER et al. 1961). MAO inhibitors without a hydrazine residue, however, do not interfere with the classical DAO and methylamine oxidase in vitro and in vivo (BURKARD et al. 1962a; COHN and SHORE 1960; PACHA and ZELLER 1959; SARKAR et al. 1960a; SHORE and COHN 1960; TABACHNIK 1960; WERNER and SEILER 1963) (Table 3).

γ) D- and ophio-amino acid oxidase (EC 1.4.3.3). These enzyme systems are not affected by iproniazid and tranylcypromine in vitro (BARSKY 1958; GUTMANN et al. 1954; SARKAR et al. 1960a).

b) Other oxidases

α) Ceruloplasmin (CURZON 1962; GELLER et al. 1959). *In vitro* the copper-α-globulin of blood plasma oxidizing aromatic amines (probably identical with para-phenylenediamine oxidase) is slightly inhibited by hydrazine derivatives regardless of their MAO inhibiting properties (HANSON et al. 1959; MARTIN et al. 1958; NAKAJIMA 1959b; NAKAJIMA and THUILLIER 1958; E. SCHMID and SCHEIFFARTH 1961; ZARAFONETIS and KALAS 1960a, 1960b). *In vivo* no inhibition has been found (NAKAJIMA 1959a; ZELLER et al. 1957b). Plasma enzymes responsible for the formation of adrenochrome are activated by iproniazid *in vivo* (BILLEWICZ-STANKIEWICZ et al. 1964).

β) Choline oxidase (EC 1.1.99.1). *In vitro* this enzyme is inhibited by harmane derivatives, but not by hydrazides like nialamide (TUNG 1960; TUNG et al. 1960). *In vivo* the activity of choline oxidase is moderately reduced by some MAO inhibitors with hydrazine structure whereas other MAO inhibitors with and without hydrazine moiety are without effect (GEY et al. 1963; GÖSCHKE et al. 1963; VIOLLIER et al. 1953).

γ) Succinate dehydrogenase (EC 1.3.99.1). *In vitro* and *in vivo* this enzyme seems to be unaffected by iproniazid (ARONSON et al. 1952; QUAY 1959; TUNG et al. 1960; VIOLLIER et al. 1953), whereas pheniprazine in high doses has been reported to decrease the activity of the enzyme in the hypothalamus (QUAY 1959).

δ) Dopamine-β-oxidase. Moderate inhibition by aralkylhydrazines has been shown *in vitro* (BLOOM 1963; CREVELING et al. 1962), but remains to be investigated *in vivo*.

ε) Various oxidoreductases. *In vitro*, hydrazines, regardless of MAO inhibiting properties, but not pargyline, markedly inhibit *α-glycerophosphate dehydrogenase* (EC 1.1.1.8) (REDETZKI and O'BOURNE 1961).

Alcohol dehydrogenase (EC 1.1.1.1) may be inhibited or not altered by MAO inhibitors (GUTMANN et al. 1954; REDETZKI and O'BOURNE 1961; SANKAR 1961; SANKAR et al. 1961).

The following enzymes are not altered *in vitro* by MAO inhibitors with hydrazine structure:

Xanthine oxidase (EC 1.2.3.2) (GUTMANN et al. 1954).

L-Lactate dehydrogenase (EC 1.1.1.27) (GEY and PLETSCHER 1960b; GUTMANN et al. 1954; HEGGLIN et al. 1960; NARANJO 1959; REDETZKI and O'BOURNE 1961).

L-Malate dehydrogenase (EC 1.1.1.37) (GUTMANN et al. 1954).

Aldehyde dehydrogenase (EC 1.2.1.3) (LOVENBERG et al. 1962a)

D-Glyceraldehyde-3-phosphate dehydrogenase (EC 1.2.1.12) (GUTMANN et al. 1954).

L-Glutamate dehydrogenase (EC 1.4.1.3) (REDETZKI and O'BOURNE 1961; (SANKAR et al. 1961).

Isocitrate dehydrogenase (EC 1.1.1.41) (GUTMANN et al. 1954).

D-Glucose-6-phosphate dehydrogenase (EC 1.1.1.49) (GUTMANN et al. 1954).

Cytochrome-c-oxidase (EC 1.6.2.1; 1.9.3.1) (GUTMANN et al. 1954; KAMIJO et al. 1956).

Tryptophan/phenylalanine hydroxylase (EC 1.99.1.4) (BURKARD, unpubl.).

ζ) Peroxidases. *In vitro catalase* (EC 1.11.1.6) and *peroxidase* (EC 1.11.1.7) are inhibited by iproniazid and by hydrazines not interfering with MAO (ANDEREJEW et al. 1959; ARONSON et al. 1952; BLASCHKO 1935; GRINSTEINS and VILLERE 1958; MAHER et al. 1958; TIRUNARAYANAN and VISCHER 1956). *In vivo*, on the other hand, the activity of serum catalase seems to be increased by iproniazid (VALENTI et al. 1958). *Tryptophan pyrrolase* (EC 1.11.1.4) is also activated *in* *vivo* by iproniazid (CANAL and MAFFAI-FACCIOLI 1959a) probably indirectly via hypophysis and adrenals (CANAL and MAFFEI-FACCIOLI 1959a; MAICKEL and BRODIE 1960). Hydrazine-free MAO inhibitors are without effect (MARTEL et al. 1962).

c) Hydrolases

Guanine deamidase of bacteria (EC 3.5.44) has been found to be inhibited by iproniazid, but also by isoniazid (ZELLER et al. 1952c).

Iproniazid and tranylcypromine do not seem to inhibit *adenosine-triphosphatase* (ATP-ase) (EC 3.6.1.3) (BAGDON and ROE, unpubl.; BRUBACHER and WISS, unpubl.; GUTMANN et al. 1954), *tributyrase* (EC 3.1.1.3) (VIOLLIER et al. 1953), *chymotrypsin* (EC 3.4.4.5) (SARKAR et al. 1960a), and *cathepsin* (EC 4.4.4.9) (SARKAR et al. 1960a). *Cholinesterases* (EC 3.1.1.8; 3.1.1.9) have been reported not to be affected by iproniazid, but by some alkylhydrazines (BARSKY 1958; HAAS and APPEL 1962; MAZZONE and SOZIO 1961; SARKAR et al. 1960a; VIOLLIER et al. 1953; ZELLER et al. 1952a, 1952b). Iproniazid protects, however, the enzyme against typical inhibitors like tabun (SCAIFE 1960).

In vitro, *diphosphopyridine nucleotidase* (DPN-ase) (EC 3.2.2.5) is slightly inhibited by iproniazid, but also by nicotinamide and isonicotinamide derivatives without MAO inhibiting properties, e.g. isoniazid (KAPLAN 1960; KAPLAN et al. 1959; RANDALL et al. 1960; ZATMAN et al. 1952, 1953, 1954b). This might be due to formation of unnatural DPN-isomers (KAPLAN et al. 1959; ZATMAN et al. 1954a, 1954b). Iproniazid-DPN, however, seems to interfere only with a few DPN-dependent dehydrogenases in vitro (e.g. with D-glyceraldehyde-3-phosphate dehydrogenase (EC 1.2.1.12) (KAPLAN et al. 1957). Iproniazid in large doses has been reported to reduce the total level of DPN in brain and liver (BURTON 1960).

Carbonic anhydrase (EC 4.2.1.1) seems not to be affected by nialamide (FINGER 1960).

Iproniazid in high oral doses increases the activity of *peptidases* (EC 3.4) in urine, liver, and kidney of animals, possibly indirectly by alteration of the histamine metabolism (KELLER 1960a, 1960b). Activation of proteolytic enzymes might explain the reduction of protein-labelling by iproniazid when ^{14}C-mezcaline or a ^{14}C-thiobarbiturate is incubated with liver homogenate (BLOCK 1961).

d) Enzymes related to pyridoxal-5'-phosphate

Alkyl- and aralkylhydrazines may combine with pyridoxal-5'-phosphate to hydrazones and thus interfere with several enzymes containing pyridoxal-5'-phosphate as cofactor.

In vitro inhibition of *L-glutamate decarboxylase* (EC 4.1.1.15) and *L-cysteine-sulphinate decarboxylase* (EC 4.1.1.29) is induced by alkyl- or aralkylhydrazines with and without acyl residue. In vivo at moderate doses only alkylhydrazines are inhibitory (CANAL and GARATTINI 1957; DAVISON 1956, unpubl.; ERNSTING et al. 1960; HEILBRONN 1960; ROSEN 1959; TABACHNICK 1959). In vitro MAO inhibitors of the hydrazine type with or without acyl group slightly inhibit *DCA* (EC 4.1.1.25; 4.1.1.26—28) (BRODIE et al. 1958b; FINGER 1960; GONNARD and NGUYEN-CHI 1958b; GREIG et al. 1959; HAGEN and WELCH 1956; SCHULER and WYSS 1960) and *L-histidine decarboxylase* (EC 4.1.1.22) (WANTON 1956). In vivo, however, at a moderate dosage a slight and presumably unimportant reduction of enzyme activity in brain is induced only by MAO inhibitors of the hydrazine type without acyl residue (BRODIE et al. 1959a; DUBNICK et al. 1959a, 1962a; GEY et al. 1963; HANSSON and CLARK 1962b; SANDLER and WEST 1958) (see also chapter III: Decarboxylase Inhibitors).

MAO inhibitors with hydrazine moiety do not seem to alter various *transaminases* in plasma, brain, and liver of young and adult animals and humans in vitro and in vivo (BAXTER and ROBERTS 1958; BONAVITA 1959; FINGER 1960; GREENBLATT and KAHN 1959; KATZ et al. 1959; NARANJO 1959; ROSEN 1959). In the liver of the chick embryo, however, hydrazides with or without MAO inhibiting properties cause a slight decrease of *aspartate transaminase* (EC 2.6.1.1) activity, but a strong and long-lasting activation of *alanine transaminase* (EC 2.6.1.2) (KOIVUSALO et al. 1963).

Hydrazines with and without MAO inhibiting properties inhibit *pyridoxal kinase* (EC 2.7.1.35) in vitro (McCORMICK and SNELL 1959, 1960).

e) Other enzymes

Catecholamine-O-methyltransferase is not altered by hydrazine derivatives in vitro and probably not in vivo either (AXELROD 1958a, 1959b; AXELROD and LAROCHE 1959; UDENFRIEND et al. 1959). Iproniazid does not inhibit *carboxylase* (EC 4.1.1.1) in vitro (GUTMANN et al. 1954).

f) Respiration and glycolysis

Iproniazid does not alter the respiration of liver and brain (BAGDON, unpubl.; ERNSTING et al. 1960) in vitro and that of heart muscle in vitro and in vivo (PLETSCHER et al. 1960a). Aryl- and alkylhydrazines, however, may decrease oxygen consumption of liver in vitro (BAGDON, unpubl.; DICKENS 1934). Iproniazid in low concentrations increases the oxidation of glucose by rat brain homogenates in vitro, but rather diminishes that of pyruvate (D. V. S. SANKAR 1961). This might indicate an acceleration of the EMBDEN-MEYERHOF pathway, possibly due to the following mechanisms:

α) Formation of hydrazones with physiological α-keto compounds, e.g. acetaldehyde, triosephosphate, pyruvate, α-ketoglutarate, as shown in vitro and in vivo (CARBON et al. 1958; HORITA 1962a, 1963; McISAAC et al. 1958; NEUBERG and FORREST 1953; W. SCHMID 1960).

β) Reduced availability of energy-rich phosphates. Thus addition of ATP abolishes the effect of iproniazid on glucose oxidation (D. V. S. SANKAR 1961). Total ATP of brain, however, has been found to be either increased (LEWIS and PETTEN 1963; PETTEN and LEWIS 1962), decreased (BERNSOHN et al. 1960; ESTLER 1962) or unchanged (GEY and PLETSCHER, unpubl.) in rats treated with MAO inhibitors of the hydrazine type. In the brain, creatine phosphate was reported to be unchanged or increased, whereas inorganic phosphate remained unaffected (ESTLER 1962; PETTEN and LEWIS 1962). In human blood platelets, however, therapy with iproniazid increases the ATP content (GIRARD 1963).

γ) Diminution of total diphosphopyridine nucleotides which was seen in brain and liver after large doses of iproniazid (BURTON et al. 1960).

δ) Facilitation of the formation of cyclic 3′,5′-adenosine monophosphate (MEYER 1961c) which is known to activate not only phosphorylase, but also phosphofructokinase.

In vitro, iproniazid enhances the epinephrine-induced activation of *glycogen phosphorylase* (EC 2.4.1.1) in liver slices (MEYER 1961a, 1961b). In vivo, however, the percentage of active phosphorylase in brain and heart is not significantly increased by iproniazid or isocarboxazid (BECKENBRIDGE and NORMAN 1962; BELFORD and FEINLIEB 1961; LACROIX and LEUSEN 1961; LACROIX et al. 1962a). The tyramine-induced activation of myocardial phosphorylase, however, is enhanced by iproniazid (LACROIX et al. 1962b). Iproniazid pretreatment of mice does not markedly affect the *hexokinase* activity in brain (ESTLER 1962).

In slices of anterior pituitary the stimulation of glucose-1-^{14}C-oxidation to $^{14}CO_2$ induced by various amines is blocked by MAO inhibitors (BARONDES 1962; BARONDES et al. 1961).

5. Effects on metabolism

a) Monoamines

α) Endogenous monoamines. *Metabolism in tissues.* MAO inhibitors with and without hydrazine moiety increase the total content of endogenous monoamines in various tissues of animals and humans, e.g. 5-HT, NE, dopamine, normetanephrine, and octopamine in brain, 5-HT and NE in autonomic ganglia, NE in the heart and adipose tissues, 5-HT in blood platelets and in small intestine, phenylethylamine in various tissues (AXELROD 1958b; BARTLET 1960; BERNHEIMER et al. 1963; BIEL et al. 1958; BONNYCASTLE et al. 1957; CANAL and

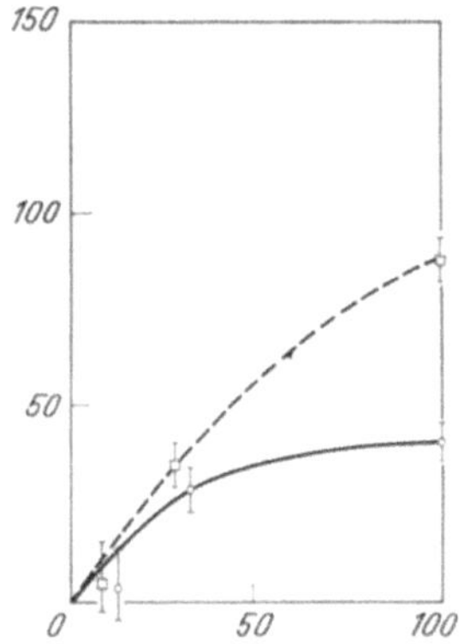

Fig. 1. *Influence of iproniazid on the content of catecholamines and 5-hydroxytryptamine in whole brain of rats. Ordinate:* Increase of the amines in percent of untreated controls. *Abscissa:* Dose of iproniazid in mg/kg. Iproniazid was administered i.p. 16 hours before decapitation. ——— catecholamines; - - - - 5-hydroxytryptamine. Each point represents an average of 4—20 spectrophotofluorimetric determinations with standard error (PLETSCHER 1957b)

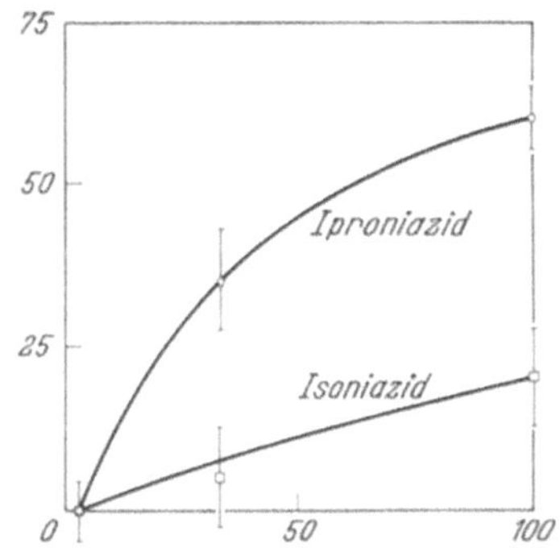

Fig. 2. *Influence of iproniazid and isoniazid on th content of catecholamines in the heart of guinea pigs Ordinate:* Increase of catecholamines in percent o untreated controls. *Abscissa:* Dose of the drugs in mg/kg. The drugs were administered i.p. 16 hours before spectrophotofluorimetric determination of the catecholamines. The points represent averages of 4—30 determinations with standard error (PLETSCHER 1958a)

MAFFEI-FACCIOLI 1959b; CANAL et al. 1959; CARLSSON et al. 1959a; CASTRÉN et al. 1958; CHESSIN et al. 1959; W. G. CLARK 1960; COSTA 1959; CROUT et al. 1960, 1961; DOMENJOZ and SCHELLENBERG 1962; EHRINGER et al. 1960; EVERETT and WIEGAND 1961; FINGER 1960; FREEDMAN and GIARMAN 1962; GAL and DREWES 1962; GANROT et al. 1962a; GEY and PLETSCHER 1959b; H. GREEN and ERICKSON 1960, 1962; HIMWICH and COSTA 1960; HOLZER and HORNYKIEWICZ 1959; JOYCE 1962; KAKIMOTO and ARMSTRONG 1960, 1962; LEROY and SCHAEPDRYVER 1961; MARSHALL et al. 1960; R. A. MAXWELL et al. 1962; MAYNERT and KLINGMAN 1960, 1962; MUSCHOLL 1959; NAKAJIMA et al. 1964; PEKKARINEN et al. 1959; PLETSCHER 1956a, 1956b, 1957a, 1957b, 1958a; PLETSCHER and BERNSTEIN 1958; PLETSCHER and GEY 1958a, 1958b, 1960a; PLETSCHER et al. 1960c; PSCHEIDT and HIMWICH 1963; PSCHEIDT and MORPURGO 1960; ROWE et al. 1959b; RUDZIK and MILLER 1963; SANAN and VOGT 1962; SCHMID 1962; SCHNEIDER et al. 1959; SHORE and BRODIE 1958; SHORE et al. 1958; S. SPECTOR et al. 1958a, 1959, 1960b, 1960d; STOCK and WESTERMANN 1963; UDENFRIEND et al. 1957a, 1957b; WIEGAND and PERRY 1961a, 1961b; ZBINDEN et al. 1960) (Fig. 1, 2, 3, 8).

The effect of MAO inhibitors on endogenous monoamines depends on the *species* (Table 4); catecholamines seem, for instance, to be less influenced in the brain of cats and dogs than of rodents and monkeys. In cats, catecholamines of the heart are even decreased by tranylcypromine, pargyline, and iproniazid, whereas in rats an increase of these amines occurs. This is probably due to a different metabolism of the catecholamines in the two species (see below). The heart of humans probably reacts similarly to that of rats (BRODIE et al. 1959a; GOLDBERG and SHIDEMAN 1961, 1962; GÖSCHKE 1961; MALING et al. 1962; PLETSCHER et al. 1961; PSCHEIDT and HIMWICH 1963; PSCHEIDT and MORPURGO 1960; SANAN and VOGT 1962; SCHOEPKE and WIEGAND 1963; SHIDEMAN and GOLDBERG 1961; SPECTOR 1963; SPECTOR et al. 1959; VOGT 1959).

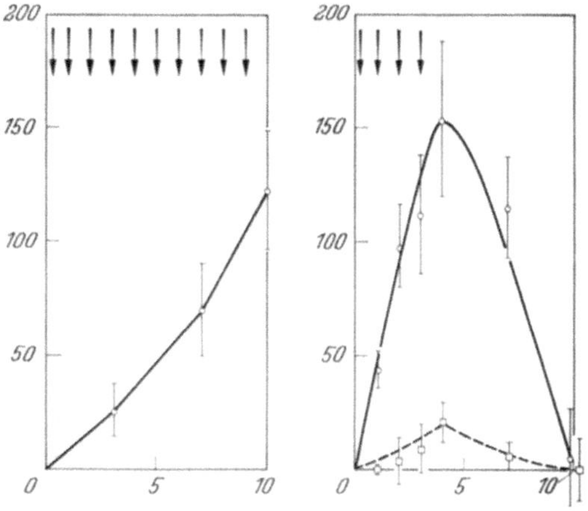

Fig. 3. *Influence of iproniazid and isoniazid on the content of 5-hydroxytryptamine of blood. Ordinate:* Percentage increase of 5-hydroxytryptamine. *Abscissa:* Days. Left hand graph: Isolated platelets of 5 humans. Daily oral administration of 5—8 mg/kg iproniazid (arrows). Right hand graph: Whole blood of 4 rabbits for each drug; ——— 30 mg/kg iproniazid i.v. (arrows); – – – – 23 mg/kg isoniazid (equimolar to iproniazid) i.v. (arrows). The percentage increase of 5-hydroxytryptamine was calculated for each individual; the values before injection of the drugs served as controls. Spectrophotofluorimetric determination of 5-hydroxytryptamine. The points represent averages with standard error (PLETSCHER and BERNSTEIN 1958)

MAO inhibitors influence the *various monoamines* to a different extent. In the brain, 5-HT is often more markedly increased than NE (PLETSCHER et al. 1960c) (Fig. 1), and differences may exist between dopamine, NE, and normetanephrine (CARLSSON et al. 1959a; WEIL-MALHERBE et al. 1961a). Tryptamine could not be rised in brain and heart by iproniazid and tranylcypromine (H. GREEN and SAWYER 1960b; HESS et al. 1959c).

The *intensity of action* of MAO inhibitors expressed by the dose causing a 50—100% increase of monoamines depends considerably on the chemical structure.

Table 4. *Dose of the monoamine oxidase inhibitors* which cause a 50% increase of brain 5-hydroxytryptamine 16 hours after i.p. administration of the drugs (ED_{50}) in various mammalian species*

	Iproniazid	Isocarboxazid	Pivaloylbenzyl-hydrazine	Tranyl-cypromine	Methyl-benzyl-propinylamine
Mouse	540 (280—930)	44 (37—49)	76 (67—84)	23 (20—26)	405 (350—475)
Rat	176 (157—196)	28 (17—37)	139 (67—178)	6 (2—9)	81 (56—112)
Guinea pig	64 (36—98)	14 (8—20)	18 (16—20)	28 (14—48)	244 (143—303)
Rabbit	290 (150—400)	74 (30—107)	425 (258—555)		

Figures in parentheses: fiducial limits for 95% probability (PLETSCHER et al. 1961)
* mg/kg.

Several hydrazine derivatives have no influence on the monoamine content, others are 10—15 times more effective than iproniazid (BIEL et al. 1958; CHESSIN et al. 1959; PLETSCHER et al. 1960c). The non-hydrazines pargyline and tranylcypromine are very effective inhibitors, the latter is at least as potent as the strongest MAO inhibitor of the hydrazine series (Table 4).

The *time course* of the monoamine increase in tissues generally reaches a maximum 6—16 hours after administration of MAO inhibitors of the hydrazide type (PLETSCHER et al. 1960c). Hydrazines like pheniprazine and phenelzine seem to act more quickly than iproniazid on the brain 5-HT; the pheniprazine-induced increase of NE is, however, slower than that of 5-HT (BRODIE et al. 1958b; CHESSIN et al. 1959; S. SPECTOR et al. 1960d). The non-hydrazine MAO inhibitors pargyline and tranylcypromine generally rise the brain amines more rapidly than the hydrazine derivatives (H. GREEN and ERICKSON 1960). The monoamine increase in the tissue after one single dose of a MAO inhibitor lasts several days depending on the animal species and the amine involved (H. GREEN and ERICKSON 1960; H. GREEN et al. 1962; PLETSCHER 1956a, 1956b, 1957b; SHORE and BRODIE 1958; S. SPECTOR et al. 1958a; WIEGAND and PERRY 1961a). Monoamine accumulation is of shorter duration than the MAO inactivation, because partial inhibition of the enzyme can still be detected 1—2 weeks after administration of the inhibitor (BURKARD et al. 1960; CHESSIN et al. 1959; HORITA 1958b, 1959; RANDALL and BAGDON 1959). Evidence exists that MAO has to be inhibited to at least 85% before the monoamine content of brain and possibly other tissues increases (CHESSIN et al. 1959; GEY and PLETSCHER 1959a, 1961b; PLETSCHER et al. 1960c) (Fig. 4 and 8).

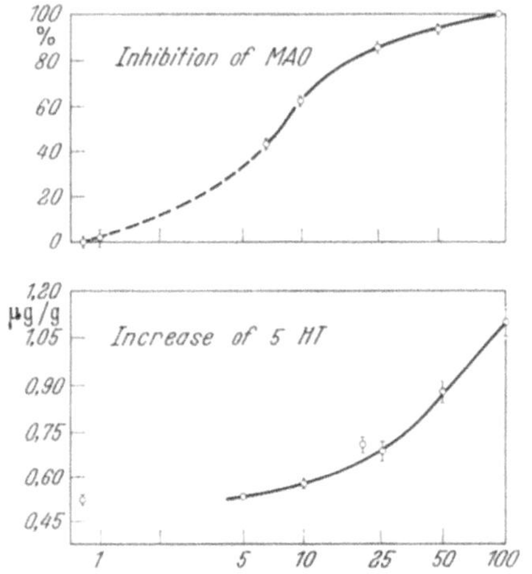

Fig. 4. *Influence of increasing doses of iproniazid on MAO activity and 5-hydroxytryptamine content of rat brain. Ordinate:* Decrease of MAO activity in percent of controls. 5-Hydroxytryptamine content of whole brain in µg/g fresh tissue. *Abscissa:* Dose of iproniazid in mg/kg. Manometric measurement of MAO activity in brain mitochondria and spectrophotofluorimetric determination of 5-hydroxytryptamine in total brain 16 hours after iproniazid i.p. The points represent averages of 2—25 experiments each with standard error. With 25 mg/kg iproniazid only the 5-hydroxytryptamine starts to rise significantly ($p < 0.01$), whereas MAO inhibition is almost 100% (PLETSCHER et al. 1960c)

The long duration of action explains the *cumulative effect* of MAO inhibitors. It is possible to cause a pronounced increase of 5-HT in brain and blood by repeated administration of low single doses of iproniazid having per se no measurable effect. In brain, this increase is about equal to that produced by the total dose administered in one single injection (PLETSCHER and BERNSTEIN 1958; PLETSCHER et al. 1960c; SHORE et al. 1958).

It has not been elucidated whether MAO inhibitors preferentially increase *free or bound monoamines* in vivo, probably because of methodological difficulties. Most investigators agree that various MAO inhibitors do not considerably or consistently change the distribution of monoamines between the high speed supernatant and particulate fraction of tissue homogenates (BERTLER et al. 1960; COHEN et al. 1962; GIARMAN 1961; GIARMAN and SCHANBERG 1961; GLUCKMAN 1960; H. GREEN and SAWYER 1960a; H. GREEN et al. 1959; W. A. HIMWICH et al. 1961; LEVI and MAYNERT 1964; MICHAELSON and WHITTAKER 1963; WEIL-MALHERBE et al. 1961a).

The effect of MAO inhibitors on *monoamine metabolites* in tissues has not been fully investigated thus far. It is known that 5-hydroxyindoleacetic acid, homovanillic acid, and 3,4-dihydroxyphenylacetic acid, which occur naturally in the brain, decrease after several MAO inhibitors, whereas the 5-hydroxyindolacetic acid of the human cerebro-spinal fluid remains unchanged (ANDÉN et al. 1963a, 1963b, 1964b; ROOS 1962, 1963; ROSENGREN 1960b).

Urinary excretion. In humans the excretion of catecholamines is not markedly changed by MAO inhibitors, but in guinea pigs iproniazid enhances the elimination of epinephrine and NE (CARLSSON et al. 1959b; PEKKARINEN et al. 1960; PSCHEIDT et al. 1961; SJOERDSMA et al. 1959c). MAO inhibitors increase the urinary output of normetanephrine and metanephrine as well as of other endogenous monoamines, i.e. tryptamine, ortho-, meta-tyramine, phenylethylamine, octopamine and its N-methyl-derivative (synephrine) (E. J. DAVIS and ROPP 1960; JEPSON et al. 1960; KAKIMOTO and ARMSTRONG 1960; OATES and ZALTZMAN 1959; PISANO et al. 1961; SJOERDSMA et al. 1959c, 1959d, 1960a; UDENFRIEND 1959a). Enhanced tryptamine excretion seems to be a sensitive indicator for MAO inhibition in vivo and has been proposed as a clinical test (BALDRIDGE et al. 1962; KRAUPP et al. 1962; OATES and ZALTZMAN 1959; SJOERDSMA et al. 1959d; UDENFRIEND 1959a). In children with phenylketonuria iproniazid causes a marked increase of the urinary content of phenylethylamine (JEPSON et al. 1960). MAO inhibitors thus enhance above all the excretion of monoamines which are preferentially metabolized by MAO (e.g. tyramine, tryptamine). The elimination of monoamines, for which alternative metabolic pathways exist (e.g. catecholamines) is, however, not or little influenced by the inhibitors.

The urinary excretion of 5-hydroxyindoleacetic acid, the major metabolic end product of 5-HT, is decreased by MAO inhibitors in humans (including patients with carcinoids) and in animals. In general a marked diminution of the acid occurs only after long-term application of the inhibitors, possibly because 5-hydroxyindoleacetic acid is also formed by transamination of 5-HTP followed by decarboxylation (BLASCHKO 1958; HAAVALDSEN 1962; SANDLER et al. 1960; R. P. SPENCER and ZAMCHEK 1960). In consequence of MAO inhibition, other metabolic pathways are activated, e.g. formation of 5-HT-O-glucuronide (ACHESON et al. 1961c; CRANE and WOLFMAN 1960; GRANOWITZ and PLETSCHER 1957; KABAKOW et al. 1959; LAUER et al. 1958; LOPES DO ROSÁRIO and FRAGOSO MENDES 1959; VOELKEL 1959; WEISSBACH et al. 1958; ZELLER 1958). The excretion of metabolic end products of catecholamines, e.g. 3-methoxy-4-hydroxymandelic acid, is also reduced to a considerable extent by MAO inhibitors (BALDRIDGE et al. 1962; GOTTFRIES 1960; STUDNITZ 1959a).

β) Exogenous monoamines and monoamine precursors. *Metabolism in tissues.* MAO inhibitors in general do not influence the biological half life time of *injected monoamines*, such as *catecholamines*, in the whole body and the blood. The inhibitors do not modify or delay the disappearance of *5-HT* possibly depending on the dose of the amine. The content of injected catecholamines in various organs, e.g. liver, spleen, adrenals, kidney, is not influenced either by MAO inhibitors. In the heart an increase or no change of exogenous catecholamines has been reported, probably depending on differences in animal species and dose of the catecholamines. MAO inhibitors, however, elevate the content of injected 5-HT in the heart and spleen and of injected NE in the hypophysis as well as in the skeletal muscle of cats. In contrast, MAO inhibitors of the hydrazine type inhibit the uptake of 5-HT by platelets in vitro, but presumably by an unspecific mechanism. The biological half life time and the content of exogenous *tyramine and tryptamine* in various tissues is increased by MAO inhibitors (AXELROD and INSCOE 1963; AXELROD et al. 1961b, 1961c; CARLSSON and HILLARP 1962; CARLSSON et al. 1963; CROUT et al. 1960, 1961; FRIEND et al. 1958; GEY and PLETSCHER 1959b; GOLDSTEIN and GERTNER 1960; GOLDSTEIN et al. 1960a, 1960c; HERTTING et al. 1961a, 1961b; LONG and LESSIN 1962; MANGER et al. 1959; PLETSCHER et al. 1963b; RAAB and GIGEE 1958; SCHAEPDRYVER 1959; SCHAEPDRYVER and KIRSHNER 1961a, 1961b, 1961c; SCHAEPDRYVER et al.

1960; Schayer et al. 1954; Udenfriend et al. 1957a, 1957d, 1959; Weil-Malherbe et al. 1961b; Weissbach et al. 1961a).

The *increase of monoamines due to injection of monoamine precursors*, e.g. dopa, 5-HTP, tryptophan, ortho-, meta-tyrosine, phenylalanine, is enhanced by MAO inhibitors. This has been shown in various organs for catecholamines, 5-HT, tryptamine, ortho- and meta-tyramine, and phenylethylamine (Fig. 5). The accumulation is probably due to inhibition of the deamination of the monoamines formed by decarboxylation. In the brain of animals pretreated with MAO inhibitors, dopa seems to increase dopamine more than NE, possibly because of a relatively low rate of dopamine-β-hydroxylation. Besides, some MAO inhibitors of the hydrazine type might inhibit dopamine-β-oxidase, an effect which has been demonstrated in vitro (see above) (Bartlet 1960; Carlsson 1959; Carlsson et al. 1958; W. G. Clark and Pogrund 1961; Costa et al. 1961a; Creveling et al. 1962; Goldstein and Musacchio 1963; Hess and Doepfner 1961; Hess et al. 1959b, 1959c; Kako et al. 1961; Mitoma et al. 1957; Nakajima et al. 1964; Paasonen et al. 1961; Pletscher 1957b; Pletscher and Gey 1960a, 1960b, unpubl.; Pletscher et al. 1960b; Schildkraut et al. 1963; Udenfriend et al. 1957a, 1957c; Vogt 1959; Wegmann et al. 1961; Weil-Malherbe et al. 1961a; Wiegand and Perry 1961a, 1961b).

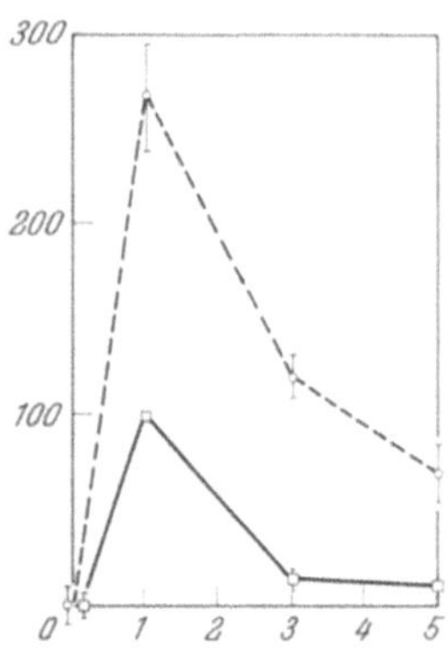

Fig. 5. *Enhancement of the 5-hydroxytryptophan-induced increase of 5-hydroxytryptamine in brain of rats by iproniazid. Ordinate:* Percentage increase of 5-hydroxytryptamine in the whole brain as compared to untreated controls. *Abscissa:* Hours after 5-hydroxytryptophan i.p. ——— 75 mg/kg 5-hydroxytryptophan alone; ---- 75 mg/kg 5-hydroxytryptophan 16 hours after 100 mg/kg iproniazid i.p. The points represent average values of 4 spectrophotofluorimetric determinations of 5-hydroxytryptamine with standard error (Pletscher and Gey 1960b)

MAO inhibitors increase the level of *O-methylated catecholamines* and decrease the content of *metabolic end products,* such as 3-methoxy-4-hydroxymandelic acid, 3,4-dihydroxymandelic acid, and 3-methoxy-4-hydroxyphenylglycols in organs of animals treated with labelled catecholamines. Furthermore, the dopa-induced increase of phenolcarboxylic acids, e.g. 3,4-dihydroxyphenylacetic acid, in various tissues is reduced by MAO inhibitors (Axelrod 1958b; Carlsson and Hillarp 1962; Goldstein and Gertner 1960; Goldstein et al. 1960a; Hertting et al. 1961a, 1961b; Pletscher and Gey 1964; Schaepdryver and Kirshner 1961a, 1961b, 1961c).

Urinary excretion. MAO inhibitors lower the enhanced urinary excretion of 5-hydroxyindoleacetic acid due to exogenous 5-HT and correspondingly increase the elimination of 5-HT, 5-HT-O-glucuronide, as well as -O-sulphate. The diminution of the excretion of 5-hydroxyindoleacetic acid after 5-HT application has been used to determine MAO inhibition in man. This effect of MAO inhibitors on the excretion of 5-hydroxyindoleacetic acid may, however, not be exclusively-due to MAO inhibition. Thus, iproniazid and isocarboxazid (but not phenelzine and nialamide) also diminish the urinary excretion of orally administered 5-hydroxyindoleacetic acid. (J. A. Anderson et al. 1958; Chadwick and Wilkinson 1960; Corne and Graham 1957; Feldstein et al. 1961; Kirberger 1963; McIsaac and Page 1959; Praag and Leijnse 1962; Sanner and Wortman 1962; Sjoerdsma et al. 1958, 1959a; Weissbach et al. 1958, 1961a).

MAO inhibitors generally enhance the urinary excretion of exogenous NE, epinephrine, and dopamine as well as the dopa-induced elimination of dopamine. The effects on urinary NE and epinephrine are not spectacular, because except immediately after the infusion, only low amounts of these amines are excreted as such (about 5% in the 24-hour urine). The excretion of phenylethylamine and tyramine after administration of phenylalanine and tyrosine does not seem to be increased by iproniazid. MAO inhibitors influence, however, the urinary elimination of the major metabolites of catecholamines, e.g. they enhance the excretion of O-methylated catecholamines after administration of epinephrine, NE, their 3-O-methyl ethers, and dopa. Correspondingly, the elimination of 3-methoxy-4-hydroxymandelic and homovanillic acid after injection of catecholamines decreases. In addition, MAO inhibitors diminish the catecholamine-induced rise of urinary 3,4-dihydroxyphenylglycol, 3-methoxy-4-hydroxyphenylglycol, and 3-methoxy-4-hydroxyphenylethanol as well as of some quantitatively less important acids, i.e. 3,4-dihydroxymandelic and 3,4-dihydroxyphenylacetic acid. Furthermore, N-acetylated amines appear in the urine of rats pretreated with iproniazid after administration of normetanephrine and dopamine (AXELROD 1958a, 1959a, 1959b; AXELROD et al. 1958a, 1958b; BALZER and HOLTZ 1956; CORNE 1956; CORNE and GRAHAM 1957; ELMADJIAN 1959; FRIEND 1962; FRIEND et al. 1958; GLUCKMAN 1960; GOLDSTEIN and MUSACCHIO 1962, 1963; GOLDSTEIN et al. 1959, 1960a, 1960b, 1960d; KIRSHNER et al. 1959, 1961; KOPIN et al. 1961; KRAUPP et al. 1962; LABROSSE 1961; McGOODALL 1959; McGOODALL et al. 1958, 1964; POGRUND et al. 1961; RESNICK 1959; RESNICK and FREEMAN 1962; RESNICK et al. 1958, 1960a; ROSEN and McGOODALL 1961, 1962; SCHAEPDRYVER and KIRSHNER 1961a, 1961b; SCHAYER and SMILEY 1953; SCHAYER et al. 1954, 1955; A. SMITH and WORTIS 1960, 1962; WEISSBACH et al. 1961a; C. M. WILLIAMS et al. 1960).

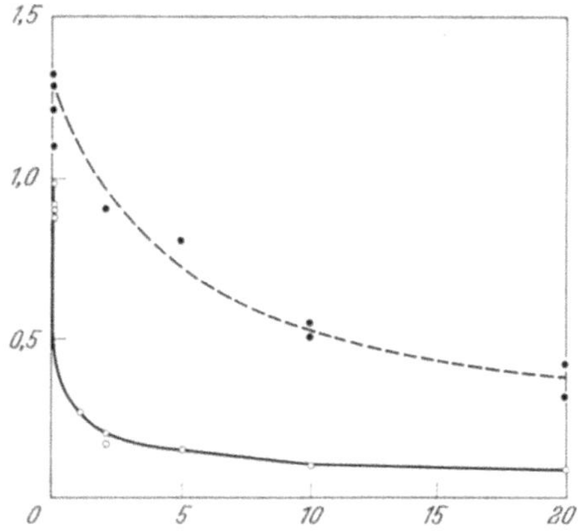

Fig. 6. *Counteraction by iproniazid of the reserpine-induced decrease of 5-hydroxytryptamine in brain of mice. Ordinate:* Content of 5-hydroxytryptamine in μg/g fresh brain. *Abscissa:* Dose of reserpine in mg/kg. Spectrophotofluorimetric determination of 5-hydroxytryptamine 16 hours after reserpine i.p. ——— No pretreatment with iproniazid (reserpine alone); – – – – 100 mg/kg iproniazid s.c. 10 hours before reserpine. For each determination of 5-hydroxytryptamine pools of 5 brains were used (PLETSCHER 1956a)

γ) Counteraction against monoamine releasers. Pretreatment with MAO inhibitors *in vivo* counteracts the monoamine decrease in the tissues due to certain *Rauwolfia alkaloids*, e.g. reserpine, and *benzoquinolizines* (e.g. tetrabenazine[1]). This has been shown for NE, dopamine, 5-HT in brain, NE and 5-HT in the blood, NE in the heart, as well as for 5-HT in the gastrointestinal tract. The interference is still seen 24 hours and more after administration of the inhibitors. The antagonism seems to be more marked in the brain than in the heart, intestine, and other organs. In the hypothalamus of cats, however, iproniazid has been found to have no effect on the decrease of NE due to reserpine (Fig. 6) (BARTLET 1960; BRODIE and SHORE 1957; BRODIE et al. 1956; CARLSSON et al. 1957b; DUBNICK et al. 1959b; FINGER 1960; H. GREEN and ERICKSON 1962; H. GREEN and SAWYER 1960a; JÄÄTELÄ and PAASONEN 1961; KRONEBERG and SCHÜMANN 1960; PAASONEN and KÄRKI 1959; PEKKARINEN et al. 1959; PLETSCHER 1956a, 1956b, 1957b; PLETSCHER et al. 1959a, 1962; SCHAEPDRYVER and PREZIOSI 1959a, 1959b; SCHAEPDRYVER and PIETTE 1961; SHORE and BRODIE 1957; S. SPECTOR et al. 1960c; M. VOGT 1959; WEIL-MALHERBE et al. 1961a; ZBINDEN

[1] 2-keto-3-isobutyl-9,10-dimethoxy-hexahydrobenzo[a]quinolizine.

et al. 1957, 1959). MAO inhibitors also diminish the rise in the urinary excretion of epinephrine and 5-hydroxyindoleacetic acid due to reserpine (BICKEL et al. 1961; SCHNITZER 1958). Furthermore, the reserpine-induced decrease of the histochemical reactivity of the enterochromaffine cells and of the adrenal medulla is partly counteracted by iproniazid (CAMMANI et al. 1960; STUDER 1961; STUDER and ZBINDEN 1960; ZBINDEN and STUDER 1958a; ZBINDEN et al. 1957) (Fig. 7).

In vitro monoamine releasers may also be counteracted by MAO inhibitors. Pretreatment of rabbits with isocarboxazid or addition of pheniprazine to platelet-rich plasma partly inhibits the 5-HT release from platelets due to the addition of reserpine or tetrabenazine to the plasma. Furthermore, the reserpine-induced catecholamine depletion of the isolated rat iris is inhibited by preincubation with isocarboxazid (CSILIK 1964; PAASONEN 1961b; PAASONEN and PLETSCHER 1960).

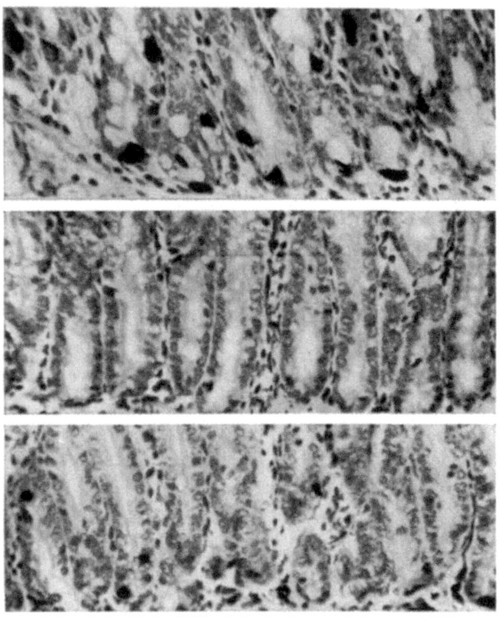

Fig. 7. *Influence of reserpine or iproniazid + reserpine on the histochemical reactivity of the enterochromaffine cells in the duodenum of guinea pigs* (formaline 10%, silver method according to MASSON. Enlargement 180×). *Top:* Untreated animal. *Middle:* 24 hours after 10 mg/kg reserpine i.p. The argentaffinity has completely disappeared. *Bottom:* 100 mg/kg iproniazid i.p. 16 hours before 10 mg/kg reserpine i.p. Decapitation 24 hours after reserpine. The argentaffinity though decreased in intensity remains visible. (Experiments carried out by Dr. A. STUDER, Department of Experimental Medicine, F. Hoffmann-La Roche & Co. Ltd., Basel.)

Some *other effects of reserpine*, e.g. the stimulation of the anterior pituitary and the adrenal cortex as well as the decrease of γ-aminobutyric acid in the brain, are also attenuated by MAO inhibitors. The inhibitors have, however, no effect on the reserpine-induced decrease of histamine in the rat stomach and do not antagonize reserpine in prolonging the nicotinamide-induced DPN-elevation in liver of mice (BALZER et al. 1961; EECHAUTE et al. 1962; KIM and SHORE 1963; MARTEL and MAICKEL 1961; MARTEL et al. 1962; PALM et al. 1961a, 1961b, 1962c; WESTERMANN 1961).

Administration of *MAO inhibitors subsequent to maximal monoamine release* accelerates the recovery of the endogenous monoamines and increases the uptake of exogenous NE by tissues. The first effect has been especially investigated in brain. Pheniprazine, isopropylhydrazine, tranylcypromine, and pargyline act faster then iproniazid. 5-HT is more rapidly normalized than the NE which might be due to a differnet turnover rate of the amines (BRODIE et al. 1958b; CANAL and MAFFEI-FACCIOLI 1959b; CANAL et al. 1959; CARLSSON et al. 1963; COSTA 1959; H. GREEN and ERICKSON 1962; KUNTZMAN et al. 1962b; PALM 1958; PLETSCHER 1957a; PLETSCHER et al. 1960c; SHORE et al. 1958; S. SPECTOR et al. 1960a).

MAO inhibitors also counteract *monoamine depletion by other compounds*, e.g. by insuline, histamine, tetramethylammonium, and nicotine, in the adrenal medulla. Pheniprazine has also been shown to partially antagonize the release of ^{3}H-NE from the rat heart induced by *guanethidine* and *α-methyltyrosine;* the amphetamine-induced release of the amine was, however, not influenced. The antagonism against guanethidine seems to be dissociated from MAO inhibition. MAO inhibitors, however, do not counteract or even enhance the 5-HT-, 5-HTP-, and tyramine- induced decrease of epinephrine. They have no inhibitory effect on the epinephrine secretion due to electrical stimulation. Monoamine depletors possibly act by several mechanisms, e.g. by inhibition of the storage capacity or by stimulation of the active secretion of monoamines. MAO inhibitors might interfere only with the first mechanism. (BALZER et al. 1961; GATGOUNIS et al. 1964; GESSA et al. 1962c, 1963; HARRISON et al. 1961; HOLTZ et al. 1957a; KRONEBERG and SCHÜMANN 1960; MIRKIN 1961; POTTER and AXELROD 1963; ROSENKRANTZ and LAFERTE 1960; SCHAEPDRYVER 1959a; SCHAEPDRYVER and PREZIOSI 1959a, 1959b; WESTERMANN 1961).

δ) Interaction of short- and long-acting MAO inhibitors. Short-acting ("reversible") MAO inhibitors, like 7-methoxyharmanes (harmine, harmaline, tetrahydroharmine) induce a marked increase of monoamines in brain, which lasts only a few hours. Pretreatment with these drugs attenuates the 5-HT, NE, and dopamine increase in the brain due to long-acting ("irreversible") MAO inhibitors, e.g. of the hydrazine type. The effect of iproniazid on the reserpine-induced decrease of 5-HT in brain (see above) is also antagonized by pretreatment with harmaline. If MAO inhibitors of the hydrazine type are administered before harmaline, its injection does not influence the hydrazine-induced monoamine increase in brain.

MAO inhibitors of the irreversible and the reversible type probably compete for the active center of MAO, as shown in vitro (see above). The inhibitor administered first prevents the second inhibitor from occupying the enzyme. This theory is supported by the findings that 7-hydroxyharmanes and isoniazid, which are no MAO inhibitors, do not counteract the monoamine increase in brain due to MAO inhibitors of the hydrazide type (HOLZER and HORNYKIEWICZ 1959; PLETSCHER and BESENDORF 1959; PLETSCHER and GEY, unpubl.; PLETSCHER et al. 1959a, 1960c; TABACHNICK and RUBIN 1959; UDENFRIEND et al. 1958b).

ε) Mechanism of action. The mechanisms to be mainly discussed are inhibition of oxidative deamination and interference with storage of monoamines.

Inhibition of oxidative deamination. The *accumulation of endogenous and exogenous monoamines* in tissues as well as the change in the excretion pattern of monoamines due to MAO inhibitors may partly be explained by their interference with oxidative deamination. Accumulation of monoamines probably occurs only if oxidative deamination is a major pathway and if the accumulation cannot be compensated by enhanced conjugation with glucuronic and sulfuric acid as well as by enhanced N-acetylation. These criteria seem to be fulfilled for several monoamines, e.g. tryptamine, tyramine, which accumulate in various tissues as well as in urine. Several monoamines increase, however, only in some tissues, because other metabolic pathways independent from MAO are probably dominant; in brain of many species, for instance, MAO inhibitors cause accumulation of 5-HT and catecholamines, whereas in blood the half life time of injected 5-HT and NE is not always prolonged. The accumulation of monoamines induced by MAO inhibitors may also vary according to the species, e.g. the NE of heart in rats and cats (see above).

The *attenuation of the reserpine- and benzoquinolizine-induced decrease of monoamines* by MAO inhibitors has also been attributed to inhibition of oxidative deamination. According to this hypothesis reserpine and tetrabenazine after pretreatment with MAO inhibitors might still be able to release the amines from the tissue stores; the metabolic transformation of the liberated monoamines would, however, be diminished because of MAO inhibition. This possibly leads to a relative increase of the free monoamines without major changes of the total monoamine content. This hypothesis is supported by the findings that monoamine releasers after pretreatment with MAO inhibitors no longer cause sedation, miosis, ptosis, hypothermia, but rather excitation, mydriasis, hyperthermia, signs of sympathetic stimulation (see below). Increase of free monoamines after administration of MAO inhibitors + monoamine releasers has, however, thus far only been proven in blood plasma (PAASONEN 1961a; PAASONEN and PLETSCHER 1959), whereas experiments on the intracellular distribution of monoamines have not been conclusive (R. A. COHEN et al. 1962; GIARMAN 1961; GIARMAN and SCHANBERG 1958; H. GREEN and SAWYER 1960a; H. GREEN et al. 1959; SCHANBERG and GIARMAN 1962; WEIL-MALHERBE and BONE 1959; WEIL-MALHERBE et al. 1961).

Interference with the storing or release of monoamines. The assumption that MAO inhibitors increase the uptake or inhibit the release of monoamines is based on the following experimental findings:

— Administration of MAO inhibitors beyond the doses which cause complete MAO inhibiton induces an additional rise of 5-HT in brain (CANAL et al. 1959; DUBNICK et al. 1959b; FUNDERBURK et al. 1962; H. GREEN et al. 1962; PLETSCHER and GEY, unpubl.).

— Histochemical investigations show that the reserpine-induced monoamine depletion in the enterochromaffine granules and the adrenal medulla is counteracted by MAO inhibitors (ZBINDEN and STUDER 1958a; ZBINDEN et al. 1957) (Fig. 7).

— MAO inhibitors counteract the release of 5-HT from blood platelets by reserpine and tetrabenazine in vitro as well as the reserpine-induced catecholamine release from isolated atria of guinea pigs (PAASONEN 1961b; PAASONEN and PLETSCHER 1960; PEPEU et al. 1961).

— MAO inhibitors block the spontaneous and reserpine-induced release of ^{3}H-labelled NE from the heart (AXELROD et al. 1961a).

— The MAO inhibitors prevent the NE decrease in brain due to electroshock (LEVI and MAYNERT 1964; MAYNERT and LEVI 1963, 1964); they also diminish the release from the isolated heart induced by nerve stimulation (HUKOVIC and MUSCHOLL 1962).

— The reserpine-induced relative increase of monoamines in the supernatant as compared to the particulate fraction of tissue homogenates is attenuated or abolished by MAO inhibitors (GIARMAN 1961; GIARMAN and SCHANBERG 1958; H. GREEN and SAWYER 1960a). Experiments of other investigators with reserpine as well as with MAO inhibitors + reserpine are, however, hardly in agreement with these findings (R. A. COHEN et al. 1962; WEIL-MALHERBE and BONE 1959; WEIL-MALHERBE et al. 1961a).

It remains to be investigated whether inhibition of MAO is directly responsible for the interference with monoamine storing. The finding that incubation in nitrogen atmosphere inhibits the tretabenazine-induced 5-HT release from isolated platelets (PAASONEN 1961b) tends to support this assumption.

b) Other metabolic effects

α) Carbohydrate metabolism and oxygen consumption. In *humans*, according to most investigators, MAO inhibitors decrease fasting blood sugar and *blood glucose*. Furthermore, MAO inhibitors induce hypoglycemic tolerance curves after infusion of glucose (but not after fructose and galactose) and prolong the hypoglycemic effect of insulin (AKSEL 1960; BARONI et al. 1957; COOPER and KEDDIE 1964; HEGGLIN et al. 1960; I. J. GREENBLATT and KAHN 1959; LEAK and DORMANDY 1961; OEZAYDIN and KOPTAGEL 1960; REYMOND et al. 1960; WEISS et al. 1959, 1960; WICKSTRÖM and PETTERSON 1964). Dependent on the therapeutic effect of MAO inhibitors in patients with angina pectoris, the level of *pyruvate* in blood is increased (HEGGLIN et al. 1960; MARQUILLO et al. 1962).

In fed but not in starved *animals* MAO inhibitors in reasonable doses decrease blood sugar and *blood glucose*. MAO inhibitors diminish the hyperglycemia caused by NE, epinephrine, reserpine, and morphine in unanesthetized, but not in narcotized animals (BOER et al. 1959; GEY and PLETSCHER, unpubl.; JORI et al. 1959; LAMESTA et al. 1960; MARQUARDT and KRAUSE 1962; MAZZONE et al. 1959; RANDALL and HALL, unpubl.; SCHMITT and SPÄTH 1963; SOULAIRAC et al. 1961). Iproniazid enhances the insulin-induced hypoglycemia in normal rats, whereas in reserpinized animals it has a protective effect against hypoglycemia due to insulin (MAZZONE et al. 1960; SCHAEPDRYVER and PREZIOSI 1959a; SOULAIRAC et al. 1960, 1961). In blood of rats, *lactate* and *pyruvate* are increased by MAO inhibitors of various types simultaneously with the monoamines in tissue (GEY and PLETSCHER 1960b, 1961a) (Fig. 8). The elevation of lactate and pyruvate in blood due to exogenous NE and 5-HT is enhanced by iproniazid (GEY and PLETSCHER 1960b). In the brain, however, no change of lactate and pyruvate was found (ESTLER 1962).

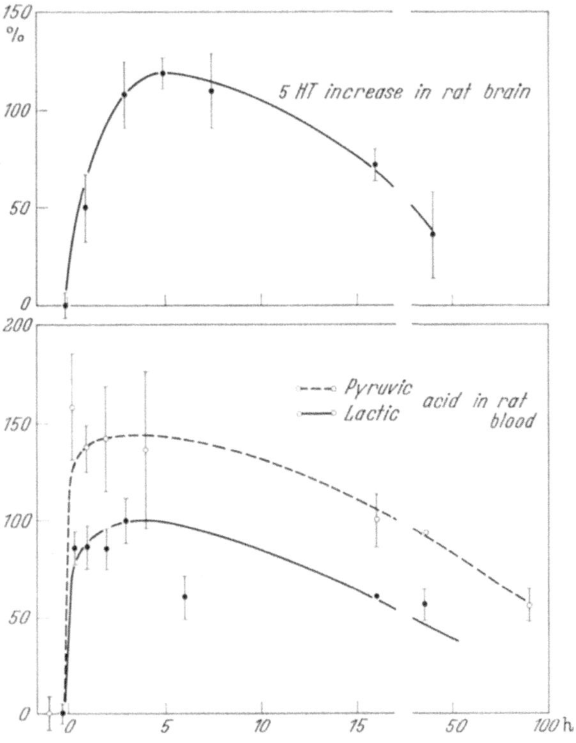

Fig. 8. *Increase of 5-hydroxytryptamine in brain as well as of pyruvic and lactic acid in blood of rats after administration of phenylcyclopropylamine. Ordinate:* Increase in percent of controls. *Abscissa:* Time in hours after i.p. injection of the MAO inhibitor. Doses of cis-trans-phenylcyclopropylamine: for 5-hydroxytryptamine in brain: 3 mg/kg; for the acids in blood: 30 mg/kg. Each point represents an average of 4—11 experiments with standard error (GEY and PLETSCHER 1961a)

The hypoglycemic action of MAO inhibitors together with the increase of pyruvate and lactate in blood might indicate an acceleration of the anaerobic glycolysis in glucose-consuming tissues. In the anesthetized perfused brain and in the heart in vivo, MAO inhibitors have indeed been found to increase the CO_2-formation from labelled glucose although in the heart the uptake of glucose might have been reduced (GEIGER et al. 1960; TEMPERO and KIEN 1964). Stimulation of aerobic glycolysis has also been postulated based on arterio-venous differences in brain (CAHN 1961; HÉROLD and CAHN 1961).

Whether MAO inhibitors also stimulate glycogenolysis, e.g. by enhancing the glycogenolytic effects of monoamines, remains unknown. A slight increase of brain glycogen after iproniazid (ESTLER 1962) might rather indicate the contrary or an enhanced glycogen formation. In any case, phosphorylase activity in the heart and brain is not influenced by iproniazid and isocarboxazid (see above).

According to some but not all investigators, iproniazid decreases *oxygen consumption of intact animals;* the drug also seems to rise the resistance of the isolated perfused heart to anoxia. This is consistent with the assumption that MAO inhibitors activate glycolysis. The 5-HT- induced reduction of oxygen consumption is prolonged and the NE-induced increase of oxygen consumption is enhanced by the MAO inhibitor (CAHN and HÉROLD 1960a, 1960b; CAHN et al. 1961b; ESTLER 1962; FÖLDES and PÁLINKÁS 1960; G. E. JOHNSON and SELLERS 1960; SETNIKAR and RAVASI 1960; SETNIKAR et al. 1960a; VIZI et al. 1963). A reduction of oxygen consumption might also be related to an increase of ATP as found by some (but not all) authors in brain and thrombocytes (see above). Iproniazid in combination with reserpine, however, increases oxygen consumption in rats, although reserpine alone has no effect (VIZI et al. 1963).

β) Diamines and other amines. Several MAO inhibitors of the hydrazine type, e.g. iproniazid, also inhibit DAO and are thus likely to interfere with the metabolism of diamines. Iproniazid indeed increases the toxicity of *spermidine* (TABOR and ROSENTHAL 1956).

The effect of MAO inhibitors on the metabolism of *histamine* in vivo has not been fully elucidated. In animals iproniazid (and partly isoniazid) modifies the metabolic pattern in the urine after ^{14}C-histamine. It increases histamine in blood and urine as well as histamine excretion due to the histamine liberator 48/80 and it decreases urinary ^{14}C-methylimidazoleacetic acid after administration of ^{14}C-methylhistamine. In mice injected with ^{14}C-histamine, pheniprazine slows the disappearance of ^{14}C-methylhistamine but not of ^{14}C-histamine (KELLER 1959; ROTHSCHILD and SCHAYER 1958; SCHAYER 1953a; SNYDER and AXELROD 1964a; WASER and ITZBICKI 1959). Furthermore, iproniazid enhances the hypotensive effect of histamine injected into the renal artery (LINDELL 1957). In man this hydrazide inhibits the oxidation of ^{14}C-histamine and methylhistamine to the corresponding carboxylic acids (LINDELL et al. 1960). MAO inhibitors have, however, been found to be without effect on histamine excretion in humans, on the histamine content of various animal tissues, on the insuline-induced histamine increase of the rat stomach, on the LD^{50} of histamine, and on the effect of the amine on blood pressure in cats as well as on isolated rabbit intestine (ANGELAKOS and LÖW 1957, 1958; BURKHALTER et al. 1959; KIM and SHORE 1963; MITCHELL 1956). These discrepancies might be due to the predominance of different metabolic pathways (e.g. primary N-methylation, primary oxidative deamination) depending on the species, tissue, and the techniques used.

In animals hydrazine derivatives with and without MAO inhibition, in contrast to non-hydrazine MAO inhibitors (harmine, tranylcypromine, pargyline), reduce the oxidative deamination of *methylamine* (E. J. DAVIS and ROPP 1960, 1961; WERNER and SEILER 1963; WERNER et al. 1961).

In patients with liver damage, iproniazid unlike isoniazid rises the arteriovenous difference of *ammonia* and reduces the increased arterial ammonia levels. This effect might be due to decreased peripheral ammonia production in consequence of MAO inhibition (DAWSON and SHERLOCK 1958).

γ) Vitamin B_6. Interference with pyridoxal-5′-phosphate which acts as a coenzyme in various enzyme systems (e.g. decarboxylases, transaminases) may be the cause of some pharmacological or clinical effects of MAO inhibitors especially of the hydrazine type (BIEHL and VILTER 1954; CORIANDOLI et al. 1959; ROSEN 1955, 1959; H. L. WILLIAMS and ABDULIAN 1956). Direct evidence that MAO inhibitors markedly interfere with vitamin B_6 is, however, lacking. Thus, an increased elimination of vitamin B_6 in the urine was obtained only with sublethal doses of iproniazid and other hydrazides (PLETSCHER et al. 1960c; WEBER and WISS, unpubl.).

From indirect evidence it would seem that iproniazid influences vitamin B_6 relatively little and probably less than other hydrazides such as isoniazid. The latter may, for instance, cause convulsions and peripheral neuritis, effects which are probably due to interference with vitamin B_6. MAO inhibitors of the hydrazine type induce no convulsions or have even an anticonvulsive action. Furthermore, iproniazid is less effective in causing peripheral neuritis than isoniazid (JENNEY and PFEIFFER 1958; JENNEY et al. 1953; REILLY et al. 1953; ZBINDEN 1960b; ZBINDEN and STUDER 1955a, 1955b). The acute toxicity of MAO inhibitors of the hydrazine type has been reported not to be influenced or to be increased by pyridoxine deficiency depending on the species or strain and to be increased by 4-desoxypyridoxine (vitamin B_6 antagonist). Administration of vitamin B_6 does not influence the 5-HT increase in brain due to MAO inhibitors of the hydrazine type (LEESON et al. 1959; PLETSCHER et al. 1960c).

δ) Varia. Certain hydrazine derivatives may inhibit the *decarboxylation of aromatic amino acids* in vivo (see below). MAO inhibitors of the hydrazine type have also been shown to delay the degradation of barbiturates in the intact animal and in the isolated perfused liver as well as of amphetamine in spiders (FOUTS and BRODIE 1950; FUJIMOTO et al. 1960; MATTHIES et al. 1962; PEARCE et al. 1959; WITT et al. 1961). This might be due to inhibition of *amphetamine oxidase*, an enzyme responsible for barbiturate oxidation (see above).

Furthermore, MAO inhibitors cause the following effects on *tissue metabolites:*

— Increase of acetylcholine and free alanine in the brain (HAAS and APPEL 1962; ROPP and SNEDEKER 1961) without changes of phosphocreatine and inorganic phosphate (PETTEN and LEWIS 1962).

— Decrease of the level of various α-amino acids in rat brain, but probably no change or an increase of γ-aminobutyric acid; enhancement of the transfer of α-aminoisobutyric acid into the brain (BALZER and PALM 1962; ELLIOT and GELDER 1960; ERNSTING et al. 1960; FERRARI and ARNOLD 1961; LOVELL et al. 1963; MAYNERT and KAJI 1962; MUSSINI and MARCUCCI 1962; PALM et al. 1962c; ROPP and SNEDEKER 1961).

— Alterations of the ascorbic acid and cholesterol content in the adrenals (GEORGES and HÉROLD 1958; MITCHELL 1956; SCHAEPDRYVER and PREZIOSI 1959a).

— Effect on connective tissue, mineral, and lipid metabolism, e.g. the potentiation of the cold-induced mobilisation of unesterified fatty acids (BLACK et al. 1958; HÉROLD et al. 1961; KATZ et al. 1959; PSCHEIDT 1962; QUADBECK 1960; REYNOLDS et al. 1959; STOCK and WESTERMANN 1962b).

— Decrease of the hydrogen bonding in the ribosomal ribonucleic acid of brain cortex (DATTA and GHOSH 1964).

These effects of MAO inhibitors are difficult to interprete at the present time.

6. Pharmacodynamic effects

MAO inhibitors show a great variety of pharmacodynamic actions which differ with the individual compound. The changes may be either due to MAO inhibition or to other mechanisms, e.g. interference with other enzyme systems, direct effects on pharmacological receptors. The present review is mainly concerned with actions apparently related to MAO inhibition. The other effects will only be briefly summarized.

a) Effects mainly connected with monoamine oxidase inhibition

α) Modification of the action of exogenous monoamines and their precursors

MAO inhibitors modify various effects of monoamines and their precursors on the *central nervous system.* They enhance hyperthermia induced by various monoamines, the convulsive effect of tryptamine, the central nervous stimulating effect of desoxyephedrine, the action of NE and epinephrine injected into the cerebral ventricles, as well as the 5-HT- and tryptamine-induced prolongation of barbiturate or chloral hypnosis. Behavioural, autonomic and other effects of the monoamine precursors 3,4-dihydroxyphenylalanine (dopa), 5-HTP, tryptophan, ortho- and meta-tyrosine, etc. (e.g. motor excitation, arousal reaction, tremors, hyperthermia, mydriasis, hypertension) are increased by pretreatment with MAO inhibitors. Pretreatment with pargyline followed by imipramine enhances the central nervous effects of dopa in mice more markedly than pargyline alone Isoniazid, a weak MAO inhibitor, is in general, devoid of these actions (APRISON and FERSTER 1961; BLASCHKO and CHRUŚCIEL 1960; BRIMBLECOMBE and GREEN 1962; BUCHEL et al. 1960b; A. BURGER et al. 1961; CARLSSON et al. 1957a; COSTA et al. 1961a; DAT-XUONG et al. 1962; DENYS et al. 1961; EVERETT et al. 1959, 1963; FERSTER and APRISON 1959; H. GREEN and SAWYER 1960b; GYLYS and OSBORNE 1962; GYLYS et al. 1963; HOLTZ et al. 1957b; HORITA 1959; G. E. JOHNSON et al. 1962; KOBINGER 1958; LESSIN 1959b; J. LÉVY and MICHEL-BER 1960a, 1960c; MITOMA et al. 1957; NASHOLD et al. 1962; OATES and SJOERDSMA 1960; PLETSCHER and GEY, unpubl.; POLLIN et al. 1961; RANDALL and BAGDON 1959; R. P. ROWE 1959; R. P. ROWE et al. 1959a, 1959b; SCHILDKRAUT et al. 1963; SCHNEIDER et al. 1959; D. H. TEDESCHI et al. 1959a, 1959b, 1960a; WADA 1961; ZBINDEN et al. 1960).

Some effects of monoamines on the central nervous system are, however, decreased or not influenced by MAO inhibitors. In rabbits iproniazid and other MAO inhibitors of the hydrazine type counteract the blood pressure rise (but not the increased spontaneous motility of the uterus) due to local application of epinephrine on the fronto-parietal cerebral cortex. This effect might be connected with inhibition of the epinephrine-induced vasopressine release by MAO inhibitors or with an increased content of endogenous monoamines in the brain as a consequence of MAO inhibition (see below) (MINZ 1960; MINZ and WALASZEK 1959).

MAO inhibitors do not uniformly influence the effects of monoamines on the *cardiovascular system and the nictitating membrane* possibly depending on the species, the individual amine, and the experimental technique. Most investigators report that MAO inhibitors enhance, for instance, the contraction of the nictitating membrane, the changes in blood pressure and heart action due to dopa and monoamines like tyramine, tryptamine, phenylethylamine, dopamine, 5-HT, 4-hydroxyphenylethanolamine, isoproterenol. Correspondingly, aromatic amines like tyramine (and possibly aromatic amino acids) contained in certain cheeses may cause hypertension in patients and animals receiving MAO inhibitors, e.g. tranylcypromine. The tyramine- and tryptamine-induced rise of blood pressure in dogs is distinctly enhanced after combined treatment with iproniazid + reserpine, possibly because of disturbances of the NE metabolism in the vessel wall. A few authors found that MAO inhibitors also enhance different effects of NE and epinephrine, nicotine, vasopressine, etc., especially the blood pressure rise in animals and humans, the contraction of the isolated aorta and of the decentralized nictitating membrane, the constriction of the peripheral arteries as well as of the mesenteric capillaries. According to most investigators, however, the cardiovascular activity of NE and epinephrine does not seem to be markedly modified or is even counteracted by MAO inhibitors, e.g. the blood pressure rise, the positive inotropic effect on the heart, the contraction of the nictitating membrane and of the small mesenteric, cutaneous, and digital blood vessels, as well as of the isolated aorta (Table 5). Myocardial necroses due to isoproterenol are also diminished by MAO inhibitors of the hydrazine type. Furthermore, the latter counteract the positive inotropic effect, the rise of blood pressure, as well as other cardiovascular effects of various drugs, e.g. nicotine and acetylcholine, which probably act by stimulating the adrenal medulla (ARAI et al. 1961; ASATOOR et al. 1963; BÄCHTOLD and PLETSCHER 1959; BALOURDAS 1964; BALZER and HOLTZ 1956; BARAC 1961; BURFORD and WALASZEK 1960; BURFORD et al. 1960; BURN et al. 1954; W. G. CLARK and POGRUND 1961; CORNE and GRAHAM 1957; CROUT 1961; DAVEY et al. 1962; DEGKWITZ et al. 1960; DEOREO and STOUGHTON 1961; EBLE 1962; FABRE et al. 1962; FREY 1963; FRIEND et al. 1958; FONTANINI et al.

Table 5. *Decrease of the norepinephrine-induced contraction of the isolated aorta by iproniazid*

The maximal contraction of aortic strips on addition of the amines to the bath fluid was measured. Rabbits pretreated with twice 50 mg/kg iproniazid or isoniazid i.v. 44 and 20 hours before sacrifice were compared to non-treated animals. The values indicate percents of controls and represent averages from 12—15 animals with standard error.

		Petreatment with	
		Iproniazid	Isoniazid
Norepinephrine	1 μg	*37 ± 7**	93 ± 13
	5 μg	*41 ± 4**	135 ± 25
5-Hydroxytryptamine	10 μg	78 ± 22	90 ± 19

* Significant decrease of the amplitude of contraction as compared to non-treated animals ($p < 0.01$) (BÄCHTOLD and PLETSCHER 1959).

1960; FURCHGOTT 1955; FURCHGOTT et al. 1955; GATGOUNIS and AYCOCK 1961, 1963; GATGOUNIS et al. 1959; GITLOW et al. 1959; GOLDBERG and SJOERDSMA 1959; GRIESEMER et al. 1953, 1955; GYLYS and OSBORNE 1962; GYLYS et al. 1959, 1963; HAZARD et al. 1960, 1961; HERMANN and MORNEX 1960; HORNYKIEWICZ 1958; HORWITZ et al. 1960a, 1960b, 1964; IMAIZUMI et al. 1959; IZQUIERDO et al. 1960; KOBINGER and FRIIS 1961; LACROIX and LEUSEN 1961; LACROIX et al. 1962b; LEE et al. 1961; LEUSEN 1959b; MARIANI and MORTARI 1960; R. A. MAXWELL et al. 1962; McCUBBIN et al. 1960; MOUQUIN and MILOVANOVICH 1962; NAKMURA and SHIMAMOTO 1960; PALOL and LEMBERG 1962; PEPEU et al. 1961; PISANTY et al. 1959b; REDISCH et al. 1960; RYALL 1961; SCHAIN 1961; SCHMITT and GONNARD 1955, 1956; TEDESCHI and FELLOWS 1964; VANOV 1962; VOTAVA and LAMPLOVÁ 1961; ZBINDEN 1960a, 1961, 1962; ZBINDEN et al. 1960; ZWEIFACH and CASCARANO 1959).

Various *other effects* of monoamines are enhanced by MAO inhibitors, e.g. the tryptamine-induced contraction of fundal strips of rat stomach; the anorexogenic action of dopa; the NE-induced rise in the metabolic rate of animals; the effects of 5-HT on connective tissue; cataracts caused by 5-HT, NE, and epinephrine; the acute toxicity of tryptamine, NE, tyramine, phenylethylamine, etc. The toxicity of epinephrine seems to be either enhanced or not influenced by MAO inhibitors (BOROWITZ and NORTH 1959a, 1959b; GUM et al. 1960; ERNST et al. 1961; G. E. JOHNSON and SELLERS 1960; MANTEGAZZA and RIVA 1961; R. A. MAXWELL et al. 1962; McLEAN and BERRY 1960a, 1960b; PISANTY et al. 1959b; REBHUN et al. 1954; SCHERBEL et al. 1960; SHANAMAN et al. 1961; SMYTH et al. 1962).

The *mechanism* by which MAO inhibitors influence the pharmacological effects of endogenous monoamines and their precursors is only partly understood.

The *enhancement* of the central nervous and cardiovascular effects of some monoamines and precursors might be due to decreased inactivation because of MAO inhibition. This would explain that MAO inhibitors increase the effects of the amines that are mainly metabolized by MAO (e.g. tryptamine, tyramine, as well as 5-HT in the brain). In organs with other major metabolic pathways (e.g. O-methylation for catecholamines, glucuronide formation for 5-HT and catecholamines), MAO inhibition has probably little influence on the inactivation of monoamines and thus on their pharmacological action.

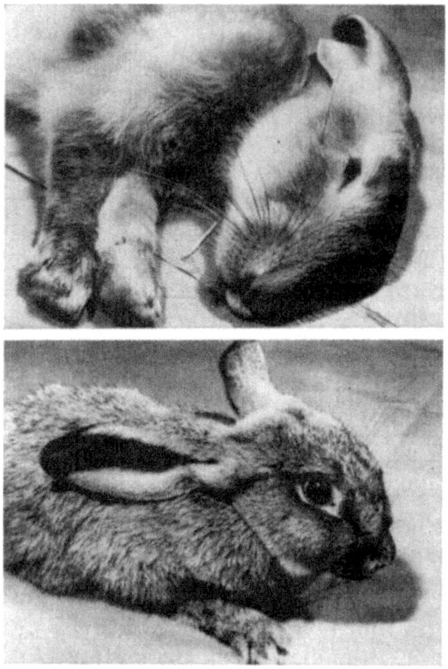

Fig. 9. *Reversal of the sedative effect of a monoamine releaser (tetrabenazine) by iproniazid. Above:* 15 minutes after 40 mg/kg tetrabenazine (benzoquinolizine derivative) i.v.; *below:* Pretreatment with 100 mg/kg iproniazid i.v. 16 hours before tetrabenazine (PLETSCHER 1959)

The fact that MAO inhibitors *counteract* some effects of monoamines, especially the cardiovascular actions of NE and epinephrine, remains to be further elucidated. In principle, two possibilities are being discussed:

— Certain MAO inhibitors, because of structural similarities with catecholamines, might compete for the same pharmacological receptor sites and therefore cause adrenergic blockade. Such an antiadrenergic effect has been shown for various MAO inhibitors of the hydrazine type by in vitro experiments with aortic strips and seminal vessels (BURFORD et al. 1960; DAY 1962; GRIESEMER et al. 1955; KAMIJO et al. 1956; KOBINGER and FRIIS 1961; KOELLE 1958; ZBINDEN et al. 1960).

— The stimulatory effect of exogenous NE and epinephrine on certain organs, e.g. blood vessels and cerebral cortex, might depend on their content of endogenous monoamines. Thus, drugs decreasing the endogenous monoamines (e.g. reserpine, tetrabenazine) enhance the sensitivity of organs, such as the cerebral cortex and the blood vessels, for NE and epinephrine. MAO inhibitors which increase the content of endogenous monoamines in various tissues might have the opposite effect (BÄCHTOLD and PLETSCHER 1959; BURN and RAND 1958a, 1958b; DUBNICK et al. 1963; MINZ and WALASZEK 1959; PLETSCHER et al. 1960c).

β) Counteraction of monoamine releasers. *Pretreatment with MAO inhibitors* counteracts or reverses various pharmacological effects of monoamine releasers. Thus, in several species reserpine and benzoquinolizine derivatives injected subsequently to MAO inhibitors no longer cause sedation, hypothermia, miosis, ptosis, but on the contrary motor excitation, hyperthermia, mydriasis, piloerection (Fig. 9). The potentiation of ethanol, barbiturates, and chloral by reserpine and benzoquinolizine derivatives is also antagonized by MAO inhibitors (BESENDORF and PLETSCHER 1956; BOVET-NITTI et al. 1961; BRODIE et al. 1956; BUCHEL and LÉVY 1960b; G. CHEN and BOHNER 1959; 1961; COSTA and PSCHEIDT 1960, 1961; DAVISON et al. 1957; ELTHERINGTON and HORITA 1960; EVERETT et al. 1959; FINGER et al. 1962; GARATTINI et al. 1960; GENOVESE et al. 1959; H. GREEN and ERICKSON 1962; H. GREEN et al. 1961; GYLYS and OSBORNE 1962;

Holtz et al. 1957b; Kobinger 1958; Kuntzman et al. 1961a; Kuznets et al. 1961; Lévy and Michel-Ber 1960a, 1960c; Pletscher et al. 1958, 1962; R. P. Rowe 1959; R. P. Rowe et al. 1959a, 1959b; Schneider et al. 1959; Shore and Brodie 1957; R. E. Tedeschi et al. 1959a, 1959b; Zbinden et al. 1960).

With some exceptions, the following effects of monoamine releasers are also counteracted or reversed by MAO inhibitors:

— The hypotensive action of reserpine (Chessin et al. 1956, 1957, 1959; Eltherington 1961; Eltherington and Horita 1960; Franco-Browder et al. 1958; Garattini et al. 1960; Gylys and Osborne 1962; Gylys et al. 1963; R. A. Maxwell et al. 1957; Mortari et al. 1962). In cats, the reserpine reversal by iproniazid seems to diminish with increasing doses of the MAO inhibitor (Hull and Horita 1964).

— The reserpine- and benzoquinolizine-induced facilitation of convulsive seizures due to electroshock, metrazol, audiogenic stimuli, hexafluorodiethyl ether, etc. (Balzer et al. 1961; G. Chen and Bohner 1959; 1961; Gylys and Osborne 1962; Hertting 1958; Lehmann and R. G. Busnel 1961, 1962; Palm et al. 1961a; Prockop et al. 1959a, 1959b; R. P. Rowe 1959; R. P. Rowe et al. 1959a, 1959b; Schneider et al. 1959; Spoerlein and Ellman 1961; Truitt and Ebersberger 1959; L. R. Weiss et al. 1960).

— The reserpine- and tetrabenazine-induced enhancement of the respiratory and circulatory effects of metrazol- and electroshock (Kobinger 1958; Piette and Reuse 1960; Reuse 1960a, 1960b; Schaepdryver and Piette 1961; Schneider et al. 1959).

— The enhanced toxicity of metrazol due to monoamine releasers in mice (Lessin and Parkes 1959).

— The reserpine- and benzoquinolizine-induced inhibition of conditioned reflexes (Heise and Boff 1960; Knoll and Knoll 1961; Orsingher 1961; Stein and Ray 1960).

— Certain effects of reserpine on the spontaneous EEG and on the EEG after electrical stimulation (Bignami et al. 1962; Cahn and Hérold 1960c; Savoldi et al. 1960).

— The reserpine-induced decrease of morphine and methadone analgesia (Buchel et al. 1960a; Schaumann 1958, 1960; Schumacher 1959).

— Gastric ulcers, gastro-intestinal hemorrhages, increase of gastrointestinal motility and gastric secretion induced by reserpine (Blackman et al. 1959; Bonfils et al. 1960; Franco-Browder et al. 1959; Leusen et al. 1959; Pletscher et al. 1960c; Studer and Zbinden 1960; Thoenen et al. 1962; Zbinden et al. 1958, 1959) (Table 6).

— The antiemetic effect of reserpine in dogs and cats, the emetic action of the alkaloid in pigeons (Förster and Kunze 1961; Gupta and Dhawan 1960).

— The reserpine-induced increase of the adrenal weight and the enhancement of adrenal and pituitary function (Canal et al. 1961; Kruger et al. 1960; Thoenen et al. 1962).

— The reserpine-induced decrease of the group toxicity of amphetamine in mice (Halpern and Drudi-Baracco 1961; Halpern et al. 1962a, 1962b, 1962c, 1962d).

— The reserpine-induced decrease of the hyperthermic effect of bacterial pyrogen (Kroneberg and Kurbjuweit 1959).

— The reserpine-induced pseudogestation (Bignami 1960; Bignami et al. 1962; Bovet-Nitti and Bignami 1961).

Several effects of Rauwolfia alkaloids and tetrabenazine are *not influenced* by pretreatment with MAO inhibitors, e.g. the reserpine-induced elevation of blood glucose (FINGER et al. 1962), the inhibitory action of reserpine on the hypertensive response to eserine in rats (LEŠIĆ and VARAGIĆ 1961; VARAGIĆ et al. 1961), the antiemetic effect of rescinamine (FÖRSTER and KUNZ 1961). Furthermore, pretreatment with pargyline does not influence the sedative effect of the NE releaser oxypertine (1-[5,6-dimethoxy-2-methyl-3-indole]ethyl-4-phenylpiperazine), although the MAO inhibitor counteracts the NE decrease in brain (S. SPECTOR et al. 1962). Some actions of monoamine releasers are even *enhanced* by MAO inhibitors, e.g. the antiemetic effects of tetrabenazine in rats (FÖRSTER and KUNZ 1961), the hypertensive action of reserpine in rats deprived of their adrenal medulla (SCHMITT and SCHMITT 1961), the reserpine-induced increase of free fatty acids in blood (SCHNEIDER et al. 1962), the radioprotective effect of reserpine (BRENK and ELLIOTT 1958). In the isolated atrium of guinea pig hearts the depressant effect of reserpine is influenced differently by iproniazid and pheniprazine, whereas the the action of nicotine is antagonized by both MAO inhibitors (PEPEU et al. 1961).

Injection of *MAO inhibitors after reserpine* (e.g. of iproniazid, N^1-phenylisopropyl-N^2-isopropylhydrazine, pargyline) at the time of maximal monoamine depletion and sedation accelerates the recovery of normal behaviour. This effect in general occurs only several hours after administration of the inhibitors. Some compounds, e.g. tranylcypromine, however, counteract the reserpine sedation rapidly (H. GREEN and ERICKSON 1962; PLETSCHER 1957a; PLETSCHER et al. 1960c; R. P. ROWE et al. 1961; S. SPECTOR et al. 1960a; R. E. TEDESCHI et al. 1959b), probably owing in part to additional amphetamine-like stimulation of the central nervous system.

The interaction between monoamine releasers and MAO inhibitors with regard to the pharmacological effects is probably connected with changes in monoamine metabolism. This may be concluded from the following findings:

— Only hydrazine derivatives inhibiting MAO in vivo counteract reserpine and benzoquinolizines. Hydrazides which are not MAO inhibitors, e.g. isoniazid, do not show this effect. Furthermore, non-hydrazine MAO inhibitors (derivatives of harmane, tranylcypromine, pargyline) also antagonize reserpine and benzoquinolizines (PLETSCHER et al. 1960c).

— The accelerated behavioural recovery of animals treated with MAO inhibitors subsequent to monoamine releasers parallels the enhanced restoration of the monoamine content in the brain (see above) (COSTA and PSCHEIDT 1961; H. GREEN et al. 1961; PLETSCHER 1957a; PLETSCHER et al. 1960c; S. SPECTOR et al. 1960a; STEIN and RAY 1960).

— The action of chlorpromazine which like reserpine is sedative and hypothermic, but does not influence the total monoamine content of brain, is not counteracted by iproniazid (BÄCHTOLD and PLETSCHER 1957; PLETSCHER et al. 1960c).

The mechanisms responsible for the decrease or reversal of the pharmacological effects of monoamine releasers are not yet fully understood. Hypotheses are mainly based on the assumption that release of stored monoamines is essential for some pharmacological effects of reserpine and benzoquinolizine derivatives. The following possibilities have to be considered:

— Subsequent to MAO inhibition, reserpine and benzoquinolizine derivatives cause an increase of free monoamines which leads to motor excitation, hypertension, and sympathomimetic effects (see above). This hypothesis is supported by the findings that these actions are antagonized by adrenergic blocking agents (e.g. phenoxybenzamine, phentolamine) as well as adrenalectomy (FRANCO-BROWDER et al. 1958; GARATTINI et al. 1960a; SICUTERI et al. 1962). Furthermore, dopa, 5-HTP, 5-HT, tryptamine, and dopamine, especially after MAO inhibition, counteract some pharmacological effects of Rauwolfia alkaloids, e.g. sedation, ptosis (BLASCHKO and CHRUŚCIEL 1960; CARLSSON et al. 1957a; G. CHEN and BOHNER 1961; CHRUŚCIEL 1961; EVERETT 1961; GARATTINI et al. 1960b; WEISS et al. 1960).

— MAO inhibitors reduce the reserpine- and benzoquinolizine-induced release of stored monoamines and in consequence some pharmacological effects of the monoamine releasers (see above).

The first hypothesis would not only explain the attenuation of some effects of monoamine releasers, but also their reversal by MAO inhibitors (e.g. excitation instead of sedation, hyperthermia instead of hypothermia). The second hypothesis may explain some attenuating effects of MAO inhibitors.

It has not yet been fully elucidated which of the monoamines involved has the most important function in the antagonism between MAO inhibitors and monoamine releasers. Motor stimulation and hypertension after treatment with MAO inhibitors followed by monoamine releasers is, according to most investigators, due to excess of NE or dopamine (CARLSSON 1961; CARLSSON et al. 1957a; COSTA and BRODIE 1961a; COSTA et al. 1962; ELTHERINGTON 1961; EVERETT 1961; FRANCO-BROWDER et al. 1958; KUNTZMAN et al. 1961a; SICUTERI et al. 1962; G. B. SMITH and DEWS 1962; S. SPECTOR 1963; S. SPECTOR et al. 1960d, 1963). The accelerated behavioural recovery after MAO inhibitors subsequent to reserpine has been attributed to enhanced restoration of 5-HT (COSTA and PSCHEIDT 1960, 1961; H. GREEN and ERICKSON 1962; H. GREEN et al. 1961; S. SPECTOR et al. 1960a) or catecholamines (CARLSSON 1961; MATSUOKA et al. 1964; SEIDEN and CARLSSON 1964; S. SPECTOR et al. 1963; STEIN and RAY 1960).

γ) Anticonvulsant effect. MAO inhibitors seem to counteract several types of convulsions and not to influence or even enhance others. Most authors agree that MAO inhibitors diminish the frequency of convulsive seizures due to supramaximal electroshock and increase the threshold current required to produce seizures especially in normal rats (but not in rats pretreated with X-rays) (BUCHEL and LÉVY 1960c; CHOW and HENDLEY 1959; FROMMEL et al. 1960; HAAS and APPEL 1962; KEASLING et al. 1962; P'AN et al. 1961; PICCHINONI et al. 1962; PROCKOP et al. 1959a, 1959b; ROSENTHAL and TIMIRAS 1961). Furthermore, the protective action of various drugs (e.g. of diphenylhydantoine) against electroshock is increased by MAO inhibitors in rats and mice (P'AN et al. 1961; YEN et al. 1960). — MAO inhibitors also reduce seizures due to audiogenic stimuli (BUCHEL and LÉVY 1960c; LEHMANN and M.-C. BUSNEL 1959; LEHMANN and R. G. BUSNEL 1959, 1961; WERBOFF et al. 1961a), raise the convulsive threshold of hexafluorodimethylether (LEUSEN 1960), counteract the bulbocapnine-induced enhancement of metrazol-shock (KOBINGER 1959), and delay the onset of tremorine tremors (P. STERN and GAŠPAROVIC 1961).

With respect to the effect of MAO inhibitors on metrazol-seizures controversial results have been reported, i.e. protection (LOPES DO ROSARIO 1959/60; PROCKOP et al. 1959b; L. R. WEISS et al. 1960), no effect or facilitation (BONNYCASTLE et al. 1957; EVERETT et al. 1959; FROMMEL et al. 1960; HERTTING 1958; KOBINGER 1958; REUSE 1960b; SANSONE and DELL'OMODARME 1963; SPOERLEIN and ELLMAN 1961). Convulsions due to caffeine and strychnine are not influenced by MAO inhibitors (PROCKOP et al. 1959a; SCHMIDT 1961). The latter even enhance cocaine- and tryptamine-induced seizures (PROCKOP et al. 1959a; SCHMIDT 1961; TEDESCHI et al. 1960a) and activate chronic experimental epilepsy in cats and monkeys (WADA 1961). In rats intraventricular administration of iproniazid and isoniazid causes convulsions (SINCLAIR 1960).

These discrepancies might be due to different mechanisms of action of the various convulsive agents (e.g. electroshock and tryptamine) and to differences in experimental procedures and animal species.

The following findings are in favour of a relationship between the anticonvulsive effects of MAO inhibitors and changes of monoamine metabolism in the central nervous system:

— The time course of the anticonvulsant action parallels the monoamine increase in brain according to some authors (PICCHINONI et al. 1962; PROCKOP et al. 1959a, 1959b).

— Increase of monoamines in brain by combined administration of iproniazid + dopa or 5-HTP counteracts tonic convulsions induced by hydrazides, like semicarbazide, or metrazol (BALZER et al. 1960; KOBINGER 1958).

— Isoniazid, a chemical congenere of iproniazid, but without effect on cerebral monoamines, has no anticonvulsant action and may even cause convulsions (PLETSCHER et al. 1960c; PROCKOP et al. 1959a, 1959b).

— The counteraction of the reserpine-induced facilitation of electroshock by MAO inhibitors parallels the reduction of the reserpine-induced monoamine decrease (see above) (PROCKOP et al. 1959b).

— Drugs lowering the monoamine content in brain (e.g. reserpine, tetrabenazine) enhance the effects of electroshock (G. CHEN et al. 1954; PLETSCHER et al. 1962) in contrast to MAO inhibitors which increase cerebral monoamines.

Other findings shed some doubts on the hypothesis that the anticonvulsive effects of MAO inhibitors are due to changes in the cerebral monoamine metabolism. Thus, the increase of monoamines in brain by pheniprazine, 5-HTP, and dopa respectively shows no relationship to the anticonvulsant action and does not influence the response to electroshock and its facilitation by reserpine (E. G. ANDERSON et al. 1962; BONNYCASTLE et al. 1957; PROCKOP et al. 1959a).

δ) Synaptic and neural transmission. At present it seems likely that at least high doses of MAO inhibitors interfere somehow with *ganglionic transmission*. Thus, MAO inhibitors diminish transmission in the perfused superior cervical ganglion of the cat as well as in the isolated cervical ganglion of the rat. The inhibition due to hydrazine derivatives is partially irreversible, whereas harmine has a reversible action. Parenteral administration of large doses of iproniazid and harmine in dogs and cats has also been found to inhibit transmission through sympathetic ganglia, whereas parasympathetic ganglia remained unaffected; in contrast pargyline causes only a transient blockade of the superior cervical ganglion in cats, but also diminishes the effects of vagal stimulation (DACOSTA and GOLDBERG 1961; KALBERMATTEN 1962; GERTNER 1959a, 1959b, 1961; L. I. GOLDBERG and DACOSTA 1960a, 1960b). Other authors, however, found no interference of parenterally administered MAO inhibitors with the transmission in the cervical, stellate, parasympathetic and other ganglia. Furthermore, pheniprazine, in contrast to iproniazid, has been reported to reduce ganglionic stimulation by a quarternary ammonium salt (McN-A-343). Moreover, various MAO inhibitors, but not isoniazid, attenuate the adrenal medullary responsiveness to nicotine and tetramethylammonium (BENSON et al. 1952; DAVEY et al. 1962; T. N. FISHER 1962; GATGOUNIS and AYCOCK 1963; B. LÉVY and AHLQUIST 1962; MENDEZ 1960; PELLMONT, unpubl.; PLETSCHER et al. 1960c; RANDALL 1958). These discrepancies might be due to differences in the doses and in the experimental techniques.

Several experimental findings support the assumption that the inhibiting effect of MAO inhibitors on ganglionic transmission may be connected with MAO inhibition:

— Only hydrazines inhibiting MAO decrease ganglionic transmission; isoniazid, for instance, is devoid of such an effect (GERTNER 1959a, 1959b, 1961).

— MAO inhibitors of various chemical structure (hydrazines, pargyline, phenylcypromine) cause ganglionic blockade (DACOSTA and GOLDBERG 1961; GERTNER 1959a, 1959b, 1961; L. I. GOLDBERG and DACOSTA 1960a, 1960b).

— Reserpine (decreasing NE in the ganglia) as well as adrenergic blocking agents facilitate ganglionic transmission. Reserpine after pretreatment with pargyline (increase of free monoamines) induces a pronounced diminution of ganglionic transmission (COSTA and BRODIE 1961b; COSTA et al. 1961b, 1961c).

The mechanism of inhibition of ganglionic transmission by MAO inhibitors does not seem to depend on the acetylcholinesterase system (GERTNER 1961). Endogenous NE in the sympathetic ganglia might have a modulating effect; increase of the amine by MAO inhibitors conceivably inhibits, whereas decrease of NE by reserpine facilitates ganglionic transmission (BRODIE and COSTA 1961; COSTA and BRODIE 1961b; COSTA et al. 1961b, 1961c).

Various MAO inhibitors also interfere with *synaptic transmission in the central nervous system* as indicated by a decrease of mono- and polysynaptic reflexes or by a decrease in the monosynaptic activity of the spinal cord. Furthermore, a reduction in the height of transcallosally evoked cortical potentials has been obtained which correlated well with MAO inhibition and a rise of 5-HT in the brain and which could also be observed after minute amounts of 5-HT (E. G. ANDERSON and BERK 1964; EMELE et al. 1960; FURGIUELE et al. 1962; GLUCKMAN et al. 1957; MARAZZI 1957, 1962; MARAZZI et al. 1961). This indicates that the cerebral synaptic inhibition might be causally connected with MAO inhibition and an increased 5-HT content. Other possibilities to be considered are: direct effect of the drugs on synapses, interference with other monoamines, etc.

Interference of MAO inhibitors with the function of *peripheral nerves* has been reported, e.g. decrease of irritability (resembling the effect of local anesthetics), interference with impulse conduction in peripheral nerve (CONDOURIS 1959, 1962). An analgesic effect of MAO inhibitors in the phenylquinone writhing, the hot plate and other tests has been found by some (EMELE et al. 1959, 1961; SALVA and MONTELEONE 1962), but not by all investigators (EVANS 1961; FROMMEL et al. 1960) and is difficult to interprete.

MAO inhibitors of different chemical structure seem to block *neuromuscular transmission* in the isolated nerve-muscle preparation as well as the response of the chronically denervated hemidiaphragm to acetylcholine (AMMANN and ANDERSON 1961; E. G. ANDERSON 1959; E. G. ANDERSON and AMMANN 1963). The NE output in a nerve-muscle preparation (cat spleen) during postganglionic sympathetic stimulation is not influenced by iproniazid (E. G. ANDERSON 1959; L. BROWN 1958).

b) Effects of doubtful connection with monoamine oxidase inhibition

α) Behaviour. The action of MAO inhibitors on *locomotor activity* is not uniform. Animal species, chemical constitution, and dose of the inhibitor as well as experimental techniques seem to be of importance. In general, MAO inhibitors, especially those with phenylethylamine-like structure, cause an increase of spontaneous motor activity, enhance irritability and aggressivity. This is specially evident after repeated administration of the inhibitors. Decrease of motor activity, however, has also been observed (ACHESON et al. 1961b; BIGNAMI et al. 1962; BRODIE et al. 1959a; B. B. BROWN 1960; BUCKLEY et al. 1960; DELGADO 1961; DOBKIN 1960; ELTHERINGTON and HORITA 1960; EVERETT 1961; EVERETT and WIEGAND 1961; EVERETT et al. 1959; FUNDERBURK et al. 1962; FURGIULE et al.

1962; GENOVESE et al. 1959; H. GREEN et al. 1962; E. N. GREENBLATT and OSTERBERG 1961a; GYLYS and MUCCIA 1964; GYLYS and OSBORNE 1962; HEIMSTRA 1962; W. A. HIMWICH and PETERSEN 1961; IRWIN 1959; IRWIN and TABACHNICK 1961; LIBERSON 1960; MAFFII and CONSTANTINI 1961; MELANDER and GLINIECKE 1961; MONNIER 1960; MÜLLER-CALGAN and HOTOVY 1961; R. P. ROWE et al. 1959b; SANAN and VOGT 1962; SCHALLEK and WALZ 1954; SCHUMANN et al. 1961; STEINER, unpubl.; STEVENS et al. 1961; TISSOT and MONNIER 1958; VANE et al. 1961).

Various conditioned reflexes are attenuated or not affected in a characteristic way by MAO inhibitors (e.g escape responses in animals, a psychogalvanic reflex in humans) (ALEXANDER 1961; ALEXANDER and HORNER 1961; ALEXANDER and LIPSETT 1959; MAFFII and CONSTANTINI 1961; PELLMONT and STEINER 1960; PLETSCHER et al. 1959b; R. P. ROWE 1959; STEINER, unpubl.). Various other effects of MAO inhibitors on behaviour have been reported, e.g. decrease of sexual activity in monkeys by iproniazid, changes in food intake by rats, counteraction of the depressant effects of cinnamic alcohol in hamsters, changes in rope climbing performance, decrease of emotional defecation in rats, etc. (ACHESON et al. 1961b; BRIMBLECOMBE and GREEN 1962; LIBERSON 1960; SOULAIRAC and SOULAIRAC 1960; WIRTH et al. 1960). Furthermore, in rats iproniazid inhibits electrical self-stimulation of various brain parts by implanted electrodes (EIDUSON 1959). Rats trained to perform self-injection of drugs into the hypothalamus inject iproniazid and epinephrine more frequently than other drugs or saline (OLDS and OLDS 1958).

There is no general agreement whether the behavioural effects of MAO inhibitors are causally connected with MAO inhibition and with changes in cerebral monoamine metabolism. The following facts are in favour of a relationship between monoamine metabolism and increased motor activity:

— Increase of the monoamine content in the brain and enhanced motor activity or irritability seem to be correlated (FUNDERBURK et al. 1962; BRODIE et al. 1959a, 1959b; IRWIN and TABACHNICK 1961).

— Monoamine precursors, e.g dopa, especially after pretreatment with MAO inhibitors cause motor excitation which is of similar quality to that produced by repeated administration of MAO inhibitors.

— The behavioural effects of monoamine precursors, e.g. in pigeons, depend on the degree of MAO inhibition (APRISON and FERSTER 1961).

The problem is complicated by the fact that some MAO inhibitors (e.g. tranylcypromine, pheniprazine), owing to their amphetamine-like structure, may produce sympathetic stimulation which is not connected with MAO inhibition (ELTHERINGTON and HORITA 1960; J. N. SPENCER et al .1960). It is therefore conceivable that these compounds increase motor activity by a dual mechanism of action, i.e. by a direct effect and via MAO inhibition.

According to various investigators, enhanced motor activity is rather connected with changes in the metabolism of catecholamines than with those of 5-HT and tryptamine (ACHESON et al. 1961a; BLASCHKO and CHRUŚCIEL 1960; BRODIE et al. 1959a, 1959b; EVERETT 1961; HESS and DOEPFNER 1961; S. SPECTOR et al. 1960d, 1963). This hypothesis needs, however, further confirmation, because it is not shared by other authors (FUNDERBURK et al. 1962; J. LÉVY and MICHEL-BER 1962; SANAN and VOGT 1962).

The importance of MAO inhibition for other behavioural effects (e.g. conditioned reactions) is rather doubtful (PLETSCHER et al. 1960c).

The relation between behavioural effects of MAO inhibitors in animals and the antidepressive action in man remains to be elucidated.

β) Electroencephalogram (EEG). At present, it is hardly possible to indicate a typical pattern for the effect of MAO inhibitors on the spontaneous EEG and the EEG-changes due to electrical stimulation. The alterations described in the literature are manyfold and often contradictory. Among others, the following changes of the spontaneous EEG have been described: increase of the electrical activity after a lag period; desynchronization, synchronization or lacking effects in various brain parts; increase, decrease, or no change of the arousal reaction; low voltage; slowing of the electrical activity in the reticular formation; appearance of spikes, waves, and spindles in hippocampus, cortex, and other brain parts. The threshold for electrical stimulation of the reticular formation has been found to be increased, decreased or unchanged. The after-discharge in various brain parts (e.g. hippocampus, amygdala) may be prolonged or reduced. The individual MAO inhibitors probably act differently from each other and their effect seems to vary depending on animal species and experimental techniques (electrocorticogram, implanted electrodes, cerveau isolé, anesthesia, etc.). The drugs probably affect various brain structures. (CAHN and HÉROLD 1960c; DACOSTA et al. 1960; EMELE et al. 1960; EVERETT 1961; FUNDERBURK and DRAKONTIDES 1960; FUNDERBURK et al. 1962; W. A. HIMWICH and PETERSEN 1961; H. E. HIMWICH et al. 1958, 1959; LIBERSON 1960; MONNIER 1960; PLAS and NAQUET 1961; SAVOLDI et al. 1960; SCHALLEK 1960; SCHALLEK and KUEHN 1959, 1960a, 1960b; SCHALLEK and WALZ 1954; SCHALLEK et al. 1962; TISSOT and MONNIER 1958; TRZEBSKI 1960).

There is no agreement whether some effects of MAO inhibitors on the electrical activity of the brain are causally connected with MAO inhibition. It seems, however, likely that other mechanisms are involved, because individual MAO inhibitors induce different EEG-changes.

MAO inhibitors enhance the effects of 5-HTP and dopa on the spontaneous EEG, decrease the convulsive threshold of metrazole and diminish the epileptogenic activity of strychnine topically applied on the cortex (REVZIN and DACOSTA 1960; SAVOLDI et al. 1960). These effects as well as the antagonism between MAO inhibitors and reserpine in the EEG are probably at least in part related to MAO inhibition (see above).

γ) Cardiovascular effects. MAO inhibitors cause a great variety of effects on the cardiovascular system which vary according to the individual inhibitor, animal species, and experimental procedure. At present, these actions cannot be attributed to a common mechanism and in most cases it is rather doubtful whether they are causally connected with MAO inhibition. Numerous, preferentially acute cardiovascular effects of MAO inhibitors have been reported:

— Increase, decrease, or no change of arterial pressure, depending on the chemical structure of the compounds. For instance, MAO inhibitors with a phenylalkylamine structure (pheniprazine, phenelzine, tranylcypromine) generally cause an acute rise in arterial pressure (ACEVES et al. 1960; BENSON et al. 1952; CAHN et al. 1961a; Chessin et al. 1959; DAVEY et al. 1962; ELTHERINGTON and HORITA 1960; GATGOUNIS and AYCOCK 1963; L. I. GOLDBERG 1959; GROVES and JENKINS 1961; GYLYS et al. 1963; HERMANN and MORNEX 1960; LEUSEN 1959b; PELLMONT 1960; PELLMONT, unpubl.; PLETSCHER et al. 1960c; R. P. ROWE 1959; SCHNEIDER et al. 1959; SCHOEPKE and WIEGAND 1963; SCHULER and WYSS 1960; J. N. SPENCER et al. 1960).

— Attenuation of carotid sinus reflexes (ELTHERINGTON and HORITA 1960; LEUSEN 1959b; PISANTI et al. 1959b).

— Increase, decrease, or no change of coronary flow in the isolated perfused heart, in the heart in situ as well as in the peripheral arteries (ACEVES et al. 1960;

ALLMARK et al. 1953; ARAI et al. 1961; BEN et al. 1959, 1960; BING et al. 1959; GAVEND et al. 1960; MENDEZ et al. 1960; MERCIER et al. 1958; 1962; MOUQUIN and MILOVANOVICH 1962; NEILL et al. 1960; PELLMONT 1960, unpubl.; PLETSCHER 1956b; PLETSCHER and PELLMONT 1958; G. G. ROWE et al. 1961: SHORE et al. 1958).

— Enhancement, diminution, or no change of the contraction force of the myocardium in isolated preparations or in situ. The positive inotropic effect of certain MAO inhibitors, especially those with phenylethylamine structure, can be inhibited by agents interfering with the physiological action or the storage of NE (e.g. dichloroisoproterenol, reserpine). This might indicate that catecholamines are involved (ACEVES et al. 1960; GATGOUNIS and AYCOCK 1963; L. I. GOLDBERG 1959; N. D. GOLDBERG and SHIDEMAN 1962; GYLYS et al. 1963; LEE et al. 1961; LEUSEN 1959a; MCCARTY and SHIDEMAN 1960; MENDEZ et al. 1960; PELLMONT 1960, unpubl.; PLETSCHER and PELLMONT 1958; SCHANBERG et al. 1959; SHIDEMAN and GOLDBERG 1961).

— Changes of the amplitude and frequency of the isolated heart and of the frequency of the heart in situ (ACEVES et al. 1960; ALLMARK et al. 1953; MENDEZ et al. 1960; PELLMONT 1960, unpubl.; PLETSCHER and PELLMONT 1958; SCHANBERG et al. 1959).

— Changes in the atrioventricular conduction time (ACEVES et al. 1960).

— Diminution of different vascular lesions and of the permeability of the small vessels due to various forms of injurious stimuli (CREMA and BERTÈ 1960; FABRE et al. 1962; GIÃO and RICO 1960; W. G. SPECTOR and WILLOUGHBY 1960a, 1960b; WILLOUGHBY and SPECTOR 1961). The 5-HT-induced increase of capillary permeability has not been found to be changed by MAO inhibitors (VOTAVA and LAMPLOVÁ 1961).

— Reduction of left ventricular oxygen consumption; enhancement and delayed recovery of hypoxia-induced ST-depression in the electrocardiogram (ECG); attenuation of ECG-changes due to hypoproteinemia; beneficial effect in experimental hypoxia of skeletal muscles (ARROYO and BERNARD 1961; CAHN and HÉROLD 1962; MELVILLE et al. 1960; PISANTY et al. 1959a).

— Beneficial effects in experimental coronary occlusion in dogs and pigs including accelerated normalization of the ECG in dogs (PISANTY et al. 1959a, 1960; REGELSON et al. 1959; TODD et al. 1959); improvement of cerebral hemodynamics in patients with cerebral sclerosis (KLEIN 1962b).

— Increase or no change of the survival time of the heart in curarized mice (HÉROLD et al. 1961; PELLMONT 1960).

— Antinicotinic action on isolated atria of guinea pigs (TIMSIT and LÉVY 1962).

— No change of the increased contractibility of the heart following premature beats (MEIJLER and DURRER 1962).

These preferentially acute effects hardly explain the clinical actions of MAO inhibitors (e.g. hypotension, antistenocardic effect) which appear only after prolonged administration and persist for some time after discontinuation of the medication (PLETSCHER et al. 1960; SJOERDSMA 1960). The mechanism of action of MAO inhibitors in arterial hypertension and in angina pectoris remains therefore speculative.

δ) Gastrointestinal tract. The action of MAO inhibitors on *gastric secretion* is not uniform and depends on the species. In humans, some authors found an increase in the production of hydrochloric acid after iproniazid administration, others could not observe a constant effect of the drug. In animals the secretion of total gastric juice is increased, decreased or not changed by iproniazid. Pheniprazine enhances the secretion of pepsine and diminishes the acidity of gastric juice in dogs (BRODY and GOETZ 1958; HAVERBACK and BRODY 1958; IVY et al. 1956; LIEPIENS et al. 1958; PLETSCHER et al. 1960c; WEISS et al. 1959; WHITE et al. 1959; ZBINDEN et al. 1958) (Table 6). The mechanism by which MAO inhibitors influence gastric secretion is not known for sure. Interference with 5-HT or histamine metabolism may be considered (PLETSCHER et al. 1960c).

Iproniazid has also been shown to counteract the formation of *gastric ulcers*, due to reserpine (see above), to exclusive feeding with glucose, or in the Shay rat. The ulcerogenic effect of 5-HT is not diminished by the MAO inhibitor (LEUSEN et al. 1959; NIKODIJEVIĆ and TRAJKOV 1961; THOENEN et al. 1962; ZBINDEN et al. 1959). The mechanism of the inhibitory action of MAO inhibitors on ulcer

Table 6. *Effect of iproniazid, reserpine, and iproniazid + reserpine on the secretion of gastric juice in guinea pigs*

Drug	Dose mg kg i.v.	Animal number	Amount of gastric juice (ml)	p
None	—	15	5.7	
Iproniazid	50	5	5.4	> 0.05[1]
Reserpine	1	10	16.2	< 0.01[1]
Iproniazid + Reserpine	50 / 1	9	5.4	> 0.05[1] / < 0.01[2]

Immediately before injecting the drugs the pylorus was ligated; measurement of the total volume of gastric juice secreted during the following 5 hours. In the last experiment iproniazid was injected 15 hours before reserpine (ZBINDEN et al. 1958).

[1] As compared to untreated controls.

[2] Comparison between animals treated with reserpine alone and those with combined iproniazid-reserpine treatment.

formation might be connected with inhibition of the reserpine-induced 5-HT release or with diminution of free 5-HT by increasing its storage (PLETSCHER et al. 1960c) (see above).

Iproniazid seems to inhibit *gastric motility* in humans. In the isolated rabbit intestine only big doses of the drug decrease peristalsis, and in rats a single injection of a large dose of iproniazid causes long-lasting constipation. The reserpine-induced increase of peristalsis is counteracted by iproniazid (BENSON et al. 1952; BRODY and GOETZ 1958; HAVERBACK and BRODY 1958; ZBINDEN et al. 1958). It is conceivable that the effects of MAO inhibitors on intestinal motility are connected with changes in the 5-HT metabolism (e.g. inhibited release or increased storing of the amine).

ε) Influence on the action of various drugs. Various MAO inhibitors, if administered shortly (up to a few hours) before *barbiturates*, prolong and enhance the hypnotic action. The intensity of this effect depends on the individual MAO inhibitor and the particular barbiturate used. If administered at a long interval (20—40 hours) before barbiturates, the MAO inhibitors of the hydrazide type may even counteract the hypnotic effect. The anticonvulsant action of phenobarbital is not affected by chronic administeration of phenelzine (ARRIGONI-MARTELLI and KRAMER 1959; O'BRIEN and DAVISON 1958; BUCHEL and STURTZ-MOURY 1957; CAHN and HÉROLD 1960c; EBERHOLST et al. 1958; ELTHERINGTON and HORITA 1960; FOUTS and BRODIE 1956; FROMMEL et al. 1960; FUJIMOTO et al. 1960; GENOVESE et al. 1959; GOLDIN et al. 1955; HÉROLD et al. 1959; HOLTZ et al. 1958; KRAUSE 1960; LAROCHE 1960; LECHAT and LEMEIGNAN 1961; LESSIN 1959b; MATTHIES et al. 1962; PEARCE et al. 1959; PENNEFATHER et al. 1958; R. P. ROWE 1959; R. P. ROWE et al. 1959a; RÜMKE 1961; RÜMKE and BOUT 1960; SCHUMANN et al. 1961; SERRONE and FUJIMOTO 1961, 1962; SHANAMAN et al. 1961; STOCK and WESTERMANN 1962a; STURTEVANT 1956; WESTERMANN and STOCK 1962).

Enhancement of barbiturate hypnosis is probably not related to MAO inhibition. The two effects have a different duration. Furthermore, not all MAO inhibitors potentiate barbiturates, and some hydrazides which are not MAO inhibitors (e.g. isoniazid) also prolong barbiturate sleeping time (ALLMARK et al. 1953; GOLDIN et al. 1955; LAROCHE and BRODIE 1960; PLETSCHER et al. 1960c).

Potentiation of barbiturates by MAO inhibitors is probably due to inhibition of the unspecific oxidase of microsomes (amphetamine oxidase) which inactivates the hypnotics. MAO inhibitors have indeed been shown to delay the degradation of barbiturates in the intact animal as well as in the isolated perfused liver (FOUTS and BRODIE 1956; MATTHIES et al. 1962; PEARCE et al. 1959).

The *decrease* of the action of barbiturates, if administered long after MAO inhibitors, might be due to direct interaction with the adrenergic receptors in the central nervous system or to activation of amphetamine oxidase. A relation with MAO inhibition is unlikely (HOLTZ et al. 1957b; MATTHIES et al. 1962; SERRONE and FUJIMOTO 1961; WESTERMANN and STOCK 1962) (see above).

MAO inhibitors have also been reported to cause the following alterations of other drug effects:

— Changes of chloral narcosis as with barbiturates; counteraction against hypnosis due to tribromoethanol (BUCHEL and LÉVY 1960a; HOLTZ et al. 1957b; J. LÉVY and MICHEL-BER 1960a).

— Enhancement of depression of the central nervous system by ethanol and chlorpromazine. Thereby the alcohol clearance from blood is delayed and in vitro the ethanol metabolism by liver slices is inhibited (ASTON and CULLUMBINE 1960; BÄCHTOLD and PLETSCHER 1957; M. E. SMITH et al. 1961).

— Decrease of the toxicity of octamethyl-pyrophosphorodiamide and tetramethyllead. The first compound is oxidized in the liver to a highly toxic cholinesterase inhibitor by amphetamine oxidase (GHERARDI and SALVI 1961; E. N. GREENBLATT and OSTERBERG 1961b; LESSIN 1959b).

— Increase of the analgesic effect of methadone, a pethidine derivative, and acetylsalicylic acid; enhancement or no change of morphine analgesia (BIANCHI and DAVID 1960; BUCHEL et al. 1960a; FROMMEL et al. 1960; SHANAMAN et al. 1961).

— Increase of the action of amphetamine in spiders (WITT et al. 1961).

ζ) Other effects. According to various authors, some MAO inhibitors influence the *genital system*, preferentially of the female. Thus certain MAO inhibitors interrupt pregnancy in mice and rats, especially when given in an early period, and suppress fertility probably by inhibition of ovular implantation. They furthermore produce degeneration of deciduomata in mice and may delay sexual maturity of mice and rats. Most investigators attribute these effects to interference with production or function of sex hormones and not to toxicity of the drugs on the gonads (BOTROS and ROBSON 1960; BOTROS et al. 1961; BOVET-NITTI and BIGNAMI 1961; LINDSAY et al. 1961a, 1961b; POULSON and ROBSON 1963; POULSON et al. 1960a, 1960b; ROBSON and BOTROS 1961; W. G. SPECTOR 1960; TUCHMANN-DUPLESSIS and MERCIER-PAROT 1962). According to other authors, iproniazid does not affect fertility and oestrus cycle in mice as well as pseudogestation due to irritation of the collum uteri in rats (BIGNAMI 1960; BIGNAMI et al. 1962; FLÜCKIGER and SALZMANN 1961; SCHAEPDRYVER and PIETTE 1961).

Other effects on the *endocrinal system* are: Stimulation of the neurosecretory hypothalamo-hypophyseal system (KIVALO and RINNE 1961); hypertrophy of the adrenal cortex; increase of the basophil cells of the hypophysis (ROBSON and

BOTROS 1961; TUCHMANN-DUPLESSIS and MERCIER-PAROT 1961, 1962); change of 17-hydroxycorticosteroids in blood of monkeys (decrease or biphasic effect) (HARWOOD and BIGELOW 1960), but no change of urinary corticoid excretion in man (LOPES DO ROSÁRIO 1959/60; SCHÜLLER 1960); inhibition of mammary secretion (MIZUNO et al. 1964); potentiation of the anti-inflammatory effect of corticosteroids (KNICK 1962); suppression of melanocyte dispersion in frogs probably by inhibition of the secretion of the melanocyte stimulating hormone of the hypophysis (SCOTT 1962); increase of iodine uptake by the thyroid (SCHWERT 1959; SCHWERT and HAWLIZEK 1961); enhancement of the blood pressure effects of dissicated thyroid (PSCHEIDT and HIMWICH 1963).

Nialamide seems to prevent *agglutination and sticking of platelets* to injured vascular endothelium. 5-HT intensifies this effect. In consequence, nialamide and to a greater extent nialamide + 5-HT inhibit intravascular thrombus formation without affecting blood coagulation. Accordingly the formation and the size of thrombi in rabbits due to epinephrine, high molecular substances, mechanical damage of the intima, etc. was found to be diminished. Nialamide and iproniazid also prevent the vascular endothelial reaction due to several atherogenic substances (e.g. epinephrine, cholesterol, other lipids). Furthermore, nialamide potentiates phenindione in preventing experimental intravascular thrombosis and counteracts the shortening of the prothrombin time due to various agents, e.g. epinephrine, cholesterol, fresh cream and butter in rabbits and humans (BAUMGARTNER et al. 1963, 1964; BERNARDI and SIDERI 1960; KLEIN 1962a; FABRE et al. 1964; SHIMAMOTO 1960a, 1960b, 1960c, 1961a, 1961b; SHIMAMOTO et al. 1960, 1961b, 1962a, 1962b, 1962c). Other changes described for blood cells are: Thrombocytosis, decrease or increase of eosinophils, prevention of stress-induced eosinopenia, etc. (KOTHARI et al. 1961; PLETSCHER and BERNSTEIN 1958; ZBINDEN and STUDER 1958b).

Various *further effects* of MAO inhibitors have been reported: Decrease of the tyramine- and heat-induced activation of ^{14}C-mezcaline incorporation and enhancement of the incorporation of a thiobarbiturate into proteins of liver homogenate (BLOCK 1961); enhancement of the gain in body weight of young adult male rats (ELLISON and SCOTT 1964); inhibition of the growth and respiration of tetrahymena pyriformis (KREZANOSKI 1961); potentiation of the anti-5-HT effect of lysergic acid diethylamide (LSD) and a derivative (VOTAVA and LAMPLOVÁ 1961); enhancement of the rise in body temperature due to injection of a bacterial pyrogen which is antagonized by dibenamine and reserpine (GÖING 1959; 1960; GENDEREN and DURVILLE 1959); protection against X-ray irradiation in mice if given before reserpine (BRENK and ELLIOTT 1958); decrease of bromsulfaleine clearance (FUJIMOTO et al. 1960); impairment of kidney function possibly in connection with the hypotensive effect of MAO inhibitors (DUPASQUIER and REUBI 1959); influence on anaphylactic shock (GERSHON and ROSS 1962); fibroplastic action (BEACH and STEINETZ 1961; COEN and WHITEHEAD 1962; S. G. COHEN and SAPP 1960; KRUEGER and SMITH 1960; ROSENBLATT et al. 1960; SMYTH et al. 1961, 1962; TEIXEIRA 1962).

η) Toxicity. MAO inhibitors have been reported to induce toxic alterations in various organ systems. A connection of the toxicity with MAO inhibition can be excluded for some effects, for others it remains to be elucidated.

General toxicity

The acute toxicity of MAO inhibitors (expressed as dosis letalis 50% [LD_{50}]) varies markedly according to the individual compound and to the animal species. Some MAO inhibitors increase neonatal mortality in animals if administered in pregnancy. Certain compounds, especially those which increase motor activity and body temperature (e.g. pheniprazine), are more toxic to grouped than to single mice. For other derivatives (e.g. phenelzine) such a difference does not exist. Methane sulfonic acid derivatives of hydrazines have a higher LD_{50} than the corresponding bases. The acute toxicity is probably not due to MAO inhibition, because, for instance in the mouse, iproniazid i.v. has an LD_{50} of 700 mg/kg, whereas the LD_{50} of isoniazid is only 150 mg/kg. Interference with vitamin B_6 metabolism might be involved, because it could be shown that pyridoxine has a protective effect (BENSON et al. 1952; BIEL et al. 1959c; BONATI 1958; CHESSIN et al. 1959; DELAHUNT and PEPIN 1959a, 1959b; DUBNICK et al. 1960; ELLISON and SCOTT 1964; GREENBLATT and OSTERBERG 1961b; GRUNBERG 1952; LEESON et al. 1959; LOGEMANN et al. 1960; RANDALL and BAGDON 1959; WERBOFF et al. 1961a, 1961b).

Organ toxicity

Blood: Hemolysis is a typical effect of hydrazine derivatives, e.g. phenylhydrazine. High daily doses of various MAO inhibitors of the hydrazine type may induce hemolytic anemia which does not parallel the degree of MAO inhibition (BENSON et al. 1952; LÄUPPI and PILLER 1960; MERMOD et al. 1953; NOËL and PALMER 1962; PSCHEIDT and HIMWICH 1963; RANDALL 1958; RANDALL and BAGDON 1959; ZBINDEN and STUDER 1959).

Nervous system: Chronic administration of hydrazine derivatives may cause degeneration of the myeline sheaths of peripheral nerves. Some MAO inhibitors, e.g. pheniprazine and JB-835 (4-phenyl-2-isobutylhydrazine), also produce degenerative changes in the inferior olivary nucleus, the pyriform lobe, the cerebellar roof nuclei, and the subcortical white matter. Some of these alterations probably explain the peripheral neuritis occasionally observed in humans after hydrazide medication and various neurological symptoms in animals (e.g. ataxia, impairment of motor coordination). Neurotoxicity might also be the cause of the red/green blindness observed in some humans treated with pheniprazine. The neurotoxicity is probably not due to MAO inhibition, but possibly at least in part to interference with vitamin B_6 metabolism. Thus, in rats nervous degeneration is more marked after isoniazid than after iproniazid and attenuated by vitamin B_6. Other hydrazine derivatives which are strong MAO inhibitors have no effect on peripheral nerves at all (ELTHERINGTON and HORITA 1960; HIGHMAN and MALING 1962; LÄUPPI and PILLER 1960; MALING et al. 1961; 1962; NOËL and PALMER 1962; SANAN and VOGT 1962; ZBINDEN 1960; ZBINDEN and STUDER 1955a, 1955b, 1959).

Liver: Patients treated with MAO inhibitors occasionally develop hepatocellular icterus and liver necrosis which cannot be distinguished from viral hepatitis. In animals, however, it has hardly been possible to reproduce this type of liver damage. The liver toxicity of MAO inhibitors seems to be dependent on the mode of application. On injection or on administration in the food only few hydrazine derivatives, e.g. N^1-L-leucinoyl-N^2-isopropylhydrazine, ethionyl-(benzylethyl)-hydrazine, induce fatty infiltration and necrosis of liver cells in rodents. Thereby, degenerative changes and fatty infiltration occur also in the kidney. The pathological picture is similar to that in intoxication with allyl alcohol. Various other hydrazine derivatives, e.g. iproniazid, pheniprazine, do not cause necrotic alterations of the liver, although they decrease blood flow in the central part of the liver lobules. In contrast, degenerative changes and spotty necroses in the liver of rodents can be seen after repeated administration of very high single doses of MAO inhibitors, including iproniazid, by stomach tube. Iproniazid orally has also been reported to induce liver necroses in dogs. Liver damage induced by ethionine, phenylhydrazine, allyl alcohol is not influenced by iproniazid. Some MAO inhibitors of the hydrazide type enhance, however, the liver toxicity of carbon tetrachloride (DELAHUNT and PEPIN 1959b; LÄUPPI and PILLER 1960; LÄUPPI et al. 1960; POPPER 1958, 1959; SCHNEIDER et al. 1959; STEBBINS and MULROY 1959; ZBINDEN and STUDER 1959; ZWEIFACH and CASCARANO 1959).

It is very doubtful whether the toxic effects of MAO inhibitors observed in the liver of animals are connected with MAO inhibition and whether they are due to the same pathogenetic mechanisms as the changes seen in humans.

Genital system: Long-term administration of high doses of MAO inhibitors to rats causes atrophy of the testes and impairment of spermatogenesis as well as keratinization of the vagina, atrophy of uterus and ovaries. The hormone-producing LEYDIG cells of the testes are not impaired (ELLISON and SCOTT 1964; TUCHMANN-DUPLESSIS and MERCIER-PAROT 1961, 1962; ZBINDEN 1960b; ZBINDEN and STUDER 1959).

Other effects

According to various authors, MAO inhibitors reduce, enhance, or do not influence the injurious effects of bacterial endotoxines (mostly of E. coli) in rodents (AUSMAN et al. 1960; R. B. DAVIS 1962; LASKER and FOX 1960a, 1960b; McLEAN and BERRY 1960a, 1960b; PREZ et al. 1961; ZWEIFACH and CASCARANO 1959).

The toxicity of NE, 5-HT, hexamethonium, ephedrine, amphetamine, digitoxine, etc. is enhanced by MAO inhibitors (JACOB and ECHINARD-GARIN 1961; SHANAMAN et al. 1961) (see above). According to some, but not to all investigators, certain MAO inhibitors have lathyrogenic action and increase the toxicity of β-aminopropionitril (GROSS et al. 1960; JUVA et al. 1959; LEVENE 1961; MOORE 1964; ROY et al. 1959).

7. On the mode of action of monoamine oxidase inhibitors in human disease

The main therapeutic indications for MAO inhibitors are mental depression, arterial hypertension, and angina pectoris. At present, there exists no definite proof that MAO inhibition is the main cause for the clinical effectiveness. The following findings are in favour of such a relation:

— All the hydrazine derivatives inhibiting MAO markedly in vivo have also a beneficial effect in the above mentioned diseases. Derivatives which show no or only weak interference with MAO have no or only little therapeutic action in these diseases (e.g. isoniazid).

— Long-acting MAO inhibitors not belonging to the hydrazine group, e.g. pargyline, tranylcypromine, have similar clinical effects as MAO inhibitors of the hydrazine type.

— The time course of MAO inhibition and of the clinical effects is similar. Clinical improvement as well as marked MAO inhibition appear only slowly or after repeated therapeutic doses of MAO inhibitors, but persist both for some time after discontinuation of the drugs.

— Alterations of other enzymes, e.g. DCA, DPN-ase, DAO, choline oxidase, etc., are probably not related to the clinical effects of MAO inhibitors. Thus, isoniazid and some other hydrazides inhibit these enzymes to the same extent or even more than iproniazid, but lack the mentioned clinical action.

— In humans, some but not all investigators report a reasonable correlation between *hypotensive* effect and MAO inhibition (as measured by the excretion of tryptamine or 5-HT in the urine or by direct estimation of MAO in jejunal mucosal biopsies) (LEVINE and SJOERDSMA 1962a; M. H. MAXWELL et al. 1963; ORVIS and TAMAGNA 1963; PLETSCHER et al. 1960c; SJOERDSMA 1960, 1961). A correlation between the action of MAO inhibitors in *mental depression* and MAO inhibition (as estimated on the basis of the content of amines and metabolites in urine and blood) has been found by some investigators, but not by others (BRUNE and HIMWICH 1961; CRANE and WOLFMAN 1960; DEWHURST and PARE 1961; FELDSTEIN et al. 1960; PLETSCHER et al. 1960c; PRAAG and LEIJNSE 1963a, 1963b; RESNICK 1959; RESNICK et al. 1958, 1960b). Such a lack of correlation is, however, no argument against a causal connection between antidepressive effect and MAO inhibition. Thus, measurements in man as mentioned above may mainly indicate MAO inhibition in the extracerebral tissues which does not necessarily correlate with MAO inhibition in brain (GOGERTY and HORITA 1960; MCGRATH and HORITA 1962; PLETSCHER and GEY, unpubl.; PLETSCHER et al. 1960c; E. SCHMID 1962; TABACHNICK and RUBIN 1959).

In conclusion it seems likely that interference with MAO is somehow related to some clinical effects of MAO inhibitors. The exact mechanism of action, however, remains to be elucidated. The following possibilities have to be considered:

a) Antidepressive effect

— Unspecific central stimulation by accumulation of endogenous sympaticomimetic amines in the central nervous system without modifying the biochemical defect responsible for causing mental depression.

— Correction of a metabolic disturbance occurring in mental depression.

b) Hypotensive effect

— Inhibition of ganglionic transmission; diminution of vascular resistance (M. H. MAXWELL et al. 1962).

— Decrease of the NE sensitivity of the arterial wall.

— Inhibition of physiological catecholamine release at the adrenergic nerve endings or in the arterial wall (possibly bretylium-like effect) (BRODIE and BEAVEN 1963; GESSA et al. 1963; HUKOVIC and MUSCHOLL 1962); diminished availability of the sympathetic transmitter (DAVEY et al. 1963).

— Preferential accumulation of dopamine or octopamine (weak pressor agents) which might compete whith NE at receptors involved in the regulation of blood pressure (KOPIN et al. 1964; SJOERDSMA 1960).

— Formation of hypotensive heterocycles by condensation of a catecholamine with the corresponding aldehyde, as shown in vitro for dopamine (HOLTZ et al. 1964a, 1964b).

— Decrease of the mechanical efficiency of the heart (CAHN and HÉROLD 1960a; CAHN et al. 1961b; KOPIN et al. 1964; NEILL et al. 1960).

c) Antistenocardic effect

— Coronary dilatation by a direct action of the drugs on the vessel wall or indirectly by increase of 5-HT (a "benign" coronary dilator) in the blood (CRUMPTON et al. 1959; G. M. MAXWELL et al. 1959).

— Decrease of the mechanical efficiency of the heart (CAHN et al. 1961b; NEILL et al. 1960).

— Psychostimulation.

— Analgesic effect similar to that observed in other pathological conditions, e.g. carcinoma, RAYNAUD's and rheumatic disease (BATEMAN 1958; M. N. FISHER et al. 1952; LEUSEN 1960; PLETSCHER et al. 1960c; SCHERBEL et al. 1958).

— Attenuation of the hemodynamic response to exercise (L. I. GOLDBERG et al. 1962; HORWITZ and SJOERDSMA 1963; HORWITZ et al. 1961).

— Inactivation of catecholamines by their enhanced storage in the myocardium (PLETSCHER and GEY 1961a; PLETSCHER et al. 1960c).

— Oxygen sparing, e.g. by activation of glycolysis.

— Improvement of myocardial energy production in consequence of increased supply of substrates easily utilized (e.g. pyruvate from the blood) (see above) (LEAK and DORMANDY 1961; MERCIER et al. 1962; NEILL et al. 1960; PLETSCHER and GEY 1961a).

C. Summary

MAO is a mitochondrial enzyme which catalyzes the transformation of primary and secondary amines into the corresponding aldehydes with liberation of ammonia and formation of hydrogen peroxide. Some physiological substrates are tryptamine, 5-HT, tyramine, catecholamines and their 3-O-methyl ethers.

In vitro the enzyme is inhibited by numerous classes of compounds among which α-alkylated aralkylamines, α-alkylated indolylalkylamines, aryl ethers of choline, harmane derivatives, and amidines also show some effect in vivo. Potent inhibition, long-lasting in vivo and irreversible in vitro, has been described for four types of compounds:

a) *Alkyl- or aralkyl-hydrazines* including N^2-acylated derivatives. The latter seem to undergo hydrolysis prior to their action on MAO.

b) *2-Phenylcyclopropylamine.*

c) *N-Benzyl-N-methyl-propargylamine.*

d) *2-Methyl-3-piperidinopyrazine.*

Hydrazine derivatives may also inhibit other enzymes in vitro and in vivo, e.g. amphetamine oxidase, DAO, DCA, ceruloplasmin, choline oxidase.

The most important metabolic and pharmacodynamic effects of strong in vivo inhibitors of MAO are:

a) Increase of endogenous monoamines (e.g. 5-HT, catecholamines, normetanephrine) in various tissues.

b) Enhanced excretion of monoamines (e.g. tryptamine, tyramine, O-methylated catecholamines); diminished elimination of indol- and phenolcarbonic acids (e.g. 5-hydroxyindolacetic acid, 3-methoxy-4-hydroxymandelic acid, 3,4-dihydroxymandelic acid, homovanillic- and 3,4-dihydroxyphenylacetic acid.)

c) Enhancement of the monoamine increase in various tissues subsequent to administration of monoamines (e.g. tryptamine, 5-HT) and their precursors (e.g. tryptophan, 5-HTP, dopa); increase of the pharmacodynamic effect of some exogenous monoamines and their precursors.

d) Counteraction of the monoamine decrease due to monoamine releasers (e.g. reserpine, benzoquinolizine derivatives); attenuation or reversal of some pharmacodynamic actions of monoamine releasers, e.g. sedation, arterial hypotension, miosis, intestinal hypermotility.

e) Increase of lactate and pyruvate in blood.

f) Anticonvulsive action and inhibition of synaptic transmission.

These effects are probably in principle connected with MAO inhibition.

Other metabolic and pharmacodynamic actions of some MAO inhibitors (e.g. the hydrazine derivatives) are probably not or only in part connected with MAO inhibition, e.g. the metabolic alterations of diamines, vitamin B_6, and cholesterol; the effects on behaviour, EEG, cardiovascular system, gastrointestinal tract; the modification of the effect of various drugs, e.g. barbiturates.

The therapeutic action of MAO inhibitors in man seems to be mainly connected with MAO inhibition.

III. Decarboxylases of aromatic amino acids[1]

A. Biochemistry of the enzyme

Since the beginning of this century, several rather specific decarboxylases of α-amino acids have been demonstrated in bacteria (ACKERMANN 1908, 1910a, 1910b; BARGER and WALPOLE 1909; BERTHOLET and BERTRAND 1912; ELLINGER 1898, 1900; GALE 1940a, 1940b, 1940c, 1941, 1946; HANKE and KOESSLER 1922, 1924a, 1924b, 1924c; KOESSLER and HANKE 1919; MELLANBY and TWORT 1912). In animal tissues decarboxylases of histidine, tyrosine, tryptophan, and dopa were discovered in 1936—1938 (BLOCH and PINÖSCH 1936; HOLTZ 1937, 1941; HOLTZ and HEISE 1937a, 1937b; HOLTZ and JANISCH 1937; HOLTZ et al. 1938a, 1942a; WERLE 1936; WERLE and HERRMANN 1937; WERLE and MENNICKEN 1937), and a decarboxylase of 5-HTP was described in 1953 (UDENFRIEND et al. 1953); relatively specific decarboxylases of aliphatic amino acids have also been found (UTTER 1961). Mammalian enzymes differ from those of bacterial origin (BLASCHKO 1950; FERRINI and GLÄSSER 1964).

The present survey deals mainly with decarboxylases of aromatic L-amino acids, such as dopa, 5-HTP, and tyrosine in mammalian tissues. These enzymes have already been reviewed (BLASCHKO 1945, 1961; W. G. CLARK 1963; W. G. CLARK and POGRUND 1961; R. A. COHEN et al. 1962; ERSPAMER 1961; GARATTINI and VALZELLI 1962; HAGEN and WELCH 1956; HOLTZ 1941, 1960; KRAYER 1959; MEISTER 1957; PELLERIN et al. 1958; SCHALES 1951; SOURKES and D'IORIO 1963; WERLE 1942/44, 1943, 1947, 1951; WERLE and KOCH 1949). Because of their possible identity the general term "decarboxylase of aromatic L-amino acids" (DCA) has been suggested (LOVENBERG et al. 1962b).

1. Reaction formula

DCA decarboxylates aromatic L-α-amino acids according to the general formula:

$$R\text{—}CH(NH_3^+)\text{—}COO^- \rightarrow R\text{—}CH_2\text{—}N^+H_3 + CO_2$$

The stereospecificity of the enzyme suggests that three groups of the asymmetric α-carbon of the substrate are involved in the reaction (BELLEAU and BURBA 1960; BLASCHKO 1950; MANDELES et al. 1954; METZLER et al. 1954; PERAULT et al. 1961; SNELL 1958).

2. Differentiation

The assumption that several aromatic α-amino acids are decarboxylated by the same enzyme is based on the following findings:

— The distribution of dopa- and 5-HTP-DCA in different tissues and within one organ, e.g. brain, is the same (BERTLER and ROSENGREN 1959b; HAGEN and LEE 1958; KUNTZMAN et al. 1962a; REID and SHEPHERD 1964; WESTERMANN et al. 1958).

— Decarboxylation of dopa is competitively inhibited by 5-HTP and vice versa. Mixtures of 5-HTP and dopa are decarboxylated at a rate laying between that of the individual substrates (BERTLER and ROSENGREN 1959b; ROSENGREN 1960a; YUWILER et al. 1959a).

— After purification of DCA the relative rate of decarboxylation of dopa and 5-HTP remains constant (AWAPARA et al. 1962a, 1962b; FELLMANN 1959b; LOVENBERG et al. 1962b: ROSENGREN 1960a; WERLE and AURES 1959).

— DCA inhibitors reduce the decarboxylation rate of various substrates to a comparable degree (LOVENBERG et al. 1962b; ROSENGREN 1960a; WESTERMANN et al. 1958; YUWILER et al. 1959a, 1960) (see below).

Histidine might differ from aromatic amino acids, such as dopa, 5-HTP, tyrosine, etc., since it is not only decarboxylated by DCA, but also by more specific decarboxylases (BLASCHKO et al. 1955; ERSPAMER 1961; GADDUM et al. 1962; GANROT et al. 1961; GARATTINI and VALZELLI 1962; HAGEN 1962; HÅKANSON 1963; HOLTZ et al. 1939b; KAMESWARAN and WEST 1961; KAMESWARAN et al. 1961; MACKAY and SHEPHERD 1962; MACKAY et al. 1961; MEISTER 1957; REID and SHEPHERD 1964; REID et al. 1964; B. ROBINSON and SHEPHERD 1961, 1962; SCHALES 1951; TABOR 1954, 1955; WEISSBACH et al. 1961b; WERLE and AURES 1959, 1960).

3. Substrates

Numerous phenol-, indol-, and imidazol derivatives of L-alanine and erythro- or threoserine are decarboxylated by DCA, but with marked differences in affinity. Substitution on the amino residue, replacement of the α-hydrogen and of the phenolic hydroxy group diminish decarboxylation (AWAPARA et al. 1962a, 1962b; BEYER et al. 1950; BLASCHKO 1939, 1942,

[1] DCA; Carboxy-lyases of aromatic amino acids; EC 4.1.1.22, 4.1.1.26—28 (Int. Union Biochem. 1961)

1950; BLASCHKO and CHRUŚCIEL 1960; BLASCHKO and HOLTON 1950; BLASCHKO et al. 1949; W. G. CLARK and POGRUND 1961; ERSPAMER 1961; ERSPAMER and NOBILI 1962; ERSPAMER et al. 1960b, 1961a, 1961b; FERRINI and GLÄSSER 1964; FRETER et al. 1957; HAGEN 1962; HARTMANN et al. 1955b; HOLTZ and WESTERMANN 1956b; LOVENBERG et al. 1962b; SHAW et al. 1957; SOURKES 1954b, 1955/56; SOURKES et al. 1952; UDENFRIEND et al. 1960; WEISSBACH et al. 1960a; WERLE and AURES 1960; WERLE and PESCHEL 1949; WERLE and SELL 1954; WERLE et al. 1955; YUWILER et al. 1959a). The relative rate of decarboxylation of some presumably physiological substrates may approximately be as follows:

High (100%): dopa.
Medium (40—10%): 5-HTP, ortho-, meta-tyrosine.
Low (10—1%): tryptophan, L-3,4-dihydroxyphenylserine, para-hydroxyphenylserine.
Extremely low (< 1%): para-tyrosine, histidine, 5-methoxytryptophan.

4. Tissue distribution

DCA occurs widely in *animal tissues* showing the following approximative order of activity:

High (> 100 $\mu l\ CO_2/g/h$): kidney, liver, adrenal medulla.

Medium (<100, > 10 $\mu l\ CO_2/g/h$): intestine, brain, pancreas, spleen, sympathetic ganglia, heart, testis.

Low (<10 $\mu l\ CO_2/g/h$): thrombocytes, skin, lung, serum, placenta, embryo, muscle, spinal cord.

This classification is, however, limited by many exceptions, because the enzyme activity varies widely according to the substrate and the species. Liver of humans, in contrast to that of mammals, contains, for instance, very little DCA activity (BLASCHKO 1942, 1945; BLASCHKO and CHRUŚCIEL 1960; BOULLIN 1963; C. T. CLARK et al. 1954; W. G. CLARK 1960; DALGLIESH and DUTTON 1957; V. E. DAVIS 1963; V. E. DAVIS and AWAPARA 1960b; DEMIS et al. 1956; DIETRICH 1953; GADDUM and GIARMAN 1956; GEY and MESSIHA 1964; GIARMAN 1956; HÅKANSON and MÖLLER 1963; HOLTZ 1941, 1942, 1959, 1960; HOLTZ and BACHMANN 1952; HOLTZ and WESTERMANN 1956a; HOLTZ et al. 1939a, 1939b, 1942b; KIZER and CHAN 1960, 1961; KUSS and JÄGER 1962; LANGEMANN 1951, 1958; LANGENDORFF and HAGEN 1963; LANGENDORFF et al. 1964; MÜLLER and LANGEMANN 1962; PAGE 1945; PRICE and WEST 1960; REID and SHEPHERD 1964; REID et al. 1963; SACKS 1961; SCHAPIRA 1946; SCHÜMANN 1958; SLOANE-STANLEY 1949; S. E. SMITH 1963; SNYDER and AXELROD 1964; SOURKES 1961; SOURKES et al. 1952; TACHIBANA 1963; UUSPÄÄ et al. 1962; WEBER and WISS 1963; WEST 1958a, 1958b; WESTERMANN 1957).

DCA activity *within one organ* may vary markedly. In the central nervous system, for instance, the enzyme activity is relatively high in the brain stem, especially in the caudate nucleus (ACKERMANN and LANGEMANN 1960; APRISON et al. 1964; BERNHEIMER and HORNYKIEWICZ 1962; BERTLER and ROSENGREN 1959a, 1959b; BOGDANSKI et al. 1957; W. G. CLARK 1959; CREVELING and UDENFRIEND 1959; HOLTZ 1960; HOLTZ and WESTERMANN 1957; KUNTZMAN et al. 1961b; LABOUESSE et al. 1959; LANGEMANN and ACKERMANN 1961; LOVENBERG et al. 1962b; POLONOVSKY et al. 1946b; SKILLEN et al. 1961; UDENFRIEND et al. 1957b) and nearly absent in the cerebral cortex (GADDUM and GIARMAN 1956; HOLTZ and WESTERMANN 1956a, 1957).

Investigations on the *intracellular distribution* showed that DCA of most organs occurs mainly in the cytoplasmatic fraction, i.e. in the supernatant of ultracentrifuged homogenates (BLASCHKO 1961; BLASCHKO et al. 1955; GIARMAN 1956; HAGEN et al. 1960; MÜLLER and LANGEMANN 1962). In rat brain, however, 50% of the enzyme activity were found in the particulate fraction, i.e. mostly in nerve endings (LORES ARNAIZ and ROBERTIS 1964).

5. Purification and properties

DCA has been *purified* up to 360 fold by heat, adsorption, ammonium sulfate fractionation, etc. (AWAPARA et al. 1962a, 1962b; C. T. CLARK 1954; V. E. DAVIS and AWAPARA 1960a; FELLMANN 1959b; HARTMANN et al. 1960; LOVENBERG et al. 1962b, 1963; WERLE and AURES 1959; WERLE and HEITZER 1938). Crude supernatant (BURKARD, unpubl.; DENGLER et al. 1962) in contrast to purified DCA (WERLE and AURES 1960) is relatively stable, e.g. at —20° C.

DCA has relatively high *substrate affinity* (C. T. CLARK et al. 1954). Thus, at optimal pH the *Michaelis-Menten-constant* is about 5×10^{-4} to 4×10^{-5} M for 5-HTP (HUANG and HSIA 1963; YUWILER 1960), 5×10^{-2} to 5×10^{-4} M for dopa (FELLMANN 1959b; HARTMANN et al. 1955a; SCHOTT and CLARK 1952), 6×10^{-4} M for ortho-tyrosine (FELLMANN 1959b), and 1×10^{-2} M for para-tyrosine (LOVENBERG et al. 1962b).

The *pH optimum* of DCA is 6.6—7.5 with dopa (AWAPARA et al. 1962a; C. T. CLARK et al. 1954; HAGEN et al. 1960; HARTMANN et al. 1960; LOVENBERG et al. 1962b; WERLE 1951; WERLE and AURES 1960; YUWILER et al. 1960) and 6.5—9.0 with 5-HTP (AWAPARA et al. 1962a; BUZARD and NYTCH 1957; C. T. CLARK et al. 1954; HAGEN et al. 1960; HARTMANN et al. 1960; LOVENBERG et al. 1962b; PRICE and WEST 1960; YUWILER et al. 1960), as well as with tyrosine (AWAPARA et al. 1962a; HARTMANN et al. 1960; LOVENBERG et al. 1962b).

Intact sulfhydril groups may be essential for DCA activity (BUZARD and NYTCH 1957; HARTMANN et al. 1955a; LOVENBERG et al. 1962b; PAGE 1945; STEENSHOLT 1955). The enzyme seems to be unaffected by Mg^{++} and Mn^{++} (FELLMANN 1959b; HARTMANN et al. 1955; LOVENBERG et al. 1962b), whereas Cu^{++}, Zn^{++}, Fe^{+++}, and Cd^{+++} may be inhibitory (BUZARD and NYTCH 1957; FELLMANN 1959b; STEENSHOLT et al. 1955). Chelating agents have no effect at least with dopa as substrate (FELLMANN 1959b; HARTMANN et al. 1955a; LOVENBERG et al. 1962b; PERRY et al. 1955), but with 5-HTP they might inhibit DCA weakly (BEILER and MARTIN 1954; WEISSBACH et al. 1961b). Cyanide reduces dopa decarboxylation slightly (BEILER and MARTIN 1954; BLASCHKO 1942; CLEGG and SEALOCK 1949; HOLTZ 1938, 1939; HOLTZ et al. 1938a, 1939c; HORITA 1962b; IMIYA 1941; SCHROEDER 1957; TOMOKICHI 1941) possibly by inactivation of the cofactor through the formation of a cyanohydrin (P. P. COHEN 1939; SCARDI and BONAVITA 1957a, 1957b).

DCA is not markedly affected by bisulfite (BEILER and MARTIN 1954; IMIYA 1941; TOMOKICHI 1941; WERLE and HEITZER 1938), aldehydes, ascorbic acid, glutathione (GONNARD 1949, 1951; HARTMANN et al. 1955a), thiopropionate (H. M. PERRY et al. 1955), thiocyanate H. M. PERRY et al. 1955; SCHROEDER 1957), pyrophosphate (HARTMANN et al. 1955a; H. M. PERRY et al. 1955), fluoride (BUZARD and NYTCH 1957; GONNARD 1951; HARTMANN et al. 1955a), arsenite, iodide, sulfate (HARTMANN et al. 1955a), borate (WERLE and AURES 1960). Phosphate and possibly arsenate activate DCA (GONNARD 1951; HARTMANN et al. 1955a). Furthermore, DCA does not seem to be affected by carbon monoxide (BLASCHKO 1942), azide (BLASCHKO 1942; H. M. PERRY et al. 1955), urea, urethane, acetamide, malonate (GONNARD 1951), ortho-toluidine (GONNARD 1950), 2,4-dinitrophenol (HARTMANN et al. 1955b), pyrogallol (GONNARD 1951), sulfhydryl compounds, i.e. dimercaprol (WENZEL and BECKLOFF 1958), chlorpromazine (GEY et al. 1961), imipramine (MARSHALL et al. 1960), reserpine (AIRAKSINEN and UUSPÄÄ 1961; BERTLER 1961; BERTLER et al. 1961; BRODIE et al. 1957; CHRUŚCIEL 1962; KUNTZMAN and SPECTOR 1960; SCHROEDER 1957; UUSPÄÄ et al. 1962; WEST 1958a), bretylium, guanethidine (CHRUŚCIEL 1961, 1962), nucleotides like ATP, adenosine-5′-monophosphate, etc. (BUZARD and NYTCH 1957), and estradiol (CHATAGNER et al. 1959; LABOUESSE et al. 1959).

Organic solvents such as acetone, octylalcohol, benzene, pyridine, chloroforme, toluene, etc. may be inert, activate or inactivate the enzyme, depending on the substrate (GONNARD 1950, 1958; HOLTZ et al. 1938a; LOVENBERG et al. 1962b; PAGE 1945; WEISSBACH et al. 1961b).

Coenzyme

Pyridoxal-5′-phosphate acts as coenzyme of DCA (BLASCHKO 1950; BLASCHKO et al. 1948, 1951; BUXTON and SINCLAIR 1956; BUZARD and NYTCH 1957; HOLTZ and PALM 1964; METZLER et al. 1954; POGRUND et al. 1961; UDENFRIEND et al. 1957b; WEBER and WISS 1963; WEISSBACH et al. 1957b). The activation by the coenzyme differs according to the substrates and the preincubation period (LOVENBERG et al. 1963). The Michaelis-Menten-constant of the apoenzyme-coenzyme complex is 9×10^{-8} M. The coenzyme can be separated from the apoenzyme by dialysis if dopa, but not 5-HTP, is used as substrate (BEILER and MARTIN 1954; BURKARD, unpubl.; C. T. CLARK et al. 1954; WERLE and AURES 1960). This difference has not been explained (AWAPARA et al. 1962a, 1962b; V. E. DAVIS 1963).

The substrate probably combines with the pyridoxal-5′-phosphate by forming a Schiff base (BELLEAU and BURBA 1960; KOSOWER 1962; MANDELES et al. 1954; METZLER et al. 1954; PELLERIN and D'IORIO 1956; PERAULT et al. 1961; SNELL 1958). If the substrate (and one of its analogues respectively) or the coenzyme is in excess, a tetrahydroisoquinoline derivative might be formed by ring closure (FRETER et al. 1958; HEYL et al. 1952; HOLTZ and PALM 1964; HOLTZ and WESTERMANN 1957; MACKAY and SHEPHERD 1962; SCHOTT and CLARK 1952; SOURKES 1954a, 1955/56; WERLE and AURES 1959; YUWILER et al. 1959a, 1960). This reaction possibly explains why DCA is inhibited by excess of either substrate (BLASCHKO 1942; GONNARD 1950; POLONOVSKI et al. 1946b; SCHAPIRA 1946; SCHOTT 1951; WERLE and AURES 1960), reaction products (e.g. NE) (BUZARD and NYTCH 1959), or cofactor (BURKARD 1964c; HOLTZ et al. 1952a, 1952b; LOVENBERG et al. 1963; SCHOTT and CLARK 1951; WERLE and KOCH 1949).

Deficiency of pyridoxal-5′-phosphate in rats reduces the apoenzyme in liver and kidney, but not in brain (V. E. DAVIS 1963).

6. Determination

DCA can be measured *in vitro* according to various principles, i.e. by determination of:

— *CO_2 formation* in Warburg manometers (BLASCHKO 1942; HARTMANN et al. 1960; HUANG et al. 1960) by colorimetry (SCHEUERBRANDT 1964), or by trapping the $^{14}CO_2$ derived from carboxyl-^{14}C-amino acids (DREYFUS and HAUSER 1964; KOBAYASHI 1962; MAYNARD and SCHENKER 1964; McCAMAN 1962; MORAN et al. 1963; SACKS 1961).

— *Formation of amines* which are assayed by biological methods (e.g. dopamine) (W. G. CLARK 1959; HOLTZ et al. 1942b), by photometry (e.g. 5-HT) (BOGDANSKI et al. 1956; C. T. CLARK et al. 1954; V. E. DAVIS and AWAPARA 1960b; HORITA 1962b; KUNTZMAN et al. 1961b; LORES ARNAIZ and ROBERTIS 1964; UDENFRIEND et al. 1953, 1955b), or by radioactive isotopes (SNYDER and AXELROD 1964; SOMERVILLE 1964).

In vivo direct determination is performed by measuring *CO_2 expiration* subsequent to administration of carboxyl-^{14}C-amino acids provided that unspecific phenomena (e.g. transamination) can be excluded (BURKARD et al. 1964c; HANSSON and CLARK 1962a, 1962b; HANSSON et al. 1963; IORIO and BOUTHILLIER 1950; MAYNARD and SCHENKER 1964; MORAN et al. 1963; NOVAK 1952). Furthermore, DCA activity may be estimated indirectly by *amine accumulation* in tissues subsequently to administration of aromatic amino acids, e.g. 5-HTP (GEY and PLETSCHER 1960a; PLETSCHER and GEY 1961b; UDENFRIEND et al. 1957a).

7. Physiological role

Decarboxylation presumably represents the last step in the formation of biogenic amines like 5-HT, tryptamine, tyramine, dopamine, 4-hydroxyphenylethanolamine (octopamine), etc. It is uncertain, however, to which extent DCA activity regulates the total monoamine content of tissues. Thus, some but no strict parallelism exists between DCA activity and amine content of different tissues (ERSPAMER 1961; GADDUM and GIARMAN 1956; GIARMAN 1956; KLINGMAN et al. 1964; SCHÜMANN 1960; SANDLER and WEST 1958) and within one organ, e.g. brain (BOGDANSKY et al. 1957). Furthermore, pronounced DCA inhibition in brain induces only a moderate reduction of the total monoamine content, but possibly a more marked decrease of free monoamines (PLETSCHER and GEY 1963). In consequence, it remains uncertain whether *changes of DCA activity* are of physiological or pathophysiological importance. A decrease of enzyme activity, for instance, might occur in phenylketonuria (NADLER and HSIA 1961; T. L. PERRY 1962; REICHLE et al. 1961), after hypophysectomy (ROSSI 1960; SKILLEN et al. 1961), adrenalectomy (W. G. CLARK 1959; PAGE and REED 1945), hepatectomy together with colchicine treatment (HAWKINS and WALKER 1951, 1952), immunosympathectomy (KLINGMAN 1964), transsection of the lower spinal cord (ANDÉN et al. 1964), in tryptophan deficiency (REID and SHEPHERD 1964), after excess of isoleucine (YUWILER et al. 1964), after thyroxine and during hunger (BERGERET et al. 1958; CHATAGNER et al. 1960; V. E. DAVIS 1963; V. E. DAVIS et al. 1961; HOLTZ and WESTERMANN 1956a; HOLTZ et al. 1956; JOLLES-BERGERET et al. 1960; SKILLEN et al. 1962; WESTERMANN 1956), in PARKINSON's disease (BARBEAU and JASMIN 1961), during seasonal variations (CARDEAU 1963; POLONOVSKY et al. 1946a), after X-rays (C. T. ANDERSON et al. 1951; CHERNOV and MOROZOVSKAYA 1962; LANGENDORFF and HAGEN 1963; LANGENDORFF et al. 1964), and after U.V. irradiation (MØLLER 1964). An increase of DCA activity has been reported in prolonged hypertension (GIORDANO 1961; GIORDANO et al. 1960b), in carcinoid tissue (CURZON 1957; LANGEMANN 1958; McISAAC and PAGE 1958; PAGE et al. 1955; SANDLER and WEST 1958; SJOERDSMA et al. 1957; SNOW et al. 1955; UDENFRIEND et al. 1955a; WESTERMANN et al. 1958), in phaeochromocytoma and neuroblastoma (ARMSTRONG and McMILLAN 1959; M. BURGER and LANGEMANN 1956; ENGEL and EULER 1950; HAGEN 1962; KÄSER 1961; KÄSER and STUDNITZ 1961; KRAUPP et al. 1959; LABROSSE et al. 1958; LABROSSE and KARON 1962; LANGEMANN et al. 1962; PARE et al. 1958; PELLERIN et al. 1958; R. ROBINSON and SMITH 1962; SANDLER et al. 1960; SJOERDSMA 1959, 1961; SJOERDSMA and UDENFRIEND 1961; STUDNITZ 1959b; WEIL-MALHERBE 1956; WESTERMANN et al. 1958), in mastocytoma (ADAMS-RAY et al. 1964; BIRT et al. 1961; W. G. CLARK 1960; HAGEN and LEE 1958; HAGEN et al. 1960; LAGUNOFF and BENDITT 1959; SCHINDLER 1958; SJOERDSMA et al. 1957; STURM and STÜTTGEN 1962; WEISSBACH et al. 1960a, 1961b), with aging (HUANG et al. 1960; KÄRKI et al. 1960, 1962; PAGE 1945; S. E. SMITH et al. 1961), and possibly after cortisone (V. E. DAVIS 1963; V. E. DAVIS et al. 1961; HICKS and WEST 1958a, 1958b; PRICE and WEST 1960). DCA activity in the pineal gland rises after light exposure of the animals (SNYDER and AXELROD 1964) and after denervation of the gland (IRALDI and LORES ARNAIZ 1964; S. H. SNYDER et al. 1964). In females, liver and brain show higher DCA activity than in males (W. G. CLARK 1959; LABOUESSE et al. 1959; POLONOVSKY et al. 1946b; SKILLEN et al. 1961).

B. Inhibitors of decarboxylase of aromatic l-amino acids

Numerous substances belonging to various chemical classes inhibit DCA in vitro, but most inhibitors have not been investigated extensively in vivo. The following compounds have been reported to cause inhibition of the enzyme: *Nitroferricyanide* and *thiocyanate* (BEILER and MARTIN 1954); *methylene blue* (GONNARD 1951); *trypan blue* (BLASCHKO 1942; WERLE 1940); *hydroxybenzylidineaminorhodanines* (STRUBE 1960); *aromatic amines*, e.g. tyramine (GONNARD 1950; POLONOVSKY et al. 1946b) or *indolalkylamines* (HESTER et al. 1964); *α-methylated aralkylamines* like α-methyltryptamine (GREIG et al. 1959, 1961b; LOVENBERG et al. 1963; METER et al. 1960); *2,5-dihydroxy-DL-tryptophan* (FRETER et al. 1958); *para-phenylendiamine* (MARTIN et al. 1942; RILEY 1958a, 1958b); *aromatic hydroxylamine derivatives* (SCHUMANN et al. 1964); *phenoxybenzamine* (CHRUŚCIEL 1961, 1962); *nicotinic, isonicotinic acid* and *nicotinamide* (GONNARD and NIGUYEN CHI 1958); *isoxazolidones* like D-cycloserine (DENGLER et al. 1962); *suramine* (BLASCHKO 1942, MARTIN et al. 1950); *ethanol* (MAYNARD and SCHENKER 1964); *catechol* (MARTIN et al. 1942); *phenylalanine and metabolites* like phenylpyruvate and phenyllactate (BOYLEN and QUASTEL 1961; DAVISON and SANDLER 1958; FELLMANN 1956; HUANG and HSIA 1963; HUANG et al. 1963; S. E. SMITH 1963; YI-YUNG HSIA 1963); *quinone* and possibly *hydroquinone* (GONNARD 1951; IMIYA 1941; TOMOKICHI 1941); *folic acid antagonists* (GONNARD 1951; MARTIN and BEILER 1947, 1948; MARTIN et al. 1948; SCHALES 1949); *deoxypyridoxine* (DIETRICH and SHAPIRO 1955); *sulfonylureas* such as carbutamide (GONNARD and NGUYEN CHI 1958b; GONNARD et al. 1958, 1959); *morphine* (MAYNARD and SCHENKER 1964; NAITO 1957); *conjugated estrogens* (M. MASON 1961); *jatamanzone* (ARORA et al. 1962); a non-dialysable *substance from salivary gland* of octopus (HARTMANN et al. 1960).

The present review will mainly be concerned with three types of compounds which inhibit DCA not only in vitro but also markedly in vivo; they are: α-alkylated amino acids, derivatives of hydrazine and some isosters, as well as derivatives of hydroxycinnamic acid.

1. α-Alkylated aromatic amino acids

a) Chemistry and action on the enzyme

Various α-alkylated DL-aromatic amino acids inhibit DCA *in vitro*, e.g. in supernatant of tissue homogenates. The L-form seems to be the active isomere (PÜTTER and KRONENBERG 1964). Phenylalanine analogues show decreasing potency in the following order: α-methyl-meta-tyrosine, α-methyldopa, α-ethyldopa, α-methyltyrosine, α-methylphenylalanine. α-Methyl-5-HTP is about as potent as α-methyldopa (LEVINE and SJOERDSMA 1964; LOVENBERG et al. 1962b, 1963; SOURKES 1954a). The inhibition is competitive or non-competitive depending on the preincubation period (LOVENBERG et al. 1962b, 1963). In the presence of substrates of high affinity like dopa, for instance, α-methyldopa and α-methyl-meta-tyrosine reduce DCA activity less than with substrates of low affinity like tryptophan and tyrosine (DRAIN et al. 1962; LOVENBERG et al. 1962b; PORTER et al. 1962). The inhibition is reversible by addition of the coenzyme pyridoxal-5′-phosphate (HIRSCH et al. 1962a; S. E. SMITH 1960a; UDENFRIEND et al. 1960; WESTERMANN et al. 1958).

α-Methylated amino acids are not only inhibitors, but also substrates of DCA; their rate of decarboxylation is, however, 100—1000 times lower than that of the corresponding physiological amino acids (LOVENBERG et al. 1962b; UDENFRIEND et al. 1960; WEISSBACH et al. 1960a). Furthermore, a non-enzymatic decarboxylation of α-alkylated amino acids in the presence of pyridoxal-5′-phosphate has been described (KALYANKAR and SNELL 1962; LOVENBERG et al. 1963).

Administration of α-alkylated amino acids to *intact animals* also inhibits DCA as measured in tissue homogenates (BURKARD et al. 1962c; R. A. DAVIS et al. 1963; HESS et al. 1960, 1961a; LEVINE and SJOERDSMA 1964; S. E. SMITH 1959, 1960b; WEISS 1963; WESTERMANN et al. 1958) (Fig. 10). The degree of inhibition varies according to the organ. In the kidney of rats α-methyldopa i.p. causes, for instance, 50% inhibition in doses about 100 times lower than in brain if no pyridoxal-5′-phosphate is added (BURKARD, unpubl.). These differences might be due to variations in the tissue distribution of the inhibitor (see below).

Single i.p. doses of α-methylated aromatic amino acids induce maximal inhibition of DCA in brain and kidney of rats within 15 minutes, which lasts for several hours and is abolished after about one day. In brain α-methyldopa is more potent than α-methyl-5-HTP. As in vitro, the inhibitory effect seems to be restricted to the L-isomers of α-methylated amino acids (BURKARD et al. 1962c; HANSSON and CLARK 1962a, 1962b; HESS et al. 1961a; PORTER et al. 1961; WEISS 1963).

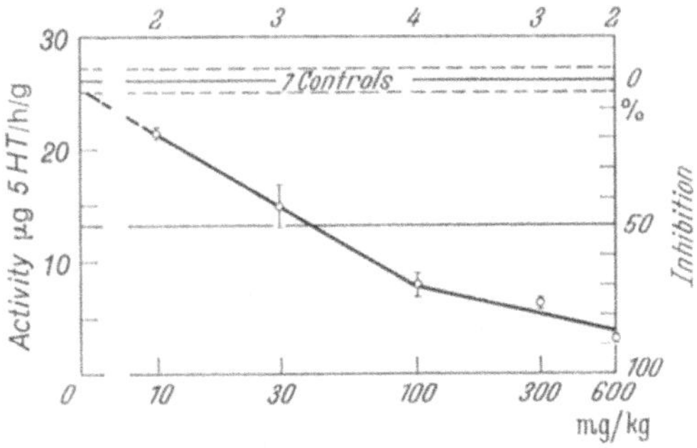

Fig. 10. *Inhibition of 5-hydroxytryptophan decarboxylation in rat brain by α-methyldopa. Ordinate.* Left: Enzyme activity (formation of 5-hydroxytryptophan in µg/g/h) without addition of the coenzyme to the incubation medium. With addition of pyridoxal-5′-phosphate, no significant reduction of the enzyme activity was measurable. Right: Inhibition in per cent as compared to untreated controls. *Abscissa:* Dose of α-methyldopa i.p. 1 hour prior to decapitation (logarithmic scale). *Vertical lines:* Standard errors of mean values which are derived from several experiments each (as indicated on the top) (BURKARD unpublished; BURKARD et al. 1962c)

b) *Effect on other enzymes*

α-Methylated aromatic amino acids decrease *histidine decarboxylation* in kidney supernatant, mast cells, growing tissues, and in bacteria. Discrepancies reported by several authors might be due to the fact that histidine is decarboxylated by at least two enzymes (e.g. DCA and histidine decarboxylase) which are possibly inhibited differently (CLARK 1963; DAY 1962; GANROT and ROSENGREN 1961; KAHLSON et al. 1962, 1963; MACKAY and SHEPHERD 1960, 1962; MACKAY et al. 1961; REID and SHEPHERD 1963; B. ROBINSON and SHEPHERD 1961, 1962; SCHAYER 1963; WERLE 1961).

In vitro and after i.p. application, α-methyldopa and related compounds strongly inhibit the *hydroxylase of tryptophan and phenylalanine* in rat liver (BURKARD et al. 1964a, 1964b; ROSS and HALJASMAA 1964). α-Methyldopa also considerably reduces the activity of *tyrosine hydroxylase* in vitro (BURKARD, unpubl.; NAGATSU et al. 1964). *Dopamine-β-oxidase* is not inhibited by α-methylated aromatic amino acids in vitro or in vivo, but by α-methylated amines like α-methyldopamine (GOLDSTEIN and CONTRERA 1962; HESS et al. 1961a, 1961b). α-Methylated aromatic amino acids, contrary to their decarboxylation products, do not inhibit *MAO* in vitro (SHARMAN and SMITH 1962). *Tryptophan pyrrolase* is activated by α-methyltryptophan in vivo (MORAN and SOURKES 1963; SANKOFF and SOURKES 1962; SOURKES and TOWNSEND 1955), whereas α-methylated aromatic amino acids do not markedly affect *tyrosine transaminase* in vitro (JACOBY and LA DU 1964; MORAN et al. 1963).

c) *Tissue distribution and metabolism*

Distribution studies have been carried out mainly with α-methyldopa. In *man*, after i.v. administration, the drug is cleared from the plasma within about 12 hours, the half-life time being less than 2 hours. After oral administration, peak plasma levels occur within 3—6 hours. A few percent of the drug pass into the erythrocytes. About 50% of the drug and its metabolites are eliminated in the urine within 24 hours; small amounts are still excreted on the second day. In *animals* (e.g. rats, guinea pigs, mice) after i.p. administration, α-methyldopa penetrates into various organs, e.g. kidney, brain (mainly grey matter), liver, adrenal medulla, spleen. In the kidney of guinea pigs the concentration of the drug is higher than in the brain and heart. It remains relatively constant for 90—120 minutes in brain and kidney; in the other organs the level is highest immediately following injection, thereafter declining. The blood content of the L-form is higher than that of the D-isomer, probably due to faster urinary elimination of the latter (DOLLERY and HARINGTON 1962; DUHM et al. 1963; GILLESPIE et al. 1962; HESS 1961a; HOGANS and PORTER 1961; PORTER and TITUS 1963; PORTER et al. 1961; SANKOFF and SOURKES 1962; SJOERDSMA et al. 1963; SOURKES and MURPHY 1960, 1961; SOURKES et al. 1962).

The *metabolism* of α-methylated aromatic amino acids and of the corresponding amines respectively in *animals* and *humans* is similar to that of the physiological analogs. It includes decarboxylation of the L-isomers, 3-O-methylation, β-hydroxylation, deamination and conjugation. Thus, in rats injected with carboxyl-^{14}C-α-methyldopa, $^{14}CO_2$ rapidly appears in the expired air. Furthermore, after administration of α-methyldopa, O-methylated and O-conjugated derivatives of α-methyldopa and α-methyldopamine as well as α-methyldopamine and desaminated metabolites are excreted in the urine. The main urinary product is, however, unchanged α-methyldopa. In addition, in various tissues, e.g. brain and heart, α-methyldopamine and α-methyl-NE have been found after application of α-methyldopa and formation of α-methyl-meta-tyramine and metaraminol (meta-hydroxynorephedrine) from α-methyl-meta-tyrosine could be demonstrated. The rate of decarboxylation of α-methylated amino acids is probably slower than that of the non-methylated amino acids (see above). The α-methylated amines, especially those with α-hydroxy groups, however, remain longer in the tissues than the corresponding unbranched amines, since the α-methyl group impedes deamination by MAO. In the brain of mice, for instance, α-methyl-NE and metaraminol can still be detected 24 hours after administration of the corresponding α-methylated amino acids; in the brain of rabbits the α-methylated amines (e.g. α-methyl-meta-tyramine) remain even for several days (CARLSSON and LINDQVIST 1962; GESSA et al. 1962a; GILLESPIE 1960; GILLESPIE et al. 1962; PORTER and TITUS 1963; PORTER et al. 1962; SJOERDSMA et al. 1963; SOURKES et al. 1962; UDENFRIEND et al. 1961; YOUNG and EDWARDS 1964).

d) *Effects on metabolism*

α) Endogenous monoamines. In normal animals various α-alkylated aromatic amino acids (e.g. α-methyldopa, α-methyl-meta-tyrosine) decrease endogenous monoamines (NE, dopamine, 5-HT) in different tissues, e.g. brain, heart, adrenal medulla, blood platelets, isolated iris. The degree of the amine diminution varies according to the animal species, the drug, and the individual amine. The effect of the drugs on brain 5-HT is rather weak, even high single (up to 600 mg/kg) and repeated doses do not decrease the amine by more than about 50% within 1—3 hours (Fig. 11). Repeated administration of high doses of α-methyldopa

(400 mg/kg) lowers the intestinal 5-HT to about 60%. The content of dopamine in brain is more markedly decreased than that of 5-HT. High doses of α-methyl-dopa and α-methyl-meta-tyrosine may diminish the levels of this amine by 60 to 80%. The decrease of both 5-HT and dopamine is of relatively short duration, the original values of 5-HT being reached after 8—12 hours, those of dopamine within about 24 hours (BRODIE et al. 1962a; CARLSSON and LINDQVIST 1962; COSTA et al. 1962; CSILIK 1964; DRAIN et al. 1962; GIARMAN 1961; GIARMAN and SCHANBERG 1961; GIRARD 1963; L. I. GOLDBERG et al. 1960; HESS et al. 1960, 1961a; LEROY 1961; PORTER et al. 1960, 1961; ROOS and WERDINIUS 1963; SJOERDSMA and UDENFRIEND 1961a; S. E. SMITH 1959, 1960a; SOURKES and MURPHY 1961; SOURKES et al. 1961).

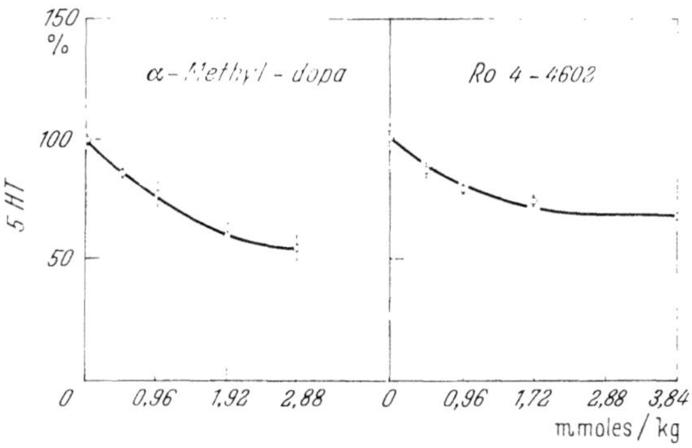

Fig. 11. *Decrease of the endogenous 5-hydroxytryptamine in brain of rats after various doses of α-methyldopa and Ro 4-4602* respectively. Ordinate:* 5-Hydroxytryptamine content in percent of untreated controls. *Abscissa:* I.p. dose of the drugs in m moles kg. Spectrophotofluorimetric determination of 5-hydroxytryptamine 1 and 2 hours after Ro 4-4602 and α-methyldopa respectively (time of maximal 5-hydroxytryptamine decrease). The points represent averages of 4—8 experiments each with standard error (KUNZ 1964)

The diminution of NE by α-methyl-meta-tyrosine and α-methyldopa is more marked and persists for a longer period of time than that of 5-HT and dopamine. In brain and heart NE may be decreased by 90% within 4—10 hours, returning to the norm only after 2—6 days. NE ist still markedly diminished when DCA activity has already been normalized (e.g. after 16 hours) (BRODIE et al. 1962a; CARLSSON and LINDQVIST 1962; COSTA and BRODIE 1961a; COSTA et al. 1962; GESSA et al. 1962a; HESS et al. 1960, 1961a; PORTER et al. 1960, 1961; SJOERDSMA and UDENFRIEND 1961a; SOURKES and MURPHY 1961; SOURKES et al. 1961; STONE et al. 1961).

Brain amines are also decreased by α-methyltryptophan and α-methyl-5-HTP, whereas α-methyl-ortho-tyrosine and α-methylphenylalanine have no effect. α-Methyl-5-HTP is in general less potent than α-methyldopa and α-methyl-meta-tyrosine. α-Methylated aromatic amines e.g. α-methyl-meta-tyramine, α-methyldopamine, and α-methyl-β-hydroxy-meta-tyramine, have also been shown to decrease NE in some tissues, e.g. in the heart (GESSA et al. 1962a; PORTER et al. 1961; SOURKES and MURPHY 1961). The order of potency of some α-methylated amino acids and amines concerning the decrease of endogenous NE in mice is the following (PORTER et al. 1961):

Brain: DL-α-methyl-meta-tyrosine $>$ DL-α-methyldopa $=$ DL-α-methyl-meta-tyramine.

Heart: DL-α-methyl-meta-tyramine $>$ DL-α-methyl-meta-tyrosine $>$ DL-α-methyldopamine $>$ L-α-methyldopa $>$ DL-α-methyldopa $>$ D-α-methyldopa (inactive).

DCA inhibition does not seem to be the main mechanism by which α-methylated aromatic amino acids decrease endogenous NE and possibly dopamine. It is rather likely that the drugs act primarily through liberation of the endogenous amines from their storage sites in the tissues. The following findings support this hypothesis:

* N^1-DL-seryl-N^2-(2,3,4-trihydroxybenzyl)hydrazine

— The decrease of NE in heart and brain after a single dose of an α-methylated amino acid lasts longer than the inhibition of DCA (HESS et al. 1961a; SOURKES et al. 1961).

— The decrease of endogenous monoamines is probably not caused by the α-methylated aromatic amino acids, but rather by metabolites, i.e. the corresponding α-methylated amines which do not inhibit DCA markedly (see below).

— The biosynthesis of endogenous NE (and also 5-HT) is not substantially impaired by doses of α-methylated amino acids decreasing these amines. Thus, after α-methyl-meta-tyrosine, during the period of marked NE diminution, MAO inhibitors (e.g. harmaline, pheniprazine, pargyline) still cause a rapid increase of NE and epinephrine in heart and brain as well as of 5-HT in brain (COSTA et al. 1962; HESS et al. 1961a, 1961b).

— The potent DCA inhibitors of the hydrazine type (e.g. Ro 4-4602) causing no major monoamine release, decrease endogenous amines less than α-methylated aromatic amino acids (see below).

— Experiments with ^{3}H-NE demonstrate that α-methyl-meta-tyrosine diminishes the storing of this amine in the heart (HESS 1961, 1962; HESS et al. 1961a; PAULSON and HESS 1962).

— α-Methyldopa enhances the urinary excretion of stored ^{3}H-NE and its desaminated metabolites (KOPIN and GORDON 1963).

The decrease of endogenous monoamines is probably not due to α-methylated aromatic amino acids as such, but rather to their decarboxylation products, i.e. the corresponding α-methylated amines. This is supported by the following findings:

— Decarboxylation of α-methylated amino acids to the corresponding α-methylated amines and in part subsequent β-hydroxylation has been demonstrated in brain and heart (see above).

— α-Methylated amino acids, e.g. α-methyl-meta-tyrosine and α-methyldopa, no longer diminish NE if their decarboxylation is inhibited by pretreatment with strong DCA inhibitors of the hydrazine type, e.g. NSD 1024, 1034, 1055 (GESSA et al. 1962a; LEVINE and SJOERDSMA 1964; ROSSUM and HURKMANS 1963).

— α-Methylated aromatic amines are strong NE liberators in the heart (GESSA et al. 1962; HARRISON et al. 1963; PORTER et al. 1961, 1962a; SOURKES and MURPHY 1961).

α-Methylated amines probably act in principle by displacement of the endogenous catecholamines. A stoichiometrical relation between the displacing and the displaced amines seems to exist. Whether α-methylated amines also impair the binding of NE remains to be elucidated (ANDÉN 1964; CARLSSON and LINDQVIST 1962; GESSA et al. 1962b; HESS 1962; PAULSON and HESS 1962; SCHÜMANN and GROBECKER 1964; SHORE and ALPERS 1964; SOURKES et al. 1961; UDENFRIEND and ZALTZMAN-NIRENBERG 1964; UDENFRIEND et al. 1961).

It remains to be further investigated whether α-methylated amino acids also liberate 5-HT in the brain. It must also be considered that they decrease the cerebral 5-HT by interference with the 5-HT biosynthesis, i.e. by inhibiting the 5-hydroxylation of tryptophan or by decreasing the uptake of 5-HTP. Thus, α-methyldopa, in contrast to reserpine, decreases the cerebral content of metabolic end products of 5-HT such as 5-hydroxyindolacetic acid (ASHCROFT and SHARMAN 1961; PLETSCHER et al. 1964a; ROOS and WERDINIUS 1963; ROOS et al. 1964; SHARMAN and SMITH 1962). Furthermore, α-methyldopa inhibits the 5-hydroxylation of tryptophan in vitro (BURKARD et al. 1964a). In addition, in cultures of neoplastic mast cells α-methyldopa inhibits the uptake of

5-HTP, whereas with brain slices the findings have been controversial (DAY and GREEN 1962b; SCHANBERG 1963; S. E. SMITH 1963; WARTBURG 1962).

According to preliminary investigations in patients with *carcinoid*, α-methyldopa enhances the urinary excretion of 5-HTP and diminishes the output of 5-HT and possibly also of 5-hydroxyindolacetic acid (BLUMBERG et al. 1962; R. B. DAVIS et al. 1961; OATES et al. 1960a; SJOERDSMA 1960; SJOERSDMA et al. 1960b). Patients with *pheochromocytoma* show decreased urinary output of catecholamine metabolites (e.g. 3-methoxy-4-hydroxymandelic acid) during therapy with α-methyldopa (SCHAUB et al. 1962; SJOERDSMA 1960). In *hypertension* α-methyldopa may lower the urinary excretion of 3-methoxy-4-hydroxymandelic acid (CANNON et al. 1962; SCHAER et al. 1963; SCHAUB et al. 1962). Other authors could not find a decrease of this acid with hypotensive doses of α-methyldopa (BUHS et al. 1964; RUGE and HARTMANN 1963; SJOERDSMA et al. 1963). In *phenylketonuria*, the phenylethylamine formation is markedly reduced by α-methyldopa (OATES et al. 1963). Most of these effects can probably be explained by DCA inhibition.

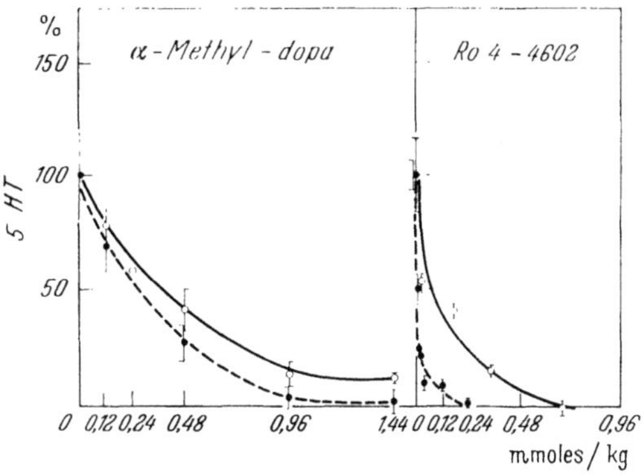

Fig. 12. *Diminution of the 5-hydroxytryptophan-induced increase of 5-hydroxytryptamine in brain and heart of rats by α-methyldopa or Ro 4-4602**. 75 mg/kg 5-hydroxytryptophan were administered s.c. 2 and 1 hour after α-methyldopa and Ro 4-4602 respectively. Spectrophotofluorimetric measurement of 5-hydroxytryptamine ½ hour after 5-hydroxytryptophan. *Ordinate:* 5-Hydroxytryptophan-induced increase of 5-hydroxytryptamine in percent of controls which had received 5-hydroxytryptophan alone (in the experiments with brain the animals were pretreated with 100 mg/kg of the MAO inhibitor pargyline i.p. 16 hours before administration of the decarboxylase inhibitors). *Abscissa:* Dose of α-methyldopa and Ro 4-4602 respectively in μ moles/kg i.p. ——— heart; – – – – brain. The points represent averages of 4—10 experiments each with standard error (KUNZ 1964)

β) Exogenous aromatic amino acids. In various organs α-methylated amino acids reduce the *monoamine increase due to* administration of the corresponding monoamine *precursors*, e.g. the 5-HTP-induced increase of 5-HT in kidney, brain, and heart, the dopa-induced increase of dopamine in brain, lungs, heart, as well as the dopa-induced rise of NE in brain (Fig. 12). In the *kidney* of mice the potency of the α-methylated amino acids decreases in the following order: DL-α-methyl-2,3-dihydroxyphenylalanine = L-α-methyldopa > DL-α-methyldopa > DL-α-methyl-meta-tyrosine; the corresponding α-methylated amines as well as the D-form of α-methyldopa have no effect. The action of α-methylated amino acids is of long duration (more than 16 hours), probably because the acids remain in the kidney for a considerable period of time. In the *brain* only α-methyldopa and α-methyl-meta-tyrosine counteract the dopa-induced increase of dopamine and correspondingly enhance the accumulation of dopa, whereas α-methyl-3-hydroxy-4-methoxyphenylalanine and α-methyl-3-methoxyphenylalanine have no effect (KUNZ 1964; MURPHY and SOURKES 1961; PORTER et al. 1961; SOURKES and MURPHY 1960). In mice with *melanosarcoma*, α-methyldopa enhances the incorporation of ^{3}H-dopa into the tumors (HEMPEL and DEIMEL 1963).

α-Methylated aromatic amino acids also reduce the *excretion of monoamines* after administration of aromatic amino acids. Thus, in humans the enhanced urinary elimination of 5-HT, tryptamine, phenylethylamine, tyramine, dopamine,

* N^{1}-DL-seryl-N^{2}-(2,3,4-trihydroxybenzyl)hydrazine

subsequent to oral intake of the corresponding amino acids is diminished by daily doses of 1—6 g α-methyldopa. The activity resides mainly in the L-isomer of the DCA inhibitor. In rats α-methyl-meta-tyrosine, α-methyl-5-HTP, α-methyldopa decrease the urinary excretion of dopamine due to injection of dopa (GILLESPIE et al. 1962; MURPHY and SOURKES 1961; OATES et al. 1960a, 1960b, 1963; PORTER et al. 1960; SJOERDSMA 1960, 1961; SJOERDSMA and UDENFRIEND 1961; SOURKES and MURPHY 1961).

The above effects of α-methylated aromatic amino acids on the metabolism of exogenous amino acids can probably in the main be explained by DCA inhibition. This is supported by recent findings in mice according to which α-methylated aromatic amino acids decrease the content of $^{14}CO_2$ in the expired air after administration of carboxyl-^{14}C-dopa and carboxyl ^{14}C-5-HTP. Thereby, α-methyldopa and α-methyl-meta-tyrosine are more potent than α-methyl-5-HTP and α-methyltryptophan, whereas DL-α-methyl-3-methoxyphenylalanine and α-methyl-histidine are without effect (HANSSON and CLARK 1962a, 1962b; HANSSON et al. 1964).

γ) Exogenous monoamines. In the heart of guinea pigs α-methyl-meta-tyrosine decreases the storage of injected ^{3}H-NE and counteracts the uptake of the labelled amine. The uptake of 5-HT by heart and kidney, however, is not markedly changed by α-methyldopa (HESS 1961, 1962; HESS et al. 1961a; PAULSON and HESS 1962; PLETSCHER and GEY, unpubl.; PORTER et al. 1961). The effect of α-methyldopa on NE uptake is probably due to α-methylated amines formed from the amino acid in vivo. Thus, α-methyldopamine and α-methyl-NE inhibit the uptake of NE by tissue slices and blood platelets in vitro (DENGLER 1964; IMAIZUMI et al. 1964).

In *conclusion*, α-alkylated amino acids inhibit DCA in vivo, but the decrease of endogenous monoamines is probably mainly due to their enhanced liberation.

δ) Other metabolic effects. α-Methyldopa does not decrease the urinary elimination of histamine in rats and mice or the histamine content of whole mice (WEISSBACH et al. 1961b; WERLE 1961). Furthermore, the drug has no influence on the level of substance P in the brain (P. STERN and KOCIC-MITROVIC 1960).

e) Pharmacodynamic effects

α) Cardiovascular effects. α-Alkylated amino acids, especially α-methyldopa, lower the *blood pressure* in animals, e.g. in dogs and in rats with experimental hypertension. α-Methyldopa is being used in high doses (several grams per day) in the treatment of hypertension including patients with carcinoid. In general the effect appears only several hours after i.v. administration of the drug. As with other hypotensives the effect is primarily orthostatic, but may also be present in the recumbant position. The drug affects mainly the systolic and less the diastolic pressure. The hypotensive activity of α-methyldopa resides in the L-isomer (ARNOLD 1962; BAYLISS and HARVEY-SMITH 1962; BREST et al. 1961; CANNON et al. 1962; GILLESPIE 1960; GILLESPIE et al. 1961, 1962; L. I. GOLDBERG et al. 1960; IRVINE et al. 1962; KIRKENDALL and WILSON 1962; LEROY 1961; OATES et al. 1960a; SCHAUB et al. 1962; SJOERDSMA 1960, 1961; SJOERDSMA and UDENFRIEND 1961; STONE et al. 1961).

The hypotensive effect of α-methyldopa is probably not related to DCA inhibition. Thus, no parallelism exists between the duration of the hypotensive action and DCA inhibition. Furthermore, the DCA inhibition induced by hypotensive doses of α-methyldopa is probably inadequate to cause an impairment of the synthesis of endogenous catecholamines (DAVIS et al. 1963; HORWITZ and SJOERDSMA 1964; SCHAUB et al. 1962; SJOERDSMA 1961; SJOERDSMA et al. 1963). The following mechanisms of action of α-methyldopa seem to be more likely:

aa) *Depletion of the monoamine stores in consequence of monoamine release.* This might lead to a lack of transmitter substance (NE) at the sympathetic nerve endings. This hypothesis is supported by the findings that the hypotensive effect of α-methyldopa parallels the NE decrease in the tissues (HORWITZ and SJOERDSMA 1964; SJOERDSMA 1961) and that other monoamine releasers (e.g. reserpine and guanethidine) also cause hypotension. On the other hand, various investigators have shown that depletion of the NE stores by α-methyldopa, in contrast to the depletion by reserpine, does not markedly interfere with sympathetic nervous transmission. In addition, α-methyl-meta-tyrosine seems to be less hypotensive, although it depletes NE more markedly than α-methyldopa (CARLSSON 1964; DAY and RAND 1963; GAFFNEY et al. 1963; GILLESPIE et al.1962; GOLDBERG L. I. et al. 1960; HORWITZ and SJOERDSMA 1964; PLETSCHER and GEY 1964; STONE et al. 1961, 1962). The differences of action of α-methyldopa and reserpine on sympathetic transmission can possibly be explained by the effect of the drugs on different amine pools. Thus, α-methyldopa, in contrast to reserpine, might deplete a pool not essential for neurohumoral transmission (CARLSSON 1964).

bb) *Replacement of liberated catecholamines by α-methylated amines*, especially α-methyl-NE, derived from the α-methylated aromatic amino acids. Such ,,unphysiological transmitters'', which have been shown to be formed in vivo (see above) and to replace NE, might be liberated instead of NE from the sympathetic nerve endings during nerve stimulation, but might have less physiological activity than NE (DAY and RAND 1963, 1964). This hypothesis is attractive, because storage and liberation of α-methyl-NE as well as of metaraminol has been shown in vivo, e.g. in the heart and the spleen (CROUT and SHORE 1964; MAÎTRE and STAEHELIN 1963; MUSCHOLL and MAÎTRE 1963; THOENEN, personal comm.). Since the relative biological activity of α-methyl-NE and NE seems to vary with the organ and the species (DAY and RAND 1964; MAÎTRE and STAEHELIN 1963; THOENEN, personal comm.), more experimental data are required. Furthermore, possible quantitative differences in the liberation and storage of NE and its α-methylated congenere have to be investigated.

α-Methyldopa has also been reported to cause bradycardia in man, whereas in dogs it does not seem to change heart rate. The drug also decreases cardiac output without increasing the peripheral vascular resistance. Furthermore, α-methyldopa antagonizes reserpine in attenuating the cardiovascular effects of tyramine (L. I. GOLDBERG et al. 1960; KIRKINDALL and WILSON 1962; KRONEBERG and STOEPEL 1963; VARMA and BENEFEY 1963; VARMA et al. 1963; WILSON et al. 1961).

β) Effects on the central nervous system. High doses of α-methyldopa and lower doses of α-methyl-meta-tyrosine may cause sedation, miosis, narrowing of the palpebral fissures, hypothermia, etc. In humans the sedative effect seems to be particularly pronounced during the first 48—72 hours of treatment. High doses of α-methyl-meta-tyrosine induce central nervous stimulation in humans and dogs, probably due to its decarboxylation to α-methyl-meta-tyramine, but in mice this α-methylated amino acid is unable to counteract reserpine sedation. α-Methyldopa, however, antagonizes some effects of reserpine, e.g. emesis and prolongation of hexobarbital hypnosis. In contrast to monoamine releasers (e.g. reserpine and the benzoquinolizine Ro 4-1284), α-methyl-meta-tyrosine has no effect on hippocampal potentials evoked by electrical stimulation of the basolateral amygdaloid complex (BAYLISS and HARVEY-SMITH 1962; GESSA et al. 1962b; GILLESPIE 1960; GILLESPIE et al. 1962; HORWITZ and SJOERDSMA 1964; KIRKINDALL and WILSON 1962; L. I. GOLDBERG et al. 1960; LEROY 1961; OATES et al. 1960a, 1960b; PLETSCHER et al. 1964b; REVZIN et al. 1961; ROSSUM and HURKMANS 1963; SCHAUB et al. 1962; SJOERDSMA 1960, 1961; SJOERDSMA and UDENFRIEND 1961; S. E. SMITH 1960a; STONE et al. 1962; VARMA et al. 1963).

The sedative effect of α-methyldopa, similar to that of reserpine, may be related to the depletion of endogenous monoamines in the brain. Liberation and delayed metabolism of endogenous monoamines might furthermore explain the central nervous stimulation if α-methyldopa is combined with the MAO inhibitor pargyline (ROSSUM and HURKMANS 1963).

γ) Interference with exogenous monoamines, monoamine precursors, and drugs. α-Methylated amino acids diminish some pharmacological effects of *aromatic amino acids*. Thus, α-methyldopa couteracts the *blood pressure* changes due to dopa and 3,4-dihydroxyphenylserine in various animal species. In dogs, it also diminishes the positive inotropic effect of dopa and meta-tyrosine on the *heart*; this diminution roughly parallels DCA inhibition. Furthermore, α-methyldopa attenuates several actions of 5-HTP, e.g. bronchoconstriction, excitation of the central nervous system including tremors, shortening of hexobarbital anesthesia, and oxytoxic activity. Some phamacological effects of 5-HT, however, (e.g. bronchoconstriction, edema) are not changed by α-methyldopa (DENGLER and REICHEL 1957/58, 1958; DRAIN et al. 1962; L. I. GOLDBERG et al. 1960; LOVAŠEN et al. 1961; PORTER et al. 1961; WESTERMANN et al. 1958). It is therefore likely that the α-methylated amino acids decrease the pharmacological actions of aromatic amino acids by DCA inhibition.

In dogs α-methyldopa, α-methyl-meta-tyrosine, as well as the corresponding amines prevent the cardiovascular action of certain *amines* like phenylethylamine and amphetamine, but not that of NE, dopamine, and tyramine (L. I. GOLDBERG et al. 1960; STONE et al. 1961, 1962). Furthermore, various pharmacological effects of reserpine are antagonized by pretreatment with α-methyldopa, e.g. sedation, ptosis, depletion of adrenal cholesterol and ascorbic acid, decrease of the threshold for metrazole seizures (NEČINA 1962).

α-Methylated amino acids have also been reported to induce the following alterations of *drug* effects:

— Increase of the frequency of tonic convulsions and death due to hexafluorodiethylether without change of the threshold for clonic convulsions (TRUITT and EBERSBERGER 1961, 1962).

— Acceleration of tremorine-induced tremors, increase of the toxicity of strychnine, decrease of convulsions due to picrotoxine (HÉROLD et al. 1962a; P. STERN and GAŠPAROVIC 1961).

— Increase of the effect of amphetamine and L-dopa on locomotor activity; this enhancement seems to follow the time course of NE depletion in brain (C. B. SMITH 1962).

— Decrease of the amphetamine toxicity in aggregated mice (MOORE 1964).

— Prolongation of barbiturate sleeping time (HÉROLD et al. 1962b; S. E. SMITH 1960a).

The influence of α-methylated aromatic amino acids on various pharmacological actions of exogenous monoamines and of drugs is probably not due to DCA inhibition, but rather to a displacement of endogenous monoamines from the tissues.

δ) Other effects. α-Methyldopa delays gastric emptying and intestinal passage of meals (S. E. SMITH 1960a). Furthermore, it has a protective effect in anaphylactic shock (GERSHORN and ROOS 1962). α-Methyl-DL-tryptophan reduces body weight in mice (SANKOFF and SOURKES 1962). It is doubtful whether these effects are connected with DCA inhibition.

2. Hydrazine derivatives and oxygen isosters

a) Chemistry and action on the enzyme

Carbonyl trapping agents, such as hydrazine and derivatives, may inhibit DCA by inactivation of the coenzyme, i.e. by forming a hydrazone or by interfering with pyridoxal-5'-phosphate kinase (responsible for the phosphorylation of pyridoxal) (McCormick and Snell 1959). Their inhibitory action on DCA is, however, in general rather weak. Even without addition of pyridoxal-5'-phosphate, concentrations as high as 10^{-2} to 10^{-3} M of the hydrazines are required in order to decrease DCA activity by 50%.

The following compounds cause some inhibition *in vitro:*

Hydrazine (Holtz 1959; McCormick and Snell 1959); most *orthosubstituted phenylhydrazines* (Schumann et al. 1961); *phenylisopropylhydrazine* (Hartmann 1963; Ozaki 1959; Wartburg 1962); *semicarbazide* (Beiler and Martin 1954; C. T. Clark et al. 1954; Clegg and Sealock 1949; Dengler et al. 1962; Fellmann 1959b; Greig et al. 1961b; Langemann 1951; Weissbach et al. 1957b); *hydroxylamine* (Buzard and Nytch 1957; C. T. Clark et al. 1954); *aminoguanidine* (Werle et al. 1955); *isoniazid* (Canal and Maffei-Faccioli 1961; Davison 1956; Gonnard and Nguyen Chi 1958b; Palm 1958; Schroeder 1957); *hydrazinophtalazines* (Apresolin, Nepresol) (H. M. Perry et al. 1955; Schroeder 1957, 1959; Schuler and Wyss 1960; Werle et al. 1955); *2-hydrazino-5-phenylpyridazine* (H. M. Perry et al. 1955). Isoniazid has, however, also been shown to activate DCA, probably because the isonicotinoylhydrazone of pyridoxal-5'-phosphate may function as a coenzyme under certain experimental conditions (Gonnard 1958, 1962; Gonnard and Boigné 1961; Gonnard and Fenard 1962; Gonnard and Nguyen Chi 1958a, 1959a, 1959b; Gonnard et al. 1964a, 1964b; Palm 1958).

Some *hydrazine derivatives inhibiting MAO* are also weak inhibitors of DCA, e.g. iproniazid (Davison 1956; Gonnard and Nguyen Chi 1958b; Greig et al. 1959; Hagen and Welch 1956; J. Lévy and Michel-Ber 1960b; Schuler and Wyss 1960); pheniprazine (Brodie et al. 1958a; Schuler and Wyss 1960); phenelzine (Dubnick et al. 1959a, 1962a; Tabachnick 1959).

In vivo, i.e. after application to intact animals, the following hydrazines cause some DCA inhibition:

Hydrazine (Hansson and Clark 1962b); *isoniazid* (Burkard et al. 1962c; Canal 1961); *phenelzine* (Dubnick et al. 1959a, 1962a); *semicarbazide* (Hansson and Clark 1962b; Weissbach et al. 1957b); *thiosemicarbazide* (Wiss and Weber 1958, 1963).

The compounds mentioned above are of limited interest as inhibitors of DCA, because their potency in vivo is rather low.

New and potent DCA inhibitors. Some *hydroxyphenylalkylhydrazines* and *oxygen isosters* have been found to be potent inhibitors of DCA in vitro and in vivo. They are listed in Table 7 and will be the main topic of chapter 2.

These substances strongly inhibit DCA *in vitro.* They are at least 100 times more effective than α-methyldopa. NSD 1034 seems to inhibit the enzyme competitively (Hirsch et al. 1962a). With Ro 4-4602 it has been shown that the inhibition is independent from coenzyme addition and irreversible by dialysis (Burkard et al. 1962b). The inhibition by Ro 4-5127 (trihydroxybenzylhydrazine) seems to be pseudoirreversible and competitive (Burkard et al. 1964c). DCA inhibition by Ro 4-4602 increases if the compound is preincubated with the enzyme before addition of the substrate. This is probably due to hydrolysis into the free hydrazine (Ro 4-5127) which seems to be the effective part of

Table 7. *Inhibition of DCA by hydrazine derivatives and isosters*

No.	Structure	In vitro 50% inhibition[1,2,4,5,8,9]		In vivo[3,6,7,10]		
		molar concentration	relative molarity *	% inhibition after 100 mg/kg	ED_{50} mg/kg	ED_{50} µm/kg
NSD 1024	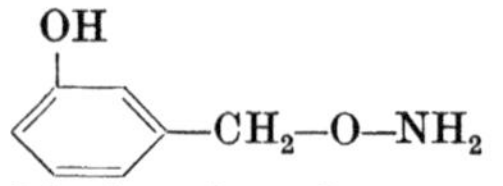 3-hydroxybenzyloxy-amine	1×10^{-6}– 2×10^{-8}	7×10^{4}	34.3	2.2	12.5
NSD 1034	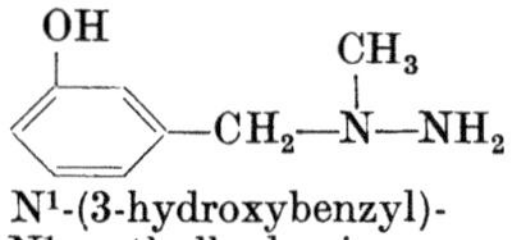 N^1-(3-hydroxybenzyl)-N^1-methylhydrazine	4×10^{-6}	2×10^{3}	85.6	—	
NSD 1055	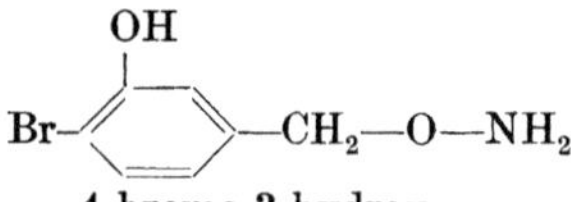 4-bromo-3-hydroxy-benzyloxyamine	4×10^{-9}	4×10^{6}	20.1	—	—
NSD 485	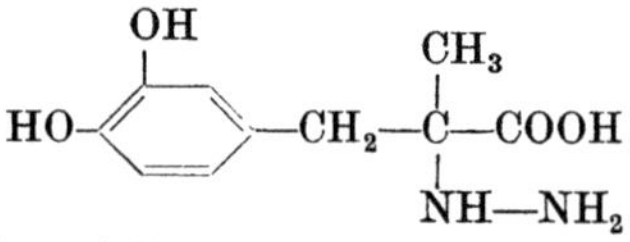 DL-α-hydrazino-α-methyl-3,4-dihydroxyphenyl-propionic acid	2×10^{-7}	2×10^{4}	93.7	1.8	7.6
Ro 4-4602	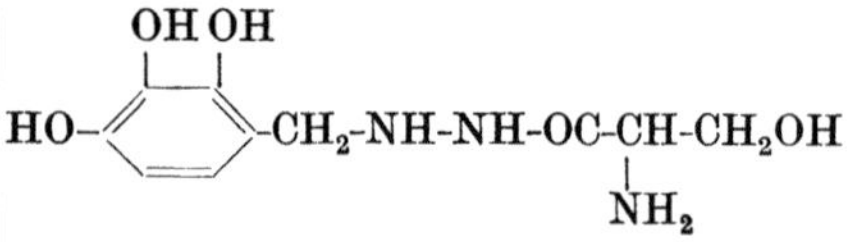 N^1-DL-seryl-N^2-(2,3,4-trihydroxy-benzyl)hydrazine	4×10^{-6} **	4×10^{4} **	91.5	2.1	10.0
Ro 4-5127	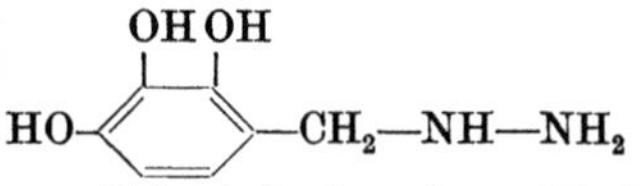 (2,3,4-trihydroxybenzyl)hydrazine	2×10^{-6}	2×10^{4}	—	—	—
α-methyl-dopa	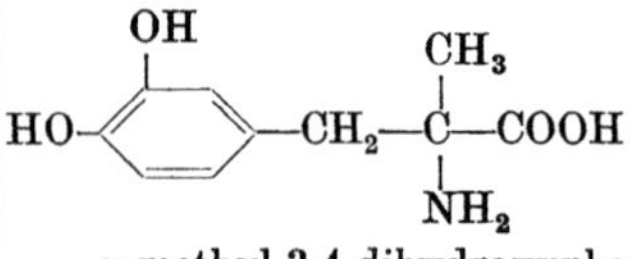 α-methyl-3,4-dihydroxyphenylalanine	1×10^{-3}	3×10^{1}	42.0	—	—

$$* \text{ relative molarity}^7 = \frac{\text{molar concentration of inhibitor}}{\text{molar concentration of substrate}}$$

** if preincubated with enzyme without substrate

[1] Drain et al. 1962
[2] Burkard et al. 1964c
[3] Hansson and Clark 1962b
[4] Lovenberg et al. 1962
[5] Porter et al. 1962
[6] Hansson and Clark 1962a
[7] Hartmann et al. 1955a
[8] S. E. Smith 1963
[9] Sletzinger et al. 1963
[10] Burkard, unpubl.

the molecule and inhibits DCA independently from the preincubation period (Burkard et al. 1962b, 1964c).

In the series of ***aralkylhydrazino acids***, phenolic groups in position 3 and particularly in both 3 and 4 enhance the potency, whereas the α-methylation is practically without effect. MK 485 and its demethylated anologue inhibit DCA 1500 times more strongly than α-methyldopa (Porter et al. 1962; Sletzinger et al. 1963).

In vivo these hydrazines and some isosters seem to be about 100 times more potent than α-methyldopa if the DCA activity is measured in the supernatant of tissue homogenates (R. A. Davis et al. 1963; Burkard et al. 1964c; Drain et al. 1962). Thereby DCA in kidney is more markedly inhibited than that in brain; within 1 hour, for instance, a 50% inhibition is obtained by 12 mg/kg Ro 4-4602 in brain (Fig. 13) as compared to 0.1 mg/kg in kidney (Burkard et al. 1962b). In order to get complete inhibition in brain, however, very high doses are needed (> 200 mg/kg) (Brodie et al. 1962b; Burkard et al. 1962b; Hirsch et al. 1962a; Pletscher et al. 1963a). After single i.p. injection of Ro 4-4602 the enzyme activity in brain as well as in kidney is maximally reduced within 15 minutes and restored after about 60 hours. Addition of the coenzyme to the incubation mixture has no effect on the degree of inhibition (Burkard et al. 1962b, 1964c) (Fig. 13). The DCA inhibition by NSD 1039 in rat brain is enhanced by α-methyldopa (R. A. Davis et al. 1963). In intact animals the difference between hydrazines and α-methyldopa seems to be less marked if the expiration of $^{14}CO_2$ is measured after application of carboxyl-^{14}C-dopa (Table 7) (Hansson and Clark 1962a, 1962b; Hansson et al. 1964; Moran et al. 1963).

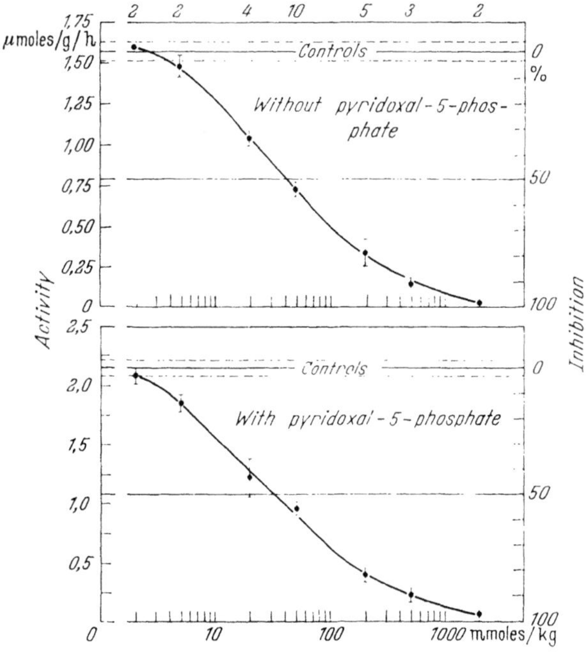

Fig. 13. *Inhibition of 3,4-dihydroxyphenylalanine decarboxylation in rat brain in vivo with and without coenzyme addition to the incubation medium. Ordinate*: Left: Enzyme activity (formation of dopamine in μ moles/g/h); Right: Inhibition in per cent as compared to untreated controls. *Abscissa:* I.p. dose of Ro 4-4602* 1 hour prior to decapitation (logarithmic scale). *Vertical lines:* Standard errors of mean values. The mean values are derived from 2—10 experiments (as indicated on the top), each with 5 pooled brains (Burkard et al. 1962b)

b) Effects on other enzymes

Histidine decarboxylase is inhibited by most carbonyl trapping agents, e.g. semicarbazide (Kahlsson and Rosengren 1959; Rothschild and Schayer 1939; Werle and Heitzer 1938), hydroxylamine (Buzard and Nytch 1957), hydrazine (B. Robinson and Shepherd 1962; Waton 1956), phenylhydrazine (Werle 1940) and NSD 485 (Sletzinger et al. 1963). NSD 1024, NSD 1034 and

* N^1-DL-seryl-N^2-(2,3,4-trihydroxybenzyl)hydrazine

NSD 1055 have also been shown to inhibit this enzyme in vitro (W. G. CLARK 1962; REID and SHEPHERD 1963), but not in vivo (HANSSON and CLARK 1962b).

MAO: Several DCA inhibitors of the hydrazine type also decrease the activity of MAO. For instance, 50 and 200 mg/kg NSD 1034 i.v. inhibit MAO of mouse brain by 14 and 34% respectively after 1 hour (BRODIE et al. 1962b), whereas Ro 4-4602 i.p. (300 mg/kg) is without significant influence on MAO in rat brain within 16 hours. The analogue of Ro 4-4602 lacking the acyl moiety, Ro 4-5127, inhibits, however, cerebral MAO to some extent (BURKARD et al. 1962b).

DAO may also be affected by hydrazine derivatives. Ro 4-4602, for instance, decreases the enzyme activity slightly in rat intestine (BURKARD unpubl.).

Dopamine-β-oxidase is inhibited by NSD 1024, 1034, 1055 and similar compounds in vitro and in vivo (HESS et al. 1961b; NIKODIJEVIC et al. 1963). In vitro, concentrations of 10^{-4} M reduce the enzyme activity markedly. Without preincubation the inhibition is competitive, but uncompetitive and more potent after preincubation (HIRSCH et al. 1962b; KUNTZMAN et al. 1962a; SCHOOT et al. 1963).

Tyrosine transaminase, phenylalanine hydroxylase, and *tyrosine hydroxylase* do not seem to be affected in vitro (BURKARD unpubl.; MORAN et al. 1963).

c) Tissue distribution and metabolism

Only investigations with labelled α-hydrazino-α-methyl-3,4-dihydroxyphenylpropionic acid (MK 485) have been published. After i.v. administration the ^{14}C-labelled drug is taken up by various organs except by brain, highest concentrations being found in kidney and lung which still retain measurable radioactivity after 24 hours. Part of the drug undergoes decarboxylation which is more marked after oral than after i.p. administration (PORTER et al. 1962).

d) Effects on metabolism

α) Endogenous monoamines. The potent DCA inhibitors of the hydrazine class diminish the total content of endogenous monoamines in animals only to a small extent. In the brain of several species high single doses (200—800 mg/kg) decrease 5-HT, NE, and dopamine by not more than 50% (Fig. 11). This effect is only transitory, normal levels having recovered after 4—8 hours. In the heart of guinea pigs and rats, however, Ro 4-4602 decreases the NE content to about 50% for more than 24 hours. Repeated administration of this drug does not seem to intensify the NE and 5-HT decrease as compared with high single doses except in the adrenal medulla, where the catecholamines are lowered by about 70% (BURKARD et al. 1962; DRAIN et al. 1962; KUNZ 1963; PLETSCHER and GEY 1963).

The rise of endogenous monoamines in the brain due to a MAO inhibitor (pargyline) is counteraceted by NSD 1034, but even high doses of the latter (320 mg/kg) inhibiting DCA almost completely cause only a 50% reduction of the 5-HT and dopamine rise. The NE increase, however, is completely inhibited by doses as low as 6.3 mg/kg, probably due to additional inhibition of dopamine-β-hydroxylase (KUNTZMAN et al. 1962).

The recovery of 5-HT and NE after their depletion from the tissue by a monoamine releaser (e.g. Ro 4-1284) can be completely prevented by repeated administration of high doses of Ro 4-4602 (PLETSCHER and GEY 1963).

β) Exogenous aromatic amino acids. DCA inhibitors of the hydrazine type may completely counteract the monoamine increase due to injection of monoamine precursors. In the kidney MK 485 is 60—80 times more potent than α-methyldopa in inhibiting the 5-HTP-induced 5-HT rise. The relative potency of other aromatic hydrazino acids corresponds to that found in vitro (see above). In heart and brain Ro 4-4602 is very effective in lowering the 5-HTP-induced 5-HT rise; doses as low as 0.5 and 10 mg/kg respectively cause 50% reduction (Fig. 12). This difference between heart and brain might be due to dissimilar penetration of the drug into these organs. MK 485, which hardly enters the brain, counteracts the 5-HTP-induced 5-HT rise in this organ only to a small extent. Ro 4-4602 inhibits also the rise in cerebral 5-HT caused by tryptophan. The urinary excretion of 5-HT after administration of 5-HTP is markedly influenced by MK 485, i.e. oral doses as low as 1.5 mg/kg cause 50% diminution in rats (Brodie et al. 1962b; Drain et al. 1962; Hirsch et al. 1962; Hodge et al. 1964; Kuntzman et al. 1962; Pletscher et al. 1964b; Porter et al. 1962). These results are probably a direct consequence of DCA inhibition. This is supported by the findings that the hydrazine derivatives decrease the expiration of $^{14}CO_2$ after administration of carbonyl-^{14}C-amino acids (Burkard et al. 1964c; Hansson and Clark 1962b; Porter et al. 1962).

In conclusion, DCA inhibitors of the hydrazine type have a weak action on endogenous monoamines, but a rather marked effect on the decarboxylation of exogenous amino acids (e.g. 5-HTP). This discrepancy might be due to the fact that decarboxylation is no rate limiting step in the formation of endogenous monoamines. Therefore, even with a high degree of DCA inhibition the remaining enzyme activity may be sufficient for normal formation of monoamines.

Some other hydrazides have also been described to change the metabolism of exogenous monoamines as a consequence of DCA inhibition. Thus, certain MAO inhibitors of the hydrazine type, e.g. phenelzine, pheniprazine, iproniazid, as well as apresoline, have been shown to decrease the formation of 5-HT from injected 5-HTP in brain and kidney respectively under certain experimental conditions (Dubnick et al. 1959a, 1962a; Porter et al. 1961). In addition, isoniazid further reduces the conversion of dopa to dopamine in pyridoxine-deficient rats, and in combination with a tryptophan-deficient diet this hydrazine diminishes the excretion of 5-hydroxyindoleacetic acid (R. B. Davis et al. 1961; Sourkes and Murphy 1961). The content of endogenous amines in the organs is, however, not decreased by isoniazid (Pletscher et al. 1960c).

e) *Pharmacodynamic effects*

The arterial pressure is at the most lowered to a moderate degree by NSD 1024, 1034, 1039 (N^1-(2-hydroxybenzyl)-N^1-methylhydrazine), and 1055 in anesthetized rabbits. Ro 4-4602 has no or only slight effect in normotensive animals or in experimental hypertension due to desoxycorticosterone or renine. Motor activity either is not markedly affected by the inhibitors: they do especially not induce sedation and have no effect on ethanol narcosis. NSD 1024, 1034, and 1055 have been reported to cause muscular hypotonia, piloerection, and hypothermia in mice (Besendorf, unpubl.; Cahn et al. 1962a, 1962b; Davis et al. 1963; Pletscher et al. 1964b; Sjoerdsma et al. 1963; Steiner et al., unpubl.).

Various DCA inhibitors, e.g. NSD 1024, 1034, and Ro 4-4602, counteract tremors, and Ro 4-4602 prevents diarrhea induced by 5-HTP. The minimal effective doses are, depending on the compound and the route of administration, 0.5—10 mg/kg. The hydrazine derivatives are 50—500 times more effective than α-methyldopa. NSD 1024, 1034, and 1055 have also been shown to reduce motor stimulation induced by dopa in mice. Furthermore, various effects of tryptophan are counteracted by Ro 4-4602, e.g. neurological symptoms (such as excitation) in humans as well as the hyperpyretic and toxic action in guinea pigs. These effects of the hydrazine derivatives are probably due to reduction of the monoamine increase because of DCA inhibition (BESENDORF, unpubl.; CAHN et al. 1962a; DRAIN et al. 1962; HANSSON et al. 1964; HODGE et al. 1964).

The following effects of DCA inhibitors of the hydrazine type, probably in part related to DCA inhibition, have also been reported:

— Enhancement of barbiturate and ethanol potentiation due to tetrabenazine (BESENDORF, unpubl.; HÉROLD et al. 1962b).

— Increase of strychnine toxicity, decrease of picrotoxine-induced convulsions (HÉROLD et al. 1962b).

— Beneficial effect in patients with carcinoid (BLUMBERG et al. 1962; DUBACH and GSELL 1962).

— Antagonism of NE-induced behavioural stimulation (SCHECKEL and BOFF 1964).

3. Derivatives of hydroxycinnamic acid

a) Chemistry and action on the enzyme

The effect of some 200 compounds on DCA has been compared in vitro, e.g. in supernatant of kidney homogenates (GRIESEMER et al. 1961; HARTMANN and CLARK 1953; HARTMANN et al. 1955a). The most active inhibitors show the following structure:

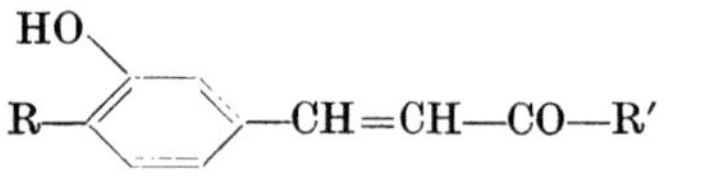

R=H or OH

The potency decreases with the following substituents: R′ = aryl > alkyl > O-alkyl > OH. The most powerful inhibitor is 5-(3,4-dihydroxycinnamoyl)salicylic acid (3,4,4′-trihydroxy-3′-carboxychalcone) (YUWILER et al. 1959a, 1960):

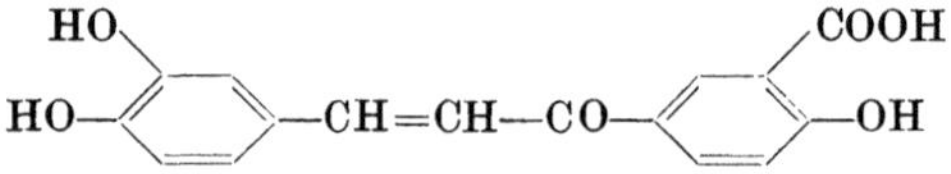

10^{-6} M of this compound cause 50% inhibition of dopa decarboxylation. Preincubation increases the degree of inhibition (GRIESEMER et al. 1961) which is competitive (W. G. CLARK 1955; HARTMANN and CLARK 1953; HARTMANN et al. 1955a; POGRUND and CLARK 1956; YUWILER et al. 1959b, 1960), pseudoirreversible (HARTMANN et al. 1955a), and relatively specific, i.e. without effect on bacterial decarboxylases, mammalian tyrosinase, and succinate dehydrogenase, respiration of liver slices (W. G. CLARK and POGRUND 1961). In adrenal slices 5-(3-hydroxycinnamoyl)salicylic acid decreases the formation of catecholamines from labelled tyrosine (W. G. CLARK and POGRUND 1961; DRELL 1957).

Measurements of DCA activity after administration of derivatives of hydroxycinnamic acid to intact animals have not been reported.

b) Tissue distribution and metabolism

After i.v. administration of caffeic acid to cats, the blood level decreases to unmeasurable values within 30 minutes, while unchanged drug and a glucuronide appear in the urine. In rabbits 5-(3-hydroxycinnamoyl)salicylic acid is partly metabolized to 5-(3-hydroxyhydrocinnamoyl)salicylic acid. Other derivatives have not been investigated (W. G. CLARK 1959).

c) Effect on monamine metabolism

The metabolism of endogenous monoamines is at best slightly affected by derivatives of hydroxycinnamic acid. Thus, repeated administration of caffeic acid inhibits the recovery of the insuline-induced depletion of the adrenal medulla. A decrease of the normal content of endogenous monoamines has not been reported and seems rather doubtful (W. G. CLARK 1959; W. G. CLARK and POGRUND 1961; DRELL 1957; POGRUND et al. 1961).

Derivatives of hydroxycinnamic acid, e.g. 5-(3,4-dihydroxycinnamoyl)salicylic acid, diminish the excretion of dopamine and tyramine following the administration of dopa and meta-tyrosine respectively. 5-(3,4-Dihydroxycinnamoyl)salicylic acid also decreases the amount of urinary tyramine formed from injected meta-hydroxyphenylpyruvic acid which is presumably transaminated to meta-tyrosine (W. G. CLARK 1959; W. G. CLARK and POGRUND 1961; POGRUND et al. 1955, 1961). Exhalation of $^{14}CO_2$ after administration of ^{14}C-carboxyl-dopa in mice, however, is inhibited only to a small degree by 100 mg/kg 5-(3,4-dihydroxycinnamoyl)-salicylic acid (HANSSON and CLARK 1962b).

d) Pharmacodynamic effects

Derivatives of hydroxycinnamic acid reduce the rise of blood pressure caused by exogenous dopa and tyrosine as well as by meta-hydroxyphenylpyruvate and 3,4-dihydroxyphenylpyruvate. The pyruvic acid derivatives are probably transaminated to meta-tyrosine and dopa respectively. According to a Lineweaver-Burk plot of the blood pressure, the effect of 5-(3,4-dihydroxycinamoyl)salicylic acid is probably competitive (W. G. CLARK 1959; W. G. CLARK and POGRUND 1961; POGRUND and CLARK 1956; POGRUND et al. 1961).

Among a great number of derivatives, 5-(3-hydroxycinnamoyl) salicylate is one of the most active compounds on blood pressure. The ED_{50} of the active compounds varies between 1 and 50 mg/kg i.v. and is much lower than the acute toxicity. The duration of action is relatively short (30—60 minutes) probably due to rapid metabolism of the drugs (see above) (W. G. CLARK 1959; W. G. CLARK and POGRUND 1961; POGRUND et al. 1961).

Hydroxycinnamic acids probably diminish the rise in blood pressure induced by exogenous aromatic amino acids in consequence of DCA inhibition. This is supported by the finding that the drugs do not counteract the effect of corresponding amines. It is, however, rather doubtful whether hydroxycinnamic acids markedly interfere with the synthesis of endogenous monoamines, e.g. at nerve endings. Thus, these drugs do not diminish the contraction of the nictitating membrane following repeated electrical stimulation (W. G. CLARK 1959; W. G. CLARK and POGRUND 1961).

A strict quantitative parallelism between DCA inhibition in vitro and decrease of dopa-induced blood pressure rise has not been found, but substances inactive in vitro have mostly no or only weak effect in vivo either. Exceptions might be explained by metabolic conversion to active structures, e.g. by esterase action on acetylated derivatives (W. G. CLARK 1959; W. G. CLARK and POGRUND 1961).

5-(3,4-Dihydroxycinnamoyl)salicylic acid also reduces tremors and motor excitation induced by 5-HTP and dopa respectively; furthermore, it potentiates barbiturate narcosis (CAHN et al. 1962a; HÉROLD et al. 1962b).

In conclusion, some hydroxycinnamic acid derivatives are potent DCA inhibitors in vitro. In vivo their potency to inhibit the formation of endogenous monoamines from endogenous sources is, however, rather weak, although they may be effective in counteracting the rise in monoamines and blood pressure due to the administration of aromatic amino acids.

C. Summary

DCA catalyzes the formation of indolyl- and phenylalkylamines (e.g. 5-HT, dopamine) from the corresponding amino acids (e.g. 5-HTP, dopa). Thereby, pyridoxal-5′-phosphate acts as a coenzyme. In vitro, the enzyme is inhibited by various types of compounds, but a definite action in vivo has only been found for the following classes:

a) α-Alkylated aromatic amino acids, e.g. α-methyldopa, α-methyl-meta-tyrosine. Their effect on the enzyme can be reversed by the coenzyme. In vivo they are decarboxylated to the corresponding α-methylated amines which displace endogenous monoamines, especially NE, in various tissues. The increase of monoamines in tissues and urine due to precursors as well as some pharmacodynamic effects of monoamine precursors are antagonized by α-methylated amino acids, probably in consequence of DCA inhibition. The lowering of blood pressure by α-methylated amino acids, however, seems to be unrelated to interference with this enzyme.

b) Hydrazine derivatives and isosters, e.g. N^1-DL-seryl-N^2-(2,3,4-trihydroxybenzyl)hydrazine (Ro 4-4602), 3-hydrobenzyloxyamine (NSD 1024). Their effect on the enzyme in vitro and in vivo is at least 100 times stronger than that of α-methyldopa and seems to be independent from the coenzyme. In the intact animal the hydrazine derivatives in general decrease the endogenous monoamines relatively little if at all. They counteract, however, the monoamine increase due to monoamine precursors as well as some pharmacodynamic effects of monoamine precursors more markedly than the α-methylated amino acids. Unlike the latter, DCA inhibitors of the hydrazine type do not seem to have a pronounced effect on blood pressure.

c) Derivatives of hydroxycinnamic acid, e.g. 5-(3,4-dihydroxycinnamoyl)salicylic acid. These are relatively weak inhibitors in vitro and in vivo. In the intact animal they have probably no marked action on endogenous monoamines, but they counteract some effects of exogenous monoamine precursors (e.g. the dopa-induced rise of blood pressure).

IV. Concluding remarks

The attempts to interfere with the metabolism of monoamines, e.g. indolyl- and phenylalkylamines, have lead to the development of interesting compounds. Thus, inhibitors of MAO and DCA are valuable tools for studying the metabolism, the physiological and pathophysiological role of monoamines. Inhibition of MAO seems to be of therapeutic value in some human diseases like mental depression, angina pectoris, hypertension. Reduction of DCA activity may be of value in the treatment of diseases with excessive production of endogenous monoamines, e.g. in carcinoid and pheochromocytoma. It is, however, unlikely that DCA inhibition represents a useful principle in the therapy of other diseases, e.g. arterial hypertension. Further studies with inhibitors of MAO and DCA might yield new information on the pathogenesis of some human diseases.

Acknowledgements

The authors wish to thank Dr. A. Jenni and Dr. R. Silberschmidt for their valuable suggestions as well as Miss M.-J. Imhof for technical assistance in preparing the manuscript.

References

Aceves, J., P. Pulido, and R. Mendez: The comparative action of Marsilid and its derivative Tersavid upon the cardiovascular system. Cardiologia (Basel) **37**, Suppl. II, 29 (1960).

Acheson, R. M., J. Cole, D. P. Dearnaley, and E. J. Dearnaley: Attempted correlations between behavioural and biochemical changes in rats following reserpine and chronic administration of amine-oxydase inhibitors. Psychopharmacologia (Berl.) **2**, 277 (1961a).

ACHESON, R. M., J. COLE, D. P. DEARNALEY, and P. GLEES: Some effects on perfomance and behaviour of the daily administration of amine oxidase inhibitors in trained rats. In: Neuropsychopharmacology, vol. 2, p. 139, edit. E. ROTHLIN. Amsterdam: Elsevier Publ. Co. 1961b.

— — — — Changes in aromatic excretion pattern of rats during chronic administration of amine oxidase inhibitors. In: Neuropsychopharmacology, vol. 2, p. 455, edit. E. ROTHLIN. Amsterdam: Elsevier Publ. Co. 1961c.

ACKERMANN, D.: Ein Fäulnisversuch mit Arginin. Hoppe-Seylers Z. physiol. Chem. **56**, 305 (1908).

— Ueber den bakteriellen Abbau des Histidins. Hoppe-Seylers Z. physiol. Chem. **65**, 504 (1910a).

— Ueber ein neues, auf bakteriellem Wege gewinnbares, Aporrhegma. Hoppe-Seylers Z. physiol. Chem. **69**, 273 (1910b).

—, u. H. LANGEMANN: Aminosäuren-Decarboxylase im menschlichen Gehirn. Helv. physiol. pharmacol. Acta **18**, C 5 (1960).

ADAMS-RAY, J., A. DAHLSTRÖM, K. FUXE, and N.-Å. HILLARP: Mast cells and monoamines. Experientia (Basel) **20**, 80 (1964).

AEBI, H.: Mitochondrial structure as a controlling factor of monoamine oxidase activity and the action of monoamine oxidase inhibitor. Biochem. Pharmacol. **9**, 135 (1962).

—, J. QUITT u. A. HASSAN: Uricase, Xanthinoxydase und Monoaminoxidase als H_2O_2-Donoren peroxydatischer Umsetzungen. Helv. physiol. pharmacol. Acta **20**, 148 (1962a).

— F. STOCKER u. M. EBERHARDT: Abhängigkeit der Monoaminoxydase-Aktivität und peroxydatischen Umsetzungen von der Mitochondrienstruktur. Biochem. Z. **336**, 526 (1962b).

AGIN, H. V.: The use of JB-516 in psychiatry. Ann. N. Y. Acad. Sci. **80**, 705 (1959).

AIRAKSINEN, M. M., and V. J. UUSPÄÄ: Is urinary 5-hydroxytryptamine formed in the kidney? Biochem. Pharmacol. **8**, 46 (1961).

AKSEL, I. S.: Die antidepressiven Drogen und ihre Wirkung auf den Glukosestoffwechsel. Wien. med. Wschr. **110**, 713 (1960).

ALBERT, A., and C. W. REES: The destruction of isonicotonic acid hydrazide in the presence of haemin. Biochem. J. **61**, 128 (1955).

ALEXANDER, L.: Objective evaluation of antidepressant therapy by conditional reflex technique. Dis. nerv. Syst. **22**, Suppl. 5, 14 (1961).

—, and S. R. HORNER: The effect of drugs on the conditional psychogalvanic reflex in man. J. Neuropsychiat. **2**, 246 (1961).

—, and S. R. LIPSETT: Effect of amine oxidase inhibitors on the conditional psychogalvanic reflex in man. Dis. nerv. Syst. **20**, Suppl. 26 (1959).

ALLEGRETTI, N., and D. VUKADINOVIČ: Atebrin inhibition of the oxidation of adrenaline by monoamine oxidase. Arh. Kem. (Zagreb) **22**, 191 (1950).

ALLES, G. A., and E. V. HEEGARD: Substrate specificity of amine oxidase. J. biol. Chem. **147**, 487 (1943).

ALLEVA, J. J.: Metabolism of tranylcypromine-C^{14} and dl-amphetamine-C^{14} in the rat. J. med. Chem. **6**, 621 (1963).

ALLMARK, M. G., F. C. LU, E. CARMICHAEL, and A. LAVALLEE: Some pharmacological observations on isoniazid and iproniazid. Amer. Rev. Tuberc. **68**, 199 (1953).

AMMANN, A., and E. G. ANDERSON: The neuromyal blocking action of the monoamine oxidase inhibitors. Pharmacologist **3**, 73 (1961).

ANDÉN, N.-E.: On the mechanism of noradrenaline depletion by α-methyl metatyrosine and metaraminol. Acta pharmacol. (Kbh.) **21**, 260 (1964).

— T. MAGNUSSON, and E. ROSENGREN: On the presence of dihydroxyphenylalanine decarboxylase in nerves. Experientia (Basel) **20**, 328 (1964).

— B.-E. ROOS, and B. WERDINIUS: On the occurrence of homovanillic acid in brain and cerebrospinal fluid and its determination by a fluorimetric method. Life Sci. **2**, 448 (1963a).

— — — 3,4-Dihydroxyphenylacetic acid in rabbit corpus striatum normally and after reserpine pretreatment. Life Sci. **2**, 319 (1963b).

— — — Effects of chlorpromazine, haloperidol and reserpine on the levels of phenolic acids in rabbit corpus striatum. Life Sci. **3**, 149 (1964b).

ANDEREJEW, A., C. GERNEZ-RIEUX et A. TACQUET: Action de l'INH et de la D-cyclosérine sur la peroxydase purifiée et sur l'activité peroxydasique des bacilles tuberculeux. Ann. Inst. Pasteur **96**, 145 (1959).

ANDERSON, C. T., H. BLASCHKO, J. H. BURN, and R. A. MOLE: The pressor amines in the adrenal medulla after irradiation. Brit. J. Pharmacol. **6**, 342 (1951).

ANDERSON, E. G.: Monoamine oxidase inhibitors and neuromyal block. Pharmacologist **1**, 82 (1959).

ANDERSON, E. G., and A. AMMANN: The effects of monoamine oxidase inhibitors on neuromyal transmission. J. Pharmacol. exp. Ther. **140**, 179 (1963).
—, and L. BERK: The effects of some monoamine oxidase (MAO) inhibitors on spinal synaptic activity. Fed. Proc. **23**, 248 (1964).
— S. D. MARKOWITZ, and D. D. BONNYCASTLE: Brain 5-hydroxytryptamine and anticonvulsant activity. J. Pharmacol. exp. Ther. **136**, 179 (1962).
ANDERSON, F. E., D. KAMINSKI, B. DUBNICK, S. R. KLUTCHKO, W. A. CETENKO, J. GYLYS, and J. A. HART: Chemistry and pharmacology of monoamine oxidase inhibitors: hydrazine derivatives. J. med. pharm. Chem. **5**, 221 (1962).
ANDERSON, J. A., M. R. ZIEGLER, and D. DOEDEN: Banana feeding and urinary excretion of 5-hydroxy-indoleacetic acid. Science **127**, 236 (1958).
ANGELAKOS, E. T., and E. R. LÖW: Histamine toxicity in mice and rats following treatment with histaminase inhibitors. J. Pharmacol. exp. Ther. **119**, 444 (1957).
— — Influence of histaminase inhibitors on certain pharmacological effects of histamine. Arch. int. Pharmacodyn. **117**, 277 (1958).
APRISON, M. H., and C. B. FERSTER: Neurochemical correlates of behavior. II. Correlation of brain monoamine oxidase activity with behavioural changes after iproniazid and 5-hydroxytryptophan administration. J. Neurochem. **6**, 350 (1961).
— R. TAKAHASHI, and T. L. FOLKERTH: Biochemistry of the avian central nervous system.— I. The 5-hydroxytryptophan decarboxylase-monoamine oxidase and cholineacetylase-acetylcholinesterase systems in several discrete areas of the pigeon brain. J. Neurochem. **11**, 341 (1964).
ARAI, A.: Studies on monoamine oxidase, report 2: p-methyl-phenyl hydrazine, a potent and selective monoamine oxidase inhibitor. Jap. J. Pharmacol. **9**, 159 (1960).
— Y. OZAWA, H. WAKAMATSU, T. TAKIUCHI, T. FUJIMAKI, and K. KAMIJO: Influence of p-methylphenyl hydrazine (MPH) on the peripheral blood vessel of rabbit. Showa Igakkai Zasshi **21**, 265 (1961). [Psychopharmacologia (Berl.) Abstr. **1**, 546 (1961).]
ARAI, Y.: Critical studies on the significance of serotonin in the mechanism of anaphylaxis. II. The changes in serotonin level and monoamine oxidase activity in the tissue after anaphylactic shock. Arerugi **12**, 380 (1963) [Chem. Abstr. **59**, 3553d (1964)].
ARIOKA, I., and H. TANIMUKAI: Histochemical studies on monoamineoxidase in the midbrain of the mouse. J. Neurochem. **1**, 311 (1957).
ARMIN, J., R. T. GRANT, R. H. S. THOMPSON, and A. TICKNER: An explanation for the heightened vascular reactivity of the denervated rabbit's ear. J. Physiol. (Lond.) **121**, 603 (1953).
ARMSTRONG, M. D., and A. MCMILLAN: Studies on the formation of 3-methoxy-4-hydroxy-D-mandelic acid, a urinary metabolite of norepinephrine and epinephrine. Pharmacol. Rev. **11**, 394 (1959).
ARNOLD, O. H.: Die Bedeutung des α-Methyldopa für die Behandlung der chronischen Hypertonie. Dtsch. med. Wschr. **87**, 844 (1962).
ARONSON, J. D., S. L. EHRLICH, and W. FLAGG: Effects of isonicotinic acid derivatives on tubercle bacilli. Proc. Soc. exp. Biol. (N. Y.) **80**, 259 (1952).
ARORA, R. B.: Mechanism of action of monoamine oxidase inhibitors in experimental myocardial infarction in the pig. Ann. N.Y. Acad. Sci. **107**, 1152 (1963).
—, M. SINGH, and Y. R. SAXENA: A biochemical approach to the mechanism of action of Jatamansone. Life Sci. **1962**, 571.
ARRIGONI-MARTELLI, E., E. GENOVESE e G. F. GOLDWURM: Azione della iproniazide sull' aumento di motilità spontanea da stimolanti centrali. Boll. Soc. ital. Biol. sper. **34**, 1576 (1958).
—, u. M. KRAMER: Einfluß von Iproniazid und von Beta-phenylisopropylhydrazin (JB 516) auf die narkotische Wirkung und den Abbau von Hexobarbital und Thiopental. Med. exp. (Basel) **1**, 45 (1959).
ARROYO, H., et A. BERNARD: A propos de l'action de l'iproniazide sur certaines myocardoses métaboliques. Presse méd. **69**, 586 (1961).
ARVY, L.: Contribution à l'histoenzymologie de la glande surrénale chez Bos taurus L. adulte. C.R. Acad. Sci. (Paris) **251**, 2782 (1960).
— Histochimie. — Contribution à l'histoenzymologie de la surrénale des sus scrofa L., (Suidae, Gray, 1821), var, domestique. C.R. Acad. Sci. (Paris) **252**, 467 (1961).
ASATOOR, A. M., A. J. LEVI, and M. D. MILNE: Tranylcypromine and cheese. Lancet **1963 II**, 733.
ASHCROFT, G. W., and D. F. SHARMAN: The effect of reserpine on the concentration of 5-OR indolyl compounds in the caudate nucleus and the cerebrospinal fluid of the dog. J. Physiol. (Lond.) **158**, 32P (1961).
ASTON, R., and H. CULLUMBINE: The effects of combinations of ataraxics with hypnotics, LSD and iproniazid in the mouse. Arch. int. Pharmacodyn. **126**, 219 (1960).

AUSMAN, R. K., R. B. DAVIS, W. R. MEEKER, and D. G. MCQUARRIE: Effect of amine oxidase inhibitors on E. coli endotoxin mortality in mice. Fed. Proc. **19**, 279 (1960).

AWAPARA, J., R. SANDMAN, and C. HANLY: Activation of DOPA decarboxylase by pyridoxal phosphate. Arch. Biochem. **98**, 520 (1962a).

— — — Purification of DOPA decarboxylase from rat liver. Fed. Proc. **21**, 228 (1962b).

AXELROD, J.: Studies on sympathomimetic amines. II. The biotransformation and physiological disposition of D-amphetamin, D-P-hydroxyamphetamin and D-methamphetamin. J. Pharmacol. exp. Ther. **116**, 315 (1954).

— The enzymatic deamination of amphetamin (Benzedrine). J. biol. Chem. **214**, 753 (1955).

— O-methylation of epinephrine and other catechols in vitro and in vivo. Science **126**, 400 (1957).

— Discussion remark to FRIEND et al.: The effect of iproniazid on the inactivation of norepinephrine in the human. J. clin. exp. Psychopath. **19**, Suppl. 1, 68 (1958a).

— Presence, formation and metabolism of normetanephrine in the brain. Science **127**, 754 (1958b).

— Discussion remark. Ann. N. Y. Acad. Sci. **80**, 624 (1959a).

— The metabolism of catecholamines in vivo and in vitro. Pharmacol. Rev. **11**, 402 (1959b).

— Metabolism of epinephrine and other sympathomimetic amines. Physiol. Rev. **39**, 751 (1959c).

— G. HERTTING, and R. W. PATRICK: Inhibition of H^3-norepinephrine release by monoamine oxidase inhibitors. J. Pharmacol. exp. Ther. **134**, 325 (1961a).

—, and J. K. INSCOE: The uptake and binding of circulating serotonin and the effect of drugs. J. Pharmacol. exp. Ther. **141**, 161 (1963).

— — S. SENOH, and B. WITKOP: O-methylation, the principal pathway for the metabolism of epinephrine and norepinephrine in the rat. Biochim. biophys. Acta (Amst.) **27**, 210 (1958a).

—, and M.-J. LAROCHE: Inhibitor of O-methylation of epinephrine and norepinephrine in vitro and in vivo. Science **130**, 800 (1959).

— J. REICHENTHAL, and B. B. BRODIE: Mechanism of the potentiating action of β-diethylaminoethyl diphenylpropylacetate. J. Pharmacol. exp. Ther. **112**, 49 (1954).

— S. SENOH, and B. WITKOP: O-methylation of catecholamines in vivo. J. biol. Chem. **233**, 697 (1958b).

— L. G. WHITBY, and G. HERTTING: Effect of psychotropic drugs on the uptake of H^3-norepinephrine by tissues. Science **133**, 383 (1961b).

— — — and I. J. KOPIN: Studies on the metabolism of the catecholamines. Circulat. Res. **9**, 715 (1961c).

BÄCHTOLD, H. P., u. A. PLETSCHER: Einfluß von Isonicotinsäurehydraziden auf den Verlauf der Körpertemperatur nach Reserpin, Monoaminen und Chlorpromazin. Experientia (Basel) **13**, 163 (1957).

— — Abschwächung der Noradrenalin-Wirkung auf die isolierte Aorta bei Hemmung der Monoaminoxydase. Experientia (Basel) **15**, 265 (1959).

BAGDON, R. E.: Unpublished results.

—, and M. D. ROE: Unpublished results.

BAKER, J., and S. CHAYKIN: The metabolism of trimethylamine-N-oxide. Fed. Proc. **20**, 47 (1960).

BALDRIDGE, E. T., L. V. MILLER, J. HAVERBACK, and S. BRUNJES: Amine metabolism after an overdose of a monoamine oxidase inhibitor. New Engl. J. Med. **269**, 421 (1962).

BALOURDAS, T. A.: Vascular hypersensitivity and potentiation of catecholamines induced by monoamine oxidase inhibition. Fed. Proc. **23**, 231 (1964).

BALZER, H., u. P. HOLTZ: Beeinflussung der Wirkung biogener Amine durch Hemmung der Aminoxydase. Nauyn-Schmiedebergs Arch. exp. Path. Pharmak. **227**, 547 (1956).

— — u. D. PALM: Untersuchungen über die biochemischen Grundlagen der konvulsiven Wirkung von Hydraziden. Naunyn-Schmiedebergs Arch. exp. Path. Pharmak. **239**, 520 (1960).

— — — Reserpin und γ-Aminobuttersäuregehalt des Gehirns. Experientia (Basel) **17**, 38 (1961).

—, u. D. PALM: Über den Mechanismus der Wirkung des Reserpins auf den Glykogengehalt der Organe. Naunyn-Schmiedebergs Arch. exp. Path. Pharmak. **243**, 65 (1962).

BARAC, G.: Sur le métabolisme de l'hydroxyphényl-méta-éthanol-amine chez le chien. C.R. Soc. Biol. (Paris) **155**, 1598 (1961).

BARBATO, L. M., and L. G. ABOOD: The inhibition of mitochondrial monoamine oxidase (MAO) by phenantroline (PTL) and phenylcyclopropylamine (PCP). Fed. Proc. **20**, 237 (1961).

— — Purification and properties of monoamineoxidase. Biochim. biophys. Acta (Amst.) **67**, 531 (1963).

BARBEAU, A., et G. JASMIN: Dosage de l'acide 5-hydroxyindolacétique urinaire dans la maladie de PARKINSON. Rev. canad. Biol. **20**, 837 (1961).
BARBOUR, B. H., and M. H. WEIL: Treatment of hypertension with alpha methyl dopa. Circulation **24**, 880 (1961).
BARGER, G., and G. S. WALPOLE: Isolation of the pressor principles of putrid meat. J. Physiol. (Lond.) **38**, 343 (1909).
BARLOW, R. B.: Effects on amine oxidase of substances which antagonize 5-hydroxytryptamine more than tryptamine on the rat fundus strip. Brit. J. Pharmacol. **16**, 153 (1961).
— H. BLASCHKO, J. M. HIMMS, and U. TRENDELENBURG: Observations on Ω-amino-polymethylene trimethylammonium compounds. Brit. J. Pharmacol. **10**, 116 (1955).
BARONDES, S. H.: The influence of neuroamines on the oxidation of glucose by the anterior pituitary. I. The role of monoamine oxidase. J. biol. Chem. **237**, 204 (1962).
— P. JOHNSON, and J. B. FIELDS: Stimulation of anterior pituitary glucose oxidation by neurohumeral agents. Clin. Res. Proc. **9**, 175 (1961).
BARONI, V., N. LUKINOVICH e N. DI MARCO: Sull' azione ingrassante dell' isopropilderivato dell' isonicotiniledrazide Marsilid "Roche". Gazz. med. ital. **1957**, 371.
BARSKY, J.: Reactive site of monoamine oxidase. Ph. D. Diss. (Northwestern University, Chicago, Ill., 1958), Univ. Microfilm Ann Arbor, L. C. No. Mic. 58-5741.
— W. L. PACHA, S. SARKAR, and E. A. ZELLER: Amine oxidases. XVII. Mode of action of 1-isonicotinyl-2-isopropylhydrazine on monoamine oxidase. J. biol. Chem. **234**, 389 (1959).
BARTLET, A. L.: The 5-hydroxytryptamine content of mouse brain and whole mice after treatment with some drugs affecting the central nervous system. Brit. J. Pharmacol. **15**, 140 (1960).
BATEMAN, J.: The role of Marsilid in patients with far advanced cancer. J. clin. exp. Psychopath. **19**, Suppl. 1, 123 (1958).
BAUDHIN, P., H. BEAUFAY, Y. RAHMAN-LI, O. Z. SELLINGER, R. WATTIAUX, P. JACQUES, and C. DE DUVE: Tissue fractionation studies. 17. Intracellular distribution of monoamine oxidase, aspartate aminotransferase, alanine aminotransferase, D-amino acid oxidase and catalase in rat-liver tissue. Biochem. J. **92**, 179 (1964).
BAUMGARTNER, H.-R., A. STUDER u. K. REBER: Über Methoden zur Erzeugung experimenteller Thrombosen am Kaninchenohr und die Bedeutung von 5-Hydroxytryptamin bei deren Entstehung. Thrombos. Diathes. haemorrh. (Stuttg.) **9**, 485 (1963).
— — — Influence of 5-hydroxytryptamine, 5-hydroxytryptophan, dopamine, noradrenaline and reserpine on the thrombotic deposits in the rabbits. Thrombos. Diathes. haemorrh. (Stuttg.) **12**, 169 (1964).
BAXTER, C. F., and E. ROBERTS: The γ-aminobutyric acid-α-ketoglutaric acid transaminase of beef brain. J. biol. Chem. **233**, 1135 (1958).
BAYLISS, R. I. S., and E. A. HARVEY-SMITH: Methyldopa in the treatment of hypertension. Lancet **1962 I**, 763.
BEACH, V. L., and B. G. STEINETZ: Quantitative measurement of evans blue space in the tissues of the rat: influence of 5-hydroxytryptamine antagonists and phenelzine on experimental inflammation. J. Pharmacol. exp. Ther. **131**, 400 (1961).
BEAVAN, G. H., and J. C. WHITE: Oxidation of phenylhydrazines in the presence of oxyhaemoglobin and the origin of Heinz bodies in erythrocytes. Nature (Lond.) **173**, 389 (1954).
BECKENBRIDGE, B. M., and J. H. NORMAN: Glycogen phosphorylase in brain. J. Neurochem. **9**, 383 (1962).
BEER, A. G.: Beiträge zur Pharmakologie des extrapyramidalen Systems. Naunyn-Schmiedebergs Arch. exp. Path. Pharmak. **193**, 393 (1939).
BEILER, J. M., and G. J. MARTIN: Inhibition of 5-hydroxytryptophan decarboxylase. J. biol. Chem. **211**, 39 (1954).
BELFORD, J., and M. R. FEINLIEB: Phosphorylase activity in heart and brain after reserpine, iproniazid and other drugs affecting the central nervous system. Biochem. Pharmacol. **6**, 189 (1961).
BELLEAU, B., and J. BURBA: The stereochemistry of the enzymic decarboxylation of amino acids. J. Amer. chem. Soc. **82**, 5751 (1960).
— — M. PINDELL, and R. REIFFENSTEIN: Effect of deuterium substitution of sympathomimetic amines on adrenergic amines on adrenergic responses. Science **133**, 102 (1961).
— M. FANG, J. BURBA, and J. MORAN: The absolute optical specificity of monoamine oxidase. J. Amer. Soc. **82**, 5752 (1960).
—, and J. MORAN: The mechanism of action of the 2-phenylcyclopropylamine type of monoamine oxidase inhibitors. J. med. pharm. Chem. **5**, 215 (1962).
— — Deuterium isotope effects in relation to the chemical mechanism of monoamine oxidase. Ann. N.Y. Acad. Sci. **107**, 822 (1963).

BEN, M., M. R. WARREN, V. P. DRINNON, and C. C. SCOTT: Cardiovascular activity of β-phenylethylhydrazine (Phenelzine). Pharmacologist 1, 82 (1959).
— — — — Cardiovascular activity of β-phenylethylhydrazine (Phenelzine). Angiology 11, 62 (1960).
BENSON, W. M., P. L. STEFKO, and M. D. ROE: Pharmacologic and toxicologic observations on hydrazine derivatives of isonicotinic acid (Rimifon, Marsilid). Amer. Rev. Tuberc. 65, 376 (1952).
BERGERET, B., J. LABOUSSE et F. CHATAGNER: Répercussion de la thyroidectomie et d'injections de tyrosine sur l'activité de quelques décarboxylases d'acides aminés chez le rat. Bull. Soc. Chim. biol. (Paris) 40, 1923 (1958).
BERNARDI, R., e G. SIDERI: Isonicotinil-isopropilidrazide ed emocoagulazione. Gazz. med. ital. 119, 91 (1960).
BERNHEIM, F.: Note on the action of copper and phenylhydrazine on certain dehydrogenases. J. biol. Chem. 133, 485 (1940).
— The effect of propamidine on bacterial metabolism. Science 98, 223 (1943).
—, and M. L. C. BERNHEIM: The oxidation of mescaline and certain other amines. J. biol. Chem. 123, 317 (1938).
— — The inactivation of tyramine by heart muscle in vitro. J. biol. Chem. 158, 425 (1945).
BERNHEIM, M. L. C.: Tyramine oxidase. II. The course of the oxidation. J. biol. Chem. 93, 299 (1931).
BERNHEIMER, H., W. BIRKMAYER u. O. HORNYKIEWICZ: Verhalten der Monoaminoxydase im Gehirn des Menschen nach Therapie mit Monoaminoxydase-Hemmern. Wien. klin. Wschr. 74, 558 (1962).
— — — Zur Biochemie des Parkinson-Syndroms des Menschen. Einfluß der Monoaminoxydase-Hemmer-Therapie auf die Konzentration des Dopamins, Noradrenalins und 5-Hydroxytryptamins im Gehirn. Klin. Wschr. 41, 32 (1963).
—, u. O. HORNYKIEWICZ: Das Verhalten einiger Enzyme im Gehirn normaler und Parkinsonkranker Menschen. Naunyn-Schmiedebergs Arch. exp. Path. Pharmak. 243, 295 (1962).
BERNSOHN, J., and I. LOZAITYTE: Effect of iproniazid supplemented with various growthfactors on brain serotonin and monoamine oxidase. Fed. Proc. 17, 189 (1958).
— L. POSSLEY, and J. T. CUSTOD: Alternations in brain adenine nucleotides and creatinine phosphate in vivo after the administration of chlorpromazine, JB-516, Dilantin, and Ro 5-0650 (Librium). Pharmacologist 2, 67 (1960).
BERNSTEIN, J., K. A. LOSEE, C. SMITH, and B. RUBIN: A novel resolution of 1-phenyl-2-propylhydrazin. J. Amer. chem. Soc. 81, 4433 (1959).
BERTACCINI, G.: Tissue 5-hydroxytryptamine and urinary 5-hydroxyindoleacetic acid after partial or total removal of the gastrointestinal tract in the rat. J. Physiol. (Lond.) 153, 239 (1960).
BERTHOLET, A., et D.-M. BERTRAND: Recherches sur la flore intestinale. Isolement d'un microbe capable de produire de la β-imidazoléthylamine aux dépens de l'histidine. C.R. Acad. Sci. (Paris) 154, 1643, 1826 (1912).
BERTLER, Å.: Effect of reserpine on the storage of catecholamines in brain and other tissues. Acta physiol. scand. 51, 75 (1961).
— N.-Å. HILLARP, and E. ROSENGREN: "Bound" and "free" catecholamines in the brain. Acta physiol. scand. 50, 113 (1960).
— — — Effect of reserpine on the storage of new-formed catecholamines in the adrenal medulla. Acta physiol. scand. 52, 44 (1961).
—, and E. ROSENGREN: Occurrence and distribution of catechol amines in brain. Acta physiol. scand. 47, 350 (1959a).
— — On the distribution in brain of monoamines and of enzymes responsible for their formation. Experentia (Basel) 15, 382 (1959b).
BESENDORF, H.: Unpublished results.
—, u. A. PLETSCHER: Beeinflussung zentraler Wirkungen von Reserpin und 5-Hydroxytryptamin durch Isonicotinsäurehydrazide. Helv. physiol. pharmacol. Acta 14, 384 (1956).
BEYER, K. H.: The relation of molecular configuration to the rate of deamination of sympathomimetic amines by aminase. J. Pharmacol. exp. Ther. 79, 85 (1943).
— Sympathomimetic amines: the relation of structure to their action and inactivation. Physiol. Rev. 26, 169 (1946).
— H. BLASCHKO, J. H. BURN, and H. LANGEMANN: Enzymic formation of noradrenaline in mammalian tissue extracts. Nature (Lond.) 165, 926 (1950).
—, and H. S. MORRISON: Relation of structure to deamination of sympathomimetic amines. Industr. Engin. Chem. 37, 143 (1945).
—, and S. H. SHAPIRO: The excretion of conjugated epinephrine related compounds. Amer. J. Physiol. 144, 321 (1945).

BEYER, K. H., and J. T. SKINNER: The detoxication and excretion of beta-phenylisopropylamine (Benzedrin). J. Pharmacol. exp. Ther. 68, 419 (1940).
BHAGVAT, K., H. BLASCHKO, and D. RICHTER: CLXIII. Amine oxidase. Biochem. J. 33, 1338 (1939).
BIANCHI, C., and A. DAVID: Analgesic properties of 4-ethoxycarbonyl-1-(2-hydroxy-3-phenoxypropyl) 4-phenylpiperidine (BDH 200) and some related compounds. J. Pharm. Pharmacol. 12, 449 (1960).
BICKEL, M. H., A. CARPI, and D. BOVET: Action of reserpine and monoamine oxidase inhibitors on the urinary excretion of catecholamines in the rat. Helv. physiol. pharmacol. Acta 19, 279 (1961).
BIEHL, J. P., and R. W. VILTER: Effect of isoniazid on vitamin B_6 metabolism; its possible significance in producing isoniazid neuritis. Proc. Soc. exp. Biol. (N.Y.) 85, 389 (1954).
BIEL, J. H., A. C. CONWAY, F. DI PERO, A. E. DRUKKER, and P. A. NUHFER: Synthesis and physiological properties of the D- and L-isomers of α-methylphenethylhydrazine (JB 515)' a potent monoamine oxidase (MAO) inhibitor. J. Amer. chem. Soc. 81, 4995 (1959a).
— A. E. DRUKKER, T. F. MITCHELL, E. P. SPRENGELER, P. A. NUHFER, A. C. CONWAY, and A. HORITA: Central stimulants. Chemistry and structure — activity relationships of aralkyl hydrazines. J. Amer. chem. Soc. 81, 2805 (1959b).
— —, P. A. SHORE, S. SPECTOR, and B. B. BRODIE: Effect of 1-phenyl-2-hydrazinopropane, a potent monoamine oxidase (MAO) inhibitor, on brain levels of norepinephrine and serotonin. J. Amer. chem. Soc. 80, 1519 (1958).
— A. HORITA, and A. E. DRUKKER: Monoamine oxidase inhibitors (hydrazines). In: Psychopharmacological Agents, vol. 1, edit. M. GORDON, New York: Academic Press Inc. 1964.
— P. A. NUHFER, and A. C. CONWAY: Structure and activity relationships of monoamine oxidase inhibitors. Ann. N.Y. Acad. Sci. 80, 568 (1959c).
— —, A. E. DRUKKER, T. E. MITCHELL, A. C. CONWAY, and A. HORITA: A new class of potent MAO inhibitors. Chemistry and structure-activity relationships of aminoalkylhydrazines. J. org. Chem. 26, 3338 (1961).
BIGNAMI, G.: Action de quelques dérivés inhibiteurs des monoaminooxydases sur le cycle oestral de la ratte normale et traitée par la réserpine. R.C. Acad. Sci. (Paris) 250, 3731 (1960).
— F. BOVET-NITTI, and A. P. CORRADO: Central action of two new monoamine oxidase inhibitors: N-(1,4-benzodioxan-2-yl)-methylhydrazine (2520 I.S.) and N-(1,4-benzodioxan-2-yl)-methyl-N-benzyl-hydrazine (2596 I.S.). Sci. Rep. Ist. Super. Sanità 2, 170 (1962).
BILLERVICZ-STANKIEWICZ, J., Z. SZCZEKALA u. W. TYBURCZYK: Beeinflussung der „Adrenalin-Oxydasen" des Blutplasma in vivo durch biogene Monoamine und Neuropharmaca. Experientia (Basel) 20, 85 (1964).
BING, R. J.: Amine oxidase inhibitors: discussion remarks. Ann. N.Y. Acad. Sci. 80, 1030 (1959).
BIRKHÄUSER, H.: Fermente im Gehirn geistig normaler Menschen. (Cholin-esterase, Mono- und Diamin-oxydase, Cholin-oxydase). Helv. chim. Acta 23, 1071 (1940).
— Cholinesterase und Mono-Aminoxydase im zentralen Nervensystem. Schweiz. med. Wschr. 71, 750 (1941).
BIRT, A. R., P. HAGEN, and E. ZEBROWSKI: Amino acid decarboxylase of urticaria pigmentose mast cells. J. invest. Derm. 37, 273 (1961).
BLACK, J. W., E. W. FISCHER, and A. N. SMITH: The effect of 5-hydroxytryptamin on gastric secretion in anaesthetized dogs. J. Physiol. (Lond.) 141, 27 (1958).
BLACKMAN, J. G., D. S. CAMPION, and E. N. FASTIER: Mechanism of action of reserpine in producing gastric haemorrhage and erosion in the mouse. Brit. J. Pharmacol. 14, 112 (1959).
BLACKWELL, B.: Hypertensive crisis due to monoamine-oxidase inhibitors. Lancet 1963 II, 849.
—, and E. MARLEY: Interaction between cheese and monoamine-oxidase inhibitors in rats and cats. Lancet 1964 I, 530.
BLANKSMA, L. A.: Substrate and inhibitor patterns of monoamine oxidase. Diss. Northwestern Univ. Chicago 1962 [Diss. Abstr. 23, 3103 (1963)].
BLASCHKO, H.: CCLXXIII. The mechanism of catalase inhibitions. Biochem. J. 29, 2302 (1935).
— Amine oxidase and ephedrine. J. Physiol. (Lond.) 93, 7P (1938).
— The specific action of 1-dopa decarboxylase. J. Physiol. (Lond.) 96, 50P (1939).
— Amine oxidase and benzedrine. Nature (Lond.) 145, 26 (1940).
— The activity of 1(—)-DOPA decarboxylase. J. Physiol. (Lond.) 101, 337 (1942).
— The amino acid decarboxylase of mammalian tissue. Advanc. Enzymol. 5, 72 (1945).

BLASCHKO, H.: Substrate specificity of amino-acid decarboxylases. Biochim. biophys. Acta (Amst.) **4**, 130 (1950).
— Amine oxidase and amine metabolism. Pharmacol. Rev. **4**, 415 (1952).
— Remarks on the location of histamine in mammalian tissues. CIBA Foundation, Symposium on Histamine, p. 375. London: J. & A. Churchill Ltd.
— Biological inactivation of 5-hydroxytryptamine. In: 5-Hydroxytryptamine, p. 50, edit. G. P. LEWIS. London: Pergamon Press Ltd. 1958.
— The role of dopa-decarboxylase in the formation of catecholamines. The Second Hahnemann Symposium on Hypertensive Disease, p. 330. Philadelphia: Lea & Febiger 1961.
— The amine oxidases of mammalian blood plasma. Advanc. comp. Physiol. Biochem. **1**, 67 (1962).
— Amine oxidase. In: The Enzymes, vol. 8, p. 337, edit. P. D. BOYER, H. LARDY and K. MYRBÄCK. New York and London: Academic Press Inc. 1963.
— J. H. BURN, and C. W. CARTER: L-dopa decarboxylase and pressor amine formation in the adrenal medulla. J. Physiol. (Lond.) **115**, 37P (1951).
— C. W. CARTER, J. R. P. O'BRIEN, and G. H. SLOANE STANLEY: Pyridoxin in relation to amine formation in the mammalian liver. J. Physiol. (Lond.) **107**, 18P (1948).
—, and T. L. CHRUŚCIEL: Observations on the substrate specificity of amine oxidases. Brit. J. Pharmacol. **14**, 364 (1959).
— — The decarboxylation of amino acids related to tyrosine and their awakening action in reserpine-treated mice. J. Physiol. (Lond.) **151**, 272 (1960).
—, and R. DUTHIE: The inhibition of amine oxidase by amidines. Biochem. J. **39**, 347 (1945a).
— — Substrate specificity of amine oxidases. Biochem. J. **39**, 478 (1945b).
— P. J. FRIEDMAN, R. HAWES, and K. NILSSON: The amine oxidase of mammalian plasma. J. Physiol. (Lond.) **145**, 384 (1959).
— P. HAGEN, and A. D. WELCH: Observations on the intracellular granules of the adrenal medulla. J. Physiol. (Lond.) **129**, 27 (1955).
—, and J. HAWKINS: Enzymic oxidation of aliphatic diamines. Brit. J. Pharmacol. **5**, 625 (1950).
—, and K. HELLMANN: Pigment formation from tryptamin and 4-hydroxytryptamin in tissues: a contribution to the histochemistry of amine oxidase. J. Physiol. (Lond.) **122**, 419 (1953).
—, and J. M. HIMMS: The inhibition of amine oxidase and spermin oxidase by amidines. Brit. J. Pharmacol. **10**, 451 (1955).
—, and P. HOLTON: Enzymic formation of other tyramine (O-hydroxyethylamine). J. Physiol. (Lond.) **110**, 482 (1950).
— — and G. H. SLOANE-STANLEY: Enzymic formation of pressor amines. J. Physiol. (Lond.) **108**, 427 (1949).
—, and F. J. PHILPOT: Enzymic oxidation of tryptamin derivatives. J. Physiol. (Lond.) **122**, 403 (1953).
—, and P. PRATESI: Specificity of amine oxidase for optically active substrates and inhibitors. Brit. J. Pharmacol. **14**, 256 (1959).
— D. RICHTER, and H. SCHLOSSMANN: CCLXVIII. The oxidation of adrenaline and other amines. Biochem. J. **31**, 2187 (1937a).
— — — The inactivation of adrenaline. J. Physiol. (Lond.) **90**, 1 (1937b).
— — — Enzymic oxidation of amines. J. Physiol. (Lond.) **91**, 13P (1937c).
—, and B. C. R. STRÖMBLAD: The inhibition of human amine oxidase by the two isomers of amphetamine. Arzneimittel-Forsch. **10**, 327 (1960).
BLOCH, W., u. H. PINÖSCH: Die Umwandlung von Histidin in Histamin im tierischen Organismus. Hoppe-Seylers Z. physiol. Chem. **239**, 236 (1936).
BLOCK, W.: Der Einbau von Barbituraten und Thiobarbituraten in Proteine. Arzneimittel-Forsch. **11**, 122 (1961).
BLOOM, B. M.: Some structural considerations regarding compounds that influence monoamine oxidase. Ann. N.Y. Acad. Sci. **107**, 878 (1963).
BLUM, S. W., B. DUBNICK, and J. M. APGAR: Distribution and metabolism of modaline (2-methyl-3-piperidino-pyrazine, W 3207). Fed. Proc. **23**, 490 (1964).
BLUMBERG, A., U. C. DUBACH, W. KREIS u. H. R. MÜLLER: Klinische und biochemische Untersuchungen beim Carcinoidsyndrom. Dtsch. med. Wschr. **87**, 921 (1962).
BOER, B. DE, O. ENGELSTADT, and D. GRAY: Inhibition of morphine hyperglycemia. Fed. Proc. **18**, 382 (1959).
BOGDANSKI, D. F., A. PLETSCHER, B. B. BRODIE, and S. UDENFRIEND: Identification and assay of serotonin in brain. J. Pharmacol. exp. Ther. **117**, 82 (1956).
— H. WEISSBACH, and S. UDENFRIEND: The distribution of serotonin, 5-hydroxytryptophan decarboxylase and monoamine oxidase in brain. J. Neurochem. **1**, 272 (1957).

BONATI, F.: Confronto degli stereoisomeri della cicloserina quali detossicanti della isoniazide. Boll. Soc. ital. Biol. sper. **34**, 956 (1958).
BONAVITA, U.: Purification and properties of glutamic-oxaloeacetic transaminase from human brain. J. Neurochem. **4**, 275 (1959).
BONFILS, S., M. DUBRASQUET et A. LAMBLING: Les utilisations de la technique de l'ulcère de contrainte du rat blanc comme test pharmacodynamique. Thérapie **15**, 1096 (1960).
BONNYCASTLE, D. D., N. J. GIARMAN, and M. K. PAASONEN: Anticonvulsant compounds and 5-hydroxytryptamine in rat brain. Brit. J. Pharmacol. **12**, 228 (1957).
BORN, G. V. R., G. I. C. INGRAM, and R. S. STACEY: The relationship between 5-hydroxytryptamine and adenosine triphosphate in blood platelets. Brit. J. Pharmacol. **13**, 62 (1958).
BOROWITZ, J. L., and W. C. NORTH: Iproniazid on the toxicity of epinephrine, norepinephrine and serotonin. Fed. Proc. **18**, 370 (1959a).
— — Potentiation of epinephrine and norepinephrine by iproniazid. Science **130**, 710 (1959b).
BOSE, B. C., and R. VIJAYVARGYA: Observations on the mechanism of action of tranquilisers — a study of their effect on monoamine oxidase, D- and L-amino acid oxidase and catalase. J. Pharm. Pharmacol. **12**, 99 (1960).
BOTROS, M., D. LINDSAY, E. POULSON, and J. M. ROBSON: Mode of action of 5-HT and iproniazid on pregnancy. Biochem. Pharmacol. **8**, 102 (1961).
—, and J. M. ROBSON: The effects of 5-hydroxytryptamine and iproniazid on sexual development. J. Endocr. **20**, X (1960).
BOULLIN, D. J.: Behaviour of rats depleted of 5-hydroxytryptamine by feeding a diet free of tryptophan. Psychopharmacologia (Berl.) **5**, 28 (1963).
BOVET-NITTI, F., et G. BIGNAMI: Action de quelques dérivés du 2-amino-méthyl-benzodioxan sur l'équilibre hormonal du cycle, de la pseudo grossesse et de la grossesse chez la ratte. Biochem. Pharmacol. **8**, 3 (1961).
— O. ORSINGER, R. LANDI-VITTORY et D. BOVET: Pharmacologie. Un nouvel inhibiteur des monoamino oxydases: le N'-(1,4-benzodioxan-2-méthyl)-N'-benzyl-hydrazine (2596 IS). C.R. Acad. Sci. (Paris) **252**, 614 (1961).
BOYLEN, J. B., and J. H. QUASTEL: Effects of L-phenylalanine and sodium phenylpyruvate on the formation of adrenaline from L-tyrosine in adrenal medulla in vitro. Biochem. J. **80**, 644 (1961).
BRENK, H. A. S., VAN DEN, and K. ELLIOTT: Radioprotective action of 5-hydroxytryptamine. Nature (Lond.) **182**, 1506 (1958).
BREST, A. N., G. ONESTI, and J. H. MOYER: Alpha-methyl dopa in the treatment of hypertension. Circulation **24**, 892 (1961).
BRIMBLECOMBE, R. W., and A. L. GREEN: Effect of monoamine oxidase inhibitors on the behaviour of rats in Hall's Open Field. Nature (Lond.) **194**, 983 (1962).
BRODIE, B. B., and M. A. BEAVEN: Neurochemical transducer systems. Med. exp. **8**, 320 (1963).
—, and E. COSTA: Role of norepinephrine in autonomic ganglia in regulation of blood pressure. The Second Hahnemann Symposium on Hypertensive Disease, p. 354. Philadelphia: Lea & Febiger 1961.
— G. L. GESSA, and E. COSTA: Association between reserpine syndrome and blockade of brain serotonin storage processes. Life Sci. **1962**a, 551.
— J. R. GILETTE, and B. N. LA DU: Enzymatic metabolism of drugs and other foreign compounds. Ann. Rev. Biochem. **27**, 427 (1958a).
— R. KUNTZMAN, C. W. HIRSCH, and E. COSTA: Effects of decarboxylase inhibition on the biosynthesis of brain monoamines. Life Sci. **1962**b, 81.
— A. PLETSCHER. and P. A. SHORE: Possible role of serotonin in brain function and in reserpine action. J. Pharmacol. exp. Ther. **116**, 9 (1956).
—, and P. A. SHORE: A concept for a role of serotonin and norepinephrine as chemical mediators in the brain. Ann. N.Y. Acad. Sci. **66**, 631 (1957).
— S. SPECTOR, R. KUNTZMAN, and P. A. SHORE: Rapid biosynthesis of brain serotonin before and after reserpine administration. Naturwissenschaften **45**, 243 (1958b).
— — and P. A. SHORE: Interaction of monoamine oxidase inhibitors with physiological and biochemical mechanism in brain. Ann. N.Y. Acad. Sci. **80**, 609 (1959a).
— — — Interaction of drugs with norepinephrine in the brain. Pharmacol. Rev. **11**, 548 (1959b).
— E. G. TOMICH, R. KUNTZMAN, and P. A. SHORE: On the mechanism of action of reserpine: effect of reserpine on capacity of tissues to bind serotonin. J. Pharmacol. exp. Ther. **119**, 461 (1957).
BRODY, M., and F. GOETZ: Studies on the gastrointestinal effects of Marsilid. J. clin. exp. Psychopath. **19**, Suppl. 1, 146 (1958).
BROWN, B. B.: DNS drug actions and interaction in mice. Arch. int. Pharmacodyn. **128**, 391 (1960).

Brown, B. G., and P. Hey: Substituted choline aryl ethers as inhibitors of amine oxidase. J. Physiol. (Lond.) **118**, 15P (1952).
— — Choline phenyl ethers as inhibitors of amine oxidase. Brit. J. Pharmacol. **11**, 58 (1956).
Brown, L.: Esperimenti sulla trasmissione adrenergica. Boll. Soc. ital. Biol. sper. **34**, 1979 (1958).
Brubacher, G. B., and O. Wiss: Unpublished results.
Brune, G. G., and H. E. Himwich: Biphasic action of reserpine and isocarboxazid on behavior and serotonin metabolism. Science **133**, 190 (1961).
Brusova, L. V., V. Z. Gorkin, D. K. Zhelyazkov, N. A. Kitrosskii, G. A. Leont'eva, and I. S. Severina: New spectrometric method for the estimation of monoamine oxidase activity in rat liver homogenates. Vop. med. Khim. **10**, 83 (1963) [Chem. Abstr. **60**, 13509f. (1964)].
Buchel, L., et J. Lévy: Contribution à l'étude des effets sur le système nerveux central de l'hydrazino-2-phényl-3-propane (PIH) comparés à ceux de la 1-isonicotinyl-2-isopropylhydrazine (iproniazide). I. Influence sur le sommeil expérimental. Anesth. et Analg. **17**, 289 (1960a).
— — Contribution à l'étude des effets sur le système nerveux centıal des inhibiteurs de la monoaminoxydase, hydrazino-2-phényl-3-propane (PIH), isopropyl-hydrazide de l'acide isonicotinique (iproniazide). II. Influence sur la potentialisation du sommeil expérimental par la réserpine. Anesth. et Analg. **17**, 313 (1960b).
— — Contribution à l'étude des effets sur le système nerveux central de l'hydrazino-2-phényl-3-propane (PIH), comparés à ceux de la 1-isonicotinyl-2-isopropylhydrazide (iproniazide). III. Action anticonvulsivante. Anesth. et Analg. **17**, 329 1960c).
— — et N. Mathieu: Contribution à l'étude des effets sur le système nerveux de l'hydrazino-2-phényl-3-propane (PIH) comparés à ceux de la 1-isonicotinyl-2-isopropylhydrazide (iproniazide). IV. Influence sur l'analgésie provoquée par la 1-méthadone. Anesth. et Analg. **17**, 339 (1960a).
— — et O. Tanguy: Influence de la sérotonine et du d,l 5-hydroxy-tryptophane sur le sommeil expérimental en présence ou non d'iproniazide. Agressologie **1**, 389 (1960b).
—, et J. Sturtz-Moury: Prolongation et renforcement de la narcose sous l'influence d'esters-amines et de leurs iodométhylates dérivés de l'acide 1-bicyclohexyl-1-carboxylique. Anesth. et Analg. **14**, 921 (1957).
Buckley, J. P., A. R. Furgiuele, and W. J. Kinnard: The pharmacology of β-phenylisopropylhydrazine. Fed. Proc. **19**, 278 (1960).
Buffoni, F., and H. Blaschko: Benzylamine oxidase and histaminase: studies of a crystalline preparation of the amine oxidase of pig plasma. Biochem. J. **89**, 111 (1963).
Bülbring, E., F. J. Philpot, and F. Basanquet: Amine oxidase, pressor amines and cholinesterase in brain tumours. Lancet **1953 I**, 865.
Buhs, R. P., J. L. Beck, O. C. Speth, J. L. Smith, N. R. Trenner, P. J. Cannon, and J. H. Laragh: The metabolism of methyldopa in hypertensive human subjects. J. Pharmacol. exp. Ther. **143**, 205 (1964).
Burford, H., J. Leick, and E. J. Walaszek: Modification of the effects of biogenic amines on the heart by iproniazid. Arch. int. Pharmacodyn. **128**, 39 (1960).
—, and E. J. Walaszek: Modification of the pressor effects of tyramine and tryptamine by iproniazid and reserpine. Fed. Proc. **19**, 124 (1960).
Burger, A., C. S. Davis, H. Green, D. H. Tedeschi, and C. L. Zirkle: 1-Methyl-2-phenylcyclopropylamine. J. med. pharm. Chem. **4**, 571 (1961).
Burger, M., u. H. Langemann: Bestimmungen von Adrenalin und Noradrenalin sowie von Decarboxylase- und Aminoxydase-Aktivitäten in Zellfraktionen von Phäochromocytomen. Klin. Wschr. **34**, 941 (1956).
Burkard, W. P.: Unpublished results.
— K. F. Gey, and A. Pletscher: Inhibition of diamine oxidase in vivo by hydrazine derivatives. Biochem. Pharmacol. **3**, 249 (1960).
— — — Differentiation of monoamine oxidase and diamine oxidase. Biochem. Pharmacol. **11**, 177 (1962a).
— — — A new inhibitor of decarboxylase of aromatic amino acids. Experientia (Basel) **18**, 411 (1962b).
— — — Diamine oxidase in the brain of vertebrates. J. Neurochem. **10**, 183 (1963).
— — — Inhibition of the hydroxylation of tryptophan and phenylalanine by α-methyl-dopa and similar compounds. Life Sci. **3**, 27 (1964a).
— — — Hemmung der Tryptophan-Hydroxylase durch α-Methyl-dopa. Helv. physiol. pharmacol. Acta **22**, C 7 (1964b).
— — — Inhibition of decarboxylase of aromatic amino acids by 2,3,4-trihydroxybenzylhydrazine and its seryl derivative. Arch. Biochem. **107**, 187 (1964c).
— R. Pavlin, A. Pletscher and K. F. Gey: Effect of psychotropic drugs on decarboxylase of aromatic amino acids in rat brain. Int. J. Neuropharmacol. **1**, 233 (1962c).

BURKHALTER, A.: Histamine formation by fetal rat liver. Fed. Proc. **20**, 257 (1961).
— The formation of histamine by fetal rat liver. Biochem. Pharmacol. **11**, 315 (1962).
— V. H. COHN, and P. A. SHORE: Studies on histamine in mammalian organs. Fed. Proc. **18**, 373 (1959).
BURN, J. H., F. J. PHILPOT, and U. TRENDELENBURG: Effect of denervation on enzymes in iris and blood vessels. Brit. J. Pharmacol. **9**, 423 (1954).
—, and M. J. RAND: Noradrenaline in artery walls and its dispersal by reserpine. Brit. med. J. **1958a I**, 903.
— — The action of sympathomimetic amines in animals treated with reserpine. J. Physiol. (Lond.) **144**, 314 (1958b).
—, and J. ROBINSON: Effect of denervation on amine oxidase in structures innervated by the sympathetic. Brit. J. Pharmacol. **7**, 304 (1952).
BURTON, R. M.: In: E. ROBERT et al.: Inhibition of the nervous system and GABA, p. 253. New York: Pergamon Press 1960.
BUXTON, J., and H. M. SINCLAIR: Pyridoxal phosphate as a coenzyme of 5-hydroxytrytophan decarboxylase. Biochem. J. **62**, 27P (1956).
BUZARD, J. A., and P. D. NYTCH: Some characteristics of rat kidney 5-hydroxytryptophan decarboxylase. J. biol. Chem. **227**, 265 (1957).
— — The effect of norepinephrine on the 5-hydroxytryptophan decarboxylase activity of rat kidney. J. biol. Chem. **234**, 884 (1959).
BYGDEMAN, M., and L. STJÄRNE: Effects of 1,4-dihydrazinophthalazine on organ content and adrenal medullary secretion of catechol amines. Nature (Lond.) **184**, 1646 (1959).
CAHN, J.: L'action du Marsilid et du Marplan sur le métabolisme cérébrale. In: Neuropsychopharmacology, vol. **2**, p. 450, edit. E. ROTHLIN. Amsterdam: Elsevier Publ. Co. 1961.
—, et M. HÉROLD: Effets cardio-vasculaires comparés des inhibiteurs de la mono-amine-oxydase: Effets pharmacologiques — Action sur la dynamique et le métabolisme cardiaque. Agressologie **1**, 579 (1960a).
— — Recherches préliminaires sur les effets pharmacologiques et biochimiques des inhibiteurs de la monoamine-oxydase sur le coeur. Cardiologia (Basel) **37**, Suppl. 2, 52 (1960b),
— — Etude pharmacologique du Ro 1—9569 (Tétrabenazine). Psychiat. et Neurol. (Basel) **140**, 210 (1960c).
— — Effets cardio-vasculaires comparés des inhibiteurs de la mono-amine-oxydase. Effets pharmacologiques. Action sur la dynamique et le métabolisme cardiaque. Chemotherapie **4**, 262 (1962).
— — J. ALANO, N. BARRE, P. ESPAGNOL, E. GAUTHIER, C. HELBECQUE, O. KABACOFF, G. MATHIAS et O. MATHIAS: Un nouvel inhibiteur de la MAO: l'isopropyl-hydrazide de l'acide 4-hydroxybutyrique (PC 614). Agressologie **2**, 687 (1961a).
— — N. BARRE, O. KABACOFF, and I. BAMBERGER: Mode of action of inhibitors of monoamine oxidase on the cardio-vascular system. Relationship to chemical structure. Biochem. Pharmacol. 8, 134 (1961b).
— — C. HELBECQUE, T. LASJAUMIAS et A.-M. JUILLARD: Effets comparés de différents inhibiteurs de la L-dopa décarboxylase chez le rat et la souris. C. R. Soc. Biol. (Paris) **156**, 1094 (1962a).
— — et O. MATHIAS: Effets de différents inhibiteurs de la L-dopa décarboxylase sur le système cardiovasculaire chez le lapin. C. R. Soc. Biol. (Paris) **156**, 1090 (1962b).
CAMANNI, F., O. LOSANA, G. M. MOLINATTI et M. OLIVETTI: Effet de la réserpine sur le contenu en catécholamines de la médullaire surrénale du rat, après administration d'iproniazide ou dénervation de la glande. Arch. int. Pharmacodyn. **123**, 430 (1960).
CANAL, N., and S. GARATTINI: Isonicotinylhydrazide, hepatic respiratory quotient and inhibition of some enzymatic systems with pyridoxal coenzyme. Arzneimittel-Forsch. **7**, 158 (1957).
—, e A. MAFFEI-FACCIOLI: Variazioni della triptofanoperossidasi-ossidase (TPO) epatica indotta da alcuni farmaci. Distribuzione della triptofano-perossidasi-ossidase (TPO) in alcune specie animali. Boll. Soc. ital. Biol. sper. **35**, 302 (1959a).
— — Reversal of the reserpine-induced depletion of brain serotonin by a monoamine oxidase inhibitor. J. Neurochem. **5**, 99 (1959b).
— — The in vitro and in vivo inhibitory action of isonicotinic acid hydrazide on 5-hydroxytryptophan decarboxylase. Rev. esp. Fisiol. **16**, Suppl. 2, 234 (1960). [Chem. Abstr. **55**, 4755 (1961)].
— — e B. MANZINI: Su alcune nuove sostanze bloccanti le monoamino-ossidasi. Boll. Soc. ital. Biol. sper. **34**, 1525 (1958).
— — e T. SCAMAZZO: Sulla varietà di effetti biochimici e farmacologici osservabili in seguito ad inibizione della monoaminossidasi (MO). Boll. Soc. ital. Biol. sper. **35**, 436 (1959).
— G. GIULIANI, A. MAFFEI-FACCIOLI, and T. SCAMAZZO: On the mechanism of the adrenal cortex stimulation by reserpine. Biochem. Pharmacol. 8, 130 (1961).

CANNON, P. J., R. T. WHITLOCK, R. C. MORRIS, M. ANGERS, and J. H. LARAGH: Effect of alpha-methyl dopa in severe and malignant hypertension. J. Amer. med. Ass. **179**, 673 (1962).

CARBON, J. A., W. P. BURKARD u. E. A. ZELLER: Über die Wirkungen von symmetrischen 1,2-Dialkyl-hydrazinen auf Cargonylverbindungen und Amin-oxydasen. Helv. chim. Acta **41**, 1883 (1958).

CARDOT, J.: Décarboxylation in vitro du 5-hydroxytryptophane par le tissue nerveux du Mollusque Gastéropode Helix pomatia. C. R. Acad. Sci. (Paris) **256**, 1036 (1963).

CARISSIMI, M.: Su alcuni nuovi derivati dell'iproniazide. Farmaco, Ed. sci. **13**, 817 (1958).

CARLSSON, A.: The occurrence, distribution and physiological role of catecholamines in the nervous system. Pharmacol. Rev. **11**, 490 (1959).

— Discussion remark. In: Adrenergic Mechanisms, p. 558, edit. J. R. VANE, G. E. W. WOLSTENHOLME and M. O'CONNOR. London: J. & A. Churchill Ltd. 1960.

— Brain monoamines and psychotropic drugs. In: Neuropsychopharmacology, vol. 2, p. 417, edit. E. ROTHLIN. Amsterdam: Elsevier Publ. Co. 1961.

— Functional significance of drug-induced changes in brain monoamine levels. In: Progress in Brain Research, vol. 8, p. 9, edit. H. E. HIMWICH and W. A. HIMWICH. Amsterdam: Elsevier Publishing Co. 1964.

— H. CORRODI u. B. WALDECK: α-Substituierte Dopacetamide als Hemmer der Catechol-O-methyl-transferase und der enzymatischen Hydroxylierung aromatischer Aminosäuren. In den Catecholamin-Metabolismus eingreifende Substanzen. Helv. chim. Acta **46**, 2271 (1963).

—, and N.-Å. HILLARP: Formation of phenolic acids in brain after administration of 3,4-dihydroxyphenylalanine. Acta physiol. scand. **55**, 95 (1962).

—, and M. LINDQVIST: In vivo decarboxylation of α-methyldopa and α-methylmetatyrosine. Acta physiol. scand. **54**, 87 (1962).

— — and T. MAGNUSSON: 3,4-Dihydroxyphenylalanine and 5-hydroxytryptophan as reserpine antagonists. Nature (Lond.) **180**, 1200 (1957a).

— — — The effect of monoamine oxidase inhibitors on the metabolism of the brain catecholamines. Simpésio internacional sobre Nialamida, Lisboa. J. Soc. Ciénc. méd. Lisboa **123**, Suppl., 96 (1959a).

— — — and B. WALDECK: On the presence of 3-hydroxytyramine in brain. Science **127**, 471 (1958).

— E. B. RASMUSSEN, and P. KRISTJANSEN: The urinary excretion of adrenaline and noradrenaline by depressive patients during iproniazid treatment. J. Neurochem. **4**, 321 (1959b).

— E. ROSENGREN, Å. BERTLER, and J. NILSSON: Effect of reserpine on the metabolism of catecholamines. In: Psychotropic Drugs, p. 363. Amsterdam: Elsevier Publ. Co. (1957b).

—, and B. WALDECK: On the role of the liver catechol-O-methyl transferase in the metabolism of circulating catecholamines. Acta pharmacol. (Kbh.) **20**, 47 (1963).

CARRIER, R. N., and P. V. BUDAY: The influence of thyroid feeding on the pharmacologic actions of some monoamine oxidase inhibitors. Arch. int. Pharmacodyn. **145**, 18 (1963).

CESARMAN, T.: Serendipitia y angina de pecho. Informe preliminare sobre un hallazgo terapeutico. Arch. Inst. Cardiol. Mex. **27**, 563 (1957).

CHADWICK, B. T., and J. H. WILKINSON: Some aspects of the metabolism of 5-hydroxytryptamine. Biochem. J. **76**, 102 (1960).

CHALMERS, J. G.: The metabolism of isoniazid in rats and mice. Biochem. J. **84**, 56P (1962).

CHATAGNER, F., B BERGERET et J. LABOUESSE: Influence d'hormones ovariennes et thyroidiennes sur deux décarboxylases d'acides aminés dans le foie du rat. Mise en évidence de l'existence de deux régulations indépendantes. Biochim. biophys. Acta (Amst.) **35**, 231 (1959).

— — and J. LABOUESSE-MERCOUROFF: Comparison of the behavior of two amino acid decarboxylases of rat liver under the influence of injections of hypoxine and under the influence of a deficiency of pyridoxine. Rev. esp. Fisiol. **16**, Suppl. 2, 225 (1960). [Chem. Abstr. **55**, 4674 (1961).]

CHEN, G., and B. BOHNER: A comparison of the anti-reserpine effects of certain centrally acting agents. Fed. Proc. **18**, 376 (1959).

— — The anti-reserpine effects of certain centrally acting agents. J. Pharmacol. exp. Ther. **131**, 179 (1961).

— C. R. ENSOR, and B. BOHNER: A facilitation action of reserpine on the central nervous system. Proc. Soc. exp. Biol. (N. Y.) **86**, 507 (1954).

CHEN, K. K., C. K. WU, and E. HENRIKSEN: Relationship between the pharmacological action and the chemical constitution and configuration of the optical isomers of ephedrine and related compounds. J. Pharmacol. exp. Ther. **36**, 363 (1929).

CHERNOV, G. A., and L. M. MOROZOVSKAYA: Mechanism of disturbed formation of serotonin during acute radiation sickness. Med. Radiol. **6**, 59 (1961) [Chem. Abstr. **57**, 13206 (1962)].

CHESSIN, M., B. DUBNICK, E. R. KRAMER, and C. C. SCOTT: Modification of pharmacology of reserpine and serotonin by iproniazid. Fed. Proc. **15**, 409 (1956).
— — G. LEESON, and C. C. SCOTT: Biochemical and pharmacological studies of β-phenylethylhydrazine and selected related compounds. Ann. N. Y. Acad. Sci. **80**, 597 (1959).
— E. R. KRAMER, and C. C. SCOTT: Modifications of the pharmacology of reserpine and serotonin by iproniazid. J. Pharmacol. exp. Ther. **119**, 453 (1957).
CHIDSEY, C. A., and D. C. HARRISON: Studies on the distribution of exogenous norepinephrine in the sympathetic neurotransmitter store. J. Pharmacol. exper. Ther. **140**, 217 (1963).
CHODERA, A., V. Z. GORKIN u. L. I. GRIDNIEVA: Über den Wirkungsmechanismus einiger Monoaminoxydase-Hemmer. Acta biol. med. germ. **13**, 101 (1964).
CHOW, M.-I., and C. D. HENDLEY: Effect of monoamine oxidase inhibitors on experimental convulsions. Fed. Proc. **18**, 376 (1959).
CHRUŚCIEL, T. L.: Sympatholytic drugs and the dopa awakening effect. Lancet **1961 I**, 676.
— Sympatholytic drugs and some enzymes involved in the metabolism of catecholamines. Int. J. Neuropharmacol. **1**, 137 (1962).
CLARK, C. T., H. WEISSBACH, and S. UDENFRIEND: 5-Hydroxytryptophan decarboxylase: preparation and properties. J. biol. Chem. **210**, 139 (1954).
CLARK, W. G.: Studies on inhibition of L-dopa decarboxylase in vitro and in vivo. Pharmacol. Rev. **11**, 330 (1959).
— Amine content and biosynthesis in mastocytomas and octopus salivary glands. Fed. Proc. **19**, 9 (1960).
— Personal communications 1962.
— Inhibition of amino acid decarboxylase. In: Metabolic Inhibitors, vol. **1**, p. 315, edit. R. M. HOCHSTER and J. H. QUASTEL. London and New York: Academic Press 1963.
—, and R. S. POGRUND: Inhibition of dopa-decarboxylase in vitro and in vivo. Circulat. Res. **9**, 721 (1961).
— — R. I. AKAWIE, W. DRELL, and W. J. HARTMANN: Inhibition of 3,4-dihydroxyphenylalanine (DOPA) decarboxylation in vivo. Abstr. Comm. XX. Int. Physiol. Congr., Brussels 1955, p. 179.
CLEGG, R. E., and R. R. SEALOCK: The metabolism of dihydroxyphenylalanine by guinea pig kidney extracts. J. biol. Chem. **179**, 1037 (1949).
COEN, E. D., and R. W. WHITEHEAD: Certain MAO inhibitors as protectors of total body X-irradiation of mice. Fed. Proc. **21**, 423 (1962).
COHEN, P. P.: Transamination in pigeon breast muscle. Biochem. J. **33**, 1478 (1939).
COHEN, R. A., W. F. BRIDGERS, J. AXELROD, H. WEIL-MALHERBE, E. H. LABROSSE, W. E. BUNNEY jr., P. V. CARDON jr., and S. S. KETY: The metabolism of the catecholamines (clinical implications). Clinical Staff Conference. Ann. intern. Med. **56**, 960 (1962).
COHEN, S. G., and T. M. SAPP: Serotonin- and histamine-affecting agents and experimental vascular sensitization. J. Allergy **31**, 248 (1960).
COHN, V. H., and P. A. SHORE: Effect of monoamine oxidase inhibitors on diamine oxidase (histaminase). Fed. Proc. **19**, 283 (1960).
CONDOURIS, G. A.: Depressant action of JB-516 (Catron) on peripheral nerve. Pharmacologist **1**, 81 (1959).
— Block of nerve conduction by MAO inhibitors. Pharmacologist **4**, 175 (1962).
CONWAY, E. J.: Microdiffusion Analysis and Volumetric Error. London: Lockwood & Son Ltd. 1957.
COOPER, A. J., and K. M. G. KEDDIE: Hypotensive collapse and hypoglycemia after Mebamazine — a monoamine oxidase inhibitor. Lancet **1964 I**, 1133.
— R. V. MAGNUS, and M. J. ROSE: A hypertensive syndrome with tranylcypromine medication. Lancet **1964 I**, 527.
COOPER, J. R., J. AXELROD, and B. B. BRODIE: Inhibitory effects of β-dietylaminoethyl diphenylpropylacetate on a variety of drug metabolic pathways in vitro. J. Pharmacol. exp. Ther. **112**, 55 (1954).
COQ, M. H., et C. BARON: Solubilisation de la monoamineoxydase des mitochondries de foie de rat. Experientia (Basel) **20**, 374 (1964).
CORIANDOLI, E. M., R. BOLDRINI, and C. CITTERIO: Different effects exerted by isoniazid upon the coenzyme A and pyridoxine contents of the host's tumour and tissues. Biochem. Pharmacol. **1**, 238 (1959).
CORNE, S. J.: The effect of inhibition of amine oxidase on the excretion of administered adrenaline and noradrenaline in cats. J. Physiol. (Lond.) **133**, 13P (1956).
—, and J. D. P. GRAHAM: The effect of inhibition of amine oxidase in vivo on administered adrenaline, noradrenaline, tyramine and serotonin. J. Physiol. (Lond.) **135**, 339 (1957).
COSTA, E.: In vivo inhibition of monoamineoxidase by 2-phenylcyclopropylamine (SKF 385). Pharmacologist **1**, 82 (1959).

COSTA, E., and B. B. BRODIE: The effect of drugs on storage and release of serotonin and catecholamines in brain. Biochem. Pharmacol. 8, 81 (1961a).
— — A role for norepinephrine in ganglionic transmission. J. Amer. Geriat. Soc. **9**, 419 (1961b).
— G. L. GESSA, C. HIRSCH, R. KUNTZMAN, and B. B. BRODIE: On current status of serotonin as a brain neurohormone and in action of reserpinelike drugs. Ann. N.Y. Acad. Sci. **96**, 118 (1962).
— W. A. HIMWICH, and H. E. HIMWICH: 5-HT content of brain structures of dogs given 5-HTP (5-hydroxytryptophan) compared with the degree of behavioral and neurological changes. In: Neuropsychopharmacology, vol. **2**, p. 475, edit. E. ROTHLIN. Amsterdam: Elsevier Publ. Co. 1961a.
—, and G. R. PSCHEIDT: Reserpine ptosis is unrelated to brain catecholamine levels. Fed. Proc. **19**, 279 (1960).
— — Correlations between active eyelid closure and depletion of brain biogenic amines by reserpine. Proc. Soc. exp. Biol. (N.Y.) **106**, 693 (1961).
— — W. G. VAN METER, and H. E. HIMWICH: Brain concentrations of biogenic amines and EEG patterns of rabbits. J. Pharmacol. exp. Ther. **130**, 81 (1960).
— A. M. REVZIN, R. KUNTZMAN, S. SPECTOR, and B. B. BRODIE: Evidence that norepinephrine in sympathetic ganglia modulates sympathetic synaptic transmission. Fed. Proc. **20**, 319 (1961b).
— — — — — Role for ganglionic norepinephrine in sympathetic synaptic transmission. Science **133**, 1822 (1961c).
COTZIAS, G. C., and V. P. DOLE: Metabolism of amines. I. Microdetermination of monoamine oxidase in tissues. J. biol. Chem. **190**, 665 (1951a).
— — Metabolism of amines. II. Mitochondrial localization of monoamine oxidase. Proc. Soc. exp. Biol. (N.Y.) **78**, 157 (1951b).
— — The activity of histaminase in tissues. J. biol. Chem. **196**, 235 (1952).
—, and J. J. GREENOUGH: Concomitant analysis for oxygen uptake and ammonia evolution during the monoamine oxidase reaction. Arch. Biochem. **75**, 15 (1958).
— — Quantitative estimation of amineoxidase. Nature (Lond.) **183**, 1732 (1959).
— — Dependence of periodic activation and inhibition of monoaminoxidase by aliphatic compounds upon chainlength. Nature (Lond.) **185**, 384 (1960).
— I. SERLIN, and J. J. GREENOUGH: Preparation of soluble monoamine oxidase. Science **120**, 144 (1954).
CRANE, G. E., and M. WOLFMAN: Studies on the urinary excretion of 5-hydroxyindol-acetic acid and 17-hydroxycorticosteroids in patients treated with Marsilid. J. nerv. ment. Dis. **130**, 134 (1960).
CREASEY, N. H.: Factors which interfere in the manometric assay of monoamine oxidase. Biochem. J. **64**, 178 (1956).
CREDNER, K., G. RENWANZ u. H.-J. HINZE: Untersuchungen über das Verhalten des m-Hydroxyphenyl(1)-äthanol(1)-amin(2)-hydrochlorids im Organismus. Naunyn-Schmiedebergs Arch. exp. Path. Pharmak. **243**, 85 (1962).
CREMA, A., e F. BERTE: L'azione di alcuni inibitori delle monoamine-ossidasi sull'edema sperimentale della zampa di ratto. Boll. Soc. ital. Biol. sper. **36**, 1069 (1960).
CREVELING, C. R., J. W. DALY, B. WITKOP, and S. UDENFRIEND: Substrates and inhibitors of dopamine-β-oxidase. Biochim. biophys. Acta (Amst.) **64**, 125 (1962).
—, and S. UDENFRIEND: Conversion of 3,4-dihydroxyphenylalanine to norepinephrine by brain homogenates. Fed. Proc. **18**, 379 (1959).
CROUT, J. R.: Effect of inhibiting both catechol-0-methyl transferase and monoamine oxidase on cardiovascular responses to norepinephrine. Proc. Soc. exp. Biol. (N.Y.) **108**, 482 (1961).
— C. R. CREVELING, and D. CATON: Metabolism of norepinephrine by rat brain and heart. Fed. Proc. **19**, 297 (1960).
—, and P. A. SHORE: Release of metaraminol (Aramine) from the heart by sympathetic nerve stimulation. Clin. Res. **12**, 180 (1964).
— — S. UDENFRIEND: Norepinephrine metabolism in rat brain and heart. J. Pharmacol. exp. Ther. **132**, 269 (1961).
CROWTHER, A. F., A. SPINKS, and E. H. P. YOUNG: The relation between structure and central nervous action of some hydrazine derivatives. Int. J. Neuropharmacol. **1**, 141 (1962).
CRUMPTON, C. W., C. A. CASTILLO, G. G. ROWE, and G. M. MAXWELL: Serotonin and the dynamics of the heart. Ann. N.Y. Acad. Sci. **80**, 960 (1959).
CSILIK, B.: Histochemical model experiments on the effect of various drugs on the catecholamine content of adrenergic nerve terminals. J. Neurochem. **11**, 351 (1964).

Culley, W. J., R. N. Saunders, D. H. Jolly, and E. T. Mertz: Reduction of brain serotonin levels in rats fed phenylpyruvic acid. Fed. Proc. **21**, 364 (1962).
Curzon, G.: The excretion of indoles in argentoffinoma. Arch. Biochem. **66**, 497 (1957).
— Coeruloplasmin. In: Genetic defects of biologically active proteins, p. 109, edit. F. Linneweh. München u. Berlin 1962.
Dacosta, F. M., and L. J. Goldberg: Depression of ganglionic transmission by MO-911 (N-methyl-N-benzyl-2-propynylamine hydrochloride), a non-hydrazine monoamine oxidase inhibitor Fed. Proc. **20**, 318 (1961).
Dalgliesh, C. E., and R. W. Dutton: Biogenesis of 5-hydroxytryptophan. Brit. J. Cancer **11**, 296 (1957).
Daly, J.W., J. Axelrod, and B. Witkop: Methylation and demethylation in relation to the in vitro metabolism of mescaline. Ann. N.Y. Acad. Sci. **96**, 371 (1962).
Dandiya, P. C., H. Cullumbine, and E. A. Sellers: Studies on acorus calamus. (IV): Investigations on mechanism of action in mice. J. Pharmacol. exp. Ther. **126**, 334 (1959).
Datta, R. K., and J. J. Ghosh: Effect of strychnine sulphate and nialamide on hydrogen bonded structure of ribonucleic acid of brain cortex ribosomes. J. Neurochem. **11**, 357 (1964).
Dat-Xuong, N., M. Duchene-Marullaz, J. Vacher et N. P. Buu-Hoi: Activité anti-monoamineoxydase de divers dérivés des nicotinyl- et isonicotinylhydrazines. Med. exp. (Basel) **7**, 85 (1962).
Davey, M. J., J. B. Farmer, and H. Reinert: Hypotension and monoaminoxydase inhibitors. Chemotherapia (Basel) **4**, 314 (1962).
— — — The effects of nialamide on adrenergic functions. Brit. J. Pharmacol. **20**, 121 (1963).
Davis, E. J., and R. S. de Ropp: The effect of some monoamine oxidase inhibitors on amine excretion in the rat. Biochem. biophys. Res. Commun. **2**, 361 (1960).
— — Metabolic origin of urinary methylamine in the rat. Nature (Lond.) **190**, 636 (1961).
Davis, R. A., D. J. Drain, M. Horlington, R. Lazare, and A. Urbanska: The effect of L-α-methyl dopa and N-2-hydroxybenzyl-N-hydrazine (NSD 1039) on the blood pressure of renal hypertensive rats. Life Sci. **2**, 193 (1963).
Davis, R. B., C. S. Alexander, and A. Adicoff: Metabolic studies in carcinoid syndrome: observations on use of α-methyl dopa, isonicotinic acid hydrazide and selective tryptophan deficiency. Metabolism **10**, 1035 (1961).
— B. W. Brown, W. R. Meeker, R. K. Ausman, and W. L. Bailey: Effects of amine oxidase inhibition on E. coli endotoxin mortality in mice. Proc. Soc. exp. Biol. (N.Y.) **109**, 412 (1962).
Davis, V. E.: Effect of cortisone and thyrosine on aromatic amino acid decarboxylation. Endocrinology **72**, 33 (1963).
—, and J. Awapara: Mammalian ortho-tyrosin decarboxylase. Fed. Proc. **19**, 5 (1960a).
— — A method for the determination of some amino acid decarboxylases. J. biol. Chem. **235**, 124 (1960b).
— C. Hanly, and J. Awapara: Decarboxylation of o-tyrosine and 5-hydroxytryptophan by tissues of rats treated with cortisone and tyroxine. Biochem. Pharmacol. 8, 127 (1961).
Davison, A. N.: The mechanism of the inhibition of decarboxylases by isonicotinyl hydrazide. Biochim. biophys. Acta (Amst.) **19**, 131 (1956).
— The mechanism of the irreversible inhibition of rat-liver monoamine oxidase by iproniazid (Marsilid). Biochem. J. **67**, 316 (1957).
— The irreversible inhibition of monoamine oxidase in vivo. Arch. Biochem. **77**, 368 (1958a).
— Inhibition of brain monoamine oxidase. Bull. Soc. Chim. biol. (Paris) **40**, 1737 (1958b).
— Physiological role of monoamine oxidase. Physiol. Rev. **38**, 729 (1958c).
— Unpublished results.
— A. W. Lessin, and M. W. Parkes: The antagonism of reserpine hypothermia by iproniazid. Experientia (Basel) **13**, 329 (1957).
—, and M. Sandler: Monoamine oxidase activity in the argentaffin carcinoma syndrome. Clin. chim. Acta **1**, 450 (1956).
— — Inhibition of 5-hydroxytryptophan decarboxylase by phenylalanine metabolites. Nature (Lond.) **181**, 186 (1958).
Dawson, A. M., and S. Sherlock: The effect of the amine oxidase inhibitor Marsilid on ammonium metabolism in liver disease. Clin. Sci. **17**, 587 (1958).
Day, M.: Effect of sympathomimetic amines on the blocking action of guanethidine, bretylium and xylocholine. Brit. J. Pharmacol. **18**, 421 (1962).
— — The uptake of biogenic amines by neoplastic mast cells in culture. J. Physiol. (Lond.) **164**, 227 (1962b).
—, and J. P. Green: The uptake of amino acids and the synthesis of amines by neoplastic mastcells in cultures. J. Physiol. (Lond.) **164**, 210 (1962a).

DAY, M., and M. J. RAND: A hypothesis for the mode of action of α-methyldopa in relieving hypertension. J. Pharm. (Lond.) **15**, 221 (1963).
— — Some observations on the pharmacology of α-methyl dopa. Brit. J. Pharmacol. **22**, 72 (1964).
DEGKWITZ, R., R. FROWEIN, C. KULENKAMPFF u. U. MOHS: Über die Wirkung des L-Dopa beim Menschen und deren Beeinflussung durch Reserpin, Chlorpromazin, Iproniazid und Vitamin B_6. Klin. Wschr. **38**, 120 (1960).
DELAHUNT, C. S., and J. PEPIN: Toxicology of nialamide, a monoamine oxidase inhibitor. Fed. Proc. **18**, 474 (1959a).
— — Toxicology of nialamide, a new psychotherapeutic agent. Toxicol. appl. Pharmacol. **1**, 524 (1959b).
DELGADO, J. M. R.: Pharmacological modifications of social behaviour. Biochem. Pharmacol. **8**, 131 (1961).
DEMIS, D. J., H. BLASCHKO, and A. D. WELCH: The conversion of dihydroxyphenylalanine-2-C^{14} (DOPA) to norepinephrine by bovine adrenal medullary homogenates. J. Pharmacol. exp. Ther. **117**, 208 (1956).
DENGLER, H. J.: Die Wirkung des α-Methyldopa auf die Aufnahme und den Stoffwechsel von markiertem Noradrenalin. Naunyn-Schmiedebergs Arch. exp. Path. Pharmak. **247**, 296 (1964).
—, E. RAUCHS u. W. RUMMEL: Zur Hemmung der L-Glutaminsäure- und L-Dopadecarboxylase durch D-Cycloserin und andere Isoxazolidone. Naunyn-Schmiedebergs Arch. exp. Path. Pharmak. **243**, 366 (1962).
—, u. G. REICHEL: Die Beeinflussung der Blutdruckwirkung von Dopa und Dops durch einen Decarboxylase-Inhibitor. Naunyn-Schmiedebergs Arch. exp. Path. Pharmak. **232**, 324 (1957/1958).
— — Hemmung der Dopadecarboxylase durch α-methyl-dopa in vivo. Naunyn-Schmiedebergs Arch. exp. Path. Pharmak. **234**, 275 (1958).
DENYS, A., J. LÉVY et E. MICHEL-BER: Comparaison, chez la souris, d'effets antidepresseurs centraux provoqués par l'administration aiguë et chronique d'un inhibiteur de la monoamine-oxydase (hydrazino-2-octane, D-1514), d'un précurseur des amines catéchiques (Dopa) et de leur association. J. Physiol. (Paris) **53**, 327 (1961).
DEOREO, G. A., and R. B. STOUGHTON: Monoamine oxidase and catechol O-methyl transferase inhibitors. Arch. Derm. **84**, 972 (1961).
DEWHURST, W. G., and C. M. B. PARE: A clinical and biochemical study of monoamine oxidase inhibition in depressed patients. II. 5-Hydroxytryptamine tolerance before and after nialamide. J. ment. Sci. **107**, 244 (1961).
DICKENS, F.: LXXVII. The metabolism of normal and humor tissue. XII. The action of phenylhydrazine on the Pasteur reaction and on tissue respiration. Biochem. J. **28**, 537 (1934).
DIETRICH, L. S.: A rapid method for the determination of dihydroxyphenylalanine decarboxylase in animal tissues. J. biol. Chem. **204**, 587 (1953).
—, and D. M. SHAPIRO: Testosterone augmentation of deoxypyridoxine antagonism of various vitamin B_6-containing enzyme systems in tumor and host tissue. Cancer Res. **15**, 133 (1955).
DISCHLER, W.: Der Einfluß langdauernder Behandlung mit Reserpin, Iproniazid und 5-Oxytryptamin auf den Oestrus-Zyklus von Mäusen erbreiner Stämme. Naturwissenschaften **47**, 401 (1960).
DOBKIN, A. B.: Drugs which stimulate affective behaviour. 2. Comparison of the analeptic effect of dl-amphetamine, bemigride with amiphenazole, methylphenidyl-acetate, iproniazid (micoren) and RP 8228. Anaesthesia **15**, 146 (1960).
DOLLERY, C. T., and M. HARINGTON: Methyldopa in hypertension: clinical and pharmacological studies. Lancet **1962 I**, 759.
DOMENJOZ, R., u. H. SCHELLENBERG: Pharmakologische Untersuchungen am 5-Hydroxytryptamin-Stoffwechsel des Mastocytom P-815. Schweiz. med. Wschr. **92**, 1185 (1962).
DRAIN, D. J., M. HORLINGTON, R. LAZARE, and G. A. POULTER: The effect of α-methyl dopa and some other decarboxylase inhibitors on brain 5-hydroxytryptamine. Life Sci. **1962**, 93.
— J. G. B. HOWES, R. LAZARE, A. M. SALAMAN, R. SHADBOLT, and H. W. R. WILLIAMS: Monoamine oxidase inhibitors. The synthesis and evaluation of a series of substituted alkylhydrazines. J. med. pharm. Chem. **6**, 63 (1963).
DRELL, W.: Separation of catecholamines from catechol acids by alumina. Fed. Proc. **16**, 174 (1957).
DREYFUS, P. M., and G. HAUSER: A simple micromethod for the collection of radioactive carbon dioxide in decarboxylation experiments. Mikrochim. ichnoanal. Acta **1964**, 150.
DUBACH, U., and O. GSELL: Carcinoid syndrome: alleviation of diarrhoea and flushing with „Deseril" and Ro 5-1025. Brit. med. J. **1962 I**, 1390.

DUBNICK, B., G. A. LEESON, and G. E. PHILLIPS: In vivo inhibition of serotonin synthesis in mouse brain by β-phenylethylhydrazine, an inhibitor of monoamine oxidase. Fed. Proc. 18, 218 (1959a).
— — — An effect of monoamine oxidase inhibitors on brain serotonin possibly in addition to that resulting from inhibition of monoamine oxidase. Pharmacologist 1, 74 (1959b).
— — — In vivo-inhibition of serotonin synthesis in mouse brain by β-phenylethylhydrazine, an inhibitor of MAO. Biochem. Pharmacol. 11, 45 (1962a).
— — — An effect of monoamine oxidase inhibitors on brain serotonin of mice in addition to monoamine oxidase. J. Neurochem. 9, 299 (1962b).
— — C. C. SCOTT: Effect of forms of vitamin B_6 on acute toxicity of hydrazines. Toxicol. appl. Pharmacol. 2. 403 (1960).
— D. F. MORGAN, and G. E. PHILLIPS: Inhibition of monoamine oxidase (MAO) by 2-methyl-3-piperidinopyrazine. Pharmacologist 4, 177 (1962c).
— — — Inhibition of monoamine oxidase by 2-methyl-3-piperidinopyrazine. Ann. N.Y. Acad. Sci. 107, 914 (1963).
DUHM, B., W. MAUL, H. MEDENWALD, K. PATZSCHKE, and L.-A. WEGNER: Tierexperimentelle Untersuchungen mit radioaktiv markiertem α-Methyldopa. Naunyn-Schmiedebergs Arch. exp. Path. Pharmak. 246, 10 (1963).
DUPASQUIER, E., et F. REUBI: Les répercussions de l'iproniazide (Marsilid) sur la tension artérielle et l'hémodynamique rénale. Cardiologia (Basel) 35, 256 (1959).
DUVE, C. DE, H. BEAUFAY, P. JACQUES, Y. RAHMAN-LI, O. Z. SELLINGER, R. WATTIAUX, and S. DE CONINCK: Intracellular localization of catalase and some oxidases in rat liver. Biochim. biophys. Acta (Amst.) 40, 186 (1960).
DVORNIK, D., M. KRAML, J. DUBUC, H. TOM, and T. ZSOTER: The effect of some inhibitors of the postganglionic sympathetic mechanism on monoamine oxidase. Biochem. Pharmacol. 12, 229 (1963).
EBERHOLST, I., I. HUUS u. R. KOPF: Zum Wirkungsmechanismus der Potenzierung von Hexobarbital durch Captodiamin. Arzneimittel-Forsch. 8, 379 (1958).
EBERSON, L. E., and K. PERSSON: Studies on monoamine oxidase inhibitors. I. The autoxidation of β-phenylisopropylhydrazine as a model reaction for irreversible monoamine oxidase inhibition. J. med. pharm. Chem. 5, 738 (1962).
EBERTS jr., F. S.: Metabolic studies with 3-(2-aminobutyl-1-C^{14}) indole acetate (Monase-C^{14}). I. Distribution and excretion in rat, dog and man. J. Neuropsychol. 2, 146 (1961).
—, and E. G. DANIELS: Metabolism of 3-(2-aminobutyl-1-C^{14}) indole acetate (etryptamine acetate) by man. Fed. Proc. 21, 180 (1961).
EBLE, J. N.: The depressor effect of tryptamine in the chicken: Absence of tachyphylaxis and reversal following monoamine oxidase inhibitors. Fed. Proc. 21, 330 (1962).
EBNÖTHER, A., E. JUCKER, A. LINDEMANN, E. RISSI, R. STEINER, R. SÜESS u. A. VOGEL: Neue basisch substituierte Hydrazin-Derivate. Helv. chim. Acta 42, 533 (1959).
EDER, M.: Der histochemische Nachweis des Fermentes Monoaminoxydase; Entwicklung einer Nachweismethode und deren Anwendung. Beitr. path. Anat. 117, 343 (1957).
EECHAUTE, W., E. LACROIX, I. LEUSEN et J. J. BOUCKAERT: L'activité du cortex surrénalien sous l'influence de la réserpine et de l'iproniazide. Arch. int. Pharmacodyn. 139, 403 (1962).
EHRINGER, H., O. HORNYKIEWICZ u. K. LECHNER: Die Wirkungen des Chlorpromazins auf den Katecholamin- und 5-Hydroxytryptamin-Stoffwechsel im Gehirn der Ratte. Naunyn-Schmiedebergs Arch. exp. Path. Pharmak. 239, 507 (1960).
— — — Die Wirkung von Methylenblau auf die Monoaminoxydase und den Catecholamin- und 5-Hydroxytryptamin-Stoffwechsel des Gehirns. Naunyn-Schmiedebergs Arch. exp. Path. Pharmak. 241, 568 (1961).
EIDUSON, S.: Effects of dopa, 5-HTP and iproniazide on self-stimulation of the brain. Fed. Proc. 18, 221 (1959).
ELLINGER, A.: Bildung von Putrescin (Tetramethylendiamin) aus Ornithin. Ber. dtsch. chem. Ges. 31, 3183 (1898).
— Die Konstitution des Ornithins und des Lysins. Zugleich ein Beitrag zur Chemie der Eiweißfäulnis. Hoppe-Seylers Z. physiol. Chem. 29, 334 (1900).
ELLIOT, K. A. C., and N. M. VAN GELDER: The state of factor I in rat brain: The effects of metabolic conditions and drugs. J. Physiol. (Lond.) 153, 423 (1960).
ELLISON, T., and C. C. SCOTT: Effects in the rat of chronic dietary supplementation with a monoamine oxidase inhibitor, tranylcypromine. Toxicol. appl. Pharmacol. 6, 411 (1964).
ELMADJIAN, F.: Excretion and metabolism of epinephrine. Pharmacol. Rev. 11, 409 (1959).
ELTHERINGTON, L. G.: A possible role of dopamine in cardiovascular "reserpine reversal". Fed. Proc. 20, 89 (1961).
—, and A. HORITA: Some pharmacological actions of β-phenylisopropylhydrazine (PIH). J. Pharmacol. exp. Ther. 128, 7 (1960).

EMELE, J. F., J. E. SHANAMAN, and M. R. WARREN: Phenelzine — a neuropharmacological study. Fed. Proc. **19**, 277 (1960).
— — — The analgesic activity of phenelzine and other compounds. J. Pharmacol. exp. Ther. **134**, 206 (1961).
— — — Analgesic activity of monoamine oxidase inhibitors. Fed. Proc. **18**, 387 (1959).
ENGEL, A., and U. S. VON EULER: Diagnostic value of increased urinary output of noradrenaline and adrenaline in phaeochromocytoma. Lancet **1950 II**, 387.
EPPS, H. M. R.: The development of amine oxidase activity by human tissues after birth. Biochem. J. **39**, 37 (1945).
ERNST, A. M., H. VAN ANDEL u. G. A. CHARBON: Beruht die experimentelle Katatonie durch Tryptamin auf einer Verdrängung des 5-Hydroxytryptamin? Psychopharmacologie **2**, 425 (1961).
ERNSTING, M. J. E., W. F. KAFOE, W. T. NAUTA, H. K. OOSTERHUIS, and C. DE WAART: Biochemical studies on psychotropic drugs. I. The effect of psychotropic drugs on γ-aminobutyric acid and glutamic acid in brain tissue. J. Neurochem. **5**, 121 (1960).
— — — and P. A. ROUKEMA: Investigation into the effect of orphenadrine hydrochloride (Disipal) on the monoamine oxidase in the brain and liver of rats and guinea pigs. Med. exp. (Basel) **7**, 119 (1962).
ERSPAMER, V.: Recent research in the field of 5-hydroxytryptamine and related indolealkylamines. In: Progress in Drug Research, vol. 3, p. 151, edit. E. JUCKER. Basel: Birkhäuser 1961.
—, and G. BERTACCINI: Observations on the antidiuretic action and the fate of 5-hydroxy-DL-tryptophan in the rat organism. Arch. int. Pharmacodyn. **137**, 6 (1962).
— R. FERRINI, and A. GLÄSSER: A note on the oxidative deamination of isomers of 5-hydroxytryptamine and other indolealkylamines. J. Pharmacol. **12**, 761 (1960a).
— A. GLÄSSER, and M. B. NOBILI: The fate of 5-hydroxy-N-acetyltryptophan and 5-acetoxy-N-acetyltryptophan in the rat organism. Arch. Biochem. **93**, 673 (1961a).
— — — and C. PASINI: The fate of 4-hydroxytryptophan in the rat organism. Experientia (Basel) **16**, 506 (1960b).
— — C. PASINI, and G. STOPPANI: In vitro decarboxylation of tryptophan by mammalian decarboxylase. Nature (Lond.) **189**, 483 (1961b).
—, and M. B. NOBILI: Observations on the fate of 4-hydroxy-DL-tryptophan in the organism. of the rat and man. Arch. int. Pharmacodyn. **137**, 24 (1962).
ESTLER, C.-J.: Untersuchungen über die Wirkung von Iproniazid auf einige Funktionen und Metaboliten des Gehirns weißer Mäuse und über die Modifizierung der Reserpinwirkung durch Iproniazid. Med. exp. **7**, 335 (1962).
EULER, U. S. VON, and S. HELLNER-BJÖRKMAN: Effect of amine oxidase inhibition on the noradrenaline and adrenaline content of cat organs. Acta physiol. scand. **33**, Suppl. 118, 21 (1955).
—, and I. ORWÉN: Preparation of extracts of urine and organs for estimation of free and conjugated noradrenaline and adrenaline. Acta physiol. scand. **33**, Suppl. 118, 1 (1955).
EVANS, W. O.: A new technique for the investigation of some analgesic drugs on a reflexive behavior in the rat. Psychopharmacologia (Berl). **2**, 318 (1961).
EVERETT, G. M.: Some electrophysiological and biochemical correlates of motor activity and aggressive behaviour. In: Neuropsychopharmacology, vol. 2, p. 479, edit. E. ROTHLIN. Amsterdam: Elsevier Publ. Co. 1961.
— J. C. DAVIN, and J. E. P. TOMAN: Pharmacological studies of monoamine oxidase inhibitors. Fed. Proc. **18**, 388 (1959).
—, and R. G. WIEGAND: Non-hydrazide monoamine oxidase inhibitors and their effects on central amines and motor behaviour. Biochem. Pharmacol. 8, 163 (1961).
— — and F. U. RINALDI: Pharmacologic studies of some nonhydrazine MAO inhibitors. Ann. N.Y. Acad. Sci. **107**, 1068 (1963).
EWINS, A. J., and P. P.LAIDLAW: The fate of parahydroxyphenylethylamine in the organism. J. Physiol. (Lond.) **41**, 78 (1910/11).
— — II. The fate of indolethylamine in the organism. Biochem. J. **7**, 18 (1913).
FABRE, J., M. RUDHARDT et B. MICHEL: L'action d'un inhibiteur de la monoamineoxydase sur l'extension des thromboses veineuses et artérielles. Schweiz. med. Wschr. **94**, 894 (1964).
— — — G. LACOURT et J. JEANDET: Action d'un inhibiteur de la monoamine-oxydase (Niamid) sur diverses lésions vasculaires expérimentales chez le lapin (artérite allergique, nécroses myocardiques par l'isoprotérénol, médionécrose aortique, thromboses veineuses et artérielles). Chemoterapia **4**, 237 (1962).
FASTIER, F. N., and J. HAWKINS: Inhibition of amine oxidase by isothiourea derivatives. Brit. J. Pharmacol. **6**, 256 (1951).

FELDSTEIN, A., H. HOAGLAND, and H. FREEMAN: Monoamine oxidase, psychoenergizers and tranquilizers. Science **130**, 500 (1959).
— — M. R. RIVIERA, and H. FREEMAN: A preliminary report on MAO inhibition and clinical effectiveness in the treatment of depressed patients with phenelzine. J. Neuropsychiat. **2**, 12 (1960).
— — — — The effect of monoamine oxidase inhibitors on the metabolism of serotonin and epinephrine. J. Neuropsychiat. **3**, 83 (1961).
FELLMANN, J. H.: Inhibition of DOPA decarboxylase by aromatic acids associated by phenylpyruvic oligophrenia. Proc. Soc. exp. Biol. (N.Y.) **93**, 413 (1956).
— The oxidation of 3,4-dihydroxyphenylacetaldehyde. Biochim. biophys. Acta (Amst.) **35**, 530 (1959a).
— Purification and properties of adrenal L-DOPA decarboxylase. Enzymologia **20**, 366 (1959b).
FELLOWS, E. J., and F. BERNHEIM: The effect of a number of aralkylamines on the oxidation of tyramine by amine oxidase. J. Pharmacol. exp. Ther. **100**, 94 (1950).
FERRARI, R. A., and A. ARNOLD: The effect of central nervous system agents on rat-brain γ-aminobutyric acid level. Biochim. biophys. Acta (Amst.) **52**, 361 (1961).
FERRINI, R., and A. GLÄSSER: In vitro decarboxylation of new phenylalanine derivatives. Biochem. Pharmacol. **13**, 798 (1964).
FERSTER, C. B., and M. H. APRISON: Increased behavioral effects of 5-hydroxytryptophan by iproniazid pretreatment. Pharmacologist **1**, 75 (1959).
FINGER, K. F.: Biochemical aspects of the action of nialamide. Fed. Proc. **19**, 278 (1960).
— J. N. PEREIRA, and J. A. SCHNEIDER: The influence of nialamide on the reserpine induced mobilization of fat and carbohydrate stores. Fed. Proc. **21**, 175 (1962).
FINKELSTEIN, J., J. A. ROMANO, E. CHIANG, and J. LEE: Monoamine oxidase inhibitors. IV. Some dialkylaminophenylalkylhydrazines and related compounds. J. med. Chem. **6**, 153 (1963).
FISHER, M. N., E. R. MAMLOK, A. TENDLAU, E. H. TEBROCK, A. E. DRUMM, and A. SPIEGELMAN: Isonicotinic acid hydrazide and its derivatives in tuberculosis. An evaluation of the side-effects in relation to peripheral circulation. N.Y. St. J. Med. **12**, 1519 (1952).
FISHER, T. N.: Current concepts of monoamine oxidase inhibitors. Marquette med. Rev. **27**, 86 (1962). [Chem. Abstr. **56**, 14865 (1962).]
FLÜCKIGER, E., and R. SALZMANN: Effect of iproniazid on pregnancy. Experientia (Basel) **17**, 130 (1961).
FLURY, F.: Beiträge zur Pharmakologie der Steppenraute (Peganum Harmala). Naunyn-Schmiedebergs Arch. exp. Path. Pharmak. **64**, 105 (1911).
FÖLDES, I., u. J. PÁLINKÁS: Weitere Untersuchungen über die Wirkung von Serotonin (5-Hydroxytryptamin) auf den Gasstoffwechsel weißer Ratten. Arch. int. Pharmacodyn. **127**, 331 (1960).
FÖRSTER, W., u. M. KUNZE: Der Einfluss von Iproniazid auf die antiemetische Wirkung von Reserpin, Rescinnamin, Raubasin (Ajmalicin), Tetrabenazin und Chlorpromazin bei Hunden und Katzen. Naunyn-Schmiedebergs Arch. exp. Path. Pharmak. **241**, 195 (1961).
FOLKERTH, T. L., and M. H. APRISON: Comparison of the recovery of monoamine oxidase activity after treatment with trans-2-phenylcyclopropylamine (SKF 385) and beta phenylisopropyl hydrazine (JB 516). Pharmacologist **4**, 169 (1962).
FONTANINI, F., P. L. PRATI e U. BARBIERI: Influenza dell'iproniazide sull'effetto permeabilizzante capillare della 5-idrossitriptamina. Boll. Soc. med.-chir. Modena **58**, 240 (1958). [Excerpta med. (Amst.), Sect. II **13**, 124 (1960).]
FOUTS, J. R.: Monoamines as substrates of diamine oxidase. Fed. Proc. **13**, 210 (1954).
— L. A. BLANKSMA, J. A. CARBON, and E. A. ZELLER: XIII. Monoamines as substrates of diamine oxidase. J. biol. Chem. **225**, 1025 (1957).
—, and B. B. BRODIE: Inhibition of drug metabolic pathways by the potentiating agent, 2,4-dichloro-6-phenyl-phenoxyethyl diethylamine. J. Pharmacol. exp. Ther. **115**, 68 (1955).
— — On the mechanism of drug potentiation by iproniazid (2-isopropyl-1-isonicotinyl hydrazine). J. Pharmacol. exp. Ther. **116**, 480 (1956).
FRANCIS, C. M.: Histochemical demonstration of amine oxidase in liver. Nature (Lond.) **171**, 701 (1953).
FRANCO-BROWDER, S., G. M. C. MASSON, and A. C. CORCORAN: Pharmacologic characterization of reserpine responses in rats pre-treated with iproniazid. Proc. Soc. exp. Biol. (N.Y.) **97**, 778 (1958).
— — — Induction of acute gastric lesions by histamine liberators in rats. J. Allergy **30** 1 (1959).
FREEDMAN, D. X., and N. J. GIARMAN: LSD-25 and the status and level of brain serotonin. Ann. N.Y. Acad. Sci. **96**, 98 (1962).

FRETER, K., H. WEISSBACH, B. G. REDFIELD, S. UDENFRIEND, and B. WITKOP: Oxindole analogs of (5-hydroxy)-tryptamine and -tryptophan, as inhibitors of the biosynthesis and breakdown of serotonin. J. Amer. chem. Soc. **80**, 983 (1958).
— — S. UDENFRIEND, and B. WITKOP: Biochemical and pharmacological studies with D- and L-5-hydroxytryptophan. Proc. Soc. exp. Biol. (N.Y.) **97**, 725 (1957).
FREY, H.-H.: Monoamine oxidase inhibition and sensitivity of the nictitating membrane to noradrenaline. Acta pharmacol. (Kbh.) **20**, 90 (1963).
FREYBURGER, W. A., B. E. GRAHAM, M. M. RAPPORT, P. H. SHAW, W. M. GOVIER, O. F. SWOAP, and M. J. VAN DER BROOK: The pharmacology of 5-hydroxytryptamine (serotonin). J. Pharmacol. exp. Ther. **105**, 80 (1952).
FRIEDENWALD, J. S., and H. HERRMANN: The inactivation of amine oxidase by enzymatic oxidative products of catechol and adrenalin. J. biol. Chem. **146**, 411 (1942).
FRIEDHOFF, A. J., and M. GOLDSTEIN: Part. I. Studies of experimental psychoses and neurohormones. New developments in metabolism of mescaline and related amines. Ann. N.Y. Acad. Sci. **96**, 5 (1962).
FRIEND, D. G.: The metabolism of dihydroxyphenylalanine in man before and after administration of psychotropic drugs. Ann. N.Y. Acad. Sci. **96**, 152 (1962).
— M. S. ZILELI, J. T. HAMLIN, and F. J. REUTER: The effect of iproniazid on the inactivation of norepinephrine in the human. J. clin. exp. Psychopath. **19**, Suppl. 1, **61** (1958).
FROMMEL, Ed., C. FLEURY, J. SCHMIDT-GINSKEY et M. BÉGUIN: De la pharmacodynamie différentielle thymoanaleptique et des substances "neuroleptiques" en expérimentation animale. Thérapie **15**, 1175 (1960).
FUJIMOTO, J. M., K. B. PEARCE, and G. L. PLAA: Barbiturate metabolism as affected by certain agents acting on the liver. J. Pharmacol. exp. Ther. **129**, 139 (1960).
FUJIMURA, H., and K. OHATA: Effect of several analeptics on brain amine oxidase activity and respiration. Yakugaku Zasshi **78**, 1054 (1958) [Chem. Abstr. **53**, 1547d (1959).]
FUNDERBURK, W. H., and A. B. DRAKONTIDES: Effects of nialamide on the electroencephalogram. Fed. Proc. **19**, 278 (1960).
— F. K. FINGER, A. B. DRAKONTIDES, and J. A. SCHNEIDER: EEG and biochemical findings with MAO inhibitors. Ann. N.Y. Acad. Sci. **96**, 289 (1962).
FURCHGOTT, R. F.: The pharmacology of vascular smooth muscle. Pharmacol. Rev. **7**, 183, 234 (1955).
— P. WEINSTEIN, H. HÜBEL, P. U. BOZORGMEHRI, and R. MENSENDIEK: Effect of inhibition of monoamine oxidase on response of rabbit aortic strips to sympathicomimetic amines. Fed. Proc. **14**, 341 (1955).
FURGIUELE, A. R., W. J. KINNARD, and J. P. BUCKLEY: Central effects of β-phenylisopropylhydrazine and iproniazid. J. Pharmacol. exp. Ther. **137**, 356 (1962).
GADDUM, J. H.: Bioassay procedures. Pharmacol. Rev. **11**, 241 (1959).
—, and N. J. GIARMAN: Preliminary studies on the biosynthesis. Brit. J. Pharmacol. **11**, 88 (1956).
— R. W. SCHAYER, G. KAHLSON, P. HAGEN, J. L. MONGAR, and C. F. CODE: Histamine metabolism. Proc. int. Union physiol. Sci., Leiden, Part II, 847 (1962).
GAFFNEY, T. E., W. ROUSSEAU, S. WORONKOW, and J. PEAGLER: Reserpine, methyl-dopa and adrenergic nerve blockade. Pharmacologist **5**, 260 (1963).
GAL, E. M., and P. A. DREWES: Studies on the metabolism of 5-hydroxytryptamine (Serotonin). I. Effect of starvation and thiamine deficiency. Proc. Soc. exp. Biol. (N.Y.) **106**. 295 (1961).
— — Studies on the metabolism of 5-hydroxytryptamine (Serotonin). II. Effect of tryptophan deficiency in rats. Proc. Soc. exp. Biol. (N.Y.) **110**, 368 (1962).
GALE, E.F.: The production of amines by bacteria. I. The decarboxylation of amino-acids by strains of bacterium coli. Biochem. J. **34**, 392 (1940a).
— The production of amines by bacteria. II. The production of tyramine by streptococcus faecalis. Biochem. J. **34**, 846 (1940b).
— The production of amines by bacteria. III. The production of putrescine from l(+)arginine by bacterium coli in symbiosis with streptococcus faecalis. Biochem. J. **34**, 853 (1940c).
— Production of amines by bacteria. IV. The decarboxylation of amino-acids by organisms of the groups clostridium and proteus. Biochem. J. **35**, 66 (1941).
— The bacterial amino acid decarboxylases. Advanc. Enzymol. **6**, 1 (1946).
GANROT, P. O., C. G. GOTTFRIES, and E. ROSENGREN: Effects of some psychotropic drugs on the metabolism of catecholamines and 5-HT in human brain. Manuscript (1962a).
— A. M. ROSENGREN, and E. ROSENGREN: On the presence of different histidine decarboxylating enzymes in mammalian tissues. Experientia (Basel) **17**, 263 (1961).
—, and E. ROSENGREN: Isolation of a mitochondrial fraction containing monoamine oxidase. Med. exp. (Basel) **6**, 315 (1962).
— — and C. G. GOTTFRIES: Effect of iproniazid on monoamines and monoamine oxidase in human brain. Experientia (Basel) **18**, 260 (1962b).

GARATTINI, S., P. FRESIA, A. MORTARI, and V. PALMA: The pressor effect of reserpine after monoamine-oxidase inhibitors. Med. exp. (Basel) **2**, 252 (1960a)
— A. GIACHETTI, L. PIERI, and R. RE: Antagonists of reserpine induced eyelid ptosis. Med. exp. (Basel) **3**, 315 (1960b).
—, and L. VALZELLI: Biochemistry and pharmacology of serotonin in the central nervous system. In: Monoamines et système nerveux central, p. 59. Genève: George & Co. S.A. 1962.
GARDNER, T. S., E. WENIS, and J. LEE: Monoamine oxidase inhibitors. I. 1-Alkyl- and 1-aralkyl-2-(picolinoy) and 5-methyl-3-isoxazolylcarbonyl hydrazines. J. med. pharm. Chem. **2**, 133 (1960).
— — — Monoamine oxidase inhibitors. II. Some amino and dialkylaminobenzyl hydrazines and their acyl derivatives. J. med. pharm. Chem. **3**, 241 (1961).
— — — Monoamine oxidase inhibitors. III. Structural variations in 1-alkyl and 1-aralkyl-1(or 2)-acyl-hydrazines. J. med. pharm. Chem. **5**, 503 (1962).
GATGOUNIS, J., and J. AYCOCK: Influence of MAO inhibitors on the adrenal medullary responses to chemical stimulation. Fed. Proc. **20**, 89 (1961).
— — Effects of monoamino oxidase inhibitors on adrenal medullary responses to nicotine and tetramethylammonium. J. Pharmacol. exp. Ther. **140**, 50 (1963).
— L. I. GOLDBERG, and W. G. WHITLOCK: Influence of monoamine oxidase inhibitors on the cardiovascular effects of sympathomimetic amines. Pharmacologist **1**, 57 (1959).
— J. A. RICHARDSON, and J. A. CLAYTON: Effect of an MAO inhibitor on adrenal catecholamine content to nicotine stimulation of the adrenal glands. Fed. Proc. **23**, 230 (1964).
GAUDETTE, L. E., and B. B. BRODIE: Relationship between the lipid solubility of drugs and their oxidation by liver microsomes. Biochem. Pharmacol. **2**, 89 (1959).
—, and G. R. COATNEY: A possible mechanism of prolonged antimalarial activity. Amer. J. trop. Med. Hyg. **10**, 321 (1961).
GAVEND, M., M.-R. GAVEND et J. MERCIER: Action du nialamide sur la circulation coronaire. L'influence exercée par un antagoniste de la sérotonine sur l'action du nialamide et de l'iproniazide. C. R. Soc. Biol. (Paris) **154**, 2089 (1960) .
GEIGER, A., V. AGUILAR, G. GOMBOS, W. SCRUGGS, and G. WHITNEY: Effect of isoniazide and iproniazide on the pathways of glucose utilization in the perfused brain. Fed. Proc. **19**, 277 (1960).
GELLER, E., S. EIDUSON, and A. YUWILER: Oxidation of p-phenylenediamine and adrenaline in enzymic and copper-catalysed reactions. J. Neurochem. **5**, 73 (1959).
GENDEREN, H. VAN, and H. H. M. DURVILLE: The role of histamine and serotonin in the production of fever by bacterial pyrogens in rabbits. Acta physiol. pharmacol. neerl. **8**, 116 (1959).
GENOVESE, E., E. ARRIGONI-MARTELLI e P. FRESIA: Proprietà farmacologiche di un nuovo inibitore delle monoaminossidasi, la beta-fenil-isopropil-idrazina. Farmaco, Ed. sci. **14**, 516 (1959).
GEORGES, G., et M. HÉROLD: Influence de la sérotonine et du Marsilid sur la réactivité de l'axe hypothalamo-hypophyso-surrénalien chez le rat. C. R. Soc. Biol. (Paris) **152**, 436 (1958).
GERSHON, M. D., and L. L. ROSS: Studies on the relationship of 5-hydroxytryptamine and the enterochromaffin cell to anaphylactic shock in mice. J. exp. Med. **115**, 367 (1962).
GERTNER, S. B.: Monoamine oxidase inhibitors and ganglionic block. Fed. Proc. **18**, 393 (1959a).
— Ganglionic block and monoamine oxidase inhibitors. Nature (Lond.) **183**, 750 (1959b).
— The effects of monoamine oxidase inhibitors on ganglionic transmission. J. Pharmacol. exp. Ther. **131**, 223 (1961).
GESSA, G. L., E. COSTA, R. KUNTZMAN, and B. B. BRODIE: On the mechanism of norepinephrine release by α-methyl-metatyrosine. Life Sci. **1962**a, 353.
— — — — Evidence that the loss of brain catecholamine stores due to blockade of storage does not cause sedation. Life Sci. **1962**b, 441.
— E. CUENCA, and E. COSTA: A bretylium-like action of monoamine oxidase inhibitors. Pharmacologist **4**, 179 (1962c).
— — — On the mechanism of hypotensive effects of MAO inhibitors. Ann. N.Y. Acad. Sci. **107**, 935 (1963).
GEY, K. F., W. P. BURKARD u. A. PLETSCHER: Hemmung der Diaminoxydase „in vivo" durch Hydrazinderivate. Helv. physiol. pharmacol. Acta **18**, C 27 (1960).
— — — Influence of chlorpromazine on the decarboxylases of aromatic amino acids. Biochem. Pharmacol. **8**, 383 (1961).
— — — Altersbedingte Veränderungen des Catecholaminstoffwechsels im Rattenherzen. Helv. physiol. pharmacol. Acta **22**, C 17 (1964).
— — — Unpublished results.

GEY, K. F., and F. MESSIHA: Einfluß von Dopa-Transaminierung auf die Dopa-Decarboxylierung in vitro. Experientia (Basel) **20**, 498 (1964).
—, u. A. PLETSCHER: Ueber Bedeutung der Monoaminoxydase-Aktivität für die Monoaminkonzentration tierischer Gewebe. Chimia **13**, 300 (1959a).
— — Ueber die Herkunft verschiedener biogener Monoamine in Herz und Gehirn. Tagg. der Ges. für Physiologische Chemie, Berlin 24. 9. 1959 (b).
— — Post mortem increase of 5-hydroxytryptamine in rat brain after 5-hydroxytryptophan administration. Experientia (Basel) **16**, 372 (1960a).
— — Vermehrung der Serum-Milchsäure durch Monoaminoxydase-Hemmer. Helv. physiol. pharmacol. Acta **18**, C 70 (1960b).
— — Biochemical methods for the investigation of amine metabolism in vivo. Int. Meeting on the Techniques for the Study of Psychotropic Drugs, Bologna June 1960 (c).
— — Increase of pyruvic and lactic acid in rat blood by inhibitors of monoamine oxidase. Experientia (Basel) **17**, 25 (1961a).
— — Activity of monoamine oxidase in relation to the 5-hydroxytryptamine and norepinephrine content of the rat brain. J. Neurochem **6**, 239 (1961b).
— — Influence of chlorpromazine and chlorprothixene on the cerebral metabolism of 5-hydroxytryptamine, norepinephrine and dopamine. J. Pharmacol. exp. Ther. **133**, 18 (1961c).
— — Effect of α-alkylated tryptamine derivatives on 5-hydroxytryptamine metabolism in vivo. Brit. J. Pharmacol. **19**, 161 (1962).
— — Unpublished results.
— —, and W. P. BURKARD: Effect of inhibitors of monoamine oxidase on various enzymes and on the storage of monoamines. Ann. N.Y. Acad. Sci. **107**, 1147 (1963).
GHERARDI, M., e G. SALVI: Azione di alcuni inibitori enzimatici sull' intossicazione acuta sperimentale da composti tetra-alchi-lici di piombo. Folia med. (Napoli) **44**, 987 (1961). [Chem. Abstr. **56**, 14880 (1962).]
GIÃO, T., et J. M. RICO: Sur l'emploi des radioisotopes dans l'étude expérimentale des actions antiphlogistiques. C. R. Soc. Biol. (Paris) **154**, 218 (1960).
GIARMAN, N. J.: Biosynthesis of 5-hydroxytryptamine (serotonin, enteramine). Fed. Proc. **15**, 428 (1956).
— Effects of hallucinogenic drugs in man (Discussion). Fed. Proc. **20**, 897 (1961).
—, and M. DAY: Presence of biogenic amines in the bovine pineal body. Biochem. Pharmacol. **1**, 235 (1959).
—. and S. M. SCHANBERG: The intracellular distribution of 5-hydroxytryptamine (5-HT, Serotonin) in the rat's brain. Biochem. Pharmacol. **1**. 301 (1958).
— — Drug-induced alterations in the intracellular distribution of 5-hydroxytryptamine in rat's brain. Biochem. Pharmacol. **8**, 6 (1961).
GILLESPIE jr., L.: Clinical pharmacology of newer antihypertensive agents, monoamine oxidase and decarbocylase inhibitors, bretylium tosylate, and guanethidine. Ann. N. Y. Acad. Sci. **88**, 1011 (1960).
— J. A. OATES, J. R. CROUT, and A. SJOERDSMA: Further clinical evaluation of α-methyldopa. Circulation **24**, 940 (1961).
— — — — Clinical and chemical studies with α-methyl-dopa in patients with hypertension. Circulation **25**, 281 (1962).
GIORDANO, C.: Activity of some enzymes in experimental hypertension in the rabbit. Experientia (Basel) **17**, 558 (1961).
— J. BLOOM, and J. P. MERRILL: Preparation of monoaminoxydase. Experientia (Basel) **16**, 346 (1960a).
— — — Effects of urea on physiologic systems. I. Studies on monoamine oxidase activity. J. Lab. clin. Med. **59**, 396 (1962).
— A. H. SAMIA, J. BLOOM, F. W. HAYNES, and J. P. MERRILL: Studies on experimental renal hypertension in rabbits. Fed. Proc. **19**, 100 (1960b).
GIRARD, J.-P.: Le rôle de l'adénosine triphosphorique (ATP) dans la fixation intraplaquettaire de la sérotonine. Schweiz. med. Wschr. **93**, 1456 (1963).
GITLOW, S., M. MENDLOWITZ, and N. NAFTCHI: Effect of iproniazid on digital vascular norepinephrine sensitivity. The first Hahnemann Symposium on Hypertensive Disease, p. 409. Philadelphia and London: W. B. Saunders Co. 1959.
GLENNER, G. G., H. J. BURTNER, and G. W. BROWN: The histochemical demonstration of monoamine oxidase activity by tetrazolium salts. J. Histochem. Cytochem **5**, 591 (1957).
GLUCKMAN, M. I.: Cerebral free and bound serotonin (5-HT) after iproniazid (IH) and reserpine (R). Fed. Proc. **19**, 265 (1960).
— A. DANIELS, and A. S. MARRAZZI: Intracellular distribution and iproniazid inhibition of monoamine oxidase in rat brain and liver. J. Pharmacol. exp. Ther. **122**, 25A (1958).

GLUCKMAN, M. I., E. R. HART, and A. S. MARRAZZI: Cerebral synaptic inhibition by serotonin and iproniazid. Science **126**, 448 (1957).
—, and Z. HOROVITZ: Limiting factors in monoamine oxidase (MAO) inhibition. Pharmacologist **1**, 81 (1959).
—, and A. S. MARRAZZI: Reversal of iproniazid inhibition of monoamine oxidase. Fed. Proc. **17**, 371 (1958).
GÖING, H.: Beeinflussung der Fieber erzeugenden Wirkung bakterieller Pyrogene durch Iproniazid, Reserpin und Dibenamin. Arzneimittel-Forsch. **9**, 793 (1959).
— Die Wirkungsweise von pyrogenen und bakteriellen Endotoxinen. Klin. Wschr. **38**, 1069 (1960).
GÖSCHKE, H.: Spezies-Unterschiede bei der Wirkung von Monoaminoxydase-Hemmern. Arch. int. Pharmacodyn. **133**, 245 (1961).
— W. P. BURKARD, K. F. GEY u. A. PLETSCHER: Hemmung der Cholinoxydase in vivo durch Neuropharmaca Med. exp. 8, 256 (1963).
GOGERTY, J. H., and A. HORITA: A comparison of the in vivo monoamine oxidase inhibitory properties of iproniazid and beta-phenylisopropyl-hydrazine. Fed. Proc. **18**, 395 (1959).
— — A comparison of the in vivo inhibition of brain and liver monoamine oxidase as produced by beta-phenylisopropylhydrazine (PIH) and iproniazid. J. Pharmacol. exp. Ther. **129**, 357 (1960).
GOLDBERG, L. I.: Iproniazid and other MAO inhibitors. Ann. N. Y. Acad. Sci. **80**, 639 (1959).
—, and F. M. DACOSTA: Selective block of sympathetic transmission by iproniazid and harmine in the intact animal. Pharmacologist **2**, 95 (1960a).
— — Selective depression of sympathetic transmission by intravenous administration of iproniazid and harmine. Proc. Soc. exp. Biol. (N. Y.) **105**, 223 (1960b).
— — and M. OZAKI: Actions of the decarboxylase inhibitor, α-methyl-3,4-dihydroxyphenylalanine, in the dog. Nature (Lond.) 188, 502 (1960).
— D. HORWITZ, and A. SJOERDSMA: Attenuation of cardiovascular responses to exercise as a possible basis for effectiveness of monoamine oxidase inhibitors in angina pectoris. J. Pharmacol. exp. Ther. **137**, 39 (1962).
—, and A. SJOERDSMA: Effects of several monoamine oxidase inhibitors on the cardiovascular actions of naturally occurring amines in the dog. J. Pharmacol. exp. Ther. **127**, 212 (1959).
GOLDBERG N. D., and F. E. SHIDEMAN: A species difference in the depletion of myocardial catecholamines by a monoamine oxidase inhibitor. Fed. Proc. **20**, 128 (1961).
— — Species differences in the cardiac effects of a monoamine oxidase inhibitor. J. Pharmacol exp. Ther. **136**, 142 (1962).
GOLDIN, A., D. DENNIS, J. M. VENDITTI, and S. R. HUMPHREYS: Potentiation of pentobarbital anesthesia by isonicotinic acid hydrazide and related compounds. Science **121**, 364 (1955).
GOLDSTEIN, M., and J. F. CONTRERA: The substrate specificity of phenylamine-β-hydroxylase. J. biol. Chem. **237**, 1898 (1962).
— A. J. FRIEDHOFF, S. POMERANTZ, and S. B. GERTNER: The distribution and metabolism of simultaneously infused norepinephrine-7-H^3 and epinephrine-1-C^{14}. Fed. Proc. **19** 295, (1960a).
— — — and C. SIMMONS: The characterization of a new metabolite of dopamine. Biochim. biophys. Acta (Amst.) **39**, 189 (1960b).
— — and G. SANDLER: The relative metabolic rates of norepinephrine-7-H^3 and epinephrine-1-C^{14}. Experientia (Basel) **16**, 211 (1960c).
— — and C. SIMMONS: Metabolic pathways of 3-hydroxytyramine. Biochim biophys. Acta (Amst.) **33**, 572 (1959).
— — — and N. N. PROCHOROFF: Indirect evidence of synthesis of norepinephrine from 3-hydroxytyramine-1-C^{14} in vivo. Proc. Soc. exp. Biol. (N.Y.) **103**, 137 (1960d).
— — S. B. WORTIS, and S. B. GERTNER: The differences in the accumulation and metabolism of catecholamines in heart and liver. Experientia (Basel) **16**, 369 (1960e).
—, and S. B. GERTNER: Formation of a new metabolite of epinephrine and norepinephrine in liver and kidney. Nature (Lond.) **187**, 147 (1960).
—, and J. M. MUSACCHIO: The formation in vivo of N-acetyl-dopamine and N-acetyl-3-methoxydopamine. Biochim. biophys. Acta (Amst.) **58**, 607 (1962).
— — Effects of monoamine oxidase inhibition on biogenic amine metabolism. Ann. N.Y. Acad. Sci. **107**, 840 (1963).
GONNARD, P.: Oxydation et activité dopadécarboxylasique. Bull. Soc. Chim. biol. (Paris) **31**, 194 (1949).
— Action d'amines cycliques et acycliques sur la dopadécarboxylation. Bull. Soc. Chim. biol. (Paris) **32**, 535 (1950).

GONNARD, P.: Action de quelques composés minéraux et organiques sur la dopadécarboxylation. Bull. Soc. Chim, biol. (Paris) **33**, 14 (1951).
— L'isonicotylhydrazone de phosphopyridoxal, rôle co-enzymatique. C. R. Acad. Sci. (Paris) **246**, 3539 (1958).
— Effect of hydrazides and hydrazones of pyridoxal-5-phosphate on the cerebral glutamic decarboxylase and pyridoxal phosphokinase. Abstr. Int. Neurochem. Symp. on "Enzymic activity of the CNS", p. 28. Göteborg (Sweden) June 17—21, 1962.
—, et N. BOIGNÉ: Rôle co-enzymatique d'hydrazones de phospho-5-pyridoxal cynuréninase et hydrazides cycliques. Bull. Soc. Chim. biol. (Paris) **43**, 609 (1961).
—, M. CAMIER et H. BOIGNÉ: Etude chromatographique du phosphate de pyridoxal, de l'isoniazide et de l'isonicotyl hydrazone de phospho-5'-pyridoxal. Bull. Soc. chim. Biol. (Paris) **46**, 407 (1964b).
— — et C. NGUYEN-PHILIPPN: Etude sur la stabilité de l'isonicotyl hydrazone de phospho-5'-pyridoxal en présence de pyridaxoloenzymes. Bull. Soc. chim. Biol. **46**, 323 (1964a).
—, et S. FENARD: Décarboxylase glutaminique et hydrazones de phospho-5-pyridoxal. J. Neurochem. **9**, 135 (1962).
—, et J. P. NGUYEN CHI: Action de l'hydrazide et des composés de structure voisine sur la dopadécarboxylase. Bull. Soc. Chim. biol. (Paris) **40**, 16 (1958a).
— — Action de l'hydrazide isonicotinique et de composés de structure voisine sur la dopadécarboxylase. Bull. Soc. Chim. biol. (Paris) **40**, 485 (1958b).
— — Rôle co-enzymatique d'hydrazones de phosphopyridoxal vis-à-vis de la dopadécarboxylase. Bull. Soc. Chim. biol. (Paris) **41**, 1455 (1959a).
— — Activation de la dopadécarboxylase par l'isonicotinyl hydrazone de phospho-pyridoxal. Enzymologia **20**, 237 (1959b).
— A. PELOU et C. N. PHILIPPON: Action de la carbutamide (BZ55) sur l'adrénalinogénèse. IV. Int. Congr. Biochem., Vienna 1958, Suppl. Int. Abstr. biol. Sci. **10**, 185 (1958).
— — — Action de la carbutamide (BZ55) sur l'adrénalinogénèse. Bull. Soc. Chim. biol. (Paris) **41**, 127 (1959).
GOODALL, M., and N. KIRSHNER: Biosynthesis of adrenaline and noradrenaline in vitro. J. biol. Chem. **226**, 213 (1957).
GORKIN, V. Z.: Some properties of mitochondrial monoamino oxidase of rat liver and brain. Biokhimija **24**. 758 (1959) [Engl. Ed.].
— Partial separation of rat liver mitochondrial amine oxidases. Nature (Lond.) **200**, 77 (1963).
— On the multiplicity of mitochondrial amine oxidases. In: Proc. 6th. Int. Congr. Biochem., p. 309, IV—58. New York 1964.
— Personal communication.
— L. I. GRIDNEVA, L. A. ROMANOVA, and I. S. SEVERINA: Spectrophotometric determination of monoamine oxidase activity in mitochondria. Biochimija (Mosc.) (Engl. Ed.) **27**, 852 (1963).
— N. A. KITROSSKY, L. B. KLYASHTORIN, N. V. KOMISAROVA, G. A. LEONTYEVA, and V. A. POOCHKOV. Biochimija (Mosc.) in press (1964a).
— N. V. KOMISAROVA, M. I. LERMAN, and I. V. VERYOVKINA: The inhibition of mitochondrial amine oxidases in vitro by proflavine. Biochem. biophys. Res. Commun. **15**, 383 (1964b).
GOTTFRIES, C. G.: Versuche mit Marsilid und Marsilid-Analogen. Psychiat. et Neurol. (Basel) **140**, 115 (1960).
GOVIER, W. M., M. E. GRELIS, N. S. YANZ, and K. H. BEYER: Studies on the mechanism of action of sympathomimetic amines. J. Pharmacol. exp. Ther. **87**, 149 (1946).
— B. G. HOWES, and A. J. GIBBONS: The oxidative deamination of serotonin and other 3-(beta-aminoethyl)-indoles by monoamine oxidase and the effect of these compounds on the deamination of tyramine. Science **118**, 596 (1953).
GRANA, E., and L. LILLA: The inhibition of amine oxidase and the central stimulating action of the steroisomeric amphetamines and l-phenyl-ethylamines. Brit. J. Pharmacol. **14**, 501 (1959).
GRANOWITZ, E., u. A. PLETSCHER: Die diagnostische Bedeutung der 5-Hydroxyindolessigsäure-Ausscheidung im Urin. Helv. med. Acta **24**, 21 (1957).
GREEN, A. L.: The inhibition of monoamine oxidase by arylalkylhydrazine. Biochem. J. **84**, 217 (1962).
— Studies on the mechanism of inhibition of monoamine oxidase by hydrazine derivatives. Biochem. Pharmacol. **13**, 249 (1964).
—, and T. M. HAUGHTON: The estimation of monoamine oxidase. Biochem. J. **76**, 44P (1960).
— — A colorimetric method for the estimation of monoamine oxidase. Biochem. J. **78**, 172 (1961).

GREEN, H., and R. W. ERICKSON: Effect of trans-2-phenylcyclopropylamine upon norepinephrine concentration and monoamine oxidase activity of rat brain. J. Pharmacol. exp. Ther. **129**, 237 (1960).

— — Further studies with tranylcypromine (monoamine oxidase inhibitor) and its interaction with reserpine in rat brain. Arch. int Pharmacodyn. **135**, 407 (1962).

— — and J. L. SAWYER: Biochemical correlates of pharmacologic activity. Pharmacologist **3**, 61 (1961).

—, and J. L. SAWYER: Intracellular distribution of norepinephrine in rat brain. I. Effect of reserpine and the monoamine oxidase inhibitors, trans-2-phenylcyclopropylamine and l-isonicotinyl-2-isopropylhydrazine. J. Pharmacol. exp. Ther. **129**, 243 (1960a).

— — Correlation of tryptamine-induced convulsions in rats with brain tryptamine concentration. Proc. Soc. exp. Biol. (N. Y.) **104**, 153 (1960b).

— — and R. ERICKSON: Intracellular distribution of noradrenaline in rat brain. Pharmacologist **1**, 75 (1959).

— — — and L. COOK: Effect of repeated oral administration of monoamine oxidase inhibitors on rat brain amines. Proc. Soc. exp. Biol. (N. Y.) **109**, 347 (1962).

GREEN, J. P.: Binding of some biogenic amines in tissues. Advanc. Pharmacol. **1**, 349 (1962).

—, and A. V. FURANO: Two pools for amines in neuroplastic mast cells. Biochem. Pharmacol. **11**, 1049 (1962).

GREENBLATT, E. N., and A. C. OSTERBERG: Effect of drugs on maintenance of exploratory behavior in mice. Fed. Proc. **20**, 397 (1961a).

— — Correlations of activating and lethal effects of excitatory drugs in grouped and isolated mice. J. Pharmacol. exp. Ther. **131**, 115 (1961b).

GREENBLATT, I. J. and A. KAHN: Clinical toxicity studies of a monoamine oxidase inhibitor. Ann. N. Y. Acad. Sci. **80**, 947 (1959).

GREIG, M. E., and A. J. GIBBONS: The effect of DL-α-ethyltryptamine acetate on serotonin metabolism. Arch. int. Pharmacodyn. **136**, 147 (1962).

— — J. P. DA VANZO, and O. K. SEBEK: Comparative effects of α-ethyltryptamine isomers on certain systems in vitro and in vivo. Biochem. Pharmacol. **8**, 32 (1961a).

— P. H. SEAY, and FREYBURGER: The pharmacology of etryptamine. J. Neuropsychiat. **2**, 131 (1961b).

— R. A. WALK, and A. J. GIBBONS: The effect of three tryptamine derivatives on serotonin metabolism in vitro and in vivo. J. Pharmacol. exp. Ther. **127**, 110 (1959).

GRIESEMER, E. C., J. BARSKY, C. A. DRAGSTEDT, J. A. WELLS, and E. A. ZELLER: Potentiating effect of iproniazid on the pharmacological action of sympathomimetic amines. Proc. Soc. exp. Biol. (N. Y.) **84**, 699 (1953).

— C. A. DRAGSTEDT, J. A. WELLS, and E. A. ZELLER: Adrenergic blockade by iproniazid. Experientia (Basel) **11**, 182 (1955).

— R. M. FLEMING, W. J. HARTMANN, and W. G. CLARK: Competitive inhibition of dihydroxyphenylalanine (DOPA) decarboxylase in vitro. Pharmacologist **3**, 77 (1961).

— and J. A. WELLS: Abolition of epinephrine inactivating properties of liver by inhibitors of monoamine oxidase. J. Pharmacol. exp. Ther. **116**, 282 (1956).

GRINSTEINS, V., and G. VILLERE: Effect of some derivatives of dibenzofuran and carboxylic acid hydrazides on enzymes system. Zinatniskie Raksti, Latv. Univ. **9**, 143 (1956). [Chem. Abstr. **52**, 10248a (1958).]

GROSS, J., C. I. LEVENE, and S. ORLOFF: Fragility and extractable collagen in the lathyritic chick embryo. An assay for lathyrogenic agents. Proc. Soc. exp. Biol. (N. Y.) **105**, 148 (1960).

GROVES, W. G., and H. J. JENKINS: Investigation of the cardiovascular response of the dog to l-phenyl-2-hydrozinopropane. J. pharm. Sci. **50**, 502 (1961).

GRUNBERG, E.: Studies on the activity of hydrazine derivatives of isonicotinic acid in the experimental tuberculosis of mice. Quart. Bull. Sea View Hosp. **13**, 3 (1952).

GUGGENHEIM, M., u. W. LÖFFLER: Das Schicksal proteinogener Amine im Tierkörper. Biochem. Z. **72**, 325 (1916).

GUM, O. B., C. J. SMYTH, P. K. HAMILTON jr., and C. MOENS: Effect of intraarticular serotonin and other amines on connective tissue proliferation of rabbit joints. Arthr. and Rheum. **3**, 447 (1960).

GUPTA, G. P., and B. N. DHAWAN: Blockade of reserpine emesis in pigeons. Arch. int. Pharmacodyn. **128**, 481 (1960).

GUTMANN, N., S. FELTON, and F. M. HUENNEKENS: Effect of isonicotinic hydrazides on enzymes systems. Biochim. biophys. Acta (Amst.) **14**, 282 (1954).

GYLYS, J. A., M. CHESSIN, and M. R. WARREN: Effects of beta-phenylethylhydrazine and related compounds on response of rabbit aortic strips to sympathomimetic amines. Pharmacologist **1**, 82 (1959).

—, and P. M. R. MUCCIA: Effect of modaline HCl (W 3207A) on locomotor activity in the mouse. Fed. Proc. **23**, 198 (1964).

GYLYS, J. A., P. M. R. MUCCIA, and M. K. TAYLOR: Pharmacological and toxicological properties of 2-methyl-3-piperidinopyrazine, a new antidepressant. Ann. N.Y. Acad. Sci. **107**, 899 (1963).

—, and M. W. OSBORNE: Antagonism between a pyrazine derivative, W3207A, and reserpine as compared to phenelzine and imipramine. Pharmacologist **4**, 117 (1962).

HAAS, H., u. W. APPEL: Vergleichende Untersuchungen mit 6-methyl-2-heptylhydrazin und anderen Monoaminoxydase-Hemmern. Arzneimittel-Forsch. **12**, 352 (1962).

HAAVALDSEN, R.: Transamination of aromatic amino-acids in nervous tissue. Nature (Lond.) **196**, 577 (1962).

HAGEN, P.: The substrate specificity of amine oxidase of mouse mastocytoma. Fed. Proc. **18**, 399 (1959).

— Observations on the substrate specificity of dopa decarboxylase from ox adrenal medulla, human phaeochromocytoma and human argentaffinoma. Brit. J. Pharmacol. **18**, 175 (1962).

—, and F. L. LEE: Amino acid decarboxylases of mouse mast cells. J. Physiol. (Lond.) **143**, 7 (1958).

—, and N. WEINER: Enzymic oxidation of pharmacologically active amines. Fed. Proc. **18**, 457, 1005 (1959).

— — S. ONO, and F.-L. LEE: Amino acid decarboxylases of mouse mastocytoma tissue. J. Pharmacol. exp. Ther. **130**, 9 (1960).

—, and A. D. WELCH: The adrenal medulla and the biosynthesis of pressor amines. Recent Progr. Hormone Res. **12**, 27 (1956).

HALPERN, B. N., C. DRUDI-BARACCO: Suppression by iproniazide of the antagonistic action of reserpine on amphetamine "group toxicity". Biochem. Pharmacol. **8**, 9 (1961).

— — et D. BESSIRARD: Toxicité de groupe par l'amphétamine et action de la réserpine, de la chlorpromazine et des inhibiteurs de la monoamineoxydase. C. R. Soc. Biol. (Paris) **156**, 769 (1962a).

— — — Toxicité de groupe par l'amphétamine et action de la réserpine, de la chlorpromazine et des inhibiteurs de la monoamineoxydase. Presse méd. **70**, 1365 (1962b).

— J. C. MORARD et C. DRUDI-BARACCO: Action protectrice de la réserpine sur les lésions de dégénérescence myocardique aiguë provoquées par la DL-amphétamine et suppression de cette action par les inhibiteurs de la monoamineoxydase. C. R. Soc. Biol. (Paris) **156**, 773 (1962c).

— — — Action protectrice de la réserpine sur les lésions de dégénérescence myocardique aiguë provoquées par la DL-amphétamine et suppression de cette action par les inhibiteurs de la monoamine-oxydase. Presse méd. **70**, 1365 (1962d).

HANKE, M. T., and K. K. KOESSLER: Studies on proteinogenous amines. XII. The production of histamine and other imidazoles from histidine by the action of microorganisms. J. biol. Chem. **50**, 131 (1922).

— — Studies on proteinogenous amines. XVII. On the faculty of normal intestinal bacteria to form toxic amines. J. biol. Chem. **59**, 835 (1924a).

— — Studies on proteinogenous amines. XVIII. On the production of histamine, tyramine and phenol in common laboratory media by certain intestinal microorganisms. J. biol. Chem. **59**, 855 (1924b).

— — Studies on proteinogenous amines. XIX. On the factors involved in the production of phenol by the colon group. J. biol. Chem. **59**, 867 (1924c).

HÅKANSON, R.: Histidine decarboxylase in the fetal rat. Biochem. Pharmacol. **12**, 1289 (1963).

—, and H. MÖLLER: Dopa decarboxylase activity in the skin. Acta derm.-venereol. (Stockh.) **43**, 485 (1963).

HANSON, K. M., D. C. AUSTIN, and M. H. APRISON: In vitro effect of nonindole compounds on oxidative activity of ceruloplasmin. J. appl. Physiol. **14**, 363 (1959).

HANSSON, E., and W. G. CLARK: A rapid method for screening dopa decarboxylase inhibitors in vivo. Pharmacologist **4**, 149 (1962a).

— — Studies on dopa decarboxylase inhibitors in vivo by use of $C^{14}O_2$ carboxyl labelled dopa. Proc. Soc. exp. Biol. (N. Y.) **111**, 793 (1962b).

— R. M. FLEMING, and W. G. CLARK Effect of some benzylhydrazines and benzyloxyamines on dopa and 5-hydroxytryptophan decarboxylase in vivo. Int. J. Neuropharmacol. **3**, 177 (1964).

HARDEGG, W.: Zur Messung der Monoaminoxydase-Aktivität. Pflügers Arch. ges. Physiol. **274**, 25 (1961).

—, u. E. HEILBRONN: Oxydation von Serotonin und Tyramin durch Rattenlebermitochondrien. Biochim. biophys. Acta (Amst.) **51**, 553 (1961).

HARE, M. L. C.: CXXI. Tyramine oxidase. I. A new enzyme system in liver. Biochem. J. **22**, 968 (1928).

HARRIS, E. S.: Studies on rat liver monoamine oxidase. Fed. Proc. **19**, 25 (1960).

HARRIS, S. C., L. M. SEARLE, and A. C. IVY: The excretion of amphetamine. J. Pharmacol. exp. Ther. **89**, 92 (1947).
HARRISON, D. C., C. A. CHIDSEY, and E. BRAUNWALD: The release of norepinephrine from the heart by vasoactive amines. Clin. Res. Proc. **9**, 328 (1961).
— — — Studies on the mechanism of action of metaraminol (Aramine). Ann. intern. Med. **59**, 297 (1963).
HARTMANN, W. J.: Unpublished [cit. D. T. MASUOKA, H. F. SCHOTT, and L. PETRIELLO: Formation of catecholamines by various areas of cat brain. J. Pharmacol. exp. Ther. **139**, 73 (1963)].
— R. W. AKAWIE and W. G. CLARK: Competitive inhibiton of 3,4-dihydroxyphenylalanine (dopa) decarboxylase in vitro. J. biol. Chem. **216**, 507 (1955a).
—, and W. G. CLARK: Competitive inhibition of dihydroxy phenylalanine (dopa) decarboxylase. Fed. Proc. **12**, 62 (1953).
— — S. D. CYR, A. L. JORDAN, and R. A. LEIBHOLD: Pharmacologically active amines and their biogenesis in the octopus. Ann. N. Y. Acad. Sci. **90**, 637 (1960).
— R. S. POGRUND, W. DRELL, and W. G. CLARK: Studies on the biosynthesis of arterenol. Enzymatic decarboxylation of diastereoisomers of hydroxyphenylserines. J. Amer. chem. Soc. **77**, 816 (1955b).
HARWOOD, C. T. and Wm. M. BIGELOW: Endocrine effects of psychic energizers and CNS stimulants. Pharmacologist **2**, 93 (1960).
HAUSCHILD, F.: Orale Wirksamkeit, Abbau und chemische Konstitution in der Ephedrin-Adrenalin-Reihe. Klin. Wschr. **20**, 363 (1941).
HAVERBACK, B. J., and M. BRODY: Results reported at the Marsilid Symposium, San Francisco 1958.
HAWKINS, J.: The localization of amine oxidase in the liver cell. Biochem. J. **50**, 577 (1952a).
— Amine oxidase activity of rat liver in riboflavin deficiency. Biochem. J. **51**, 399 (1952b).
—, and J. M. WALKER: The effect of colchicine on L-dopa decarboxylase and on the pressor amine content of rat adrenals. J. Physiol. (Lond). **115**, 38 P (1951).
— — The effect of colchicine on the enzyme content of regenerating rat liver and on the pressor amine content of the adrenal. Brit. J. Pharmacol. **7**, 152 (1952).
HAZARD, R., M. BEAUVALLET, J. HAZARD, P. MOUILLÉ et M. SOLIER: Effets des sensibilisateurs de l'adrénaline sur la teneur en hormone du plasma au cours de perfusions intraveineuses continues. C. R. Soc. Biol. (Paris) **154**, 1366 (1960).
— — E. C. SAVINI et S. LARNO: Variations dans la teneur en adrénaline du liquide ayant perfusé l'oreille isolée de lapin. I. Etude de l'action des adrénalino-sensibilisateurs. Biochem. Pharmacol. 8, 66 (1961).
HEEGARD, E. V., and G. A. ALLES: Inhibitor specificity of amine oxidase. J. biol. Chem. **147**, 505 (1943).
HEGGLIN, R., E. LÜTHY, U. ISLER u. G. FORSTER: Stoffwechseluntersuchungen bei mit Tersavid behandelten Angina-pectoris-Kranken. Cardiologia (Basel) **37**, Suppl. II, 230 (1960).
HEILBRONN, E.: Effect of certain hydrazines and amines on monoamine oxidase and some pyridoxal phosphate-requiring enzymes. Biochem. J. **76**, 45 P (1960).
HEIM, F.: Die Bedeutung der experimentellen Änderung der Aminooxydase-Aktivität für die Adrenalinwirkung. Naunyn-Schmiedebergs Arch. exp. Path. Pharmak. **204**, 520 (1947).
— Über den Einfluss verschiedener Ester auf die fermentative Oxydation von Adrenalin und Adrenalinderivaten. Naunyn-Schmiedebergs Arch. exp. Path. Pharmak. **209**, 181 (1950a).
— Über den Einfluss von Alkohol auf den enzymatischen Abbau des Tyramins. Naunyn-Schmiedebergs Arch. exp. Path. Pharmak. **210**, 16 (1950b).
—, u. K. DIEMER: Über quantitative Wirkungsunterschiede zwischen 1-Isonicotinoyl-2-isopropylhydrazin (Iproniazid) und Isopropylhydrazin auf die Monoaminoxydase. Med. exp. (Basel) **3**, 249 (1960).
HEIMSTRA, N. W.: Social influence on the response to drugs. II. Chlorpromazine and iproniazid. Psychopharmacol. **3**, 72 (1962).
HEISE, G. A., and E. BOFF: Behavioral determination of time and dose parameters of monoamine oxidase inhibitors. J. Pharmacol. exp. Ther. **129**, 155 (1960).
HEMPEL, K., u. M. DEIMEL: Einfluß des Dopa-Decarboxylase-Hemmers α-Methyl-Dopa auf die Umwandlung von Dopa in Melanin und Brenzcatechinamine. Naunyn-Schmiedebergs Arch. exp. Path. Pharmak. **246**, 203 (1963).
HERMANN, M., et R. MORNEX: Etude expérimentale des effets cardiovasculaires de l'iproniazide. Thérapie **15**, 993 (1960).
HÉROLD, M., et J. CAHN: Premier essai d'interprétation du mécanisme d'action des inhibiteurs de la monoamine-oxydase. Rev. Agréssologie **2**, 679 (1961).

HÉROLD, M., J. CAHN, C. HELBECQUE et O. KABACOFF: Action de quelques inhibiteurs de la L-dopa décarboxylase à l'égard de différents types de convulsions. C. R. Soc. Biol. (Paris) **156**, 1273 (1962a).
— — — T. LASJAUNIAS et A.-M. JUILLARD: Action de quelques inhibiteurs de la L-dopa décarboxylase sur la durée de la narcose barbiturique chez la souris. C. R. Soc. Biol. (Paris) **156**, 1270 (1962b).
— G. GEORGES et C. CAHN: Quelques aspects de l'action de l'iproniazide sur le système nerveux central. In: Neuro-Psychopharmacology, vol. **1**, p. 324, edit. E. ROTHLIN. Amsterdam: Elsevier Publ. Co. 1959.
— O. KABACOFF, O. MATHIAS, G. MATHIAS et J. CAHN: Variations du temps de survie du coeur chez la souris prétraitée par les inhibiteurs de la monoamineoxydase. C.R. Soc. Biol. (Paris) **155**, 2111 (1961).
HERTTING, G.: Über den Einfluss des Serotoninstoffwechsels auf die Metrazolkrampfschwelle bei Mäusen. Wien. klin. Wschr. **70**, 190 (1958).
—, and J. AXELROD: Fate of tritiated noradrenaline at the sympathetic nerve-endings. Nature (Lond.) **192**, 172 (1961).
— — and L. G. WHITBY: Effect of drugs on the uptake and metabolism of H^3-norepinephrine. J. Pharmacol. exp. Thei. **134**, 146 (1961a).
— — —, and R. W. PATRICK: Effect of drugs on the uptake of circulating H^3-norepinephrine by tissues. Fed. Proc. **20**, 167 (1961b).
— I. J. KOPIN, and E. GORDON: The uptake, release and metabolism of norepinephrine-7-H^3 in the isolated perfused rat heart. Fed. Proc. **21**, 331 (1962).
—, and E. H. LABROSSE: Biliary and urinary excretion of metabolites of 7H-epinephrine in the rat. J. biol. Chem. **237**, 2291 (1962).
HESS, S. M.: The releasing action of α-methyl-3-hydroxyphenylalanine (α-methyl-meta-tyrosine). Pharmacologist **3**, 77 (1961).
— The releasing action of α-methyl-3-hydroxyphenylalanine (α-methyl-meta-tyrosine). Arch. int. Pharmacodyn. **138**, 584 (1962).
— R. H. CONNAMACHER, M. OZAKI, and S. UDENFRIEND: The effects of α-methyl-dopa and α-methyl-meta-tyrosine on the metabolism of norepinephrine and serotonin in vivo. J. Pharmacol. exp. Ther. **134**, 129 (1961a).
— —, and S. UDENFRIEND: Effect of α-methylamino acids on catecholamines and serotonin. Fed. Proc. **20**, 344 (1961b).
—, and W. DOEPFNER: Behavioral effects and brain amine content in rats. Arch. int. Pharmacodyn. **134**, 89 (1961).
— —, and S. UDENFRIEND: Lack of correlation between excitement and brain amine content after monoamine oxidase inhibitors and amine precursors in rats. Pharmacologist **1**, 83 (1959a).
— M. OZAKI, and S. UDENFRIEND: The effects of α-methyl-dopa and α-methyl-meta-tyrosine on the metabolism of serotonin and norepinephrine. Pharmacologist **2**, 81 (1960).
— B. G. REDFIELD, and S. UDENFRIEND: Tryptamine in animal tissues following administration of iproniazid. Fed. Proc. **18**, 402 (1959b).
— — — The effect of monoamine oxidase inhibitors and tryptophan on the tryptamine content of animal tissues and urine. J. Pharmacol. exp. Ther. **127**, 178 (1959c).
—, and H. WEISSBACH: Marsilid metabolism. Fed. Proc. **17**, 377 (1958).
— — B. G. REDFIELD, and S. UDENFRIEND: The relationship between iproniazid metabolism and the duration of its effect on monoamine oxidase. J. Pharmacol. exp. Ther. **124**, 189 (1958).
HESTER, J. B., M. E. GREIG, W. C. ANTHONY, R. V. HEINZELMAN, and J. SZMUSZKOVICZ: Enzyme inhibitory activity of 3-(2-aminobutyl) indol derivatives. J. med. Chem. **7**, 274 (1964).
HEYL, D., E. LUZ, S. A. HARRIS, and K. FOLKERS: Chemistry of vitamin B_6. VIII. Additional pyridoxylideneamines and pyridoxylamines. J. Amer. chem. Soc. **74**, 414 (1952).
HICKS, R., and G. B. WEST: Adrenal cortical hormones and the formation of histamine and 5-hydroxytryptamine. Nature (Lond.) **181**, 1342 (1958a).
— — Adrenalectomy and tissue amines. Nature (Lond.) **182**, 401 (1958b).
HIGHMAN, B., and H. M. MALING: Neuropathologic lesions in dogs after prolonged administration of phenylisopropylhydrazine (JB 516) and phenylisobutylhydrazine (JB 835). J. Pharmacol. exp. Ther. **137**, 344 (1962).
HIMWICH, H. E., E. COSTA, G. R. PSCHEIDT, and W. G. VAN METER: MAO and mechanisms in brain. Ann. N.Y. Acad. Sci. **80**, 614 (1959).
— — W. G. VAN METER, and H. OWENS: Results reported at the Roche Symposium on MAO inhibitors. Chicago 1958.

HIMWICH, W. A., and E. COSTA: Behavioral changes associated with changes in concentrations of brain serotonin. Fed. Proc. 19, 838 (1960).
— —, and H. E. HIMWICH: Brain serotonin in relation to imipramine interaction with a monoamine oxidase inhibitor. In: Neuropsychopharmacology, vol. 2, p. 485, edit. E. ROTHLIN. Amsterdam: Elsevier Publ. Co. 1961.
—, and J. C. PETERSEN: Effect of the combined administration of imipramine and a monoamine oxidase inhibitor. Amer. J. Psychiat. 117, 928 (1961).
HIRSCH, C. W., R. KUNTZMAN, and E. COSTA: Effects of dopa-5-HTP decarboxylase inhibition on synthesis of brain amines. Fed. Proc. 21, 364 (1962a).
— — —, and B. B. BRODIE: Inhibition of the biosynthesis of brain norepinephrine in mice. Pharmacologist 4, 179 (1962b).
HODGE, J. V., J. A. OATES, and A. SJOERDSMA: Reduction of the central effects of tryptophan by a decarboxylase inhibitor. Clin. Pharmacol. Ther. 5, 149 (1964).
HOFFMANN, C., J. FROSSARD, K. MAI-XUAN et I. KARADAVIDOFF: Hydrazines N_1N_2 disubstituées et monoamino oxydase. Ann. pharm. franç. 20, 539 (1962).
HOGANS, A. F., and C. C. PORTER: Excretion of the optical isomers of α-methyl-dopa. Fed. Proc. 20, 113 (1961).
HOLMSTEDT, B., and R. THAM: A spectrophotometric method for determination of diamine oxidase (DAO) activity. Acta physiol. scand. 45, 152 (1959).
HOLTZ, P.: Über die Entstehung von Histamin und Tryramin im Organismus. Klin. Wschr. 16, 1561 (1937).
— Über die Bildung einer blutdrucksteigernden Substanz aus Dioxyphenylalanin durch tierisches Gewebe. Naunyn-Schmiedebergs Arch. exp. Path. Pharmak. 190, 178 (1938).
— Dopadecarboxylase. Naturwissenschaften 27, 724 (1939).
— Fermentative Aminbildung aus Aminosäuren. Ergebn. Physiol. 44, 230 (1941).
— Über das Vorkommen der Dopadecarboxylase im Pankreas. Naunyn-Schmiedebergs Arch. exp. Path. Pharmak. 199, 145 (1942).
— Role of L-dopa decarboxylase in the biosynthesis of catecholamines in nervous tissue and the adrenal medulla. Pharmacol. Rev. 11, 317 (1959).
— Aminosäurendecarboxylasen des Nervengewebes. Psychiat. et Neurol. (Basel) 140, 175 (1960).
—, u. F. BACHMANN: Aktivierung der Dopadecarboxylase des Nebennierenmarks durch Nebennieren-Rindenextrakt. Naturwissenschaften 39, 116 (1952).
— — u. C. CARSTEN: Einfluss von Vitamin B_6 (Pyridoxin) und Pyridoxalphosphat auf die Dopadecarboxylase tierischer Organe. Naturwissenschaften 39, 235 (1952a).
— H. BALZER u. E. WESTERMANN: Die Beeinflussung der Reserpinwirkung auf das Nebennierenmark durch Hemmung der Monoaminoxydase. Naunyn-Schmiedebergs Arch. exp. Path. Pharmak. 231, 361 (1957a).
— — — Beeinflussung der Narkosedauer durch Hemmung der Cholinesterase des Gehirns. Naunyn-Schmiedebergs Arch. exp. Path. Pharmak. 233, 438 (1958).
— — — E. WEZLER: Beeinflussung der Evipannarkose durch Reserpin, Iproniazid und biogene Amine. Naunyn-Schmiedebergs Arch. exp. Path. Pharmak. 231, 333 (1957b).
—, u. K. CREDNER: Decarboxylierung von Dioxyphenylalanin (DOPA) und Histidin in vivo. Naturwissenschaften 29, 649 (1941).
— — u. W. KOEPP: Die enzymatische Entstehung von Oxytyramin im Organismus und die physiologische Bedeutung der Dopadecarboxylase. Naunyn-Schmiedebergs Arch. exp. Path. Pharmak. 200, 356 (1942a).
— — u. A. REINHOLD: Aminbildung durch Darm. Naunyn-Schmiedebergs Arch. exp. Path. Pharmak. 193, 688 (1939a).
— — u. C. STRÜBING: Über das Vorkommen der Dopadecarboxylase im Pancreas. Naunyn-Schmiedebergs Arch. exp. Path. Pharmak. 199, 145 (1942b).
— — u. H. WALTER: Über die Spezifität der Aminsäuredecarboxylasen. Hoppe-Seylers Z. physiol. Chem. 262, 111 (1939b).
— A. ENGELHARDT u. G. THIELECKE: Aktivierung und Hemmung der Histidindecarboxylase durch Vitamin B_6 (Pyridoxin). Naturwissenschaften 39, 266 (1952b).
—, u. R. HEISE: Über die Entstehung von Histamin im Organismus. Naturwissenschaften 25, 201 (1937a).
— — Über Histaminbildung im Organismus. Naunyn-Schmiedebergs Arch. exp. Path. Pharmak. 186, 377 (1937b).
— — u. K. LÜDTKE: Fermentativer Abbau von l-Dioxyphenylalanin (DOPA) durch Niere. Naunyn-Schmiedebergs Arch. exp. Path. Pharmak. 191, 87 (1938a).
— — u. W. SPREYER: Fermentative Bildung und Zerstörung von Histamin und Tyramin. Naunyn-Schmiedebergs Arch. exp. Path. Pharmak. 188, 580 (1938b).
—, u. H. JANISCH: Über Tyraminbildung im Organismus. Naunyn-Schmiedebergs Arch. exp. Path. Pharmak. 186, 684 (1937).

HOLTZ, P., and D. PALM: Pharmacological aspects of vitamin B_6. Pharmacol. Rev. **16**, 113 (1964).
— A. REINHOLD u. K. CREDNER: Fermentativer Abbau von L-Dioxyphenylalanin (DOPA) durch Leber und Darm. Hoppe-Seylers Z. physiol. Chem. **261**, 278 (1939c).
—, and K. STOCK: Formation of tetrahydropapaveroline from dopamine in vitro. Nature (Lond.) **203**, 656 (1964a).
— — u. E. WESTERMANN: Über den Einfluß des Thyroxins und des Hungerns auf die Aktivität der Monoaminoxydase und Dopadecarboxylase der Leber. Naunyn-Schmiedebergs Arch. exp. Path. Pharmak. **228**, 322 (1956).
— — — Pharmakologie des Tetrahydropapaverolins und seine Entstehung aus Dopamin. Naunyn-Schmiedebergs Arch. exp. Path. Pharmak. **248**, 387 (1964b).
—, u. E. WESTERMANN: Über die Dopadecarboxylase und Histidindecarboxylase des Nervengewebes. Naunyn-Schmiedebergs Arch. exp. Path. Pharmak. **227**, 538 (1956a).
— — Über die Vorstufe des Nor-adrenalins im Nebennierenmark und Nervengewebe. Biochem. Z. **327**, 502 (1956b).
— — Hemmung der Glutaminsäuredecarboxylase des Gehirns durch Brenzcatechinderivate. Naunyn-Schmiedebergs Arch. exp. Path. Pharmak. **231**, 311 (1957).
HOLZER, G., u. O. HORNYKIEWICZ: Über den Dopamin-(Hydroxytyramin-) Stoffwechsel im Gehirn der Ratte. Naunyn-Schmiedebergs Arch. exp. Path. Pharmak. **237**, 27 (1959).
HOPE, D. B., and A. D. SMITH: Distribution and activity of monoamine oxidase in mouse tissues. Biochem. J. **74**, 101 (1960).
HORITA, A.: Beta-phenylisopropylhydrazine, a monoamine oxidase inhibitor. Fed. Proc. **17**, 379 (1958a).
— Beta-phenylisopropylhydrazine, a potent and long acting monoamine oxidase inhibitor. J. Pharmacol. exp. Ther. **122**, 176 (1958b).
— Pharmacology of JB-516 (PIH). Ann. N.Y. Acad. Sci. **80**, 590 (1959).
— Route of administration of the hydrazines as a determinant in the selective inhibition of brain and liver monoamine oxidase. Fed. Proc. **19**, 279 (1960).
— The route of administration of some hydrazine compounds as a determinant of brain and liver monoamine oxidase inhibition. Toxicol. appl. Pharmacol. **3**, 474 (1961).
— The influence of pH on serotonin metabolism by rat tissue homogenates. Biochem. Pharmacol. **11**, 147 (1962a).
— A possible source of error in the measurement of 5-hydroxytryptophan decarboxylase activity in rat tissues. Biochem. Pharmacol. **11**, 672 (1962b).
— Some antagonists of the monoamine oxidase inhibitors. Ann. N.Y. Acad. Sci. **107**, 951 (1963a).
— The influence of drug-tissue interactions on the inhibition of monoamine oxidase by pheniprazine and iproniazid. J. Pharmacol. exp. Ther. **142**, 141 (1963b).
—, and C. CHINN: An analysis of the interaction of reversible and irreversible monoamine oxidase inhibitors. Biochem. Pharmacol. **13**, 371 (1964).
—, and C. MATSUMOTO: The antagonism of hydrazine-type inhibitors of monoamine oxidase by sodium pyruvate. Life Sci. **1962**, 491.
—, and W. R. MCGRATH: The interaction between reversible and irreversible monoamine oxidase inhibitors. Biochem. Pharmacol. **3**, 206 (1960a).
— — Specific liver and brain monoamine oxidase inhibition by alkyl- and arylalkylhydrazines. Proc. Soc. exp. Biol. (N.Y.) **103**, 753 (1960b).
—, and R. G. PARKER: Comparison cf monoamine oxidase inhibitory effects of iproniazid and its phenyl congener. Proc. Soc. exp. Biol. (N.Y.) **99**, 617 (1958).
HORNYKIEWICZ, O.: The action of dopamine on the arterial blood pressure of the guinea-pig. Brit. J. Pharmacol. **13**, 91 (1958).
HOROWITZ, Z. P.: A biochemical and pharmacological correlation of the effects of certain monoamine oxidase inhibitors. Diss. Pittsburgh (Pa.) 1960.
HORWITZ, D., L. I. GOLDBERG, and A. SJOERDSMA: Effects of monoamine oxidase inhibitors on the pressor actions of norepinephrine and dopamine in man. Clin. Res. Proc. 8, 21 (1960a).
— — — Increased blood pressure responses to dopamine and norepinephrine produced by monoamine oxidase inhibitors in man. J. Lab. clin. Med. **56**, 747 (1960b).
— — — Possible hemodynamic basis for beneficial effects of a monoamine oxidase inhibitor in angina pectoris. Circulation **24**, 959 (1961).
—, W. LOVENBERG, K. ENGELMANN, and A. SJOERDSMA: Monoamine oxidase inhibitors, tyramine, and cheese. J. Amer. med. Ass. **188**, 1108 (1964).
—, and A. SJOERDSMA: A basis for the use of monoamine oxidase inhibitors in angina pectoris. Ann. N.Y. Acad. Sci. **107**, 1033 (1963).
— — Effects of alpha-methyl-meta-tyrosine intravenously in man. Life Sci. **3**, 41 (1964).

HUANG, I., S. TANNENBAUM, and D. Y.-Y. HSIA: Development of 5-hydroxytryptophan decarboxylase activity in rat kidney. Nature (Lond.) **186**, 717 (1960).
—, and D. Y.-Y. HSIA: Studies on inhibition of 5-hydroxytryptophan decarboxylase by phenylalanine metabolites. Proc. Soc. exp. Biol. (N.Y.) **112**, 81 (1963).
HUKOVIC, S., and E. MUSCHOLL: Die Noradrenalin-Abgabe aus dem isolierten Kaninchen-Herzen bei sympathischer Nervenreizung und ihre pharmakologische Beeinflussung. Naunyn-Schmiedebergs Arch. exp. Path. Pharmak. **244**, 81 (1962).
HULL, L. D., and A. HORITA: Reserpine reversal response by iproniazid: a dose-dependent phenomenon. Nature (Lond.) **202**, 604 (1964).
HUSZTI, Z., and J. BORSY: The effect of diethyltryptamine and its derivatives on moonamine oxidase. Biochem. Pharmakol. **13**, 1151 (1964).
IIDA, N.: Inhibitory effect of quinine on the oxidation of adrenaline. Nippon Yakurigaku Zasshi **54**, 648 (1958) Brevaria 31. [Chem. Abstr. **53**, 18290c (1959).]
IISALO, E.: In the enzymatic destruction of adrenaline and noradrenaline in smooth muscle tissues. Acta physiol. scand. **42**, Suppl. 145, 75 (1957).
— Enzyme action on noradrenaline and adrenaline studies on bovine and guinea-pig tissues in vitıo with special reference to monoamine oxidase. Acta pharmacol. (Kbh.) **19**, Suppl. 1, 5 (1962).
—, and A. PEKKARINEN: On the enzymatic destruction of adrenaline and noradrenaline in the heart muscle. Acta physiol. scand. **31**, Suppl. 114, 25 (1954).
— — Enzyme action on adrenaline and noradrenaline. Studies on heart muscle in vitro. Acta pharmacol. (Kbh). **15**, 157 (1958).
IMAIZUMI, R., M. OKA, and T. OHUCHI: Mechanism of the antihypertensive effect of α-methyldopa. Nature (Lond.) **203**, 982 (1964).
—, K. OMORI, A. UNOKI, K. SANO, Y. WATARI, J. NAMBA, and K. INUI: Physiological significance of monoamine oxidase. Jap. J. Pharmacol. 8, 87 (1959).
IMIYA, T.: On the problem of precursors of adrenalin. VI. Especially on dopa decarboxylase and hydroxytryptamine. J. Osaka med. Sch. **40**, 1494 (1941). [CLARK, W. G., Pharmacol. Rev. **11**, 330 (1959).]
IORIO, A. D', et L.-P. BOUTHILLIER: Métabolisme de la DL-histidine ($C^{14}OOH$) radioactive chez le rat. Rev. canad. Biol. **9**, 388 (1950).
IRALDI, A. P. DE, and G. R. DE LORES ARNAIZ: 5-Hydroxytryptophan-decarboxylase in normal and denervated pineal gland of rats. Life Sci. **3**, 589 (1964).
—, and E. DE ROBERTIS: Action of reserpine, iproniazid and pyrogallol on nerve endings of the pineal gland. Int. J. Neuropharmacol. **2**, 231 (1963).
IRVINE, R. O. H., K. P. O'BRIEN, and J. D. K. NORTH: Alpha methyl dopa in treatment of hypertension. Lancet **1962 I**, 300.
IRWIN, S.: Behavioral effects of chronic iproniazid administration. Fed. Proc. 18, 406 (1959).
—, and I. I. A. TABACHNICK: Correlation between locomotor stimulant and brain monoamine-oxidase-inhibitory activity of iproniazid, nialamide and pheniprazine in the rat. Fed. Proc. **20**, 396 (1961).
IVY, A. D., T. M. LIN, E. K. IVY, and E. KARVINEN: Effect of histaminase inhibitors on gastric secretion. Amer. J. Physiol. **186**, 239 (1956).
IZQUIERDO, J. A., A. M. BISCARDI, and J. A. CARIZZONI: Detection of catechol amines through (vaıiation of) carotid pressure in rats previously treated with iproniazid. An. Farm. Quim. S. Paulo **11**, 43 (1960). [Chem. Abstr. **56**, 1959d (1962).]
JÄÄTELÄ, A. J., and M. K. PAASONEN: Effect of pyrocatechol on the change of noradrenaline content induced in rat brain by raunescine. Acta pharmacol. (Kbh.) 18, 95 (1961).
JACKSON, R. L., D. B. MEYERS, and J. W. MARTIN jr.: Effects of four phenylsubstituted 1:2:4-triazoles on various enzymic and respiratory activities, in vitro. Fed. Proc. **21**, 174 (1962).
JACOB, J., and P. ECHINARD-GARIN: Increased toxicity of digitaline in the guinea pig due to iproniazid and phenylisopropylhydrazine. Biochem. Pharmacol. 8, 108 (1961).
JACOBI, H. P., J. HAGGSTROM, D. ROSENBERG, M. KELLY and M. J. CARVER: Effects of phenothiazine derivatives on enzyme activity. Abstr. V. Int. Congr. Biochem., Moscow 18.70.2037 (1961).
JACOBY, G. A., and B. N. LA DU: Studies on the specificity of tyrosine-α-ketoglutarate transaminase. J. biol. Chem. **239**, 419 (1964).
JAKUBOVIČ, A., u. J. NEČINA: Der Einfluß von Methylenblau auf die Aktivität der Monoaminoxydase in Leber und Gehirn von Ratten nach verschiedener Applikation. Arzneimittel-Forsch. **13**, 134 (1963).
JENNEY, E. H., and C. C. PFEIFFER: The convulsant effect of hydrazides and the antidotal effect of anticonvulsants and metabolites. J. Pharmacol. exp. Ther. **122**, 110 (1958).

JENNEY, E. H., R. P. SMITH, and C. C. PFEIFFER: Pyridoxine as an antidote to semicarbazide seizure. Fed. Proc. **12**, 333 (1953).
JENNI, A., u. A. PLETSCHER: Monoaminoxydase-Hemmer. Schweiz. Apoth.-Ztg **100**, 177 (1962).
JEPSON, J. B., W. LOVENBERG, P. ZALTZMAN, J. A. OATES, A. SJOERDSMA, and S. UDENFRIEND: Amine metabolism, studied in normal and phenylketonuric humans by monoamine oxidase inhibition. Biochem. J. **74**, 5 P (1960).
JOHNSON, G. E., E. GORDON, and E. A. SELLERS: The influence of iproniazid and pyrogallol on the thermogenic effects of noradrenaline. Canad. J. Biochem. **40**, 631 (1962) [Psychopharmacol. Abstr. **2**, 477 (1962)].
— and E. A. SELLERS: The effects of reserpine, noradrenaline and inhibitors on the metabolic rate of rats. Fed. Proc. **19**, 297 (1960).
JOHNSON, P. C., and G. SEVELIUS: Effect of nitroglycerin, pentaerythritol tetranitrate and a new monoamine oxidase inhibitor on coronary blood flow and cardiac minute volume. Clin. Res. Proc. 8, 74 (1960).
JOLLES-BERGERET, B., J. LABOUESSE et F. CHATAGNER: Influence des hormones thyroidiennes sur la désulfuration de la cystéine par le foie de rat. Comparaison du comportement de la désulfuration avec celui d'autres réactions enzymatiques nécessitant le phosphate de pyridoxal. Bull. Soc. Chim. biol. (Paris) **42**, 51 (1960).
JORI, A., A. BUONACCORSI, L. VALZELLI, and S. GARATTINI: New orally active monoamine oxidase inhibitors. Life Sci. **1963**, 611.
— L. LAMESTA, e A. VALSECCHI: Variazioni glicemiche indotte dalla serotonina e da sostanze capaci di modificare il contenuto di serotoninia. Boll. Soc. ital. Biol. sper. **35**, 716 (1959).
JOYCE, D.: Changes in the 5-hydroxytryptamine content of rat, rabbit and human brain after death. Brit. J. Pharmacol. **18**, 370 (1962).
JUCKER, E.: Neuartige, basisch substituierte Hydrazine und ihre Anwendung in der Arzneimittelsynthese. Angew. Chem. **71**, 321 (1959).
JUVA, K., L. MIKKONEN, T. TUOMINEN, and E. KULONEN: Iproniazid and experimental lathyrism. Experientia (Basel) **15**, 350 (1959).
KABAKOW, B., B. WEINSTEIN, G. ROSS, and M. TRESSER: A clinical and metabolic study of metastatic carcinoid. Amer. J. Med. **26**, 636 (1959).
KADZIELAWA, K.: Mechanism of action of guanethidine. Brit. J. Pharmacol. **19**, 74 (1962).
KÄRKI, N., R. KUNTZMAN, and B. B. BRODIE: Norepinephrine and serotonin brain levels at various stages of ontogenetic development. Fed. Proc. **19**, 282 (1960).
— — — Storage, synthesis and metabolism of monoamines in the developing brain. J. Neurochem. **9**, 53 (1962).
KÄSER, H.: Die Bedeutung der 3-Methyoxy-4-hydroxy-mandelsäure (MHMS) für die Differentialdiagnostik neutraler Tumoren im Kindesalter. Schweiz. med. Wschr. **91**, 586 (1961).
—, and W. von STUDNITZ: Urine of childern with sympathetic tumors. Amer. J. Dis. Child. **102**, 199 (1961).
KAHLSON, G., and E. ROSENGREN: Inhibition of histamine formation and some of its consequences. J. Physiol. (Lond.) **149**, 66P (1959).
— — and S. E. SVENSSON: Inhibition of histamine formation in vivo. Nature (Lond.) **194**, 876 (1962).
— — and R. THUNBERG: Observations on the inhibition of histamine formation. J. Physiol. (Lond.) **169**, 467 (1963).
KAKIMOTO, Y., and M. D. ARMSTRONG: Identification of octopamine in animals treated with monoamine oxidase inhibitors. Fed. Proc. **19**, 295 (1960).
— — On the identification of octopamine in mammals. J. biol. Chem. **237**, 422 (1962).
KAKO, K., A. CHRYSOHOU, and R. J. BING: Factors affecting myocardial storage and release of catecholamines. Circulat. Res. **9**, 295 (1961).
KALBERMATTEN, J. P. DE: Effet de la sérotonine sur l'hypersensibilité de dénervation du ganglion sympathique cervical isolé du rat. Helv. physiol. pharmacol. Acta **20**, 294 (1962).
KALIMAN, P. A.: Enzymatic oxidation of adrenaline, noradrenaline and tyramine in the liver and heart of rabbits. Biokhimiya **26**, 256 (1961) [Engl. Ed.].
KALYANKAR, G. D., and E. E. SNELL: Pyridoxal-catalyzed decarboxylation of amino acids. Biochemistry **4**, 594 (1962).
KAMESWARAN, L., J. M. TELFORD, and G. B. WEST: Histamine formation in the rat. J. Physiol. (Lond.) **157**, 23P (1961).
—, and G. B. WEST: Histidine decarboxylase in rat hepatoma. J. Pharm. Pharmacol. **13**, 191 (1961).
KAMIJO, K., G. B. KOELLE, and H. H. WAGNER: Modification of the effect of sympathomimetic amines and of adrenergic nerve stimulation by 1-isonicotinyl-2-isopropylhydrazine (IIH) and isonicotinic acid hydrazide (INH). J. Pharmacol. exp. Ther. **117**, 213 (1956).

KAMINSKI, D., B. DUBNICK, and F. E. ANDERSON: Monoamine oxidase inhibitors. Hydrazine derivatives. J. med. Chem. **7**, 367 (1964).
KANAOKA, Y., H. WEISSBACH, T. E. SMITH, and B. WITKOP: Oxidation of kynuramine derivatives by monoamine oxidase and the enzymatic conversion of dihydronorkynuramine to indigo. J. Amer. chem. Soc. **83**, 732 (1961).
KAPELLER-ADLER, R., u. J. KRAEL: Untersuchungen über die Stickstoffverteilung in den Muskeln verschiedener Tierklassen. Biochem. Z. **221**, 437 (1930).
— — Über das Schicksal der mit der Nahrung aufgenommenen Alkylamine und über deren angebliche Entmethylierung im Organismus sowie über das Vorkommen von Monomethylamin im normalen Harn. Biochem. Z. **235**, 394 (1931).
—, and H. MACFARLANE: Purification and identification of hog-kidney histaminase. Biochim. biophys. Acta (Amst.) **67**, 542 (1963).
KAPLAN, N. O.: Coenzyme metabolism of the brain. In: The Neurochemistry of nucleotides and amino acids, p. 70, edit. R. O. BRADY and D. B. TOWER. New York: Wiley 1960.
— M. M. CIOTTI, J. VAN EYS, and R. M. BURTON: Effect of pyridine derivatives on animal tissue, diphosphopyridine nucleotitidases. J. biol. Chem. **234**, 134 (1959).
— — and F. E. STOLZENBACH: Studies on the interaction of diphosphopyridine nucleotide analogs with dehydrogenases. Arch. Biochem. **69**, 441 (1957).
KATZ, R., J. KLINGER, L. SILVA, J. RODRIGUEZ, and H. DUCCI: Serial hepatic study in patients treated with iproniazid. Ann. N.Y. Acad. Sci. **80**, 898 (1959).
KEASLING, H. H., R. R. RUSSEL, and H. J. TREIZENBERG: The comparative effects of etryptamine, pheneline and isocarboxazide on electroshock thresholds. Pharmacologist **4**, 182 (1962).
KEGLEVIĆ, D., Z. SUPEK, S. KVEDER, S. JSKRIĆ, S. KEČKEČ, and A. KISIČ: The metabolism of exogenous ^{14}C-labelled 5-hydroxytryptamine in rats. Biochem. J. **73**, 53 (1959).
KELLER, R.: Der Einfluß von Iproniazid auf den Histamin-Stoffwechsel der Albinoratte in vivo. Arzneimittel-Forsch. **9**, 346 (1959).
— Histaminfreisetzung und proteolytische Aktivität unter verschiedenen Versuchsbedingungen. Helv. physiol. pharmacol. Acta **18**, C 85 (1960a).
— Beeinflussung der proteolytischen Aktivität in Geweben durch Iproniazid. Naturwissenschaften **47**, 379 (1960b).
KIM, K. S., and P. A. SHORE: Mechanism of action of reserpine and insulin on gastric amines and gastric acid secretion, and the effect of monoamine oxidase inhibition. J. Pharmacol. exp. Ther. **141**, 321 (1963).
KIRBERGER, E.: Variable action of monoamine oxidase-inhibiting hydrazines on serotonin metabolism. Nature (Lond.) **197**, 1211 (1963).
KIRKENDALL, W. M., and W. R. WILSON: Pharmacodynamics and clinical use of guanethidine, bretylium and methyldopa. Amer. J. Cardiol. **9**, 107 (1962).
KIRSHNER, N., C. MCGOODALL, and L. ROSEN: The effect of iproniazid on the metabolism of DL-epinephrine-2-C^{14} in the human. J. Pharmacol. exp. Ther. **127**, 1 (1959).
— L. TERRY, and D. D. POLLARD: The metabolism of DL-adrenaline-2-C^{14} in the cat. I. Urinary catabolites. Arch. int. Pharmacodyn. **131**, 421 (1961).
KISHI, S., B. ASANO, S. ICHII, and K. ASHIKAWA: Monoamine oxidase activity in the liver of rats fed on hepatic carcinogen. Gann **47**, 223 (1956). [Excerpta med. (Amst.), Sect. V, **10**, Abstr. Nr. 627 (1957).]
KIVALO, E., and U. K. RINNE: Activity of the hypothalamo-neurohypophysical neurosecretory system after iproniazid treatment. Ann. Med. exp. Fenn. **39**, 50 (1961).
— — and H. KARINKANTA: The effect of imipramine on the 5-hydroxytryptamine content and monoamine oxidase activity of the rat brain and on the excretion of 5-hydroxyindole acetic acid. J. Neurochem. 8, 105 (1961).
KIZER, D. E., and S. K. CHAN: The effect of azo-dye carcinogenesis on rat liver 5-hydroxytryptophan decarboxylase. Proc. Amer. Ass. Cancer Res. **3**, 126 (1960).
— — The effect of hepatocarcinogenesis upon 5-hydroxytryptophan decarboxylase and serotonin deaminase. Cancer Res. **21**, 489 (1961).
KLEIN, K.: Klinisch-experimentelle Untersuchungen über die Wirkung von Niamid auf Haemodynamik und Gerinnung. Chemotherapia (Basel) **4**, 203 (1962a).
— Dynamographische Untersuchungen über die Beeinflussung zerebraler Kreislaufgrößen durch den „Monoaminoxydase-Hemmer" Niamid. Med. Klin. **57**, 1089 (1962b).
KLINGMAN, G. I.: Effects of immunosympathectomy on catecholamine levels and dopa decarboxylase activity in peripheral tissues of the rat. Fed. Proc. **23**, 455 (1964).
— S. KARDAMAN, and J. HABER: Amine levels, monoamine oxidase and dopa-decarboxylase activities in the gastro-intestinal tract of the rat. Life Sci. **3**, 1355 (1964).
KNICK, B.: Klinische und experimentelle Daten zu den neurohumoralen Gefäß- und Gewebswirkungen von Nialamid bei cardiovasculären und Stoffwechselerkrankungen. Chemotherapia (Basel) **4**, 297 (1962).

KNOLL, J., and B. KNOLL: Reserpine: modification of its tranquilizer effect and analysis of its central mode of action. Arch. int Pharmacodyn. **133**, 310 (1961).
KOBAYASHI, Y.: A histamine metabolizing enzyme system of mouse liver. Arch Biochem. **71**, 352 (1957).
— Effect of x-irradiation on histidine decarboxylase of rat stomach and intestine. Fed. Proc. **21**, 424 (1962).
—, and T. OKUYAMA: Recovery of diamine oxidase activity inhibited by isonicotinic acid hydrazide and its derivatives. Biochem. Pharamocol. **11**, 949 (1962).
—, and R. W. SCHAYER: Action of rat liver monoamine oxidase on multiple substrates. Arch. Biochem. **58**, 181 (1955).
KOBINGER, W.: Beeinflussung der Cardiazolkrampfschwelle durch veränderten 5-Hydroxytryptamin-gehalt des Zentralnervensystems. Naunyn-Schmiedebergs Arch. exp. Path. Pharmak. **233**, 559 (1958).
— Förderung von Streckkrämpfen und experimentelle Katatonie. Naunyn-Schmiedebergs Arch. exp. Path. Pharmak. **236**, 123 (1959).
—, u. N. F. FRIIS: Beeinflussung von Gefäßreaktionen am isolierten Kaninchenohr durch Monoaminoxydasehemmkörper. Naunyn-Schmiedebergs Arch. exp. Path. Pharmak. **242**, 238 (1961).
KOECHLIN, B. A., and V. ILIEV: Metabolism of iproniazid. Ann. N. Y. Acad. Sci. **80**, 864 (1959).
— M. A. SCHWARTZ, and W. E. OBERHAENSLI: Metabolism of C^{14}-iproniazid and C^{14}-isocarboxazid in man. J. Pharmacol. exp. Ther. **138**, 11 (1962).
KOELLE, G. B.: Pharmacologic significance of inhibition of monoamine oxidase. J. clin exp. Psychopath. **19**, Suppl. **1**, 37 (1958).
— Possible mechanisms for the termination of the physiological actions of catecholamines. Pharmacol. Rev. **11**, 381 (1959).
—, and A. DE T. VALK jr.: Physiological implications of the histochemical localization of monoamine oxidase. J. Physiol. (Lond.) **126**, 434 (1954).
KOESSLER, K. K., and M. T. HANKE: Studies on proteinogenous amines. IV. The production of histamine from histidine by bacillus coli communis. J. biol. Chem. **39**, 539 (1919).
KOHN, H. I.: CCXII. Tyramine oxidase. Biochem. J. **31**, 1693 (1937).
KOHN, R.: Methylamin als Zwischenprodukt des Glykokollabbaues in der überlebenden Leber. Hoppe-Seylers Z. physiol. Chem. **200**, 191 (1931).
KOIVUSALO, M., I. PENTILLÄ, A. RAINA, and R. TENHUNEN: Effect of hydrazides on liver alanine and aspartate transaminase and lactate dehydrogenase in developing chick embryo. Acta physiol. scand. **57**, 454 (1963).
KOPIN, I. J.: Technique for the study of alternate metabolic pathways; epinephrine metabolism in man. Science **131**, 1372 (1960).
— Storage and metabolism of catecholamines: the role of monoamine oxidase. Pharmacol. Rev. **16**, 179 (1964).
—, and J. AXELROD: The metabolic fate of epinephrine in the rat. Fed. Proc. **19**, 295 (1960).
— —, and E. K. GORDON: The metabolic fate of H^3-epinephrine and C^{14}-metanephrine in the rat. J. biol. Chem. **236**, 2109 (1961).
— J. E. FISCHER, J. MUSACCHIO, and W. D. HORST: Induction of false neurochemical transmitters as a mechanism for the sympathetic blocking action of monoamine oxidase inhibitors (MAOI). Pharmacologist **6**, 175 (1964).
— — — — Evidence for a false neurochemical transmitter as mechanism for the hypotensive effect of monoamine oxidase inhibitors. Proc. nat. Acad. Sci. (Wash.) **52**, 716 (1964).
—, and E. K. GORDON: Metabolism of administered and drug-released norepinephrine-7-H^3 in the rat. J. Pharmacol. exp. Ther. **140**, 207 (1963).
— G. HERTTING, and E. K. GORDON: Fate of norepinephrine-H^3 in the isolated perfused rat heart. J. Pharmacol. exp. Ther. **138**, 34 (1962).
KORY, M., and E. MINGIOLI: Volatile amine oxidase inhibitor from hydrazine derivative. Biochem. Pharmacol. **13**, 577 (1964).
KOSOWER, E. M.: Molecular Biochemistry, p. 71. New York: McGraw-Hill Book Co. Inc. 1962.
KOTHARIN, N. J., J. C. SAUNDERS, and N. S. KLINE: Effect of phenothiazines and hydrazines on pituitary-adrenal-cortical response. Psychopharmacologia (Berl.) **2**, 22 (1961).
KRAUPP, O., H. BERNHEIMER, P. HEISTRACHER, D. PAPISTAS u. Th. SCHIEFTHALER: Die Wirkung von Iproniazid sowie i.p. Zufuhr von Catecholaminen und ihrer O-Methylderivate auf die renale Ausscheidung von Metanephrin und Normetanephrin an der Ratte. Naunyn-Schmiedebergs Arch. exp. Path. Pharmak. **243**, 459 (1962).
— H. STORMANN, H. BERNHEIMER u. H. OBENAUS: Vorkommen und diagnostische Bedeutung von Phenolsäuren im Harn beim Phaeochromocytom. Klin. Wschr. **37**, 76 (1959).
KRAUSE, D.: Der Einfluß von Iproniazid und l-Phenyl-2-hydrazinopropan auf die Wirkung von Hexobarbital. Naunyn-Schmiedebergs Arch. exp. Path. Pharmak. **240**, 21 (1960).

KRAYER, O.: In: Symposium on Catecholamines. Pharmaccl. Rev. **11**, 233 (1959).
KREZANOSKI, J. Z.: Effects of iproniazid on tetrahymena pyriformis. J. pharm. Sci. **50**, 421 (1961).
KRISHNA, N., M. J. MANN, and J. H. LEOPOLD: Manometric determination of monoamine oxidase in ocular tissues. Arch. Ophthal. **65**, 338 (1961).
KRONEBERG, G. u. H. G. KURBJUWEIT: Die Beeinflussung von experimentellem Fieber durch Reserpin und Sympathicolytica am Kaninchen. Arzneimittel-Forsch. **9**, 556 (1959).
—, H. J. SCHÜMANN: Der Einfluß von Iproniazid auf die durch Reserpin gesteigerte Sekretion des Kaninchennebennierenmarks. Naunyn-Schmiedebergs Arch. exp. Path. Pharmak. **239**, 29 (1960).
—, u. K. STOEPEL: Zum Wirkungsmechanismus von α-Methyldopa. Naunyn-Schmiedebergs Arch. exp. Path. Pharmak. **246**, 11 (1963).
KRUEGER, A. P., and R. F. SMITH: The biological mechanisms of air ion action. I. 5-Hydroxytryptamine as the endogenous mediator of positive air ion effects on the mammalian trachea. J. gen. Physiol. **43**, 533 (1960).
KRUEGER-THIEMER, E.: Chemismus der Isoniazidspaltung durch Hämin. Naturwissenschaften **42**, 47 (1955).
KRUGER, S., W. C. STANDEFFER, and F. W. SCHUELER: Some effects of reserpine on normal and leukemic mice. Arch. int. Pharmacodyn. **129**, 395 (1960).
KUBIKOWSKI, P., and J. WYSOKOWSKI: The influence of some hypotensive drugs and diuretics on the level of catecholamines and monoamine oxidase activity in brain and in blood. Biochem. Pharmacol. **12**, Suppl., 31 (1963).
KUNTZMAN, R., E. COSTA, G. L. GESSA, C. W. HIRSCH, and B. B. BRODIE: Combined use of α-methyl meta-tyrosine (MMT) and reserpine to associate norepinephrine (NE) with excitation and serotonin (5-HT) with sedation. Fed. Proc. **20**, 308 (1961a).
— — C. R. CREVELING, C. W. HIRSCH, and B. B. BRODIE: Blockade in vivo of dopamine β-hydroxylase by NSD 1024 and NSD 1034, isosteres of α-methyl-m-tyramine. Fred. Proc. **21**, 365 (1962a).
— — — — — Inhibition of norepinephrine synthesis in mouse brain by blockade of dopamine-β-oxidase. Life Sci. **1962** b, 85.
—, and M. M. JACOBSON: Monoamine oxidase inhibition by a series of compounds structurally related to bretylium and guanethidine. J. Pharmacol. exp. Ther. **141**, 166 (1963a).
— — The inhibition of monoamine oxidase by benzyl and phenethylguanidines related to bretylium and guanethidine. Ann. N.Y. Acad. Sci. **107**, 945 (1963b).
— P. A. SHORE, D. BOGDANSKI, and B. B. BRODIE: Microanalytical procedures for fluorometric assay of brain dopa-5-HTP decarboxylase, norepinephrine and serotonin, and a detailed mapping of decarboxylase activity in brain. J. Neurochem. **6**, 225 (1961b).
—, and S. SPECTOR: Impairment of catecholamine binding sites in brain by reserpine. Fed. Proc. **19**, 282 (1960).
KUNZ, E.: Vergleichende Wirkung von zwei Decarboxylasehemmern auf den Metabolismus von endogenem und exogenem 5-Hydroxytryptamin. Arch. int. Pharmacodyn. **147**, 1 (1964).
KUSS, E., u. R. JÄGER: Zur Frage der Geburtsauslösung durch Serotonin. Klin. Wschr. **40**, 917 (1962).
KUZNETS, E. I., V. S. SHASHKOV, M. N. TER-VAR-TANIAN, N. N. PREOBRAZHENSKAIA, T. P. SUVOROV, T. P. SYCHEVA, and M. N. SHCHUKINA: Variations in activity of some monoamine oxidase inhibitors in vitro and in vivo. Psychopharmacol. Abstr. **1**, 414 (1961). [Dokl. Akad. Nauk SSSR **136**, 1231 (1961).]
LABOUESSE, J., F. CHATAGNER et B. BERGERET: Comparaison de la régulation, in vivo, par les hormones ovariennes du taux de deux décarboxylases d'acides aminés dans le foie du rat. Biochim. biophys. Acta (Amst.) **35**, 226 (1959).
LABROSSE, E. H.: Effect of iproniazid and amino acid loads on urinary excretion of tryptamine and indole acetic acid by schizophrenic patients. Fed. Proc. **20**, 169 (1961).
— J. AXELROD, I. J. KOPIN, and S. KETY: Metabolism of 7-H^3-epinephrine-d-bitartrate in normal young men. J. clin. Invest. **40**, 253 (1961).
— — and A. SJOERDSMA: Urinary excretion of normetanephrine by man. Fed. Proc. **17**, 386 (1958).
—, and M. KARON: Metabolism of 2-C^{14}-Dopa in a patient with neuroblastoma. Fed. Proc. **21**, 360 (1962).
LACROIX, E., et I. LEUSEN: Action inotrope des amines sympathomimétiques et activité phosphorylasique du coeur de rat isolé. Arch. int. Pharmacodyn **133**, 89 (1961).
— P. VANHOUTTE et I. LEUSEN: L'activité phosphorylasique du myocarde sous l'influence de la réserpine. Arch. int. Pharmacodyn. **138**, 329 (1962a).
— J. WEYNE et I. LEUSEN: Influence de la tyramine sur l'activité phosphorylasique cardiaque chez le rat traité par l'iproniazide. C. R. Soc. Biol. (Paris) **156**, 972 (1962b).

La Du, B. N., L. E. Gaudette, N. Trousof, and B. B. Brodie: Enzymatic dealkylation of aminopyrine (Pyramidon) and other alkylamines. J. biol. Chem. **214**, 741 (1955).
Läuppi, E. u. M. Piller: Bemerkungen zur Toxizität von „Tersavid" und analoger Derivate. Cardiologia (Basel) **37**, Suppl. II. 87 (1960).
— K. Schärer u. A. Studer: Zur Frage einer eventuell bestehenden Lebertoxizität von Iproniazid. Psychiat. et Neurol. (Basel) **140**, 241 (1960).
Lagnado, J. R.: Unpublished results; mentioned in T. L. Sourkes: Oxidative pathways in the metabolism of biogenic amines; Rev. canad. Biol, **17**, 328 (1958).
—, and T. L. Sourkes: The enzymatic reduction of tetrazolium salts by amines. Canad. J. Biochem. **34**, 1095 (1956a).
— — Inhibition of amine oxidase by metal ions and by sulphydryl compounds. Canad. J. Biochem. **34**, 1185 (1956b).
— — Cofactor requirements of amine dehydrogenase system of rat liver and brain. II. The effects of some purines and purine derivatives on amine dehydrogenase (AD) activity. Rev. canad. Biol. **15**, 258 (1956c).
— — Further observations on the enzymatic reduction of tetrazolium salts by monoamines. Canad. J. Biochem **36**, 587 (1958).
Lagunoff, D., and E. P. Benditt: 5-Hydroxytryptophan decarboxylase activity in rat mast cells. Amer. J. Physiol. **196**, 993 (1959).
Lamesta, L., A. Valsecchi e L. Valzelli: Variazioni glicemiche indotte dalla reserpina e da alcuni suoi nuovi derivati. Boll. Soc. ital. Biol. sper. **36**, 683 (1960).
Langemann, H.: Weitere Untersuchungen über das Vorkommen der Cholinesterase und der Monoaminoxydase in menschlichen Organen. 3. Mitteilung über Bestimmungen der Fermentaktivität in normalen und pathologisch veränderten Organen. Helv. physiol. pharmacol. Acta **2**, 367 (1944).
— Enzymes and their substrates in the adrenal gland of the ox. Brit. J. Pharmacol. **6**, 318 (1951).
— Aminoacid decarboxylase and amine oxidase in carcinoid tumor. In: 5-Hydroxytryptamin, p. 153, edit. G. P. Lewis, London and New York: Pergamon Press 1958.
—, u. H. Ackermann: Über die Aktivität der Aminosäuren-Decarboxylasen im Gehirn des Menschen. Helv. physiol. pharmacol. Acta **19**, 399 (1961).
— A. Boner u. P. B. Müller: Aminosäurendecarboxylase in Phäochromocytom- und Karzinoidgewebe. Schweiz. med. Wschr. **92**, 1621 (1962).
— F. Roulet u. E. A. Zeller: Fermentuntersuchungen an gesunden und tuberkulösen menschlichen Lungen. Klin. Wschr. **22**, 644 (1943).
Langendorff, H., u. U. Hagen: Die Wirkung einer Röntgenbestrahlung auf die Aktivität der 5-Hydroxytryptophan-Decarboxylase. Naturwissenschaften **50**, 665 (1963).
— G. Scheuerbrandt, C. Streffer u. H.-J. Melching: Die Wirkung einer Ganzkörperbestrahlung von Mäusen auf die Aktivität der Decarboxylase aromatischer Aminosäuren in Leber und Milz. Naturwissenschaften **51**, 290 (1964).
Laroche, M.-J., and B. B. Brodie: Lack of relationship between inhibition of monoamine oxidase and potentiation of hexobarbital hypnosis. J. Pharmacol. exp. Ther. **130**, 134 (1960).
Lasker, S. E., and C. L. Fox jr.: Protective effect of histamine: L-histidine and their metabolites on E. coli endotoxin shock in mice. Clin. Res. Proc. **8**, 31 (1960a).
— — The comparative protective action of histamine, l-histidine and their metabolites on endotoxin and thermal shock in mice. Fed. Proc. **19**, 103 (1960b).
Lauer, J. W., W. M. Inskip, J. Bernsohn, and E. A. Zeller: Observations on schizophrenic patients after iproniazid and tryptophan. Arch. Neurol. Psychiat. (Chic.) **80**, 122 (1958).
Lazanas, J. C., and E. A. Zeller: On the active site of diamine oxidases. 134th Meeting Amer. chem. Soc., Abstr. 1c (1958).
Leak, D., and T. L. Dormandy: Possible relations of hypoglycaemia induced by monoamine oxidase inhibition and angina pectoris. Proc. Soc. exp. Biol. (N. Y.) **108**, 597 (1961).
Lechat, P., et M. Lemeignan: Inhibiteurs de la monoaminoxydase et potentialisation du sommeil expérimental. Biochem. Pharmacol. **8**, 7 (1961).
Lee, W. C., Y. H. Shin, and F. E. Shideman: Cardiac activities of several monoamine oxidase inhibitors. J. Pharmacol. exp. Ther. **133**, 180 (1961).
Leeper, L. C., H. Weissbach, and S. Udenfriend: Studies on the metabolism of norepinephrine and their O-methyl analogs by partially purified enzyme preparations. Arch. Biochem. **77**, 417 (1958).
Leeson, G. A., B. Dubnick, and C. C. Scott: Effect of forms of vitamin B_6 on acute toxicity of β-phenylethylhydrazine. Fed. Proc. **18**, 414 (1959).
Lehmann, A., et M.-C. Busnel: Antagonismes entre la réserpine, la tétrabenazine, le carbamate de méthylpentynol et leur association avec l'iproniazide étudiés avec le test de la crise audiogène de la souris. In: Neuropsychopharmacology ,vol. **2**, p. 348, edit. E. Rothlin. Amsterdam: Elsevier Publ. Co. 1959.

LEHMANN, A., et R. G. BUSNEL: Etude sur la crise audiogène. Arch. Sci. physiol. **31**, 193 (1959).
— — A new test for MAOI detecting effects. Biochem. Pharmacol. 8, 8 (1961).
— — A new test for detecting MAO inhibitor effects. Int. J. Neuropharmacol. **1**, 61 (1962).
LEROY, J. G.: 5-Hydroxytryptamine levels in brain of mice pretreated with α-methyldopa. Arch. int. Pharmacodyn. **134**, 492 (1961).
—, and A. F. DE SCHAEPDRYVER: Catecholamine levels of brain and heart in mice after iproniazid syrosingopine and 10-methoxy-deserpidine. Arch. int Pharmacodyn. **130**, 231 (1961).
LEŠIĆ, R., and V. VARAGIĆ: Factors influencing the hypertensive effect of eserine in the rat. Brit. J. Pharmacol. **16**, 99 (1961).
LESPAGNOL, A., D. BAR, R. OSTEUX, A. ROBELET et C. MIZON-CAPRON: Action de phénylhydrazines sulfamidées sur la monoaminoxydase et la diaminoxydase. Ann. pharm. franç. **22**, 417 (1964).
LESSIN, A. W.: The pharmacological evaluation of monoamine oxidase inhibitors. Biochem. Pharmacol. **2**, 296 (1959a).
— Pharmacological methods of estimating inhibition of drug oxidation in the mouse. Brit. J. Pharmacol. **14**, 251 (1959b).
—, and M. W. PARKES: The effects of reserpine and other agents upon leptazol convulsions in mice. Brit. J. Pharmacol. **14**, 108 (1959).
LEUSEN, I.: Discussion of the paper: Iproniazid and other MAO inhibitors. Ann. N. Y. Acad. Sci. **80**, 636 (1959a).
— Discussion of the paper: Serotonin and the heart. Ann. N. Y. Acad. Sci. **80**, 963 (1959b).
— Pharmacological effects of monoamine oxidase inhibitors. Cardiologia (Basel) **37**, Suppl. 2, 18 (1960).
—, E. LACROIX, and G. DEMEESTER: Influence of iproniazid pretreatment on formation of gastric ulcers by reserpine in the rat. Experientia (Basel) **15**, 73 (1959).
— H. THOENEN et E. LACROIX: L'iproniazide et l'hypersécrétion gastrique postréserpinique. Arch. int. Pharmacodyn. **141**, 190 (1963).
LEVENE, C. I.: Structural requirements for lathyrogenic agents. J. exp. Med. **114**, 295 (1961).
LEVI, R., and E. W. MAYNERT: The subcellular localization of brain-stem norepinephrine and 5-hydroxytryptamine in stressed rats. Biochem. Pharmacol. **13**, 615 (1964).
LEVINE, R. J.: Inhibition of monoamine oxidase activity in sympathetic ganglia of the cat. Biochem. Pharmacol. **11**, 395 (1962).
—, and A. SJOERDSMA: Direct measurement of monoamine oxidase (MAO) inhibition in humans. Fed. Proc. **21**, 179 (1962a).
— — Monoamine oxidase acticity in human tissues and intestinal biopsy specimens. Proc. Soc. exp. Biol. (N. Y.) **109**, 225 (1962b).
— — Direct measurement of monoamine oxidase inhibition in humans. Clin. Pharmacol. Ther. **4**, 22 (1963a).
— — Estimation of monoamine oxidase activity in man: Techniques and applications. Ann. N.Y. Acad. Sci. **107**, 966 (1963b).
— — Dissociation of the decarboxylase-inhibiting and norepinephrine-depleting effects of α-methyl-dopa, α-ethyl-dopa, 4-bromo-3-hydroxyl-benzyloxyamine and related substances. J. Pharmacol. exp. Ther. **146**, 42 (1964).
LÉVY, B., and R. P. AHLQUIST: A study of sympathetic ganglionic stimulants. J. Pharmacol. exp. Ther. **137**, 219 (1962).
LÉVY, J., et E. MICHEL-BER: Hypothèse sur les mécanismes d'action des inhibiteurs de la monoamino-oxydase au niveau du système nerveux central. C. R. Acad. Sci. (Paris) **250**, 415 (1960a).
— — Antagonisme pharmacologique entre le pyridoxal-5-phosphate (activateur de la dopa-décarboxylase) et certains hydrazines (inhibiteurs de la monoamine-oxydase). C. R. Acad. Sci. (Paris) **250**, 4061 (1960b).
— — Mécanismes d'action des inhibiteurs de la monoamine-oxydase (hydrazides et hydrazines) au niveau du système nerveux central: faits expérimentaux et hypothèses. J. Physiol. (Paris) **52**, 789 (1960c).
— — Sur les relations entre le mécanisme d'action de quelques substances psychotropes et le taux cérébral des amines biogènes ou de leurs précurseurs. Encéphale **51**, 132 (1962).
LEWIS, J. J., and G. R. VAN PETTEN: The effect of antidepressive drugs and some related compounds on the levels of adenine nucleotides, inorganic phosphate and phosphocreatine in the rat brain. Brit. J. Pharmacol. **20**, 462 (1963).
LIBERMANN, D., et J. D. DENIS: Sur quelques nouveaux isopropylhydrazides inhibiteurs de la monoamino-oxydase, synthétisés à partir d'action physiologiquement active. Bull. Soc. chim. Fr. **1961**, 1952.
LIBERSON, W. T.: Electroencephalography. Amer. J. Psychol. **116**, 584 (1960).

LIEPINS, K. W., A. C. IVY, and R. SUZUCKI: Effect of certain histaminase inhibitors on gastric secretion. Amer. J. Physiol. **195**, 209 (1958).
LINDAHL, K. M., S. E. LINDELL, H. WESTLING, and T. WHITE: Histamine degradation in tissue extracts form the cat. Acta physiol. scand. **38**, 280 (1957).
LINDBERG, S., and H. WESTLING: Placental monoamine-oxidase activity and toxaemia of pregnancy. Lancet **1962** II, 46.
LINDELL, S. E.: The effect of iproniazid on the blood pressure responses in dogs to histamine injected into the renal artery. Acta physiol. scand. **41**, 255 (1957).
— K. NILSSON, B.-E. ROSS, and H. WESTLING: The effect of enzyme inhibitors of histamine catabolism in man. Brit. J. Pharmacol. **15**, 351 (1960).
—, and H. WESTLING: Enzymic oxidation of some substances related to histamine. Acta physiol. scand. **39**, 370 (1957).
LINDSAY, D., E. POULSON, and J. M. ROBSON: Effects of 5-hydroxytryptamine and of an amineoxidase inhibitor on decidual tissue. J. Endocr. **22**, V (1961a).
— — — The effect of 5-hydroxytryptamine and of an amine oxidase inhibitor on experimental deciduomata in mice. J. Endocr. **23**, 209 (1961b).
LOGEMANN, W., F. LAURIA, and D. ARTINI: Methanesulphonic acid derivatives of central stimulant drugs. Nature (Lond.) **185**, 532 (1960).
LONG, R. F.: Some studies with reversible monoamineoxidase inhibitors. Biochem. J. **82**, 3P (1962a).
— Reversible inhibition of brain monoamine oxidase in vitro and in vivo. Int. Neurochem. Symposium on Enzyme Activity of the Central Nervous System, Göteborg 1962b, p. 27.
— Unpublished results.
—, and A. W. LESSIN: Inhibition of 5-hydroxytryptamine uptake by platelets in vitro and in vivo. Biochem. J. **82**, 4P (1962).
LOOMER, H. P., J. C. SAUNDERS, and N. S. KLINE: A clinical and pharmacodynamic evaluation of iproniazid as a psychic energizer. Psychiat. Res. Rep. Amer. psychiat. Ass. **8**, 129 (1958).
LOPES DO ROSÁRIO, J. A.: Influence of an inhibitor of amine oxidase on the urinary elimination of neutral 17-keto steroids and hydroxy corticosteroids. Arch. port. Bioquim. **4**, 237 (1959/60). [Chem. Abstr. **56**, 904h (1962).]
—, and J. M. FRAGOSO MENDES: Urinary excretion of 5-hydroxyindolacetic acid in cases of depression treated with nialamide. Simpósio internacional sobre Nialamida, J. Soc. Ciénc. méd Lisboa **123**, Suppl., 136 (1959).
LORES ARNAIZ, R. G. DE, and E. DE ROBERTIS: Cholinergic and non-cholinergic nerve endings in the rat brain. II. Subcellular localization of monoamine oxidase and succinate dehydrogenase. J. Neurochem. **9**, 503 (1962).
— — 5-Hydroxytryptophan decarboxylase activity in nerve endings of the rat brain. J. Neurochem. **11**, 213 (1964).
LOTLIKAR, P. D., and R. S. MCCUTCHEON: Inhibition of mitochondrial monoamine oxidase of canine spleen and liver by l-isonicotinyl-2-isopropylhydrazine (Iproniazid). J. pharm. Sci. **50**, 568 (1961).
LOVAŠEN, Ž., Z. SUPEK, and M. RANDIĆ: The oxytoxic activity of DL-5-hydroxytryptophan. J. Pharm. Pharmacol. **13**, 565 (1961).
LOVELL, R. A., S. J. ELLIOTT, and K. A. C. ELLIOTT: The γ-aminobutyric acid and factor I content of brain. J. Neurochem. **10**, 479 (1963).
LOVENBERG, W., J. BARCHAS, H. WEISSBACH, and S. UDENFRIEND: Characteristics of the inhibition of aromatic L-amino acid decarboxylase by α-methyl amino acids. Arch. Biochem. **103**, 9 (1963).
— R. J. LEVINE, and A. SJOERDSMA: Sensitive assay of monoamine oxidase activity; application to sympathetic ganglia and heart. Fed. Proc. **20**, 318 (1961).
— — — A sensitive assay of monoamine oxidase activity in vitro: application to heart and sympathetic ganglia. J. Pharmacol. exp. Ther. **135**, 7 (1962a).
— H. WEISSBACH, and S. UDENFRIEND: Aromatic L-amino acid decarboxylase. J. biol. Chem. **237**, 89 (1962b).
LUSCHINSKY, H. L.: Quantitative estimation of monoamine oxidase in placenta in normal pregnancy and toxemia. Amer. J. Obstet. Gynec. **59**, 906 (1950).
—, and H. O. SINGHER: Identification and assay of monoamine oxidase in the human placenta. Arch. Biochem. **19**, 95 (1948).
LUTWACK, R., H. F. MOWER, and C. NIEMANN: The α-chymotrypsin-catalyzed hydrolysis of a series of hydrazides. II. Evaluation of the kinetic constants for aqueous system at 25° and at the optimum pH for each specific substrate. J. Amer. chem. Soc. **79**, 5690 (1957).
MAASS, A. R., and M. J. NIMMO: A new inhibitor of serotonin metabolism. Nature (Lond.) **184**, 547 (1959).

MACKAY, D., J. F. RILEY, and D. M. SHEPHERD: Amino acid decarboxylase activities in rat hepatoma. J. Pharm. Pharmacol. **13**, 257 (1961).
—, and D. M. SHEPHERD: A study of potential histidine decarboxylase inhibitors. Brit. J. Pharmacol. **15**, 552 (1960).
— — Inhibition of histidine decarboxylase and interaction of the inhibitors with pyridoxal-5'-phosphate. Biochim. biophys. Acta (Amst.) **59**, 553 (1962).
MAFFII, G., and D. COSTANTINI: Effects of drugs on timing behaviour. Biochem. Pharmacol. **8**, 61 (1961).
MAGISTRETTI, M., and M. PEIRONE: The action of carbon disulphide on cerebral monoamine oxidase. Med. d. Lavoro **52**, 1 (1961). [Psychopharmacol. Abstr. **1**, 336 (1961).]
MAHER, J. R., J. F. SPEYER, and M. LEVINE: Studies on the mode of action of isoniazid. I. The role of trace metals in the inhibition of bovine liver catalase by isoniazid. Amer. Rev. Tuberc. **77**, 501 (1958).
MAICKEL, R. P., and B. B. BRODIE: Increase in rat liver tryptophan peroxidase as a response to pituitary-adrenal stimulation by various centrally acting drugs. Fed. Proc. **19**, 267 (1960).
MAÎTRE, L., and M. STAEHELIN: Effect of α-methyl-dopa on myocardial catecholamines. Experientia (Basel) **19**, 573 (1963).
MAJOR, R. T., and K. W. OHLY: Derivatives of hydroxylamine: central nervous system stimulants. J. med. pharm. Chem. **4**, 51 (1961).
MALAFAYA-BAPTISTA, A., J. GARRETT, W. OSSWALD u. M. F. MALAFAYA-BAPTISTA: pH-Beeinflussung der Aminoxydase-Aktivität. Naunyn-Schmiedebergs Arch. exp. Path. Pharmak. **230**, 10 (1957).
MALING, H. M., B. HIGHMAN, and S. SPECTOR: Neurologic and neuropathologic effects of prolonged administration of JB 516, JB 835 and other monoamine oxidase inhibitors. Fed. Proc. **20**, 322 (1961).
— — — Neurologic, neuropathologic and neurochemical effects of prolonged administration of phenylisopropylhydrazine (JB 516), phenylisobutylhydrazine (JB 835) and other monoamine oxidase inhibitors. J. Pharmacol. exp. Ther. **137**, 334 (1962).
MANDELES, S., R. KOPPELMAN, and M. E. HANKE: Deuterium studies on the mechanism of enzymatic amino acid decarboxylation. J. biol. Chem. **209**, 327 (1954).
MANGER, W. M., K. G. WAKIM, and J. L. BOLLMAN: Chemical quantitation of epinephrine and norepinephrine in plasma, p. 309. Springfield (Ill.): Ch. C. Thomas 1959.
MANN, P. J. G.: Purification and properties of the amine oxidase of pea seedlings. Biochem. J. **59**, 609 (1955).
—, and J. H. QUASTEL: Benzedrin and brain metabolism. Nature (Lond.) **144**, 943 (1939).
— — Benzedrine (β-phenylisopropylamine) and brain metabolism. Biochem. J. **34**, 414 (1940).
—, and W. R. SMITHIES: Plant enzyme reactions leading to the formation of heterocyclic compounds. I. The formation of unsaturated pyrrolidine and piperidine compounds. Biochem. J. **61**, 89 (1955a).
— — Plant enzyme reactions leading to the formation of heterocyclic compounds. II. The formation of indole. Biochem. J. **61**, 101 (1955b).
MANTEGAZZA, P., and M. RIVA: Anorexigenic activity of l(—)dopa in animals pretreated with MAO inhibitor. Med. exp. (Basel) **4**, 367 (1961).
MANUKHIN, B. N.: Urea inhibition of thiol enzymes using monoamine oxidase. Biokhimiya **23**, 225 (1958). [Chem. Abstr. **52**, 12004i (1958).]
MARAZZI, A. S.: The effects of certain drugs on cerebral synapses. Ann. N. Y. Acad. Sci. **66**, 496 (1957).
— Synaptic and behavioral correlates of psychotherapeutic and related drug actions. Ann. N. Y. Acad. Sci. **96**, 211 (1962).
— E. R. HART, M. I. GLUCKMAN, and Z. HOROVITZ: Cerebral synaptic inhibitory action of in situ serotonin. Fed. Proc. **20**, 324 (1961).
MARIANI, L., e A. MORTARI: Analisi degli effetti pressori della serotonina nel ratto. Atti Accad. med. lombarda **15**, 210 (1960).
MARQUARDT, P., u. I. KRAUSE: Die Blutzucker-Wirkung des Adrenalins nach Vorbehandlung mit Sympathicolytica. Arzneimittel-Forsch. **12**, 843 (1962).
MARQUILLO, Q. I. L., M. T. ESPERBEN, and E. LASALVIA: Variation of pyruvic acid in enzymatic inhibition of monoamine oxidase. Chemotherapia (Basel) **4**, 580 (1962).
MARSHALL, E. F., G. S. STIRLING, A. C. TAIT, and A. TODRICK: The effect of iproniazid and imipramine on the blood platelet 5-hydroxytryptamine level in man. Brit. J. Pharmacol. **15**, 35 (1960).
MARTEL, R., and R. P. MAICKEL: Inhibition of the reserpine-induced ACTH hypersecretion with a monoamine oxidase inhibitor (N-methyl-N-benzylpropynylamine). Pharmacologist **3**, 56 (1961).

MARTEL, R. R., E. O. WESTERMANN, and R. P. MAICKEL: Dissociation of reserpine-induced sedation and ACTH hypersecretion. Life Sci **1962**, 151.
MARTIN, G. J., and J. M. BEILER: Inhibition of the action of dopa decarboxylase. Arch. Biochem. **15**, 201 (1947).
— — The effect of folic acid analogues on the action of dopa decarboxylase. J. Amer. pharm. Ass., sci. Ed. **37**, 32 (1948).
— R. BRENDEL, and J. M. BEILER: Biochemical and pharmacological effects of structural analogues of tyrosine and related compounds. Exp. Med. Surg. **8**, 5 (1950).
— — — J. MOSS, S. AVAKIAN, H. URIST, L. TOLMAN, and S. ALPERT: Studies of pteroylglutamic acid displacing agents. Amer. J. Pharm. **120**, 189 (1948).
— N. ERIKSEN, and E. P. BENDITT: Oxidation of 5-hydroxytryptamine by human serum and its inhibition by iproniazid. Fed. Proc. **17**, 447 (1958).
— C. T. ICHNIOWSKI, W. A. WISANSKY, and S. ANSBACHER: Oxidases, pressor amines and hypertension. Amer. J. Physiol. **136**, 66 (1942).
MASAMI, M., Y. HIROSHI, and I. REJI: Effect of pyrogallol on the catecholamine content of the rabbit brain. Biochem. Pharmacol. **11**, 1109 (1962).
MASON, H. S.: Mechanisms of oxygen metabolism. Advanc. Enzymol. **19**, 79 (1957a).
— Mechanisms of oxygen metabolism. Science **125**, 1185 (1957b).
MASON, M.: Inhibition of B_6-enzymes by free and conjugated estrogens. Fed. Proc. **20**, 200 (1961).
MATSUOKA, M., H. YOSHIDA, and R. IMAIZUMI: Correlation between brain catecholamine and sedative action of reserpine. Nature (Lond.) **202**, 198 (1964).
MATTHIES, H., L. DECESI u. J. SCHMIDT: Über den Mechanismus der Narkosebeeinflussung durch Iproniazid. Biochem. Pharmacol. **11**, 502 (1962).
MAXWELL, D. R., W. R. GRAY, and E. M. TAYLOR: Relative activity of some inhibitors of monoamine oxidase in potentiating the action of tryptamine in vitro and in vivo. Brit. J. Pharmacol. **17**, 310 (1961).
MAXWELL, G. M., C. A. CASTILLO, J. E. CLIFFORD, C. W. CRUMPTON, and G. G. ROWE: Effect of serotonin (5-hydroxytryptamine) on the systemic and coronary vascular bed of the dog. Amer. J. Physiol. **197**, 736 (1959).
MAXWELL, M. H., H. C. GONICK, L. SCADUTO, N. L. PEARCE, and C. R. KLEEMAN: Hemodynamic studies of a monoamine oxidase inhibitor, DL-serine-N^2-isopropylhydrazide (Ro 4—1038). Mechanism of hypotensive action. Circulation **16**, 1279 (1962).
— S. I. ROTH, H. C. GONICK, and C. R. KLEEMAN: Clinical experience with the monoamine oxidase inhibitor dl-serine-N^2-isopropylhydrazide (Ro 4-1038) in the treatment of hypertension. Amer. Heart J. **66**, 151 (1963).
MAXWELL, R. A., A. I. DANIEL, H. SHEPPARD, and J. H. ZIMMERMAN: Some interactions of guanethidine, cocaine, methylphenidate and phenylalkylamines in rabbit aortic strips. J. Pharmacol. exp. Ther. **137**, 31 (1962).
— A. J. PLUMMER, J. J. PAYTAS, S. D. ROSS, and A. I. DANIEL: Influence of adrenergic blokkade and an amine oxidase inhibitor on reserpine hypotension. Proc. Soc. exp. Biol. (N.Y.) **95**, 539 (1957).
MAYNARD, L. S., and V. J. SCHENKER: Monoamine oxidase inhibition by ethanol in vitro. Nature (Lond.) **196**, 575 (1962).
— — Decarboxylase activity in vivo: Effects of morphine and ethanol pretreatment in mice. Int. J. Neuropharmacol. **2**, 303 (1964).
MAYNERT, E. W., and H. K. KAJI: On the relationship of brain γ-aminobutyric acid to convulsion. J. Pharmacol. exp. Ther. **137**, 114 (1962).
—, and G. I. KLINGMAN: Tolerance to morphine. I. Effects on catecholamines in the brain and adrenal glands. J. Pharmacol. exp. Ther. **135**, 285 (1962). [Fed. Proc. **19**, 270 (1960).]
—, and R. LEVI: Effect of drugs on the stress-induced release of brain norepinephrine. Biochem. Pharmacol. **12**, Suppl., 113 (1963).
— — Stress-induced release of brain norepinephrine and its inhibition by drugs. J. Pharmacol. exp. Ther. **143**, 90 (1964).
MAZZONE, R., e N. SOZIO: Il meccanismo di azione di taluni neuroplegici sulla sindrome reattiva allo "stress". Ricerche con il test dell'attività colinesterasica del siero. Boll. Soc. ital. Biol. sper. **37**, 253 (1961).
— — e N. PADOLECCHIA: Indigini circa l'influsso dell'iproniazide sul tasso glucemico. Boll. Soc. ital. Biol. sper. **35**, 1275 (1959).
— — — Influenza della deplezione tessutale di catecolamine sul potere di autoregolazione omeostatica. Boll. Soc. ital. Biol. sper. **36**, 160 (1960).
MCCAMAN, R. E.: A new micromethod for monoamine oxidase. Fed. Proc. **20**, 344 (1961).
— A microradiometric method for 5-hydroxytryptophan decarboxylase. Fed. Proc. **21**, 365 (1962).

McCarty, L. P. and F. E. Shideman: The cardiostimulant actions of β-phenylethylhydrazine (Phenelzine). Angiology **11**, 58 (1960).
McColl, J. D., and W. B. Rice: A new stimulant: 5-phenyl-2-imino-4-oxo oxazolidine (FWH—352). Fed. Proc. **19**, 269 (1960).
McCormick, D. B., and E. E. Snell: Pyridoxal kinase of human brain and its inhibitors by hydrazine derivatives. Proc. nat. Acad. Sci. (Wash.) **45**, 1371 (1959).
— — Purification and properties of pyridoxal kinase from rat liver. Fed. Proc. **19**, 413 (1960).
McCoubrey, A.: Inhibition of monoamine oxidase by l-phenyl-ethylamines. Biochem. Pharmacol. **2**, 264 (1959).
McCubbin, J. W., Y. Kaneko, and I. H. Page: Ability of serotonin and norepinephrine to mimic the central effects of reserpine on vasomotor activity. Circulat. Res. **8**, 849 (1960).
McEwen, C. M., and J. D. Cohen: An amine oxidase in normal human serum. J. Lab. clin. Med. **62**, 766 (1963).
McGeer, P., E. McGeer, A. Feldstein, H. Hoagland, M. R. Riviera, and H. Freeman: Metabolism of radioactive serotonin in psychotics treated with a MAO inhibitor. J. Neuropsychiat. **1**, 274 (1960).
McGoodall, C.: Metabolic products of adrenaline and noradrenaline in human urine. Pharmacol. Rev. **11**, 416 (1959).
— H. Alton, and L. Rosen: Normetadrenaline metabolism in man. Biochem. Pharmacol. **13**, 703 (1964).
— N. Kirshner, and L. Rosen: Metabolism of noradrenaline in the human. J. clin. Invest. **38**, 707 (1959).
— L. Rosen, and N. Kirshner: Catabolites of dl-adrenaline-2-C^{14} and effect thereon of Marsilid. Fed. Proc. **17**, 56 (1958).
McGrath, W. R. and A. Horita: Differential inhibition of liver and brain monoamine oxidase by a series of arylalkylhydrazines. Toxicol. appl. Pharmacol. **4**, 178 (1962).
McIsaac, W. M., and I. H. Page: New metabolites of serotonin in carcinoid urine. Science **128**, 537 (1958).
— — The metabolism of serotonin (5-hydroxytryptamine). J. biol. Chem. **234**, 858 (1959).
— D. V. Parke, and R. T. Williams: Studies in detoxication. The metabolism of phenylhydrazine and some phenylhydrazones. Biochem. J. **70**, 688 (1958).
McLean, R. A., and L. J. Berry: Adrenergic inhibition and lethal effect of bacterial endotoxin in mice. Fed. Proc. **19**, 245 (1960a).
— — Adrenergic inhibition and lethal effect of bacterial endotoxin in mice. Proc. Soc. exp. Biol. (N. Y.) **105**, 91 (1960b).
—, and G. Chen: Elevation by propinylamines of rat tissue norepinephrine-levels and reserpine antagonism in mice. Nature (Lond.) **200**, 686 (1963).
Meijler, F. L., and D. Durrer: Influence of monoamine oxidase inhibitor on contractility of isolated rat hearts. Amer J. Physiol. **202**, 1152 (1962).
Meister, A.: Biochemistry of the amino acid. New York: Academic Press Inc. Publ. 1957.
Melander, B., and G. Gliniecke: Amphetamine, diethylpropion and tranylcypromin, a psychopharmacological study in the relation between structure and activity. Acta pharmacol. (Kbh.) **18**, 239 (1961).
Mellanby, E., and F. W. Twort: On the presence of β-imidazolethylamine in the intestinal wall; with a method of isolating a bacillus from the alimentary canal which converts histidine into this substance. J. Physiol. (Lond.) **45**, 53 (1912).
Meltzer, H. Y.: The effect of thiamine on monoamine oxidase. Biochem. Pharmacol. **7**, 277 (1961a).
— A new class of inhibitors of monoamine oxidase (MAO). Fed. Proc. **20**, 227 (1961b).
— The effect of pyridine aldoxine dodecyliodide on monoamine oxidase and bound amines. Biochem. Pharmacol. **11**, 617 (1962).
Melville, K. I., D. R. Varma, and H. E. Shister: Cardiovascular responses to hypoxia after iproniazid or reserpine treatment. Pharmacologist **2**, 81 (1960).
Mendez, R., J. Aceves y P. Pulido: Accion de la iproniacida sobre el corazon. Symposium Internacional sobre Aterosclerosis y enfermedad coronaria, Mexico, p. 395. Mexico: Editorial Interamericana 1960.
Mercier, F., A. Jouve, M. Gavend, M.-R. Gavend, J. Gerin et J. Mercier: Action énergétique et métabolique cardiaque de l'iproniazide (Marsilid). C. R. Soc. Biol. (Paris) **152**, 1556 (1958).
Mercier, J., M. Gavend et M.-R. Gavend: Influence exercée par deux inhibiteurs de la MAO (l'iproniazide et le nialamide) sur la circulation coronaire. Analyse du mécanisme de cette action. Chemotherapia (Basel) **4**, 248 (1962).
Mermod, G., P. L. Stefko, M. D. Roe, and W. B. Benson: Microscopic pathologic changes in tissues of rats and dogs given hydrazine derivatives of isonicotinic acid. Amer. J. Med. **14**, 518 (1953).

METER, W. G. VAN, G. F. AYALA, E. COSTA, and H. E. HIMWICH: Biochemical and EEG changes caused by (+) α-methyltryptamine (IT 403). Fed. Proc. **19**, 265 (1960).

METZLER, D. E., M. IKAWA, and E. E. SNELL: A general mechanism for vitamin B_6 catalyzed reactions. J. Amer. chem. Soc. **76**, 684 (1954).

MEYER, M. F.: Etude sur le mode d'action des biguanides hypoglycémiants. C. R. Acad. Sci. (Paris) **251**, 1928 (1960).

— Sur l'action adrénergique de l'iproniazide, inhibiteur de la monoamineooxydase. C. R. Acad. Sci. (Paris) **252**, 2616 (1961a).

— A propos du mode d'action de l'iproniazide inhibiteur de la monoamino-oxydase. Experientia (Basel) **17**, 563 (1961b).

— Rapport de l'Institut de Biologie Physico-Chimique, Fond. Edm. de Rothschild, p. 39. Paris 1961c.

MICHAELSON, I. A., and V. P. WHITTAKER: The subcellular localization of 5-hydroxytryptamine in guinea pig brain. Biochem. Pharmacol. **12**, 203 (1963).

MICHOTTE, L. J., u. M. de VAHIA: Die Störung der Cortison-Noradrenalin-Homeostasis bei der primär chronischen Polyarthritis. Z. Rheumaforsch. **17**, 501 (1958).

MILNE, M. D.: Biochemical effect of phenylacetic acid. Lancet **1959 II**, 467.

MINATOYA, H.: In vivo effects of an in vitro active non-hydrazine monoamine oxidase inhibitor. Pharmacologist **5**, 259 (1963).

MINKOWSKI, O.: Über Spaltungen im Tierkreis. Naunyn-Schmiedebergs Arch. exp. Path. Pharmak. **17**, 445 (1883).

MINZ, B.: Effects of reserpine and iproniazid on hypothalamic neurosecretion. Fed. Proc. **19**, 263 (1960).

—, and E. J. WALASZEK: Effects of amine oxidase inhibitors on cerebral cortical responses to epinephrine. Ann. N. Y. Acad. Sci. **80**, 617 (1959).

MIRKIN, B. L.: The effect of synaptic blocking agents on reserpine-induced alterations in adrenal medullary and urinary catecholamine levels. J. Pharmacol. exp. Ther. **133**, 34 (1961).

MITCHELL, R. G.: The effect of enzyme inhibitors on the excretion of free histamine in human urine. Brit. J. Pharmacol. **11**, 467 (1956).

MITOMA, C., H. S. POSNER, D. F. BOGDANSKI, and S. UDENFRIEND: Biochemical and pharmacological studies on o-tyrosine and its META and PARA analogues. A suggestion concerning phenylketonuria. J. Pharmacol. exp. Ther. **120**, 188 (1957).

MIZUNO, H., P. K. TALWALKER, and J. MEITES: Inhibition of mammary secretion in rats by iproniazid. Proc. Soc. exp. Biol. (N.Y.) **115**, 604 (1964).

MØLLER, H.: Uptake and metabolism of noradrenaline in acute inflammation of rabbit skin induced by ultraviolet light. Nature (Lond.) **201**, 1233 (1964).

MONNIER, M.: Actions électro-physiologiques des stimulants du système nerveux central. I. Systèmes adrénergiques, cholinergiques et neurohumeurs sérotoniques. Arch. int. Pharmacodyn. **124**, 281 (1960).

MOORE, K. E.: The role of endogenous norepinephrine in the toxicity of d-amphetamine in aggregated mice. J. Pharmacol. exp. Ther. **144**, 45 (1964).

MORAN, J. F., and T. L. SOURKES: Induction of tryptophan pyrrolase by α-methyltryptophan and its metabolic significance in vivo. J. biol. Chem. **238**, 3006 (1963).

— — and B. CHAVEZ: Inhibitory effects of decarboxylase inhibitors on the metabolism of tyrosine-C^{14} in the rat. Canad. J. Biochem. **41**, 2376 (1963).

MORTARI, A., F. MARCUCCI e L. LAMESTA: Ulteriori ricerche sulla ipertensione da reserpina in ratti con blocco delle monoaminoossidasi. Boll. Soc. ital. Biol. sper. **37**, 1256 (1962).

MOSSO, U.: Quantitative Untersuchungen über die Ausscheidung der Salicylsäure und der Umwandlungsprodukte des Benzylamins aus dem tierischen Organismus. Naunyn-Schmiedebergs Arch. exp. Path. Pharmak. **26**, 267 (1890).

MOUQUIN, M., et J. B. MILOVANOVICH: Contribution à l'étude clinique et expérimentale en cardiologie de la nialamide. Presse méd. **70**, 1189 (1962).

MÜLLER, P. B., u. H. LANGEMANN: Decarboxylierung von Dopa durch Herzmuskel von Meerschweinchen. Klin. Wschr. **40**, 911 (1962).

MÜLLER-CALGAN, H. u. R. HOTOVY: Verhaltensänderungen der Katze durch verschiedene zentralerregend wirkende Pharmaka. Arzneimittel-Forsch. **11**, 775 (1961).

MURPHY, G. F., and T. L. SOURKES: The action of antidecarboxylases on the conversion o 3,4-dihydroxyphenylalanine to dopamine in vivo. Arch. Biochem. **93**, 338 (1961).

MUSCHOLL, E.: The effect of nialamide on the concentrations of norepinephrine and adrenalin in the cardiac muscle and in the brain. Simpósio Internacional sobre Nialamida. J. Soc. Ciénc. méd. Lisboa **123**, Suppl., 76 (1959).

—, and L. MAÎTRE: Release by sympathetic stimulation of α-methyl-noradrenaline stored in the heart after administration of α-methyldopa. Experientia (Basel) **19**, 658 (1963).

MUSSINI, E., and F. MARCUCCI: Free amino acids in brains after treatment with psychotropic drugs. In: Amino Acid Pools, p. 486, edit. J. T. HOLDEN. Amsterdam: Elsevier Publ. Co. 1962.
MUSTAKALLIO, K. K., E. LEVONEN, and J. RAEKALLIO: Histochemical demonstration in rat of monoamine oxidase inhibition by β-phenyl-isopropyl hydrazine. Science **134**, 344 (1961).
NACHMIAS, V. T.: Amine oxidase and 5-hydroxytryptamine in developing rat brain. J. Neurochem. **6**, 99 (1960).
NADLER, H. L., and D. Y.-Y. HSIA: Epinephrine metabolism in phenylketonuria. Proc. Soc. exp. Biol. (N. Y.) **107**, 721 (1961).
NAGATSU, T., M. LEVITT, and S. UDENFRIEND: Tyrosine hydroxylase, the initial step in norepinephrine biosynthesis. J. biol. Chem. **239**, 2910 (1964).
NAIR, V.: The fate of ^{14}C-labelled iproniazid in the rat. Biochem. Pharmacol. **3**, 78 (1959).
— A. HANNGREN, H. LAL, and L. J. ROTH: Whole body autoradiography of C^{14}-iproniazid in mouse. Fed. Proc. **19**, 352 (1960).
— H. LAL, and L. J. ROTH: A demonstration of the early entry of iproniazid into the central nervous system. Int. J. Neuropharmacol. **1**, 361 (1962).
NAITO, T.: The histidine decarboxylase activity of the central nervous system and the effects of anesthetics and central stimulants on it. Nippon Yakurigaku Zasshi **53**, 1064 (1957). [Chem. Abstr. **52**, 18872 (1958).]
NAKAI, K.: Serotonin metabolism in herbivores. Nature (Lond.) **181**, 1734 (1958).
NAKAJIMA, H.: Contribution à l'étude des oxydases sériques et de la céruloplasmine en psychiatrie expérimentale. Encéphale **48**, 313 (1959a).
— Studies on amine oxidase: effects of chlorpromazine and its analogues. J. Biochem. (Tokyo) **46**, 559 (1959b).
— Contribution à l'étude des oxydases sériques et de la céruloplasmine en psychiatrie expérimentale. J. Neurol. Psychiat. **48**, 313 (1959c).
—, et J. THUILLIER: Action de la céruloplasmine sur certaines amines biologiques — considérations physico-pathologiques. 3e Symposium Internat. de Neurochimie, Strasbourg August 1958.
NAKAJIMA, T., Y. KAKIMOTO, and I. SANO: Formation of β-phenylethylamine in mammalian tissue and its effect on motor activity in the mouse. J. Pharmacol. exp. Ther. **143**, 319 (1964).
NAKMURA, K., and K. SHIMAMOTO: The effects of reserpine on the responses of the nictitating membrane in the cat. Jap. J. Pharmacol. **9**, 150 (1960).
NANTKA-NAMIRSKI, P., S. KURZEPA, J. DUSZKA, J. KAZIMIERCZYC, and H. KIERYLOWICZ: Untersuchungen über den Wirkungsmechanismus der MAO-Blockierung durch einige Pyridinderivate. Biochem. Pharmacol. **12**, Suppl., 70 (1963).
NARANJO, R.: Chemico-metabolic considerations of isonicotinic acid hydrazine derivatives: with particular reference to nialamide. J. Soc. Ciénc. med. Lisboa **123**, Suppl., 79 (1959).
—, and N. S. PALACIOS: Inhibition of monoamine oxidase. Mechanism of action. Rev. Invest. Biol. Univ. Guadalajara **1**, 3 (1961). [Chem. Abstr. **56**, 14887b (1962).]
NASHOLD jr., B. S., E. MANNARINO, and M. WUNDERLICH: Pressor-depressor blood pressure responses in the cat after intraventricular injection of drugs. Nature (Lond.) **193**, 1297 (1962).
NATOFF, I. L.: Cheese and monoamine oxidase inhibitors. Interaction in anaesthetised cats. Lancet **1964 I**, 532.
NEČINA, J.: Antagonism between L-α-methyl dopa and reserpine. Life Sci. **1962**, 301.
NEILL, W. A., R. J. WAGMAN, J. V. MESSER, H. J. LEVINE, and R. GORLIN: The effect of a monoamine oxidase inhibitor (β-phenylethylhydrazine) on coronary blood flow and myocardial oxygen metabolism in dogs. Clin. Res. Proc. 8, 189 (1960).
NEUBERG, C., and I. S. FORREST: Action of isonicotinic acid in microbial metabolism. Arch. Biochem. **45**, 237 (1953).
NICKERSON, M., and S. S. PARMAR: Criteria of the nature of enzyme inhibition. Studies on monoamine oxidase and cholinesterase inhibitors. Fed. Proc. **20**, 165 (1960).
NIKAIDO. T.: Chemical changes in brain tissues produced by sleep-deprivation in the rat. Seishin Shinkeigaku Zasshi **63**, 246 (1961). [Psychopharmacol. Abstr. **1**, 348 (1961).]
NIKODIJEVIĆ, B., C. R. CREVELING, and S. UDENFRIEND: Inhibition of dopamine β-oxidase in vivo by benzyloxyamine and benzylhydrazine analogs. J. Pharmacol. exp. Ther. **140**, 224 (1963).
— and T. TRAJKOV: Mechanism of ulcerogenic action of 5-hydroxytryptamine in rat's stomach. Biochem. Pharmacol. **8**, 169 (1961).
NOËL, P. R. B., and A. C. PALMER: Toxicity of some monoamine-oxidase inhibitors in dogs. Lancet **1962 I**, 1050.
NOVAK, A.: Effect of ACTH on incorporation of labeled-histidine into tissue proteins in male adult mice. Amer. J. Physiol. **168**, 121 (1952).

NOVICK jr., W. J.: The effect of age and thyroid hormones on the monoamine oxidase of rat heart. Endocrinology **69**, 55 (1961 a).
— The effect of oxygen tension on monoamine oxidase (MAO). Fed. Proc. **20**, 237 (1961 b).
OATES, J. A., L. GILLESPIE, J. R. CROUT, and A. SJOERDSMA: Inhibition of aromatic amino acid decarboxylation in man and associated pharmacological effects. J. clin. Invest. **39**, 1015 (1960 a).
— — S. UDENFRIEND, and A. SJOERDSMA: Decarboxylase inhibition and blood pressure reduction by α-methyl-3,4-dihydroxy-DL-phenylamine. Science **131**, 1890 (1960 b).
— P. Z. NIRENBERG, J. B. JEPSON, A. SJOERDSMA, and S. UDENFRIEND: Conversion of phenylalanine to phenethylamine in patients with phenylketonuria. Proc. Soc. exp. Biol. (N.Y.) **112**, 1078 (1963).
—, and A. SJOERDSMA: Neurologic effects of tryptophan in patients receiving a monoamine oxidase inhibitor. Neurology (Minneap.) **10**, 1076 (1960).
—, and P. ZALTZMAN: Discussion remark to SJOERDSMA A., GILLESPIE L., UDENFRIEND S., A method for measurement on monoamine oxidase inhibition in man: application to studies on hypertension. Ann. N. Y. Acad. Sci. **80**, 977 (1959).
O'BRIEN, R. D., and A. N. DAVISON: Antagonists to schradan poisoning in mice. Canad. J. Biochem. **36**, 1203 (1958).
OEZAYDIN, S., u. G. KOPTAGEL: Depressif hallerde Marsilid'in (iproniazid) glikoz metabolizmasi uezerine tesiri. Yeni Tip Alemi **9**, 3 (1960).
OGAWA, Y., and A. KUROSAWA: Inhibition of monoamine oxidase of the rat liver mitochondria by some inhibitors. Biochem. Pharmacol. **12**, Suppl., 40 (1963).
— K. YAMAMOTOIK, T. YOSHIZIRA, A. KUROSAWA, M. KISHIGAMI, R. HIROTA, T. IWATA, T. KITAKAZE, H. TAKASE, T. DOZAKI, and T. MINESITA: Monoamine oxidase inhibitors: a series of hydrazine derivatives. Part II. Biochemical studies on hydrazine derivatives, 1-benzyl-2-[3-(4,5,6,7-tetrahydroisoxazolyl) carbonyl]-hydrazine hydrochloride (03—1037) and 1-benzyl-(3-methyl-5-isoxazolylcarbonyl) hydrazine (03—1087). Ann. Rep. Shionogi Res. Lab. **14**, 50 (1964).
OKUDA, K. Y., and T. O. OKADA: Inhibitory mechanism of chlortetracyline on D-amino acid oxidase. Science **124**, 273 (1956).
OKUMURA, T.: Enzymological and pharmacological studies on serotonin; influences of various inhibitors upon enzymic decomposition and several biological actions of serotonin. Bull. Osaka med. Sch. **6**, 58 (1960).
OLDS, J., and M. E. OLDS: Positive reinforcement produced by stimulating hypothalamus with iproniazid and other compounds. Science **127**, 1175 (1958).
ORSINGHER, O. A.: The effect of monoamine oxidase inhibitors on the deconditioning action of reserpine in rats. Psychopharmacologia (Berl.) **2**, 326 (1961).
ORVIS, H. H., and I. G. TAMAGNA: Correlation of hypotensive effects and urinary tryptamine levels during pargyline therapy. Ann. N.Y. Acad. Sci. **107**, 958 (1963).
ORZECHOWSKI, G.: Über die Wirkungsweise der Sympathicomimetica. IX. Die stoffliche Blockade spezifischer Grenzflächen als Ursache der Tachyphylaxie der Sympathicomimetica. Beeinflussung der Adrenalinoxydase. Naunyn-Schmiedebergs Arch. exp. Path. Pharmak. **198**, 27 (1941).
OSWALD, E. O., and C. F. STRITTMATTER: Comparative studies in the characterization of monoamine oxidases. Proc. Soc. exp. Biol. (N.Y.) **114**, 668 (1963).
OTSUKA, S., and Y. KOBAYASHI: A radioisotopic assay for monoamine oxidase determinations in human plasma. Biochem. Pharmacol. **13**, 995 (1964).
OZAKI, M.: Inhibitors of the enzyme involved in the metabolism of serotonin. Nippon Yakurigaku Zasshi **55**, 1131 (1959). [Chem. Abstr. **55**, 643 (1961).]
— H. WEISSBACH, A. OZAKI, B. WITKOP, and S. UDENFRIEND: Monoamine oxidase inhibitors and procedures for their evaluation in vivo and in vitro. J. med. pharm. Chem. **2**, 591 (1960).
PAASONEN, M. K.: Inactivation of 5-hydroxytryptamine by mammalian blood platelets. Biochem. Pharmacol. **8**, 241 (1961 a).
— Influence of β-phenylisopropylhydrazine on the ability of blood platelets to retain 5-hydroxytryptamine. Biochem. Pharmacol. **8**, 301 (1961 b).
—, and N. T. KÄRKI: Increase of 5-hydroxytryptamine in the rat brain by raunescine. Brit. J. Pharmacol. **14**, 164 (1959).
— — and S. MOLKKA: Influence of iproniazid and 5-hydroxytryptamine content in the gastrointestinal tract and thyroid gland of rats. Ann. Med. exp. Fenn. **39**, 405 (1961).
—, and E. KIVALO: The inactivation of 5-hydroxytryptamine by blood platelets in mental deficiency with elevated serum 5-hydroxytryptamine. Psychopharmacologia (Berl.) **3**, 188 (1962).
—, and A. PLETSCHER: Increase of free 5-hydroxytryptamine in blood plasma by reserpine and a benzoquinolizine derivative. Experientia (Basel) **15**, 477 (1959).

PAASONEN, M. K., and A. PLETSCHER: Inhibition of 5-hydroxytryptamine release from blood platelets by N^2-isopropyl isonicotinic acid hydrazide. Experientia (Basel) **16**, 30 (1960).
— E. SOLANTUTURI, and E. KIVALO: Monoamine oxidase activity of blood platelets and their ability to store 5-hydroxytryptamine in some mental deficiencies. Psychopharmacologia (Berl.) **6**, 120 (1964).
PACHA, W. L., and E. A. ZELLER: Purification of hog kidney diamine oxidase. 136th Meeting Amer. Chem. Soc., Abstr. 38 C, 1959.
PAGE, E. W.: The dopa decarboxylase activity of human and animal tissues. Arch. Biochem. 8, 145 (1945).
—, and R. REED: Hypertensive effect of L-dopa and related compounds in the rat. Amer. J. Physiol. **143**, 122 (1945).
PAGE, I. H., A. C. CORCORAN, S. UDENFRIEND, A. SJOERDSMA, and H. WEISSBACH: Argentaffinoma as endocrine tumor. Lancet **1955 I**, 198.
PAGET, C. J., and C. S. DAVIS: Synthesis and in vitro activity of some aryl diaziridines as potential monoamine oxidase inhibitors. J. med. Chem. **7**, 626 (1964).
PALM, D.: Über die Hemmung der Dopa-Decarboxylase durch Isonicotinsäurehydrazid. Naunyn-Schmiedebergs Arch. exp. Path. Pharmak. **234**, 206 (1958).
— H. BALZER, and P. HOLTZ: Amino-acid and carbohydrate metabolism of brain after reserpine. Biochem. Pharmacol. 8, 34 (1961a).
— — — Reserpin und γ-Aminobuttersäuregehalt des Gehirns. Naunyn-Schmiedebergs Arch. exp. Path. Pharmak. **241**, 190 (1961b).
— — — Amino acid and carbohydrate metabolism of brain after reserpine. Int. J. Neuropharmacol. **1**, 173 (1962c).
PALOL, J. DE, and A. LEMBERG: Iproniazid and experimental hypertension in rabbits. Nature (Lond.) **194**, 482 (1962).
P'AN, S. Y., W. H. FUNDERBURK, and K. F. FINGER: The anticonvulsant effect of nialamide and diphenylhydantoin. Proc. Soc. exp. Biol. (N. Y.) **108**, 680 (1961). [Fed. Proc. **20**, 323 (1961).]
PANT, M. C., S. S. PARMAR, and K. P. BHARGAVA: Inhibition of monoamine oxidase by an anticholinesterase (Demecarium bromide). Canad. J. Biochem. **42**, 1114 (1964a).
— — — Role of polymethylene chain in derivatives of demecarium bromide on the inhibition of monoamine oxidase. J. Pharm. Pharmacol. **16**, 503 (1964b).
PARE, C. M. B., M. SANDLER, and R. S. STACEY: Decreased 5-hydroxytryptophan decarboxylase activity in phenylketonuria. Lancet **1958 II**, 1099.
PARKES, M. W., A. W. LESSIN, and R. F. LONG: A hypothesis for the mechanism of a central stimulant action of α-methyl-tryptamine. Proc. XXII. Int. Congr. Physiol. Sci. Leiden **2** 1231 (1962a).
— — — (In press) (1962b).
PARMAR, S. S., and M. NICKERSON: Further studies on monoamine oxidase inhibitors. Biochem. Pharmacol. 8, 8 (1961).
PAULSEN, E. C., and S. M. HESS: Mechanism of depletion of catecholamines (CA) in guinea pigs. Pharmacologist **4**, 168 (1962).
PAVLIN, R., i. A. O. ŽUPANČIČ: Inbilejui Zbornik Med. Fak. **1945—1955**, 165 (1956).
PEARCE, K. B., J. M. FUJIMOTO, and G. L. PLAA: Inhibition of hexobarbital metabolism by JB-516 (β-phenylisopropylhydrazine). Pharmacologist **1**, 64 (1959).
PEKKARINEN, A., O. CASTRÉN, and E. IISALO: Effect of iproniazid, reserpine and ganglionic blocking substances on the noradrenaline content of tissues. Abstr. IV. Int. Congr. Biochem., Wien 1958, p. 106.
— — — Effect of iproniazid and ganglionic blocking substances on the noradrenaline content of tissues. Symposium on the Catecholamines in the Cardiovascular Pathology, Burlington, Vermont, August 23—25, 1959.
— N. NIEMELÄ, and E. SOTANIEMI: The effect of dogs and Marsilid on the excretion of adrenaline and noradrenaline in guinea pigs. Acta physiol. scand. **50**, Suppl. 175, 116 (1960).
PELLERIN, J., and A. D'IORIO: Metabolism of DL-3,4-Dihydroxyphenylalanine-α-C^{14} in bovine adrenal homogenates. Rev. canad. Biol. **15**, 274 (1956).
— J. LEDUC, and A. D'IORIO: Biogenesis and metabolism of catecholamines. Rev. canad. Biol. **17**, 267 (1958).
PELLMONT, B.: Pharmakologische Untersuchungen mit Tersavid (Ro 4—1634) unter besonderer Berücksichtigung der Kreislaufdynamik. Cardiologia (Basel) **37**, Suppl. II, 44 (1960).
— Unpublished results.
—, u. F. A. STEINER: Beeinflussung eines bedingten Reflexes durch Pharmaka mit Wirkung auf den Monoaminstoffwechsel im Zentralnervensystem. Psychiat. et Neurol. (Basel) **140**, 216 (1960).

PENNEFATHER, J. N., and R. H. THORP: The influence of β-tetrahydronaphthylamine and a derivative on the central effects of 5-hydroxytryptamine, reserpine and iproniazid. J. Pharm. Pharmacol. **10**, 249 (1958).

PEPEU, G., M. ROBERTS, S. M. SCHANBERG, and N. J. GIARMAN: Differential action of iproniazid (Marsilid) and β-phenylisopropylhydrazine (Catron) on isolated atria. J. Pharmacol. exp. Ther. **132**, 131 (1961).

PERAULT, A.-M., B. PULLMAN, and C. VALDEMORO: Electronic aspects of the reactions of pyridoxal phosphate enzymes. Biochim. biophys. Acta (Amst.) **46**, 555 (1961).

PERRY jr., H. M., S. TEITLEBAUM, and P. L. SCHWARTZ: Effects of antihypertensive agents on amino acid decarboxylation and amine oxidation. Fed. Proc. **14**, 113 (1955).

PERRY, T. L.: Urinary excretion of amines in phenylketonuria and mongolism. Science **136**, 879 (1962).

PETERS, J. H.: Studies on the metabolism of isoniazid. I. Development and application of a fluorometric procedure for measuring isoniazid in blood plasma. Amer. Rev. resp. Dis. **81**, 485 (1960).

PETTEN, G. VAN, and J. J. LEWIS: The effect of anti-depressive drugs on the phosphate metabolism of rat brain in vivo. Biochem. J. **83**, 13P (1962).

PFEIFER, A. K., E. SATORY u. I. PATAKY: Pharmakologische und biochemische Wirkung des Diaethyltryptamins (DET). Naunyn-Schmiedebergs Arch. exp. Path. Pharmak. **241**, 196 (1961).

PHILLIPS, A. W., H. R. NEWCOMB, F. A. RUPP, and R. LACHAPELLE: Nutritional and microbial effects on liver monoamine oxidase and serotonin in the chick. J. Nutr. **76**, 119 (1962).

PHILPOT, F. J.: The oxidation of tyramine in the liver. Biochem. J. **31**, 856 (1937).

— The inhibition of adrenaline oxidation by local anaesthetics. J. Physiol. (Lond.) **97**, 301 (1940).

PICCHINONI, A. L., L. CHIN, and G. BREITNER: Relationship between brain levels of 5-hydroxytryptamine (5-HT) and norepinephrine (NE) and susceptibility to electrically-induced seizures. Fed Proc **21**, 416 (1962).

PIETTE, Y., et J. J. REUSE: Action de l'iproniazide sur les réponses cardiovasculaires et respiratoires au cours de l'életrochoc chez le lapin réserpiné. C. R. Soc. Biol. (Paris) **154**, 842 (1960).

PINSON jr., R., B. M. BLOOM, and C. J. BUCK: Some central nervous system drugs designed from metabolic considerations. Ann. N. Y. Acad. Sci. **96**, 336 (1962).

— J. CHIAINI, and D. BAUMGARTNER: The fate and excretion of d-amphetamine in man. Pharmacologist **3**, 81 (1961).

PISANO, J. J., J. A. OATES, A. KARMEN, A. SJOERDSMA, and S. UDENFRIEND: Identification of p-hydroxy-α-(methylaminomethyl) benzyl alcohol (synephrine) in human urine. J. biol. Chem. **236**, 898 (1961).

PISANTY, J., A. PIÑEYRO, R. MOREIRA, and L. E. TODD: Pharmacological studies on nialamide in: I. experimental myocardial infarction; II. ischemia of striated muscle; III. convulsions induced by metrazol. Simpósio internacional sobre Nialamida, J. Soc. Ciénc. méd. Lisboa **123**, Suppl., 58 (1959a).

— — — — Further pharmacological studies on nialamide: IV. with respect to diamine oxidase; V. with respect to the chemical mediators of the autonomic nervous system. Simpósio internacional sobre Nialamida, J. Soc. Ciénc. méd. Lisboa **123**, Suppl., 99 (1959b).

— — — — Effects of amine oxidase inhibition during acute coronary occlusion. Cardiologia (Basel) **37**, Suppl. 2, 74 (1960).

PLAS, R., et R. NAQUET: Contribution à l'étude neurophysiologique de l'iproniazide. C. R. Soc. Biol. (Paris) **155**, 547 (1961).

PLETSCHER, A.: Beeinflussung des 5-Hydroxytryptaminstoffwechsels im Gehirn durch Isonikotinsäurehydrazide. Experientia (Basel) **12**, 479 (1956a).

— Wirkung von Isonicotinsäurehydraziden auf den 5-Hydroxytryptaminstoffwechsel in vivo. Helv. physiol. pharmacol. Acta **14**, C76 (1956b).

— Alteration of some biochemical and pharmacological effects of reserpine by iproniazid. In: Psychotropic drugs, p. 468, edit. S. GARATTINI and V. GHETTI. Amsterdam: Elsevier Publ. Co. 1957a.

— Wirkung von Isopropyl-isonicotinsäurehydrazid auf den Stoffwechsel von Catecholaminen und 5-Hydroxytryptamin im Gehirn. Schweiz. med. Wschr. **87**, 1532 (1957b).

— Einfluß von Isopropyl-isonikotinsäurehydrazid auf den Catecholamingehalt des Myokards. Experientia (Basel) **14**, 73 (1958a).

— On the mode of action of monoamine oxidase inhibitors in the brain. Proc. IV. Internat. Congr. Biochem. Vienna (New York) **3**, 124 (1958b).

— Alterations of monoamine metabolism caused by drugs acting on the central nervous system. In: Psychopharmacology Frontiers, p. 395. Boston 6 Mass.: Little Brown & Co. 1959.

PLETSCHER, A. and A. BERNSTEIN: Increase of 5-hydroxytryptamine in blood platelets by isopropylisonicotinic acid hydrazide. Nature (Lond.) **181**, 1133 (1958).
—, and H. BESENDORF: Antagonism between harmaline and long-acting monoamine oxidase inhibitors concerning the effect on 5-hydroxytryptamine and norepinephrine metabolism in the brain. Experientia (Basel) **15**, 25 (1959).
— — u. H. P. BÄCHTOLD: Benzo [a] chinolizine, eine neue Körperklasse mit Wirkung auf den 5-Hydroxytryptamin- und Noradrenalin-Stoffwechsel des Gehirns. Naunyn-Schmiedebergs Arch. exp. Path. Pharmak. **232**, 499 (1958).
— — — u. K. F. GEY: Über pharmakologische Beeinflussung des Zentralnervensystems durch kurzwirkende Monoaminoxydasehemmer aus der Gruppe der Harmala-Alkaloide. Helv. physiol. pharmacol. Acta **17**, 202 (1959a).
— A. BROSSI, and K. F. GEY: Benzoquinclizine derivatives, a new class of monoamine decreasing drugs with psychotropic action. Int. Rev.Neurobiol. **4**, 275 (1962).
— W. P. BURKARD, and K. F. GEY: Effect of monoamine releasers and decarboxylase inhibitors on endogenous 5-hydroxyindole derivatives in brain. Biochem. Pharmacol. **13**, 385 (1964a).
—, u. K. F. GEY: Beeinflussung des Monoaminstoffwechsels in vivo durch Alkylhydrazide von Aminosäuren. Helv. physiol. pharmacol. Acta **16**, C26 (1958a).
— — Stereospecificity of monoamine oxidase inhibitors. Science **128**, 900 (1958b)..
— — Pharmakologische Beeinflussung des 5-Hydroxytryptaminstoffwechsels im Gehirn und Monoaminoxydasehemmung in vitro. Helv. physiol. pharmacol. Acta **17**, C35 (1959).
— — Über den Metabolismus von Noradrenalin und Dopamin im Gehirn. Helv. physiol. pharmacol. Acta **18**, C42 (1960a).
— — Zur Biochemie der Pharmaka, welche den Monoaminstoffwechsel im Gehirn beeinflussen. Psychiat. et Neurol. (Basel) **140**, 165 (1960b).
— — On the mechanism of action of monoamine oxidase inhibitors in angina pectoris. J. Amer. Geriat. Soc. **9**, 410 (1961a).
— — Assay of 5-hydroxytryptophan decarboxylation in intact brain. Nature (Lond.) **190**, 918 (1961b).
— — The effect of a new decarboxylase inhibitor on endogenous and exogenous monoamines. Biochem. pharmacol. **12**, 223 (1963).
— — The effect of psychotropic drugs on the metabolism of exogenous dl-2-C^{14}-3,4-dihydroxyphenylalanine. Med. exp. **11**, 169 (1964).
— — Unpublished results.
— — and W. P. BURKARD: Beeinflussung des cerebralen Stoffwechsels von 5-Hydroxytryptamin durch Decarboxylasehemmung. Helv. physiol. pharmacol. Acta **21**, C 46 (1963a).
— — y B. PELLMONT: Posibles mecanismos de accion de los inhibidores de la monoaminooxidasa en la angina de pecho. Symposium Internacional sobre Aterosclerosis y Enfermedad Coronaria, Mexico, p. 391. Mexico: Editorial Interamericana 1960a.
— — u. H. THÖLEN: Über Monoaminstoffwechsel nach Tersavid und mögliche Beziehungen zu Angina pectoris. Cardiologia (Basel) **37**, Suppl. 2, 11 (1960b).
— — u. P. ZELLER: Monoaminoxydase-Hemmer. Chemie — Biochemie — Pharmakologie — Klinik. In: Progress in drug research, vol. **2**, p. 417, edit. E. JUCKER. Basel: Birkhäuser 1960c.
— H. GÖSCHKE, K. F. GEY, and H. THÖLEN: Species differences in the action of monoamine oxidase inhibitors. Med. exp. (Basel) **4**, 113 (1961).
— E. KUNZ, H. STAEBLER, and K. F. GEY: The uptake of tryptamine by brain in vivo and its alteration by drugs. Biochem. Pharmacol. **12**, 1065 (1963b).
—, and B. PELLMONT: Biochemical and pharmacologic actions of Marsilid on the heart. J. clin. exp. Psychopath. **19**, Suppl. 1, 163 (1958).
— M. DA PRADA, and F. STEINER: Inhibition of cerebral decarboxylase and behaviour. J. Neuropharmacol., **3**, 559 (1964b).
— F. A. STEINER, and A. VOELKEL: Discussion remark to W. MAYER-GROSS, A. D. HARRIS and F. LETEMENDIA: Comparison of abnormal behavioural states induced by psychotropic drugs in animals and man. In: Neuropsychopharmacology, vol. 2, p. 138, edit. E. ROTHLIN. Amsterdam: Elsevier Publ. Co. 1959.
POGRUND, R. S., and W. G. CLARK: Decarboxylation of 3,4-dihydroxyphenylalanine (dopa) and its competitive inhibition. Fed. Proc. **15**, 145 (1956).
— W. DRELL, and W. G. CLARK: Transamination of 3-hydroxyphenylpyruvic acid in vivo. Fed. Proc. **14**, 116 (1955).
— — — Metabolism of 3-hydroxy- and 3,4-dihydroxyphenylpyruvic acids in vivo. J. Pharmacol. exp. Ther. **131**, 294 (1961).
POHL, J.: Über die Oxydation des Methyl- und Aethylalkohols im Tierkörper. Naunyn-Schmiedebergs Arch. exp. Path. Pharmak. **31**, 281 (1893).

POLLIN, W., P. V. CARDON jr., and S. S. KETY: Effects of amino acid feedings in schizophrenic patients treated with iproniazid. Science **133**, 104 (1961).

POLONOVSKI, M., P. GONNARD, H. SCHMITT et A. PELOU: Inhibition de l'aminooxydase et potentialisation de l'action hypertensive des sympathicomimétiques par la cocaine. C. R. Soc. Biol. (Paris) **147**, 1979 (1953).

— — et G. SCHAPIRA: Variations saisonniers et facteurs écologiques d'activité diasbasique: étude de la dopa-décarboxylase rénale d'un mammifère. C. R. Soc. Biol. (Paris) **140**, 280 (1946a).

— G. SCHAPIRA et P. GONNARD: Constitution chimique et inhibition enzymatique; dopa-décarboxylase et amines inhibitrices. Rapports entre dopa-décarboxylase et amine-oxydase. Bull. Soc. Chim. biol. (Paris) **27**, 735 (1946b).

POPPER, H.: Pathological findings in jaundice associated with iproniazid therapy. J. Amer. med. Ass. **168**, 2235 (1958).

— Hepatic injury in patients who had received iproniazid. Ann. N. Y. Acad. Sci. **80**, 928 (1959).

PORTER, C. C., and D. C. TITUS: Distribution and metabolism of methyldopa in the rat. J. Pharmacol. exp. Ther. **139**, 77 (1963).

— J. A. TOTARO, and C. M. LEIBY: Effect of decarboxylase inhibitors on serotonin and catecholamine levels in mice. Pharmacologist **2**, 81 (1960).

— — — Some biochemical effects of α-methyl-3,4-dihydroxyphenylalanine and related compounds in mice. J. Pharmacol. exp. Ther. **134**, 139 (1961).

— —, and C. A. STONE: Effect of some dopamine derivatives upon tissue catecholamines. Pharmacologist **4**, 149 (1962a).

— L. S. WATSON, D. C. TITUS, J. A. TOTARO, and S. S. BYER: Inhibition of dopa decarboxylase by the hydrazino analog of α-methyldopa. Biochem. Pharmacol. **11**, 1067 (1962b).

POTTER, L. T., and J. AXELROD: Studies on the storage of norepinephrine and the effect of drugs. J. Pharmacol. exp. Ther. **140**, 199 (1963).

POULSON, E., M. BOTROS, and J. M. ROBSON: The effects of 5-hydroxytryptamine and iproniazid on pregnancy. J. Endocr. **20**, XI (1960a).

— — — Effect of 5-hydroxytryptamine and iproniazid on pregnancy. Science **131**, 1101 (1960b).

—, and J. M. ROBSON: The effect of amine oxidase inhibitors on pregnancy. J. Endocr. **27**, 147 (1963).

PRAAG, H. M. VAN, and B. LEIJNSE: The influence of so-called monoamine-oxidase-inhibiting hydrazines on oral loading-tests with serotonin and 5-hydroxyindoleacetic acid. Psychopharmacologia (Berl.) **3**, 202 (1962).

— — Die Bedeutung der Monoaminoxydasehemmung als antidepressives Prinzip. I. Psychopharmacologia (Berl.) **4**, 1 (1963a).

— — Die Bedeutung der Monoaminoxydasehemmung als antidepressives Prinzip. II. Psychopharmacologia (Berl.) **4**, 91 (1963b).

PRATESI, P., and H. BLASCHKO: Specificity of amine oxidase for optically active substrates and inhibitors. Brit. J. Pharmacol. **14**, 256 (1959).

PREZ, R. M. DES, N. FALLON, and E. W. HOOK: Modification of lethal effect of bacterial endotoxin by substances altering the metabolism of 5-hydroxytryptamine. Proc. Soc. exp. Biol. (N. Y.) **107**, 529 (1961).

PRICE, S. A. P., and G. B. WEST: Further studies on the biosynthesis of 5-hydroxytryptamine. J. Pharm. Pharmacol **12**, 617 (1960).

PROCKOP, D. J., P. A. SHORE, and B. B. BRODIE: Anticonvulsant properties of monoamine oxidase inhibitors. Ann. N. Y. Acad. Sci. **80**, 643 (1959a).

— — — An anticonvulsant effect of monoamine oxidase inhibitors. Experientia (Basel) **15**, 145 (1959b).

PSCHEIDT, G. R.: Excretion of minerals and biogenic amines in dogs receiving trifluoperazine and monoamine oxidase inhibitors. Fed. Proc. **21**, 417 (1962).

— Monoamine oxidase inhibitors. In: Int. Rev. Neurobiol., vol. 7, p. 191, edit. C. C. PFEIFFER and J. R. SMYTHIES. New York and London: Academic Press 1964.

— G. BRUNE, and H. E. HIMWICH: Uniform response of biogenic amines to psychotropic drugs in selected schizophrenic patients. Fed. Proc. **20**, 305 (1961).

—, and H. E. HIMWICH: Reserpine, monoamine oxidase inhibitors, and distribution of biogenic amines in monkey brain. Biochem. Pharmacol. **12**, 65 (1963).

—, and C. MORPURGO: Comparison of chemical and biological determination of brain catechol amines. Fed. Proc. **19**, 294 (1960).

PÜTTER, J., u. G. KRONENBERG: Untersuchungen über die Stereospezifität der decarboxylasehemmenden Wirkung von α-Methyldopa. Naunyn-Schmiedebergs Arch. exp. Path. Pharmak. **249**, 470 (1964).

PUGH, C. E. M., and J. H. QUASTEL: XLI. Oxidation of aliphatic amines by brain and other tissues. Biochem. J. **31**, 286 (1937a).

— — Oxidation of aliphatic amines by brain and other tissues. Biochem. J. **31**, 2306 (1937b).

QUADBECK, G.: Der Einfluß von Nitoman und Iproniazid auf die Blut-Hirnschrankenpermeabilität der Ratte. Psychiat. et Neurol. (Basel) **140**, 29 (1960).

QUAY, W. B.: Effects of amines and monoamine oxidase inhibitors on hypothalamic succinic dehydrogenase activity. Proc. Soc. exp. Biol. (N. Y.) **101**, 230 (1959).

RAAB, W., and W. GIGEE: Uptake and breakdown of catecholamines in vascular tissue. Angiology **9**, 283 (1958).

RALL, T. W., and E. W. SUTHERLAND: Action of epinephrine and norepinephrine in broken cell preparations. Pharmacol. Rev. **11**, 464 (1959).

RANDALL, L. O.: Oxidation of phenethylamine derivatives by amine oxidase. J. Pharmacol. exp. Ther. **88**, 216 (1946).

— Toxicology of Marsilid. J. clin. exp. Psychopath. **19**, Suppl. 1, 178 (1958).

— N. ATKINSON, and V. ILIEV: The effect of psychostimulants and psychodepressants on DPN synthesis in the liver. Arch. int. Pharmacodyn. **129**, 434 (1960).

—, and R. E. BAGDON: Toxicology of Marsilid and other amine oxidase inhibitors. Dis. nerv. Syst. **19**, 539 (1958).

— — The pharmacology of iproniazid and other amine oxidase inhibitors. Ann. N. Y. Acad. Sci. **80**, 626 (1959).

—, and F. HALL: Unpublished results.

— B. KAPPELL, C. K. CALLAHAN, M. GOWER, E. KOLAR, and V. ILIEV: Unpublished results.

REBER, K., and A. STUDER: Unpublished results.

REBHUN, J., S. M. FEINBERG, and E. A. ZELLER: Potentiating effect of iproniazid on action of some sympathicomimetic amines. Proc. Soc. exp. Biol. (N. Y.) **87**, 218 (1954).

REDETZKI, H., and F. O'BOURNE: Action of monoamine oxidase inhibitors on dehydrogenases. Arch. int. Pharmacodyn. **130**, 299 (1961).

REDISCH, W., K. DE CRINIS, J. M. STEELE, and W. BROWN: Studies on vasoactivity of catecholamines in man. Amer. J. Cardiol. **5**, 660 (1960).

REGELSON, W., F. S. HOFFMEISTER, and H. RUBIN: Effect of iproniazid on survival in the dog following acute coronary occlusion. Ann. N. Y. Acad. Sci **80**, 981 (1959).

REICHLE, F. A., R. C. BALDRIGE, J. DOBBS, and M. TROMPETTER: Tryptophan metabolism in phenylketonuria. J. Amer. med. Ass. **178**, 171 (1961).

REID, J. D., J. F. RILEY, and D. M. SHEPHERD: Histological and enzymatic changes in the livers of rats fed the hepatic carcinogen diethylnitrosamine. Biochem. Pharmacol. **12**, 1151 (1963).

—, and D. M. SHEPHERD: Inhibition of histidine decarboxylases. Life Sci. **1963**, 5.

— — Decarboxylase activities in tissues of tryptophan-deficient rats. Biochim. biophys. Acta (Amst.) **81**, 560 (1964).

REILLY, R. H., K. F. KILLAM, E. H. JENNEY, W. H. MARSHALL, T. TAUSIG, N. S. APTER, and C. C. PFEIFFER: Convulsant effects of isoniazid. J. Amer. med. Ass. **152**, 1317 (1953).

RESNICK, O.: The influence of amine oxidase inhibitors on epinephrine metabolism in man. Ann. N. Y. Acad. Sci. **80**, 726 (1959).

—, and H. FREEMAN: Epinephrine metabolism in normal and psychotic man. Arch. gen. Psychiat. **6**, 388 (1962).

— M. HAGOPIAN, and H. FREEMAN: The alteration of epinephrine metabolism in man. Fed. Proc. **19**, 277 (1960a).

— — H. HOAGLAND, and H. FREEMAN: An in vivo test for measuring monoamine oxidase inhibition in human subjects. Arch. gen. Psychiat. **2**, 459 (1960b).

— J. M. WOLFE, H. FREEMAN, and F. ELMADJIAN: Iproniazid treatment and metabolism of labeled epinephrine in schizophrenics. Science **127**, 1116 (1958).

REUSE, J. J.: Effets de la tétrabénazine sur les manifestations cardiovasculaires et respiratoires au cours de convulsions tonicocloniques chez le lapin. Arch. int. Pharmacodyn. **126**, 478 (1960a).

— Inhibition, par l'iproniazide, de l'action de la réserpine sur les effets du pentétrazol, à doses convulsivantes, chez le lapin. C. R. Soc. Biol. (Paris) **154**, 447 (1960b).

REVZIN, A. M., and E. COSTA: The effects of monoamine oxidase substrates and inhibitors on evoked potentials. Fed. Proc. **19**, 265 (1960).

— S. SPECTOR, and E. COSTA: Relationship between reserpine-induced facilitation of evoked potentials in the limbic system and change in brain serotonin level. Biochem. Pharmacol. **8**, 39 (1961).

REYMOND, Cl., P.-A. ROSSEL et J.-L. RIVIER: Traitement à l'iproniazide et métabolisme intermédiaire des hydrates de carbone. Cardiologia (Basel) **36**, 216 (1960).

REYNOLDS, B. L., J. B. CODINGTON, A. R. MANSBERGER, and R. W. BUXTON: Discussion remarks to D.M.BOSWORTH: Iproniazid: a brief review of its introduction and clinical use. Ann. N.Y. Acad. Sci. **80**, 812 (1959).
RICHTER, D.: Adrenaline and amine oxidase. Biochem. J. **31**, 2022 (1937).
— CCXXIX. Elimination of amines in man. Biochem. J. **32**, 1763 (1938).
— M. H. LEE, and D. HILL: The rate or removal of amines from the blood. Biochem. J. **35**, 1225 (1941).
—, and A. H. TINGEY: Amine oxidase and adrenaline. J. Physiol. (Lond.) **97**, 265 (1939).
RILEY, V.: Demonstration of differences between normal and tumor-bearing animals. Proc. Soc. exp. Biol. (N.Y.) **97**, 169 (1958a).
— Synergistic reaction between p-phenylenediamine and melanoma components. Proc. Soc. exp. Biol. (N.Y.) **98**, 57 (1958b).
RITTER, E. DE, L. DREKTEN, J. SCHEINER, and S. H. RUBIN: Urinary excretion of hydrazine derivatives of isonicotinic acid in normal humans. Proc. Soc. exp. Biol. (N.Y.) **79**, 654 (1952).
ROBINSON, B., and D. M. SHEPHERD: Inhibition of histidine decarboxylase. Biochim. biophys. Acta (Amst.) **53**, 431 (1961).
— — The inhibition of the L-histidine decarboxylases of guinea pig kidney and rat hepatoma. J. Pharm. Pharmacol. **14**, 9 (1962).
ROBINSON, J.: Amine oxidase in the iris and nictitating membrane of the cat and the rabbit. J. Pharmacol. **7**, 99 (1952).
ROBINSON, R., and P. SMITH: Urinary amines in phaeochromocytoma. Clin. chim. Acta **7**, 29 (1962).
ROBSON, J. M., and M. BOTROS: The effect of 5-hydroxytryptamine and of monoamine oxidase inhibitors on sexual maturity. J. Endocr. **22**, 165 (1961).
ROONEY, C. S., E. J. CRAGOE jr., C. C. PORTER, and J. M. SPRAGUE: Synthesis of sulfonylhydrazine derivatives with monoamine oxidase inhibitory activity. J. med. pharm. Chem. **5**, 155 (1962).
ROOS, B.-E.: On the occurrence and distribution of 5-hydroxyindoleacetic acid in brain. Life Sci. **1962**, 25.
— The effect of monoamine oxidase inhibitors on the level of 5-hydroxyindoleacetic acid in human cerebrospinal fluid. Life Sci. **1963**, 1.
— N.-E. ANDÉN, and B. WERDINIUS: Effect of drugs on the levels of indole and phenolic acids in the central nervous system. Int. J. Neuropharmacol. **3**, 117 (1964).
—, and B. WERDINIUS: The effect of α-methyl dopa on the metabolism of 5-hydroxytryptamine in brain. Life Sci. **2**, 92 (1963).
ROPP, R. S. DE, and E. H. SNEDEKER: Effect of drugs on amino levels in brain: excitants and depressants. Proc. Soc. exp. Biol. (N.Y.) **106**, 696 (1961).
ROSEN, F.: Effect of isonicotinic acid hydrazide on niacin and pyridoxin metabolism in rats. Proc. Soc. exp. Biol. (N.Y.) **88**, 243 (1955).
— The relationship of certain vitamin deficiencies to the toxicity of iproniazid. Ann. N.Y. Acad. Sci. **80**, 885 (1959).
ROSEN, L., and C. MCGOODALL: The effect of iproniazid on the metabolism of DL-noradrenaline-2-C^{14} in the human. Fed. Proc. **20**, 182 (1961).
— — Effect of iproniazid on metabolism of noradrenaline in man. Amer. J. Physiol. **202**, 883 (1962).
ROSENBLATT, S., J. D. CHANLEY, H. SOBOTKA, and M. R. KAUFMANN: Interrelationships between electroshock, the blood-brain barrier, and catecholamines. J. Neurochem. **5**, 172 (1960).
ROSENFELD, G.: Inhibitory influence of ethanol on serotonin metabolism. Proc. Soc. exp. Biol. (N.Y.) **103**, 144 (1960).
ROSENGREN, E.: Are dihydroxyphenylalanine decarboxylase and 5-hydroxytryptophan decarboxylase individual enzymes? Acta physiol. scand. **49**, 364 (1960a).
— On the role of monoamine oxidase for the inactivation of dopamine in brain. Acta physiol. scand. **49**, 370 (1960b).
— Formation of histamine in the pregnant mouse. Experientia (Basel) **18**, 176 (1962).
ROSENKRANTZ, H., and R. O. LAFERTE: Further observations on the relationship between serotonin and the adrenal. Endocrinology **66**, 832 (1960).
ROSENTHAL, F., and P. S. TIMIRAS: Electroshock seizure responses to psychopharmacological agents after 500 r Wholebody X-irradiation in rats. Biochem. Pharmacol. 8, 50 (1961).
ROSS, S. B., and Ö. HALJASMAA: Inhibition of the enzymatic hydroxylation of phenylalanine and tryptophan by rat liver extract in vitro. Life Sci. **3**, 579 (1964).
ROSSI, C. A.: Dopa decarboxylase in the hypophysectomized animal. Ric. Sci. **25**, Suppl. G. Biochim. Italo-Franco-Elvetiche, **422** (1955) [Chem. Abstr. **54**, 11196 (1960).]

ROSSUM, J. M. VAN, and J. A. T. M. HURKMANS: Reversal of the effect of α-methyldopa by monoamine oxidase inhibitors. J. Pharm. (Lond.) **15**, 493 (1963).
ROTH, M., and J. RIEDER: Unpublished results 1960.
— — Untersuchungen über das Schicksal einiger Alkylhydrazin-Derivate und von Benzylhydrazin im Tierkörper. Helv. physiol. pharmacol. Acta (1963).
ROTHSCHILD, A. M., and R. W. SCHAYER: Characterization of histidine decarboxylase from rat peritoneal fluid mast cells. Biochim. biophys. Acta (Amst.) **34**, 392 (1959).
ROTHSCHILD, Z., and R. W. SCHAYER: Synthesis and metabolism of a histamine metabolite, 1-methyl-4-(β-aminoethyl)-imidazole. Biochim. biophys. Acta (Amst.) **30**, 23 (1958).
ROWE, G. G., S. ALFONSO, C. J. CHELIUS, H. P. GURTNER, and CH. W. CRUMPTON: Systemic and coronary hemodynamic effects of an amine oxidase inhibitor. J. clin. Invest. **40**, 1077 (1961). [Psychopharmacol. Abstr. **1**, **344** (1961).]
ROWE, R. P.: A pharmacologic summary of nialamide. Dis. nerv. Syst. **20**, 5 (1959).
— B. M. BLOOM, S. Y. P'AN, and K. F. FINGER: The pharmacological characterization of the antidrepessant, nialamide. Fed. Proc. **18**, 441 (1959a).
— — — — Pharmacological studies with nialamide, a new antidepressant agent. Proc. Soc. exp. Biol. (N.Y.) **101**, 832 (1959b).
— S. L. LOFGREN, and A. KELLEY: Reversal of reserpine sedation with some MAO inhibitors and analeptics. Fed. Proc. **20**, 396 (1961).
ROY, D. N., S. H. LIPTON, F. M. STRONG, and H. R. BIRD: Potentiation of lathyrogenic effect of beta aminopropionitrile in turkey poults. Proc. Soc. exp. Biol. (N.Y.) **102**, 767 (1959).
RUBIN, S. H., L. DREKTEN, J. SCHEINER, and E. DE RITTER: Determination of blood plasma levels of hydrazine derivatives of isonicotinic acid. Dis. Chest. **21**, 439 (1952).
RUDZIK, A. D., and J. W. MILLER: The effect of administration of various phenylalkyl hydrazines on the catecholamine content and rate of contractions of the rat uterus. J. Pharmacol. exp. Ther. **139**, 69 (1963).
RÜMKE, C. L.: The influence of drugs given 1—72 hours previously upon hexobarbital-narcosis and upon bemegride-induced convulsions in mice. Biochem. Pharmacol. 8, 48 (1961).
—, u. J. BOUT: Die Beeinflussung der Hexobarbitalnarkose durch vorher verabfolgte Pharmaka. Naunyn-Schmiedebergs Arch. exp. Path. Pharmak. **240**, **218** (1960).
RUGE, W., u. F. HARTMANN: Phenolsäuren- und Indolausscheidung im Urin bei Gabe von α-Methyldopa. Klin. Wschr. **41**, 856 (1963).
RYALL, R. W.: Effects of cocaine and antidepressant drugs on the nictitating membrane of the cat. Brit. J. Pharmacol. **17**, 339 (1961).
SACKS, W: A cerebral decarboxylase for 5-hydroxytryptophane in humans. J. appl. Physiol. **16**, 1050 (1961).
SAKOMOTO, Y., Y. OGAWA, and K. HAYASHI: Monoamine oxidase. J. Biochem. (Tokyo) **54**, 292 (1963) [Chem. Abstr. **60**, 13507f. (1964)].
SALVA, S. J. DE, and V. J. MONTELEONE: Local anesthetic property of MAO inhibitors. Pharmacologist **4**, 155 (1962).
SANAN, S., and M. VOGT: Effect of drugs on the noradrenaline content of brain and peripheral tissues and its significance. Brit. J. Pharmacol. **18**, 109 (1962).
SANDLER, M., and H. G. CLOSE: Biochemical effect of phenylacetic acid in patient with 5-hydroxytryptophansecreting carcinoid tumor. Lancet **1959 II**, 316.
—, and J. COVENEY: Placental monoamine oxidase activity in toxaemia of pregnancy. Lancet **1962 I**, 1096.
— A. DAVIES, and C. RIMINGTON: Effect of phenylacetic acid on the carcinoid syndrome. Lancet **1959 II**, 318.
—, and C. R. J. RUTHVEN: 3-Methoxy-4-hydroxymandelic acid excretion in phaeochromocytoma. In: Ciba Foundation, Symposium on Adrenergic Mechanism, p. 40. London: J. & A. Churchill Ltd. 1960.
—, and P. J. D. SNOW: An atypical carcinoid tumour secreting 5-hydroxytryptophan. Lancet **1958 I**, 137.
— R. G. SPECTOR, C. R. J. RUTHVEN, and A. N. DAVISON: The occurrence and adaptive increase of 5-hydroxytryptophan-α-oxoglutarate transaminase in rat liver. Biochem. J. **74**, 42P (1960).
—, and G. B. WEST: Biosynthesis of 5-hydroxytryptamine. J. Physiol. (Lond.) **140**, 9P (1958).
SANKAR, D. V. S.: Effect of psychopharmacological drugs on main oxidative activity. J. Neuropsychiat. **3**, 123 (1961).
— E. GOLD, E. SANKAR, and N. MCRORIE: Effect of psychopharmacological agents of DPN-dependent enzymes. Fed. Proc. **20**, 394 (1961).
SANKOFF, I., and T. L. SOURKES: The weight-depressing action of α-methyl-DL-tryptophan in the rat. Canad. J. Biochem. **40**, 739 (1962).

SANNER, E., and B. WORTMAN: Tubular excretion of serotonin 5-hydroxytryptamine in the chicken. Acta physiol. scand. **55**, 319 (1962).
SANSONE, M., et G. DELL'OMODARME: Influence de l'isocarboxazide (Marplan) et de deux nouveaux inhibiteurs de la MAO sur les convulsions cloniques et sur la mortalité par métrazol. Arch. int. Pharmacodyn. **144**, 392 (1963).
SARKAR, S., R. BANERJEE, M. S. ISE u. E. A. ZELLER: Über die Wirkung von 2-Phenylcyclopropylamin auf die Monoaminoxydase und andere Enzymsysteme. 18. Mitteilung über Aminoxydasen. Helv. chim. Acta **43**, 439 (1960a).
— J. P. KALTENBACH, and E. A. ZELLER: Occurrence of monoamine oxidase in ascites tumor cells and effect of iproniazid on this enzyme. 137th Meeting Amer. Chem. Soc., Abstr. 45C (1960b).
—, and E. A. ZELLER: Characterization of two homologous monoamine oxidases. Fed. Proc. **20**, 238 (1961).
SATAKE, K.: Saikin no Kosokagu **4**, 39 (1955) quoted in Okumura 1960.
— S. ANDO, and H. FUJITA: Bacterial oxidation of some primary amines. J. Biochem. (Tokyo) **40**, 299 (1953).
SÁTORY, E., A. K. PFEIFER, I. PATAKY u. L. KEREKES: Die Wirkung von Diäthyltryptamin auf die Monoaminoxydase-Aktivität. Acta physiol. Acad. Sci. hung. **18**, Suppl., 83 (1961).
SAUNDERS, J. C., N. RADINGER, and N. S. KLINE: Results at the Meeting of the Soc. for biologic Psychiatry, Atlantic City (N.Y.) June 15, 1957.
SAVOLDI, F., G. C. MAGGI e S. NOLI: Azione degli inibitori delle monoaminoossidasi sull'attività elettrica cerebrale del coniglio. Boll. Soc. ital. Biol. sper. **36**, 1423 (1960).
SCAIFE, J. F.: Protection of human red cell cholinesterase against inhibition by tabun and 0,0-diethyl-S-2-diethylaminoethyl phosphorothiolate. Canad. J. Biochem. **38**, 301 (1960).
SCARDI, V., e V. BONAVITA: Interazione piridossal-5-fosfato-KCN ed attivazione dell'apotransaminasi. Acta vitamin. (Milano) **11**, 117 (1957a).
— — Sull'interazione tra piridossal-5-fosfato ed apotransaminasi. Boll. Soc. ital. Biol. sper. **33**, 770 (1957b).
SCHAEPDRYVER, A. F. DE: Physio-pharmacological effects on suprarenal secretion of adrenaline and noradrenaline in dogs. Arch. int. Pharmacodyn. **119**, 517 (1959a).
— Pharmacological effects on distribution and urinary excretion of radioactive adrenaline. Arch. int. Pharmacodyn. **121**, 478 (1959b).
—, W. M. BOOKER, T. WALTON, E. FISHER, and R. LINARES: Further studies on the estimation of infused adrenalin and noradrenalin, using the isolated perfused guinea pig heart. Fed. Proc. **19**, 155 (1960).
—, and N. KIRSHNER: Metabolism of adrenaline after blockade of monoamine oxydase and catechol-0-methyltransferase. Science **133**, 586 (1960).
— — Tissular metabolism of DL-adrenaline-2-C^{14} in the cat. Arch. int. Pharmacodyn. **130**, 477 (1961a).
— — The metabolism of DL-adrenaline-2-C^{14} in the act. II. Tissue metabolism. Arch. int. Pharmacodyn. **131**, 433 (1961b).
— — Metabolism of adrenaline after blockade of monoamine oxidase and catechol-0-methyltransferase. Science **133**, 586 (1961c).
—, and Y. PIETTE: Electroshock and tissue catecholamine content in reserpinized rabbits. Arch. int. Pharmacodyn. **130**, 225 (1961).
—, et P. PREZIOSI: Iproniazide et effets pharmacologiques sur la médullo-cortico-surrénale. Arch. int. Pharmacodyn. **119**, 506 (1959a).
— — Physico-pharmacological effects on suprarenal secretion of adrenaline and noradrenaline in dogs. Arch. int. Pharmacodyn. **121**, 177 (1959b).
SCHAER, H., P. LICHTLEN, and H. LANGEMANN: Influence of α-methyl-dopa on the urinary excretion of 3-methoxy-4-hydroxymandelic acid in hypertensive patients. (Manuscript) (1963).
SCHAIN, R. J.: Some effects of a monoamine oxidase inhibitor upon changes produced by centrally administered amines. Brit. J. Pharmacol. **17**, 261 (1961).
SCHALES, O.: Amino acid decarboxylases of animals. In: The Enzymes, vol. 2, p. 216, edit. J. B. SUMMER and K. MYRBÄCK. New York: Academic Press Inc. Publ. 1951.
—, and S. S. SCHALES: Dihydroxyphenylalanine decarboxylase: preparation and properties of a stable dry powder. Arch. Biochem. **24**, 83 (1949).
SCHALLEK, W.: Neurophysiological studies with monoamine oxidase inhibitors. Dis. nerv. Syst. **21**, Suppl. 3, 64 (1960).
—, and A KUEHN: Effects of drugs on spontaneous and activated EEG of cat. Arch. int. Pharmacodyn. **120**, 319 (1959).
— — Effects of drugs on limbic system of cat. Pharmacologist **2**, 79 (1960a).
— — Effects of psychotropic drugs on limbic system of cat. Proc. Soc. exp. Biol. (N.Y.) **105**, 115 (1960b).

SCHALLEK, W., A. KUEHN, and N. JEW: Effects of chlordiazepoxide (Librium) and other psychotropic agents on the limbic system of the brain. Ann. N.Y. Acad. Sci. **96**, 303 (1962).
—, and D. WALZ: Effects of isoniazid and iproniazid on the central nervous system of the dog. Amer. Rev. Tuberc. **69**, 261 (1954).
SCHANBERG, S. M.: A study of the transport of 5-hydroxytryptophan and 5-hydroxytryptamine (serotonin) into brain. J. Pharmacol. exp. Ther. **139**, 191 (1963).
—, and N. J. GIARMAN: Drug-induced alterations in the sub-cellular distribution of 5-hydroxytryptamine in rat's brain. Biochem. Pharmacol. **11**, 187 (1962).
—, G. PEPEU, and N. J. GIARMAN: Some pharmacologic actions of iproniazid on isolated atria of the guinea pig. Pharmacologist **1**, 82 (1959).
SCHAPIRA, G.: Réparation de l'amineoxydase et métabolisme de l'adrénaline. C. R. Soc. Biol. (Paris) **139**, 36 (1945).
— Dopa-décarboxylase et adrénaline. C. R. Soc. Biol. (Paris) **140**, 173 (1946).
SCHAUB, F., F. NAGER, H. SCHAER, W. ZIEGLER u. P. LICHTLEN: α-Methyl-dopa. Therapeutische Erfahrungen bei Hypertonie und biochemische Untersuchungen zu seiner Wirkungsweise. Schweiz. med. Wschr. **92**, 620 (1962).
SCHAUMANN, W.: Beeinflussung der analgetischen Wirkung des Morphins durch Reserpin. Naunyn-Schmiedebergs Arch. exp. Path. Pharmak. **235**, 1 (1958).
— Modification of the analgesic action of morphine by means of reserpine. Excerpta med. (Amst.), Sect. 2, **13**, 129 (1960).
—, u. H. G. KURBJUWEIT: Beeinflussung verschiedener Wirkungen von Thiopropazat durch ein zentrales Stimulans. Arzneimittel-Forsch. **11**, 343 (1961).
SCHAYER, R. W.: Studies on histamine-metabolizing enzymes in intact animals. J. biol. Chem. **203**, 787 (1953a).
— In vivo inhibition of monoamine oxidase studied with radioactive tyramine. Proc. Soc. exp. Biol. (N.Y.) **84**, 60 (1953b).
— Histidine decarboxylase in mast cells. Ann. N.Y. Acad. Sci. **103**, 164 (1963).
—, and R. L. SMILEY: The metabolism of epinephrine containing isotopic carbon. J. biol. Chem. **202**, 425 (1953).
— — K. J. DAVIS, and Y. KOBAYASHI: Role of monoamine oxidase in nor-adrenaline metabolism. Amer. J. Physiol. **182**, 285 (1955).
— K. Y. T. WU, R. L. SMILEY, and Y. KOBAYASHI: Studies on monoamine oxidase in intact animals. J. biol. Chem. **210**, 259 (1954).
SCHECKEL, C., and E. BOFF: Antagonism of norepinephrine-induced behavioural stimulation by a decarboxylase inhibitor (Ro 4-4602), α-methyl-meta-tyrosine or diazepam. Fed. Proc. **23**, 456 (1964).
SCHERBEL, A. L., G. H. CURTIS, and J. W. HARRISON: The effect of iproniazid ointment on trophic ulcers associated with Raynaud's phenomenon. Cleveland Clin. Quart. **25**, 92 (1958).
— R. L. MCKITTRICK, and W. A. HAWK: Lesions in rats caused by serotonin and histamine before and after amine oxidase inactivation and serotonin inhibition. J. clin. Invest. **39**, 1025 (1960).
SCHEUERBRANDT, G.: Automatische Bestimmung der Decarboxylase für aromatische Aminosäuren in Mäuseleber. Angew. Chem. **76**, 604 (1964).
SCHIATTI, P.: Osservazioni tecniche sulla metodica per il saggio di sostanze inibitrici della MAO. Boll. Soc. ital. Biol. sper. **36**, 2040 (1960).
SCHIEVELBEIN, H., u. E. WERLE: Zur Frage der Entstehung von Methylamin beim Abbau des Nikotins durch Leber und zum Abbau von Methylamin durch Leber. Arzneimittel-Forsch. **7**, 117 (1957).
SCHILDKRAUT, J. J., G. L. KLERMAN, D. G. FRIEND, and M. GREENBLATT: Biochemical and pressor effects of oral d,l-dihydroxyphenyl-alanine in patients pretreated with antidepressant drugs. Ann. N.Y. Acad. Sci. **107**, 1005 (1963).
SCHINDLER, R.: The conversion of ^{14}C-labelled tryptophan to 5-hydroxytryptamine by neoplastic mast cells. Biochem. Pharmacol. **1**, 323 (1958).
SCHMID, E.: Zum Wirkungsmechanismus von Aminoxydase-Inhibitoren. Versuche über den Serotonin-Stoffwechsel. Chemotherapia (Basel) **4**, 255 (1962).
—, u. F. SCHEIFFARTH: Zur Anwendung von Monoaminoxydase-Inhibitoren in der inneren Medizin. Arzneimittel-Forsch. **11**, 612 (1961).
SCHMID, W.: Zur Biochemie der monoaminoxydasehemmenden Substanzen. Psychiat. et Neurol. (Basel) **140**, 225 (1960).
SCHMIDT, G.: Beeinflussung zentraler Cocainwirkungen durch Reserpin und Adrenolytica. Naunyn-Schmiedebergs Arch. exp. Path. Pharmak. **241**, 510 (1961).
SCHMIEDEBERG, O.: Über Spaltung und Synthese im Tierkörper. Naunyn-Schmiedebergs Arch. exp. Path. Pharmak. **14**, 379 (1881).

SCHMITT, H., et P. GONNARD: Action de l'iproniazide sur les effets des sympathicomimétiques sur la membrane nictiante du chat. C. R. Acad. Sci. (Paris) **240**, 2573 (1955).
— — Modifications par un inhibiteur de l'aminooxydase, l'iproniazide, des effets de quelques amines sympathicomimétiques sur la membrane nictiante du chat. Arch. int. Pharmacodyn. **108**, 74 (1956).
—, et H. SCHMITT: I. Mécanismes de la potentialisation de l'hypertension réserpinique chez le rat sans moelle. Arch. int. Pharmacodyn. **132**, 97 (1961).
—, u. M. SPÄTH: Der Einfluß von Cocain, Iproniazid und Pyrogallol auf die durch Adrenalin ausgelöste Blutzuckersteigerung. Arzneimittel-Forsch. **13**, 761 (1963).
SCHNEIDER, J. A., B. M. BLOOM, C. DELAHUNT, K. F. FINGER, M. FINKELSTEIN, R. P. ROWE, R. STEBBINS, and A. WEISSMAN: Pharmacological considerations on monoamine oxidase inhibition as a therapeutic principle. Simpósio internacional sobre Nialamida. J. Soc. Ciénc. méd. Lisboa **123**, Suppl., 43 (1959).
— K. F. FINGER, u. J. N. PEREIRA: Pathophysiologische Betrachtungen über therapeutische Anwendung von Monoamin-Oxydase-Hemmern. Chemotherapia (Basel) **4**, 219 (1962).
SCHNITZER, B.: On the significance of endogenous 5-hydroxytryptamine in the regulation of water diuresis. Inaug.-Diss. Basel 1958.
SCHOEPKE, H. G., and R. G. WIEGAND: Relation between norepinephrine accumulation or depletion and blood pressure responses in the cat and rat following parygline administration. Ann. N.Y. Acad. Sci. **107**, 924 (1963).
SCHONE, H.-H., u. E. LINDER: Über die Wirkung von N-(3'-Phenyl-propyl-(2')-1,1-diphenylpropyl-(3)-amin auf den Katecholamin-Stoffwechsel. Klin. Wschr. **40**, 1196 (1962).
SCHOOT, J. B. VAN DER, E. J. ARIËNS, J. M. VAN ROSSUM, and J. A. Th. M. HURKMANS: Phenylisopropylamine derivatives, structure and action. Arzneimittel-Forsch. **12**, 902 (1962).
— C. R. CREVELING, T. NAGATSU, and S. UDENFRIEND: On the mechanism of inhibition of dopamine-β-oxidase by benzyloxyamines. J. Pharmacol. exp. Ther. **141**, 74 (1963).
SCHOTT, H. F.: Pyridoxal phosphate as accelerator for kidney DOPA decarboxylase and its inactivation by DOPA and related substances. Fed. Proc. **10**, 211 (1951).
—, and W. G. CLARK: Dopa decarboxylase inhibition through the interaction of coenzyme and substrate. J. biol. Chem. **196**, 449 (1952).
SCHROEDER, H. A.: Mechanism of Hypertension, p. 88. Springfield: Charles C. Thomas 1957.
— The pharmacology of hydralazine. The first Hahnemann Symposium on Hypertensive Disease, p. 332, edit. JOHN MOYER. Philadelphia and London: W. B. Saunders Co. 1959.
SCHÜLLER, E.: Corticosteroidausscheidung nach Nialamid-Medikation. Wien. klin. Wschr. **72**, 856 (1960).
SCHÜMANN, H. J.: Über den Hydroxytyramin- und Noradrenalingehalt der Lunge. Naunyn-Schmiedebergs Arch. exp. Path. Pharmak. **234**, 282 (1958).
— Formation of adrenergic transmitters. Ciba Foundation, Symposium on Adrenergic Mechanism, p. 6. London: J. & A. Churchill Ltd. 1960.
—, u. H. GROBECKER: Nachweis und Lokalisation von α-Methyl-Noradrenalin in Meerschweinchenorganen nach Vorbehandlung mit α-Methyl-Dopa. Naunyn-Schmiedebergs Arch. exp. Path. Pharmak. **247**, 297 (1964).
SCHULER, W., u. R. MEYER: Vergleich der aminooxydasehemmenden und der blutdrucksenkenden Wirkung von Hydrazinophthalazinen. Helv. physiol. pharmacol. Acta **13**, 106 (1955).
—, u. A. WIEDEMANN: Über die Adrenalinsynthese im Reagenzglase unter physiologischen Bedingungen. Hoppe-Seylers Z. physiol. Chem. **233**, 235 (1935).
—, u. E. WYSS: Zur Frage der Spezifität der Wirkung blutdrucksenkender und Reserpin-antagonistisch wirksamer Hydrazinderivate auf Ferment- und Metall-Katalysen biogener Amine in vitro. Arch. int. Pharmacodyn. **128**, 431 (1960).
SCHUMACHER, H.: Dtsch. Ophthalmologenkongr. Heidelberg 1959.
SCHUMANN, E. L., M. E. GREIG, R. V. HEINZELMANN, and P. H. SEAY: The synthesis and pharmacological actions of ortho-substituted phenylethylhydrazines. J. med. pharm. Chem. **3**, 567 (1961).
— R. V. HEINZELMANN, M. E. GREIG, and W. VELDKAMP: Hydroxylamine chemistry. IV. O-Aralkylhydroxylamines. J. med. Chem. **7**, 329 (1964).
SCHWARTZ, D. E., W. P. BURKARD, M. ROTH, K. F. GEY, and A. PLETSCHER: Effect of chlorpromazine on the penetration of MAO inhibitors and monoamine releasers into rat brain. Arch. int. Pharmacodyn. **141**, 135 (1963).
SCHWARTZ, M. A.: The metabolism of isocarboxazid (Marplan) in the rat. J. Pharmacol. exp. Ther. **130**, 157 (1960).
— Interrelationships between isocarboxazid (Marplan), benzylhydrazine and monoamine oxidase. Fed. Proc. **20**, 167 (1961a).

SCHWARTZ, M. A.: Isocarboxazid metabolism in rat liver homogenate. Proc. Soc. exp. Biol. (N.Y.) **107**, 613 (1961b).
— Monoamine oxidase inhibition by isocarboxazid. J. Pharmacol. exp. Ther. **135**, 1 (1962).
SCHWEPPE, J. S., E. A. ZELLER, and G. M. HIGGINS: Interrelationships between enzymes and hormones. VI. Influence of age, sex, adrenalectomy and cortisone acetate upon the concentration of monoamine oxidase in the livers of white rats. Proc. Mayo Clin. **26**, 371 (1951).
SCHWERT, J.: Effect of nialamide on thyroid function as measured by the radioactive iodine uptake test: a case study. Simpósio internacional sobre Nialamida, J. Soc. Ciênc. méd. Lisboa **123**, Suppl., 126 (1959).
—, u. F. HAWLICZEK: Jodaufnahme der Schilddrüse unter Niamid. Wien. med. Wschr. **111**, 502 (1961).
SCOTT, G. T.: Suppression of melanocyte dispersion in the frog by psychic energizers. Nature (Lond.) **193**, 552 (1962).
SEIDEN, L. S., and A. CARLSSON: Brain and heart catecholamine levels after l-dopa administration in reserpine treated mice: correlations with a conditioned avoidance response. Psychopharmacologia (Berl.) **5**, 178 (1964).
— and J. WESTLEY: Brain monoamine oxidase: mechanism of iproniazid inhibition. Fed. Proc. **21**, 416 (1962).
— — Mechanism of iproniazid inhibition of brain monoamine oxidase. Arch. int. Pharmacodyn. **146**, 145 (1963).
SEKERIS, C. E.: Zum Tyrosinstoffwechsel der Insekten. Reinigung, Eigenschaften und Substratspezifität der Dopa-Decarboxylase. Hoppe-Seylers Z. physiol. Chem. **332**, 70 (1963).
SERRONE, D. M., and J. M. FUJIMOTO: Inhibition of the metabolism cf hexobarbital in vitro. Biochem. Pharmacol. **5**, 263 (1960).
— — Components involved in the potentiating action of β-phenylisopropylhydrazine (PIH) on hexobarbital action. Fed. Proc. **20**, 171 (1961).
— — The effect of certain inhibitors in producing shortening of hexobarbital action. Biochem. Pharmacol. **11**, 609 (1962).
SETNIKAR, I., W. MURMANN, and M. J. MAGISTRETTI: Decrease in oxygen consumption of rats by chronic iproniazid treatment. Arch. int. Pharmacodyn. **129**, 172 (1960a).
— — — Retardation of sexual development in female rats due to iproniazid treatment. Endocrinolgy **67**, 511 (1960b).
—, and M. T. RAVASI: Increase in resistance of the heart to anoxia by iproniazid. Arch. int. Pharmacodyn. **124**, 116 (1960).
SHANAMAN, J., J. F. EMELE, V. C. SCOTT, W. E. ROWE, M. R. WARREN, and C. C. SCOTT: The effect of phenelzine on the pharmacology and toxicology of various drugs. Pharmacologist **3**, 60 (1961).
SHARMAN, D. F., and S. E. SMITH: The effect of α-methyldopa on the metabolism of 5-hydroxytryptamine in rat brain. J. Neurochem. **9**, 403 (1962).
SHAW, K. N. F., A. MCMILLAN, and M. D. ARMSTRONG: The metabolism of 3,4-dihydroxyphenylalanine. J. biol. Chem. **226**, 255 (1957).
SHEE, J. C.: Dangerous potentiation of pethidine by iproniazid, and its treatment. Brit. med. J. **1960**, 507.
SHIDEMAN, F. E., and N. D. GOLDBERG: A species difference in metabolism of myocardial catecholamines. Biochem. Pharmacol. **8**, 65 (1961).
SHIMAMOTO, T.: Damages of "silicone-like property" of vascular endothelium by arteriosclerogenic substances and their prevention by nialamide. Circulation **22**, 657 (1960a).
— Antithrombolic effects of a monoamine oxidase inhibitor. Circulation **22**, 687 (1960b).
— Antithrombolic effect of a monamine oxidase inhibitor (hydrazine derivative). Circulation **22**, 809 (1960c).
— Acute vascular endothelial reaction; in reference to atherogenesis. Asian med. J. **4**, 309 (1961a).
— Methods of discovering thrombotic and antithrombotic substances. Discovery of a new type of antithrombotic effect of monoamine oxidase (MAO) inhibitors. Biochem. Pharmacol. **8**, 95 (1961b).
—, and T. FUJITA: New type of antithrombotic effect of MAO inhibitor in experimental thrombosis. Proc. Jap. Acad. **37**, 104 (1961).
— T. ISHIOKA, and T. FUJITA: New type of antithrombotic effect of monoamine oxidase inhibitor compared with anticoagulant. Circulation **24**, 1040 (1961a).
— — — Antithrombotic effect of monoamine oxidase inhibitor (nialamide), comparison with prothrombinogenic anticoagulants. Circulat. Res. **10**, 647 (1962a).
— K. TAKEUCHI, and T. ISHIOKA: Preventive effectiveness of MAO inhibitor and ineffectiveness of prothrombinogenic anticoagulant against increase in plasma thrombin activity by adrenaline, cholesterol, and traumatization. Amer. Heart. J. **64**, 71 (1962b).

SHIMAMOTO, T., K. TAKEUCHI, and T. ISHIOKA: MAO inhibitor and anticoagulant in shortening of prothrombin time by adrenaline, cholesterol and traumatization. Chemotherapia (Basel) **4**, 227 (1962c).

— H. YAMAZAKI, M. INOUE, T. FUJITA, N. SAGAWA, T. SUNAGA, and T. ISHIOKA: Discovery of antithrombolic effect of nialamide protection of silicone-like property of blood vessels by nialamide. Proc. Jap. Acad. **36**, 240 (1960).

— — H. TSUCHIHASHI, T. SUNAGA, and T. ISHIOKA: Application of antithrombotic effect of nialamide in arteriosclerotic disorders including myocardial infarction. Circulation **24**, 1040 (1961b).

SHIMIZU, N., N. MORIKAWA, and M. OKADA: Histochemical studies of monoamine oxidase of the brain of rodents. Z. Zellforsch. **49**, 389 (1959).

SHORE, P. A.: Release of serotonin and catecholamines by drugs. Pharmacol. Rev. **14**, 531 (1962).

—, and H. S. ALPERS: Binding and release of metaraminol (aramine). Fed. Proc. **23**, 350 (1964).

—, and B. B. BRODIE: LSD-like effects elicited by reserpine in rabbits pretreated with iproniazid. Proc. Soc. exp. Biol. (N.Y.) **99**, 433 (1957).

— — Effect of iproniazid on brain levels of norepinephrine and serotonin. Science **127**, 704 (1958).

—, and V. H. COHN jr.: Comparative effects of monoamine oxidase inhibitors on monoamine oxidase and diamine oxidase. Biochem. Pharmacol. **5**, 91 (1960).

— L. GILLESPIE, S. SPECTOR, and D. PROCKOP: Increase in blood serotonin levels induced by iproniazid in man and rabbits. Naturwissenschaften **45**, 340 (1958).

— J. A. R. MEAD, R. G. KUNTZMAN, S. SPECTOR, and B. B. BRODIE: On the physiologic significance of monoamin oxidase in brain. Science **126**, 1063 (1957).

SICUTERI, F., S. MICHELACCI e G. FRANCHI: Contributo alla carratterizzazione della farmacologia della reserpina sul sistema nervoso centrale. Antagonismo di un bloccante adrenergico sul fenomeno della eccitazione paradossa da reserpina nel topo. Boll. Soc. ital. Biol. sper. **38**, 381 (1962).

SINCLAIR, L.: The effects of intraventricular iproniazid on the rat. J. Physol. (Lond.) **153**, 47P (1960).

SINGER, T. P., and E. S. G. BARBON: Studies on biological oxidations. XX. Sulfhydryl enzymes in fat and protein metabolism. J. biol. Chem. **157**, 241 (1945).

SJOERDSMA, A.: Catecholamine metabolism in patients with phaeochromocytoma. Pharmacol. Rev. **11**, 374 (1959).

— Newer biochemical approaches to the treatment of hypertension. Ann. N.Y. Acad. Sci. **88**, 933 (1960).

— Relationships between alterations in amine metabolism and blood pressure. Circulat. Res. **9**, 734 (1961).

— L. A. GILLESPIE, and S. UDENFRIEND: A simple method for the measurement of monoamin-oxidase inhibition in man. Lancet **1958 II**, 159.

— — — A method for measurement of monoamine oxidase inhibition in man: application to studies on hypertension (Discussion). Ann. N. Y. Acad. Sci. **80**, 969, 977 (1959a).

— A. LEEPER, L. L. TERRY, and S. UDENFRIEND: Studies on the biogenesis and metabolism of norepinephrine in patients with phaeochromocytoma. J. clin. Invest. **38**, 31 (1959b).

— W. LOVENBERG, J. A. OATES, J. R. CROUT, and S. UDENFRIEND: Alterations in the pattern of amine excretion in man produced by a monoamine oxidase inhibitor. Science **130**, 225 (1959c).

— J. A. OATES, and L. GILLESPIE jr.: Quantitation of monoamine oxidase inhibition produced with various drugs in man. Proc. Soc. exp. Biol. (N.Y.) **103**, 485 (1960a).

— — P. ZALTZMAN, and S. UDENFRIEND: Identification and assay of urinary tryptamine: application as an index of monamine oxidase inhibition in man. J. Pharmacol. exp. Ther. **126**, 217 (1959d).

— — — — Serotonin synthesis in carcinoid patients. Its inhibition by α-methyl-dopa, with measurement of associated increases in urinary 5-hydroxytryptophan. New Engl. J. Med. **263**, 585 (1960b).

— T. E. SMITH, T. D. STEVENSON, and S. UDENFRIEND: Metabolism of 5-hydroxytryptamine (serotonin) by monoamine oxidase. Proc. Soc. exp. Biol. (N. Y.) **89**, 36 (1955).

—, and S. UDENFRIEND: Pharmacology and biochemistry of α-methyldopa in man and experimental animals. Biochem. Pharmacol. **8**, 164 (1961).

— A. VENDSALU, and K. ENGELMAN: Studies on the metabolism and mechanism of action of methyldopa. Circulation **28**, 492 (1963).

— H. WEISSBACH, L. L. TERRY, and S. UDENFRIEND: Further observations on patients with malignant carcinoid. Amer. J. Med. **23**, 5 (1957).

SKILLEN, R. G., C. H. THIENES, and L. STRAIN: Brain 5-hydroxytryptamine, 5-hydroxytryptophan decarboxylase and monoamine oxidase on normal, thyroid-fed, and propylthiouracil-fed male and female rats. Endocrinology **69**, 1099 (1961).
— — — 5-Hydroxytryptamine, 5-hydroxytryptophan decarboxylase and monoamine oxidase in hearts of normal, thyroid-fed and propylthiouracil-fed male and female rats. Endocrinology **70**, 743 (1962).
SLETZINGER, M., J. M. CHEMEDERA, and F. W. BOLLINGER: Potent decarboxylase inhibitors. Analogs of methyldopa. J. med. Chem. **6**, 101 (1963).
SLOANE-STANLEY, G. H.: Amino-acid decarboxylase of rat liver. Biochem. J. **45**, 556 (1949).
SMITH, A., and S. B. WORTIS: Formation and metabolism of N-acetylnormetanephrine in rats treated with iproniazid. Fed. Proc. **19**, 294 (1960).
— — Formation and metabolism of N-acetylnormetanephrine in rats treated with iproniazid. Biochim. biophys. Acta (Amst.) **60**, 420 (1962).
SMITH, B.: The distribution of monoamine oxidase in the brain and pituitary gland of the albino rat. Acta neurol. scand. **38**, Suppl. 1, 52 (1962).
SMITH, C. B.: Enhancement by α-methyl dopa of the effect of amphetamine and l-dopa upon locomotor activity of mice. Pharmacologist **4**, 152 (1962).
—, and P. B. DEWS: Antagonism of locomotor suppressant effects of reserpine in mice. Psychopharmacol. **3**, 55 (1962).
SMITH, F. A., L. BERGER, and A. CORRAZ: Pyrid (2,1-c) oxazine derivatives. J. med. pharm. Chem. **3**, 187 (1961).
SMITH, M. E., R. L. EVANS, E. J. NEWMAN, and H. W. NEWMAN: Psychotherapeutic agents and ethyl alcohol. Quart. J. Stud. Alcohol **22**, 241 (1961).
SMITH, S. E.: Action of α-methyldopa on brain and intestinal 5-hydroxytryptamine in mice. J. Physiol. (Lond.) **148**, 18P (1959).
— The pharmacological actions of 3,4-dihydroxyphenyl-α-methylalanine (α-methyldopa), an inhibitor of 5-hydroxytryptophan decarboxylase. Brit. J. Pharmacol. **15**, 319 (1960a).
— Discussion. Ciba Foundation, Symposium on Adrenergic Mechanism, p. 25. London: J. & A. Churchill Ltd. 1960b.
— Uptake of 5-hydroxy(^{14}C)tryptophan by rat and dog brain slices. Brit. J. Pharmacol. **20**, 178 (1963).
— R. S. STACEY, and I. M. YOUNG: 5-Hydroxytryptamine and 5-hydroxytryptophan decarboxylase activity in the developing nervous system of rats and guinea pigs. Biochem. Pharmacol. 8, 32 (1961).
— — 5-Hydroxytryptamine and 5-hydroxytryptophan decarboxylase activity in the developing nervous system of rats and guinea-pigs. In: Proceedings of the First International Pharmacological Meeting, vol. 8, p. 101. London: Pergamon Press 1962.
SMITH, T. E., H. WEISSBACH, and S. UDENFRIEND: Studies on the mechanism of action of monoamine oxidase: metabolism of N,N-dimethyltryptamine and N,N,-dimethyltryptamine-N-oxide. Biochemistry **1**, 137 (1962).
— — — Studies on monoamine oxidase: The mechanism of inhibition of monoamine oxidase by iproniazid. Biochemistry **2**, 746 (1964).
SMUSZKOVICZ, J., and M. E. GREIG: A study of the inhibitory effect of various hydrazides on monoamine oxidase in vitro and in vivo. J. med. pharm. Chem. **4**, 259 (1961).
SMYTH, CH. J., O. B. GUM, and P. K. HAMILTON: Effect of intra-articular serotonin and competitive amines on connective tissue proliferation of rabbit joints. J. Lab. clin. Med. **58**, 958 (1961).
— — — Effects of intra-articular serotonin and competitive amines on connective tissue proliferation in rabbit joints. J. Lab. clin. Med. **60**, 492 (1962).
SNELL, E. E.: Chemical structure in relation to biological activities of vitamin B_6. In: Vitamins and Hormones, vol. 16, p. 77, edit. R. S. HARRIS, E. D. MARRIAN, and K. V. THIMANN. New York: Academic Press Inc. Publ. 1958.
SNOW, P. J. D., J. E. LENNARD-JONES, G. CRUZON, and R. J. STACEY: Humoral effects of metastasising carcinoid tumors. Lancet **1955 II**, 1004.
SNYDER, F. H., H. GOETZE, and F. W. OBERST: Metabolic studies on derivatives of β-phenylethylamine. J. Pharmacol. exp. Ther. **86**, 145 (1946).
—, and F. W. OBERST: Metabolic studies on β-cyclohexylethylamines. J. Pharmacol. exp. Ther. **87**, 389 (1946).
SNYDER, S. H., and J. AXELROD: Inhibition of histamine methylation in vivo by drugs. Biochem. Pharmacol. **13**, 536 (1964a).
— — A sensitive assay for 5-hydroxytryptophan decarboxylase. Biochem. Pharmacol. **13**, 805 (1964b).
— — Influence of light and the sympathetic nervous system on 5-hydroxytryptophan decarboxylase activity in the pineal gland. Fed. Proc. **23**, 206 (1964c).

SNYDER, S. H., J. AXELROD, J. E. FISCHER, and R. J. WURTMANN: Neural and photic regulation of 5-hydroxytryptophan decarboxylase in the rat pineal gland. Nature (Lond.) **203**, 981 (1964).

SOEP, H.: Determination of monoamine oxidase activity. In: Enzymes in Clinical Chemistry, p. 481. Int. Union of Pure and Applied Chemistry, London 1962.

SOMERVILLE, A. R.: The assay of aromatic amino acid decarboxylase using radioactive substrates. Biochem. Pharmacol. **13**, 1861 (1964).

SORIANO, V.: Estudios clinicos con el Marsilid en estados depresivos y en el Parkinson. Arch. urug. Med. **51**, 40 (1958).

SOULAIRAC, A., et M.-L. SOULAIRAC: Action de la réserpine, de la sérotonine et de l'iproniazide sur le comportement alimentaire du rat. C. R. Soc. Biol. (Paris) **154**, 510 (1960).

— — et J. N. VAN STEENKISTE: Action de la chlorpromazine, de l'amphétamine et de l'iproniazide sur l'hypoglycémie insulinique du rat. Ann. Endocr. (Paris) **22**, 367 (1960).

— — — Action de la chlorpromazine, de l'amphétamine et de l'iproniazide sur l'hypoglycémie insulinique du rat. Presse méd. **69**, 995 (1961).

SOURKES, T. L.: Inhibition of dihydroxyphenylalanine decarboxylase by derivatives of phenylalanine. Arch. Biochem. **51**, 444 (1954a).

— Enzymatic decarboxylation of 2,6- and 2,3-dihydroxyphenylalanine. Canad. J. Biochem. **32**, 515 (1954b).

— Substrate specificity of hydroxy-L-phenylalanine decarboxylase and related enzymes. Rev. canad. Biol. **14**, 49 (1956).

— Oxidative pathways in the metabolism of biogenic amines. Rev. canad. Biol. **17**, 328 (1958).

— Formation of dopamine in vivo: relation to the function of the basal ganglia. Rev. canad. Biol. **20**, 187 (1961).

— P. HENEAGE, and Y. TRANO: Enzymatic decarboxylation of isomeres and derivatives of dihydroxyphenylalanine. Arch. Biochem. **40**, 185 (1952).

—, and A. D'IORIO: Inhibitors of catecholamine metabolism. In: Metabolic Inhibitors, vol. 2, p. 79, edit. R. M. HOCHSTER and J. H. QUASTEL. New York and London: Academic Press Inc. 1963.

—, and J. R. LAGNADO: On the role of purines in the enzymatic reduction of tetrazolium salts. Experientia (Basel) **13**, 476 (1957a).

— — Reduction of tetrazolium salts in an amine dehydrogenating system. J. Histochem. Cytochem. **5**, 442 (1957b).

—, and G. F. MURPHY: Effects of catechclamino acids on catecholamine (CA) content of rat organs. Fed. Proc. **19**, 295 (1960).

— — Action of pyridoxine deficiency and antidecarboxylases on the metabolism of dihydroxyphenylalanine in the rat. Abstr. V. Int. Congr. Biochem. Moscow 1961.

— — B. CHAVEZ, and M. ZIELINSKA: The action of some α-methyl and other amino acids on cerebral catecholamines. J. Neurochem. **8**, 109 (1961).

— — and B. CHAVEZ-LARA: A metabolic study of α-methyl-β-(3,4-dihydroxyphenyl)-DL-alanine in man. J. med. pharm. Chem. **5**, 204 (1962).

— — and V. R. WOODFORD: Effects of deficiencies of pyridoxine, riboflavin and thiamine upon the catecholamine content of rat tissues. J. Nurt. **72**, 145 (1960).

—, and E. TOWNSEND: Effects of 2-methyl-DL-tryptophan on the oxidation of tryptophan. Canad. J. Biochem. **33**, 735 (1955).

— — and G. N. HANSEN: The oxidation of tryptamine by rat liver and other tissue suspensions. Canad. J. Biochem. **33**, 725 (1955).

SPECTOR, S.: Monoamine oxidase in control of brain serotonin and norepinephrine content. Ann. N.Y. Acad. Sci. **107**, 856 (1963).

— C. W. HIRSCH, and B. B. BRODIE: Association of behavioural effects of pargyline, a nonhydrazide MAO inhibitor with increase in brain norepinephrine. Int. J. Neuropharmacol. **2**, 81 (1963).

— R. KUNTZMAN, C. HIRSCH, and B. B. BRODIE: Delayed arousal of reserpinetreated rabbits by monoamine oxidase inhibitor. Fed. Proc. **19**, 279 (1960a).

— — — — Norepinephrine content of various ganglia after reserpine, guanethidine and JB 516. Pharmacologist **2**, 94 (1960b).

— — P. A. SHORE, and B. B. BRODIE: Evidence for release of brain amines by reserpine in presence of monoamine oxidase inhibitors: implication of monoamine oxidase in norepinephrine metabolism in brain. J. Pharmacol. exp. Ther. **130**, 256 (1960c).

— H. MALING, and P. A. SHORE: Effect of JB 516, a monoamine oxidase inhibitor, on levels of serotonin and norepinephrine in brain and spinal cord. Fed. Proc. **18**, 447 (1959).

— K. MELMON, and A. SJOERDSMA: Evidence for rapid turnover of norepinephrine in rat heart and brain. Proc. Soc. exp. Biol. (N.Y.) **111**, 79 (1962).

SPECTOR, S., D. PROCKOP, P. A. SHORE, and B. B. BRODIE: Effect of iproniazid and other monoamine inhibitors on norepinephrine and serotonin in brain. J. Pharmacol. exp. Ther. **122**, 71A (1958a).
— — — — Effect of iproniazid on brain levels of norepinephrine and serotonin. Science **127**, 704 (1958b).
— P. A. SHORE, and B. B. BRODIE: Biochemical and pharmacological effects of the monoamine oxidase inhibitors, iproniazid, 1-phenyl-2-hydrazinopropane (JB 516) and 1-phenyl-3-hydrazinobutane (JB 835). J. Pharmacol. exp. Ther. **128**, 15 (1960d).
SPECTOR, W. G.: Anti-fertility action of a monoamine oxidase inhibitor. Nature (Lond.) **187**, 514 (1960).
—, and D. A. WILLOUGHBY: The enzymic inactivation of an adrenaline-like substance in inflammation. J. Path. Bact. **80**, 271 (1960a).
— — Suppression of increased capillary permeability in injury by monoamine oxidase inhibitors. Nature (Lond.) **186**, 162 (1960b).
SPENCER, J. N., M. PORTER, H. L. FROEHLICH, and H. WENDEL: Observations on the cardiovascular effects of tranylcypromine. Fed. Proc. **19**, 277 (1960).
SPENCER, R. P., and N. ZAMCHEK: Alternate metabolic fate of 5-hydroxytryptophan. Biochem. biophys. Res. Commun. **3**, 386 (1960).
SPINKS, A., and E. H. P. YOUNG: The relation between structure and central nervous action of some hydrazine derivatives. Biochem. Pharmacol. **8**, 10 (1961).
SPOERLEIN, M. T., and A. M. ELLMAN: Facilitation of metrazol-induced seizures by iproniazid and β-phenylisopropylhydrazine in mice. Arch. int. Pharmacodyn. **133**, 193 (1961).
STARR, K. W., J. GIBBONS, and J. C. CLAUDATUS: Mono- and Di-amine oxidase activities of human tumours and host tissues. Nature (Lond.) **195**, 1010 (1962).
STEBBINS, R. B., and M. I. MULROY: Anatomic effects of nialamide, a new antidepressant. Pharmacclogist **1**, 71 (1959).
STEENSHOLT, G., M. FLIKKE, and P. E. JONER: Some properties of amino acid decarboxylases, and their mechanism of action. Abstr. III. Int. Congr. Biochem., Brussels 1955, p. 38.
STEIN, L., and O. S. RAY: Accelerated recovery from reserpine depression by monoamine oxidase inhibitors. Nature (Lond.) 188, 1199 (1960).
STEINER, F. A.: Unpublished results.
— H. BESENDORF, and H. P. BÄCHTOLD: Unpublished results.
STERN, I. J., S. WILK, and R. D. HOLLIFIELD: An internal standard for the colorimetric determination of monoamine oxidase activity. Analyt. Biochem **2**, 396 (1961).
STERN, P., and J. GAŠPAROVIC: A contribution to the pharmacology of tremorine-induced tremor. Biochem Pharmacol. **8**, 26 (1961).
—, u. D. KOCIC-MITROVIC: Wirkung des Reserpins auf die Menge der Substanz P im Rattengehirn. Naunyn-Schmiedebergs Arch. exp. Path. Pharmak. **238**, 57 (1960).
STEVENS, G. DE, P. W. STRACHAN, M. DUGHI, and A. HALAMANDARIS: Hydrazines, hydrazides and hydrazide esters. J. med. pharm. Chem. **3**, 533 (1961).
STOCK, K., u. E. WESTERMANN: Untersuchungen über den Mechanismus der narkoseverkürzenden Wirkung von Monoaminoxydase-Hemmstoffen. Naunyn-Schmiedebergs Arch. exp. Path. Pharmak **243**, 44 (1962a).
— — Über eine Wirkung von Monoaminoxydase-Hemmstoffen auf den Fettstoffwechsel der Ratte. Naunyn-Schmiedebergs Arch. exp. Path. Pharmak. **243**, 296 (1962b).
—, and E. O. WESTERMANN: Concentration of norepinephrine, serotonin, and histamine, and of amine-metabolizing enzymes in mammalian adipose tissue. J. Lipid Res. **4**, 297 (1963).
STONE, C. A., C. C. PORTER, L. S. WATSON, and C. A. ROSS: Pharmacology of decarboxylase inhibitors. Second Hahnemann Symposium on Hypertensive Disease, p. 417, edit. A. N. BREST and J. H. MOYER. Philadelphia and London: W. B. Saunders 1961.
— C. A. ROSS, H. C. WENGER, C. T. LUDDEN, J. A. GLESSING, J. A. TOTARO, and C. C. PORTER: Effect of α-methyl-3,4-dihydroxyphenylalanine (methyldopa), reserpine and related agents on some vascular responses in the dog. J. Pharmacol. exp. Ther. **136**, 80 (1962).
STRÖMBLAD, B. C. R.: Observations on amine oxidase in human salivary glands. J. Physiol. (Lond.) **147**, 639 (1959a).
— Amine-oxidase in human salivary glands. Lancet **1959** b **I**, 1100.
STRUBE, R. E.: Hydroxybenzylidineaminorhodamines. U. S. Pat. 2,957,869, Oct. 25, 1960.
STUDER, A.: Einfluß von Pharmaka auf die Histochemie des Nebennierenmarkes der Ratte. Path. et Microbiol. (Basel) **24**, 221 (1961).
—, u. G. ZBINDEN: Monoaminstoffwechsel und enterochromaffines System. Psychiat. et Neurol. (Basel) **140**, 237 (1960).
STUDNITZ, W. v.: Effect of Marsilid on excretion of 3-methoxy-4-hytroxymandelic acid in man. Scand. J. clin. Lab. Invest. **11**, 224 (1959a).
— On the excretion of 3-methoxy-4-hydroxymandelic acid in patients with serotonin producing tumours. Scand. J. clin. Lab. Invest. **11**, 309 (1959b).

STÜTTGEN, G., W. KELLER u. K. KNOBEL: Zum Einfluß von Heparin und Adenosinphosphorsäuren auf Substrate und Aktivität der Mono- und Diaminoxydasen. Z. ges. exp. Med. **134**, 446 (1961).

STURM jr. A., u. G. STÜTTGEN: Nachweis von 5-Hydroxytryptophan in menschlichen Mastzellen. Klin. Wschr. **40**, 199 (1962).

STURTEVANT, F. M.: Prolongation of hexobarbital-hypnosis in mice by iproniazid, serotonin and reserpin. Naturwissenschaften **43**, 67 (1956).

SWETT, L. R., W. B. MARTIN, J. D. TAYLOR, G. M. EVERETT, A. A. WYKES, and Y. C. GLADISH: Structure-activity relations in the pargyline series. Ann. N.Y. Acad. Sci. **107**, 891 (1963).

SYMUL, F.: Etude de la dibenzylméthylamine (566 Labaz) comme inhibiteur de l'aminoxydase. C. R. Soc. Biol. (Paris) **141**, 1269 (1947).

SZARA, S.: Hallucinogenic effects and metabolism of tryptamine derivatives in man. Fed. Proc. **20**, 885 (1961).

SZPORNY, L., and P. GÖRÖG: Investigations into the correlations between monoamine oxidase inhibition and other effects due to methylphenydate and its stereoisomers. Biochem. Pharmacol. **8**, 263 (1961).

TABACHNICK, I. I. A.: On the enzymic specificity of antidepressant monoamine oxidase (MAO) inhibitors. Pharmacologist **1**, 81 (1959).

—, and A. A. RUBIN: Some relationship between peripheral monoamine oxidase inhibition and brain 5-hydroxytryptamine levels in rats. Proc. Soc. exp. Biol. (N. Y.) **101**, 435 (1959).

TABOR, C. W., and S. M. ROSENTHAL: Pharmacology of spermine and spermidine. Some effects on animals and bacteria. J. Pharmacol. exp. Ther. **116**, 139 (1956).

— H. TABOR, and U. BACHRACH: Identification of the aminoaldehydes produced by the oxidation of spermine and spermidine with purified plasma amine oxidase. J. biol. Chem. **239**, 2194 (1964).

— — and S. M. ROSENTHAL: Purification of amine oxidase from beef plasma. J. biol. Chem. **208**, 645 (1954).

TABOR, H.: Metabolic studies on histidine, histamine and related imidazoles. Pharmacol. Rev. **6**, 299 (1954).

— Degradation of histidine. Symposium on Amino Acid Metabolism, p. 373, edit. MCELROY and GLASS. Baltimore: Johns Hopkins Press 1955.

TAKEHIKO, T.: Microbiochemical study of the development and the differentiation of the nervous system. Juzen Igakukai Zasshi **61**, 157 (1959) [Chem. Abstr. **59**, 7941 (1963)].

TAYLOR, J. D., and R. A. KRAUSE: Distribution and metabolism of the monoamine oxidase inhibitor (N-methyl-N-benzyl-2-propynylamine hydrochloride) in the rat and dog. Fed. Proc. **21**, 181 (1962).

— A. A. WYKES, Y. C. GLADISH, and W. B. MARTIN: New inhibitor of monoamine oxidase. Nature (Lond.) **187**, 941 (1960a).

— — — —, and G. M. EVERETT: A new non-hydrazide monoamine oxidase inhibitor (A 19120) (N-methyl-N-benzyl-2-propynylamine hydrochloride). Fed. Proc. **19**, 278 (1960b).

TEDESCHI, D. H., and E. J. FELLOWS: Monoamine oxidase inhibitors: augmentation of pressor effects of peroral tyramine. Science **144**, 1225 (1964).

— R. E. TEDESCHI, and E. J. FELLOWS: A pharmacological procedure for the evaluation of in vivo inhibitors of monoamine oxidase; observations on the neuropharmacological effects of tryptamine hydrochloride. Fed. Proc. **18**, 450 (1959a).

— — — The effects of tryptamine on the central nervous system, including a pharmacological procedure for the evaluation of iproniazid-like drugs. J. Pharmacol. exp. Ther. **126**, 223 (1959b).

— — — Activity of various pharmacological agents as in vivo inhibitors of monoamine oxidase. Fed. Proc. **19**, 278 (1960a).

— — — In vivo monoamine oxidase inhibition measured by potentiation of tryptamine convulsions in rats. Proc. Soc. exp. Biol. (N. Y.) **103**, 680 (1960b).

— — P. J. FOWLER, H. GREEN, and E. J. FELLOWS: N-Methyl-α-methyl-tryptamine: a potent monoamine oxidase inhibitor and tryptamine antagonist. Biochem. Pharmacol. **11**, 481 (1962).

TEDESCHI, R. E., D. H. TEDESCHI, P. L. AMES, L. COOK, P. A. MATTIS, and E. J. FELLOWS: Some pharmacological observations on tranylcypromine (SKF trans-385); a potent inhibitor of monoamine oxidase. Proc. Soc. exp. Biol. (N. Y.) **102**, 380 (1959a).

— — L. COOK, P. A. MATTIS, and E. J. FELLOWS: Some neuropharmacological observations on SKF trans 385 (2-phenyl-cyclopropylamine hydrochloride), a potent inhibitor of monoamine oxidase. Fed. Proc. **18**, 451 (1959b).

TEIXEIRA, I.: Action du benzyl-carbamyl-éthyl-isonicotinyl-hydrazide sur le développement du fémur cartilagineux d'embryon de poulet en culture in vitro. C. R. Soc. Biol. (Paris) **156**, 209 (1962).

TEMPERO, K. F., and G. A. KIEN: Effect of iproniazid on the intermediary metabolism of rabbit heart. Fed. Proc. **23**, 230 (1964).
— E. LACROIX et I. LEUSEN: Lésions gastriques postréserpiniques, rôle du cortex surrénalien. Gastroenterologia (Basel) **98**, 225 (1962).
THOENEN, H.: Personal communication.
— E. LACROIX et I. LEUSEN: Lésions gastriques postréserpiniques, rôle du cortex surrénalien. Gastroenterologia (Basel) **98**, 225 (1962).
THOMPSON, R. H. S.: Amine oxidase of blood vessels. Ciba Foundation, Symposium on Visceral Circulation, p. 100. London: J. & A. Churchill Ltd. 1952.
—, and A. TICKNER: Observations on the monoamine oxidase activity of placenta and uterus. Biochem. J. **45**, 125 (1959).
— — The occurrence and distribution of monoamine oxidase in blood vessels. J. Physiol. (Lond.) **115**, 34 (1951).
TICKNER, A.: Inhibition of amine oxidase by antihistamine compounds and related drugs. Brit. J. Pharmacol. **6**, 606 (1951).
TIMSIT, J., et J. LÉVY: Comparaison, sur l'oreillette isolée de cobaye, des actions antinicotiniques de trois inhibiteurs de la monoamineoxydase dérivés de l'hydrazine et de trois amines possédant le même squelette carboné. C. R. Soc. Biol. (Paris) **155**, 2304 (1962).
TIRUNARAYANAN, M. O., and W. A. VISCHER: Effect of isoniazid on catalase and peroxidase of tubercle bacilli in vitro. Naturwissenschaften **43**, 474 (1956).
TISSOT, R., et M. MONNIER: Suppression de l'action de la réserpine sur le cerveau par ses antagonistes: iproniazid et LSD. Helv. physiol. pharmacol. Acta **16**, 268 (1958).
TODD, L., H. VILLARREAL y J. PISANTY: Iproniazida en la anoxia tisular. II. Congr. nacional de ciencias fisologicas, Buenos Aires 1959 (Programa General y Estractos de las Communicaciones, p. 103).
TOMOKICHI, I.: On the problem of precursors of adrenalin. J. Osaka med. Sch. **40**, 1494 (1941). [W. G. CLARK, Pharmacol. Rev. **11**, 330 (1959).]
TOWNE, J. C.: Effect of ethanol and acetaldehyde on liver and brain monoamine oxidase. Nature (Lond.) **201**, 709 (1964).
TRUITT jr., E. B., G. DURITZ, and E. M. EBERSBERGER: Evidence for monoamine oxidase inhibition by myristicin and nutmeg. Proc. Soc. exp. Biol. (N.Y.) **112**, 647 (1963).
— and E. M. EBERSBERGER: The therapeutic index of hexafluorodiethyl ether (Indoklon) and its modification by reserpine and iproniazid. Pharmacologist **1**, 66 (1959).
— — Lowered convulsive thresholds to hexafluorodiethyl ether produced by drugs with differential effects on brain serotonin and norepinephrine levels. Fed. Proc. **20**, 320 (1961).
— — Decarboxylase inhibitors affect convulsion thresholds to hexafluorodiethyl ether. Science **135**, 105 (1962).
TRZEBSKI, A.: The action of adrenaline, noradrenaline and monoamine oxidase inhibitors injected directly into the reticular formation of the brain stem. Bull. Acad. pol. Sci., Sér. sci. biol. **8**, 525 (1960).
TUCHMANN-DUPLESSIS, H., et L. MERCIER-PAROT: Répercussions d'un inhibiteur de la monoamineoxydase, la niamide, sur l'appareil hypophyso-génital et la corticosurrénale de la ratte. C. R. Acad. Sci. (Paris) **252**, 3882 (1961).
— — Influence de la niamide sur la sphère sexuelle et la fertilité du rat. Chemotherapia (Basel) **4**, 304 (1962).
TUNG, Y.-C.: Studies on β-carboline derivatives. II. Synthesis of norharman, harman and 3-methyl-harman derivatives and their effects on monoamine oxidase, choline oxidase and succinoxidase. J. Formosan med. Ass. **59**, 889 (1960).
— Y.-S. HWANG, C.-C. WU, and K.-H. LING: Studies on β-carboline derivatives. I. Synthesis of 3-methyl-norharman derivatives and their effects on monoamine oxidase and choline oxidase. J. Formosan med. Ass. **59**, 550 (1960).
UDENFRIEND, S.: Urinary tryptamine in hypertensive patients treated with JB-516 and nialamide. Dis. nerv. Syst. **20**, Suppl., 14 (1959a).
— Biochemistry of serotonin and other indoleamines. Vitam. u. Horm. **17**, 133 (1959b).
— C. J. CLARK, and E. TITUS: 5-Hydroxytryptophan decarboxylase: a new route of metabolism of tryptophan. J. Amer. chem. Soc. **75**, 501 (1953).
— R. H. CONNAMACHER, and S. M. HESS: On the mechanism of release of norepinephrine by α-methyl-m-tyrosine and α-methyl-m-tyramine. Biochem. Pharmacol. **8**, 419 (1961).
— C. R. CREVELING, M. OZAKI, J. W. DALY, and B. WITKOP: Inhibitors of norepinephrine metabolism in vivo. Arch. Biochem. **84**, 249 (1959).
— W. M. LOVENBERG, and H. WEISSBACH: L-Amino acid decarboxylase activity in mammalian tissues and its inhibition by α-methyl-dopa. Fed. Proc. **19**, 7 (1960).
— E. TITUS, and H. WEISSBACH: The identification of 5-hydroxy-3-indoleacetic acid in normal urine and a method for its assay. J. biol. Chem. **216**, 499 (1955a).

UDENFRIEND, S., H. WEISSBACH and D. F. BOGDANSKI: Biochemical findings relating to the action of serotonin. Ann. N. Y. Acad. Sci. **66**, 602 (1957a).
— — — Biochemical studies on serotonin and their physiological implications. In: Hormones, Brain Function and Behavior, edit. H. HOAGLAND, p. 147. New York: Academic Press. Inc. Publ. 1957b.
— — — Increase in tissue serotonin following administration of its precursor 5-hydroxytryptophan. J. biol. Chem. **224**, 803 (1957c).
— — — Effect of iproniazid on serotonin metabolism in vivo. J. Pharmacol. exp. Ther. **120**, 255 (1957d).
— — and B. B. BRODIE: Assay of serotonin and related metabolites, enzymes and drugs. Meth. biochem. Anal. **6**, 95 (1958a).
— — and C. T. CLARK: The estimation of 5-hydroxytryptamine (serotonin) in biological tissues. J. biol. Chem. **215**, 337 (1955b).
— B. WITKOP, B. G. REDFIELD, and H. WEISSBACH: Studies with reversible inhibitors of monoamine oxidase harmaline and related compounds. Biochem. Pharmacol. **1**, 160 (1958b).
—, and P. ZALTZMAN-NIRENBERG: On the mechanism of norepinephrine depletion by aramine. Life Sci. **3**, 695 (1964).
USDIN, E. and V. R. USDIN: Effects of psychotropic compounds on enzyme systems. II. In vitro inhibition of monoamine oxidase. Proc. Soc. exp. Biol. (N. Y.) **108**, 461 (1961).
UTTER, M. F.: Nonoxidative carboxylation and decarboxylation. In: The Enzymes, vol. 5, p. 319, edit. P. D. BOYER et al. New Yerk and London: Academic Press 1961.
UUSPÄÄ, V. J., M. M. AIRAKSINEN, and V. I. UUSPÄÄ: Formation of 5-hydroxytryptamine in the kidney. Int. J. Neuropharmacol. **1**, 231 (1962).
VALENTI, S., B. TREVES, and M. KAMEL-EL-WASSY: Warburg manometric analysis of catalase activity of blood of isoniazid-treated guinea pigs. Gazz. int. Med. Chir. **63**, 860 (1958). [Chem. Abstr. **52**, 13997h (1958).]
VANE, J. R.: The relative activities of some tryptamine analogues on the isolated rat stomach strip preparation. Brit. J. Pharmacol. **14**, 87 (1959).
— H. O. J. COLLIER, S. J. CORNE, E. MARLEY, and P. B. BRADLEY: Tryptamine receptors in the central nervous system. Nature (Lond.) **191**, 1068 (1961).
VANOV, S.: Effect of monoamine oxidase inhibitors and pyrogallol on the pressor response to adrenaline, noradrenaline, normetanephrine and tyramine in the rat. Arch. int. Pharmacodyn. **138**, 51 (1962).
VARAGIĆ, V., R. LEŠIĆ, J. VUCO, and B. STAMENOVIĆ: The effect of eserine on the activity of adrenergic nerves in the rat. Biochem. Pharmacol. 8, 10 (1061).
VARMA, D. R., and B. G. BENFEY: Antagonism of reserpine-induced subsensitivity to tyramine by methyldopa. J. Pharmacol. exp. Ther. **141**, 310 (1963).
— R. A. GILLIS, and B. G. BENFEY: Antagonism of reserpine by methyldopa. Pharmacologist **5**, 256 (1963).
VEREVKINA, I. V., V. Z. GORKIN, V. M. MITYUSHIN, and I. E. EL'PINER: Effect of ultrasonic waves on monoamine oxidase associated with submicroscopic structures of mitochondria. Biofizika **9**, 503 (1964) [Chem. Abstr. **61**, 9697 g (1964)].
VINCENT, D., et G. SEGONZAC: Recherche de l'effet des alcaloides in vitro sur l'activité de l'aminoxydase du cerveau vis-à-vis de la sérotonine. Thérapie **15**, 914 (1960).
— — et M. C. MARQUES-VINCENT: Action de quelques substances anticholinestérasiques sur la monoaminoxydase du cerveau. C. R. Soc. Biol. (Paris) **115**, 2446 (1962).
VIOLLIER, G., E. QUIRING u. H. STAUB: Einfluß von oral verabreichtem Isonicotinsäurehydrazid und dessen Isopropylderivat auf den Enzymhaushalt der weißen Ratte. Helv. chim. Acta **36**, 724 (1953).
VITEK, V., and K. RYSANEK: Inhibition of monoamine oxidase by benactyzine in vitro and in vivo. Nature (Lond.) **186**, 244 (1960).
VIZI, E. Sz., A. K. PFEIFER, E. SÁTORY u. E. GALAMBOS: Die Wirkung von Reserpin und Iproniazid auf die Stoffwechselzentren. Arch. exp. Path. Pharmakol. **246**, 49 (1963).
VOELKEL, A.: Die Behandlung psychomotorischer Hemmungszustände mit dem Aminoxydasehemmer Marsilid. Klin. Wschr. **37**, 101 (1959).
VOGT, M.: Catecholamines in brain. Pharmacol. Rev. **11**, 483 (1959).
VOTAVA, Z., and I. LAMPLOVÁ: Antiserotonin activity of some ergolenyl and isoergolenyl derivatives in comparison with LSD and the influence of monoamine oxidase inhibitors on this antiserotonin effect. In: Neuropsychopharmacology, vol. 2, p. 68, edit. E. ROTHLIN. Amsterdam: Elsevier Publ. Co. 1961.
WAALKES, T. P., and H. COBURN: Conversion of serotonin (5-hydroxytryptamine) to 5-hydroxyindoleacetic acid by rabbit blood. Proc. Soc. exp. Biol. (N. Y.) **99**, 742 (1958).
WADA, J. A.: Epileptogenic cerebral electrical activity and serotonin levels. Science **134**, 1688 (1961).

WANG, H. L., V. H. HARWALKAR, and H. A. WAISMAN: Effect of dietary phenylalanine and tryptophan on brain serotonin. Arch. Biochem. **96**, 181 (1962).
WARTBURG, J. P. v.: Uptake of 5-hydroxytryptophan-3-C^{14} and its metabolism in rat brain cortex slices. Canad. J. Biochem. **40**, 1439 (1962).
—, u. H. AEBI: Der Einfluß langdauernder Aethylalkohol-Belastung auf die Catecholaminausscheidung im Harn der Ratte. Helv. physiol. pharmacol. Acta **18**, C95 (1960).
WASER, P. G., u. M. ITZBICKI: Der Einfluß verschiedener Psychopharmaka auf den Bluthistamingehalt von Ratten. Experientia (Basel) **15**, 197 (1959).
WATARI, Y.: Adrenaline dehydrogenase in blood vessel walls. Osaka Daigaku Zasshi **10**, 1075 (1958) [Chem. Abstr. **52**, 18591f (1958).]
WATON, N. G.: Studies on mammalian histidine decarboxylase. Brit. J. Pharmacol. **11**, 119 (1956).
WATTENBERG, L. W.: A histochemical study of five oxidative enzymes in carcinoma of the large intestine in man. Amer. J. Path. **35**, 113 (1959).
WEBB, J. L.: Enzyme and Metabolic Inhibitors, vol. 1, p. 545, 561. New York and London: Academic Press Inc. 1963.
WEBER, F., u. O. WISS: Über die unterschiedliche Beeinflussung des Tryptophanstoffwechsels durch Vitamin B_6-Mangel in der Ratte. Hoppe-Seylers Z. physiol. Chem. **331**, 124 (1963).
— — Unpublished results.
WEGMANN, A., K. KAKO, and A. CHRYSOHOU: Dopa uptake and catecholamine content in heart and spleen. Amer. J. Physiol. **201**, 673 (1961).
WEIKEL, J. H., and J. E. SALMON: Biochemical properties of N-benzyl-N'-isopropylhydrazine. Biochem. Pharmacol. **11**, 93 (1962).
WEIL-MAHLHERBE, H.: Phaeochromocytoma catechols in urine and tumour tissue. Lancet **1956 II**, 282.
—, and A. D. BONE: The effect of reserpine on the intracellular distribution of catecholamines in the brain stem of the rabbit. J. Neurochem. **4**, 251 (1959).
— H. S. POSNER, and G. R. BOWLES: Changes in the concentration and intracellular distribution of brain catecholamines: the effects of reserpine, β-phenylisopropylhydrazine, pyrogallol and 3,4-dihydroxyphenylalanine, alone and in combination. J. Pharmacol. exp. Ther. **132**, 278 (1961a).
— L. G. WHITBY, and J. AXELROD: The uptake of circulating (^3H) norepinephrine by the pituitary gland and various areas of the brain. J. Neurochem. **8**, 55 (1961b).
WEINER, N.: Relative activities of two particulate enzymes, monoamine oxidase and succinoxidase, in various parts of brain. Pharmacologist **1**, 81 (1959).
— Substrate specificity of brain amine oxidase of several mammals. Arch. Biochem. **91**, 182 (1960).
— The distribution of monoamine oxidase and succinic oxidase in brain. J. Neurochem. **6**, 79 (1961).
— The catecholamines: biosynthesis, storage and release, metabolism, and metabolic effects. In: The Hormones, vol. 4, p. 403, edit. G. PINCUS, K. V. THIMANN, and E. B. ASTWOOD. New York and London: Academic Press Inc. 1964.
WEISS, B.: Metabolism of dopa-C-14 in the normal and α-methyldopa treated mouse. Fed. Proc. **22**, 540 (1963).
WEISS, J., S. WEISS, and B. WEISS: The effects of iproniazid and similar compounds on the gastrointestinal tract. Ann. N. Y. Acad. Sci **80**, 854 (1959).
— — — The clinical effects of iproniazid and similar compounds on the gastrointestinal tract. Amer. J. Gastroent. **33**, 592 (1960).
WEISS, L. R., J. W. NELSON, and A. TYE: The facilitative action of reserpine on metrazol convulsions when modified by iproniazid. J. Amer. pharm. Ass., sci. Ed. **49**, 514 (1960).
WEISSBACH, H., D. F. BOGDANSKI, B. G. REDFIELD, and S. UDENFRIEND: Effectiveness of iproniazid on 5-hydroxytryptamine (serotonin) destruction in vivo. Fed. Proc. **16**, 345 (1957a).
— — — — Studies on the effect of vitamin B_6 on 5-hydroxytryptamine (serotonin) formation. J. biol. Chem. **227**, 617 (1957b).
— W. KING, A. SJOERDSMA, and S. UDENFRIEND: Formation of indole-3-acetic acid and tryptamine in animals. A method for estimation of indole-3-acetic acid in tissues. J. biol. Chem. **234**, 81 (1959).
— W. LOVENBERG, B. G. REDFIELD, and S. UDENFRIEND: In vivo metabolism of serotonin and tryptamine: effect of monoamine oxidase inhibition. J. Pharmacol. exp. Ther. **131**, 26 (1961a).
— — and S. UDENFRIEND: Enzymatic decarboxylation of α-methyl amino acids. Biochem. biophys. Res. Commun. **3**, 225 (1960a).
— — — Characteristics of mammalian histidine decarboxylating enzymes. Biochim. biophys. Acta (Amst.) **50**, 177 (1961b).

WEISSBACH, H., B. G. REDFIELD, G. G. GLENNER, and C. MITOMA: Tetrazolium reduction as a measure of monoamine oxidase activity in vitro. J. Histochem. Cytochem. **5**, 601 (1957c).
— — and S. UDENFRIEND: Soluble monoamine oxidase; its properties and actions on serotonin. J. biol. Chem. **229**, 953 (1957d).
— — — Serotonin-O-glucuronide: an alternate route of serotonin metabolism. Fed. Proc. **17**, 418 (1958).
— T. E. SMITH, J. W. DALY, B. WITKOP, and S. UDENFRIEND: A rapid spectrophotometric assay of monoamine oxidase based on the rate of disappearance of kynuramine. J. biol. Chem. **235**, 1160 (1960b).
WENZEL, D. G., and G. N. BECKLOFF: The effect of dimercaprol on amine oxidase and amino acid decarboxylase of the normotensive and hypertensive rat kidney. J. Amer. pharm. Ass., sci. Ed. **47**, 844 (1958).
WERBOFF, J., J. S. GOTTLIEB, E. L. DEMBICKI, and J. HAVLENA: Postnatal effect of antidepressant drugs administered during gestation Exp. Neurol. **3**, 542 (1961a).
— — J. HAVLENA, and T. J. WORD: Behavioral effects of prenatal drug administration in the white rat. Pediatrics **27**, 318 (1961b).
WERLE, E.: Über die Bildung von Histamin aus Histidin durch tierisches Gewebe. Biochem. Z. **288**, 292 (1936).
— Zur Kenntnis der Histidin-decarboxylase und der Histaminase. Biochem. Z. **304**, 201 (1940).
— Aminosäure-Decarboxylasen-Histaminase-Diaminoxydase. Fermentforsch. **17**, 103 (1942—1944).
— Bildung und Abbau biogener Amine. Chemie **56**, 141 (1943).
— Aminosäure-Decarboxylasen. Z. Vitamin-, Hormon- u. Fermentforsch. **1**, 504 (1947).
— Aminosäure-Decarboxylasen. Angew. Chem. **63**, 550 (1951).
— Hemmung der Histidin-Decarboxylase durch α-Methyldopa. Naturwissenschaften **48**, 54 (1961).
—, u. D. AURES: Über die Reinigung und Spezifität der Dopa-Decarboxylase. Hoppe-Seylers Z. physiol. Chem. **316**, 45 (1959).
— — Über Reinigung und Spezifität der Dopa-Decarboxylase. Psychiat. et Neurol. (Basel) **140**, 227 (1960).
—, u. K. HEITZER: Zur Kenntnis der Histidincarboxylase. Biochem. Z. **299**, 420 (1938).
—, u. E. HENNIG: Einwirkung von Aryl- und Alkylpolyglykoläthern auf Monoaminoxydase aus Schweineleber und über den Mono- und Diaminoxydasegehalt der Nieren von Foeten und ausgewachsenen Tieren. Z. Vitamin-, Hormon- u. Fermentforsch. **11**, 159 (1960).
—, u. HERRMANN: Über die Bildung von Histamin aus Histidin durch tierisches Gewebe. Biochem. Z. **291**, 105 (1937).
—, u. J. JÜNTGEN-SELL: Zur Frage der Vorstufe vor Noradrenalin im Nebennierenmark und im sympathischen Nervengewebe und zur Frage der Identität von Dopa- und Oxyphenylserindecarboxylase. Biochem. Z. **327**, 259 (1955).
—, u. W. KOCH: Zur Kenntnis der Aminosäure-Decarboxylasen und ihres Wirkungsmechanismus. Biochem. Z. **319**, 305 (1949).
—, u. G. MENNICKEN: Über die Bildung von Tryptamin aus Tryptophan und von Tyramin aus Tyrosin durch tierisches Gewebe. Biochem. Z. **291**, 325 (1937).
— — Über die Inaktivierung von Tryptamin und Tyramin durch tierisches Gewebe. Biochem. Z. **296**, 99 (1938).
—, u. E. v. PECHMANN: Zur Kenntnis der Mono- und der Diaminoxydase von tierischen Geweben. Z. Vitamin-, Hormon- u. Fermentforsch. **2**, 433 (1948—1949).
—, u. W. PESCHEL: Über den Abbau von Phenylserin und p-Oxyphenylserin durch tierisches Gewebe. Biochem. Z. **320**, 1 (1949).
—, u. F. ROEWER: Über tierische und pflanzliche Monoaminoxydasen. Biochem. Z. **322**, 320 (1952).
— A. SCHAUER u. G. HARTUNG: Einfluß von Hydrazin- und Guanylhydrazon-derivaten auf die Aktivität der Monoamin-oxydase, Diaminoxydase, Dopa-decarboxylase und Histidindecarboxylase. Klin. Wschr. **33**, 562 (1955).
—, u. J. SELL: Über die fermentative Decarboxylierung von Mono- und Dioxyphenylserinen. Biochem. Z. **326**, 110 (1954).
WERNER, G., u. N. SEILER: Untersuchungen zum Nachweis einer Methylamin-Oxydase. Biochem. Z. **337**, 383 (1963).
— — and H.-L. SCHMIDT: On the effect of monoamine oxidase inhibitors and other psychotropic substances on the oxidative degradation of methylamine in some mammals. Med. exp. (Basel) **5**, 151 (1961).
WEST, G. B.: Studies on 5-hydroxytryptamine and 5-hydroxytryptophan. J. Pharm. Pharmacol., Suppl. **10**, 92T (1958a).
— 5-Hydroxytryptamine and hyperglycaemia. Nature (Lond.) **182**, 182 (1958b).

WESTERMANN, E.: Über den Einfluß von Thyroxin in Trijodthyroxin auf die Aminoxydase- und Dopadecarboxylaseaktivität der Leber. Naunyn-Schmiedebergs Arch. exp. Path. Pharmak. **228**, 159 (1956).
— Über die Dopadecarboxylase des Nebennierenmarkes verschiedener Tierarten. Biochem. Z. **328**, 405 (1957).
— Stimulierung und Blockierung des Hypophysen-Nebennierenrinden-Systems durch Reserpin. Naunyn-Schmiedebergs Arch. exp. Path. Pharmak. **241**, 518 (1961).
— H. BALZER u. J. KNELL: Hemmung der Serotoninbildung durch α-Methyl-Dopa. Naunyn-Schmiedebergs Arch. exp. Path. Pharmak. **234**, 194 (1958).
—, u. K. STOCK: Tierexperimentelle Untersuchungen über den Mechanismus der narkoseverkürzenden Wirkung von Monoaminoxydase-Hemmstoffen. Chemotherapia (Basel) **4**, 329 (1962).
WESTLEY, J., and L. S. SEIDEN: Partial purification of monoamine oxidase from rat brain. Biochim. biophys. Acta (Amst.) **58**, 363 (1962).
WHITE, T.T., R. A. MCALEXANDER, and D. F. MAGEE: Effects of serotonin (5-HT) and serotonin precursor (5-HTP) on gastric secretion in the dog. Surg. Gynec. Obstet. **109**, 168 (1959).
WHITHY, L.-G., J. AXELROD, and H. WEIL-MAHLHERBE: The fate of H^3-norepinephrine in animals. J. Pharmacol. exp. Ther. **132**, 193 (1961).
WHITTAKER, V. P.: Sub-cellular distribution of 5-hydroxytryptamine in guinea pig brain. Nature (Lond.) **195**. 1100 (1962).
WICKSTRÖM, L., and K. PETTERSON: Treatment of diabetics with monoamine-oxidase inhibitors. Lancet **1964 II**, 995.
WIEGAND, R. E., and J. E. PERRY: Effect of L-dopa and N-methyl-N-benzyl-2-propynylamine, HCl on dopa, dopamine, norepinephrine, epinephrine and serotonin levels in mouse brain. Biochem. Pharmacol. **7**, 181 (1961a).
— — Dopa, dopamine, norepinephrine, epinephrine and serotonin; mouse brain levels after N-methyl-N-benzyl-2-propynylamine, HCl and l-dopa. Fed. Proc. **20**, 306 (1961b).
WILLIAMS, C. M., A. A. BABUSCIO, and R. WATSON: In vivo alteration of the pathways of dopamine metabolism. Amer. J. Physiol. **199**, 722 (1960).
WILLIAMS, H. L., and D. H. ABDULIAN: The effects of convulsant hydrazides, including INH, on blood levels and urinary excretion of pyridoxine. J. Pharmacol. exp. Ther. **116**, 62 (1956).
WILLOUGHBY, D. A. and W. G. SPECTOR: The local release of an adrenaline-like substance during inflammation. Biochem. Pharmacol. 8, 62 (1961).
WILSON, W. R., F. D. FISHER, and W. M. KIRKENDALL: The acute hemodynamic effects of α-methyl dopa in man. J. clin. Invest. **40**, 1089 (1961).
WIRTH, W., H. KREISKOTT u. U. SCHUMACHER: Zur Prüfung stimulierender Substanzen (Hydrazin-Derivate) an „verstimmten“ Tieren. Naunyn-Schmiedebergs Arch. exp. Path. Pharmak. **238**, 62 (1960).
WISEMAN-DISTLER, M. H., and T. L. SOURKES: The effect of riboflavin and mepacrine on the metabolism of 5-hydroxytryptamine. Biochem. J. **78**, 123 (1961).
— — The role of riboflavin in monoamine oxidase activity. Canad. J. Biochem. **41**, 57 (1963).
WISS, O., and F. WEBER: Vitamin B_6 and tryptophan metabolism. Med. J. Osaka Univ. **8**, 41 (1958).
WITT, P. N., L. BRETTSCHNEIDER, and A. P. BORIS: Sensitivity to D-amphetamine in spiders after iproniazid and imipramine. J. Pharmacol. exp. Ther. **132**, 183 (1961).
WOHLRAB, F.: Die intrazelluläre Lokalisation der Monoaminoxydase (MAO) mittels N′-thiazolyl-substituierten Tetrazoliumsalzen in Gegenwart von Metallionen. Naturwissenschaften **47**, 325 (1960).
— Der histochemische Nachweis der Monoaminooxydase mit Thiazolyl-substitutierten Tetrazoliumsalzen in Gegenwart von Metallionen. Z. Zellforsch., Abt. Histochem. **2**, 163 (1961).
WOOLLEY, D. W., and P. M. EDELMAN: Displacement of serotonin from tissues by a specific antimetabolite. Science **127**, 281 (1958).
WURTMAN, R. J., and J. AXELROD: A sensitive and specific assay for the estimation of monoamine oxidase. Biochem. Pharmacol. **12**, 1439 (1963a).
— — Sex steroids, cardiac ^3H-norepinephrine, and tissue monoamine oxidase levels in the rat. Biochem. Pharmacol. **12**, 1417 (1963b).
WYKES, A. A., Y. C. GLADISH, and J. D. TAYLOR: A screening method for the rapid detection of monoamine oxidase inhibitors in vitro. Fed. Proc. **18**, 462 (1959).
YAMADA, H., P. GEE, M. EBATA, and K. T. YASUNOBU: Monoamine oxidase. VI. Physicochemical properties of plasma monoamine oxidase. Biochim. biophys. Acta (Amst.) **81**, 165 (1964).
— and K. T. YASUNOBU: The nature of the prosthetic groups of plasma amine oxidase. Biochem. biophys. Res. Commun. 8, 387 (1962a).

YAMADA, H., and K. T. YASUNOBU: Monoamine oxidase. I. Purification, crystallization and properties of plasma monoamine oxidase. J. biol. Chem. **237**, 1511 (1962b).
— — (Di)Monoamine oxidase. II. Copper, one of the prosthetic groups of plasma (benzyl)-monoamine oxidase. J. biol. Chem. **237**, 3077 (1962c).
— — Monoamine oxidase. IV. Nature of the second prosthetic group of plasma monoamine oxidase. J. biol. Chem. **238**, 2669 (1963).
— — H. YAMANO, and H. S. MASON: Monoamine oxidase. Nature (Lond.) **198**, 1092 (1963).
YASUDA, K.: The combined demonstration of monoamine oxidase and cholinesterase in the same section. I. Observations on the skin. Okajimas Folia anat. jap. **38**, 139 (1962). [Chem. Abstr. **57**, 6255g (1962).]
YEN, H. C. Y., A. J. SILVERMAN, and A. SALVATORE: Iproniazid reinforcement of anticonvulsants. Fed. Proc. **19**, 278 (1960).
YI-YUNG HSIA, D., P. JUSTICE, J. L. BERMAN, and Y. BRENCHLEY: Brain serotonin in experimental tyrosinosis. Nature (Lond.) **202**, 495 (1964).
— K. NISHIMURA, and Y. BRENCHLEY: Mechanism for the decrease of brain serotonin. Nature (Lond.) **200**, 578 (1963).
YOUNG, J. A., and K. D. G. EDWARDS: Studies on the absorption, metabolism and excretion of methyldopa and other catechols and their influence on amino acid transport in rats. J. Pharmacol. exp. Ther. **145**, 102 (1964).
YUWILER, A., E. GELLER, and S. EIDUSON: Studies on 5-hydroxytryptophan decarboxylase. I. In vitro inhibition and substrate interaction. Arch. Biochem. **80**, 162 (1959a).
— — — Competitive inhibiton of 5-hydroxytryptophan decarboxylase. Fed. Proc. **18**, 606 (1959b).
— — — Studies on 5-hydroxytryptophan decarboxylase. II. Additional inhibition studies and suggestions on the nature of the enzymic site. Arch Biochem. **89**, 143 (1960).
— — and G. G. SLATER: Dietary isoleucine inhibition of liver tryptophan hydroxylase. Life Sci. **3**, 567 (1964).
ZAMBONI, V., and A. DEFRANCESCHI: Identification of isonicotinoylhydrazones of pyruvic and α-ketoglutaric acid in rat urine after treatment with isonicotinic acid hydrazide (isoniazid). Biochim. biophys. Acta (Amst.) **14**, 430 (1954).
ZARA, E. e R. BELSANTI: Contributo allo studio del meccanismo d'azione della fenelzina. Acta neurol. (Napoli) **16**, 313 (1961). [Psychopharmacol. Abstr. **1**, 394 (1961).]
ZARAFONETIS, C. J. D., and J. P. KALAS: Serotonin degradation by ceruloplasmin and its inhibition by isoniazid and iproniazid. Amer. J. med. Sci. **239**, 203 (1960a).
— — Effect of certain compounds on in vitro degradation of serotonin by ceruloplasmin. Proc. Soc. exp. Biol. (N. Y.) **105**, 560 (1960b).
ZATMAN, L. J., S. P. COLOWICK, N. O. KAPLAN, and M. M. CIOTTI: Action of nicotinamide and isonicotinic acid hydrazide on diphosphopyridine nucleotides; preliminary note Bull. Johns Hopk. Hosp. **91**, 211 (1952).
— N. O. KAPLAN, S. P. COLOWICK, and M. M. CIOTTI: Formation of the isonicotinic acid hydrazide analog of DPN. J. Amer. chem. Soc. **75**, 3293 (1953).
— — — — The isolation and properties of the isonicotininic acid hydrazide analogue of diphosphopyridine nucleotide. J. biol. Chem. **209**, 467 (1954a).
— — — — Effect of isonicotinic acid hydrazide on diphosphopyridine nucleotidases. J. biol. Chem. **209**, 453 (1954b).
ZBINDEN, G.: Inhibition of experimental myocardial necrosis by the monoamine oxidase inhibitor isocarboxazid (Marplan). Amer. Heart. J. **60**, 450 (1960a).
— Biochemische, funktionelle und morphologische Organveränderungen durch Beeinflussung des 5-Hydroxytryptamin-Stoffwechsels. Ergebn. allg. Path. path. Anat. **39**, 225 (1960b).
— Effect of anoxia and amine oxidase inhibitors on myocardial necrosis induced by isoproterenol. Fed. Proc. **20**, 128 (1961).
— Beeinflussung der experimentellen, durch Isoproterenol hervorgerufenen Myocardnekrose durch Aminoxydasehemmer, gefäßerweiternde und tranquilisierende Arzneimittel. Arzneimittel-Forsch. **12**, 635 (1962).
— H. BESENDORF u. A. PLETSCHER: Über die Bedeutung des endogenen 5-Hydroxytryptamin für die pharmakologische Wirkung von Iproniazid auf Magen und Darm. Gastroenterologia (Basel) **90**, 382 (1958).
— A. PLETSCHER u. A. STUDER: Hemmung der Reserpin-bedingten 5-Hydroxytryptamin-Freisetzung im enterochromaffinen System durch Isopropyl-isonicotinsäure-hydrazid. Klin. Wschr. **35**, 565 (1957).
— — — Beeinflussung experimenteller Magengeschwüre der Ratte durch Reserpin, Tetrabenazin und Iproniazid (Marsilid). Schweiz. med. Wschr. **89**, 289 (1959).
— L. O. RANDALL, and R. A. MOE: Clinical and pharmacological considerations on mode of action of MAO inhibitors. Dis. nerv. Syst. **21**, Suppl., 89 (1960).

ZBINDEN, B., u. A. STUDER: Zur Wirkung von Vitaminen der B-Gruppe auf die experimentelle Isoniazid-„Neuritis". Schweiz. Z. Path. **18**, 1198 (1955a).
— — Experimenteller Beitrag zur Frage der Isoniazid-Neuritis und ihre Beeinflussung durch Pyridoxin. Z. Tuberk. **107**, 97 (1955b).
— — Histochemische Untersuchungen über den Einfluß von Iproniazid (Marsilid) auf die durch Reserpin erzeugte Freisetzung von Adrenalin und Noradrenalin aus dem Nebennierenmark. Experientia (Basel) **14**, 201 (1958a).
— — Bluteosinophile und Thrombocyten bei Hemmung der Monoaminoxydase und weiteren Einwirkungen auf den Catecholamin- und 5-Hydroxytryptamin-Stoffwechsel. Schweiz. med. Wschr. **88**, 1067 (1958b).
— — Experimental pathology of iproniazid and related compounds. Ann. N.Y. Acad. Sci. **80**, 873 (1959).
ZELLER, E. A.: Über den enzymatischen Abbau von Histamin und Diaminen. Helv. chim. Acta **21**, 880 (1938).
— Über die Verwendung von Indigo-disulfonat in der Fermentmethodik. Helv. chim. Acta **23**, 1502 (1940a).
— Zur Mikrobestimmung von Ammoniak. Helv. chim. Acta **23**, 1509 (1940b).
— Zur Kenntnis der Mono- und Diamin-oxydase. Helv. chim. Acta **24**, 539 (1941a).
— Über eine einfache Farbreaktion als Schwangerschaftsnachweis. Schweiz. med. Wschr. **71**, 1349 (1941b).
— Diamin-oxydase. In: Advances in Enzymology, vol. 2, p. 93. New York: Interscience Publ. Inc. 1942.
— Oxidation of amines. In: The Enzymes, vol. 2, part 1, p. 536. New York: Academic Press Inc., Publ. 1951.
— On the classification and nomenclature of amine oxidase. Ciba Foundation, Symposium on Histamine, p. 258. London: J. & A. Churchill Ltd. 1956a.
— The fate of histamine in the body, with particular reference ot the enzymology of histamine oxidation. Ciba Foundation, Symposium on Histamine, p. 339. London: J. & A. Churchill Ltd. 1956b.
— Enzymologic effects of Marsilid and related hydrazine derivatives. J. clin. exp. Psychopath. **19**, Suppl. I, 27 (1958).
— The role of amine oxidase in the destruction of catecholamines. Pharmacol. Rev. **11**, 387 (1959).
— Studies on the active center of monoamine oxidase. Experientia (Basel) **16**, 399 (1960).
— Some remarks about monoamine oxidase and monoamine oxidase inhibitors. J. Neuropsychiat. **2**, 125 (1961).
— Monoamine oxidase. In: Monoamines et système nerveux central, p. 51, edit. J. DE AJURIAGUERRA, Geneva et Paris: Georg & Co. S.A. 1962.
— A new approach to the analysis of the interaction between monoamine oxidase and its substrates and inhibitors. Ann. N.Y. Acad. Sci. **107**, 811 (1963a).
— Über eutope und dystope Substratkomplexe der Monoaminoxydase. Biochem. Z. **339**, 13 (1963b).
— Diamine oxidases. In: The Enzymes, vol. 8, p. 313, edit. P. D. BOYER, H. LARDY, and K. MYRBÄCK. New York and London: Academic Press Inc. 1963c.
— Monoamine and polyamine analogues. In: Metabolic Inhibitors, vol. 2, p. 53, edit. R. M. HOCHSTER and J. H. QUASTEL. New York and London: Academic Press Inc. 1963d.
— Personal communication 1964.
— L. M. BARBATO, J. BARSKY, C. A. BLANKSMA, and J. C. LAZANAS: Study of the reactive site of amine oxidase by methoxyamines and 1,2-alkyldiamines. Fed. Proc. **17**, 342 (1958a).
—, and J. BARSKY: In vivo inhibition of liver and brain monoamine oxidase by 1-isonicotinyl-2-isopropyl hydrazine. Proc. Soc. exp. Biol. (N.Y.) **81**, 459 (1952).
— — and E. R. BERMAN: Inhibition of monoamine oxidase by 1-isonicotinyl-2-isopropyl hydrazine. J. biol. Chem. **214**, 267 (1955a).
— — — M. S. CHERKAS, and J. R. FOUTS: Degradation of mescaline by amine oxidases. J. Pharmacol. exp. Ther. **124**, 282 (1958b).
— — — and J. R. FOUTS: Action of isonicotinic acid hydrazide and related compounds on enzymes of brain and other tissues. J. Lab. clin. Med. **40**, 965 (1952a).
— — — — Action of isonicotinic acid hydrazide and related compounds on enzymes involved in the autonomic nervous system. J. Pharmacol. exp. Ther. **106**, 427 (1952b).
— — L. A. BLANKSMA, and J. C. LAZANAS: Reactive site of amine oxidases. Fed. Proc. **16**, 276 (1957a).
— — J. R. FOUTS, W. F. KIRCHHEIMER, and L. S. VAN ORDEN: Influence of isonicotinic acid hydrazide (INH) and 1-isonicotinyl-2-isopropyl hydrazide (IIH) on bacterial and mammalian enzymes. Experientia (Basel) **8**, 349 (1952c).

ZELLER, E. A., J. BARSKY, J. R. FOUTS, and J. C. LAZANAS: Structural requirements for the inhibition of amine oxidases. Biochem. J. **60**, V (1955b).
— J. BERNSOHN, W. M. INSKIP, and J. W. LAUER: On the effect of a monoamine oxidase inhibitor on the behavior and tryptophan metabolism of schizophrenic patients. Naturwissenschaften **44**, 427 (1957b).
— L. A. BLANKSMA, W. P. BURKARD, W. L. PACHA, and J. C. LAZANAS: In vitro and in vivo inhibition of amine oxidases. Ann. N.Y. Acad. Sci. **80**, 583 (1959).
— — u. J. A. CARBON: Über die Wirkung von optisch aktiven Hydraziden auf die Diaminoxydase. Helv. chim. Acta **40**, 257 (1957c).
— H. R. BUERKI, and T. ISHIMARU: Phenomenology of monoamine oxidase reaction (MOR). Fed. Proc. **21**, 246 (1961).
—, and J. R. FOUTS: Enzymes as primary targets of drug action. Ann. Rev. Pharmacol. **3**, 9 (1963).
— — J. A. CARBON, J. C. LAZANAS u. W. VOEGTLI: Über die Substratspezifität der Diamin-Oxydase. Helv. chim. Acta **39**, 1632 (1956a).
—, u. C. A. JOËL: Über das Vorkommen der Cholinesterase, der Mono- und Diaminoxydase in Sperma und Prostata, und über die Beeinflussung der Spermien-Beweglichkeit durch Fermentinhibitoren. Helv. chim. Acta **24**, 968 (1941).
— W. L. PACHA, and S. SARKAR: Further exploration of the active centre of monoamine oxidase. Biochem. J. **76**, 45P (1960).
—, and S. SARKAR: Further exploration of the active center of monoamine oxidase (MO) with cycloalkylamines. Fed. Proc. **19**, 28 (1960).
— — Amine oxidases. XIX. Inhibition of monoamine oxidase by phenylcyclopropylamines and iproniazid. J. biol. Chem. **237**, 2333 (1962).
— P. STERN, and L. A. BLANKSMA: Degradation of histamine by monoamine oxidase. Naturwissenschaften **43**, 157 (1956b).
— — u. M. WENK: Über die Diamin-Diamin-Oxydase-Reaktion. Helv. chim. Acta **23**, 3 (1940).
ZELLER, P., A. PLETSCHER, K. F. GEY, H. GUTMANN, B. HEGEDÜS, and O. STRAUB: Amino acid and fatty acid hydrazides: chemistry and action on monoamine oxidase. Ann. N.Y. Acad. Sci. **80**, 555 (1959).
ZILE, M.: Effect of thyroxine and related compounds on monoamine oxidase activity. Endocrinology **66**, 311 (1960).
— and H. A. LARDY: Monoamine oxidase activity in liver of thyroid-fed rats. Arch. Biochem. **82**, 411 (1959).
ZIRKLE, C. L., and C. KAISER: Monoamine oxidase inhibitors (nonhydrazides). In: Psychopharmacological Agents, vol. 1, edit. M. GORDON. New York: Academic Press Inc. 1964.
— —, D. H. TEDESCHI, R. E. TEDESCHI, and E. BURGER: 2-Substituted cyclopropylamines. II. Effect of structure upon monoamine oxidase-inhibitory activity as measured in vivo by potentiation of tryptamine convulsions. J. med. pharm. Chem. **1**, 1265 (1962).
ZWEIFACH, B. W., and J. CASCARANO: Changes in the intrahepatic circulation and the reticuloendothelial system induced by inhibitors of monoamine oxidase. Ann. N.Y. Acad. Sci. **80**, 939 (1959).

Chapter 13

Morphological changes caused by injections of 5-HT in animals and man

By

R. S. STACEY

With 3 Figures

The rapid inactivation of 5-HT makes it possible to give large doses to animals over many weeks; moreover tolerance rapidly develops and near lethal doses can be quickly increased. HEDINGER and VERAGUTH (1962) for example, using rats, started with daily intraperitoneal doses of 1 to 15 mg base/kg and were able to increase the dose to over 500 mg base/kg in 20 days. Similarly with guinea-pigs, starting with a dose of 40 mg base/kg i.p., the dose could be doubled every 5 days until 320 mg base/kg was being given. However when large doses are given, whether singly or repeatedly, morphological changes develop in many organs.

Blood

Changes in the numbers of blood cells are only caused by very large doses and their significance is uncertain. The injection of large single (20 to 50 mg base/kg) or repeated doses of 5-HT into rats causes an increase in the *platelet* count. After a single injection this is seen during the subsequent 4 hours (SERRA and BRUNI 1957) and with repeated doses may, in the course of 40 days, rise from 500,000/mm^3 to 1,500,00/mm^3 (HEDINGER and LANGEMANN 1955a). BALLERINI and CANTELLI (1955) found the changes in the peripheral blood to be associated with an increase in number and activity of bone megakaryocytes. A thrombocythaemia has also been produced in guinea-pigs (HUSER et al. 1959); and in rabbits it is accompanied by a leucocytosis (FERRATA and CAPPELLETTI 1959).

Large single doses of 5-HT cause *eosinopenia* in small laboratory animals (STEINER and HEDINGER 1956; SERRA and BRUNI 1957) and in man, after 50 to 100 mg 5-HT creatinine sulphate intramuscularly, reaches its greatest extent in 15 to 30 mins and returns to normal in 2 hours (ROSA et al. 1958; CENACCHI et al. 1959). This effect is said to be inhibited by the administration of antihistamines. After adrenalectomy, STEINER et al. (1957) found that a thrombocytosis still occurred but was accompanied by an eosinophilia. A reduction in the number of *basophil leucocytes* following intravenous injection in rabbits is described by BOSEILA (1959).

According to ZBINDEN and STUDER (1958) both thrombocytosis and eosinopenia follow the intravenous injection of 5-HIAA (50 mg/kg) but DAVIDSON et al. (1957) found no change in the platelet count after the daily injection of 5-HTP (200 mg/kg) for a year.

Cardiovascular system

In the malignant carcinoid syndrome (see p. 755) there is an increased synthesis of 5-HT and, in many cases, high concentrations of it in the blood. Endocardial fibrosis is a common feature of this condition and many attempts have been made to simulate it by the administration of 5-HT to animals. These have failed (LANGEMANN and KAGI 1956; FIORE-DONATI and ERSPAMER 1957; STEGER 1958; MACDONALD, ROBBINS and MALLORY 1958a; ROBERTSON et al. 1962); though in rats STEGER (1958) produced oedema of the pulmonary valve and an inflammatory infiltration of cardiac muscle, without fibrosis, by this means; and EDER and SCHAUER (1959) a perivascular oedema with fibrosis (see also SCHAUER and EDER, 1959). ROSSI et al. (1962) report a thickening of the coronary arteries and heart valves in dogs. In an attempt to simulate still closer the conditions in the malignant carcinoid syndrome, MACDONALD (1959) injected large doses of 5-HT into rats kept on a diet deficient in tryptophan and niacin. This also failed to cause cardiac lesions. DAVIDSON et al. (1957) and ANGRIST et al. (1962) were unable to produce cardiac lesions with injections or with intrahepatic pellets of 5-HTP; and GOTTLIEB et al. (1960), who transplanted mouse mast-cell tumours into mice, thereby increasing their urinary 5-HIAA excretion from 10—20 μg/day to 380—550 μg/day, also failed to cause cardiac lesions.

Pulmonary arteriocleroses was produced in rabbits by the intramuscular or intraperitoneal injection of 5 mg 5-HT every 12 hours over a period of 25 days by ROSSI and ZAMBONI (1958). In the medium and small pulmonary arteries there was a fibrous-elastic intimal hyperplasia, thickening of the walls and narrowing of the lumen. The walls of the large arteries and of the pulmonary veins were unaffected but the arteries contained a fibrous, adherent thrombus. Somewhat similar changes were produced by CARLIER et al. (1959) in dogs.

A minority of investigators thus appear to have caused cardiovascular changes by injections of 5-HT, but these do not resemble the changes in malignant carcinoid disease. Why most investigators have failed to cause even these changes is unexplained; but differences in strain, age and diet may be important as well as differences in the details of the dosage schedule.

Observations have also been made on clot formation and lysis *in vivo* using the rabbits' ear vein. BAUMGARTNER et al. (1963) report that the formation of thrombotic deposits, consisting of platelet aggregations and leucocytes, is inhibited during the first few minutes after traumatisation of the vein, by previous systemic administration of either 5-HT or an amine oxidase inhibitor. The ultimate number and size of thrombi formed is however unaffected. On the other hand KWAAN et al. (1958) find that lysis of thrombi caused by the injection of thrombin into the vein is accelerated by the subsequent infiltration of the surrounding tissue with 5-HT. The importance of these observations on clot formation cannot at present be assessed but recent work on the action of 5-HT on platelet adhesiveness (HONOUR and MITCHELL, 1963) may in time clarify them.

Gastrointestinal tract

When large doses of 5-HT (2 to 70 mg base/kg) or of 5-HTP (300 mg/kg) are injected into mice or rats a large proportion develop lesions of the stomach and colon (HAVERBACK and BOGDANSKI 1957; HEDINGER and VERAGUTH 1957 and 1962; WILHELMI 1957; WILHELMI and SCHINDLER 1959). In the stomach they are confined to the glandular part and take the form of necrosis of the mucosa, erosions and ulcers (Fig. 1). These prinicipally involve the mucosa, but may extend through the muscularis mucosa to the muscle layer. When the injections are discontinued there is a strong tendency to heal with scar formation. The lesions are not due to an increase in the volume or acidity of gastric secretion, both of which are, in fact, reduced (OWENS and MASSON 1958). Atropine and dimercaprol (4 mg/kg) diminish ulceration caused by 5-HTP injections. Ulceration by

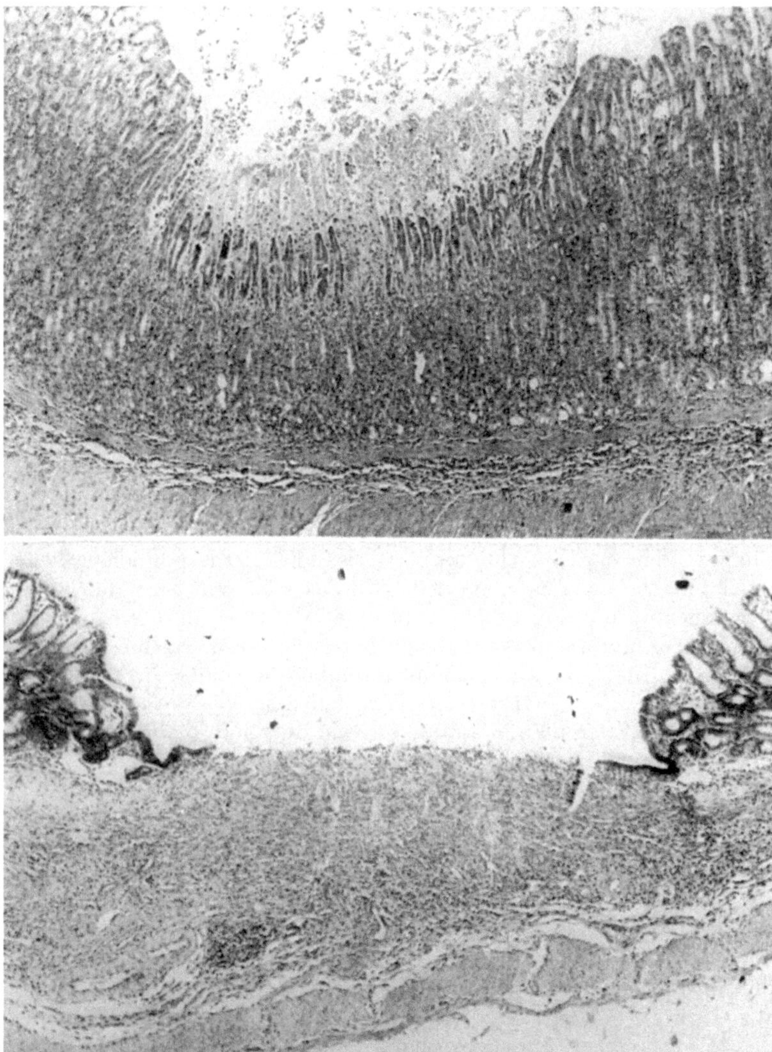

Fig. 1. Rat. Section of stomach wall showing ulcer. Killed after 20 intraperitoneal injections of 5-HT. (× 60). [From fig. 2, HEDINGER, Ch., u. F. VERAGUTH: Z. ges. exp. Med. **136**, 64 (1962).]

5-HT is prevented by vagotomy (BLACKMAN et al. 1959); its incidence in rats is diminished by lysergic acid diethylamide, methysergide, chlorpromazine, iproniazid, antazoline, promethazine, thenalidine, papaverine (WILHELMI and SCHINDLER 1959; NIKODIJEVIĆ and VANOV 1960; NIKODIJEVIĆ and TRAJKOV 1961) and chlorbenzoxamine (LEVIS and BEERSAERTS 1960).

Histamine liberators cause similar lesions (OWENS and MASSON 1958) and the inhibition of 5-HT ulceration by histamine antagonists, such as antazoline, having little antagonism to 5-HT, has led to the suggestion that histamine liberation by 5-HT (FELDBERG and SMITH 1953) may play a part in ulcer formation.

Gastric ulceration is also caused by the administration of 5 mg reserpine/kg to rats and mice (HAVERBACK and BOGDANSKI 1957; LA BARRE 1959); this ulceration is diminished by previous treatment with iproniazid (LEUSEN et al. 1959; ZBINDEN et al. 1959), which inhibits the release of 5-HT by reserpine, by atropine and hexamethonium, by vagotomy (KIM and SHORE 1963) and by the administration of an antacid mixture (BLACKMAN et al. 1959).

Kidney

The intravenous injection of quite small doses of 5-HT (70 µg base/kg) to anaesthetised rats in which a kidney has been exposed, cause visible blanching of the kidney due to constriction mainly of cortical vessels (PAGE and GLENDENING 1955). With larger single or repeated doses (1 to 20 kg base/kg) there is necrosis of the cortex involving both glomeruli and tubules; tubules being more affected than glomeruli and proximal convoluted tubules more than distal tubules (Fig. 2 and 3). The collecting tubules may escape severe damage but may be clogged with casts and there may be marked tubular dilatation (ERSPAMER 1954a; SALGADO and GREEN 1955; FIORE-DONATI and ERSPAMER 1957; HEDINGER and VERAGLUTH 1957; MACDONALD 1959; WAUGH and PEARL 1960; ANGRIST et al. 1962). MACDONALD et al. (1958a), who gave rats subcutaneous injections of 2 to 8 mg base twice daily for a year describe, in addition, tubular regeneration and wedge-shaped areas of fibrosis in the cortex (Fig. 2 and 3).

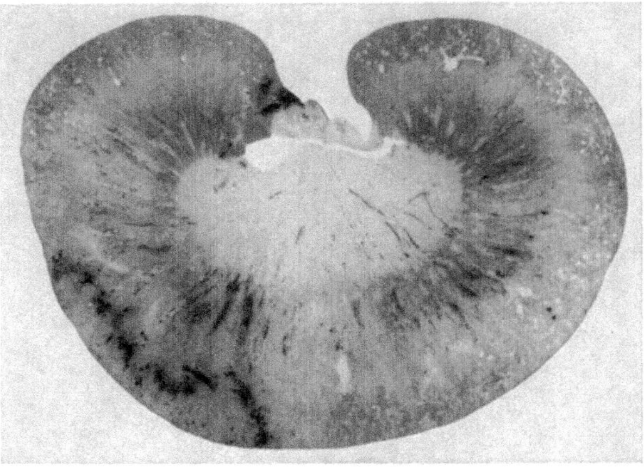

Fig. 2. Cut surface of an ischemic kidney with infarct-like area in the cortex, sharply outlined by a narrow zone of hyperemia. Rat sacrificed 10 hours after subcutaneous injection of 10 mg 5-HT/kg. Benzidine stain. × 6. [From fig. 1, FIORE-DONATI, L., and V. ERSPAMER: Amer. J. Path. **33**, 913 (1957).]

BROSMAN et al. (1959) found that either the incidence or the severity of the lesions could be diminished significantly by the simultaneous administration of hydralazine, isoprenaline, dicyclomine, sodium glutamate, sodium nitrite and by the 5-HT antagonists LSD and lysergic acid morpholide. The lesions were increased by mephenteramine, noradrenaline and adrenaline (JASMIN and BOIS 1960).

Renal changes appear to be ischaemic in origin and lesions of the same kind can be caused by large doses of adrenaline (MACDONALD 1959). Similar lesions may be produced in the rabbit, which is however less sensitive; 5-HTP and 4-HTP have an identical action (FIORE-DONATI and ERSPAMER 1957; ERSPAMER 1961).

Liver

Even very large doses of 5-HT administered to adult rats over long periods cause no obvious morphological changes in the liver, but MACDONALD et al. (1959) found that a single subcutaneous injection of 40 mg 5-HT creatinine sulphate/kg, given to young rats weighing less than 115 g., resulted in an increased formation of hepatic parenchyma cells. This was demonstrated by autoradiographic techiques employing tritiated thymidine and by histological methods which revealed an increase in mitotic figures; smaller doses caused neither changes, nor were they produced in older rats even by larger doses.

Reproductive system

Mammary hypertrophy and *lactation* occurs in rats and rabbits given daily injections of 2 to 5 mg 5-HT base/kg/day, provided these injections follow a

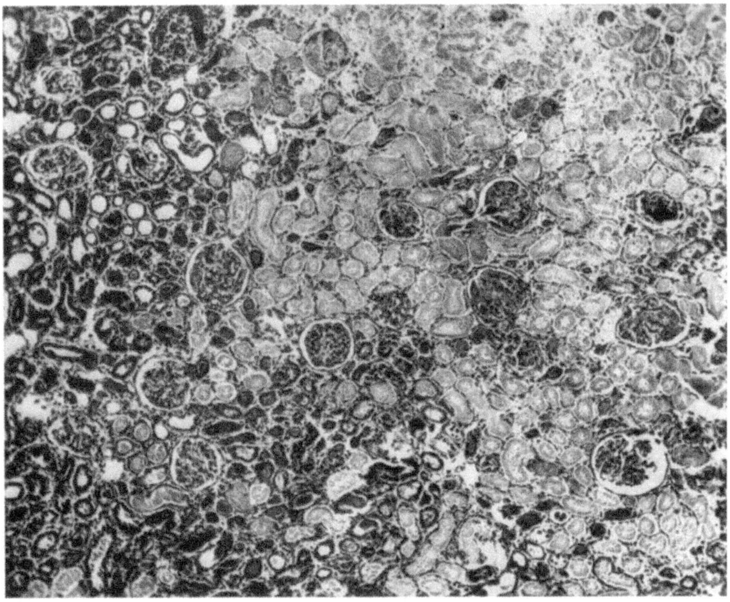

Fig. 3. Extensive area of coagulative necrosis in the kidney cortex of a rat treated with three subcutaneous injections of 10 mg 5-HT/kg each. Hematoxylin and eosin stain. × 110. [From fig. 3, FIORE-DONATI, L., and V. ERSPAMER: Amer. J. Path. **33**, 913 (1957).]

course of oestradiol injections. The effect is abolished by previous hypophysectomy and is ascribed to stimulation of prolactin secretion. Similar changes in the mammary gland are evoked by acetylcholine and adrenaline (MEITES et al. 1959, 1960).

In immature mice, 1 to 25 mg 5-HT creatinine sulphate/kg/day depresses growth of *ovaries*, *uterus* and *vagina* and delays sexual maturity (ROBSON and BOTROS 1961). *Pregnancy* is interrupted at all stages in both mice and rats and there is bleeding and disorganization of the *placenta* (POULSON et al. 1960; WAUGH and PEARL 1960; MORLUNGHI and ROMEO 1961); progesterone and prolactin antagonise this action but only during early pregnancy (LINDSAY et al. 1963). Abnormalities in the eyes, limbs, tail, skull and central nervous system of the foetus are reported after subcutaneous injection of 5-HT (POULSON et al. 1963; REDDY et al. 1963). Using radioactive sodium, ROBSON and SULLIVAN (1963) have shown that 5-HT prevents the escape of sodium from the maternal blood into the extravascular spaces in the placenta and so prevents it entering the foetal circulation. Having excluded a direct toxic effect on the foetus, contraction of the uterine muscle and constriction of the umbilical vessels as causes of the interruption of pregnancy by 5-HT, ROBSON and SULLIVAN suggest that it may be due to impaired placental function of which the transfer of sodium to the foetus is a manifestation.

SALGADO and GREEN (1955) and BOCCABELLA et al. (1962) found a reduction in weight and gross changes in the histological appearance of the *male organs of reproduction* (testicles, prostate and seminal vesicles) after the administration of 10 mg 5-HT/kg twice daily for 10 days. Spermatogenesis was markedly affected. Since the simultaneous administration of hydrallazine prevented the development of these changes, they may have been caused by testicular ischaemia. Similar results have been reported by HEDINGER (1963).

Other tissues

Necrosis of the *submaxillary gland*, starting in the inferior pole and usually extending over the whole lower half of the gland and resulting in a total destruction of the acini, follows the intraperitoneal injection of 40 mg 5-HT base/kg in rats (ERSPAMER 1961); other salivary glands are not affected (JASMIN and BOIS 1960). The digits and the tip of the *tail* may also become necrotic and *lenticular opacities* and clouding of the *aqueous humor* (JASMIN and BOIS 1960) have been described. In hamsters, intraperitoneal injections (1 to 2 mg) cause degranulation of the *mast cells* of the cheeck pouch (ASBOE-HANSEN and WEGELIUS 1956).

With subcutaneous injections, changes occur in the *skin* at the site of injection. After 5 mg 5-HT creatinine sulphate twice daily MACDONALD, ROBBINS and MALLORY (1958 b) and MACDONALD (1959) found that rats developed a progressive collagenous and fibrous proliferation within the dermis accompanied by an increased vascularity and hyperplasia of the epidermis. In the horse, an intradermal injection of histamine is followed by a local infiltration of the area with eosinophils. No such infiltration follows the injection of 5-HT (1 to 3 mg) but a wheal forms; this is prevented by the simultaneous intradermal injection of brom-lysergic acid diethylamide (ARCHER 1959). The effect of 5-HT injections on the reaction to implanted "Ivadon" sponges was studied in rats by SCHERBEL et al. (1960). They found that 1 to 30 mg 5-HT by subcutaneous injection increased the inflammatory reaction but did not alter the fibroplasia. The changes were aggravated by the simultaneous administration of an amine oxidase inhibitor and diminished by methysergide.

References

ANGRIST, A., M. OKA, and K. NAKAO: Failure to produce right-sided valve lesions by intrahepatic pellets of 5-hydroxytryptophan. Fed. Proc. **21**, 95 (1962).

ARCHER, R. K.: Eosinophil leucocytes and their reactions to histamine and 5-hydroxytryptamine. J. Path. Bact. **78**, 95—103 (1959).

ASBOE-HANSEN, G., and O. WEGELIUS: Serotonin and connective tissue. Nature (Lond.) **178**, 262 (1956).

BALLERINI, G., e T. CANTELLI: Piastrinosi sperimentale da 5-idrossitriptamina. Boll. Soc. ital. Ematol. **3**, 405—408 (1955).

BAUMGARTNER, H. R., A. STUDER u. K. REBER: Über Methoden zur Erzeugung experimenteller Thrombosen am Kaninchenohr und die Bedeutung von 5-Hydroxytryptamin bei deren Entstehung. Thrombos. Diathes. haemorrh. (Stuttg.) **9**, 485—511 (1963).

BLACKMAN, J. G., D. S. CAMPION, and F. M. FASTIER: Mechanism of action of reserpine in producing gastric haemorrhage and erosion in the mouse. Brit. J. Pharmacol. **14**, 112—116 (1959).

BOCCABELLA, A. V., E. D. SALGADO, and E. A. ALGER: Testicular function and histology following serotonin administration. Endocrinology **71**, 827—837 (1962).

BOSEILA, A.-W. A.: Influence of heparin and serotonin on basophil leucocytes of rabbit blood. Experientia (Basel) **15**, 343—344 (1959).

BROSMAN, S. A., P. F. BRADFORD, and F. W. HUGHES: Modification of renal lesions produced by 5-hydroxytryptamine (serotonin). Amer. J. Clin. Path. **32**, 457—464 (1959).

CARLIER, J., G. LEJEUNE-LEDANT et Ch. KEIL: 5-Hydroxytryptamine, lésions pulmonaires et pression artérielle pulmonaire. Med. exp. (Basel) **1**, 72—77 (1959).
CENACCHI, G. C., E. BERGAMI, D. CAVAZZONI e L. ROSA: Effetto eosinopenico della 5-ossitriptamina. Folia allerg. (Roma) **6**, 14—24 (1959).
DAVIDSON, J., A. SJOERDSMA, L. N. LOOMIS, and S. UDENFRIEND: Studies with the serotonin precursor, 5-hydroxytryptophan, in experimental animals and man. J. clin. Invest. **36**, 1594—1599 (1957).
EDER, M., u. A. SCHAUER: Morphologische und experimentelle Untersuchungen zur Fibrosierung beim Carcinoid. Beitr. path. Anat. **121**, 375—405 (1959).
ERSPAMER, V.: Pharmocology of indolealkylamines. Pharmacol. Rev. **6**, 425—487 (1954a).
— Observations on the fate of oral 4-HTP in man. Experientia (Basel) **17**, 351—352 (1961a).
— Recent research in the field of 5-hydroxytryptamine and related indolealkylamines. Fortschr. Arzneimittelforsch. **3**, 151—367 (1961b).
FELDBERG, W., and A. N. SMITH: Release of histamine by tryptamine and 5-hydroxytryptamine. Brit. J. Pharmacol. **8**, 406—411 (1953).
FERRATA, A., e G. A. CAPPELLETTI: Sulla trombocitosi da serotonina. Haematologica **44**, 501——512 (1959).
FIORE-DONATI, L. and V. ERSPAMER: Studies on the nephrotoxicity of 5-hydroxytryptamine (enteramine) in the rat. Amer. J. Path. **33**, 895—917 (1957).
GOTTLIEB, L. S., S. A. BROITMAN, J. J. VITALE, and N. ZAMCHECK: Failure of endogenous serotonin to produce lesions of the carcinoid syndrome. Studies in mouse mastocytoma. Arch. Path. **69**, 77—81 (1960).
HAVERBACK, B. J. and D. F. BOGDANSKI: Gastric mucosal erosion in the rat following administration of the serotonin precursor, 5-hydroxytryptophan. Proc. Soc. exp. Biol. (N.Y.) **95**, 392—393 (1957).
HEDINGER, C.: Hodenveränderungen bei Ratten und Meerschweinchen nach Serotonininjektionen. Path. et Microbiol. (Basel) **26**, 325—329 (1963).
—, u. H. LANGEMANN: Ausgesprochene Thrombocytose bei Ratten unter Behandlung mit 5-Oxytryptamin. Schweiz. med. Wschr. **85**, 368—370 (1955a).
— — Nierenschädigungen mit Rindennekrosen bei Ratten unter Behandlung mit 5-Oxytryptamine. Schweiz. med. Wschr. **85**, 541—544 (1955b).
—, u. F. VERAGUTH: Magengeschwüre bei Ratten unter Behandlung mit 5-Hydroxytryptamin. Schweiz. med. Wschr. **87**, 1175—1176 (1957).
— — Magengeschwüre bei Ratten und Meerschweinchen nach intraperitonealer Injektion von 5-Hydroxytryptamin (Serotonin). Z. ges. exp. Med. **136**, 64—77 (1962).
HONOUR, A. J., and J. R. A. MITCHELL: Platelet clumping *in vivo*. Nature (Lond.) **197**, 1019—1020 (1963).
HUSER, H. J., C. SANDRI u. C. HEDINGER: Thrombozytose bei Meerschweinchen unter massiver Behandlung mit 5-Hydroxytryptamin (Serotonin). Klin. Wschr. **37**, 660—662 (1959).
JASMIN, G., and P. BOIS: Effect of various agents on the development of kidney infarcts in rats treated with serotonin. Lab. Invest. **9**, 503—515 (1960).
KIM, K. S., and P. A. SHORE: Mechanism of action of reserpine and insulin on gastric amines and gastric secretion and the effect of monoamine oxidase inhibition. J. Pharmacol. exp. Ther. **141**, 321—325 (1963).
KWAAN, H. C., R. LO, and A. J. S. MCFADZEAN: On the lysis of thrombi experimentally produced within veins. Brit. J. Haemat. **4**, 51—62 (1958).
LA BARRE, J.: A propos de la pathogénèse de l'ulcère gastrique post réserpinique. C. R. Soc. Biol. (Paris) **153**, 364—366 (1959).
LANGEMANN, H., u. J. KÄGI: Oxytryptamin- und Oxyindolessigsäurebestimmungen bei einem Fall von Carcinoidsyndrom, nebst einigen anderen Untersuchungen über Oxytryptamin. Klin. Wschr. **34**, 237—241 (1956).
LEUSEN, I., E. LACROIX, and G. DEMEESTER: Influence of iproniazid on formation of gastric ulceres by reserpine in the rat. Experientia (Basel) **15**, 73 (1959).
LEVIS, S., et J. BEERSAERTS: E'tude de l'activité de la chlorbenzoxamine dans quelques types d'ulcères expérimentaux. Pharmacodyn. **126**, 359—364 (1960).
LINDSAY, D., E. POULSON, and J. M. ROBSON: The effect of 5-HT on pregnancy. J. Endocr. **26**, 85—96 (1963).
MACDONALD, R. A.: Pathogenesis of lesions induced by serotonin: nutritional, vascular, autoradiographic and comparative studies using epinephrine. Amer. J. Path. **35**, 297—313 (1959).
—, and S. L. ROBBINS: Dermal fibrosis following subcutaneous injections of serotonin creatinine sulphate. Proc. Soc. exp. Biol. (N.Y.) **97**, 334—337 (1958b).
— —, and G. K. MALLORY: Morphologic effects of serotonin (5-hydroxytryptamine). Arch. Path. **65**, 369—377 (1958a).
— R. SCHMID, T. R. HAKALA, and G. K. MALLORY: Effect of serotonin upon liver cells of young rats. Proc. Soc. exp. Biol. (N.Y.) **101**, 83—86 (1959).

MEITES, J., C. S. NICOLL, and P. K. TALWALKER: Effect of reserpine and serotonin on milk secretion and mammary growth in the rat. Proc. Soc. exp. Biol. (N.Y.) **101**, 563—365 (1959).

— P. K. TALWALKER, and C. S. NICOLL: Induction of mammary growth and lactation in rabbits with epinephrine, acetylcholine and serotonin. Proc. Soc. exp. Biol (N.Y.) **104**, 192—194 (1960).

MORLUNGHI, C. e P. ROMEO: Effetti della somministrazione cronica della 5-idrossitriptamina (serotonina) sulla coniglia gravida. Arch. Ostet. Ginec. **66**, 155—173 (1961).

NIKODIJEVIĆ, B., and T. TRAJKOV: Mechanism of ulcerogenic action of 5-hydroxytryptamine in rat's stomach. Biochem. Pharmacol. **8**, 169 (1961).

—, and S. VANOV: The influence of thenalidine on reserpine- and serotonin-induced gastric ulcers in rats. Experientia (Basel) **16**, 464—465 (1960).

OWENS, F. J., and G. M. C. MASSON: Effects of amine liberators on gastric secretions in the rat. J. Lab. clin. Med. **53**, 932—933 (1958).

PAGE, E. W., and M. B. GLENDENING: Production of renal cortical necrosis with serotonin (5-hydroxytryptamine). Amer. J. Med. **19**, 285 (1955).

POULSON, E., M. BOTROS, and J. M. ROBSON: Effect of 5-hydroxytryptamine and iproniazid on pregnancy. Science **131**, 1101—1102 (1960).

— J. M. ROBSON, and F. M. SULLIVAN: Teratogenic effect of 5-HT in mice. Science **141**, 717—718 (1963b).

REDDY, D. V., F. H. ADAMS, and C. BAIRD: Teratogenic effects of serotonin. J. Pediat. **63**, 394—401 (1963).

ROBERTSON, J. I. S., W. S. PEART, and T. M. ANDREWS: The mechanism of facial flushes in the carcinoid syndrome. Quart. J. Med. **31**, 103—123 (1962).

ROBSON, J. M., and M. BOTROS: The effect of 5-hydroxytryptamine and of monoamine oxidase inhibitors on sexual maturity. J. Endocr. **22**, 165—175 (1961).

—, and F. M. SULLIVAN: Mechanism of lethal action of 5-HT on the foetus. J. Endocr. **25**, 553—554 (1963).

ROSA, L., G. C. CENACCHI et G. BERGAMI: Les variations numériques des éosinophiles circulants après injection d'antigène, d'histamine ou de 5-hydroxytryptamine. Acta allerg. (Kbh.) **12**, 427—431 (1958).

ROSSI, P., M. STEVENSON, P. KHAKSAR, and S. BELLET: Coronary arteriosclerosis induced in young dogs by prolonged intra-aortic infusion of serotonin. Circulat. Res. **9**, 436—440 (1961).

—, and L. ZAMBONI: Pulmonary arteriosclerosis due to serotonin. Nature (Lond.) **181**, 1216—1217 (1958).

SALGADO, E. and D. M. GREEN. Renal necrosis induced in rats by serotonin. Amer. J. Physiol. **183**, 657 (1955).

SCHAUER, A., u. M. EDER: Der Fibrosierungsvorgang beim Darmcarcinoid. Klin. Wschr. **37**, 880—881 (1959).

SCHERBEL, A. L., R. L. MCKITTRICK, and W. A. HAWK: Lesions in rats caused by serotonin and histamine before and after amine oxidase inactivation and serotonin inhibition. J. clin. Invest. **39**, 1025—1026 (1960).

SERRA, U. e K. BRUNI: Comportamento delle piastrine e degli eosinofili circolante dopo somministrazione di 5-ossitriptamina in dose unica nel ratto. Folia endocr. (Roma) **10**, 657—664 (1957).

STEGER, C.: Contributo sperimentale alla conoscenza dei rapporti esisteni tra carcinoidi intestinale e lesioni del cuore destro. Arch. ital. Chir. **84**, 202 (1958).

STEINER, F. A., u. C. HEDINGER: Thromtozytose und Eosinopenie bei Ratten nach einmaliger 5-Oxytryptamininjektion. Experientia (Basel) **12**, 109—111 (1956).

— R. E. SIEBENMANN, C. SANDRI u. C. HEDINGER: Thrombozytose und Eosinophilie bei Adrenalektomierten Ratten nach einmaliger 5-Hydroxytryptamininjection. Experientia (Basel) **13**, 500—502 (1957).

WAUGH, D., and M. J. PEARL: Serotonin-induced acute nephrosis and renal cortical necrosis in rats. Amer. J. Path. **36**, 431—455 (1960).

WILHELMI, G.: Über die ulcerogene Wirkung von 5-Hydroxytryptamine am Rattenmagen und deren Beeinflussung durch verschiedene Pharmaca. Helv. physiol. acta. **15**, C, 83—84 (1957).

—, u. W. SCHINDLER: Über die gastrotrope Wirkung von 5-Hydroxytryptamine (HTA), seiner Vorstufen und der entsprechenden Isomeren bei der Ratte. Naunyn-Schmiedebergs Arch. exp. Path. Pharmak. **236**: 49—51 (1959).

ZBINDEN, G., A. PLETSCHER u. A. STUDER: Beeinflussung experimenteller Magengeschwüre durch Reserpin, Tetrabenazin und Iproniazid (Marsilid). Schweiz. med. Wschr. **89**, 289—291 (1959).

— — — Bluteosinophile und Thrombocyten bei Hemmung der Monoaminoxydase und weiteren Einwirkungen auf den Katecholamin- und 5-Hydroxytryptamin-Stoffwechsel. Schweiz. med. Wschr. **88**, 1067—1070 (1958).

Chapter 14

Clinical aspects of cerebral and extracerebral 5-hydroxytryptamine

By

R. S. Stacey

With 3 Figures

A. The distribution of 5-hydroxytryptamine in man

Estimations of the concentration of 5-HT in tissues are unreliable unless extraction and assay are carried out soon after death or biopsy: changes due to the presence, often in the same cells, of enzymes synthesizing or metabolising the substance may otherwise affect the results. Hence determinations on human tissues present special difficulties. Autopsy material must be suspect unless special precautions have been taken to ensure that changes have not occurred, and biopsy material may be affected by general or local disease. To these objections, blood is an exception. Human blood, both normal and abnormal, is readily available and more work has been done with it than with the blood of any other single species.

a) Blood

The estimation of 5-HT in blood presents certain problems: these are discussed below. The value obtained varies with the procedure used for extraction and assay, as will be seen from the results reported by different investigators given in Table 1. There is considerably less 5-HT in human blood than in the blood of most laboratory animals (rabbit, rat, mouse, hamster, cat, pig), but the blood of the dog and guinea-pig has about the same amount. Platelets contain almost the whole of the 5-HT in blood; negligible amounts can be extracted from red cells and white cells and the amount free in the plasma is probably less than 10 ng per ml normally. The greater the care taken to avoid liberation of 5-HT from platelets during the collection of blood and the separation of platelet-free plasma, the smaller the amount of free 5-HT found.

When platelet-rich plasma is incubated with added 5-HT at 37° C, the platelets take up 5-HT even if the concentration in the surrounding fluid is low. For example, if there is 1 μg 5-HT/ml in the surrounding fluid, uptake will continue for 90 to 120 minutes, after which the concentration in the platelets will remain constant at about 3 μg/10^9 platelets (260 μg/ml platelet substance), that is about 5 times as much as they originally contained (Pare et al. 1960). The rapid uptake is dependent on an active transport system and its rate varies with temperature and with the reaction and composition of the medium in which the platelets are suspended. Below 20° C it is slow, but above 30° C increases rapidly and reaches a maximum at 40° C. At pH 6.8 it is twice as fast as at pH 8 (Hardisty and Stacey 1955; Born and Gillson 1959; Born and Bricknell 1959; Stacey 1961).

The concentration of 5-HT in the blood at birth and during early infancy has been determined by MITCHELL and CASS (1959). Blood obtained from the umbilical vein contained little (53 ± 47 ng/10^9 platelets) and there was little change

Table 1. *5-Hydroxytryptamine in human blood*
(mean ± standard error of the mean; or range)

	No.	Assay method	References
Platelets (μg/10^9 platelets)			
0.57 ± 0.03	35	rat uterus	1
0.73 ± 0.03	150	rat uterus	2
0.76 (0.5 to 1.3)	8	rabbit ear	3
0.87 (0.025 to 2.2)	94	fluorimetric	4
0.65 ± 0.06	18	fluorimetric	5
(μg/ml packed platelets)			
49 ± 2.4	17	fluorimetric	6
(μg/mg platelet protein)			
0.26 to 0.63	10	fluorimetric	7
Blood (μg/ml blood)			
0.160 ± 0.01	35	rat uterus	1
0.123 ± 0.041	150	rat uterus	2
0.22 (0.025 to 0.65)	94	fluorimetric	4
0.125 (0.09 to 0.18)	10	fluorimetric	8
0.19 ± 0.02	13	fluorimetric	9
Serum (μg/ml serum)			
0.030 to 0.200	30	rat uterus	10
0.098 (0.044 to 0.247)	31	rat uterus	11
0.145 ± 0.013	16	rat uterus	12
0.210 ± 0.008	50	fluorimetric	13

[1] HARDISTY and STACEY 1955. [2] SCHMID et al. 1960c. [3] ZUCKER and BORRELLI 1955. [4] WEINER and UDENFRIEND 1957. [5] CROSTI and LUCCHELI 1962. [6] INGRAM and STACEY (unpublished). [7] SJOERDSMA et al. 1957. [8] WAALKES 1959. [9] FELDSTEIN et al. 1959. [10] ERSPAMER 1954a. [11] BARKHAM 1955. [12] PARE et al. 1960. [13] DAVIS 1959.

during the first four months of life, thereafter there was a rapid increase to adult levels (Table 2). It might be objected that blood from the umbilical vein at birth might contain less 5-HT than elsewhere in the circulation as it drains direct from the placenta. STACEY (unpublished) has therefore estimated the amount in

Table 2. *The concentration of 5-hydroxytryptamine in the blood of neonates, infants and adults* (number of samples). (From MITCHELL and CASS 1959). (Mean ± standard deviation)

	μg/10^9 platelets	μg/ml blood
Adults (6)	0.317 ±0.115	—
Children (11) $1^1/_2$ to 12 years	0.423 ±0.157	0.124 ±0.056
Infants (8) 7 to 29 weeks	0.197 ±0.212	0.098 ±0.114
Newborn (10) (blood from umbilical vein)	0.053 ±0.047	0.012 ±0.012

blood taken simultaneously from the umbilical vein and artery. The mean concentrations per ml. blood in 12 estimations were: artery 43 ng., vein 45 ng. When platelet-rich plasma from blood from the umbilical vein was incubated at 37° C with added 5-HT, giving a concentration of 1 μg 5-HT/ml, the concentration of 5-HT in the platelets reached a value of 3.11 μg/10^9 platelets, a figure similar to that reached by adult platelets. It would therefore appear that the low blood 5-HT concentration found in the neonate is not due to an inability of the platelets to absorb 5-HT, and is probably due to a low output of 5-HT from the intestine.

Note on the estimation of 5-HT in human blood. Blood must be collected into a suitable anticoagulant (sodium edetate or sodium citrate), using syringes and tubes of siliconed glass or some other unwettable material such as nylon, polystyrene or polyethylene, and kept at 4° C. When the usual methods for the extraction for 5-HT from tissues are applied to blood, part only of the 5-HT present is recovered (HARDISTY and STACEY 1955), probably due to destruction by red cells (STACEY 1956; CARGILL-THOMPSON et al. 1958). To prevent this, RODNIGHT (1958) suggested previous treatment of the blood with carbon monoxide and WAALKES (1959) described a method in which recovery is improved by the addition of large amounts of edetate. Probably the most satisfactory method, however, is to prepare platelet-rich plasma by slow centrifugation of the blood. The platelets from this are then separated by centrifugation at 2000 g for 40 mins and the 5-HT in the platelet pellet estimated either fluorimetrically or by bioassay. If the platelet count in both blood and platelet-rich plasma is known, the total platelet bound 5-HT in the blood can be calculated (HARDISTY and STACEY 1955; CROSTI and LUCCHELLI 1962. Estimation of free 5-HT is rarely needed, as it represents normally only a very small fraction of the whole, but if necessary, it can be extracted with acetone from the platelet-poor plasma; it must be assayed on the rat uterus or the rat stomach preparation, as the concentration will be too low for fluorimetric estimation.

The estimation of 5-HT in blood is thus time-consuming, subject to the errors introduced by platelet counting and in some clinical situations may be impracticable; estimation on serum has therefore often been used instead. When blood clots, 5-HT is released from platelets, but the serum which separates contains only part of the 5-HT in the blood from which it is derived (HARDISTY and STACEY 1955). Moreover the fraction recovered varies in different specimens and with the treatment of the blood before the serum is separated; agitation during clotting causes loss of 5-HT (SHARMAN and SULLIVAN 1956). Standardisation of the routine for clotting the blood and removing the serum, improves the consistency of the results, and PARE et al. (1960) obtained good agreement in specimens taken from the same subject if the blood was left for 20 minutes in an incubator at 37° C immediately after being drawn. and was then cooled in ice until the serum could be separated by centrifugation. Davis (1959) found that the addition of 6 mg ascorbic acid to each ml blood immediately after collection improved recovery. However, at best, serum 5-HT estimations provide only an approximate measure of 5-HT in blood and differences in technique are no doubt largely responsible for the differences in Table 1.

b) Central nervous system

Little work has been done on the distribution of 5-HT in human brain because of the difficulty of obtaining normal tissue by biopsy or immediately after death. The effect of storage on the 5-HT content of brain has been investigated by JOYCE (1962). She found that there was a substantial reduction in the amount of 5-HT in brain stored after removal from the skull, and that the percentage reduction varied from one part of the brain to another. The loss was less in brain stored at —17° C than at higher temperatures (Table 3). On the other hand, when the brain was left in the skull and removed immediately before extraction and assay, the losses were much smaller. Changes in the 5-HT content of the tissues are due to both enzymes synthesizing as well as those destroying 5-HT, and the relative activity of these may be affected by the temperature of storage, by the access of oxygen, by changes in pH and in the permeability of cell barriers caused by autolysis. Freezing may also lead to the destruction of cellular or intracellular barriers, and may affect the access of enzymes to the amine. Probably storage of

Table 3. *Effect of storage for 24 hours on the 5-hydroxytryptamine content of rat brain*

(The 5-HT content is expressed as a percentage of the content found immediately after death). (From JOYCE 1962)

	Temperature during storage		
	20° C	4° C	−17° C
Stored before removal from skull	116	97	95
Stored after removal from skull	57	54	86

bodies up to 24 hours at 4° C before autopsy will not affect 5-HT content greatly; if it is necessary to preserve portions of the brain after dissection, this should be done at −20° C and chemical extraction should follow immediately on thawing. The observations by COSTA and APRISON (1958) and by BERTLER (1961) on the distribution of 5-HT in human brain, given in Table 4, although made on post mortem

Table 4. *Distribution of 5-hydroxytryptamine in the human central nervous system* (µg/g tissue)

	Mean (range)[1]	[2]
Cortex		
Frontal	0.02 (0.01—0.03)	0.04
Frontal, grey matter	0.05 (0.03—0.08)	
Frontal, pole	0.01 (0.01—0.03)	
Temporal pole	0.03 (0.01—0.07)	
Occipital pole	0.02 (0.01—0.05)	0.06
Cingulate gyrus	0.06 (0.04—0.10)	
Hippocampal gyrus	0.17 (0.10—0.30)	
Uncus	0.22 (0.16—0.30)	
Sub-callosal gyrus	0.31 (0.14—0.60)	
Anterior perforated substance	0.98 (0.45—1.51)	
Hippocampus	0.09 (0.05—0.19)	0.11
Corpus striatum:		
Putamen	0.57 (0.30—0.95)	0.23
Caudatus nucleus	0.44 (0.20—0.70)	0.27
Globus pallidus	0.27 (0.10—0.73)	0.08
Fornix (anterior)	0.36 (0.06—0.55)	
Corpus callosum	0.25 (0.05—0.39)	
Amygdaloid nucleus	0.32 (0.14—0.67)	
Thalamus	0.73 (0.23—2.70)	0.23
Hypothalamus	0.82 (0.32—1.53)	0.30—0.48
Mammillary body	0.39 (0.27—0.48)	
Corp. quadrig. (ant.)	0.81 (0.05—1.02)	
Corp. quadrig. (post).	0.47 (0.29—0.81)	
Substantia nigra	1.42 (1.11—1.96)	
Cerebellum	0.03 (0.01—0.09)	
Pons	0.07 (0.52—1.03)	0.19
Medulla oblongata	0.34 (0.20—0.50)	0.31—0.50
Area postrema	0.57 (0.42—0.81)	
Cervical spinal cord	0.14 (0.09—0.21)	
Cerebrospinal fluid[3]	0.001	

[1] COSTA and APRISON (1958), bioassay. [2] BERTLER (1961), fluorimetric assay.
[3] ASHCROFT and SHARMAN (1960), fluorimetric assay.

material, should have suffered little from post mortem change. In general the results are in good agreement, though the methods of extraction and assay were different.

When the distribution in human brain is compared with that in the brain of the dog (AMIN et al. 1954; BOGDANSKI et al. 1957) and cat (KUNTZMAN et al. 1961), similarities are to be observed in the small amounts found in the isocortex, cerebellum and spinal cord, and the large amounts in the corpus striatum, amygdaloid body, thalamus, hypothalamus and in the nuclei of the midbrain. Striking differences will also be noted; but further observations are needed before these can be profitably discussed. COSTA and APRISON drew attention to the very much larger amounts of 5-HT in the human allocortex than in the isocortex.

The cerebrospinal fluid contains inappreciable amounts of 5-HT, but GIARMAN and FREEDMAN (1960), using autopsy material, found considerable amounts in the *pineal gland*. The figures ranged from 0.36 to 22.8 μg 5-HT/g (mean 4.1) and were similar to those obtained for rhesus monkeys (mean 3.28 range 1.2 to 10.0) and considerably higher than for steers (mean 0.40, range 0.20 to 0.63). The human glands examined by GIARMAN and FREEDMAN came from patients with a variety of diseases and possibly the great variability may be due to this.

c) Alimentary canal

Post mortem change in the alimentary canal is very rapid and estimations must therefore be made on material obtained at operation. This has the disadvantage that the tissue removed may not be normal. Gastrointestinal 5-HT is contained in the mucosa, which can easily be scraped off and extracted for the assay; or the whole thickness of the wall may be homogenised and extracted. Results obtained by both methods are contained in Table 5. Comparison with the amount in laboratory animals is unreliable owing to differences in technique but the values are roughly similar; the human stomach may contain rather less 5-HT than that of the dog and rat. Argentaffin cells first appear in the human embryo between the sixth and twelfth week of foetal life (COLE and McKALEN 1962).

Table 5. *Distribution of 5-hydroxytryptamine in the human gastro intestinal tract (biopsy material)*

	μg 5-HT/g. mucosa [1] range	μg 5-HT/g. tissue [2] mean ± S.D.
Stomach, body	0.7—3.5	0.7 ± 0.4
antrum	—	0.9 ± 0.4
pylorus	1.9—418	0.6 ± 0.4
Duodenum	4.8—7.8	3.7 ± 0.8
Ileum	—	2.9 ± 1.7
Appendix	1.1	0.9 ± 0.5
Colon	3.3—8.6	1.7 ± 0.7
Rectum	2.5—8.3	—
Gall bladder	0.01	—

[1] ERSPAMER (1954b), bioassay.
[2] RESNICK and GRAY (1961), fluorimetric assay.

d) Urine

Only small amounts (Table 6) of 5-HT are found in human urine (GADDUM and PAASONEN 1955; LEMBECK and NEUHOLD 1955). According to RODNIGHT (1956) the daily excretion is increased by the oral administration of L-tryptophan. He was unable to detect either N-methyl-5-hydroxytryptamine or bufotenine, although both these substances had been reported in human urine by BUMPUS and PAGE (1955). The principal hydroxyindole excreted is 5-hydroxyindoleacetic acid and this, in man, is excreted unconjugated. Excretion is partly by tubular secretion and is depressed by previous administration of probenecid, but is little affected by change in the pH of the urine (DESPOPOULOS and WEISSBACH 1957; MILNE et al. 1960). In patients with the malignant carcinoid syndrome (p. 757), N-acetyl-5-hydroxytryptamine and 5-hydroxyindoleaceturic acid have also been identified (McISAAC and PAGE 1959).

Table 6. *Daily excretion of 5-hydroxytryptamine and 5-hydroxyindoleacetic acid in human urine*

	mg/24 hours	
5-hydroxytryptamine	0.06 to 0.16	RODNIGHT and McILWAIN (1956)
5-hydroxyindoleacetic acid	2 to 9	SJOERDSMA et al. (1956)
	3 to 14	MACFARLANE et al. (1956)

Small amounts of tryptamine (mean 79, range 36 to 120 μg/day) are excreted (RODNIGHT 1956; SJOERDSMA et al. 1959) and WEISSBACH et al. (1959) have found the corresponding acid, indole-3-acetic acid (3 to 18 mg/day). Both substances are derived from tryptophan and their excretion is increased by tryptophan feeding and by changes in intestinal bacterial flora. In non-tropical sprue, WEISSBACH et al. (1959) found excretions up to 200 mg indole-3-acetic acid/day but this was reduced to 40 mg/day when neomycin was given by mouth. Bufotenine has been reported in the urine of hallucinated schizophrenics by FISCHER et al. (1961).

ELIASON (1961) found no 5-HT (< 0.5 μg/ml) in human *semen*.

B. Effects following infusions of 5-hydroxytryptamine

a) *Subjective symptoms*

When small amounts of 5-HT (< 10 μg/kg/min) are infused intravenously in man, subjective effects are mild or absent. About 50% of subjects develop a facial flush and a few notice increased intestinal motility or mild epigastric pain (BOJS 1961). With large doses, pain is experienced along the course of the vein and contraction of the wall of the vein may obstruct the infusion; thromboses in veins into which 5-HT has been infused are common. The following symptoms, in decreasing order of frequency, are noted: heaviness in the legs and arms, pressure in the head and eyes, nausea, abdominal colic and tightness across the chest (SPIES and STONE 1952; MAGALINI et al. 1956; GROVER et al. 1958; LE MESSURIER et al. 1959). In occasional subjects, there may be a sudden fall in blood pressure, bradycardia or tachycardia, nausea, sweating and pallor. All symptoms subside rapidly on discontinuing the infusion. Marked hypotension and bradycardia may be due to a von Bezold-like reflex (HARRIS et al. 1960), such as has been described in cats by DAWES and COMROE (1954), KOTTEGODA and MOTT (1955) and FASTIER et al. (1959).

b) *Cardiovascular system*

The effects on the cardiovascular system are by no means clear cut and there is considerable variation both in individual response and in results reported by different groups of workers. Differences in dosage, in techniques, in the methods used in assessing the results and the time after the commencement of the infusion when the effects are assessed, are no doubt responsible for the latter. An increase in *heart rate* starting 1 to $1^1/_2$ minutes after beginning the infusion is nearly always seen (Fig. 2), even with small doses, but systemic *blood pressure* changes vary from individual to individual. Some show a rise, some a fall, others a biphasic response (HOLLANDER et al. 1957). Some authors (BALDRIGHI and FERRARI 1955; PAGE 1958) have reported a rise in *pulmonary arterial pressure*, as is commonly observed in cats and dogs; others (NEMIR et al. 1954, HOLLANDER et al. 1957; HARRIS et al. 1960; BOJS 1961) have found no consistent change. *Cardiac output* and both *pulmonary* and *systemic vascular resistance* were unchanged in the experiments of HARRIS et al. (1960) in which doses of 1.85 to 6.5 μg/kg/min were infused, whereas GOVER et al. (1958), PAGE (1958) and BOJS (1961), who used somewhat larger doses, found an increase in cardiac output and decrease in total peripheral resistance. In BOJS' experiments both effects were maximal with doses of 4 to 6 μg/kg/min (Table 7) and were less striking when the dose had been gradually increased than when a single medium sized infusion was given. This suggests the development of tachyphylaxis, and may explain the negative results of some other workers.

Table 7. *Change in heart rate, cardiac output, total peripheral vascular resistance and left ventricular work during infusions of 5-hydroxytryptamine in man, expressed as a percentage of the values during the control period.* (From BOJS 1961)

Dose µg/kg/min	Heart rate mean increase ± S.D.	Cardiac output ± S.D.	Total peripheral vascular resistance ± S.D.	Left ventricle work ± S.D.
2.2	+ 6.0 ± 10.1	+ *9.1* ± 9.9	−6.4 ± 9.9	+*10.1* ± 10.2
4.3	+*11.5* ± 10.3	+*14.3* ± 14.8	−**10.3** ± 7.0	+*17.2* ± 22.7
6.5	+*12.8* ± 15.1	+*12.6* ± 15.9	−*13.0* ± 11.7	+10.1 ± 24.5
8.7	+*16.8* ± 11.6	+13.0 ± 14.1	−*12.2* ± 7.7	+11.5 ± 18.9
No. of subjects	13	12	12	12

The values in italics ($P < 0.05$) and in heavy type ($P < 0.001$) are significantly different from the control values.

LE MESSURIER et al. (1959) followed the changes in blood flow through the human forearm by venous occlusion plethysmography during an intravenous infusion of 0.4 to 1.3 mg 5-HT/min. They found an initial transient 3- to 4-fold increase in flow, followed by a smaller sustained increase. The pattern of the response was unaltered after blocking the nerves to the forearm with lignocaine, and the site of action was therefore thought to be peripheral. BOCK et al. (1957) obtained similar changes in muscle flow, but a reduction in skin flow. The overall forearm blood flow changes appear to be the resultant of two effects: dilatation of muscle vessels and constriction of skin vessels. This may explain the results of infusion into the brachial artery described by RODDIE et al. (1955). Blood flow in both forearm and hand was reduced, but this reduction was preceded by a transient increase in flow (Fig. 1). The low pressure capacity of the limb (GLOVER et al. 1958), determined by measuring limb swelling on occluding the veins at a pressure of 10 cms of water, decreased. The skin flushed red but subsequently the colour changed to a dusky red and finally the fingers became cyanosed. The changes were ascribed to capillary dilatation (evidenced by the flushing of the skin), constriction of the arterioles, causing a reduction in blood flow, and an increase in tone of capacity vessels, probably mainly venules and veins. With the larger doses there was evidence of oedema formation, and petechial haemorrhages developed in some subjects some hours after the infusion. More direct evidence of increase in venous tone was obtained by SHARPEY-SCHAFER and GINSBURG (1962). They measured the rate of rise of venous pressure per unit

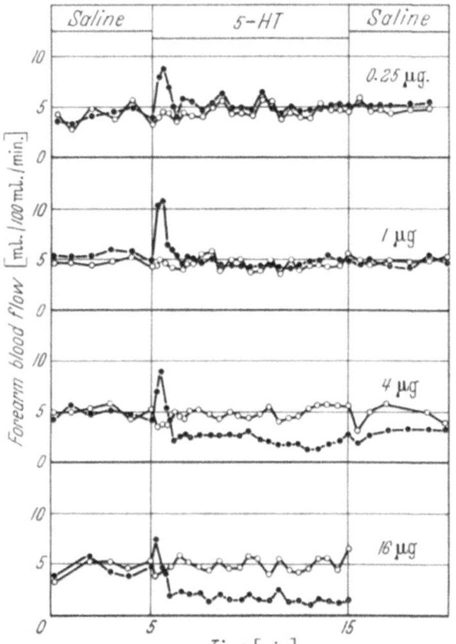

Fig. 1. Response of the forearm blood flow in one subject to four doses of 5-hydroxytryptamine (indicated at right of each frame) infused into the left brachial artery. ● Left forearm; ○ right forearm. (From RODDIE et al. 1955.)

of limb blood flow in an anticubital vein during venous occlusion. With intra-arterial infusions of 10 μg 5-HT creatinine sulphate/minute they cound a marked rise in venous tone and changes in forearm flow similar to those caused by intra-arterial infusions of adrenaline.

The vasoconstrictor action of intra-arterial infusions of 5-HT is antagonised by brom-lysergic acid diethylamide and by sodium salicylate. The latter substance needs to be given intravenously in sufficient dose to raise its serum concentration to 0.1 to 0.2 mg/ml and does not appear to have a direct local action on the vessels, as there is no antagonism when it is infused intra-arterially in doses which give a similar concentration in the arterial blood (GLOVER et al. 1957).

An analysis of the peripheral vascular actions of 5-HT is further complicated by the observation of FELDBERG and SMITH (1953) that it releases histamine. Although it is not a powerful histamine releaser, this may contribute to its vascular effects.

The human umbilical artery (SCHMERMUND et al. 1959) and vein (PANIGEL and MAYER 1959) contract to 5-HT in a concentration of 0.1 μg/ml, and the addition of 5-HT to the solution perfusing a human placenta raises the vascular resistance (ÅSTRÖM and SAMELIUS 1957). Its potency is about 10 times that of adrenaline. This action can be antagonised by a variety of substances: by drugs with adrenaline blocking actions such as phentolamine, by dihydroergotamine and yohimbine, by the antihistamine phenbenzamine, by chlorpromazine and by lysergic acid diethylamide.

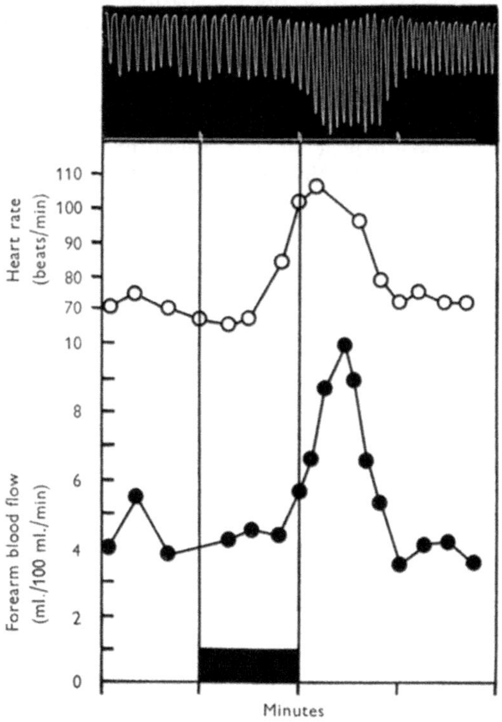

Fig. 2. Respiration, heart rate and forearm blood flow before, during and after the intravenous infusion of 5-hydroxytryptamine. Top trace: stethogram, inspiration downwards. The period of infusion is given by the black rectangle. (From PARKS et al. 1960.)

c) *Respiration*

Intravenous infusions of 5-HT increase *total pulmonary ventilation* (HOLLANDER et al. 1957a; MICHELSON et al. 1958; LE MESSURIER et al. 1959; PARKS et al. 1960; BOJS 1961) but both *tidal air* and *rate of respiration* are not increased in all cases (Fig. 2). In a large proportion of cases there is an increase in tidal air. PARKS et al. (1960) noted that the changes are less well marked after the first five minutes and this may account for the failure of HARRIS et al. (1960) to observe them. There is a small rise in *oxygen consumption* but this is insufficient to cause the respiratory stimulation, and is probably accounted for by the increased work done by the heart and respiratory muscles (BOJS 1961), and by oxygen storage (PARKS et al. 1960); there is no evidence of metabolic stimulation. Animal experiments have shown that 5-HT stimulates chemoreceptors of the carotid body, and the increased respiration is probably caused in this way. Further evidence in support of this has been obtained by SKINNER and WHELAN (1962). They found that injection of 125 μg 5-HT into the common carotid artery of 3 patients caused an immediate stimulation of respiration. Repetition after surgical removal of the carotid body failed to cause hyperpnoea. Stimulation of respiration is potentiated by mepyramine and antagonised by 1-benzyl-2,5-dimethyl tryptamine (BAS) but not by atropine, hexamethonium, phentolamine or by chlorpromazine (MICHELSON et al. 1958). *Bronchospasm* has rarely been seen during intravenous infusions in man.

d) Renal function

The effect of 5-HT on renal function in man has been investigated by ANNONI et al. (1955); NOTTER (1956); HULET and PERERA (1956); HOLLANDER et al. (1957a); CORA' et al. (1957); SCHNECKLOTH et al. (1957); CENACCHI et al. (1958); SINCLAIR (1959); AMBANELLI and SALVI (1959); BOJS (1961).

In general there is agreement that during high urine flows the i.v. injection 4 μg/kg/min and more, is usually followed by a reduction in *urine flow*, and that this is accompanied by a small reduction in *renal plasma flow* and often, but not always, by a reduction in *glomerular filtration rate*. On the other hand CORA et al. (1957) failed to detect these changes. An antidiuretic response has been obtained in patients with diabetes insipidus (BOJS 1961; ANNONI et al. 1955) and in adrenalectomised patients (BOJS 1961).

A reduction in *sodium excretion* has also usually been reported, but in the experiments of HOLLANDER et al. (1957) the reduction, though significant, was slight and might in some cases have been due to reduced urine flow and inadequate 'dead space' washout, and there was also a similar reduction in *potassium excretion*. In BOJS' experiments, sodium retention was marked and was attributed to increased tubular reabsorption, but no definite effect on potassium excretion was found.

e) Gastrointestinal tract

HENDRIX et al. (1957) have used a balloon introduced into the *jejunum* to measure changes in *intestinal tone* caused by the intravenous injection of 0.5 to 3.0 mg 5-HT in 29 subjects. Tone increased abruptly 10 to 60 secs. after the injection and remained raised for an average of 3.7 mins (range: 1 to 8 mins). Small, rapid (11/min) waves, only, were recorded during this period. For a period of 1 to 6 mins after the tone had fallen to normal, there was little rhythmic activity and the intestine failed to respond to a further injection of 5-HT. The effect of 5-HT on intestinal tone was blocked by previous administration of atropine, methantheline or BAS but unaffected by hexamethonium. However, in view of the findings of HAVERBACK and DAVIDSON (1958) and DANIEL et al. (1960) the effect of atropine needs confirmation. No reduction in the response was caused by a variety of antihistamines but, on the contrary, in 7 out of 9 subjects sensitivity to 5-HT was increased. In contrast to this usual response, in 4 subjects the injection of 4 to 30 mg 5-HT caused no change in tone. Repeated injection of 5-HT leads to the development of tachyphylaxis (HAVERBACK and DAVIDSON 1958).

Changes in tone and electrical activity in human *ileum* after the intravenous injection of 2 mg 5-HT have been recorded by DANIEL et al. (1960) in subjects with ileostomies. An initial spasm, starting within 1 min of the injection, was followed by rhythmic propulsive contractions which lasted 2 to 6 mins. Relaxation was followed, as in the case of the jejunum, by diminished motility. The initial contraction was accompanied by a burst of electrical activity, whereas during the period of rhythmic contractions electrical activity diminished. The recordings of electrical activity were made just distal to the recordings of muscle tone. Brom-lysergic acid diethylamide intravenously diminished both the mechanical and electrical response to 5-HT, but atropine, promethazine, morphine and effect. These results would be explained nalorphine intravenously were without if the human ileum possessed only the D-receptors of GADDUM and PICARELLI (1957).

Rhythmical activity of the *stomach* and *rectum* is inhibited during infusions of 5-HT.

Gastric secretion is increased in volume and decreased in acidity by intravenous infusions of 5-HT, and there is an increase in the flow of bile pigment. The volume of pancreatic juice is unchanged (SCHMID and KINZLMEIER 1959; WARNER et al. 1959). Gastric acidity is increased by the 5-HT antagonist methysergide (RESNICK et al. 1962).

f) Effect of an infusion of 5-HT on the concentration of 5-HT in the blood

BOJS (1961) has estimated the amount of 5-HT in the blood before, during and after infusions of 5-HT given into the subclavian vein. Blood samples were withdrawn from the brachial artery. During an infusion of 80 mins, in which 868 µg 5-HT were given, platelet 5-HT rose from 0.39 to 1.12 µg/10^9 platelets. No "free" 5-HT was detected in platelet poor plasma. The total amount of 5-HT which could be accounted for from the increase found in the platelets, amounted to only about 2% of that infused. The results of a similar experiment in which 4.3 µg 5-HT/kg/min was infused for 40 mins are shown in Fig 3. The amount of 5-HT in the platelats, raised during the infusion, did not decline in the succeeding 100 mins.

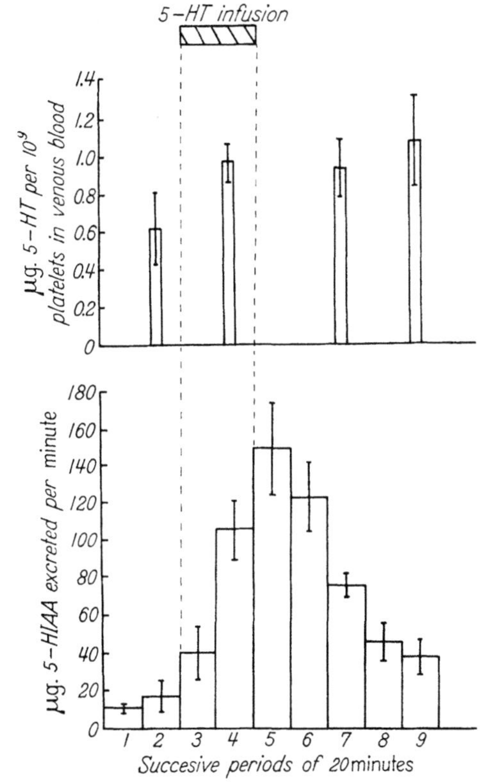

Fig. 3. Effect of an intravenous infusion of 4.3 µg 5-HT/kg/min for 40 mins on platelet 5-HT content and on the urinary excretion of 5-hydroxyindoleacetic acid. Abscissa: successive 20 min periods. The results are the mean for 5 subjects ± standard deviation. (From BOJS 1961.)

g) The metabolism and excretion of infused 5-HT

After the infusion of as much as 10 mg of 5-HT, no increase in 5-HT in the urine is found but there is a considerable increase in the excretion of 5-HIAA. The total amount recovered is equivalent to 85 to 100% of the 5-HT given (DAVIDSON et al. 1957; BOJS 1961). In man no tracer studies have been done, so that it is not known whether or not any of the extra 5-HIAA is derived from an increased secretion of endogenous 5-HT. The increased peristalsis caused by the infusion, and the effects of purgation on the concentration of 5-HT in the blood (see p. 755) make this a possibility.

h) The metabolism and excretion of 5-HT ingested orally

As much as 50 mg of 5-HT may be taken by mouth without producing any symptoms (SJOERDSMA et al. 1958) and recovery as 5-HIAA in the urine is 90 to 100% (SJOERDSMA et al. 1958; DONALDSON et al. 1960). The recovery is reduced if an active amine oxidase inhibitor has been given and this a convenient method of estimating amine oxidase inhibition in man (SJOERDSMA et al. 1958).

i) Intradermal injections of 5-HT

These cause a flare but no wheal (HERXHEIMER and SCHACHTER 1958). The injection is painful and ARMSTRONG et al. (1953) found that pain was caused by concentrations as low as 10^{-7} to 10^{-6}M, when solutions were applied to the exposed base of a human skin blister; in this it as more potent than other tryptamine derivatives tested, and more potent than both acetylcholine and histamine.

C. Effects following an infusion of 5-hydroxytryptophan (5-HTP)

Intravenous infusions of D,L-5-HTP, over a dose range of 10 mg in 10 secs to 120 mg in 60 mins, have been given by DAVIDSON et al. (1957) and HAVERBACK and DAVIDSON (1958). With all doses nausea developed after 15 to 20 mins, and was sometimes accompanied by abdominal cramps, borborygmi and vomiting. A balloon in the jejunum recorded increased intestinal activity starting 6 to 40 mins after beginning the infusion and persisting for 60 mins after it was concluded; the increased activity could be inhibited by an injection of 1 mg atropine. With similar doses of 5-HTP, SCHMID et al. (1960d) found, in addition to increased activity in the small intestine, an inhibition of rhythmical activity in the stomach and colon, and a reduction in gastric acidity. No change in pupil size, respiration, electrocardiogram, blood pressure (except for one subject who had a transient hypotension) or mental function was observed. Doses of 10 to 30 mg 5-HTP by mouth had no effect on intestinal activity.

The infusion of 50 mg D,L-5-HTP leads to an increase in the amount of 5-HT in the urine for a period of 8 hours or more. Of the infused 5-HTP 4 to 7% is recovered as 5-HT and 14 to 35% as 5-HIAA. OATES and SJOERDSMA (1961) compared the excretion of these two substances after the infusion of equal amounts of L-5-HTP and its D-isomer. Of the former, 20% was recovered as 5-HT and 40% as 5-HIAA. Of the latter, a total of 8% was excreted as 5-HT and 5-HIAA. They suggest that some of the D-acid is metabolised by D-amino acid oxidase and then transaminated to L-5-HTP, and that the kidney is the main site of this change.

D. Effect of diet and drugs on hydroxyindoles in blood and urine

a) Diet

The excretion of 5-HIAA is increased by the consumption of bananas and plantains (CROUT and SJOERDSMA 1959; PUENTE-DUANY et al. 1958) due to the large amount 5-HT in these fruits (WAALKES et al. 1958; UDENFRIEND et al. 1959). East Africans of the Buganda may eat 500 to 800 g cooked banana pulp daily, with a resulting rise in the daily excretion of 5-HIAA up to 150 mg/day (CRAWFORD 1962); and in Nigeria (FOY and PARRATT 1962) plantain meals cause a similar increase in 5-HIAA excretion. The high incidence in these two districts of endomyocardial fibrosis (DAVIES 1960), a condition in which the cardiac lesions resemble in some respects those of the malignant carcinoid syndrome (p. 758), is of interest. However, whereas both sides of the heart are affected in endomyocardial fibrosis (SHILLINGFORD and SOMERS 1961), the right is mainly affected in the malignant carcinoid syndrome.

KIRBERGER (1962) has reported the daily excretion of 100 mg 5-HIAA in the urine of a patient who eats large quantities of walnuts. In the nuts he found 17 to 34 mg 5-HT/100 g.

b) Purgatives and carbachol

The administration of magnesium sulphate or carbachol, in doses which cause hyperperistalsis, increases the amount of 5-HT in the blood. The increase was noticed 4 hours after the oral administration of magnesium sulphate and 1 hour after the subcutaneous or intramuscular injection of carbachol (O'HARA et al. 1959; ADAMS 1960; BOJS 1961). BOJS could detect no change in 5-HIAA excretion.

c) Other drugs

The amount of 5-HT in platelets is increased by the daily administration of 5 to 8 mg iproniazid/kg/day (PLETSCHER and BERNSTEIN 1958; SHORE et al. 1958; MARSHALL et al. 1960) presumably by the inhibition of mono-amine oxidase and a resulting increase in free 5-HT in the blood, though this has not been measured. *Imipramine*, in doses used for the treatment of psychiatric patients, causes a marked fall in platelet 5-HT probably due to inhibition of the absorption of 5-HT by platelets (MARSHALL et al. 1960) since concentrations of imipramine as low as 10^{-6} M appreciably inhibit 5-HT uptake by human platelets *in vitro*. A similar though weaker action is exerted by cocaine, chlorpromazine, tryptamine, chlorprothixene and a number of other drugs (STACEY 1961) including desmethylimipramine and amitriptyline (unpublished).

The administration of *reserpine* in doses of 1 mg/day is followed by a loss of virtually all the 5-HT in platelets and in their capacity to take up 5-HT when incubated with it. Recovery is slow and normal platelet 5-HT levels are only reached after 10 days or more (HARDISTY, INGRAM and STACEY 1956; STACEY 1959).

Blood 5-HT levels rise during surgical operations (STONE et al. 1961) and this is followed, during the first day after an operation by an increased excretion of 5-HIAA and of indolyl-3-acetic acid and indican (CATCHPOLE 1962; CRAWFORD and WATTS 1962). On the other hand after burns 5-HIAA excretion is low, often less than 1.0 mg/day, from shortly after the burn until convalescence (GOLDSMITH et al. 1961). There is at present no explanation of either or these findings.

The effect of cigarette smoking on 5-HIAA excretion has been investigated by SCHIEVELBEIN et al. (1962). They found that the daily excretion of smokers was considerably higher than that of non-smokers and that when non-smokers smoked 5 to 10 cigarettes daily, their daily excretion was raised from 1.82 ± 0.34 to 3.03 ± 0.56 (mean of 7 subjects $\pm$ S.E.M.). They ascribe these changes to the release of 5-HT from stores by nicotine, an effect previously described (SCHIEVELBEIN et al. 1961).

E. 5-Hydroxytryptamine in disease

1. Carcinoid disease

Carcinoid tumours of the intestinal tract were first recognised as a morphological entity by OBERNDORFER (1907) who proposed the name, Karzinoiden; but LUBARSCH (1888) had already identified them and suggested that they originated from the crypts of Lieberkühn, and nearly a century carlier they had been described by MERLING (1802) (cited by STEGER and AVONZINI, 1953/54) and later by LANGHANS (1867) and BEGER (1882).

Primary carcinoid tumours may be found anywhere along the gastrointestinal tract between the cardiac sphincter and the anus, in the appendix, MECKEL's diverticulum, biliary tract, in the larger pancreatic ducts, in the ovary or testis, and in the parotid gland (NICOD 1958). Some bronchial adenomata are morphologically very similar and will be discussed later (p. 757). The overall incidence in four large series of combined surgical and necropsy cases is given by PESKIN and ORLOFF (1959) as 0.08% (138 carcinoids in 175,891 cases). The commonest sites are the appendix and ileum, which accounted for 33% and 31% respectively of the 705 tumours collected by DAVIES (1959), but 10% were found in the rectum.

It was at first thought that tumours rarely metastasized, but it has now become apparent that malignancy is common, particularly in carcinoids of the small intestine where 50% show a tendency to spread. Only 10% of carcinoids of the appendix in DAVIES' series were classified as malignant. Spread is mainly by lymph channels; metastases may be found in regional lymph glands, liver, pancreas, ovaries, adrenal glands and other abdominal viscera, heart, lung, bone, skin, etc.

Macroscopically tumours are usually yellow but may be white, grey or orange; they are situated in the submucosa though they may invade deeper layers and more rarely, the mucosa. DAVIES (1959) comments on an apparent hypertrophy of the adjacent intestinal wall. *Microscopically* they are seen to consist of nests or columns of round or polygonal cells in a fibrous tissue stroma. When stained with haematoxylin and eosin, the nuclei are prominent and the chromatin deeply basophilic. The cytoplasm is pale, acidophilic with acidophilic granules. The appearances under the electron microscope have been described by SCHUHMACHER and SCHULZ (1963).

The origin of carcinoid tumours has been the subject of much speculation. GOSSET and MASSON (1914) showed that the cells of these tumours, and also those of the cells of Nikolai-Kultschitsky, contain granules which, after fixation in formol, stain by ammonical silver nitrate and supported the earlier suggestion of HUEBSCHMANN (1910) that carcinoid tumours were derived from the Nikolai-Kultschitzky cells (MASSON 1928).

The presence of granules led GOSSET and MASSON to the view, first suggested by CIACCIO (1906), that they had an endocrine activity, and in the following years the secretion of various substances was suggested: insulin (MASSON 1924), adrenaline, pterins (ERÖS 1933, JACOBSON, 1939), glucagon (WEISBERG and SCHAEFER 1952) and enteramine (ERSPAMER 1940). However no appreciable amounts of insulin (FEYRTER and UNNA 1936), adrenaline (WALDENSTRÖM and LJUNGBERG 1955), acetylcholine (LEMBECK 1954), substance P (LEMBECK 1954) or histamine (LEMBECK 1954, DAUGHERTY et al. 1955) were found in the tumours and no increased secretion of glucagon (FEIN and KNUDTSON 1956).

FEYRTER and UNNA (1936) and SELBERG (1940) found a pressor substance in crude extracts of tumour tissue, but the presence of 5-hydroxytryptamine was first demonstrated by LEMBECK (1953), who subsequently pointed out (RATZENHOFER and LEMBECK 1954) that the pressor effects obtained by FEYRTER and by SELBERG were probably due to this substance. During the last 10 years LEMBECK's observation has been repeatedly confirmed in many, but not in all carcinoid tumors, and the findings are discussed below (p. 761).

The early work on carcinoid disease was largely morphological but in 1953 ISLER and HEDINGER reported three cases, with a primary tumour in the ileum and secondaries in the liver, in which there was a chronic endocarditis of the right side of the heart with pulmonary stenosis and tricuspid insufficiency. They described this as a definite syndrome (see also HEDINGER and GLOOR 1954) and at about the same time ROSENBAUM et al. (1953) described a similar case. In 1952 BIÖRCK, AXÉN and THORSON had described a similar case without recognising the syndrome, but THORSON et al. (1954) subsequently reported three cases of their own and thirteen from the literature, and described most of the features now recognised as part of the malignant carcinoid syndrome. They also suggested that the symptoms and pathological changes might be due to a hormone secreted by the tumor, possibly 5-hydroxytryptamine.

Since the description of the syndrome, a retrospective review of the literature has brought to light a number of cases unrecognised at the time: CASSIDY (1930, 1931, 1934), SCHOLTE (1931), MILLMAN (1943), CURRENS, KINNEY and WHITE (1945).

About 85% of bronchial adenomata (LIEBOW, 1952) have a microscopic structure similar to carcinoids of the small intestine and have been referred to as *bronchial carcinoids.* SINCE 1958 a number of cases with a primary bronchial carcinoid but with paroxysmal attacks similar to those seen in the malignant carcinoid syndrome, and with an increased excretion of 5-HIAA in the urine has been reported. In most cases liver metastases were present, but BERNHEIMER et al. (1960) have described a case with a lung primary but without metastases. In this case cardiac lesions were confined to the left side of the heart. Bronchial carcinoids giving both argentaffin and argyrophil staining reactions (p. 759) have been reported; references are given by WILLIAMS and AZZOPARDI (1960), and by GOWENLOCK et al. (1964), who have also reported cases in which an oat cell carcinoma of lung was associated with the syndrome, and by SANDLER, SCHEUER and WATT (1961) who describe a 5-HTP secreting tumour. The histology of these tumours has been discussed recently by FEYRTER (1960) and by LANGER (1961).

2. The malignant carcinoid syndrome

The symptoms of patients with carcinoid tumours without metastases are usually related entirely to the bowel. They consist of abdominal pain and distension sometimes associated with constipation or diarrhoea and malaena; symptoms which can be explained by mechanical obstruction or ulceration of the mucosa. However in some patients in whom metastases have occurred, a number of other symptoms are also found. Prominent among these are a peculiar *episodic flush, abdominal colic* and *watery diarrhoea*, attacks of *dyspnoea* due to bronchoconstriction and *oedema* and *ascites*, due to *right heart failure.* Usually the liver contains metastases in these cases, but occasionally it has none; other abdominal viscera, lung, bones, etc. are then involved.

a) The flush

Typically this starts in the face, and in the more advanced cases spreads down the neck and over the trunk and extremities. It may be bright red at first, but soon changes to a dusky colour. It is patchy, the areas vary considerably in size, and it is associated with a burning sensation. At the beginning of the attack there is often some fall in blood pressure, but this is succeeded by a period when the blood pressure is raised and there is some tachycardia. Finally the flush becomes cyanotic before gradually fading away. Usually the whole episode is over in about 10 minutes, but signs of the flush may be visible for several hours, and cases are described (THORSON 1958) in which it never completely faded away. Migrating yellow, red and white patches surrounded by a dark red area may be seen in late cases, in which also there may be permanently dilated, tortous veins

(Waldenström 1958a). There is no itching or wheal formation. The peritoneum has been reported to participate in a flush and a rise in pulmonary arterial pressure has been found (Waldenström 1958). Sometimes there is a feeling of fullness in the head, giddiness or, rarely, loss of consciousness.

b) Intestinal symptoms

These consist of attacks of intestinal colic, watery diarrhoea, abrupt evacuation of the bowels and borborygmi and may precede, accompany or follow the flushes, but also may recur independently. There may be as many as 20 or more in a day, may occur in patients who have no intestinal lesion and result in hypokalaemia (Steel 1962).

c) Bronchoconstriction

Attacks of bronchoconstriction are less common than flushes or intestinal colic. They occurred in 25% of the 79 cases reported by Thorson (1958) and usually occur at the same time as a flush.

d) Cardiac lesions

These develop late in the disease and the principal lesion is a fibrosis of the endocardium affecting both the valves and walls of the heart (Isler and Hedinger 1953; MacDonald and Robbins 1957). It takes the form of greyish or white pads of connective tissue composed of fibroblasts, a ground substance and condensed collagenous and sometimes elastic fibrils. It is proliferative in nature, there is no destruction of underlying tissue and the endocardium is intact (Davies 1960). Present pathological opinion is that it is distinct from the cardiac lesions in any other condition. A striking feature is that the right heart is much more commonly affected than the left; when the left heart is affected the right heart is usually, though not invariably (see below) more severely affected. Tricuspid and pulmonary valves are about equally often involved; stenosis and insufficiency are equally common in the tricuspid valve but stenosis is more common than insufficiency in the pulmonary valve. Minor changes are occasionally seen in the myocardium and pericardium. The cardiac lesions result in the development of congestive cardiac failure, but Thorson (1958) found no clear correlation between valvular lesions and oedema, and concluded that other factors (low serum albumin concentration, periodic increases in venous pressure during flushing) also contributed to oedema formation.

e) Other symptoms and signs

Hyperkeratosis, with or without a greyish black pigmentation of the skin of the limbs, has been reported, and its similarity to the skin lesions of pellagra noted (Scholte 1931; McNeely and Jones 1946; Kahr 1956; Thorson 1958 and Wolfe et al. 1960). Treatment with nicotinamide may sometimes be followed by the disappearance of the skin lesions (Thorson 1958), but usually there is little improvement.

A number of other findings have been reported but the incidence of them is too low to be certain that they are not coincidental: recurrent *peptic ulcer* (see p. 765), swelling and pain in the *joints*, *localised oedema*, transient *swelling of the face*, attacks of profuse *sweating* and normal or increased excretion of *uropepsinogen* in the presence of achlorhydria.

Usually there is no *mental disturbance*, but Jenkins and Butcher (1955) and Goble et al. (1956) reported patients who were mentally confused or hallucinated, depressed and mentally labile terminally.

3. The carcinoid tumour

Chemical and biochemical observations

A number of estimations of the 5-HT content of carcinoid tissue have been published, but these are probably not very accurate as they are dependent on the methods used for preserving the tissue between biopsy and the preparation of extracts. The amount found varies from less than 1 μg to more than 2.5 mg/g fresh tissue (Lembeck 1953; Sauer et al. 1958). Normal values are given in Table 5. According to Pernow (1958) higher concentrations are usually found in primaries than in metastases. It may be significant that in a case described by Sandler and Snow (1958), in which the tumour contained a small amount (0.3 μg/g), the cells did not contain argentaffin granules. This case is further discussed on p. 761. From studies on the rate of excretion of ^{14}C labelled 5-HIAA after the administration of ^{14}C labelled 5-HTP to a patient with a malignant carcinoid tumour, Sjoerdsma et al (1957) deduced that the total pool of 5-HT in the patient was 2.8 g.

Few estimations of other amines have been made. Waldenström, Pernow and Silver (1957) report 10 μg histamine/g tissue in a tumour from a patient who was excreting large amounts of histamine in the urine (see p. 760), and Schneckloth et al. (1959) report the presence of another, unidentified, indole. Lembeck (1953) found other substances, which he did not identify but which contracted plain muscle; and Langemann (1956), Langemann et al. (1962) and Sjoerdsma et al. (1956) identified 5-HTP decarboxylase and amine oxidase in a tumour.

Note on the staining reactions of carcinoid tumours. A variety of stains has been used to characterise carcinoid tumours, and a specialised work should be consulted for details of staining methods and for a discussion of the significance to be attached to the histochemical findings (Pearse 1960). The result of staining with silver depends not only on the technique used, but also on the fixative and the speed of fixation after death or biopsy. Formol fixation is to be prefered; fixatives containing chromates are unsuitable. Granules disappear rapidly after death and can rarely be found in autopsy material. Two kinds of silver reaction must be distinguished

Argyrophil reaction (e.g. Bodian or Davenport techniques). A silver solution is used to impregnate the tissue. Silver is then precipitated in the structures that have taken it up by the use of a reducing agent.

Argentaffin reaction (e.g. Masson-Fontana, Masson-Hamperl and Gomori hexamine-silver techniques). With these stains, no external reducing agent is used, but silver precipitation is dependent on reduction by the tissues.

Carcinoid tumours may be classified into two groups: those which show a positive argyrophil reaction but a negative argentaffin reaction, and those which give both reactions. The relationship between silver staining and the *diazonium reaction*, which also demonstrates granules in some carcinoid tumours, is not definitely established, but in general, this reaction is only given by cells having a positive argentaffin reaction.

Hamperl (1952) has expressed the view that cells giving an argyrophil but not an argentaffin reaction are the precursors of cells giving an argentaffin reaction. This conception would accord with the finding that 5-hydroxytryptophan secreting tumours appear to be argentaffin negative (see p. 761).

4. The blood of patients with carcinoid tumours

a) 5-Hydroxytryptamine

The estimation of 5-HT in the blood of patients with carcinoid tumours must take account of the following facts: 1. 5-HT in blood is present in two forms: bound to platelets and free in the plasma. The estimation of the latter is of especial interest as it is probably more pharmacologically active than that bound to platelets, but its accurate estimation is difficult as liberation of even a small amount of bound 5-HT will give grossly erroneous results. 2. The concentration of 5-HT in the blood probably varies considerably from time to time with variations in the rate of discharge from the tumour; and also in samples taken at the same time from different vessels (c.f. HEGGLIN and LANGEMANN 1955; DAVIS et al. 1961; PEART et al. 1961; ROBERTSON et al. 1962; SMITH et al. 1962). Variation is particularly likely if any considerable fraction is circulating free in the plasma for it will be exposed to enzymic distruction. Thus GADDUM et al. (1953) found perfused cat's lungs removed 5-HT added to the perfusing blood.

Table 8 summarises results in published reports of cases and indicates the range of the figures; though methods of collecting samples, preparing extracts and the assay procedures used, differed.

Table 8. *Blood 5-hydroxytryptamine estimations in normal subjects and in patients with the carcinoid syndrome*

	Platelet-poor plasma μg/ml	Platelets μg/10^9	Whole blood μg/ml	Serum μg/ml
Normal[1]	trace	0.72	0.15	0.15
Carcinoid	trace to 2.7	0.8 to 3.4	0.4 to 3.0	0.05 to 6.5

[1] See Table 1.

Values within the normal range (or only a little raised) have been reported for platelets, whole blood and serum in proved cases of carcinoid syndrome with typical symptoms; but this is an exceptional finding and usually all are considerably raised. The values for platelet-poor plasma must be accepted with reserve for reasons given above. Recently PEART et al. (1961) have made a careful study of this fraction and have taken special precautions to avoid release of 5-HT after withdrawal of the blood. In one case, with a primary carcinoid in the ileum and liver metastases, they found at different times 0.02 to 0.4 μg 5-HT/ml platelet-poor plasma in blood from the inferior vena cava. The lower figure corresponded to a period when the symptoms were quiescent; the higher, during a flush. No values for platelet or whole blood 5-HT are available for this case but it would appear that, although at times a considerable fraction may be free in the plasma, the high value for blood 5-HT is usually largely due to the large amount contained in platelets. This, so far as is known, would need to be released before it could cause symptoms.

b) Other hydroxyindoles

There are few estimations on other hydroxyindoles in blood. SJOERDSMA et al. (1957) report 0.2 to 0.8 μg 5-HIAA/ml blood in a patient with the carcinoid syndrome.

c) Histamine

Only a few estimations of blood histamine have been reported. Some (SNOW et al. 1955) were normal but PERNOW and WALDENSTRÖM (1954, 1957) found 9 μg and 0.3 μg histamine/ml serum in two of their cases (normal: 0.02 to 0.08 μg/ml). The subject is further discussed below.

LEVINE and SJOERDSMA (1963) found the concentration of tryptophan in the blood to be normal or reduced and that of tyrosine normal. There are no reports of the amounts of other amines present, but an increase in the concentration of a bradykinin-like substance has been reported by OATES et al. (1964).

5. The urine of patients with the carcinoid syndrome

5-Hydroxyindoles

The amount of 5-HT found in the urine of patients with the carcinoid syndrome has varied from normal amounts of 200 μg or less in 24 hours to 4.625 mg/24 hours in a case reported by PERNOW and WALDENSTRÖM (1957). The excretion of 5-HIAA is usually but not invariably (DAVIS and ROSENBERG 1961; VON HEILMEYER and CLOTTEN 1958) raised and the increase is usually large; thus 0.5 to 1 g/day is not uncommon (normal 5 to 10 mg/day). The rate of excretion varies not only during the course of the day but also from day to day. It is therefore advisable in assessing hydroxyindole synthesis to carry out estimations on aliquots from urine collected over 24 hours and to examine more than one specimen. Complete 24 hr. saves may present difficulties in patients with severe diarrhoea and a more accurate estimate of 5-HIAA excretion can then be obtained by expressing the results as mg 5-HIAA per g. urinary creatinine. The diet during the period of collection of urine must not contain articles such as bananas, walnuts or tomatoes which may increase 5-HIAA excretion. Urine should be collected into a bottle containing 25 ml concentrated hydrochloric acid and 3 ml toluene.

The relatively small amount of 5-HT excreted is not surprising in view of the effectiveness of oxidative deamination mechanisms. SCHNECKLOTH et al. (1959) have sought chromatographically for other hydroxyindoles and found small amounts of 5-hydroxyindoleaceturic acid, but no N-acetyl-5-hydroxytryptamine.

SJOERDSMA et al. (1956) and SMITH et al. (1957) found that the addition of tryptophan to the diet of a patient with a malignant carcinoid tumour caused an increased excretion of 5-HIAA, whereas no such increase followed the administration of tryptophan to normal subjects; presumably in normal subjects 5-hydroxytryptophan synthesis is already proceeding maximally on the normal tryptophan intake. From their studies, SJOERDSMA et al. (1956, 1957) concluded that under normal circumstances only about 1% dietary tryptophan is metabolised through the 5-hydroxyindole pathway, but that in cases of the carcinoid syndrome it may be as much as 60%. In this event insufficient tryptophan may be available for protein, nicotinamide etc. synthesis (see p. 758). This was supported when it was found that patients excreting large amounts of 5-HIAA, excreted less N′-methylnicotinamide than either normal individuals or those carcinoid patients excreting smaller amounts of 5-HIAA.

In some cases 5-hydroxytryptophan is present in the urine; in others it is absent. It was first detected by SMITH et al. (1957) and thought to be due to the presence of a renal metastasis. Subsequently SANDLER and SNOW (1958) reported a case excreting 30 to 50 mg 5-HTP/day with no evidence of renal abnormality. There seems no doubt that while most cases excrete no 5-HTP (see SCHNFCKLOTH et al. 1959, SJOERDSMA et al. 1956; SMITH et al. 1957) this precursor of 5-HIAA is excreted regularly by a minority of cases (DONALDSON et al. 1959). SANDLER and SNOW suggested that some carcinoid tumours secrete 5-HTP into the blood stream and that this is partly decarboxylated elsewhere and partly excreted unchanged. In the case they described the primary tumour was in the stomach, was argyrophil but contained no argentaffin granules and little 5-HT (0.3 μg/g). Large amounts of both histamine (480 to 940 μg/day) and 5-HT (18 to 24 mg/day) were excreted in the urine in addition to 5-HTP (33 to 49 mg/day). The flush was of a brighter red than is normal, had a more patchy distribution and was diminished by anti-histamine therapy. CAMPBELL et al. (1963) have since shown that tumour tissue from this patient contained much 5-HTP but little 5-HT and no 5-HTP decarboxylase. Similar cases have been described by SANDLER, SCHEUER and WATT (1961) and by OATES and SJOERDSMA (1962). It appears, therefore, that while most patients with the syndrome have tumours which synthesise 5-HT, a minority have tumours which, because they lack 5-HTP decarboxylase, carry the synthesis only as far as 5-HTP. Platelet 5-HT may be little raised in these cases, presumably because platelets have no 5-HTP decarboxylase. An increased excretion of *tryptamine* in the urine has been reported by

Eccleston et al. (1963). A patient with extensive metastase excreted 84 mg/24 hours (normal 0.036 to 0.12). Tryptamine was also detected chromatographically in the blood. The excretion of indolyl-3-acetic acid was little raised. On the other hand, Levine and Sjoerdsma (1963) found the excretion of tryptamine to be more commonly below normal.

Increased *histamine* excretion, in one case up to 6.8 mg/day, was found in 7 out of 9 cases investigated by Pernow and Waldenström (1957), and Waldenström (1961) has suggested that there may be an association between high histamine excretion, bright red patchy flush, 5-HTP excretion and a gastric carcinoid tumour (Table 9) The possibility of this association should be kept in mind when cases of this syndrome are investigated, and if possible correlated with the staining characteristics of the carcinoid cells and the composition and enzyme activity of the tumour. The reported high incidence of peptic ulceration in the carcinoid syndrome (MacDonald, 1956 found this complication in 8 out of 21 cases) may be associated with the presence of a large amount of circulating histamine. Smith et al. (1957) commented on the high excretion of uropepsinogen in the four cases they investigated and Davis and Rosenberg (1961) noted an increased pepsin secretion in gastric juice.

Table 9. *Excretion of 5-hydroxytryptamine, 5-hydroxyindoleacetic acid and histamine in the urine of normal people and in patients with carcinoid tumours.* (Modified from Pernow 1958)

	5-HT µg/ml	5-HIAA mg/24 hrs	Histamine µg/24 hrs
Normal	0.01 to 0.02	2 to 10	6 to 19
Carcinoid	0.10 to 20.0	15 to 1,680	15 ro 2,500

The daily urinary excretion of *noradrenaline* was normal in a single case reported by Waldenström et al. (1957) and below normal in the case reported by Davis and Rosenberg (1961), but v. Studnitz (1959) found a small rise in the excretion of *3-methoxy-4-hydroxy mandelic acid* in 6 out of 7 cases he investigated and high normal excretions were also found in 3 cases by Sandler and Ruthven (1960). The high concentration of 5-hydroxytryptophan decarboxylase, now know to be identical with dopa decarboxylase, in carcinoid tissue (see p. 759) may provide an explanation for increased excretion of this end product of catecholamine metabolism.

6. Causation of symptoms

a) The flush

A number of factors have been reported as precipitating attacks of flushing and are recorded in Table 10. It has been noted that cases with flushing usually have tumours which drain directly into the vena cava and so secretions from the tumours would be able to reach the systemic circulation without first passing through the liver. On the other hand Thorson (1958) noted that in 40 patients without flushing the carcinoid tissue was drained by the portal system. Intestinal symptoms in these patients were probably due to the mechanical effect of the tumour on intestinal function. This accords with the view that the flush is caused by a secretion of the carcinoid tissue, though how this is provoked by the agents mentioned above is not clear. Possibly the ingestion of food, by causing peristalsis, may lead to compression of the tumour. Waldenström et al. (1957) found that in their case it was necessary that the food should be swallowed, taking it into the mouth and chewing it was not followed by a flush; and Snow et al. (1955) found that alcohol given intravenously failed to cause a flush in a patient in whom the same volume by mouth was effective. Robertson et al. (1962) investigated the action of adrenaline and noradrenaline in 13 patients with the syndrome. The intravenous injection of 2 to 20 μg of either amine was followed, after an interval of 40 to 100 secs., by a flush in the 11 patients who suffered from spontaneous flushing, and failed to do so in the 2 who had no spontaneous flushing. The flush and associated symptoms resembled the spontaneous attack both objectively and subjectively. Adrenaline was more effective than noradrenaline and previous treatment with phenoxybenzamine (2 mg daily for 10 days) abolished the effect of the injected amines; but spontaneous flushes persisted. Flushes could not be precipitated by injections of saline, tyramine, ephedrine, amphetamine and methylamphetamine. That the flush was not due to an abnormal reaction of blood vessels to adrenaline, but might be either reflex or due to the liberation into the circulation of a second substance, was shown by two experiments. Electrophoresis

Table 10. *Precipitation of flushing attacks in malignant carcinoid syndrome*

	References
1. Ingestion of food (in some cases especially fatty or highly seasoned food)	1, 4, 5, 12, 13, 14, 15
2. Ingestion of alcohol	7, 11, 12, 14
3. Heat	14
4. Emotion	7, 10, 12, 13
5. Adrenaline, noradrenaline, sympathomimetic amines	7, 16
6. Hypotensive drugs	9
7. Histamine	2, 14
8. Insulin	10
9. Compression of tumour	3, 6, 8

[1] Bleehan 1955. [2] Daugherty et al. 1955. [3] Dockerty and Scheifly 1955. [4] Goble et al. 1956. [5] Macfarlane et al. 1956. [6] McKusick 1956. [7] Robertson et al. 1962. [8] Sauer et al. 1958. [9] Schneckloth et al. 1957. [10] Schneckloth et al. 1959. [11] Smith et al. 1957. [12] Snow et al. 1955. [13] Waldenström and Ljungberg 1955. [14] Waldenström et al. 1957. [15] Oates and Sjoerdsma 1962. [16] Levine and Sjoerdsma 1963).

of adrenaline into the skin caused normal blanching and the intracarotid injection of noradrenaline caused ipsilateral blanching, followed after 1 minute by simultaneous bilateral flushing of the face. Intravenous infusion of 5-HT into patients in whom a flush could always be produced by adrenaline, was not always followed by a flush even though doses large enough to cause other systemic effects were given. 'Moreover the flush after 5-HT was more cyanotic than either the spontaneous flush or that provoked by adrenaline injection. Robertson et al. estimated the concentration of 5-HT in platelet poor plasma before, during and after the flush in 3 patients and found a rise, during the flush, in one case only. In this case the concentration of free plasma 5-HT in the hepatic vein and upper inferior vena cava rose from 20 to 40 ng/ml before the flush, to 400 to 1000 ng/ml during the flush. In one of the cases, where no rise was observed, specimens were taken from the right atrium and radial artery, where a rise would be expected if 5-HT was the cause of the flush, while in the second case the specimen was taken from the superior vena cava. To reach this, 5-HT from an abdominal neoplasm would have been exposed to destruction both in the lungs and in peripheral vessels.

From their observations Robertson et al. (1962) concluded that adrenaline and noradrenaline sometimes, but not always, cause a release of 5-HT in patients with carcinoid syndrome, and that the flush is due to the release of a vasoactive substance, probably not 5-HT, which they have not so far identified. Histamine, substance P and adenosine triphosphate they reject because, though all cause a flush on intravenous injection, they cause other effects not associated with either spontaneous flushes or by flushes caused by adrenaline; and nicotinic acid, was rejected because it causes a more prolonged cutaneous vasodilatation and a flush of a different colour. DEMIS and ZIMMAR (1962) find that they can imitate the carcinoid flush by the intradermal injection of a mixture 5-HT with either adrenaline or noradrenaline and believe that many of the findings of ROBERTSON et al. can be explained by the combined action of these substances. HEGGLIN and LANGEMANN (1955) found a rise in blood 5-HT during a flush, but some other workers have failed to detect changes in either free or platelet bound 5-HT during flushing (SJOERDSMA et al. 1957), while a rise in total 5-HT in peripheral venous blood from 2.2 to 3.3 μg/ml was recorded by GOBLE et al. (1955).

The interpretation of blood estimations must be doubtful because of the difficulties mentioned above (p. 759) but there is now a considerable amount of evidence that attacks of flushing do not correlate well with blood 5-HT levels. OATES et al. (1964) therefore investigated the possibility that attacks of flushing might be due to the circulation of kinins. An intravenous injection of synthetic bradykinin in patients with the carcinoid syndrome was found to cause flushing resembling the patients' spontaneous flushes and the changes in heart rate, blood pressure and respiration associated with flushing were similar. Moreover an injection of adrenaline caused an increase in the concentration of a bradykinin-like substance (assayed on the rat uterus) in the hepatic venous blood. OATES et al. also showed that extracts of liver metastases contained kalikrein activity whereas extracts of normal liver contained none. They therefore suggest that carcinoid flushing may be partly or wholly due to the release of a kinin formed by kalikrein contained in carcinoid tissue. What part this substance may play in other manifestations of the carcinoid syndrome, and how it is released, remain to be established.

b) *Gastrointestinal and respiratory symptoms*

Apart from obstruction caused by the mechanical effects of abdominal tumours, gastrointestinal symptoms can be attributed with some confidence to the action of 5-HT on the intestine. The colic and diarrhoea caused by infusions of 5-HT in normal subjects are similar to symptoms experienced by patients with carcinoid disease. The effect of 5-HT on the respiratory tract is complex. Infusions in man cause hyperventilation and feelings of constriction (p. 751) and these, together with attacks of bronchospasm, occur in the carcinoid syndrome. In animals, respiration is stimulated by the action of 5-HT on chemoreceptors in the carotid body and possibly also by a central action (GINZEL and KOTTEGODA 1954; MCCUBBIN et al. 1956) and both in animals and man it causes bronchoconstriction (HERXHEIMER 1955; KONZETT 1956).

c) *Cardiovascular lesions*

The late development of the cardiac lesions has led to the belief that they are secondary to the development of the tumour; and HEDINGER and GLOOR (1954) and RAMBO et al. (1954) suggested that they were caused by a secretion from the tumour. The finding of large amounts of 5-HT in tumours and blood made it necessary to consider if the presence of this substance could be the cause of the lesions. 5-HT is destroyed in the lungs and there is some evidence that its concentration is higher on the right side of the heart than on the left; this would accord with the common finding that lesions are confined to the right heart or are much more marked on the right side than the left. The few cases with extensive left sided lesions have usually had anatomical peculiarities which might be expected to give a high concentration in the left heart, either by the presence of a pulmonary neoplasm (BERNHEIMER et al. 1960) or by the existence of a septal defect (MCKUSIC 1956; SJOERDSMA et al. 1956). However evidence has not always been available (e.g. in McKusick's case) that there was a right to left shunt. The case of Bernheimer et al. (1960) is of especial interest as gross changes were also observed in the walls of branches of the pulmonary vein leading from tumours, but not elsewhere in the lungs. Thorson (1958), on the other hand, has reported a case in which the only metastases were in the lungs; yet the right heart was affected but not the left.

Two possibilities have been advanced to explain the mechanism by which 5-HT might cause the changes: (i) Hedinger and Gloor (1954) suggested that 5-HT may stimulate the growth of connective tissue and Thorson et al. (1954) that it causes direct damage to the endocardium, leading to the adhesion of platelets and the deposition of fibrin (Goble et al. 1956). Stacey and Wildy (unpublished observations) were unable to obtain any evidence of an increased rate of growth of chick fibroblasts in tissue culture when 5-HT in concentrations up to 5 μg/ml was added to the culture medium but extensive fibrosis, particularly in the neighbourhood of abdominal lesions, is frequently noticed Hallén (1964). (ii) Thorson (1958) suggested that the intermittent increases in pulmonary arterial pressure might contribute to the endocardial lesions by causing episodic dilatation of the right heart. As support for this, Thorson (1958) cites the aortic valvular lesions reported by Dewitsky (1912) to follow prolonged periods of intravenous adrenaline injection, and the appearance of fibrosis in various pathological conditions where raised intracardiac pressures are to be expected (Böger 1928; Hertel 1921; Allanby and Campbell 1949). However attempts to reproduce the cardiac lesions by the administration of 5-HT to animals have usually failed. These experiments are described on p. 737.

d) Other symptoms

Hyperkeratosis and pigmentation of the skin and black, furrowed tongue (Collini 1961) have been ascribed to nicotinamide deficiency, due to the diversion of dietary tryptophan from the synthesis of this vitamin. The skin changes do not always improve however when nicotinamide is given. *Recurrent peptic ulcer* may be due to increased histamine synthesis or to an increase in the amount of pepsin in gastric juice, but more evidence of the relation between these changes is needed. No explanation for the *arthralgia* reported has been advanced. *Oedema*, in some cases is no doubt due to cardiac failure, in others due to diarrhoea and low serum albumen; but Thorson (1958) concludes from an analysis of 52 cases that other factors must also be involved as well; this also needs further investigation.

Malignant carcinoid tumours have been found in association with a variety of other conditions: malabsorption syndrome (Kowlessar, Law and Sleisenger 1959), scleroderma (Zarafonetis, Lorber and Hanson 1958), adrenal hyperplasia (Davis and Kennedy, 1962; Escovitz and Reingold 1961), pancreatic carcinoma (Dengler 1959) and silicosis (Halonen et al. 1962). In the last report the authors suggest that the presence of the carcinoid tumour may have contributed to the rapid development of pulmonary fibrosis.

7. Treatment of the malignant carcinoid syndrome

a) Surgical treatment

Resection of as much as possible of the neoplastic tissue is well worth while. This is often followed by an amelioration of the symptoms and cases have been reported (e.g. Pernow and Waldenström 1954; Waldenström 1958a) where all symptoms disappeared. Surgical intravention is not without risk owing to the occasional development of severe, sometimes fatal, bronchospasm (Stacey 1957; Wolfe et al. 1960).

b) *Drug therapy*

The results of treatment with 5-HT antagonists have been disappointing. Little benefit has followed from the use of bromlysergic acid diethylamide, BAS and ergotamine.

Rather more success has followed the use of methysergide (1-methyl-D-lysergic acid butanolamide tartrate, UML 491, Deseril). Relief of diarrhoea was obtained by LANZ (1960) and by PEART and ROBERTSON (1961), but SCHNECKLOTH et al. (1959) found little benefit. BLUMBERG et al. (1962) and DUBACH and GSELL (1962) found that doses up to 6 mg/day by mouth stopped the diarrhoea but had no effect on the flushes. When Ro 5-1025 (1-[p-dimethylamino-benzyl]-2[5-methyl-3-isoxazolylcarbonyl]-hydrazine), was given at the same time as methysergide in a dose of 75 mg/day by mouth, the flushes became less intense and of shorter duration. These drugs caused no ill effects and were continued for several months. Ro 5-1025 is a hydrazine and an inhibitor of both monoamine oxidase and of aromatic amino-acid decarboxylase; but its mode of action in decreasing flushes is not clear. Depression of 5-HT synthesis was not demonstrated and it is not known if Ro 5-1025 inhibits decarboxylase directly or, like isoniazid, by trapping the coenzyme pyridoxal phosphate (LUDWIG 1960). In some patients flushing may be alleviated by phentolamine or dibenyline (LEVINE and SJOERDSMA 1963). Iproniazid exacerbates the symptoms (KABAKOW et al. 1959).

SJOERDSMA et al. (1960) introduced the use of the decarboxylase inhibitor α-methyldopa (α-methyl-3,4-dihydroxyphenylalanine) and reported on the treatment of two patients. Synthesis of 5-HT was depressed, as shown by a reduction in the urinary excretion of 5-HIAA and an increase in 5-hydroxytryptophan excretion. Usually there is little improvement in symptoms but good results have been reported (DAVIS et al. 1961; NICHOLSON et al. 1962); possibly these were with 5-hydroxytryptophan secreting tumours. The drug is sometimes poorly tolerated, somnolence, lethargy and hypothermia may be marked, and hypotension may limit the dose. Severe symptoms may develop with as little as 3 g per day and alarming mental effects have been reported (DUBACH and BLUMBERG 1961).

Phenylacetic acid, a weak inhibitor of decarboxylase, has been given (SANDLER and CLOSE 1959; SANDLER, DAVIES and RIMINGTON 1959) without convincing improvement; a reduction in 5-HIAA excretion was observed but this may have been due to reduced renal clearance (MILNE 1959).

Chlorpromazine (SJOERDSMA et al. 1959; KABAKOW et al. 1959; MUSTALA and AIRAKSINEN 1962) and promazine (WARNER and SOUTHREN 1958) may diminish the severity of the symptoms but their mode of actions is unknown. It is unlikely that it is due to 5-HT antagonism because this action is weak. Symptomatic improvement with 6-methyl prednisolone has also been reported (URELES et al. 1962).

Reserpine might be expected to exacerbate the symptoms by the release of 5-HT, but WARNER and SOUTHREN (1958) report a marginal improvement.

Some improvement on antihistamines has been reported (WALDENSTRÖM et al. 1957) but probably can only be expected in those cases secreting excessive amounts of histamine.

The possibility of tryptophan deficiency should be born in mind; the *diet* should contain adequate protein and nicotinamide supplements. Reduction of tryptophan in the diet diminishes 5-HIAA excretion but causes clinical deterioration (DAVIS et al. 1961).

Little success has attended radiotherapy (SAUER et al. 1958) or treatment with radioactive gold, with 5-fluoracil (DAVIS and KENNEDY 1962) or by regional perfusion of the liver with nitrogen mustard (DAVIS and ROSENBERG 1961).

8. Hyperserotonaemia without increased 5-HIAA excretion

Southern et al. (1959) have described a patient with an intermittent patchy erythematous rash of the face, neck and arms, ataxia, attacks of hypertension and mental confusion. The serum 5-HT varied from 4 to 30 μg/ml (normal 0.2 to 0.4 μg/ml) but the excretion of 5-HIAA was 1.09 to 3.60 mg/24 hours (normal 1—9 mg/24 hours). Excretion of 5-HIAA after infusion of 5-HIAA and of 5-HT was normal but after an infusion of 5-hydroxytryptophan, the excretion was low. No evidence of a carcinoid tumour could be found. The authors suggest that the syndrome is due to an abnormal metabolism of 5-HT and further cases have been briefly reported (Warner 1961 and 1963).

9. Other diseases of the alimentary canal

The mean blood 5-HT in a group of patients who had suffered a **resection** of the stomach was found by Schmid et al. (1960b) to be reduced, but low values were not found in every case. However resection of small and large intestine markedly reduces both blood 5-HT and the excretion of 5-HIAA (Haverback and Davidson 1958), and even removal of the large intestine alone reduces 5-HIAA excretion (Bertaccini and Chieppa 1960).

An increase both in blood 5-HT and in the excretion of 5-HIAA is found in **non-tropical sprue** (Kowlessar et al. 1958; Haverback and Davidson 1958; Pimparker et al. 1961); these changes are most marked during relapse and there is also an increase in indole-3-acetic acid excretion (see p. 749). In **peptic ulceration, ulcerative colitis** and in **chronic diarrhoea,** blood 5-HT is normal. Small reductions have been reported in acute and chronic **hepatitis** and in **cirrhosis of the liver** (Schmid et al. 1960b) and in hepatic coma (Borges et al. 1959). However, in cirrhosis the excretion of 5-HIAA is normal although the recovery of 5-hydroxytryptophan (but not of 5-HT) as 5-HIAA, after a loading dose, is greater (Donaldson and Gray, 1959). The increased excretion of 5-HIAA after loading doses of 5-HT, 5-HTP and 5-HIAA has been compared in normal subjects and in patients with severe liver damage by Donaldson and Gray (1959), Donaldson et al. (1960), Amann (1962) and Schmid et al. (1962). The results, which depend on the route of administration, the dose and the severity and nature of the liver damage, show some disagreement and their interpretation must be treated with caution.

The administration of oxytetracyline has no effect on 5-HIAA excretion (Brummer and Jaurola 1958) but the result of the administration of drugs more effectively **sterilizing the gut** has not been reported.

The concentration of 5-HT in the stomach is reported to be normal in **peptic ulceration** and in **carcinoma of the stomach** (Resnick and Gray 1961).

10. Diseases of the blood and blood forming organs

The amount of 5-HT in platelets is reduced in a number of haematological conditions (Hardisty and Stacey 1957; Schmid et al. 1960c). This cannot be explained by a reduction in the size of the platelets, and is often accompanied by an impaired capacity for binding 5-HT when the platelets are incubated with it *in vitro*. It therefore appears that a platelet defect contributes to this finding, though it is not necessarily the only cause of it. Other factors which might contribute, and which have not so far been adequately investigated, are: diminished 5-HT synthesis, accelerated platelet turnover and loss of 5-HT from platelets during circulation. There is good reason to believe that in some organs adenosine triphosphate is concerned in amine storage (Hillarp et al. 1955; Blaschko et al. 1956; Prusoff 1960). Evidence for this in platelets is less convincing but with this possibility in mind, Born, Ingram and Stacey (1958) estimated the amount of adenosine triphosphate in platelets from patients with myeloid leukaemia. They found that although the amount of 5-HT which the platelets could bind was considerably below normal, the adenosine triphosphate content of the platelets was not reduced.

Diseases in which the platelets contain less 5-HT than normally include acute leukaemia, myeloid leukaemia, myelofibrosis, pernicious anaemia in relapse, polycythaemia vera and thrombocythemia. In HODGKIN's disease and in iron deficiency anaemia the reduction in platelet 5-HT is less marked. Treatment of pernicious anaemia with cyanocobalamine is followed by a rise in platelet 5-HT (SCHMID et al. 1960c). The reduced amount of 5-HT in the blood in blood diseases does not appear to play any important part in the production of purpuric symptoms (HARDISTY and STACEY 1957). The effect of 5-HT on haemostatic mechanisms has been the subject of a considerable amount of work. Much of this is contradictory and has recently been reviewed by QUIVY (1961), but it seems unlikely that 5-HT plays any important part in the arrest of haemorrhage and the evidence for the success of 5-HT therapy in haemorrhagic conditions is unconvincing.

In the investigation of blood diseases, the ability of the platelets to take up 5-HT may be of value in assessing platelet normality (MCCLURE et al. 1965); and MELMON and SJOERDSMA (1963) have estimated platelet half-life by loading platelets with 5-HT by oral administration of the creatinine sulphate for a few days and then following the subsequent fall in platelet 5-HT. Alternatively the rate of disappearance of ^{14}C 5-HT from circulating platelets labelled with the isotope may be followed. Platelets may be labelled either by the intravenous injection of small quantities of ^{14}C 5-HT or by returning to the circulation platelets labelled *in vitro* (HEYSSEL 1961).

11. Diseases of the cardiovascular system

The complex effects of 5-HT on the cardiovascular system has led to considerable speculation as to its possible role in diseases of the circulation. No definite evidence for this has so far been found.

In patients with **neurocirculatory asthenia (effort syndrome)** (NIKKILA 1958) and with **essential hypertension** (HAVERBACK et al. 1956; POUMAILLOUX and LABIGNETTE 1959) the excretion of 5-HIAA is usually normal; but in 2 patients with **chronic glomerular nephritis,** BORGES and BESSMAN (1956) found markedly low excretions. AMERIO (1960) found high excretions in some cases of bilateral renal disease.

COMROE et al. (1953) and SMITH and SMITH (1955) were struck by the observation that the general effects of cardiac infarction and pulmonary embolism are often considerably greater than would be expected from the size of the embolus and they showed that there is a similarity between the effects in cats of injected blood clot and an injection of 5-HT. However no support has so far been found (SANDERS et al. 1959) for their suggestion that the signs and symptoms of **pulmonary thrombosis** might be due, in large measure, to release of 5-HT from the blood clot and from the infarcted area of lung, nor is there, at present, any factual basis for the suggestion of HALPERN et al. (1960) that release of 5-HT from platelets plays a part in the symptomatology of **Raynaud's disease.**

12. Mental deficiency

In **phenylketonuria** (phenylpyruvic oligophrenia) a reduction in the amount of 5-HT in the serum and a diminished excretion of 5-HIAA was reported by PARE et al. (1957, 1959) and has been confirmed by BERENDES et al. 1958, by

Baldridge et al. (1959), by Reichle et al. (1961) and by Perry (1962). The relation of this to the other biochemical changes in this inherited metabolic defect is still uncertain. Various possibilities have been suggested. The primary defect is a failure in the conversion of phanylalanine to tyrosine. The hydroxylation of both phenylalanine and tryptophan involve complex systems which are not easily studied; it is possible, though of this there is at present no evidence, that a common defect impairs both reactions, resulting in the case of tryptophan, in a deficit of 5-hydroxytryptophan, the immediate metabolic precursor of 5-HT. A second explanation is based on the observation of Davison and Sandler (1958), that three metabolic products of phenylalanine, namely, phenylpyruvic, phenyllactic and phenylacetic acids, all present in the

Table 11. *Mean serum 5-hydroxytryptamine concentration and urine 5-hydroxyindoleacetic acid excretion in normal subjects, in mental defectives, and in various other groups.* (From Pare, Sandler and Stacey 1960)

	ng 5-HT/ml serum Mean (No.) ± SE	mg 5-HIAA per g urine creatinine Mean (No.) ± SE
Normals	145 (16) ± 13	3.9 (40) ± 0.12
Cerebral palsy (normal intelligence)	136 (12) ± 12	3.5 (9) ± 0.47
Cerebral palsy (I.Q. < 50)	**351** (28) ± 26	7.7 (25) ± 0.73
Mongolism	146 (10) ± 18	7.0 (10) ± 1.2
Phenylketonuria	**79** (26) ± 10	**2.6** (26) ± 0.23
Maternal rubella	**391** (4) ± 66	6.9 (5) ± 2.18
Unclassified	**297** (30) ± 24	**6.8** (29) ± 0.47
Epilepsy (normal intelligence)	104 (4) ± 15	2.8 (4) ± 0.46
Schizophrenia	*89* (3) ± 12	— —
Dementia due to anoxia	222 (4) ± 38	— —
Dementia due to other causes	158 (5) ± 27	— —

Numbers of subjects are given in brackets. The values in italics ($P < 0.05$) and in heavy type ($P < 0.001$) are significantly different from the corresponding values for normals.

circulation in abnormally high concentrations in phenylketonuria, are 5-hydroxytryptophan decarboxylase inhibitors. The presence of these substances might thus retard the synthesis of 5-HT at the final stage. The observations of Yuwiler and Loutit (1961) that the administration of phenylalanine to rats lowers brain 5-HT concentration, and of McKean et al. (1962) and Smith (1963) that the uptake of 5-hydroxytryptophan by brain *in vitro* and *in vivo* is depressed by L-phenylalanine and certain other L-amino acids, suggests a third possible cause of impaired 5-HT synthesis in this condition. That either the accummulation of phenylalanine or its metabolites, or the overburdening of the defective hydroxylating system is linked to the low blood 5-HT level in this condition is supported by the finding of Pare et al. (1958) that when phenylketonuric children were put on a low phenylalanine diet, thus reducing the concentration of phenylalanine in the blood and the formation of its metabolic products, there was a rise in the serum 5-HT level.

As well as the changes in concentration of hydroxyindoles described above, Armstrong and Robinson (1954) and Jepson (1955) have reported an increased excretion of indoleacetic and indolelactic acid.

In a variety of other cases of mental deficiency, Pare et al. (1960) found an increase in both serum 5-HT and platelet 5-HT. (Table 11). This was sometimes associated with an increased daily excretion of 5-HIAA (estimated as 5-HIAA per g. urine creatinine). It is of interest that mentally defective children with cerebral palsy had a high serum 5-HT, while children of normal intelligence, with a like physical defect due to cerebral palsy, had a normal serum 5-HT. In mongolism, epilepsy (with normal intelligence) and schizophrenia the serum 5-HT was also normal. Similar results have been reported by SCHAIN and FREEDMAN (1961) and by PAASONEN and KIVALO (1962).

13. Other diseases of the central nervous system

a) *Schizophrenia*

Noting that some 5-HT antagonists are hallucinogens, WOOLEY and SHAW (1954) suggested that there might be a deficiency or excess (WOOLEY 1962) of 5-HT in the brain in schizophrenia. A considerable amount of work on the metabolism of hydroxyindoles in this disease followed. The results are conflicting but the evidence on the whole, is in favour of the view that 5-HIAA excretion, with and without a tryptophan load, is normal (FELDSTEIN et al. 1958; SANO et al. 1957; KOPIN 1959; TODRICK et al. 1960), and that the concentration of 5-HT in blood and CSF and its excretion in the urine are within normal limits (TURNER and MAUSS 1959; FELDSTEIN et al. 1959; JUS et al. 1958). BRUNE and PSCHEIDT (1961) however find that although *mean* daily excretions of 5-HIAA, tryptamine and indole-3-acetic acid are within the normal range, in patients with signs of high psychotic activity there is increased excretion of all three compounds. FISCHER et al. (1962) have found bufotenine in the urine of 25 out of 26 hallucinated or catatonie schizophrenics, but not in that of normal subjects or non-hallucinated schizophrenics. The administration of 5-HT and 5-hydroxytryptophan has not caused any improvement in this condition (BRENGELMANN et al. 1959).

ASHCROFT and SHARMAN (1960) found that the cerebrospinal fluid of *hydrocephalics* and of patients who had a history of *brain injury* or of brain operations had a high concentration (83 to 313 ng/ml) of hydroxyindoles but they were unable to identify 5-HT in those specimens in which they looked for it; while SOUTHREN and CHRISTOFF (1962) found an increased amount of this substance in the cerebrospinal fluid of patients with a variety of neurological conditions GRABNER and LEMBECK (1960) have reported the presence of 5-HT (1.3 to 5 μg/g) in a ganglio-neuroma and a retinoblastoma. Only small amounts of 5-HT have been found in other cerebral tumours (JOYCE 1963).

b) *Parkinsonism*

BERNHEIMER, BIRKMAYER and HORNYKIEWICZ (1961) have found that the concentration of 5-HT in certain parts of the brain of patients with Parkinson's syndrome is reduced. The greatest differences were found in the corpus striatum,

Table 12. *Concentration of 5-HT in human brain in normal subjects and in those with Parkinson's syndrome.* (From BERNHEIMER et al. 1961)

	μg 5-HT/g brain Mean (range): 4 to 6 estimations	
	normals	Parkinsonism
Putamen	0.32 (0.19 to 0.42)	0.14 (0.008 to 0.16)
Caudate nucleus	0.33 (0.20 to 0.46)	0.12 (0.11 to 0.15)
Globus pallidus	0.23 (0.19 to 0.29)	0.13 (0.07 to 0.22)
Thalamus	0.26 (0.21 to 0.35)	0.13 (0.08 to 0.18)
Hypothalamus	0.29 (0.14 to 0.51)	0.12 (0.06 to 0.21)
Substantia nigra	0.55 (0.40 to 0.85)	0.26 (0.15 to 0.36)
Mesencephalic grey matter	0.53 (0.32 to 0.84)	0.36 (0.09 to 0.85)
4th ventricle(floor) and reticular formation	0.60 (0.39 to 1.07)	0.55 (0.29 to 1.13)

thalamus and substantia nigra, where there was no overlap in the ranges of the two sets of figures (Table 12). Whether this reflects slower synthesis, increased turnover or impaired storage is not known, but there is also a reduction of brain dopamine and noradrenaline (EHRINGER and HORNYKIEWICZ 1960; HORNYKIEWICZ 1963) and of urinary dopamine excretion (BARBEAU, MURPHY and SOURKES 1961) in this condition.

14. Miscellaneous conditions

An increased excretion of 5-HIAA has been found by JOHANSSON (1960) in cases of **burns,** by VACCAREZZA and BOCHI (1963) in *asthma*, and by SKANSE and HANSON (1962) in **hyperthyroidism.** In the latter condition effective treatment with thiouracil or radioactive iodine or by thyroidectomy reduced the excretion to normal. In **rheumatoid arthritis,** blood 5-HT was raised (KERBY and TAYLOR 1959) but not in **rheumatic fever** (SCHMID et al. 1960a). In the latter

Table 13. *Excretion of 5-hydroxyindoleacetic acid (mg/24 hrs ± S.D.) and N-methylnicotinamide (mg/24 hrs ± S.D.) before and after the administration of 10 g D,L-tryptophan.* (From OLSEN et al. 1960)

	No of subjects	before tryptophan		after tryptophan	
		5-HIAA	N-methyl nicotinamide	5-HIAA	N-methyl nicotinamide
Normal subjects . . .	16	6.4 ± 1.4	11.0 ± 5.8	11.6 ± 5.7	20.8 ± 9.0
Alcoholic patients . .	34	2.5 ± 1.0	7.6 ± 2.9	5.7 ± 2.9	22.0 ± 20.4
P		0.01	N. S.	0.01	N. S.

N. S. = not significant

condition the urine has been found to contain 5-methoxytryptamine by HADDOX and SASLAW (1963). This substance is not found in normal urine and its presence is attributed by the authors to a failure in its further metabolism to 5-methoxyindole acetic acid.

OLSON et al. (1960) have found evidence for a defect in tryptophan metabolism in **chronic alcoholism.** The daily output of 5-HIAA in a group of these patients was less than half that of a group of normal subjects both before and after the administration of 10 g. D,L-tryptophan (Table 13). No evidence could be found for depression of tryptophan metabolism along the kynurenine pathway, and the authors therefore suggested that conversion of tryptophan to 5-HIAA is preferentially depressed in this condition. No improvement in 5-HIAA excretion was found in 4 patients studied after a period of alcohol abstinence lasting up to 4 months. On the other hand MURPHY et al. (1962) found no difference in the excretion of 5-HIAA by a group of normal subjects and chronic alcoholics studied by them. The administration of 0.5 to 0.7 g ethanol/kg to normal subjects in a single dose did not change 5-HIAA excretion during the subsequent 3 hours (PERMAN 1961).

Menstruation, Pregnancy, Menopausal flushing

Excretion of 5-HIAA has been reported to reach a maximum during the first day of menstruation (ROTH and RICHTER 1957) but to be normal in patients with menopausal flushing (MUNSICK 1959; ROWELL and SUMMERSCALES 1960). Reports on changes during pregnancy, and on excretion in patients with pregnancy toxaemia, need confirmation (BETTENDORF et al. 1959; CARTER, CHERNEY and CRENSHAW 1962).

In a variety of other conditions small increases in 5-HIAA excretion have been reported to occur in occasional patients (HAVERBACK et al. 1956).

15. Clinical use of 5-hydroxytryptamine antagonists

The use of 5-HT antagonists in the treatment of patients with malignant carcinoid syndrome, in whom the symptoms are largely due to the discharge into the blood stream of large quantities of 5-HT, is a logical procedure and the failure of any considerable benefit is unexplained. It is discussed on p. 765.

For a variety of reasons, which do not bear close scrutinty, a role has been ascribed to 5-HT in a number of other diseases, and the treatment of them with 5-HT antagonists attempted. These will now be considered.

A mild hypotensive effect was obtained with 1-benzyl,2-methyl, 5-methoxytryptamine (BAS) in about 25% of cases of *essential hypertension*. Sedation, abdominal cramp, bradycardia, nasal stuffiness and diminished libido also occurred (WILKINS and HOLLANDER 1957). The size of dose used was limited by the drowsiness caused.

In *migraine* (SICUTERI 1959; HEYCK 1960; FRIEDMAN 1960; KIMBALL et al. 1960; DALASSIO 1962; GRAHAM 1964) and in *rheumatoid arthritis* (SHERBEL and HARRISON 1958; JUNG 1960; MÉRIEL et al. 1960; GARELLI 1960) improvement has been reported with bromlysergic acid diethylamide and methyl lysergic acid butanolamide (methysergide, UML 491). In these conditions assessment of the value of any form of therapy is notoriously difficult, and until the results of well planned clinical trials are available, no opinion can be expressed as to its value; nor is there any evidence at present as to whether effects ascribed to the drugs are due to 5-HT antagonism or to some other action. A small but carefully designed double blind trial by SHEKELLE and OSTFIELD (1964) on patients with migraine showed a significant advantage for methysergide over dummy tablets. Typical migraine headaches are said to have been precipitated by reserpine and relieved by intravenous injections of 5-HT and 5-hydroxytryptophan (KIMBALL et al. 1960). Symptoms due to ischaemia (ischaemic pain, intermittent claudication, angina) have been reported in patients receiving methysergide: these are reviewed by URELES and ROB (1963). Patients with active rheumatoid arthritis and *systemic lupus erythematosus* are said to have an abnormal reaction to subcutaneously injected 5-HT (SCHERBEL and HARRISON 1958).

Cyproheptadine (Periactin) antagonises the action of both histamine and 5-HT and is comparable in potency to chlorpheniramine on the one hand and lysergic acid diethylamide on the other (STONE et al. 1961). It has been found to be effective in the treatment of *urticaria* (BAILEY 1961) and in some cases of *hay fever* (MILLER and FISHMAN 1961), *eczemoid dermatitis*, *pruritis*, *tension headache* (BODI et al. 1961) and very occasionally in *asthma*. In these conditions histamine antagonists are sometimes effective but whether antagonism to 5-HT plays any part is unknown.

JOHNSON et al. (1962) report subjective improvement in the postgastrectomy dumping syndrome in 10 patients treated with cyproheptadine. Methysergide and α-methyl dopa are also reported to have caused improvement (MILLER and PESKIN 1963).

16. 5-Hydroxytryptamine and anaphylaxis in man

A considerable body of animal work has accummulated on the release of 5-HT in antigen-antibody reactions and in anaphylaxis. In most species 5-HT plays a minor role and this appears also to be the case in man; though little work has been done on the subject, apart from the indirect evidence from clinical work on the effect of 5-HT antagonists on the treatment of allergic conditions. Much of this has been poorly controlled and the conclusions drawn from it are unrealiable. Reference has been made to some of the results reported in the section on 5-HT antagonists, above.

The serum of patients with allergic conditions is said to contain more 5-HT than normal subjects (MacHaffie et al. 1960), but Band et al. (1961) failed to find any abnormality in the excretion of 5-HIAA. Scherbel and Harrison (1958) observed that patients with active rheumatoid arthritis and systemic lupus erythematosus have an exaggerated response to subcutaneous injections of 5-HT characterised by erythema, swelling and cyanosis; this can be antagonised by lysergic acid diethylamide and methysergide. An increased sensitivity to intravenous injections is reported by Stone et al. (1961) in patients with collagen disease. This was shown by cardiovascular responses with doses causing no symptoms in normal subjects; there was also an exacerbation of either cutaneous or articular symptoms.

17. Administration of other indolealkylamines to man

Bufotenine (5-hydroxy-*N N*-dimethyltryptamine) is a constituent of the snuff powder, cohoba, made by Haitians from the seeds of *Piptadenia peregrina*, and used for its hallucinogenic properties. The mental effects of bufotenine are described by Fabing (1956) and by Fabing and Hawkins (1956) as consisting of visual hallucinations and mental confusion, and as being similar to those caused by mescaline and lysergic acid diethylamide, but of shorter duration. Tachycardia, tachypnoea, mydriasis, abdominal discomfort and defaecation also occur. The failure of Turner and Merlis (1959) to cause hallucinations in their patients, though they observed the peripheral actions, may have been due to their being schizophrenics.

The actions of *NN-dimethyltryptamine* and *NN-diethyltryptamine*, on injection in man, has been described by Szara (Szara 1957; Sai-Halâsz et al. 1958). by Bôszörményi 1961, by Turner and Merlis (1959) and by Rosenberg et al. (1963). Both substances are hallucinogenic and cause mydriasis and an increase in blood pressure and pulse rate. After the intramuscular injection of 75 mg of the dimethyl compound, symptoms develop in 3 to 4 minutes and persist for an hour. With the diethyl compound they take 15 minutes to develop and last 3 hours. Böszörményi and Brunecker (1957) noted that schizophrenics are apparently less sensitive than normal subjects to the hallucinogenic action of these compounds. These amines are mainly excreted as indolyl-3-acetic acid but products of 6-hydroxylation have also been detected by Szara (1961), who has suggested that these metabolites, rather than the parent amines, are responsible for the mental effects.

The *NN*-dimethyl derivate of 4-hydroxytryptamine is known as *psilocine*, the name being derived from *psilocybin*, an alkaloid isolated from the mushroom *Psilocybe mexicana* Heim by Hofmann et al. (1958). Psilocine is formed from psilocybin by the action of alkaline phosphatase and equimolecular doses of these two substances have similar effects (Wolbach et al. 1962). They cause changes of mood, disturbances of sensation and hallucinations, mental effects very similar to those caused by mescaline and lysergic acid diethylamide. The pupils are dilated and there is intense facial congestion; pulse rate and blood pressure usually fall but respiration is increased. The effects following injection have been described by Delay et al. (1959), Isbell (1959), Böszörményi (1961), Rinkel et al. (1961), Rummele and Gnirss (1961) and by Sercl et al. (1961).

Oral administration of DL-4-hydroxytryptophan in doses up to 1 g in man causes no obvious pharmacological effects. In the urine 10% was recovered as 4-hydroxyindole acetic acid, 1.3 to 2.2% as unchanged 4-hydroxytryptophan and

1% as 5-HT (ERSPAMER 1961 c). It was thought that 4-hydroxytrytophan given by this route was metabolised principally in the intestinal wall and liver.

SMITH and PROKOP (1962) gave L-tryptophan in doses of 30 to 90 mg/kg by mouth and reported drowsiness and nystagmus in all patients with the larger dose. The excretion of tryptamine rose from a mean of 28 to 347 μg/8 hr period. Somewhat similar effects are described by OATES and SJOERDSMA (1960). When they gave L-tryptophan (20 to 50 mg/kg) to patients receiving an amine oxidase inhibitor (pheniprazine), symptoms similar to those of alcoholic intoxication developed.

References

ADAMS, B. G.: Serum 5-hydroxytryptamine levels following experimental increase in gastrointestinal activity in man. Lancet **1960 I**, 207—208.

ALLANBY, K. D., and M. CAMPBELL: Congenital pulmonary stenosis with closed ventricular septum. Guy's Hosp. Rep. **98**, 18—53 (1949).

AMANN, R.: Der Serotonin-Stoffwechsel bei Leberkranken. Klin. Wschr. **40**, 981—984 (1962).

AMBANELLI, V., e G. SALVI: L'antiuresi da enteramins. G. Clin. med. **40**, 1499—1513 (1959).

AMERIO, A.: L'eliminazione urinaria dell'acido 5-idrossindolacetico nella insufficienza renale. Minerva nefrol. **7**, 1—8 (1960).

AMIN, A. H., T. B. B. CRAWFORD and J. H. GADDUM: The distribution of substance P and 5-HT in the central nervous system of the dog. J. Physiol. (Lond.) **126**, 596—618 (1954).

ANNONI, G., P. D. LUCCHELLI e G. BARBIERA: L'azione della 5-idrossitriptamina (enteramina-serotonina) sulla diuresi nell'uomo. Farmaco, Ed. sci. **10**, 306—311 (1955).

ARMSTRONG, D., R. M. L. DRY, C. A. KEELE, and J. W. MARKHAM: Observations on chemical excitants of cutaneous pain in man. J. Physiol. (Lond.) **120**, 326—351 (1953).

ARMSTRONG, M. D., and K. S. ROBINSON: On the excretion of indole derivatives in phenylketonuria. Arch. Biochem. **52**, 287—288 (1954).

ASHCROFT, G. W. and D. F. SHARMAN: 5-Hydroxyindoles in human cerebrospinal fluid. Nature (Lond.) **186**, 1050—1051 (1960).

ÅSTRÖM, A., and U. SAMELIUS: The action of 5-hydroxytryptamine and some of its antagonists on the umbilical vessels of the human plancenta. Brit. J. Pharmacol. **12**, 410—414 (1957).

BAILEY, I. S.: Cyproheptadine in treatment of urticaria. Brit. med. J. **1961 II**, 430.

BALDRIDGE, R. C., L. BOROFSKY, H. BAIRD III, F. REICHLE and D. BULLOCK: Relationship of serum phenylalanine levels and ability of phenylketonurics to hydroxylate tryptophan. Proc. Soc. exp. Biol (N.Y. **100**, 529—531 (1959).

BALDRIGHI, V., e V. FERRARI: Risposte emopressorie sistemiche e polmonari ella serotonina (5-idrossitriptamina) nell'uomo. Folia cardiol. (Milano) **14**, 7—23 (1955).

BAND, P., G. JASMIN et J. LEGER: Dosage de l'acide 5-hydroxyindol-acetique urinaire chez des patients allergiques. Rev. canad. Biol. **20**, 69—70 (1961).

BARBEAU, A., G. F. MURPHY, and T. L. SOURKES: Excretion of dopamine in diseases of basal ganglia. Science **133**, 1706—1707 (1961).

BARKHAM, P.: 5-Hydroxytryptamine activity of human serum. Values in normal subjects and in some blood coagulation disturbances. Afr. J. med. Sci. **20**, 49—55 (1955).

BEGER, A.: Ein Fall von Krebs des Wurmfortsatzes. Klin. Wschr. **19**, 616—618 (1882).

BERENDES, H., J. A. ANDERSON, M. R. ZIEGLER, and D. RUTTENBERG: Disturbance in tryptophane metabolism in phenylketonuria. Amer. J. Dis Child. **96**, 430 (1958).

BERNHEIMER, H., W. BIRKMAYER u. O. HORNYKIEWICZ: Verteilung des 5-Hydroxytryptamins im Gehirn des Menschen und sein Verhalten bei Patienten mit Parkinson-syndrom. Klin. Wschr. **39**, 1056—1059 (1961).

— H. EHRINGER, P. HEISTRACHER, Q. KRAUPP, V. LACHNIT, I. OBIDITSCH-MAYER u. M. WENZI: Biologisch aktives, nicht metastasierendes Bronchuscarcinoid mit Linksherzsyndrom. Wien. klin. Wschr. **48**, 867—873 (1960).

BERTACCINI, G. and S. CHIEPPA: Urinary excretion of 5-hydroxyindole acetic acid after removal of the large intestine in man. Lancet 1960 **I**, 881.

BERTLER, Å.: Occurrence and localization of catechol amine in the human brain. Acta physiol. scand. **51**, 97—107 (1961).

BETTENDORF, G., U. SCHANDER and H.-J. SCHMERMUND: Die Ausscheidung des Serotoninkataboliten 5-Hydroxyindolessigsäure in der Schwangerschaft. Klin. Wschr. **37**, 936 (1959).

BIÖRCK, G., O. AXEN, and Å. THORSON: Unusual cyanosis in a boy with congenital pulmonary stenosis and tricuspid insufficiency. Fatal outcome after angiocardiography. Amer. Heart J. **44**, 143—148 (1952).

Blaschko, H., G. V. R. Born, A. D'Iorio, and N. R. Eade: Obsevations on the distribution of catechol amines and adenosine triphosphate in the bovine adrenal medulla J. Physiol. (Lond). **133**, 548—557 (1956).

Bleeham, N. M.: Precipitation by fatty food of systemic disturbance from argentaffinoma. Lancet **1955 II**, 1362—1363.

Blumberg, A., U. C. Dubach, W. Kreis u. H. R. Muller: Klinische und biochemische Untersuchungen beim Carcinoidsyndrom. Dtsch. med. Wschr. **87**, 921—929 (1962).

Bock, K. D., H. Dengler, H. M. Kuhn u. K. Matthes: Die Wirkung von 5-Hydoxytryptamin auf Blutdruck, Haut- und Muskeldurchblutung des Menschen. Naunyn-Schmiedebergs Arch. exp. Path. Pharmak. **230**, 257—273 (1957).

Bodi, T., P. E. Siegler, M. Gershenfeld, E. B. Brown and J. H. Nodine: Clinical use of a new antihistamine and antiserotonin drug: cyproheptadine. Ann. Allergy **19**, 386—396 (1961).

Böger, A.: Über die Endocardsklerosen. Beitr. path. Anat. **81**, 441—472 (1928/29).

Böszörményi, Z.: Psilocybin and diethyltryptamine: two tryptamine hallucinogens. Neuro-Psychopharmacology **2**, 226—229 (1961).

—, and G. Brunecker: In: Psychotropic Drugs, edit. by S. Garattini and V. Ghetti, p. 580—581. Amsterdam: Elsevier Publ. Co. 1957.

Bogdanski, D. F., H. Weissbach, and S. Udenfriend: The distribution of serotonin, 5-hydroxytryptophan decarboxylase and monoamine oxidase in brain. J. Neurochem. **1**, 272—278 (1957).

Bojs, G.: An experimental study on serotonin (5-HT) on man, with special reference to renal function. Scand. J. clin. Lab. Invest. **13**, Suppl. 55, 1—88 (1961).

Borges, F. J., and S. P. Bessman: Urinary excretion of 5-hydroxyindoleacetic acid, a serotonin metabolite, in hypertensive renal-vascular disease. Proc. Soc. exp. Niol. (N.Y.) **93**, 513—515 (1956).

— J. K Merlis, and S. P. Bessman: Serotonin metabolism in liver disease. J. clin. Invest. **38**, 715—719 (1959).

Born, G. V. R., and J. Bricknell: The uptake of 5-hydroxytryptamine by blood platelets in the cold. J. Physiol. (Lond.) **147**, 153—161 (1959).

—, and R. E. Gillson: Studies on the uptake of 5-hydroxytryptamine by blood platelets. J. Physiol. (Lond.) **146**, 472—491 (1959).

— G. I. C. Ingram, and R. S. Stacey: The relationship between 5-hydroxytryptamine and adenosine triphosphate in blood platelets. Brit. J. Pharmacol. **13**, 62—64 (1958).

Brengelmann, J. C., C. M. B. Pare, and M. Sandler: Effects of 5-hydroxytryptophan on schizophrenia. J. ment. Sci. **105**, 770—776 (1959).

Bridges, J. M., M. Baldwin, C. Fichera, and W. Damashek: Effect of antiplatelet antibodies on the *in vitro* uptake of 5-hydroxytryptamine by blood platelets. Nature (Lond.) **197**, 364 (1963).

Brummer, P., and A. Jaurola: Excretion of 5-hydroxyindoleacetic acid in achlorhydria and the effect upon it of hydrochloric acid. Acta med. scand. **162**, 397—400 (1958).

Brune, G., and G. R. Pscheidt: Correlation between behaviour and urinary excretion of indole amines and catecholamines in schizophrenic patients. Fed. Proc. **20**, 889—893 (1961).

Bumpus, F. M., and I. H. Page: Serotonin and its methylated derivatives in human urine. J. biol. Chem. **212**, 111—116 (1955).

Campbell, A. C. P., A. H. Gowenlock, D. S. Platt, and P. J. D. Snow: A 5-hydroxytryptophan-secreting carcinoid tumour. Gut **4**, 61—67 (1963).

Cargill-Thompson, H. E. C., D. C. Hardwick, and J. M. Wiseman: Estimation of 5-HT in blood and serum. J. Physiol. (Lond.) **140**, 10—11 P (1958).

Carter, F. B., W. B. Cherney, and C. Crenshaw: Serotonin studies in abnormal pregnancies. Amer. J. Obstet. Gynec. **84**, 913—916 (1962).

Cassidy, M. A.: Abdominal carcinomatosis with probable adrenal involvement. Proc. Roy. Soc. Med. **24**, 139—141 (1930); **24**, 920—921 (1931); **27**, 220—221 (1934).

Catchpole, B. N.: Excretion of 5-Hydroxyindole acetic acid in postoperative ileus. Lancet **1962 II**, 1249.

Cenacchi, G. C., e A. Cariani: L'influenza della 5-idrossitriptamina sulla funzionalita'renale nell'uomo. Boll. Soc. ital. Biol. sper. **34**, 569—570 (1958).

Ciaccio, C.: Sur une novelle éspece cellulaire dans les glandes de Lieberkuhn. C. R. Soc. Biol. (Paris) **60**, 76—77 (1906).

Cole, J. W., and A. McKalen: Argentaffin cells in the intestinal epithelium of human embryos. Nature (Lond.) **193**, 198 (1962).

Collini, F. J.: Use of α-methyldopa in the management of the carcinoid syndrome. New Engl. J. Med. **264** 986—987 (1961).

COMROE, J. H., B. VAN LINGEN, R. C. STROUD, and A. RONCORONI: Reflex and direct cardiopulmonary effects of 5-OH-tryptamine (serotonin); their possible role in pulmonary embolism and coronary thrombosis. Amer. J. Physiol. **173**, 379 —386 (1953).

CORÀ, D., F. ABRIGNANI e S. DEBIASI: Influenza della 5-idrossitriptamina sulla diuresi; studio clinicosperimentale mediante le clearances renale. Minerva nefrol. **4**, 21—23 (1957).

COSTA, E., and M. H. APRISON: Studies on the 5-hydroxytryptamine (serotonin) content in human brain. J. nerv. ment. Dis. **126**, 289—293 (1958).

CRAWFORD, M. A.: Excretion of 5-hydroxyindoleacetic acid in East Africans. Lancet **1962 I**, 352—353.

CRAWFORD, N., and G. T. WATTS: Excretion of 5-hydroxyindolyl acetic acid after surgery, Nature (Lond.) **195**, 182 (1962).

CROSTI, P. F., and P. E. LUCCHELLI: An easy method to determine the serotonin content of human platelets. J. clin. Path. **15**, 191—193 (1962).

CROUT, J. R., and A. SJOERDSMA: The clinical and laboratory significance of serotonin and catechol amines in bananas. New Engl. J. Med. **261**, 23—26 (1959).

CURRENS, J. H., T. D. KINNEY, and P. D. WHITE: Pulmonary stenosis with intact interventricular septum. Amer. Heart J. **30**, 491—510 (1945).

DALESSIO, D. J.: On migraine headache: serotonin and serotonin antagonism: J. Amer. med. Ass. **181**, 318—321 (1962).

DANIEL, E. E., A. J. HONOUR, and A. BOGOCH: Antagonism of serotonin induced contraction and electrical activity in the ileum. Gastroenterology **39**, 62—73 (1960).

DAUGHERTY, G. W., W. M. MANGER, G. M. ROTH, E. V. FLOCK, D. S. CHILDS, and J. M. WAUGH: Malignant carcinoid with hyperserotonemia occurring spontaneously or induced by palpation of the tumour or by intravenous histamine. Proc. Mayo Clin. **30**, 595 (1955).

DAVIDSON, J., A. SJOERDSMA, L. N. LOOMIS, and S. UDENFRIEND: Studies with the serotonin precursor, 5-hydroxytryptophan, in experimental animals and man. J. clin. Invest. **36**, 1594—1599 (1957).

DAVIES, A. J.: Carcinoid tumours (argentaffinomata). Ann. roy. Coll. Surg. Engl. **25**, 277—296 (1959).

DAVIES, J. N. P.: Some considerations regarding obscure diseases affecting the mural endocardium. Amer. Heart J. **59**, 600—631 (1960).

DAVIS, R. B.: The concentration of serotonin in normal human serum as determined by an improved method. J. Lab. clin. Med. **54**, 344—351 (1959).

— C. S. ALEXANDER, and A. ADICOFF: Metabolic studies in carcinoid syndrome: observations on use of α-methyl DOPA, isonicotinic acid hydrazide and selective tryptophan deficiency. Metabolism **10**, 1035—1044 (1961).

—, and B. J. KENNEDY: Carcinoid syndrome associated with adrenal hyperplasia. Arch. intern. Med. **109**, 192—200 (1962).

—, and J. C. ROSENBERG: Carcinoid syndrome associated with hyperserotoninemia and normal 5-hydroxyindoleacetic acid excretion. Amer. J. Med. **30**, 167 —174 (1961).

DAVISON, A. N., and M. SANDLER: Inhibition of 5-hydroxytryptophan decarboxylase by phenylalanine metabolites. Nature (Lond.) **181**, 186—187 (1958).

DAWES, G. S., and J. H. COMROE: Chemoreflexes from the heart and lungs. Physiol. Rev. **34**, 167—201 (1954).

DELAY, J., P. PICHOT, T. LEMPÉRIÈRE, P. NICOLAS-CHARLES et A. M. QUÉTIN: Les effets somatiques de la psilocybine. Ann. méd.-psychol. **117**, 891—899 (1959).

DEMIS, D. J., and J. G. ZIMMER: Carcinoid flush. Lancet **1962 II**, 360—361.

DENGLER, H.: Atypisches Carcinoidsyndrom mit vermehrter Ausscheidung von 5-Hydroxyindolessigsäure bei Pancreascarcinom. Klin. Wschr. **37**, 1245—1248 (1959).

DESPOPOULOS, A., and H. WEISSBACH: Renal metabolism of 5-hydroxyindoleacetic acid. Amer. J. Physiol. **189**, 548 (1957).

DEWITSKY, W.: Über Endokardialflecken. Frankfurt. Z. Path. **9**, 82—96 (1912).

DOCKERTY, M. B., and C. H. SCHEIFLY: Metastasizing carcinoid. Amer. J. clin. Path. **25**, 770—774 (1955).

DONALDSON, R. M., and S. J. GRAY: Urinary excretion of 5-hydroxyindoleacetic acid after administration of serotonin precursor in patients with hepatic cirrhosis. Gastroenterology **36**, 7—11 (1959).

— J. G. SEYMOUR, and V. G. LETSOU: 5-Hydroxytryptophan as an intermediate of serotonin biosyntheses in malignant carcinoidosis. Lancet **1959 II**, 1002—1003.

— I. ZAIDMAN, and S. J. GRAY: The urinary excretion of 5-hydroxyindoleacetic acid after the oral administration of serotonin in various disease states. Gastroenterology **38**, 937—941 (1960).

DUBACH, U. C., u. A. BLUMBERG: Über die therapeutische Verwendung von α-Methyl-dopa beim Carcinoidsyndrom. Klin. Wschr. **39**, 973 (1961).
—, and O. R. GSELL: Carcinoid syndrome: alleviation of diarrhoea and flushing with "Deseril" and RO 5-1025. Brit. med. J. **1962 I**, 1390—1391.
ECCLESTON, D., T. B. B. CRAWFORD, and G. W. ASHCROFT: Tryptamine in the blood and urine of a patient with a carcinoid tumour. Nature (Lond.) **197**, 502—503 (1963).
EHRINGER, H., u. O. HORNYKIEWICZ: Verteilung von Noradrenalin und Dopamin (3-Hydroxytyramin)im Gehirn des Menschen und ihr Verhalten bei Erkrankungen des extrapyramidalen Systems. Klin. Wschr. **38**, 1236—1239 (1960).
ELIASSON, R.: Critical evaluation of the occurrence of 5-hydroxytryptamine in human semen. J. Urol. (Baltimore) **86**, 676—678 (1961).
ERÖS, G.: Die Bedeutung der „argentaffinen" Zellen des Magen-Darmtraktes bei der perniziösen Anämie. Wien. klin. Wschr. **46**, 1119—1121 (1933).
ERSPAMER, V.: Pharmakologische Studien über Enteramin. Naunyn-Schmiedebergs Arch. exp. Path. Pharmak. **196**, 343—365 (1940).
— Pharmacology of indolealkylamines. Pharmacol. Rev. **6**, 425—487 (1954a).
— Il sistema cellulare enterocromaffine e l'enteramina (5-idrossitriptamina). R. C. sci. Farmitalia **1**, 1—193 (1954b).
— Observations on the fate of oral 4-hydroxytryptophan in man. Experientia (Basel) **7** (8), 351—352 (1961a).
— Recent research in the field of 5-hydroxytryptamine and related indolealkylamines. Fortschr. Arzneimittelforsch. **3**, 151—367 (1961b).
—, and M. B. NOBILI: Observations on the fate of oral 4-hydroxytryptophan in man. Experientia (Basel) **17**, 351—352 (1961c).
ESCOVITZ, W. E., and I. M. REINGOLD: Functioning malignant bronchial carcinoid with Cushing's syndrome and recurrent sinus arrest. Ann. intern. Med. **54**, 1248—1259 (1961).
FABING, H. D.: On going berserk: a neurochemical inquiry. Amer. J. Psychiat. **113**, 409—415 (1956).
—, and J. R. HAWKINS: Intravenous injection of bufotenine in man. Science **123**, 886 (1956).
FASTIER, F. N., M. A. MCDOWELL, and H. WAAL: Pharmacological properties of phenyldiguanide and other amidine derivatives in relation to those of 5-hydroxytryptamine. Brit. J. Pharmacol. **14**, 527—535 (1959).
FEIN, S. B., and K. P. KNUDTSON: The malignant carcinoid syndrome. Cancer **9**, 148—151 (1956).
FELDBERG, W., and A. N. SMITH: Release of histamine by tryptamine and 5-hydroxytryptamine. Brit. J. Pharmacol. **8**, 406—411 (1953).
FELDSTEIN, A., H. HOAGLAND, and H. FREEMAN: On the relationship of serotonin to schizophrenia. Science **128**, 358 (1958).
— — — Blood and urinary serotonin and 5-hydroxyindoleacetic acid levels in schizophrenic patients and normal subjects. J. nerv. ment. Dis. **129**, 62—68 (1959).
FEYRTER, F.: Über das bronchiale und das pulmonale Karzinoid. Wien. klin. Wschr. **22**, 386—392 (1960).
—, u. K. UNNA: Über den Nachweis eines blutdrucksteigernden Stoffes in Carcinoid. Virchows Arch. path. Anat. **298**, 187—194 (1936).
FICHERA, C., J. M. BRIDGES, and M. BALDINI: Reduction in 5-hydroxytryptamine uptake by blood platelets as expression of immunological damage. Clin. Res. **10**, 215 (1962).
FISCHER, E., T. A. FERNÁNDEZ, A. J. VAZQUEZ, and A. O. DI STEFANO: A bufotenine-like substance in the urine of schizophernics. J. nerv. ment. Dis. **133**, 441—444 (1962).
— F. A. VAZQUEZ, T. A. FERNÁNDEZ, and L. LISKOWSKI: Bufotenine in human urine. Lancet **1961 I**, 890—891 .
FOY, J. M., and J. R. PARRATT: Urinary excretion of 5-hydroxyindoleacetic acid in West Africans. Lancet **1962 I**, 942—943.
FRIEDMAN, A. P.: Clinical observations with 1-methyl-lysergic acid butanolamide (UML-491) in vascular headache. Angiology **2**, 364—366 (1960).
GADDUM, J. H., C. O. HEBB, A. SILVER and A. A. B. SWAN: 5-hydroxytryptamine. Pharmacological action and destruction in perfused lungs. Quart. J. exp. Physiol. **38**, 255—262 (1953).
—, and M. K. PAASONEN: The use of same molluscan hearts for the estimation of 5-hydroxytryptamine. Brit. J. Pharmacol. **10**, 474—483 (1955).
—, and Z. P. PICARELLI: Two kinds of tryptamine receptor. Brit. J. Pharmacol. **12**, 323—328 (1957).
GARELLI, R.: Azione di un'antiserotinina sulla flogosi reumatica. Reumatismo **2**, 92—98 (1960).
GIARMAN, N. J., and D. X. FREEDMAN: Serotonin content of the pineal glands of man and monkey. Nature (Lond.) **186**, 480—481 (1960).

GINZEL, K. H., and S. R. KOTTEGODA: The action of 5-hydroxytryptamine and tryptamine on aortic and carotid sinus receptors in the cat. J. Physiol. (Lond.) **123**, 277—288 (1954).
GLOVER, W. E., A. D. M. GREENFIELD, B. S. L. KIDD, and R. F. WHELAN: The reaction of the capacity blood vessels of the human hand and forearm to vaso-active substances infused intra-arterially. J. Physiol. (Lond.) **140**, 113—121 (1958).
— R. J. MARSHALL, and R. F. WHELAN: The antagonism of the vascular effects of 5-hydroxytryptamine by BOL-148 and sodium salicylate in the human subject. Brit. J. Pharmacol. **12**, 498—503 (1957).
GOBLE, A. J., D. R. HAY, R. HUDSON, and M. SANDLER: Acquired heart disease with argentaffin carcinoma. Brit. Heart J. **18**, 544—552 (1956).
— — and M. SANDLER: 5-Hydroxytryptamine metabolism in acquired heart disease associated with argentaffin carcinoma. Lancet **1955 II**, 1016—1017.
GOLDSMITH, R. S., B. W. EVANS, and J. P. ROBERTS: Excretion of 5-hydroxyindoleacetic acid (5-HIAA) following burns. Clin. Res. **9**, 179 (1961).
GOSSET, A., et P. MASSON: Tumeurs endocrines de l'appendice. Presse méd. **22**, 237—240 (1914).
GOWENLOCK, A. H., D. S. PLATT, A. C. P. CAMPBELL and K. G. WORMSLEY: Oat-cell carcinoma of the bronchus secreting 5-hydroxytryptophan. Lancet **1964 I**, 304—306.
GRABNER, K., u. F. LEMBECK: Untersuchungen über den Gehalt cerebraler Tumoren an Substanz P and Serotonin. Naunyn-Schmiedebergs Arch. exp. Path. Pharmak. **240**, 157—161 (1960).
GRAHAM, J. R.: Methysergide for prevention of headache: experience in 500 patients over 3 years. New Engl. J. Med. **270**, 67—72 (1964).
GROVER, R. F., S. K. OLSON, and S. G. BLOUNT: Pulmonary vascular response to serotonin in man. Clin. Res. **6**, 62 (1958).
HADDOX jr., CH. H., and M. S. SASLAW: Urinary 5-methoxytryptamine in patients with rheumatic fever. J. clin. Invest. **42**, 435—441 (1963).
HÁLLEN, A.: Fibrosis in the carcinoid syndrome. Lancet **1964 I**, 746.
HALONEN, P. I., P. KOSKELO, M. H. FRICK, and L. MERENMIES: Metastatic carcinoid tumour associated with complicated silicosis. Acta med. scand. **171**, 477—482 (1962).
HALPERN, A., P. H. KUHN, H. E. SHAFTEL, S. S. SAMUELS, N. SHAFTEL, D. SELMEN, and H. G. BIRCH: Raynauds disease, Raynaud's phenomenon and serotonin. Angiology **11**, 151—167 (1960).
HAMPERL, H.: Über argyrophile Zellen. Virchows Arch. path. Anat. **321**, 482—507 (1952).
HANSON, A., and F. SERIN: Determination of 5-hydroxy-indole-acetic acid in urine and its excretion in patients with malignant carcinoids. Lancet **1955 II**, 1359—1361.
HARDISTY, R. M., G. I. C. INGRAM, and R. S. STACEY: Reserpine and human platelet 5-hydroxytryptamine. Experientia (Basel) **12**, 424—425 (1956).
—, and R. S. STACEY: 5-Hydroxytryptamine in normal human platelets. J. Physiol. (Lond.) **130**, 711—720 (1955).
— — Platelet 5-hydroxytryptamine in disorders of the blood. Brit. J. Heamat. **3**, 292—298 (1957).
HARRIS, P., H. W. FRITTS jr., and A. COURNAND: Some circulatory effects of 5-hydroxytryptamine in man. Circulation **21**, 1134—1139 (1960).
HAVERBACK, B. J., and J. D. DAVIDSON: Serotonin and the gastrointestinal tract. Gastroenterology **35**, 570—578 (1958).
— A. SJOERDSMA, and L. L. TERRY: Urinary excretion of the serotonin metabolite, 5-hydroxyindoleacetic acid, in various clinical conditions. New Engl. J. Med. **255**, 270—272 (1956).
HEDINGER, C., u. R. GLOOR: Metastasierende Dünndarmkarzinoide, Tricuspitalklappenveränderungen und Pulmonalstenose — ein neues Syndrom. Schweiz. med. Wschr. **84**, 942—946 (1954).
HEGGLIN, R., u. H. LANGEMANN: Über klinische Symptomatologie und Nachweis von 5-Oxytryptamin und der 5-Oxyindolessigsäure beim metastasierenden Dünndarmkarzinoid. Helv. med. Acta **22**, 463—469 (1955).
HEILMEYER, L. v., u. R. CLOTTEN: Metastasierendes Dünndarmkarzinoid mit zeitweise fehlender Ausscheidung von 5-Hydroxyindolessigsäure und hochgradiger Tryptophanurie. Deutsch. med. Wschr. **83**, 617—619 (1958).
HENDRIX, T. R., M. ATKINSON, J. A. CLIFTON, and F. J. INGELFINGER: The effect of 5-hydroxytryptamine on intestinal motor function in man Amer. J. Med. **23**, 886—893 (1957).
HERTEL, M. P.: Das Verhalten des Endocards bei perietaler Endokarditis und bei allgemeiner Blutdrucksteigerung. Frankfurt. Z. Path. **24**, 1—57 (1921).

HERXHEIMER, H.: The 5-hydroxytryptamine shock in the guinea-pig. J. Physiol. (Lond.) **128**, 435—445 (1955).
—, and M. SCHACHTER: Wheal and flare in human skin produced by histamine and other substances. J. Physiol. (Lond.) **145**, 34—35P (1958).
HEYCK, H.: Serotoninantagonisten in der Behandlung der Migräne und der Erythroprosopalgie Bings oder des Horton-Syndroms. Schweiz. med. Wschr. **90**, 203—209 (1960).
HEYSSEL, R. M.: Determination of human platelet survival utilising ^{14}C labelled serotonin. J. clin. Invest. **40**, 2134—2142 (1961).
HILLARP, N. Å., B. HÖGBERG, and B. WILSON. : Adenosine triphosphate in the adrenal medulla of the cow. Nature (Lond.) **176**, 1032—1033 (1955).
HOFMANN, A., R. HEIM, A. BRACK u. H. KOBEL: Psilocybin ein psychotroper Wirkstoff aus dem mexikanischen Rauschpilz *Psilocybe mexicana* Heim. Experientia (Basel) **14**, 107—109 (1958).
HOLLANDER, W., A. L. MICHELSON, and R. W. WILKINS: Serotonin and antiserotonins. I. Their circulatory, respiratory and renal effects in man. Circulation **16**, 246—255 (1957).
HORNYKIEWICZ, O.: Die topische Lokalisation und das Verhalten von Noradrenalin und Dopamin (3-Hydroxytyramin) in der Substantia nigra des normalen und Parkinsonkranken Menschen. Wien. klin. Wschr. **75**, 309—312 (1963).
HUEBSCHMANN, P.: Sur le carcinome primitif de l'appendice vermiculaire. Rev. méd. Suisse rom. **30**, 317—332 (1910).
HULET, W. H., and G. A. PERERA: Effect of serotonin or renal excretion of sodium; possible relation to rauwolfia action. Proc. Soc. exp. Biol. (N.Y.) **91**, 512—514 (1956).
ISBELL, H.: Comparison of the reactions induced by psilocybin and LSD in man. Psychopharmacologia (Berl.) **1**, 29—38 (1959).
ISLER, P., u. C. HEDINGER: Metastasierendes Dünndarmcarcinoid mit schweren, vorwiegend das rechte Herz betreffenden Klappenfehlern und Pulmonalstenose. Ein eigenartiger Symptomenkomplex? Schweiz. med. Wschr. **83**, 4—7 (1953).
JACOBSON, W.: The argentaffine cells and pernicious anaemia. J. Path. Bact. **49**, 1—19 (1939).
JENKINS, J. S., and P. J. A. BUTCHER: Malignant argentaffinoma with cyanosis and pulmonary stenosis. Lancet **1955 I**, 331—333.
JEPSON, J. B.: Paperchromatography of urinary indoles. Lancet **1955 II**, 1009—1011.
JOHANSSON, S. A.: 5-Hydroxytryptamine in burns. Acta physiol. scand. **48**, 126—132 (1960a).
— Inhibition of thrombocytopoenia and 5-hydroxytryptamine release in anaphylactic shock by heparin. Acta physiol. scand. **50**, 95—104 (1960b).
JOHNSON, L. P., R. D. SLOOP, and J. E. JESSEPH: Treatment of "Dumping" with serotonin antagonists. Preliminary report. J. Amer. med. Ass. **180**, 493—494 (1962).
JOYCE, D.: Changes in the 5-hydroxytryptamine content of rat, rabbit and human brain after death. Brit. J. Pharmacol. **18**, 370—380 (1962).
— 5-Hydroxytryptamine content of glioma. Experientia (Basel) **19**, 187—188 (1963).
JUNG, A.: Rheumatherapie auf verschiedenen Ebenen. Praxis **49**, 161—169 (1960).
JUS, A., D. LASKOWSKA et S. ZIMNY: Recherches sur le comportement de la serotonine dans le serum sanguin des chizophrenes. Ann. méd. -pschychol. **116**, 898—913 (1958).
KABAKOW, B., B. WEINSTEIN, G. ROSS, and M. TRESSER: A clinical and metabolic study of metastatic carcinoid. Amer. J. Med. **26**, 636—645 (1959).
KAHR, H.: Zur pathologischen Anatomie und Physiologie des „Karzinoidsyndroms". Klin. Med. **1956 II**, 341—349.
KERBY, G. P., and S. M. TAYLOR: The acid mucopolysaccharide and 5-hydroxytryptamine content of human thrombocytes in rheumatoid arthritic and non-arthritic individuals. J. clin. Invest. **38**, 1059—1064 (1959).
KIMBALL, R. W., A. P. FRIEDMAN, and E. VALLEJO: Effect of serotonin in migraine patients. Neurology (Minneap.) **10**, 107—111 (1960).
KIRBERGER, E.: Differentialdiagnostische Überlegungen bei vermehrter 5-Hydroxyindolessigsäure-Ausscheidung im Harn. Dtsch. med. Wschr. **87**, 929—934 (1962).
KONZETT, H.: The effects of 5-hydroxytryptamine and its antagonists on tidal air. Brit. J. Pharmacol. **11**, 289—294 (1956).
KOPIN, I. J.: Tryptophan loading and excretion of 5-hydroxyindoleacetic acid in normal and schizophrenic subjects. Science **129**, 835—836 (1959).
KOTTEGODA, S. R., and J. C. MOTT: Cardiovascular and respiratory actions of 5-hydroxytryptamine in the cat. Brit. J. Pharmacol. **10**, 66—72 (1955).
KOWLESSAR, O. D., D. H. LAW, and M. H. SLEISENGER: Malabsorption syndrome associated with metastatic carcinoid tumor. Amer. J. Med. **27**, 673—677 (1959).
— R. C. WILLIAMS, D. H. LAW, and M. S. SLEISENGER: Urinary excretion of 5-hydroxyindoleacetic acid in diarrhoeal states with special reference to non-tropical sprue. New Engl. J. Med. **259**, 340—341 (1958).

KUNTZMAN, R., P. A. SHORE, D. F. BOGDANSKI, and B. B. BRODIE: Microanalytical procedures for fluorimetric assay of brain, DOPA-5-HTP decarboxylase, norepinephrine and serotonin, and a detailed mapping of decarboxylase activity in brain. J. Neurochem. **6**, 226—232 (1961).

LANGEMANN, H.: Bestimmungen von Fermentaktivitäten in Geweben eines Falls von metastasierenden Karzinoid. Naunyn-Schmiedebergs Arch. exp. Path. Pharmak. **228**, 244—245 (1956).

— A. Boner u. P. B. MÜLLER: Aminosäurendecarboxylase in Phaochromocytom- und Karzinoidgewebe. Schweiz. med. Wschr. **92**, 27—34 (1962).

—, u. J. KÄGI: Oxytryptamin- und Oxyindolessigsäurebestimmungen bei einem Fall von Carcinoidsyndrom nebst einigen anderen Untersuchungen über Oxytryptamin. Klin. Wschr. **34**, 237—241 (1956).

LANGER: Submikroskopischer Bau des Bronchial- und das Darmcarcinoids. In: Symposium über Krebsprobleme, Ed. OBER, RAUEN, SCHOENMACKERS u. ZANDER. Berlin-Göttingen-Heidelberg: Springer 1961.

LANGHANS, T.: Über einen Drüsenpolyp im Ileum. Virchows Arch. path. Anat. **38**, 559—560 (1867).

LANZ, R.: Beobachtungen bei einem Karzinoidsyndrom. Schweiz. med. Wschr. **90**, 1046—1048 (1960).

LEMBECK, F.: 5-Hydroxytryptamine in a carcinoid tumour. Nature (Lond.) **172**, 910—911 (1953).

— Über den Nachweis von 5-Oxytryptamine (Enteramin, Serotonin) in Carcinoidmetastasen. Naunyn-Schmiedebergs Arch. exp. Path. Pharmak. **221**, 50—66 (1954).

—, u. K. NEUHOLD: Nachweis von 5-Oxytryptamin im Harn. Naunyn-Schmiedebergs Arch. exp. Path. Pharmak. **226**, 456—459 (1955).

LE MESSURIER, D. H., C. J. SCHWARTZ, and R. F. WHELAN: Cardiovascular effects of intravenous infusion of 5-hydroxytryptamine in man. Brit. J. Pharmacol. **14**, 246—250 (1959).

LEVINE, R. J., and A. SJOERDSMA: Pressor amines and carcinoid flush. Ann. intern. Med. **58**, 818—828 (1963).

LIEBOW, A. A.: Tumours of the lower respiratory tract. Atlas of tumour pathology. AFIP, Washington, Sect V, Fasc. 17 (1952).

LUBARSCH, O.: Über den primären Krebs des Ileum nebst Bemerkungen über das gleichzeitige Vorkommen von Krebs und Tuberkulose. Virchows Arch. path. Anat. **111**, 280—317 (1888).

LUDWIG, G. F.: Inhibition of 5-hydroxyindoleacetic acid excretion by isonicotinic acidhydrazide in a patient with malignant carcinoid. Clin. Res. **8**, 30 (1960).

MACDONALD, R. A.: A study of 356 carcinoids of the gastrointestinal tract. Report of four new cases of the carcinoid syndrome. Amer. J. Med. **21**, 867—878 (1956).

—, and S. L. ROBBINS: Pathology of the heart in the carcinoid syndrome. Arch. Path. **63**, 103—112 (1957).

— — and G. K. MALLORY: Dermal fibrosis following subcutaneous injection of serotonin creatine sulphate. Proc. Soc. exp. Biol. (N.Y.) **97**, 334 (1958b).

MACFARLANE, P. S., C. E. DALGLIESH, R. W. DUTTON, B. LENNOX, L. M. NYHUS, and N. A. SMITH: Endocrine aspects of argentaffinoma, with special reference to the use of urinary 5-hydroxyindoleacetic acid estimations in diagnosis. Scot. med. J. **1**, 148—155 (1956).

MACHAFFIE, R. A., L. R. MENEBROKER, D. L. MAHLER, and A. J. BARAC: Studies in allergy. II. Serotonin levels in human beings and guinea-pigs. Allergy **31**, 106—110 (1960).

MAGALINI, S. I., M. STEFANINI, and F. E. SMITH: Vasopressor effects of synthetic 5-hydroxytryptamine creatinine sulphate in man. Proc. Soc. exp. Biol. (N.Y.) **92**, 433—436 (1956).

MARSHALL, E. F., G. S. STIRLING, A. C. TAIT, and A. TODRICK: The effect of iproniazid and imipramine on the blood platelet 5-hydroxytryptamine level in man. Brit. J. Pharmacol. **15**, 35—41 (1960).

MASSON, P.: Appendicite neurogene et carcinoides. Ann. Anat. path. **1**, 3—5 (1924).

— Carcinoids (argentaffine cell tumours) and nerve hyperplasia of the appendicular mucosa. Amer. J. Path. **4**, 181—211 (1928).

MCCLURE, P., U. GLASS, G. I. C. INGRAM, and R. S. STACEY: In preparation.

MCCUBBIN, J. W., J. H. GREEN, G. C. SALMOIRAGHI, and I. H. PAGE: The chemoceptor stimulant action of serotonin in dogs. J. Pharmacol. exp. Ther. **116**, 191—197 (1956).

MCISAAC, W. M., and I. H. PAGE: The metabolism of serotonin (5-hydroxytryptamine). J. biol. Chem. **234**, 858—864 (1959).

MCKEAN, C. M., S. M. SCHANBERG, and N. J. GIARMAN: A mechanism of the indole defect in experimental phenylketonuria. Science **137**, 604—605 (1962).

MCKUSICK, V. A.: Carcinoid cardiovascular disease. Johns Hopk. Hosp. Bull. **98**, 13—36 (1956).

McNeely, R. G. D., and N. W. Jones: Secondary pellagra caused by multiple argentaffin carcinoma of the ileum and jejunum. Gastroenterology **6**, 443—448 (1946).
Melmon, K., and A. Sjoerdsma: Serotonin in platelets. Lancet **1963 II**, 316—318.
Mériel, P., R. Ruffié, A. Fournié, Ch. Ayrolles et P. Cuq: Utilisation d'une antisérotonine (UML-491) en injections intra-articulaires. Rev. Rhum. **27**, 149—155 (1960).
Michelson, A. L., W. Hollander, and F. C. Lowell: The effect of 5-hydroxytryptamine (serotonin) on the respiration of non-asthmatic and asthmatic subjects. J. Lab. clin. Med. **51**, 57—62 (1958).
Miller, J., and A. Fishman: A serotonin antagonist in the treatment of allergic and allied disorders. Ann. Allergy **19**, 164—171 (1961).
Miller, L. D., and G. W. Peskin: The postgastrectomy dumping syndrome. Amer. J. med. Sci. **245**, 218—243 (1963).
Millman, S.: Tricuspid stenosis and pulmonary stenosis complicating carcinoid of the intestine with metastases to the liver. Amer. Heart. J **25**, 391—398 (1943).
Milne, M. D.: Biochemical effect of phenylacetic acid. Lancet **1959 II**, 467—468.
— M. A. Crawford, C. B. Girão, and L. W. Loughridge: The excetion of indolylacetic acid and related indolic acids in men and the rat. Clin. Sci. **19**, 165—179 (1960).
Mitchell, R. G., and R. Cass: Histamine and 5-hydroxytryptamine in the blood of infants and children. J. clin. Invest. **38**, 595—604 (1959).
Munsick, R. A.: Serotonin and the menopausal flush. Amer. J. Obstet. Gynec. **78**, 147—151 (1959).
Murphy, G. E., S. B. Guze, and I. J. King: Urinary excretion of 5-hydroxyndoleacetic acid in cronic alcoholism. J. Amer. med Ass. **182**, 565 (1962).
Mustala, O. D., and M. M. Airaksinen: Excretion of histamine and metabolites of 5-hydroxytryptamine in a case of metastasized carcinoid tumour. Acta. med. scand. **171**, 483—489 (1962).
Nemir, P., H. H. Stone, T. N. Mackell, and H. R. Hawthorne: Studies on pulmonary embolism utilizing the method of controlled unilateral pulmonary artery occlusion. Surg. Forum **5**, 210 (1954).
Nicholson, G. I., M. C. Evans, and R. O. H. Irvine: Effect of methyldopa in carcinoid disease. Brit. med J. **1962 II**, 961—963.
Nicod, J.-L.: Carcinoide de la parotide. Bull. Ass. franç. Cancer **45**, 214—222 (1958).
Nikkila, E. A.: Urinary excretion of the serotonin metabolite 5-hydroxyindoleacetic acid in neurocirculatory asthenia. Acta med. scand. **162**, 231—235 (1958).
Notter, B.: Der Einfluß von 5-hydroxytryptamine (Serotonin) auf die Nierenfunktion beim Menschen. Schweiz. med. Wschr. **86**, 481—483 (1956).
Oates, J. A., K. Melmon, A. Sjoerdsma, L. Gillespie, and D. T. Mason: Release of a kinin peptide in the carcinoid syndrome. Lancet **1964 I**, 514—517.
— and A. Sjoerdsma: Neurologic effects of tryptophan in patients receiving a monoamine oxidase inhibitor. Neurology **10**, 1076—1078 (1960).
— — Metabolism of 5-hydroxy-D-and L-tryptophan in man: synthesis of serotonin from the D-isomer. Proc. Soc. exp. Biol. (N.Y.) **108**, 264—266 (1961).
— — A unique syndrome associated with secretion of 5-hydroxytryptophan by metastatic gastric carcinoids. Amer. J. Med. **32**, 333—341 (1962).
Oberndorfer, S.: Karzinoide Tumoren des Dünndarms. Frankfurt. Z. Path. **1**, 426 (1907).
O'Hara, R. S., R. O. Fox and J. W. Cole: Serotonin release mediated by intraluminal sucrose solutions. Surg. Forum **10**, 215 (1959).
Olson, R., D. Gursey, and J. W. Vester: Evidence for a defect in tryptophan metabolism in chronic alcoholism. New Engl. J. Med. **263**, 1169—1174 (1960).
Paasonen, M. K., and E. Kivalo: The inactivation of 5-hydroxytryptamine by blood platelets in mental dificiency with elevated serum 5-hydroxytryptamine. Psychopharmacologia (Berl.) **3**, 188—192 (1962).
Page, I. H.: Cardiovascular actions of serotonin (5-hydroxytryptamine). In: 5-Hydroxytryptamine, p. 93—108, ed. by G. P. Lewis, London: Pergamon Press 1958.
Panigel, M., et M. Mayer: Reactions vaso-motrices de la veine du cordon ombilical humain. C. R. Acad. Sc. (Paris) **248** (7), 1031—1033 (1959).
Pare, C. M. B., M. Sandler, and R. S. Stacey: 5-Hydroxytryptamine deficiency in phenylketonuria. Lancet **1957 I**, 551—553.
— — — Decreased 5-hydroxytryptophan decarboxylase activity in phenylektonuria. Lancet **1958 II**, 1099—1101.
— — — The relationship between decreased 5-hydroxyindole metabolism and mental defect in phenylketonuria. Arch. Dis. Child. **34**, 422—423 (1959).
— — — 5-Hydroxyindoles in mental deficiency. Neurol. Neurosurg. Psychiat **23**, 341—346 (1960).
Parks, V. J., A. G. Sandison, S. L. Skinner, and R. F. Whelan: The stimulation of respiration by 5-hydroxytryptamine in man. J. Physiol. (Lond.) **151**, 342—351 (1960).

PARROT, J. L., et N. FLAVIAN: Captation de la 5-hydroxytryptamine par le serum humain normal. Absence de cette captation chez les sujets allergiques. C. R. Acad. Sci. (Paris) **249**, 463—465 (1959).

PEARSE, A. G. E.: Histochemistry, theoretical and applied, 2nd Ed. London: Churchill 1960.

PEART, W. S., T. M. ANDREWS, and J. I. S. ROBERTSON: Carcinoid syndrome Serotonin release induced with intravenous adrenaline or noradrenaline. Lancet **1961 I**, 577—578.

—, and J. I. S. ROBERTSON: The effect of serotonin antagonist (UML 491) in carcinoid disease. Lancet **1961 II**, 1172—1173.

PERMAN, E. S.: Observations on the effect of ethanol on the urinary excretion of histamine, 5-hydroxyindoleacetic acid, catecholamines and 17-hydroxycorticosteroids in man. Acta physiol. scand. **51**, 62—67 (1961).

PERNOW, B.: In Modern Trends in Gastroenterology, Ed. AVERY JONES. London: Butterworth & Co. 1958.

—, and J. WALDENSTRÖM. Paroxysmal flushing and other symptoms caused by 5-hydroxytryptamine and histamine in patients with malignant tumors. Lancet **1954 II**, 951.

— — Determination of 5-hydroxytryptamine, 5-hydroxyindoleacetic acid and histamine in 33 cases of carcinoid tumour. Amer. J. Med. **23**, 16—25 (1957).

PERRY, T. L.: Urinary excretion of amines in phenylketonuria and mongolism. Science **136**, 879—880 (1962).

PESKIN, G. W., and M. J. ORLOFF: Carcinoids, the malignant carcinoid syndrome and 5-hydroxytryptamine (serotonin). Amer. J. med. Sci. **237**, 224—237 (1959).

PIMPARKER, B. D., D. SENESKY and M. H. KALSEN: Blood serotonin in non-tropical sprue. Gastroenterology **40**, 504—506 (1961).

PLETSCHER, A., and A. BERNSTEIN: Increase of 5-hydroxytryptamine in blood platelets by isopropyl-isonicotinic acid hydrazide. Nature (Lond.) **181**, 1133—1134 (1958).

POUMAILLOUX, M., et L. LABIGNETTE: Serotonine et antiserotonines. Leur role dans la pathologie cardio-vasculaire. Rev. Path. gén. **59**, 333—345 (1959).

PRUSOFF, W. H.: The distribution of 5-hydroxytryptamine and adenosine triphosphate in cytoplasmic particles of the dog's small intestine. Brit. J. Pharmacol. **15**, 520—524 (1960).

PUENTE-DUANY, G. A., W. E. RIEMER, and J. B. MIALE: Effect of banana ingestion on urinary excretion of 5-HO-indole compounds in normal adults. Proc. Soc. exp. Biol (N.Y.) **98**, 499—501 (1958).

QUIVY, D.: La serotonine intervient-elle dans l'hémostase. Hémostase **1**, 193—200 (1961).

RAMBO, O. N., I. GORE, V. K. VANCE, and H. BROWN. The syndrome of intestinal carcinoid with massive hepatic metastases and endocardial fibrosis with tricuspid and pulmonic stenosis: its recognition and significance. Amer. J. Path. **30**, 625 (1954).

RATZENHOFER, M., u. F. LEMBECK: Über den Gehalt an 5-Oxytryptamin in Carcinoiden des Darmtraktes. Z. Krebsforsch. **60**, 169—195 (1954).

REICHLE, F. A., R. C. BALDRIDGE, J. DOBBS, and M. TROMPETTER: Tryptophan metabolism in phenylketonurics. J. Amer. med. Ass. **178**, 939—941 (1961).

RESNICK, R. H., C. F. ADELARDI, and S. J. GRAY: Stimulation of gastric secretion in man by a serotonin antagonist. Gastroenterology **42**, 22—25 (1962).

—, and S. J. GRAY: Distribution of serotonin (5-hydroxytryptamine) in the human gastro-intestinal tract. Gastroenterology **41**, 119—121 (1961).

RINKEL, M., A. DIMASCIO, A. ROBEY, and C. ATWELL: Personality and reactions to psilocybine. Neuro-Psychopharmacology **2**, 273—279 (1961).

ROBERTSON, J. I. S., W. S. PEART, and T. M. ANDREWS: The mechanism of facial flushes in the carcinoid syndrome. Quart. J. Med. **31**, 103—123 (1962).

RODDIE, I. C., J. T. SHEPHERD and R. F. WHELAN: The action of 5-hydroxytryptamine on the blood vessels of the human hand and forearm. Brit. J. Pharmacol **10**, 445—450 (1955).

RODNIGHT, R.: Separation and characterization of urinary indoles resembling 5-hydroxytryptamine and tryptamine. Biochem. J. **64**, 621—626 (1956).

— Carbon monoxide saturation and the recovery of 5-hydroxytryptamine from whole blood. J. Physiol. (Lond.) **141**, 10—11 P (1958).

—, and H. MCILWAIN: Serotonin, lysergic acid diethylamide and mental status. Brit. med. J. **1956 I**, 108.

ROSENBAUM, F. F., D. G. SANTER, and D. B. CLAUDON: Essential telangiectasia, pulmonic and tricuspid stenosis and neoplastic liver disease A possible new clinical syndrome. J. Lab. clin. Med. **42**, 941—942 (1953).

ROSENBERG, D. E., H. ISBELL, and E. J. MINER: Comparison of a placebo, N-dimethyltryptamine and 6-hydroxy-N-dimethyltryptamine in man. Psychopharmacologia (Berl.) **4**, 39—42 (1963).

Roth, F., u. R. Richter: Über die Ausscheidung des Serotoninketaboliten, 5-Hydroxyindolyl-essigsäure, im Urin während des normalen Zyklus. Zbl. Gynäk. **45**, 1733—1740 (1957).
Rowell, N. R., and J. W. Summerscales: The urine excretion of 5-hydroxyindoleacetic acid in a patient with menopausal flushing. J. Clin. Path. **13**, 518 (1960).
Rummele, W., u. F. Gnirss. Untersuchungen mit Psilocybin, einer psychotropen Substanz aus Psilocybemexicana. Schweiz. Arch. Neurol. Psychiat. **87**, 365—385 (1961).
Sai-Halâsz, A., G. Brunecker u. S. Szára: Dimethyltryptamin: ein neues Psychoticum. Psychiat. et Neurol. (Basel) **135**, 285 (1958).
Sanders, R., T. P. Waalkes, J. W. Gilbert jr., and L. L. Terry: Serotonin (5-hydroxytryptamine) and pulmonary thromboembolism. Surg. Gynec. Obstet. **109**, 455—459 (1959).
Sandler, M., and H. G. Close: Biochemical effects of phenylacetic acid in a patient with a 5-hydroxytryptophan secreting carcinoid tumour. Lancet **1959 II**, 316—318.
— A. Davies, and C. Rimington: Effect of phenylacetic acid on carcinoid syndrome. Lancet **1959 II**, 318—322.
—, and C. R. J. Ruthven: In: Adrenergic Mechanisms, Ed. J. Vane. London: Churchill 1960.
— P. J. Scheuer, and P. J. Watt: 5-Hydroxytryptophan secreting bronchial carcinoid tumor. Lancet **1961 II**, 1067—1069.
—, and P. J. D. Snow: An atypical cardinoid tumour secreting 5-hydroxytrypophan. Lancet **1958 I**, 137—139.
Sano, I., Y. Kakimoto, T. Okamoto, H. Nakajima u. Y. Kudo: Über 5-Oxyindolessigsäure-Ausscheidung im Urin von Schizophrenen mit Berücksichtigung des Einflusses von Chlorpromazin und Reserpin auf den Serotoninstoffwechsel. Schweiz. med. Wschr. **87**, 214—217 (1957).
Sauer, W. G., W. H. Dearing, and E. V. Flock: Diagnosis and clinical management of functioning carcinoids. J. Amer. med. Ass. **168**, 139—147 (1958).
Schain, R. J., and D. X. Freedman: Studies on 5-hydroxyindole metabolism in autistic and other mentally retarded children. J. Pediat. **58**, 315—320 (1961).
Scherbel, A. L., and J. W. Harrison: Exaggerated reactivity to serotonin in patients with rheumatoid arthritis and related diseases. Circulation **18**, 777 (1958).
— — Rheumatoid arthritis and related diseases. Clin. Res. **6**, 402 (1958).
Schievelbein, H., U. Surberg u. E. Werle: Erhöhung der Ausscheidung von 5-Hydroxyindolessigsäure bei Rauchern. Klin. Wschr. **40**, 52 (1962).
— E. Werle u. W. Jacoby: Über die Freisetzung von 5-Hydroxytryptamin (Serotonin) aus Geweben durch Nikotin. Naturwissenschaften **48**, 602 (1961).
Schmermund, H. J., H. Rodegra u. K. Soehring: Über die Beteiligung von 5-Hydroxytryptamin beim physiologischen Verschluß der Nebelschnurgefäße post partum. Arch. Gynäk. **191**, 457 (1959).
Schmid, E., H. Haas, N. Henning, K. Meythaler jr. u. H. Schön: Untersuchungen über den Stoffwechsel von Serotonin und seiner Vorstufe 5-Hydroxytryptophan bei Gesunden und Leberkranken. Klin. Wschr. **24**, 1229—1233 (1962).
—, u. H. Kinzlmeier: Das Verhalten der Magenazidität und der Motilität im Verdauungstrakt des Menschen bei Infusion von Serotonin. Naunyn-Schmiedebergs Arch. exp. Path. Pharmak. **236**, 51—53 (1959).
— F. Scheiffarth, L. Zicha u. H. Siede: Untersuchungen über die Rolle des 5-Hydroxytryptamin bei allergischen und rheumatischen Erkrankungen sowie über die Beeinflußbarkeit des Blutserotoninspiegels durch ACTH und Glucocorticoide. Z. ges. exp. Med. **133**, 1—8 (1960a).
— I. Seng, N. Henning u. K. Heinkel: 5-Hydroxytryptamin und Erkrankungen der Verdauungsorgane. Gastroenterologia (Basel) **93**, 235—255 (1960b).
— J. Stern, S. Witte, K. T. Schricker u. N. Henning: Untersuchungen über die Thrombocytenpathologie mit Hilfe der Serotoninbestimmung. Folia haemat. N. F. **4**, 425—443 (1960c).
— L. Zicha u. F. Scheiffarth: Über die Wirkung von 5-Hydroxytryptophan auf den Magendarmtrakt des Menschen. Med. exp. (Basel) **2**, 266—269 (1960d).
Schneckloth, R. E., I. H. Page, and A. C. Corcoran: Depressed renal function in the carcinoid syndrome: Effects of serotonin in normal subjects and of an antiserotonin (Bromo-LSD). Clin. Res. Proc. **5**, 308 (1958).
— — F. del Greco, and A. C. Corcoran: Effects of serotonin antagonists in normal subjects and patients with carcinoid tumours. Circulation **26**, 523—532 (1957).
— A. M. McIsaac, and I. H. Page: Serotonin metabolism in carcinoid syndrome with metastatic bronchial adenoma. J. Amer. med. Soc. **170**, 1143—1147 (1959).
Scholte, A. J.: Ein Fall von Angioma teleangiectaticum Cutio mit chronischer Endocarditis und malignem Dünndarmcarcinoid. Beitr. path. Anat. **86**, 440—443 (1931).

SCHUHMACHER, A., u. H. SCHULZ: Licht- und elektronenmikroskopische Untersuchungen an einem metastasierenden Dünndarmcarcinoid mit Serotoninbestimmungen an Tumorzellfraktionen. Klin. Wschr. **24**, 1188—1196 (1963).

SELBERG, W.: Über das Carcinoid des Darmes. Virchows Arch. path. Anat. **306**, 467—490 (1940).

SERCL, M., J. KOVARIK u. O. JAROS: Klinische Erfahrungen mit Psilocybin. Psychiat. Neurologia (Basel) **142**, 137—146 (1961).

SHARMAN, D. F., and F. M. SULLIVAN: 5-Hydroxytryptamine in serum. Nature (Lond.) **177**, 332—333 (1956).

SHARPEY-SCHAFER, E. P., and J. GINSBURG: Humoral agents and venous tone: Effects of catecholamines, 5-hydroxytryptamine, histamine and nitrites. Lancet **1962 II**, 1337—1340.

SHEKELLE, R. B., and A. M. OSTFIELD: Methysergide in the migraine syndrome. Clin. Pharmacol. Ther. **5**, 201—204 (1964).

SHILLINGFORD, J. P., and K. SOMERS: Clinical and haemodynamic patterns in endomyocardial fibrosis. Brit. Heart J. **23**, 433—446 (1961).

SHORE, P. A., L. GILLESPIE, S. SPECTOR, and D. PROCKOP: Increase in blood serotonin levels induced by iproniazid in man and rabbits. Naturwissenschaften **14**, 340—341 (1958).

SICUTERI, F.: Prophylactic and therapeutic properties of l-methyl-lysergic acid butanolamide in migraine. Int. Arch. Allergy. **15**, 300 (1959).

SINCLAIR, J. S.: Serotonin and antidiuresis. J. roy. Coll. Surg. Edinb. **4**, 147 (1959).

SJOERDSMA, A., J. A. OATES, P. ZALTZMAN, and S. UDENFRIEND: Identification and assay of urinary tryptamine: application as an index of monoamine oxidase inhibition in man. J. Pharmacol. exp. Ther. **126**, 217—222 (1959).

— — — — Serotonin synthesis in carcinoid patients. New Engl. J. Med. **263**, 585—588 (1960).

— L. A. GILLESPIE, and S. UDENFRIEND: A simple method for the measurement of monoamineoxidase inhibition in man. Lancet **1958 II**, 159—160.

— H. WEISSBACH, and S. UDENFRIEND: A clinical physiological and biochemical study of patients with malignant carcinoid (argentaffinoma). Amer. J. Med. **20**, 520—532 (1956).

— — L. L. TERRY, and S. UDENFRIEND: Further observations on patients with malignant carcinoid. Amer. J. Med. **23**, 5—15 (1957).

SKANSE, B., and A. HANSON: Increased thyroid function and the urinary excretion of 5-hydroxyindoleacetic acid. Lancet **1962 I**, 1072.

SKINNER, S. L., and R. F. WHELAN: Carotid body stimulation by 5-hydroxytryptamine in man. J. Physiol (Lond.) **162**, 35—43 (1962).

SMITH, A. N., L. M. NYHUS, C. E. DALGLIESH, R. W. DUTTON, B. LENNOX, and P. S. MACFARLANE. Further observations on the endocrine aspects of argentaffinoma. Scot. med. J. **2**, 24 (1957).

SMITH, B. and D. J. PROCKOP: Central nervous system effects of ingestion of L-tryprophan by normal subjects. New Engl. J. Med. **267**, 1338—1340 (1962).

SMITH, G., and A. N. SMITH: The role of serotonin in experimental pulmonary embolism. Surg. Gynec. Obstet. **101**, 691—701 (1955).

SMITH, S. E.: Uptake of ^{14}C-5-hydroxytryptophan by rat and dog brain slices. Brit. J. Pharmacol. **20**, 178—189 (1963).

SNOW, P. J. D., J. E. LENNARD-JONES, G. CURZON, and R. S. STACEY: Humoral effects of metastasising carcinoid tumours. Lancet **1955 II**, 1004—1009.

SOUTHREN, A. L., and N. I. CHRISTOFF: Cerebrospinal fluid serotonin in brain tumour and other neurological disorders determined by a spectrophotofluorimetric method. J. clin. Lab. Med. **59**, 320—326 (1962).

— R. R. P. WARNER, N. I. CHRISTOFF, and H. E. WEINER: An unusual neurologic syndrome associated with hyperserotonemia. New Engl. J. Med. **260**, 1265—1268 (1959).

SPIES, T. D., and R. E. STONE: Effect of serotonin on blood pressure and lack of effect of antimetabolite. J. Amer. med. Soc. **150**, 1599—1600 (1952).

STACEY, R. S.: Red cells and 5-hydroxytryptamine. J. Physiol. (Lond.) **132**, 39—40P (1956).

— Malignant carcinoid tumours. Proc. roy. Soc. Med. **50**, 40—43 (1957).

— 5-Hydroxytryptamine and other pharmacologically active substances in the central nervous system. Acta physiol. pharm. neerl. 8, 222—239 (1959).

— Uptake of 5-hydroxytryptamine by platelets. Brit. J. Pharmacol. **16**, 284—295 (1961).

STEEL, C. W.: Malignant carcinoid. Arch. intern. Med. **110**, 763—768 (1962).

STEINER, F. A., R. E. SIEBENMANN, C. SANDRI u. C. HEDINGER: Thrombozytose und Eosinophilie bei adrenalektomierten Ratten nach einmaliger 5-Hydroxytryptamin-injection. Experientia (Basel) **13**, 500—502 (1957).

STONE, C. A., H. C. WENGER, C. T. LUDDEN, J. M. STAVORSKI, and C. A.ROSS: Antiserotonin-antihistaminic properties of cyprohepatdine. J. Pharmacol. exp. Ther. **131**, 73—84 (1961).
STONE, H. H.. S. HORIGUCHI, C. C. DONNELLY, and P. NEMIR: Changes in plasma serotonin concentration in surgical patients: a possible significance. Surg. Forum **12**, 140—142 (1961).
STUDNITZ, W. v.: On the excretion of 3-methoxy-4-hydroxymandelic acid in patients with serotonin producing tumours. Scand. J. klin. Lab. Invest. **11**, 309—310 (1959).
SZARA, S.: In: *Psychotropic Drugs*, edit. by GARATTINI and GHETTI, p. 460—467. Amsterdam: Elsevier, 1957.
— Hallucinogenic effects and metabolism of tryptamine derivatives in man. Fed. Proc. **20**, 885—888 (1961).
THORSON, Å., G. BIÖRCK, G. BJORKMAN, and J. WALDENSTRÖM: Malignant carcinoid of the small intestine with metastase to the liver, valvular disease of the right side of the heart (pulmonary stenosis and tricuspid regurgitation without spetal defects), peripheral vasomotor symptoms, bronchoconstriction, and an unusual type of cyanosis: a clinical and pathologic syndrome. Amer. Heart J. **47**, 795 (1954).
THORSON, Å. H.: Hemodynamic changes during "flush" in carcinoidosis. Amer. Heart J. **52**, 444—461 (1956).
— Studies on carcinoid disease. Acta med. scand. **161**, Supp. 334, 1—132 (1958).
TODRICK, A., A. C. TAIT, and E. MARSHALL: Blood platelet and 5-hydroxytryptamine levels in psychiatric patients. J. ment. Sci. **106**, 884—890 (1960).
TURNER, W. J., and E. A. MAUSS: Serotonin (5-hydroxytryptamine) and acetylcholine in human ventricular and spinal fluids. Arch. gen. Psychiat. **1**, 646—650 (1959).
—, and S. MERLIS: Effect of some indolealkylamines on man. Arch. Neurol. Psychiat. (Chic) **81**, 121—129 (1959).
UDENFRIEND, S., W. LOVENBERG, and A. SJOERDSMA: Physiologically active amines in common fruits and vegetables. Arch. Biochem. **85**, 487—490 (1959).
URELES, A. L., M. MURRAY, and R. WOLF: Results of pharmacologic treatment in the malignant carcinoid syndrome. New. Engl. J. Med. **267**, 435—438 (1962).
—, and C. ROB: Acute ischaemia of a limb complicating methysergide maleate therapy. J. Amer med. Ass. **183**, 1041—2 (1963).
VACCAREZZA, J. R., and A. BOCHI: Urinary determination of 5-hydroxyindoleacetic acid, catabolite of serotonin, in normal subjects and respiratory allergic patients. Ann. Allergy **21**, 448—453 (1963).
WAALKES, T. P.: The determination of serotonin (5-hydroxytryptamine) in human blood. J. Lab. clin. Med. **53**, 824—829 (1959).
— A. SJOERDSMA, C. R. CREVELING, H. WEISSBACH, and S. UDENFRIEND, Serotonin, norepinephrine and related compounds in bananas. Science **127**, 648—650 (1958).
WALDENSTRÖM, J.: In: Modern Trends in Gastro-enterology, edit. F. AVERY JONES. London: Butterworth & Co. 1958a.
— Clinical picture of carcinoidosis. Gastroenterology **35**, 565—569 (1958b).
— Cardinoidosis. Gastroenterologia (Basel) **95**, 209—219 (1961).
—, and E. LJUNGBERG: Studies on the functional circulatory influence from metastasizing carcinoid (argentaffine, enterochromaffine) tumours and their possible relation to enteramine production. Acta med. scand **152**, 293—331 (1955).
— B. PERNOW, and H. SILWER. Case of metastasizing carcinoma (argentaffinoma) of unknown origin showing peculiar red flushing and increased amounts of histamine and 5-hydroxytryptamine in blood and urine. Acta med. scand **156**, 73—83 (1957).
WARNER, R. R. P.: Symptomatic hyperserotonemia (without carcinoid) associated with diminished excretion of 5-hydroxyincoleacetic acid: a new syndrome. Clin. Res. **9**, 156 (1961).
— Hyperserotonaemia in functional gastro-intestinal disease. Ann. intern. Med. **59**, 464—476 (1963).
— H. D. JANOWITZ, and D. A. DREILING. The effect of serotonin on human gastric and pancreatic secretion and bile flow. Clin. Res. **7**, 32 (1959).
—, and A. L. SOUTHREN. Carcinoid syndrome produced by metasizing bronchial adenoma. Amer. J. Med. **24**, 903—914 (1958).
WEINER, M., and S. UDENFRIEND. Relationship of platelet serotonin to disturbances of clotting and hemostasis. Circulation **15**, 353—357 (1957).
WEISBERG, H. F., and G. L. SCHAEFER: Possible relationship between carcinoid (argentaffin) tumours and the hyperglycemic -glycogenolyticfactor (HGF). Amer. J. clin. Path. **22**, 1169—1174 (1952).
WEISSBACH, H., W. KING, A. SJOERDSMA, and S. UDENFRIEND. Formation of indole-3-acetic acid and tryptamine in animals. J. biol. Chem. **234**, 81—86 (1959).

WILKINS, R. W., and W. HOLLANDER: Serotonin and antiserotonins II. Clinical studies, especially in essential hypertension with the benzyl anelogue of serotonin (BAS). Circulation **16**, 256—262 (1957).

WILLIAMS, E. D., and J. G. AZZOPARDI: Tumours of the lung and the carcinoid syndrome. Thorax **15**, 30—36 (1960).

WOLBACH, A. B., E. J. MINER, and H. ISBELL. Comparison of psilocin with psilocybin, mescaline and LSD — 25. Psychopharmacologia (Berl.) 219—223 (1962).

WOLFE, H. R. I., A. DAVIES, A. P. MATHIAS, and M. SCHACHTER: Metastatic argentaffinoma secreting 5-hydroxytryptamine in a patient with a patent foramen ovale. Brit. med. J. **1960 I**, 925—929.

WOOLLEY, D. W.: The Biochemical Basis of Psychoses. New York: John Wiley & Sons 1962.

—, and E. Shaw: Some neurophysiological aspects of serotonin. Brit. med. J. **1954 II**, 122—126.

YUWILER, A., and R. T. LOUTTIT: Effects of phenylalanine diet on brain serotonin in the rat. Science **134**, 831—832 (1961).

ZARAFONETIS, C. J. D., S. H. LORBER, and S. M. HANSON. Association of functioning carcinoid syndrome and scleroderma. Amer. J. med. Sci. **236**, 1—14 (1958).

ZUCKER, M. B., and J. BORRELLI: Quantity, assay and release of serotonin in human platelets J. app. Physiol. **7**, 425—431 (1955).

Author Index

Page numbers in *italics* refer to the bibliography

Subject Index

(Compiled by the Sub-Editor and by Dr. G. Falconieri Erspamer with the collaboration of the individual contributors)

The following abbreviations are used, excepting as primary headings, throughout: ATP: adenosine triphosphate; BAS: benzyl analogue of serotonin (5-HT); BOL: 2-bromo-D-lysergic acid diethylamide; CNS: central nervous system; DCA: decarboxylase of aromatic L-amino acids; EC: enterochromaffin cell(s); EEG: electroencephalogram; 5-HIAA: 5-hydroxyindoleacetic acid; 5-HT: 5-hydroxytryptamine; 5-HTP: 5-hydroxytryptophan; LSD: D-lysergic acid diethylamide; MAO: monoamine oxidase.

T

U

V

W

X

Y

Z

GPSR Compliance

The European Union's (EU) General Product Safety Regulation (GPSR) is a set of rules that requires consumer products to be safe and our obligations to ensure this.

If you have any concerns about our products, you can contact us on ProductSafety@springernature.com

In case Publisher is established outside the EU, the EU authorized representative is:

Springer Nature Customer Service Center GmbH
Europaplatz 3
69115 Heidelberg, Germany

Batch number: 10838053

Printed by Printforce, the Netherlands